Forever Active O[lder Adult]
Health and Fitness Playbook

Michael PJ Bedard

Copyright © 2022
All Rights Reserved

Disclaimer

The information provided in this book is designed to provide helpful information on the subjects discussed. This book is not meant to be used, nor should it be used, to diagnose or treat any medical condition. For diagnosis or treatment of any medical problem, consult your own physician. The author is not responsible for any specific health or allergy needs that may require medical supervision, and is not liable for any damages or negative consequences from any treatment, action, application or preparation, to any person reading or following the information in this book. References are provided for informational purposes only and do not constitute endorsement of any websites or other sources. Readers should be aware that the websites listed in this book may change.

Every effort has been made to reference or acknowledge material used from other authors properly. Although the author has made every effort to ensure that the information in this book was correct at the time of publishing, the author does not assume and hereby disclaims any liability to any party for any loss, damage, or disruption caused by errors or omissions, whether such errors or omissions result from negligence, accident, or any other cause.

The author advises readers to take full responsibility for their safety and know their limits. Before practicing the exercises described in this book, be sure that your equipment is well maintained, and do not take risks beyond your level of experience, aptitude, training, and comfort level.

Table of Contents

Disclaimer i
About the Author ii
Fair Use Statement iii
Dedications iv
Endorsements for Forever Active Older Adult Health and Fitness Playbook vii
Acknowledgments viii
Suggestions for Reading this Book x
Section 1 1
Before We Begin 1
   1.0. Introduction: Before We Begin 2
   1.1. Motivation to Start 5
   1.2. Introducing the Older Adult: The Science of Aging 8
Section 2 25
The Off-Season – Studying the Opposition to Your Health 25
   2.0. Introduction: The Off-Season – Studying the Opposition to Your Health 26
   2.1. Arthritis 27
   2.2. Heart Disease, Stroke and Hypertension 36
   2.3. Cancer 47
   2.4. Diabetes 58
   2.5. Obesity 73
   2.6. Dementia 90
   2.7. Oral and Dental Health and Decay 104
   2.8. Visual Challenges and Impairments 132
   2.9. Hearing Impairments and Disorders of the Ear 149
Section 3 168
Pre-Season – Preparation Time so You Can Perform at Your Best 168
   3.0. Introduction: The Preseason: Preparation Time 169
   3.1. The Eight Golden Rules of Training 170
   3.2. Learning to Overcome the Five Internally Generated Obstacles to Exercise 179
   3.3. The Importance and Art of Goal Setting 184
   3.4. Visualization for Motivation to Promote Change 188
Section 4 190
The Offense – Getting Active the Right Way 190
   4.0. Introduction: The Offense – Getting Active The Right Way 191
   4.1.0. Introduction: Cardiovascular Health, Fitness and Training..................................... 193
      4.1.1. Cardiovascular Fitness Training 194
      4.1.2. Walking with an Activity Tracking Device: A Great Way to Get Started on the Road to Improved Health 209
      4.1.3. Monitoring Heart Rate for Effective Cardiovascular Training 212

4.2.0. Introduction: Muscular Resistance Training	220
4.2.1. Muscular Resistance Training: Developing Muscle Strength and Endurance	221
4.2.2. Core Strengthening	240
4.2.3. Whole Body Muscular Strengthening	242
4.2.4. Bodyweight Strength/Resistance Training	244
4.3. Fall Prevention: Agility, Balance and Coordination Training	247
4.4. The Value of Cross-Training	253

Section 5 260

The Defense – Protecting Your Health and Fitness 260

5.0. Introduction: The Defense – Protecting Your Health and Fitness	261
5.1.0. Introduction: Flexibility	262
5.1.1. Flexibility Defined	263
5.1.2. The Biology of Stretching	267
5.1.3. Yin Yoga: a Meditative Way to Improved Flexibility	271
5.1.4. Myofascial Self Massage: An Effective Way to Improve Flexibility	274
5.2.0. Nutrition: Introduction	278
5.2.1. Nutrition Primer	280
5.2.2. How to Read Nutritional Labels	290
5.2.3. Canadian Health Food Guide	301
5.2.4. Sugar	306
5.2.5. Salt/Sodium	313
5.2.6. Cholesterol	321
5.2.7. Gluten	328
5.2.8. Dietary Supplementation	336
5.2.9. Glycemic Index: What It Is and Its Nutritional Usefulness for Controlling Blood Glucose Levels	343
5.2.10. Weight Loss and a Review of the Most Popular Diets	349
5.3. Sleep – Don't Ignore Its Importance for Recovery and Health	381

Section 6 398

Special Teams – Mental Health: Supporting the Offense and Defense 398

6.0. Introduction: Special Teams – Mental Health – Supporting the Offense and Defense	399
6.1. Understanding and Managing Cognitive Health	401
6.2. The Six Components of Wellness	408
6.3. Understanding Depression	417
6.4. Developing Mental Fitness	424
6.5. Finding Meaning/Purpose in Life	433
6.6. Self-Compassion: The Proven Power of Being Kind to Yourself	439
6.7. Self-Leadership	447
6.8. Learn From Others Through Good Communication Techniques	456
6.9. Mindfulness and Mindfulness Meditation	466
6.10. Make Life a Joyful Journey	475
6.11. Dealing with Grief	486

- 6.12. Social Intimacy 513
- 6.13. Physical and Sexual Intimacy 518
- 6.14. Finding Zen in Your Life.. 523

Section 7 532

The Post-Season – The Playoffs and Super Bowl – Raising Your Expectations 532

- 7.0. Introduction: The Post Season – Raise Your Expectations 533
- 7.1. How to Play to Win 535

Section 8 544

Post-Season Wrap-up – Measuring Progress and Success 544

- 8.0. Evaluation of Effort – Measuring Progress and Success...................................... 545

Section 9 580

The Support Staff 580

- 9.0. Introduction: The Support Staff.. 581
- 9.1. Introduction to the Appendices... 582
- 9.1.0. Appendices 582
  - Appendix 9.1.1.0. Introduction to Cardiovascular Fitness Exercises 584
  - Appendix 9.1.1.1. Walking with Good Posture... 586
  - Appendix 9.1.1.2: Developing Proper Running/Jogging Form 589
  - Appendix 9.1.1.3. Cycling Safely: Good Sizing, Good Posture, Follow Safety Guidelines ... 593
  - Appendix 9.1.1.4. Swimming: Knowing How Makes It Easier and More Enjoyable 597
  - Appendix 9.1.2.0. Introduction to the Muscular Strengthening/Resistance Exercises........... 600
    - Appendix 9.1.2.1.0. Introduction to Core Strengthening Exercises 601
    - Appendix 9.1.2.1.1. Core Strengthening Exercises Described and Illustrated 602
    - Appendix 9.1.2.2.0. Introduction to Whole Body Muscular Strength Training Exercises 620
    - Appendix 9.1.2.2.1. Whole-Body Muscular Strength Training Exercises Described and Illustrated.. 622
    - Appendix 9.1.2.3. Introduction to Bodyweight Muscle Strength Training........................... 664
    - Appendix 9.1.2.3.1: Bodyweight Muscle Strengthening Exercises Described and Illustrated 665
  - Appendix 9.1.3.0. Introduction to Agility, Balance and Coordination Exercises........................ 689
    - Appendix 9.1.3.1. Agility, Balance and Coordination Exercises Described and Illustrated. 690
  - Appendix 9.1.4.0. Introduction to Flexibility/Stretching Exercises.. 706
    - Appendix 9.1.4.1. Stretching Exercises Described and Illustrated 707
    - Appendix 9.1.4.2. 10 Minute Dynamic and Static Stretching Routine 740
    - Appendix 9.1.4.3. Yin Yoga Poses Illustrated and Described 750
    - Appendix 9.1.4.4. Myofascial Self Massage Utilizing a Roller 761
  - Appendix 9.1.5. Resistance Band Exercises Described and Illustrated 769
  - Appendix 9.1.6. Stability Ball Exercises Described and Illustrated 784

Appendix 9.1.7. BOSU Exercises Described and Illustrated 803
Appendix 9.1.8. TRX Exercises Described and Illustrated 850
Appendix 9.1.9. Medicine Ball Exercises Described and Illustrated 870
Appendix 9.1.10. Floor Slider Exercises Described and Illustrated 883

9.2.0. Introduction: Workout Sheets 890
9.2.1. Goal Setting Worksheet (S.M.A.R.T.) 891
9.2.2. Cardiovascular Exercise and Daily Activity Recording Sheet 893
9.2.3. Muscle Resistance Workout Sheets 895

Core Workout Sheets 896
45 Minute Core Workout #1 896
45 Minute Core Workout #2 898
10 Minute Core Workout #1 900
10 Minute Core Workout #2 901
10 Minute Core Workout #3 902
10 Minute Core Workout #4 903
10 Minute Core Workout #5 904

Core and Whole-Body Workout Sheets 905
Core and Whole-Body Muscle Resistance Routine #1 905
Core and Whole-Body Muscle Resistance Routine #2 908
Core and Whole-Body Muscle Resistance Routine #3 911
Core and Whole-Body Muscle Resistance Routine #4 914
Core and Whole-Body Muscle Resistance Routine #5 917

Core and Upper-Body Workout Sheets 920
Core and Upper-Body Muscle Resistance Routine #1 920
Core and Upper-Body Muscle Resistance Routine #2 922
Core and Upper-Body Muscle Resistance Routine #3 925
Core and Upper-Body Muscle Resistance Routine #4 928

Core and Lower-Body Workout Sheets 932
Core and Lower-Body Muscle Resistance Routine #1 932
Core and Lower-Body Muscle Resistance Routine #2 934
Core and Lower-Body Muscle Resistance Routine #3 936
Core and Lower-Body Muscle Resistance Routine #4 938
Core and Lower-Body Muscle Resistance Routine #5 940

Core and Bodyweight Workout Sheets 942
Core and Bodyweight Muscle Resistance Routine #1 942
Core and Bodyweight Muscle Resistance Routine #2 945

- 9.2.4. Agility, Balance and Coordination Workout Sheets ... 947
  - Core, Leg Strengthening and Agility, Balance and Coordination Exercise Routine ... 948
  - Core and Leg Strengthening Exercise Routine To Improve Agility, Balance and Coordination (Illustrated) ... 952
  - Core and Leg Strengthening Exercise Routine to Improve Agility, Balance and Coordination ... 956
    - Agility and Coordination Exercise Routine ... 957
    - Balance Exercise Routine (Illustrated) ... 959
    - Balance Exercise Routine ... 962
- 9.2.5. Stretching to Improve Flexibility Workout Sheets ... 963
  - 45 Minute Dynamic and Static Stretching Routine ... 964
  - 10 Minute Dynamic and Static Stretching Routine (Illustrated) ... 976
  - 10 Minute Dynamic Stretching Routine (Illustrated) ... 973
  - 10 Minute Static Stretching Routine (Illustrated) ... 976
  - Yin Yoga - Upper Back, Chest and Shoulders (Illustrated) ... 980
  - Yin Yoga - Lower Back, Hips and Legs Routine (Illustrated) ... 983
  - Myofascial Self Massage Utilizing a Roller (Illustrated) ... 987
- 9.2.6. Re-Evaluation Worksheets ... 991
  - Physical Activity Re-Evaluation ... 992
  - Nutritional Balance Re-Evaluation ... 993
  - Holistic Wellness Re-Evaluation ... 994
  - Physical Fitness Re-Evaluation ... 995
  - Goal Setting Re-Evaluation ... 1020
- 9.3.0. Online Support ... 1022
- 9.4.0. Introduction: Reference Library ... 1023
  - 9.4.1. Hard Copy Reference Library ... 1024
  - 9.4.2 Online Reference Library: Healthy Links ... 1030

Section 10 ... 1031

Epilogue ... 1031

- 10. Epilogue ... 1032

About the Author

Michael graduated on the Dean's list with an Honours Bachelor of Science degree in Kinesiology from the University of Waterloo in 1975. He followed that with a Doctor of Chiropractic degree in 1983 and an MBA from Wilfrid Laurier University in 2008. In 2012, Michael became certified as a personal trainer, and started his own business, Forever Active (www.forever-active.com). As a personal trainer, he specialized in the health and fitness of older adults – people aged 50 years and older.

Michael is an avid runner with 25 complete marathons under his belt. He has run a marathon in every province in Canada as well as in Athens Greece and London England. For the London race Michael helped train and guided a blind runner.

Following his last marathon in 2017, Michael turned his attention to triathlon racing. This was again another challenge since he had no experience swimming in open water or racing on a road bike. After completing one sprint and two Olympic distance triathlons, Michael began to focus on Ironman training. In September 2021 he completed the Weymouth England half Ironman race and on November 21, 2021 Michael completed his first full Ironman race in Cozumel, Mexico.

Michael loves to travel with his wife, Ann. In the spring of 2018, Michael was fortunate to complete an expedition to the base camp of Mt. Everest with True Patriot Love which is an organization that supports mentally and physically injured military veterans.

Michael believes in developing and practising strong physical and mental health, neither of which comes easily to anyone. He feels a daily plan needs to be put into place and implemented diligently to achieve optimal health and enjoyment. This book, Forever Active Older Adult Health Fitness Playbook, is his way of giving back and hopefully helping everyone achieve a life full of health and happiness.

Michael and Ann have been married for 35 years and live in Toronto. They have two lovely children, Scott and Kelly.

Fair Use Statement

This book contains some copyrighted material, the use of which has not been specially authorized by the copyright holders. The material is made available to advance education and teaching related to personal health and fitness. There is no reason to believe that any copyrighted material used will in any way affect the market value of the copyrighted works. For this reason, it is believed that this book is clearly under current fair use copyright laws.

Dedications

I want to dedicate the writing of this book to five individuals who have been instrumental in guiding me, supporting me, and enhancing the quality of my life.

My first dedication is to my high school basketball coach and mentor, Ron Coristine. Being an adolescent can be confusing, and entering high school can be an intimidating experience. Fortunately, I navigated both of these challenges quite well, with the help of Mr. Coristine. I entered grade nine in a four-year business and commerce program. I was not disciplined in school, lacking both academically and behaviourally. Fortunately, I liked and was pretty good at sports, so I played many in high school. Mr. Coristine was one of our physical education teachers and basketball coach. To me though, he was much more than a teacher and coach. He was a true mentor. Every day, he taught me through his words and actions to treat people with respect and always keep a smile on my face. He encouraged me to pursue five-year academic classes and to control my emotions. To "take a breath" when I felt emotional so I could evaluate better and handle the situation effectively. My high school years were a tremendously positive experience. I grew as a student, athlete, and person. At a crucial time in my life, Mr. Coristine was there to guide and mentor me. He taught me how to approach each day with positive energy, and I became a much better person because of him.

My second dedication is to the late Father Jim Williams. He was an older priest in his mid to late 60s when he came to our church. He was a tremendous orator, attracting three times more attendance at Sunday masses because of his speaking skills. Over the years, we became good friends and shared many thoughts and ideas about societal issues, including the church. He told me that when he was first ordained, he used to be a very conservative priest and abided by the church's strict 'man-made' laws. Over time and with more real-world experience, he became more liberated in his views and fully embraced individuals marginalized by the traditional church teachings, such as divorcees and gays. When I experienced difficult times, he shepherded me through them, always telling me to "let things unfold as they should." He taught me tolerance, to be non-judgmental of people because everyone has a backstory of their own, and forgiveness of one's self. His teachings were and still are a guiding light to me.

My third dedication is to my good friend, Brian MacEachern. Brian is a veteran of the Canadian Arm Forces and served in Afghanistan with the 5 Combat Engineers Regiment in 2004 and Engineer Support Regiment in 2007. I met Brian when I joined The True Patriot Love Expedition to the base camp of Mt. Everest in 2018. The trip was great, but developing my friendship with Brian was the highlight. Like the other nine veterans on our expedition, Brian suffers from Post-Traumatic Stress Disorder (PTSD). Over the last three and a half years, Brian has taught me what real courage is. The horrors he and other veterans have experienced defending our freedom and way of life are unimaginable. Like all our Canadian soldiers, Brian volunteered for armed services and, unfortunately, has paid a profound price while doing his duty. Brian is physically a BIG guy but has the heart and soul of a teddy bear. He is someone who would be there if you asked for help, and would and likely be there even if you didn't ask. His desire to feel whole again, to feel normal again, can only be measured by the size of his heart and determination to make that happen. I have learned so much from Brian over these past few years. He exemplifies courage, self-sacrifice, determination, and commitment to what you believe in, even though it may cost you a lot. I love Brian, not because he needs my love or support, but because he unwaveringly opened himself up to me with the courage I had not experienced before. I dedicate this book to him because it is the only way I can sincerely thank him for all he has done to enhance my life.

My fourth dedication is to my brother Rick or, as my mother would call him, Richard. What younger brother does not admire and wants to be like their older brother? I sure did. As I grew up, Rick was my hero. Rick was three and a half years older than me but tolerated me hanging by his side. That was not an easy thing to do. He was an excellent athlete, and I am sure that helped me pursue athletics. Rick was a firefighter for over 35 years, the last ten as a Captain. One of the loveliest things about him is that Rick has a strong sense of family. He and his wife Suzanne have been married 42 years and have raised three wonderful children, each of whom has their own great families now. Rick was a tremendous role model for me growing up, and continues to be. He has helped me become a better person, husband, and father.

My fifth dedication, and certainly not least, is to my wife, Ann. Where would I be without my wife? We have been married thirty-five years and have raised two wonderful independent children, Scott and Kelly. Ann has been a rock in my life; she is the yin to my yang, ever-present as a calming influence and an inspiration for excellence. Ann has her Master's in Occupational Therapy and specialized in treating people with acquired brain injuries while in private practice for over thirty-five years. Not only was this a very specialized field, but she was the best in Canada doing it. This is not coming from me but from her professional colleagues. She has touched and helped the lives of so many people that I could only aspire to have touched. She is my life partner, and I am so much better for it.

In this dedication section, I must also mention my parents, Francis (Frank) and Frances (Fran) Bedard, and my children, Scott and Kelly.

My parents were hard-working, warm, caring, and loving. They sacrificed so my brother and I would never be in want of anything. They taught Rick and me the meaning of generosity towards others and the importance of supporting each other in times of need. They provided a strong foundation for my brother and me to grow and spread our wings. What more could you ask of your parents?

My children, Scott and Kelly, are my inspiration. They are the greatest gifts that God could have ever given to me. Ann and I are so fortunate to have kids whose behaviour never gave us a reason to be concerned through childhood and adolescence. They have grown into adults that I am very proud of. They are independent-minded, have a high level of integrity, are much more intelligent than I ever would hope to be, empathic toward those in need, and, most importantly, are just good people.

As I conclude, it is evident that I have been very fortunate to have many people grace my life at what seemed to have been a perfect time. However, these are only a small sample of the people who shaped and influenced my life. To mention each would require a book in itself. Though I will not give special mention to each of them, I want them to know how thankful I am for having them touch my life. I am better for it, and I hope those that I have touched are better for it as well.

My daughter has a quote from Shakespeare's tragedy King Lear that she likes to use and I would like to share it, "Speak what you feel, not what you ought to say."

This dedication is me speaking what I feel.

Michael Bedard

Endorsements for Forever Active Older Adult Health and Fitness Playbook

"This book is not only a guide but hopefully a motivation to find activities that are both physically and mentally challenging to maintain your "best self" as you age. The health benefits of both physical and mental activity cannot be overstated in assisting with management of chronic disease. Find activities that you enjoy and then incorporate them into your everyday life."
DH, 76, Type 1 Diabetic, Avid Walker and World Traveler

"Mike Bedard provides a bridge between the science of anti aging and the application of psychology to give the reader meaning and direction to their exercise program. A great read for anyone looking improve their fitness later in life."
Derek Murchie, Fitness Motivator, Founder Max Revolution

"Mike Bedard draws from his personal experience as a master's athlete (over 50 years of age) with 25 marathons completed and an Ironman finisher at age 65, personal trainer and science background to put together a great playbook for how to stay fit and healthy as you age."
Nigel Gray, Head Coach NRG Performance Training, 24 years of triathlon coaching experience, 25+ Ironman finishes, 3rd overall Ironman Canada 2005, 9-hour Ironman at age 48

"Mike's book offers a practical guide for those of us who are classified as 'older adults' to start or continue their fitness and wellness journey through their 60's, 70's, 80's and beyond. His concepts focus on strength, resistance training and exercise to slowly build up your fitness levels safely so as to avoid injury. As a client for 10 years, I started my fitness journey in my late 40's with hip, back and balance issues. I can attest to the fact that Mike's training regime and philosophy allowed me to gain a lot of physical strength, endurance and rectified my hip, back and balance issues. I feel stronger and more energetic than I felt in my early 40's and am ready to take on my 60's with vigor!"
E. O'Donnell, client of Mike's and Forever Active for 10years

"We don't stop playing because we grow old, we grow old because we stop playing," is a quote that struck me as I read Forever Active Older Adult Health and Fitness Playbook. As an Olympic athlete, I realize the important role that mental, physical and spiritual health play in one's lifelong happiness. Michael has captured this not only from his personal Ironman experiences, but also with detailed information from true experts in their field. The mature adult who is looking to live a longer and more active life will thoroughly enjoy this in-depth book, complete with easy-to-follow illustrations that will guide and inspire you along the way."
Karen Stemmle, Canadian Olympian – Alpine Skiing, Sarajevo, 1984

"As a fitness instructor whose primary clientele is over 50, I find Forever Active Older Adult Health and Fitness Playbook clear and instructive. Knowing how to safely continue to be active and strong (or to take up fitness later in life) is critical to maintaining or enhancing one's quality of life. This book will be an asset to instructors, trainers and clients alike."
Danielle Keystone-Adler, owner AdlerFitness Inc., Fitness Trainer

Acknowledgments

"Don't walk behind me, I may not lead.
Don't walk in front of me, I may not follow.
Just walk beside me and be my friend."

— Anonymous

Writing Forever Active Older Adult Playbook has not been a solitary effort. There have been many people that have contributed to the writing, reviewing, editing, sharing of ideas and opinions and completion of this book. In this section, I want to send a mighty thank you to the following. Without their interest, time and efforts the quality of this book would not be comparable to what has been published.

Ann Bedard, MSc. OT (Retired). Ann, my wife, wrote chapter 6.1, Understanding and Managing Cognitive Health. Ann was able to tackle this huge and complicated topic and simplify and communicate it into understandable layman's terms. Ann also edited many chapters for grammar and punctuations. Certainly not one of my strongest attributes.

Dr. Charles Tator, CM, MD, MA, PhD, FRCSC, Toronto Western Hospital who reviewed and edited chapters 2.1. Arthritis and 2.2. Heart Disease.

Dr. Caroline Chung, , MD, MSc., FRCPC, CIP, Radiation Oncology and Diagnostic Imaging, The University of Texas MD Anderson Cancer Center who reviewed and edited chapters 2.3. Cancer and 2.4. Diabetes.

Dr. Nitsa Kohut, MD, M Sc., MCFP, who reviewed and edited chapter 2.6. Dementia.

Dr. Dana Colson, D.D.S., Dentist, who reviewed and edited chapter 2.7 Oral and Dental Health and Decay.

Dr. David Ng, O.D. who reviewed and edited the chapter 2.8. Visual Challenges and Impairments.

Dr. Alexandre Osborne. MD, PhD, Otolaryngologist who reviewed and edited chapter 2.9 Hearing Impairments.

Elizabeth McLeod, BSc. RD, Dietitian, who reviewed and edited chapter 2.5 Obesity and all 10 chapters (5.2.1. to 5.2.10.) on nutrition.

Aaron Arkin, B.Sc., RP, RPSGT, President of evolutionsleep.com who reviewed and edited chapter 5.3. Sleep: Don't Ignore It.

Dr. Jeffrey Lipsitz, M.D. Founder and Medical Director, Sleep Disorders Centre of Metropolitan Toronto who reviewed and edited chapter 5.3. Sleep Don't Ignore It.

Dr. Elaine McKinnon, PhD, Clinical Psychologist who reviewed and edited chapter 6.1, Understanding and Managing Cognitive Health.

LCol. Markus Besemann, CD, MD, FRCP (C) Head of Rehabilitative Medicine, Canadian Forces Health Services who reviewed and edited chapter 6.3. Depression.

Dr. Lucinda Sykes, MD. Director, Mediation for Health and www.relaxyourstressfullmind.com, who contributed, reviewed and edited chapter 6.9. Mindfulness and Mindfulness Mediation.

Dr. Randy Gangbar, MD who reviewed and edited chapters 6.12. Social Intimacy and chapter 6.13. Physical and Sexual Intimacy.

Kathy Mott, Wenli Yang, Geoff Anderton, Gord Mott and Doug McLeod who graciously volunteered to be models so all the strength and flexibility exercises would be properly illustrated in the appendices.

Alyse Mirabelli, my one person does all. She was my photographer for all the various exercises illustrated in the appendices and my computer technologist who saved me countless times when I thought I had lost a chapter after spending hours completing it. Alyse was also my graphic designer and was instrumental in the helping the design of the front and back covers of the book. She also gave me the lead to my publisher.

Savvy Book Marketing for editing and their guidance that led to the completion and printing of this book.

To my wife, children, relatives and friends and who have loved and supported me throughout the years. Without them in my life, this book would not have been attempted, completed or have the meaning that it has for me.

Suggestions for Reading this Book

Forever Active Older Adult Health and Fitness Playbook is not meant to be read sequentially from cover to cover but rather picked apart one chapter at a time. It is my suggestion that you review the Table of Contents, pick a chapter that interests you and read it. This might mean reading a chapter in Section 2 on one of the oppositions to your health such as arthritis or a chapter in section 6 on mental health. When you are ready to create and implement your personal health and fitness plan, read the chapters in Sections 3, 4 and 5 to help you do so.

Section 8 explains how to evaluate your nutritional, physical activity and holistic health and physical fitness before you begin your health and fitness plan. There are re-evaluation work sheets in the appendix that you can use to continue to re-evaluate your progress as you continue to implement your personal plan.

Section 9 includes a very comprehensive appendix with chapters illustrating and explaining core, whole-body, body weight, flexibility, agility, balance and coordination exercises. As well, exercises utilizing resistance bands, stability balls, BOSU, TRX, medicine balls and floor sliders are illustrated and explained. The appendix also includes workout sheets with over 40 exercise routines for the core, upper and lower body, flexibility, agility, balance and coordination. Use the appendices and worksheets to help develop and implement your health and fitness plan.

Forever Active Older Adult Health and Fitness Playbook is an excellent reference book and should be utilized that way.

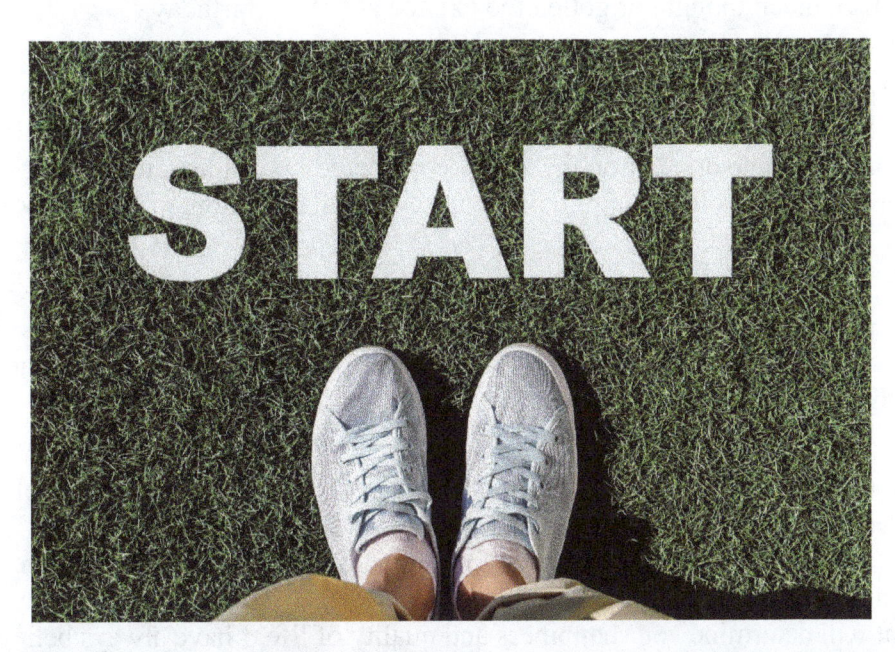

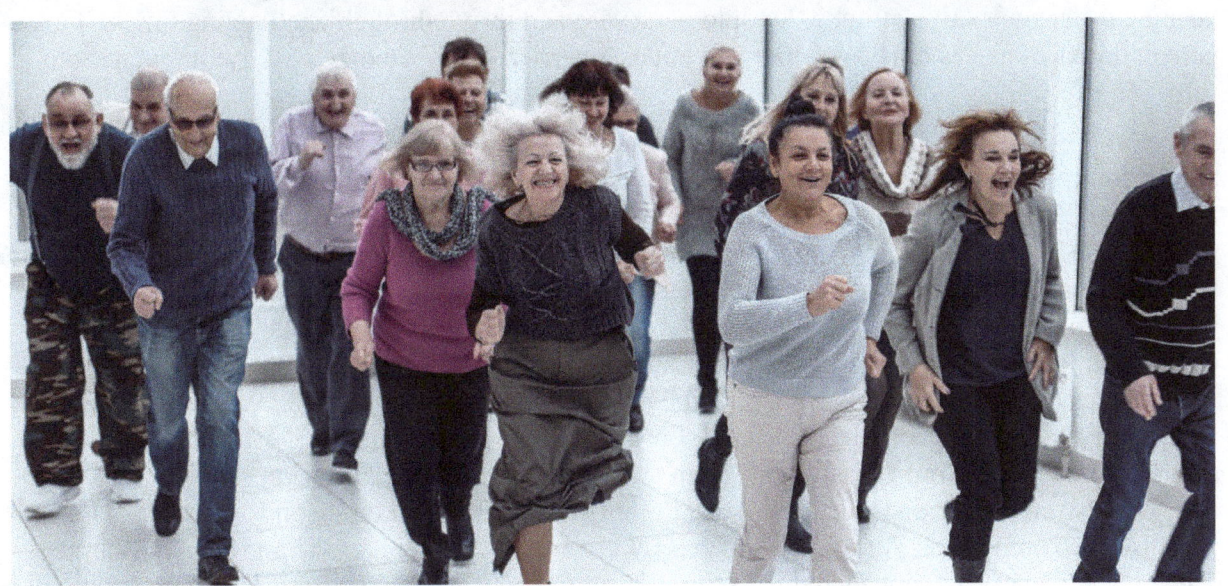

Section 1
Before We Begin

1.0. Introduction: Before We Begin

It is January 1, 2021, the world is in the middle of the Covid-19 pandemic, I am eight days away from my 65th birthday, and I can't do much about either.

To combat the virus, I can socially isolate, wear a mask when I am out and about and get a vaccine when it is my turn to do so. As for my birthday, well, birthdays come and go. In the past, I have never given much thought or gotten too excited about my birthday.

My 16th was obviously a big one since I could drive. My 18th was special as I could drink legally. When I turned 21 and was in university, I thought of myself as a young adult. At 31, married with one child and another on the way, I considered myself a mature young adult. At 40, I was not so young but not old either. At 50, I became middle-aged but did not think too much of it.

However, at 60, *bam*, all of a sudden, I began to think about my mortality. I was shocked; it just occurred to me that I was well past the midpoint of my life. Now I wonder, what thoughts and actions will my 65th birthday bring?

From a thought's perspective, I have adopted the philosophy of "You are only old when you use age as an excuse." I love the meaning of this quote and have fully embraced it. Throughout my life, I have always felt that the positivity of my mind, attitude and emotions were my biggest assets. Challenging things will happen throughout a person's lifetime, but it is how you tackle them that what will determine your happiness and quality of life. I have always believed that by keeping a strong positive attitude, I would persevere and thrive through challenging times. If a person thinks of age as only a number and not as a barrier, I believe they will live a much more fulfilling life.

As for my actions, well, first, I am training to complete my first full Ironman Triathlon in September 2021. I thought that doing an Ironman at 65 would be pretty cool. At age 61, I was a runner with 25 marathons to my credit. I had run a marathon in every province in Canada, as well as one in Greece and England. The latter, I ran as a guide for a blind runner. However, I was NOT a swimmer and only a recreational biker. Despite these skill limitations, I set a goal to complete a full Ironman (3.8 km swim, 180 km bike ride and 42.2 km full marathon) in less than 17 hours (to be considered an Ironman, you have to complete the race in 16:59:59). I plan on using every second. To complete this goal, I broke it down into attainable pieces. Three years ago, I competed in a Sprint Triathlon (750 m swim, 20 km bike ride and 5 km run). Two years ago, I did two Olympic distance triathlons (1.5 km swim, 40 km bike ride and 10 km run). Last year, I was to complete a 70.1 half Ironman (1.9 km swim, 90 km bike ride and 21.1 km run). The race, however, got cancelled due to COVID, so my coach arranged for a 111 race (1 km swim, 100 km bike ride and 10 km run).

(Yes, I have a tri coach to guide and support me through the rigors of training. As I will explain later in the book, most things are easier to accomplish if you have help doing them. Relying exclusively on yourself, in most cases, is an unnecessary burden to carry).

This year is the big one for me, the full Ironman. You will have to read the epilogue to see how I did 😊.

The second action I am taking is writing this book, 'Forever Active Older Adult Health and Fitness Playbook'. Writing a book has been on my bucket list for a number of years, and I thought that completing it while I was celebrating my 65th year would be a great achievement.

Ten years ago, I started a personal training business for older adults called Forever Active. It has been very rewarding, but I realized early on that training the older adult is a speciality upon itself. Unlike 20- and 30-year-olds, many older adults present with special needs such as arthritis in their hips and knees, chronic lower back pain, diabetes, visual and hearing impairments or being a cancer survivor. For their training to be successful, these health issues must be accommodated.

I also learned that though older adults may have been very successful in raising a family and building their careers, many are uninformed when it comes to taking care of their own physical, nutritional and mental health. It is my hope that this book fills that void for them.

I have called this book, 'Forever Active Older Adult Health and Fitness Playbook' for two reasons. First, I wanted to emphasize the word 'play'. Life presents enough challenges, so doing things to improve your health, fitness and enhance the quality of your life should be as much fun as possible.

Again, it is all about a person's mental outlook. If they perceive a thing as fun, it becomes fun. If they look upon them as a burden, they become a burden. Everyone should make taking care of their health as enjoyable as possible. I hope this book will help everyone do so.

Second, I feel the word, 'Playbook' gives the book structure. I have organized the book as if it was a football 'playbook'. Though a person may not be familiar with the X's and O's of football, almost everyone knows that there is an offense, a defense and special teams in football. The ultimate prize is getting into the playoffs winning the Super Bowl. By structuring the book this way, I feel it emphasizes what a person is trying to accomplish.

For example, by participating in cardiovascular, muscle strengthening and agility, balance and coordination exercises, a person is being 'offensive' in strengthening their heart, protecting their joints and in fall prevention. By maintaining good flexibility and following good nutritional principles and oral health, a person is 'defending' themselves from immobility, obesity, diabetes and tooth decay, which reduces a person's quality of life.

The special teams section guides a person through understanding the principles of maintaining mental and emotional health, depression, dementia, social and sexual dysfunction and mindfulness. This special team's section is necessary to support a person's offensive and defensive efforts for optimal health.

As part of any good team, there is a support staff to ensure success. Under this section are the Appendices that illustrate and describe in detail how to perform various strengthening and stretching exercises, Ying Yoga poses and self-massage 'roller' techniques in a safe and effective manner. There are also Workout Sheets that will allow you to record and monitor over 40 muscle strengthening, agility, balance and coordination, stretching workouts, as well as forms to evaluate your progress.

Because of the pandemic, 2020 and 2021 have been challenging years for everyone. It has been more of a challenge for some than for others, but everyone is doing things differently than they were prior to the pandemic.

For the older adult, doing things differently than they previously were is a daunting task. This is especially true when it comes to their health. Years of neglect to their health as they raised their family and built their career have led to seeding bad health habits, which has eventually weakened them. Whether it is due to a lack of knowledge or commitment, the goal of trying to be healthier next year than you are today often feels out of reach.

However, "If you understand the *whys*, you can overcome the *hows*." The *'whys'* are obvious. Having a healthier, stronger, more flexible body, a more positive attitude, and a better understanding of depression, dementia and grief can only enhance a person's quality of life and make their 'golden years' more enjoyable. The *'hows'* can be more elusive. How do they go about achieving a stronger body and better attitude in the face of advancing years and debilitating conditions like osteoarthritis and obesity?

It is my hope and goal that this book will assist the older adult in embracing the *why's* and understanding the *how's*; so they can develop the mindset and skills necessary to make this year and every year a better year.

1.1. Motivation to Start

Motivation can come in many forms. It can be verbal motivation through a pep talk like the great football coach Knute Rockne's speech, *'Win one for the Gipper'* or Vince Lombardi's quote, *"It's not whether you get knocked down, it's whether you get up."*

Visual motivation can come from watching a movie like Rocky. Who was not pumped up after watching that movie and his famous quote, "I know I can't beat the champ, my goal is to finish the fight." Rocky Balboa did finish the fight, and won our hearts by doing so.

We can also receive motivation by observing the courage, perseverance and accomplishments of others. Watching the Olympics is a great example of this.

Two older adults that I find as motivational figures are featured here: Ruth Bader Ginsberg and Ed Whitlock. The former is someone most people have probably heard of. Ruth was a highly respected American Supreme Court Judge and is fondly remembered as The Notorious RBG. The latter, most people probably have not heard of, but he is someone whom I refer to as the world's greatest athlete.

As you read this book and begin your journey for improved health and fitness, I encourage you to keep these two in mind and use them as inspiration when you feel the journey is getting too tough or the mountain too high for you to continue. They did not quit, and neither should you!

Ruth Bader Ginsberg (1933-2020), American Supreme Court Judge (1993-2020)

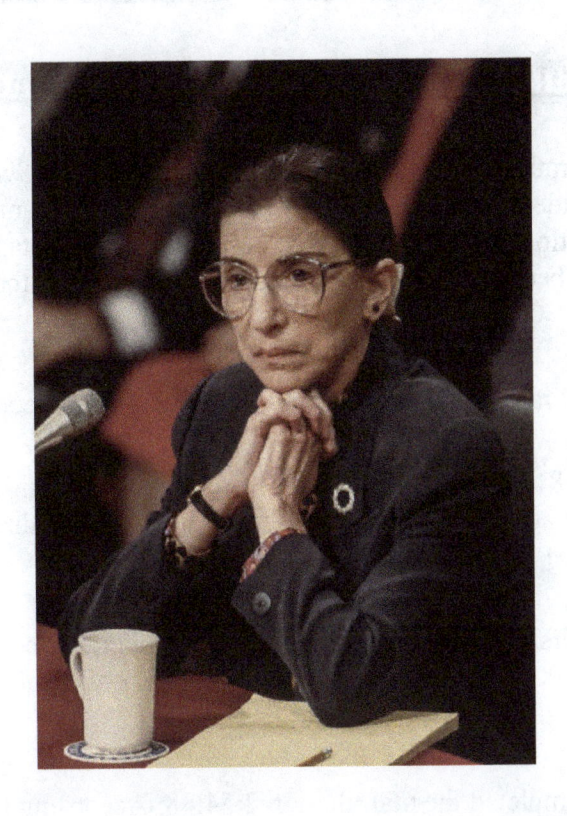

Famous Quote:
"Fight for the things that you care about, but do it in a way that will lead others to join you."

RBG, was an American Supreme Court Judge for 27 years, and during that time she was a passionate fighter for human rights.

On a personal level, she was a survivor of multiple cancers and a heart operation. After her first bout with cancer in 1999, she began to diligently work out for one hour two times a week with her personal trainer. Her workouts consisted of a series of full-body strength exercises that targeted her arms, chest, legs, back, shoulders, glutes, and abs. She continued these workouts until just a few months before she died on September 18, 2020. Ruth Bader Ginsberg was a courageous and spirited fighter right to the end.

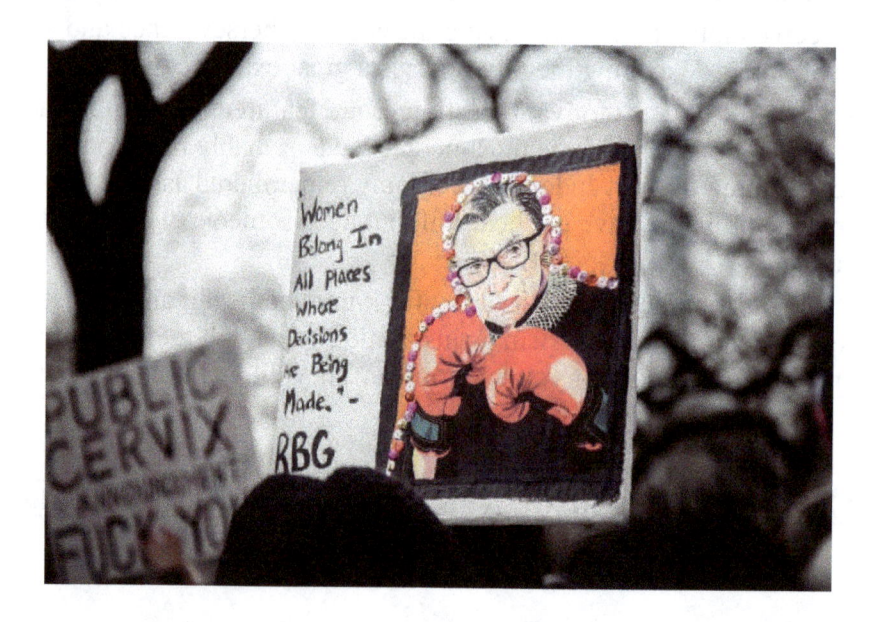

Ed Whitlock (1931-2017), Canadian Long-Distance Runner

Ed started running marathons accidentally when his youngest son, who was 14 at the time and was into running, decided he was going to run a marathon after running every day for over a year without a break. Whitlock tried to deter him, but in the end reluctantly ran the race with him. Although he had not been concentrating on training for the marathon, he ran 2:31:23 at age of 48.

After this first race, Ed ran and trained daily by running laps in a cemetery.

By 2012, at the age of 81, Ed held 15 world age group records, ranging in distance from 1500 meters to 10,000 meters in age groups 65+, 70+, 75+, 80+ as well as three age group marathon records in 70+, 75+ and 80+.

Ed Whitlock was the first person over 70 years old to run a marathon in less than three hours with a time of 2:59:10 in 2003. At the time of his death, he was the holder of all world records for marathons over age 70.

At the age of 73, he completed the marathon in 2:54:48. According to scientists, if this time was age-graded, it would be equivalent to a 20-year-old running 2:03:57, which would have been the fastest marathon run ever in 2010.

At age 85, Ed completed a marathon in 3:56:33, which is a world record.

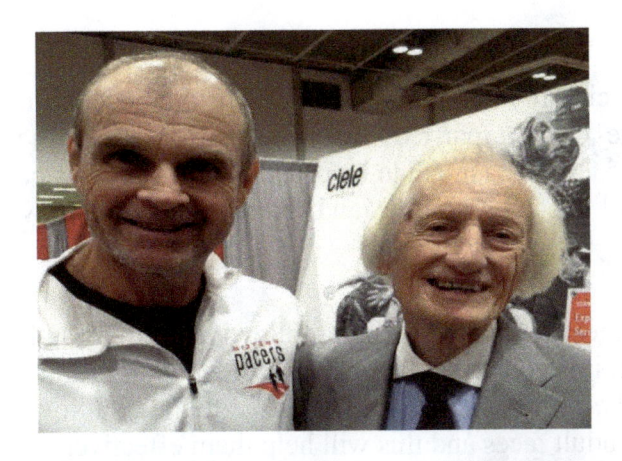

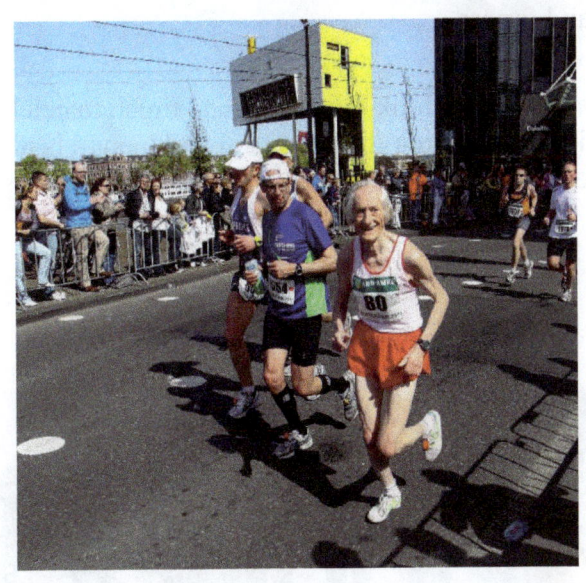

RBG and Ed are extraordinary individuals. It would not be fair to compare yourself to what they have accomplished. I would rather encourage you to use them as sources of motivation, to remember and believe in what is possible. Dream it, believe it, do it and enjoy the journey along the way.

1.2. Introducing the Older Adult: The Science of Aging

Introduction

The older adult is special. In most cases, with good health and a little luck, he or she has lived a full and active life. Getting married, raising a family, working in their occupation, or building a business for 35+ years is much to be proud of. However, as people enter their golden years, physical, emotional, mental/cognitive, and social challenges are waiting to threaten their quality of life.

Each of these challenges are dealt with in the following sections and chapters of this book. But before we get to that, it is good to define who the older adult is and the science behind how we age. Understanding the aging process will set a solid foundation for understanding the future challenges that the older adult faces and this will help them effectively deal with these challenges through improved health and fitness.

The older adult will have much to look forward to and much to celebrate in their future years if they make the right choices concerning their physical and mental health today. Understanding how a person ages will prepare that person to make those correct choices.

Human Life Cycle

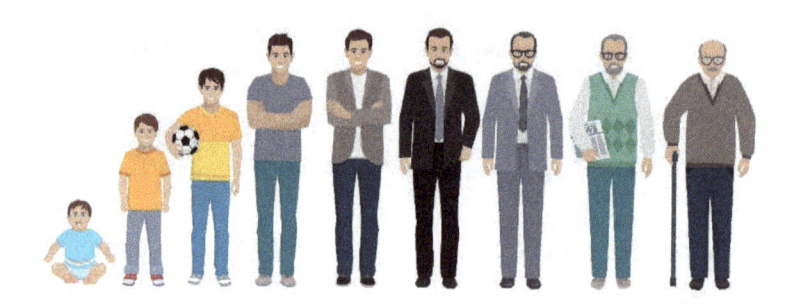

Throughout the early stages of a person's life, they grow physically and mature emotionally and mentally. Their bodies and minds are like sponges, soaking up everything, the good, the bad, and unfortunately, the ugly that is thrown their way. During childhood, adolescence, and early adulthood, a person has unbountiful energy. Their metabolism is racing, and it appears that nothing can slow them down.

Unfortunately, when a person reaches their mid-twenties and ages through their 30's and 40's, their metabolism slows down. The physical and mental tasks taken for granted in a person's younger years are no longer so easily accomplished.

As a person reaches 50 and beyond, the aging process accelerates, and the body starts to break down and atrophy (decrease in size or waste away). Chronic health problems such as arthritis, diabetes, heart disease, hearing and eye impairments, and cognitive impairment/dementia start to show their ugly head. Unfortunately, most older adults are unaware of how to deal with these issues and are physically and mentally deconditioned to do so.

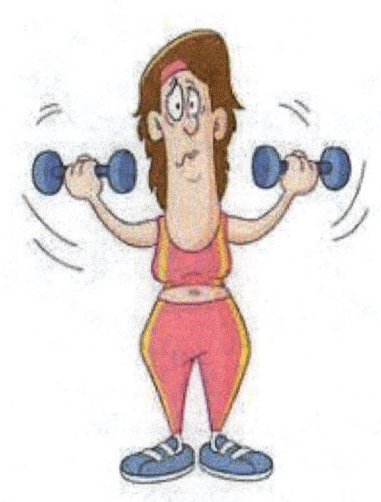

Fortunately, the last thirty years of a person's life do not have to be all doom and gloom. A person in their 50's and 60's can become functionally younger if they make healthy choices. The lifelines illustrated below reinforce this point. Chart 1 shows an individual who has continuous declining health, whereas in Chart 2, the lifeline illustrates that declining health is slowed significantly by healthy choices.

Quality of Life as You Age

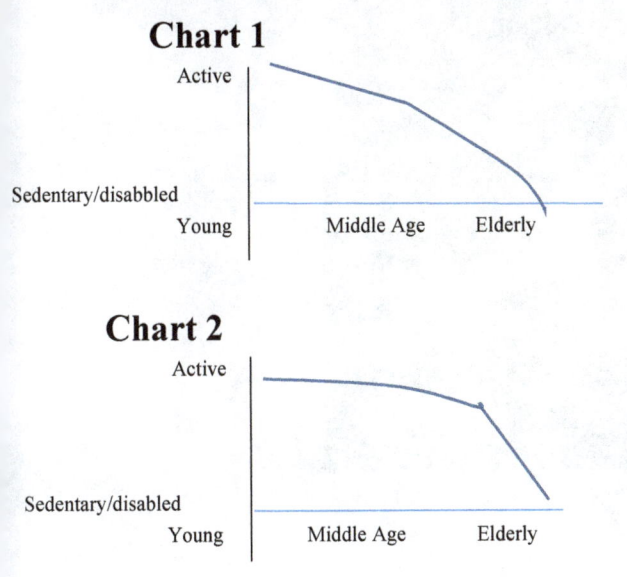

Chart 1

Chart 2

The goal for older adults is to extend their lifeline as far as possible into their later years before the disabling effects of age occur and significantly diminish their quality of life.

Defining the Older Adult

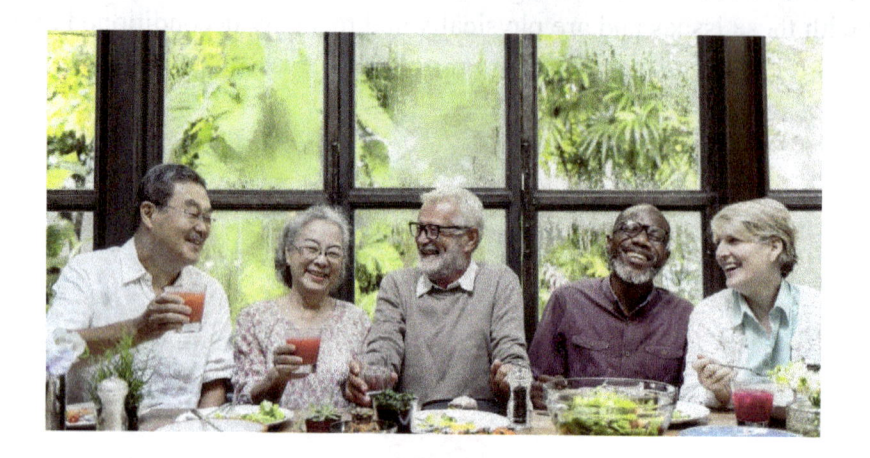

The classic definition of an older adult is based on their chronological age. This means anyone 50 years or older is considered an older adult. Realistically, a person should be viewed as an older adult based upon a broader functional, psychological and social perspective.

Functional age is determined by:

- How physically active a person is
- How well they move
- A person's agility, balance, coordination, muscular strength and cardiovascular endurance.

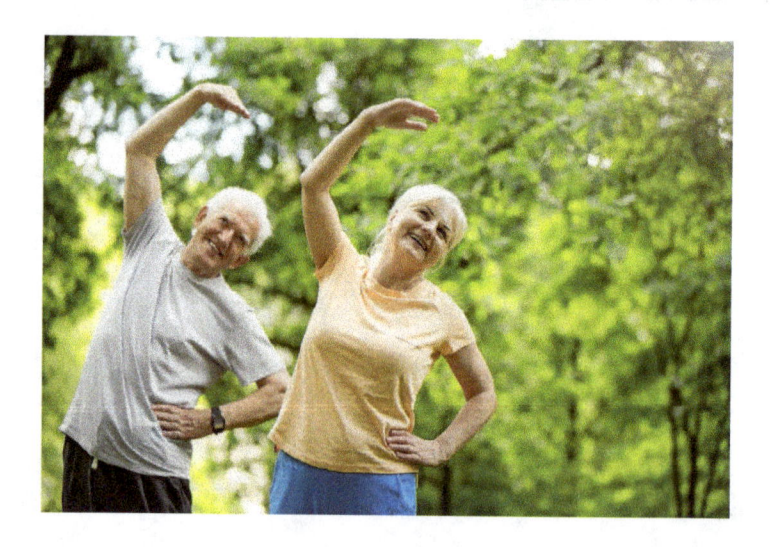

Example – Sister Madonna Buder (86)

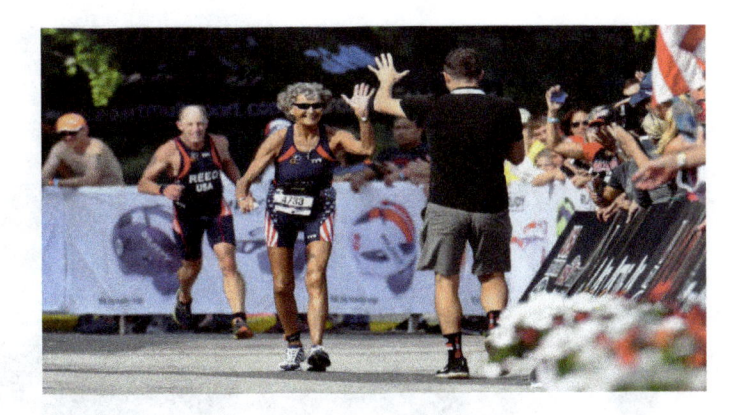

Sister Buder is known as the "Iron Nun" because of her prolific triathlon and Ironman career. She has completed over 360 triathlons and 45 Ironman's. Sister Madonna chose a cloistered life as a Roman Catholic nun, and only began running at age 48. She is the oldest person ever to finish an Ironman, and in her 80's completed an Ironman in 16 hours and 32 minutes. Sister Buder's motto is, "The only failure is not to try because your effort in itself is a success."

Psychological age is determined by:

- A person's cognitive abilities, entailing their attention span, memory and ability to think, reason, problem-solve and analyze.

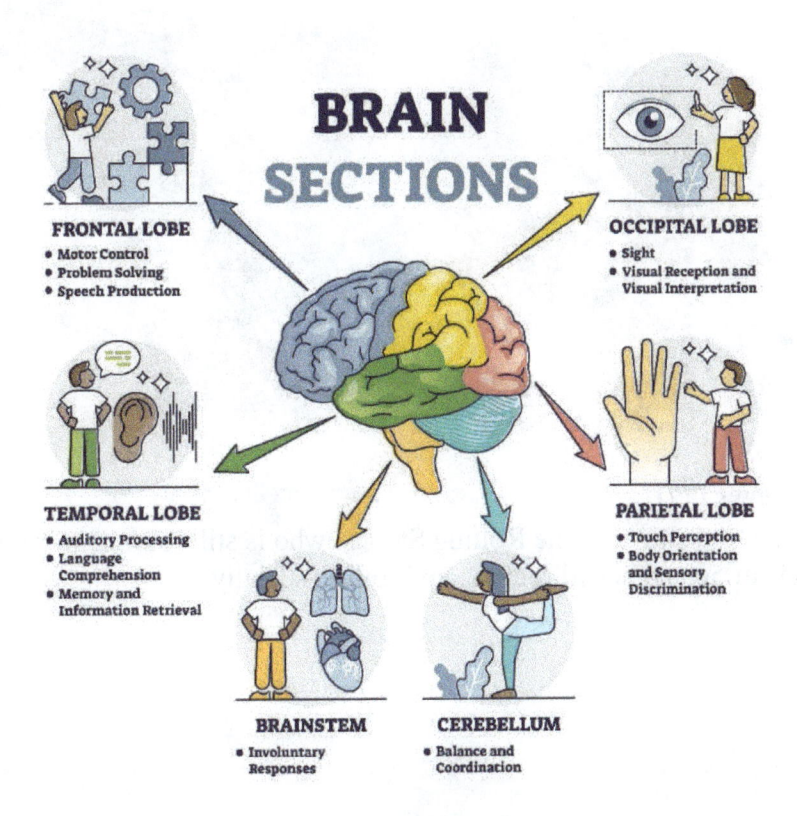

Example – Richard Branson (70)

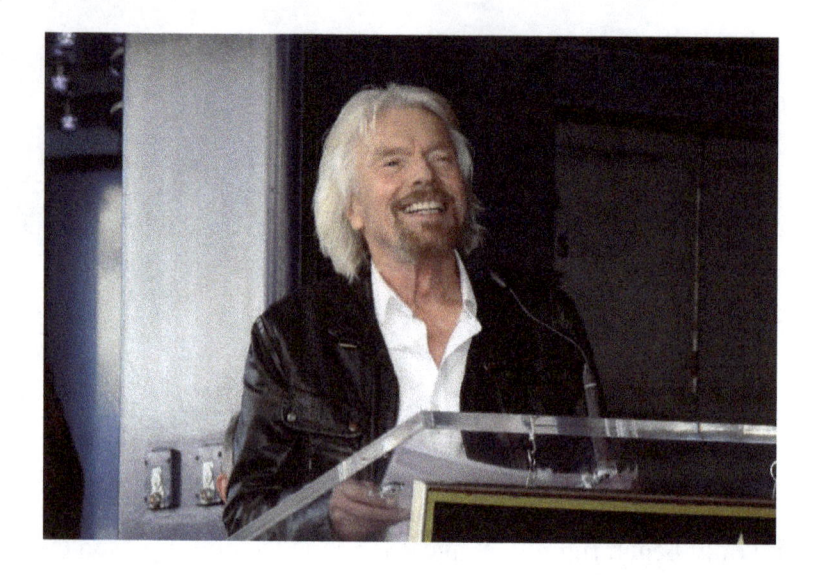

Sir Richard Branson is the founder and still active CEO of The Virgin Group with over 400 companies worldwide.

Social age is determined by:

- A person's ability and desire to socialize and interact with others.

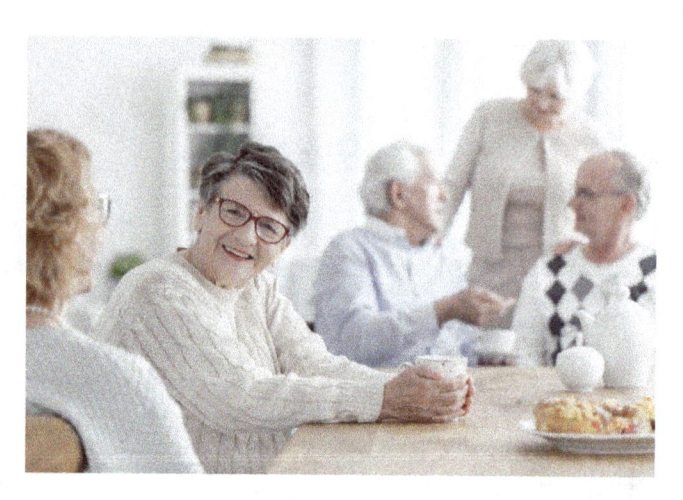

Example – Mick Jagger (77)

Mick Jagger is the lead singer of the Rolling Stones, who is still touring worldwide. He has three children after the age of 50 and is still rocking and rolling socially.

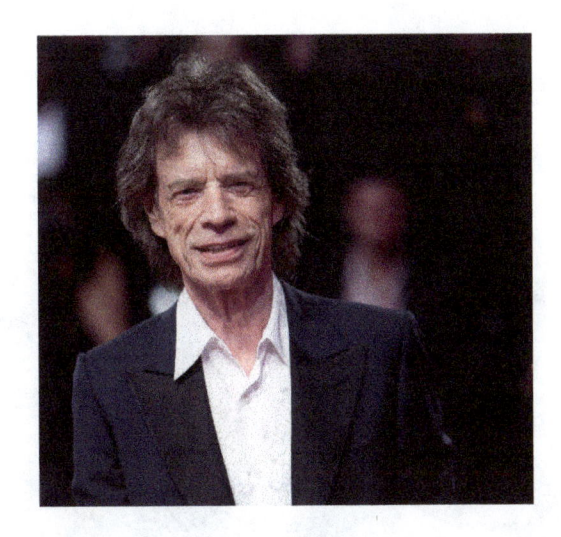

The critical point is that chronological age alone cannot define a person as an older adult. Instead, each individual must be considered from a holistic perspective (functionally, psychologically, and socially). Chronological age, in and of itself, is irrelevant.

The Science of Aging

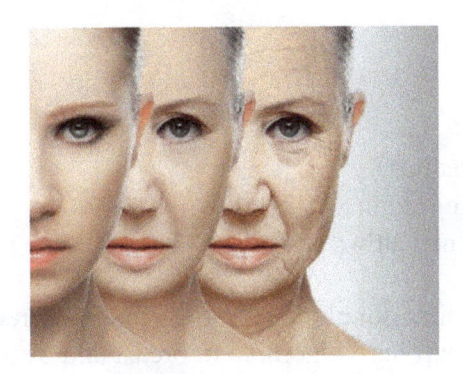

1. Theories of Aging

There are three prominent theories on aging. The aging process probably results from an interaction of each of these theories.

I. Cellular Theory
  Based on - Breakdown of cellular structure.
  Result:
  1. Destruction of DNA. (DNA carries the genetic instructions for the development, function, growth and reproduction of cells)
  2. Deterioration of the immune system.
  Causative Factor – Environmental toxins (water, food, air) resulting in cellular breakdown and cancers.
  Example – Smoking.

ANIMAL CELL STRUCTURE

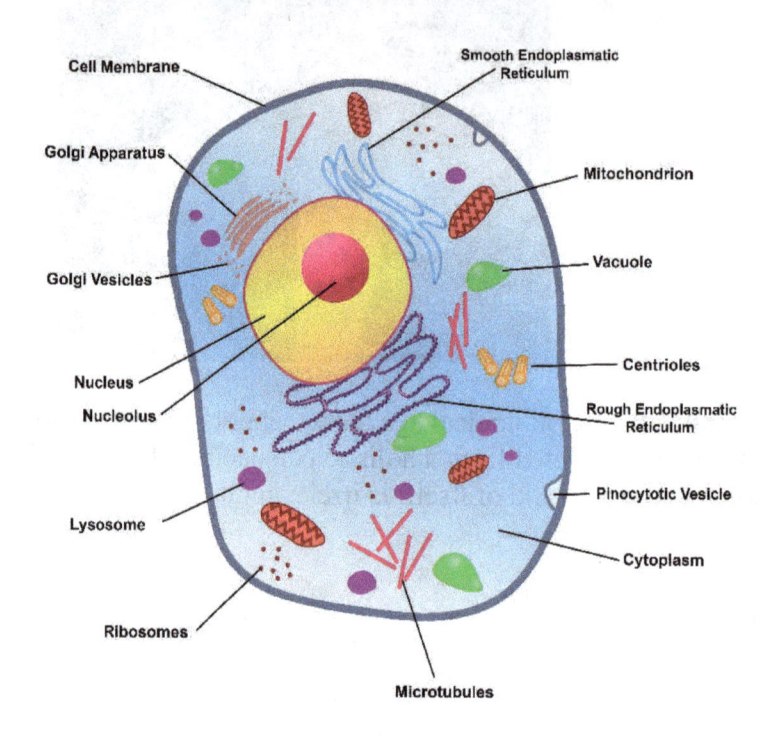

II. Genetic Theory

Based on – Role of hereditary.
Result – Genetically programmed breakdown of cells.
Causative Factor – Genetically mutated genes (Genes are made up of DNA and determine a person's individual traits).
Example – Angelina Jolie's double mastectomy and hysterectomy because she has the genes (BRCA1 and BRCA2) that left her vulnerable to breast and ovarian cancer.

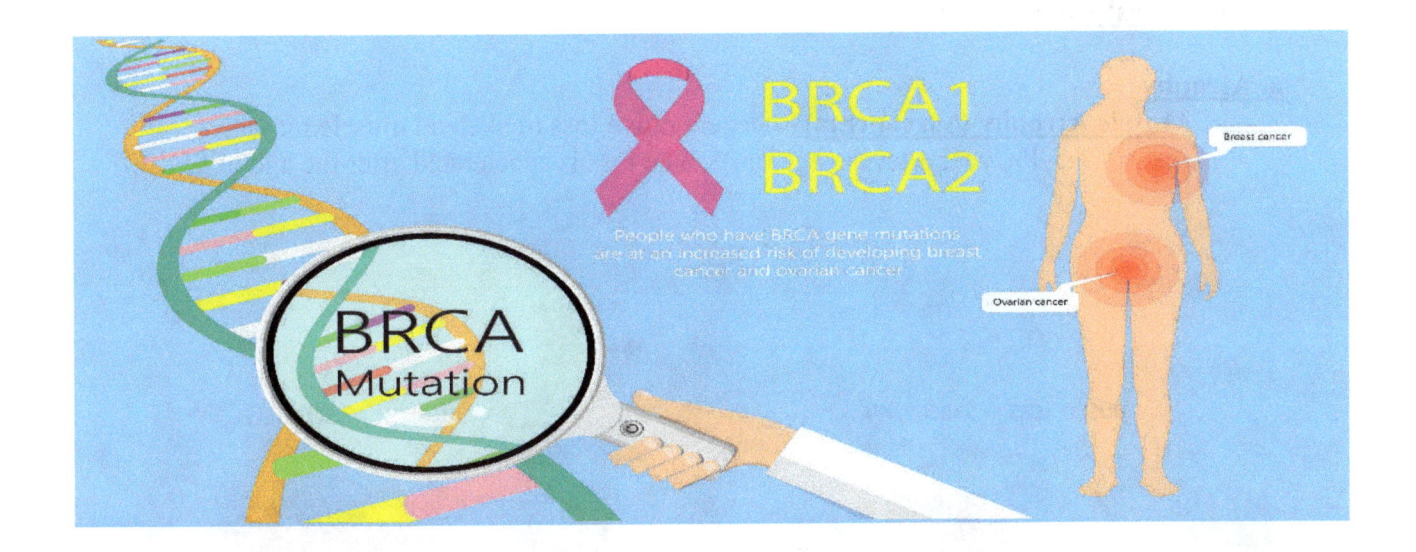

III. Control Theory

Based on – Poor regulation of the immune system.
Result – Weakened immune system cannot protect against environmental assaults resulting in damage and the accelerated aging process of cells.
Causative Factor – Poorly functioning endocrine and nervous system.
Example – Parkinson's (neurologic) and diabetes (endocrine).

2. Physical, Functional and Psychological Changes Associated with Aging

I. Physical Changes

Physical changes associated with aging can be classified as cosmetic and structural.

a. Cosmetic Changes

1. Thinning, loss and greying of hair
2. Skin becomes wrinkled, thinner, and develops "age" spots
3. Hearing loss
4. Visual acuity diminished
5. Loss of height
6. Loss of weight

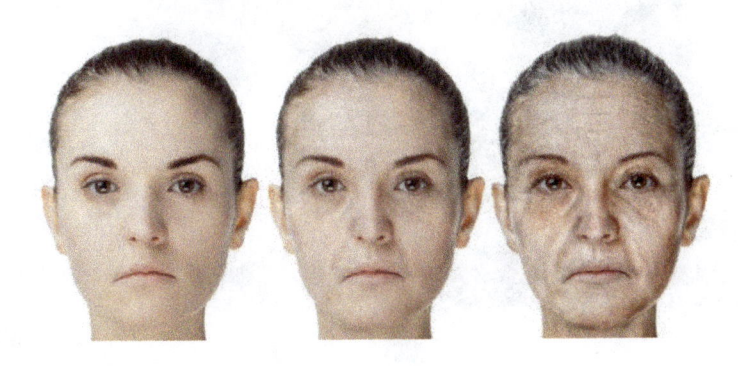

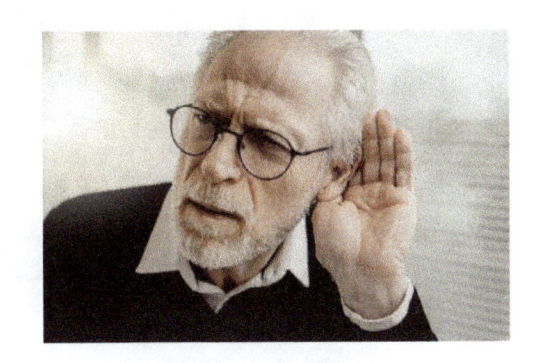

II. Structural Changes

a. Atrophy

Muscle Atrophy (Sarcopenia) – Degenerative loss of skeletal muscle mass
– .5-1%/year after the age of 25. The loss is accelerated after the age of 65.

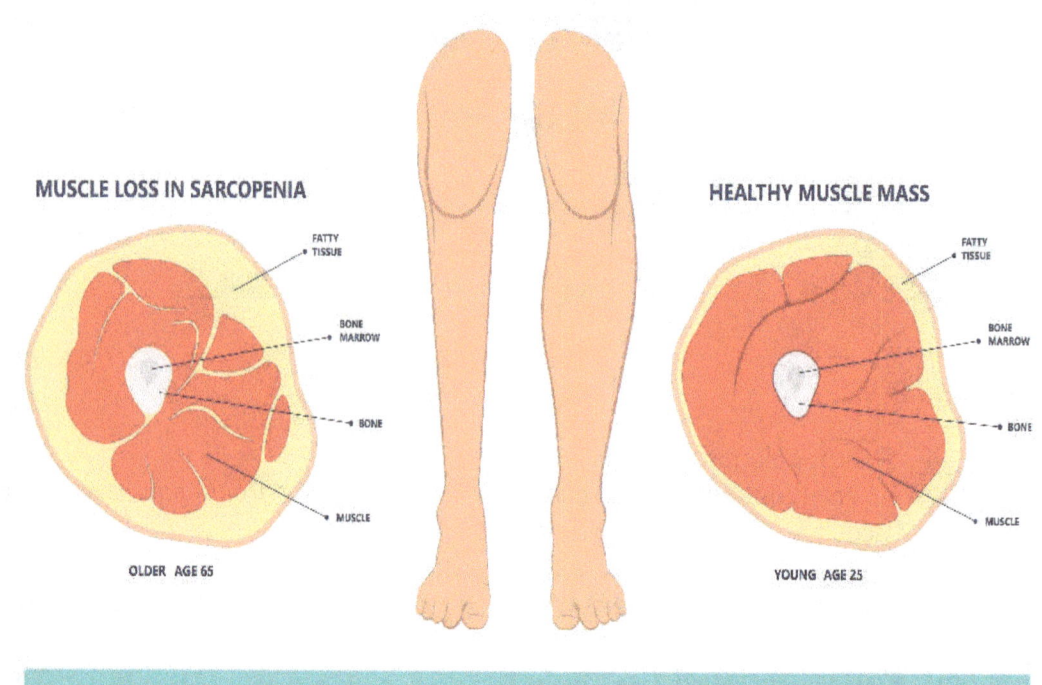

Cerebral Atrophy - Loss of neurons and the connections between them
– .5-1% of brain volume is loss/year after age 60.

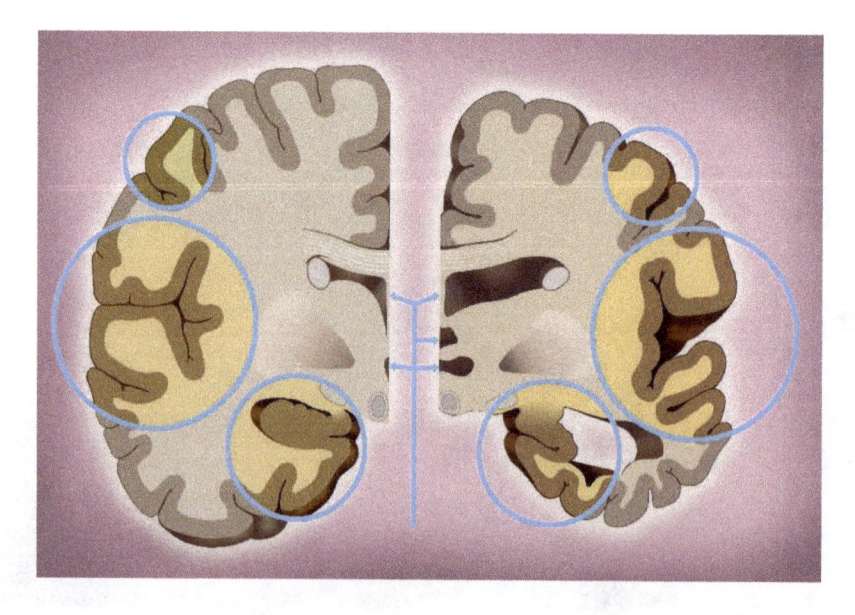

b. Edema – Abnormal excess accumulation of fluids (e.g., puffy face, hands, ankles and feet).

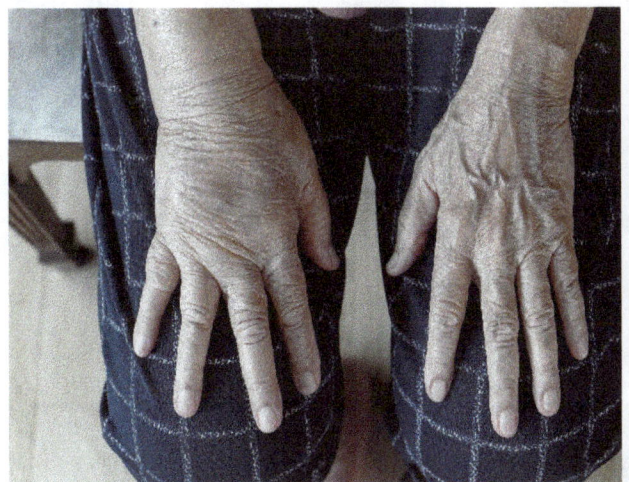

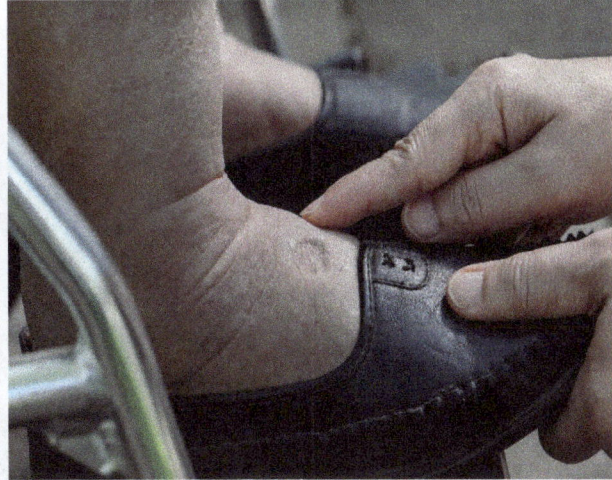

c. Inelasticity – Of muscles, connective tissue (ligaments, tendons), and fascia (e.g., stiffness bending over).

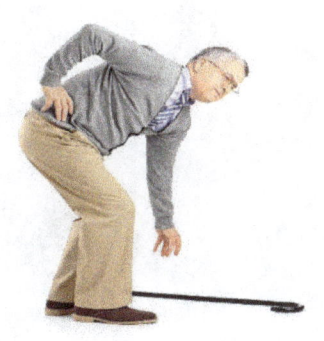

d. Osteoporosis – Demineralization of bone.

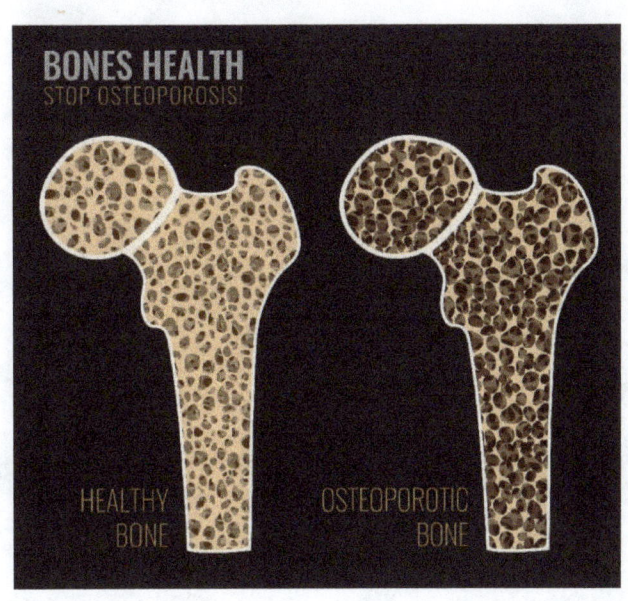

e. Demyelination – Destruction of the myelin along the peripheral nerves.
　　　　　　　　　– Slows transmission of nerve impulses.

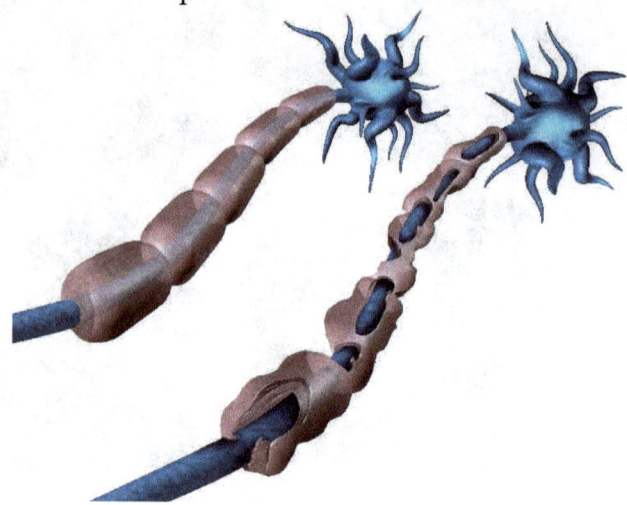

f. Neoplasm – Growing of tissues that serve no physiological function (benign and malignant tumors).

Benign Tumor　　　　　　　　　**Malignant Tumor**

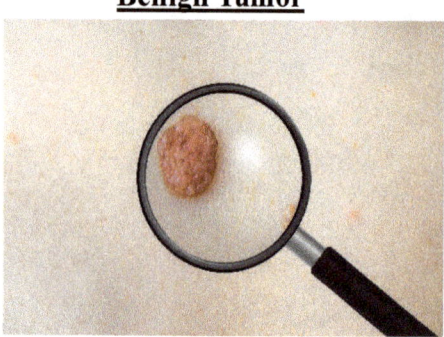

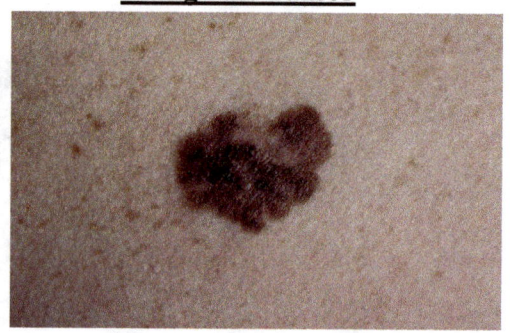

Image source: clevelandclinicmeded.com　　　　Image source: cbsnews.com

III. Functional Changes (as a result of structural changes)

a. Memory & Cognitive Decline (due to cerebral atrophy)

Result – Primarily weakened short-term memory (confusion, disorientation, frustration).

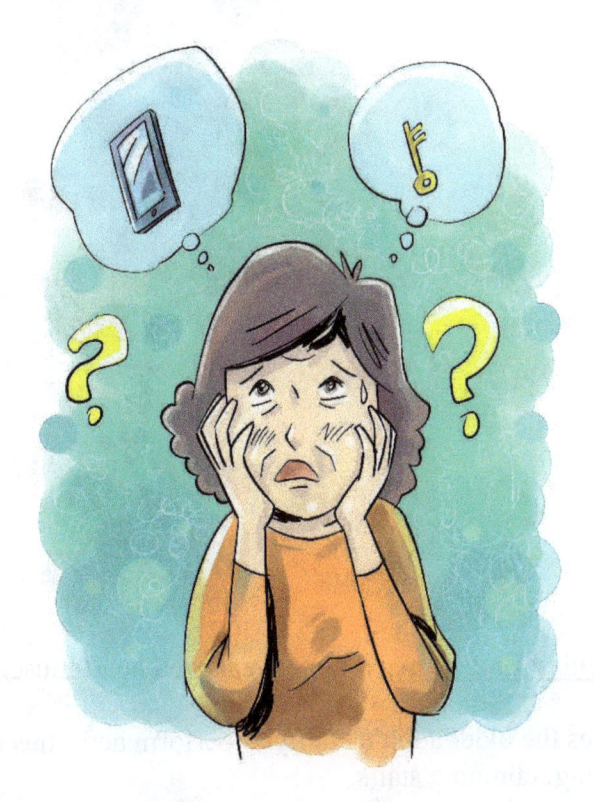

b. Slower Reflexes (due to peripheral nerve demyelination and cerebral/brain atrophy)

Result – Slow peripheral nerve transmission (peripheral demyelination)
– Slow central cerebral recognition (cerebral atrophy)

Driving accidents   **Falls**

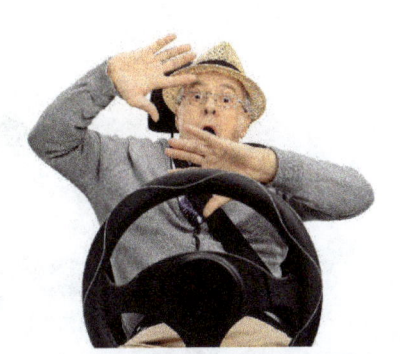

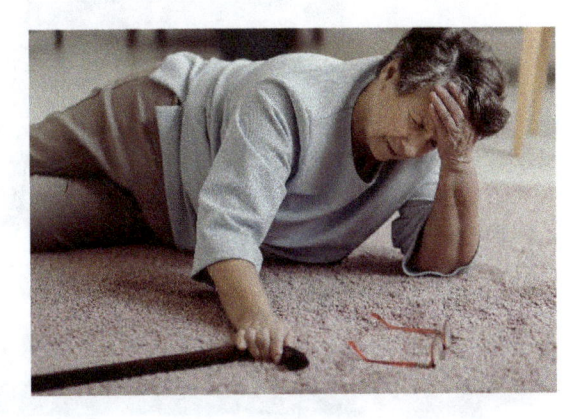

c. Loss of Flexibility (due to inelasticity of muscles and connective tissues)

Result – Increase difficulty with activities of daily living (putting on shoes, coats, combing hair, reaching above their shoulders to put things away).

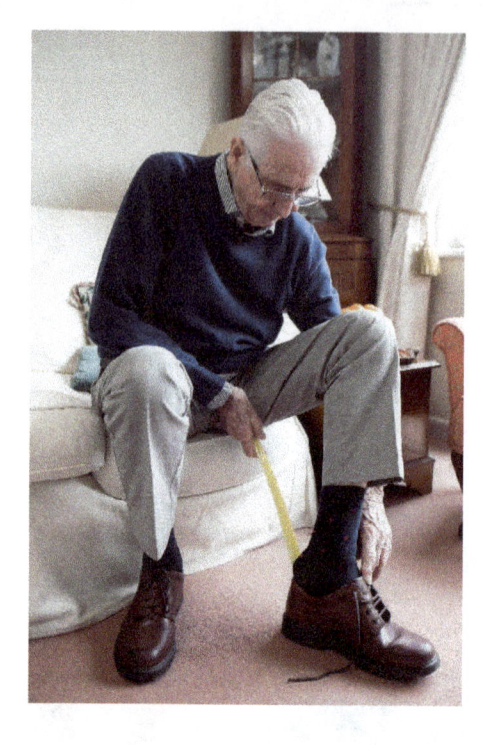

d. Loss of Cardiovascular Endurance (due to weakened heart muscle)

Result – Fatigue reduces the older adult's ability to perform activities that require sustained movement such as standing, walking, climbing stairs.

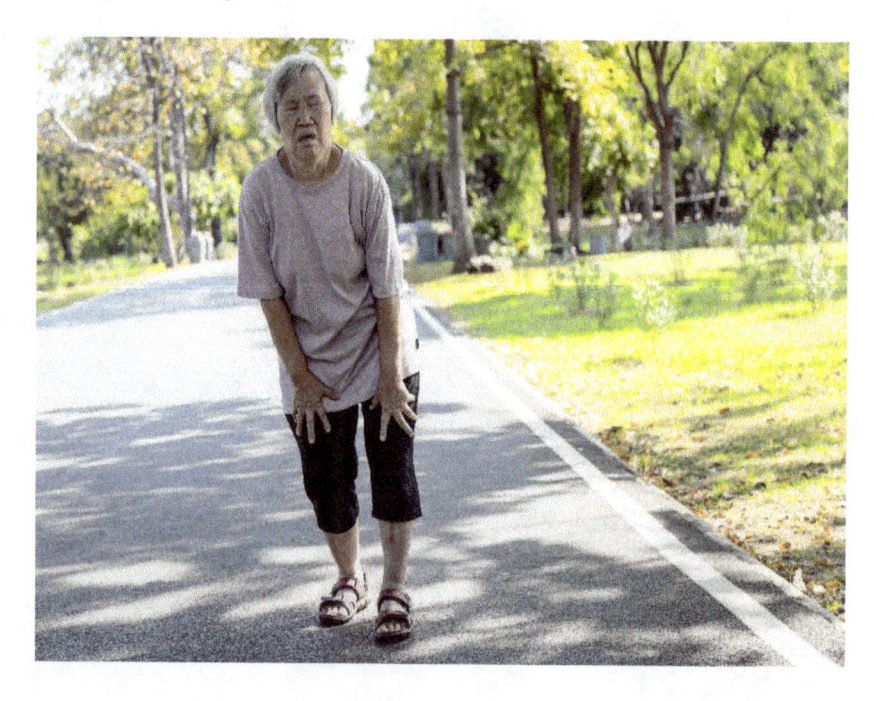

e. Loss of muscle power, strength and endurance (due to skeletal muscle atrophy (sarcopenia))

Result – Reduced ability to lift, stand, carry and perform activities requiring muscle strength and endurance.

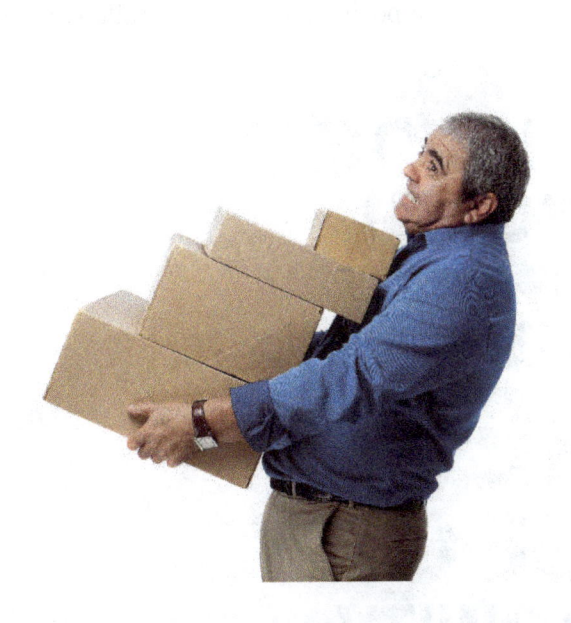

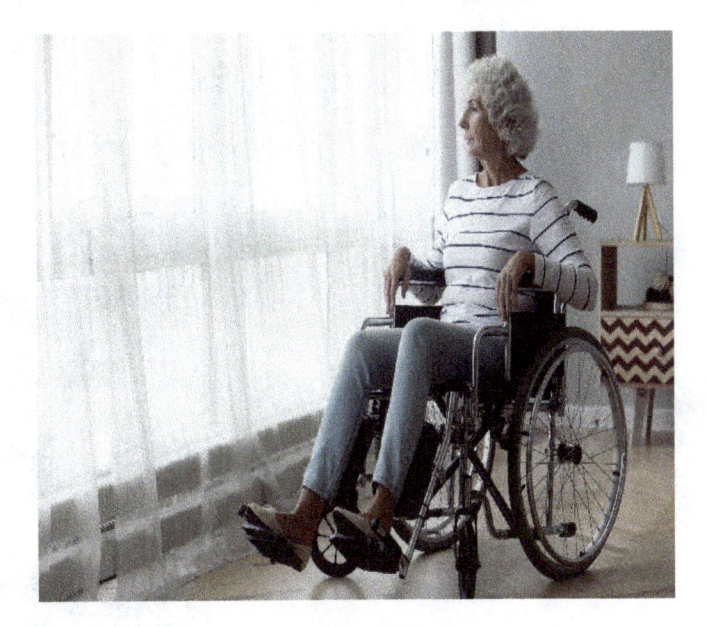

Result of Functional Changes for the Older Adult

1. Increased Risk of Falling

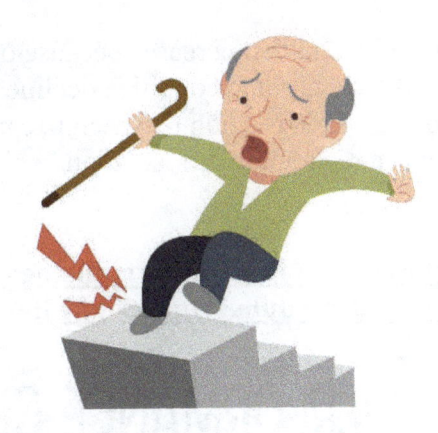

2. Diminished Quality of Life

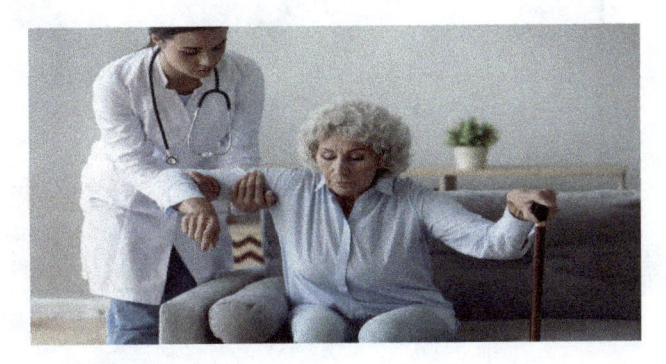

21

3. Psychological Changes with Age

Due to the cerebral structural changes that occur with aging and the resulting cognitive decline, maintaining a positive attitude by the older adult is essential to maintain function, independence, and high quality of life. However, maintaining a positive attitude is challenged by the psychological stress of aging.

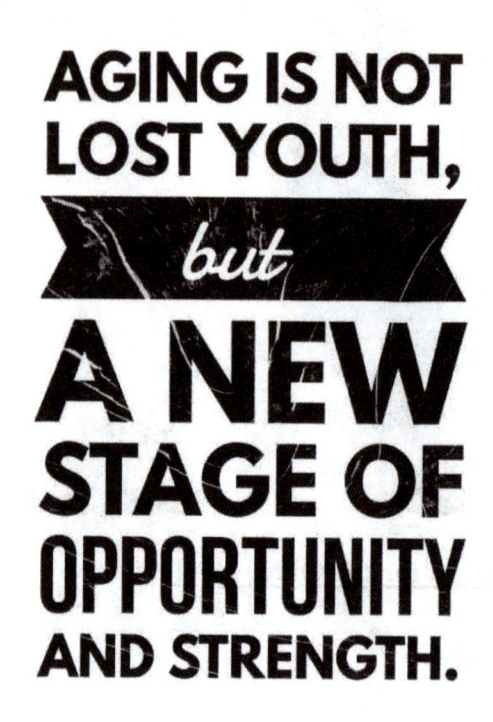

AGING IS NOT LOST YOUTH, but A NEW STAGE OF OPPORTUNITY AND STRENGTH.

Psychological stress among older adults increases because of the onset of chronic physical illnesses such as arthritis and heart disease and chronic cognitive decline in the form of diminished memory and problem-solving. As will be discussed in Section 6: Special Team: Mental Health, the psychological changes associated with aging can result in social isolation, which has devastating effects on the quality of life of the older adult.

Social Isolation (Lack of Arousal) and Excessive Psychological Stress (Due to Chronic Illness and Exhaustion) and Its Effect on Older Adults' Quality of Life

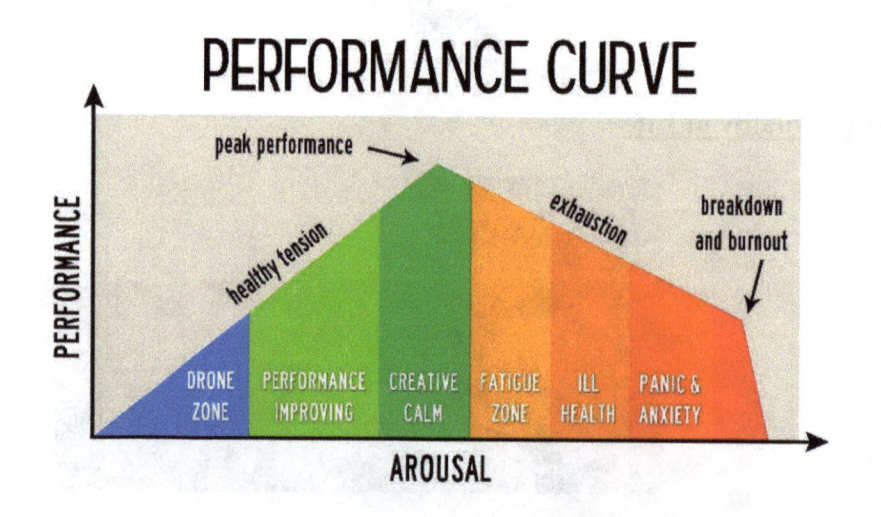

PERFORMANCE CURVE

Performance vs. Arousal curve showing zones: Drone Zone, Performance Improving (healthy tension), Creative Calm, peak performance, Fatigue Zone (exhaustion), Ill Health, Panic & Anxiety (breakdown and burnout).

Maintaining a Positive Attitude is a key component of good strong mental health

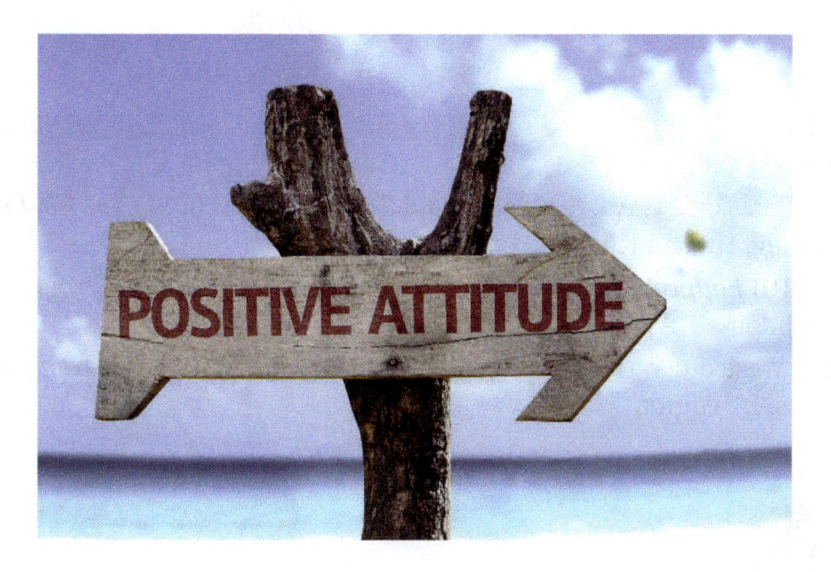

Conclusion

If a person is lucky and lives long enough, aging and its associated structural, functional, and psychological changes are inevitable. These changes, however, should be looked upon as a privilege and not a curse.

As examples of Sister Buder, Sir Richard Branson, and Sir Mick Jagger illustrate, an older adult's quality of life does not have to be significantly diminished because they crossed a chronological age threshold.

How active an older adult is, how positive their attitude is, how well they think, problem-solve, handle stress, and how much they pursue and welcome social interaction will dictate how well they will live their golden years.

The science of aging is clear; it happens, but it affects older adults in different ways. Many of the structural, functional, and psychological changes that occur with advancing age can be positively influenced to minimize their effects on older adults' quality of life. The older adult needs to manage their physical and mental health well, and that is what this book, Forever Active Older Adult Health and Fitness Playbook, is focused on.

References

www.forever-active.com

www.findingbalancealberta.ca

Hutton, J. (editor) (2003) *Can-Fit-Pro Older Adult Fitness Specialist Certification Manual*, Human Kinetics, 1st edition

Anderson, G., Bates, M., Cova, S., Macdonald, R., (editors) (2008) *Can-Fit-Pro Foundations of Personal Training*, Human Kinetics, 1st edition

Rose, D. J. (2010) *Fallproof!:A Comprehensive Balance and Training Program*. Human Kinetics, 2nd edition

Baechle, T. R., Westcott, W. L. (2010) *Fitness Professional's Guide to Strength Training the Older Adult*. Human Kinetics, 2nd edition

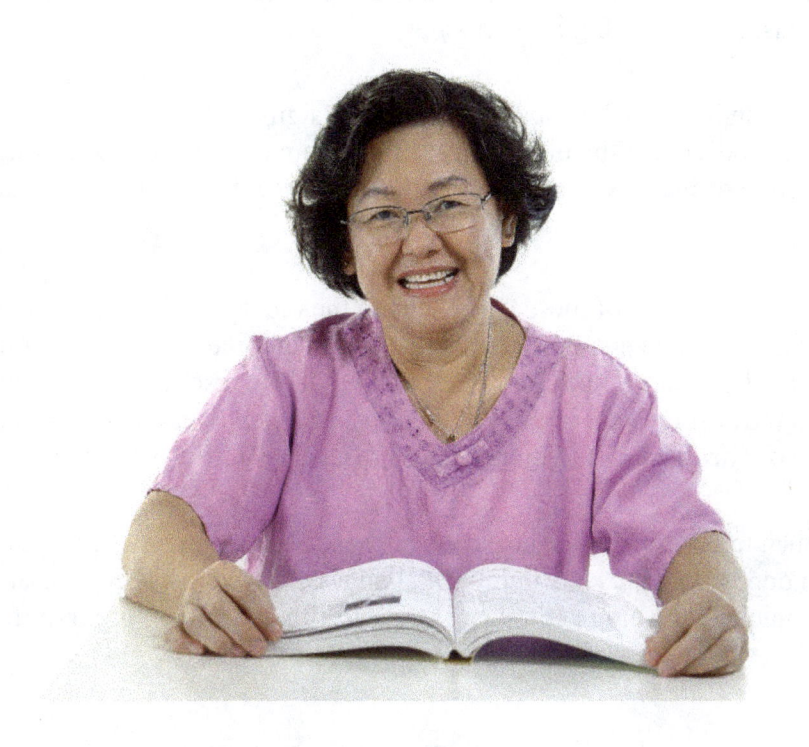

Section 2

The Off-Season – Studying the Opposition to Your Health

2.0. Introduction: The Off-Season – Studying the Opposition to Your Health

In football, the off-season is all about understanding the opponent. By getting to know their strengths and weaknesses, you can better prepare your team and to meet and overcome the challenges that they present.

Concerning your health, and especially as you are growing older, the major obstacle to a high quality of life comes from the likelihood that you will develop and suffer from one or more of the following health conditions: arthritis, heart disease, cancer, diabetes, obesity, dementia, oral and dental decay, visual and hearing impairments.

It is important to understand the causes, risk factors, signs and symptoms, complications and treatments for each condition. If the older adult suffers from one or more of them, they will need to modify the structure of their exercise and health plan to accommodate the limitations that they can impose.

This section will cover each of these opponents to the older adult's health so they can better understand what they can and cannot do to manage and overcome them. The information presented is meant to be a starting point for the older adult's investigation into how best to manage them. It is the best practice not to rely entirely on a healthcare professional's advice. The responsibility for your health and how to manage it rests on your own shoulders.

There is be much to be learned because each of these health opponents, just like in the case of a football team opposition, presents unique challenges and health concerns that will require the older adult to uniquely develop and manage their health and fitness program for success.

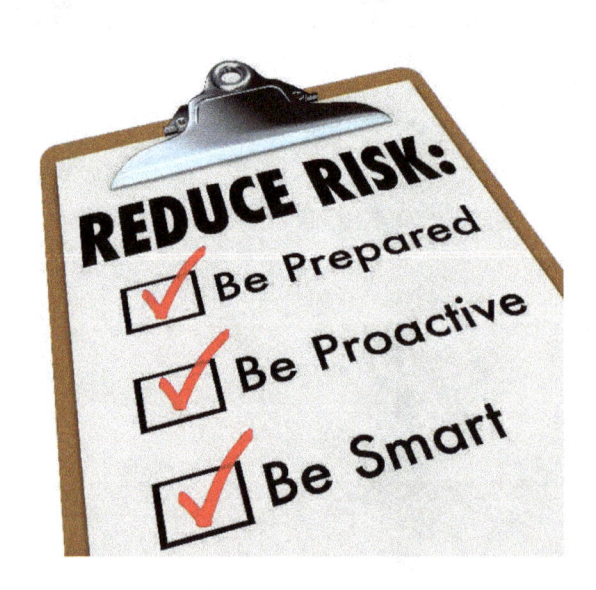

2.1. Arthritis

Introduction

Arthritis is the primary cause of physical disability in older adults. It is estimated that one in five Canadians have arthritis, and over 80% of older adults (50+ years) have some form of the disease. Arthritis affects more adults than heart disease, cancer, respiratory conditions, and spinal cord trauma combined, and severely impacts the quality of life of those afflicted. Arthritis disables two to three times more people than all other chronic conditions combined. The cost to the Canadian economy as the result of arthritis disability is estimated to be $4.4 billion/year.

Types of Arthritis

The various types of arthritis fall within two main broad categories:

I. Inflammatory arthritis

This is the autoimmune form of arthritis. In this type of arthritis, healthy joints and tissues are attacked by the body's immune system resulting in inflammation, joint stiffness, pain, joint damage and muscle atrophy (due to a lack of use). Rheumatoid Arthritis is the most common form of inflammatory arthritis and most frequently affects the small joints of the hand.

Ankylosing Spondylitis which affects the spine, Psoriatic Arthritis, where most body joints are vulnerable, and Lupus, which primarily affects joints of the extremities are other most common forms of inflammatory arthritis.

Rheumatoid Arthritis

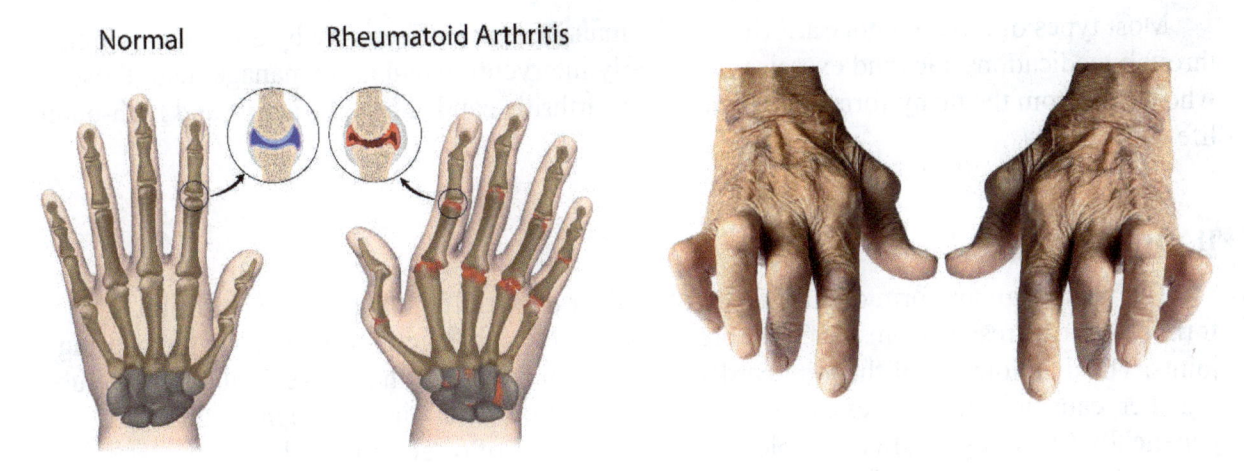

RHEUMATOID ARTHRITIS

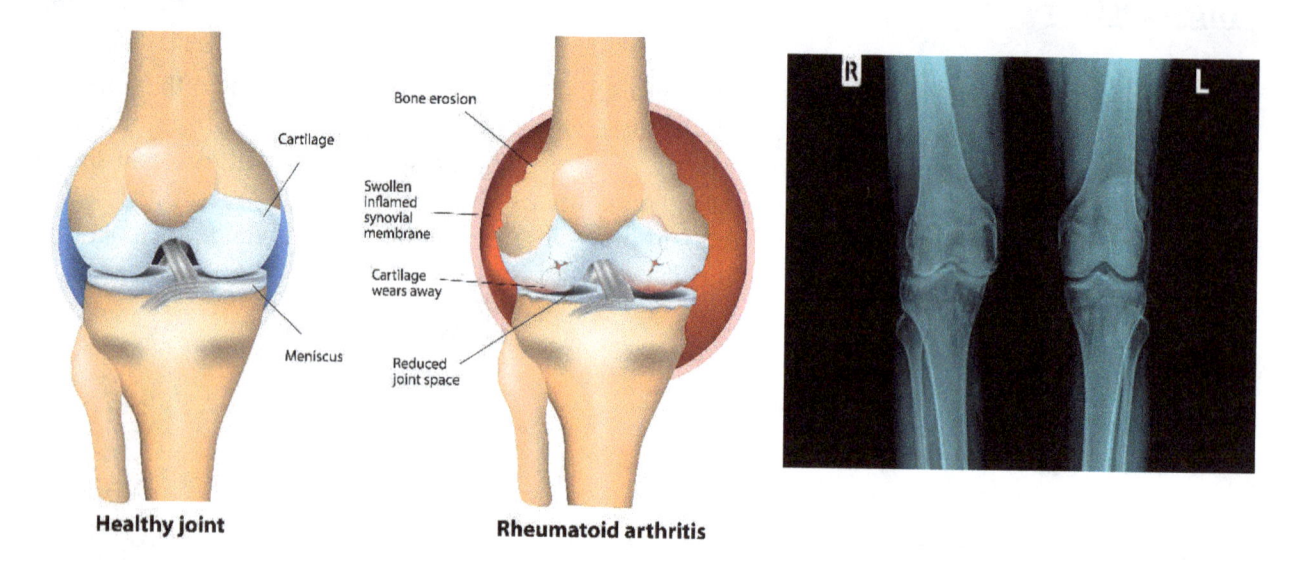

Since the origin of this form of arthritis is autoimmune, it was previously believed that there was not much that could be done to prevent its occurrence. However, current research has shown that the risk of developing rheumatoid arthritis can be lowered by:

- avoiding environmental toxins
- eating an anti-inflammatory diet (Mediterranean Diet – Chapter 5.2.10)
- sustaining a healthy weight
- minimizing chronic stress
- making sure you get sufficient sleep.

Most types of inflammatory arthritis can be managed very effectively by a Rheumatologist through medications, diet and exercise. With early intervention and good management, those who suffer from the many forms of inflammatory arthritis can lead a very active and high-quality life.

II. Osteoarthritis

The most common form of arthritis that the older adult suffers from is osteoarthritis. This form or arthritis results from structural breakdown of the cartilage in primarily weight bearing joints. The deterioration of the joint cartledge results in the bones that make up the joint to rub together, causing pain, stiffness, and eventual loss of use of the joint. Some individuals are genetically (in your genes) vulnerable to the development of osteoarthritis; however, osteoarthritis occurs most often due to previous injury, obesity, overuse, and advanced age. In the latter case, osteoarthritis is made worse due to atrophy of the muscles and weakening of the ligaments, whose function is to support and protect the joints during use. As previously mentioned, the weight-bearing joints of the body such as the neck, lower back, ankles, knees and hips, are the most vulnerable, followed by the joints of the shoulder and small joints of the hands.

Synovial joint

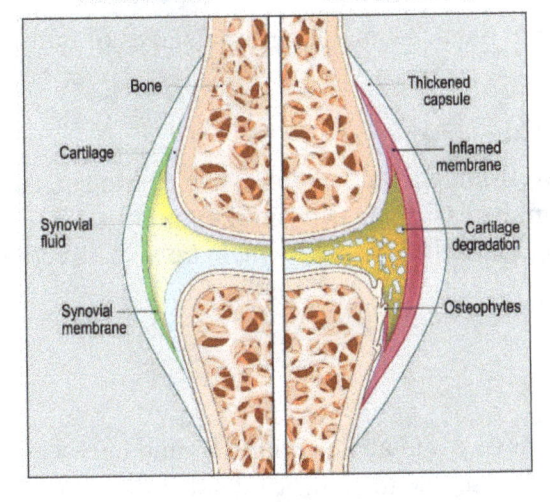

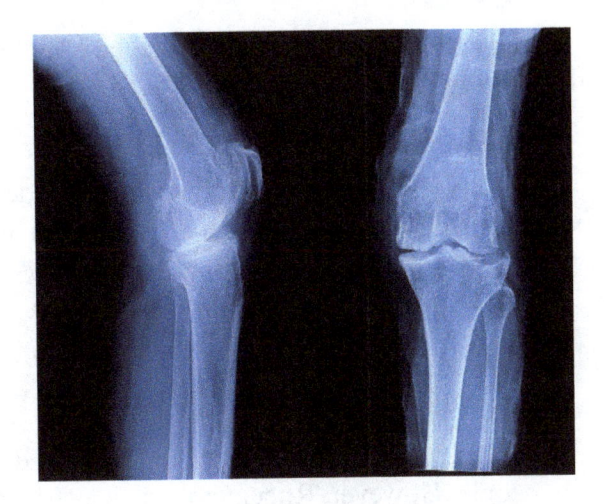

The harsh reality is that every person will develop some form of osteoarthritis if they live long enough. It is the gift a person receives for reaching the golden years. However, regular exercise, good flexibility, weight control, an anti-inflammatory diet, and avoiding contact or high-risk sports that leaves a person vulnerable to a joint injury can reduce the early onset and severity of osteoarthritis.

A special mention should be made concerning exercise and the onset and aggravation of osteoarthritis. There are many benefits of exercise such as weight control, strengthening of the muscles, ligaments, and tendons. These help prevent wear and tear on vulnerable joints, and the development of osteoarthritis. However, there is significant individual variation in how much exercise a person can tolerate before aggravating and accelerating the effects of osteoarthritis.

Everyone who has or is vulnerable to osteoarthritis due to a previous injury needs to consult their doctor before starting an exercise program. The doctor will determine which type of exercises are safe for you to participate in. The golden rule of starting and progressing low and slow (Chapter 3.1: The Eight Golden Rules of Training) should be followed by everyone as they begin any exercise program.

Treatments

I. Medications

Certain medications have shown to be effective in the acute and long-term stages of both inflammatory and osteoarthritis.

1. Nonsteroidal Anti-inflammatories (NSAIDS)

Over-the-counter anti-inflammatories include well-known medications such as Motrin, Advil (Ibuprofen) and Aspirin. These are most effective in the early stages or mild to moderately severe arthritis. Celebrex and Arthrotec are prescription-only NSAIDS which are also effective in treating the disabling effects of osteoarthritis.

2. Steroidal Medications

Corticosteroids, such as Prednisone, are used in severe and acute conditions and have helped many people. However, Rheumatologists restrict their use due to significant side effects such as suppression of the immune system resulting in high vulnerability to infection, and reduction in bone strength resulting in an increased risk of fractures, diabetes, and hypertension.

3. Anti-Rheumatic Drugs (DMARDs)

DMARDs are long-term standard treatment for Inflammatory Arthritis. Their purpose is to reduce joint damage that results from the inflammatory response associated with rheumatoid arthritis, juvenile inflammatory arthritis and psoriatic arthritis. Unfortunately, this form of medication can take one or more months to become fully effective, however, in many cases, they have been found to stop the damage from the disease.

4. Biologics

Biologics are a new and faster acting type of DMARDs. They are expensive and can result in suppressing an older adult's immune system which potentially can leave them vulnerable to infections. However, biologics have dramatically improved the function and prognosis for those who suffer from inflammatory arthritis. This is especially true for those who have not respond to treatment with traditional DMARDs.

II. Diet

Certain foods help reduce inflammation associated with arthritis. The Mediterranean Diet contains many of these foods such as; fish, nuts, fruits and vegetables, olive oil, beans, and whole grains (refer to Chapter 5.2.10 for a complete review of the Mediterranean Diet).

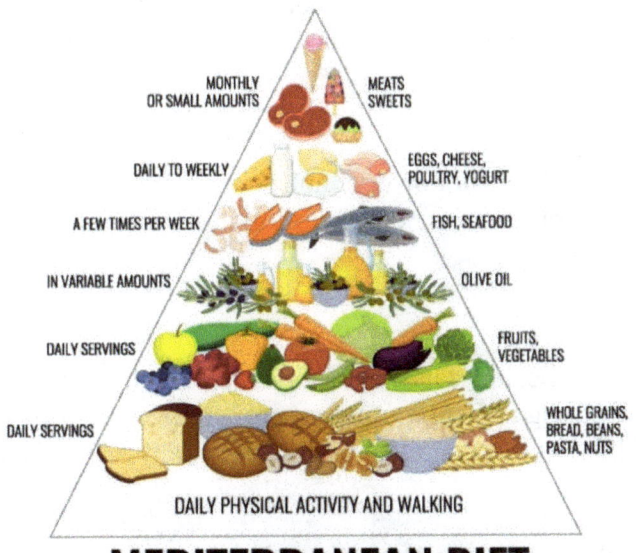

Foods that can Help Control Arthritic Inflammation

Fish

Food guides recommend fish (three to four ounces) twice a week but arthritis experts recommend more is better. Research has shown that omega-3 fatty acids fight inflammation and good sources of these are "fatty" types of fish such as salmon, tuna, and scallops. Researchers have also shown that taking 600 to 1000 mg of fish oil supplements helps reduce morning stiffness, pain and swelling in joints in those who suffer from rheumatoid arthritis (RA).

Nuts

Nuts are full of monounsaturated fat which helps reduce inflammation. You are recommended to eat 1.5 ounces (a handful and half of the nuts) daily. Multiple studies have confirmed the role of nuts in an anti-inflammatory diet. One study found that over 15 years, those who consumed a higher amount of nuts in their diet had a 51% lower risk of dying from an inflammatory disease (like RA) than those who ate the fewest nuts.

Studies have shown that weight loss is an additional benefit of consuming nuts. Although nuts are high in fat and calories, they promote weight loss because their protein, fiber and monounsaturated fats make you feel full faster so you don't feel as hungry and therefore eat less. The best sources of nuts are almonds, pistachios, walnuts, and pine nuts.

Fruits & Veggies

Research has shown that getting sufficient amounts of vitamin C and K in your diet aids in reducing inflammation markers in the blood which are associated with the presence of inflammatory arthritis. Oranges, grapefruits, and limes are rich in vitamin C while vitamin K can be found abundantly in veggies like lettuce, cabbage, kale, broccoli, and spinach. These fruits and vegetables should be part of every older adult's diet.

Fruits and vegetables are also full of antioxidants which act as a natural defense system for the body by helping neutralize free radicals (unstable molecules) that can damage cells and cause cancer.

Darker or more colourful the fruit or vegetables, the more antioxidants they contin. Good examples include cherries, blueberries, kale, broccoli and spinach.

Olive Oil

Olive oil contains heart-healthy fats and oleocanthal which if part of the family of polyphenols, which has strong anti-inflammatory properties similar to nonsteroidal anti-inflammatory drugs (NSAIDs). A couple of tablespoons daily are recommended.

Extra virgin olive oil is the best source since it is subject to less refining and processing and, as a result, retains more nutrients than standard varieties.

Beans

Beans are rich in fiber and phytonutrients and these help lower CRP, a blood indicator of inflammation. Beans are also an excellent source of protein which is essential for muscle health.

Whole Grains

Whole grains contain a lot of fiber, which helps weight management because it makes you fill fuller sooner as you eat. Research has shown that fiber can lower blood levels of the inflammatory marker CRP.

Eating foods made with the entire grain kernel, like oatmeal, brown rice, quinoa, whole-wheat flour, is recommended.

On a cautionary note, people who have been diagnosed with celiac disease or have a gluten sensitivity will need to eat gluten-free whole grains. Gluten, a protein found in wheat and other grains, has been linked to inflammation in these people.

Foods to Avoid

Research has shown that refined sugar, high-fat animal meat (beef and pork), cheese, and processed foods high in trans-fats are foods you need to avoid taking regularly.

III. Exercise

Regular exercise is necessary to maintain joint mobility. Exercise strengthens your muscles, tendons, and ligaments to protect against the wear and tear on the joints that will lead to the development of arthritis. There is controversy about what type of exercise, if any exercise at all, is best for people who already suffer from joint pain due to arthritis.

Recent research from McMaster University suggests that doing too little exercise may be as bad as doing too much exercise in the long term. The reason is that the cartilage in the joint is not inertly padded but can adapt and get stronger in response to regular use. This explanation fits with multiple long-term running studies showing that runners are less likely to develop osteoarthritis in their knees and hips than non-runners. The reasons for this are probably multifactorial.

First, running is a great aerobic exercise and valuable in controlling weight gain. Less weight means less pressure on the knees and hips. Second, running helps strengthen the supporting structures, muscles, tendons, and ligaments around the joint. The stronger the supporting tissues, the less stress/load is transmitted to the joints. Third, is the adaptation effect of the cartilage to repetitive loads. Cartilage reacts like bones and muscles; if you don't use it, you will lose it.

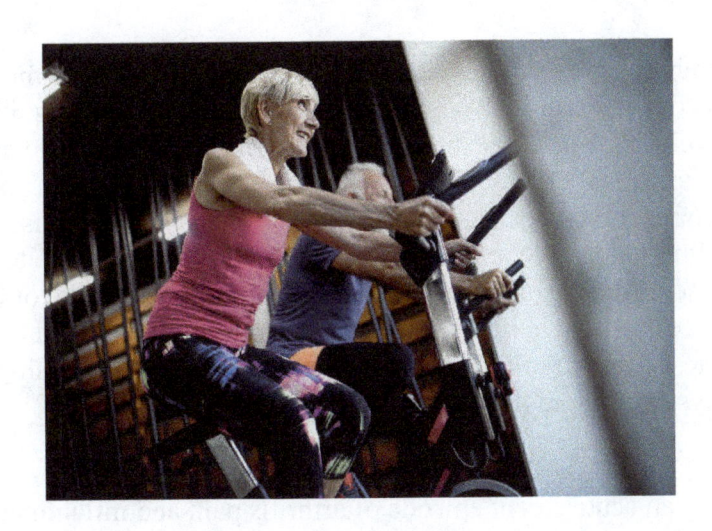

The advice for those with osteoarthritis is the same advice for the general population. Stay active by mixing strength and aerobic exercises that don't aggravate your affected joints. When you begin to exercise, you should start low and slow (Refer to Chapter 3.1: The Eight Golden Rules of Training) to give the body time to adapt to the stresses that exercise physically puts on it.

Starting low and slow means that the more unfit you are when you start, the lower the intensity of the exercise, and the slower you progress. The number one reason people stop exercising is that they hurt themselves within the first month. Not continuing to exercise a month after starting is even more true for individuals who have an injured or arthritic joint before they start. Following the golden rule of starting low and slow is even more necessary for these individuals.

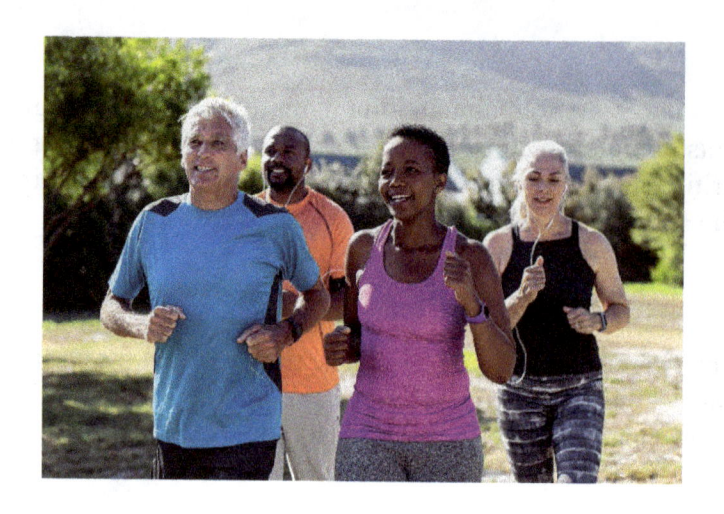

It is also important to remember that the benefit of each exercise is very specific and targeted (another Golden Rule). Even though cycling, running and walking are excellent aerobic exercises and strengthen the heart, they each strengthen the leg muscles differently. If a person has cycled for years and then decides to start running, they must begin low and slow because the muscles, tendons and ligaments are unconditioned to handle the stress of running. These soft tissues are not "work hardened" to withstand the new stress or running.

It is vital to remember that exercising is not contraindicated for those who suffer from either inflammatory arthritis or osteoarthritis. Whether the arthritis is in the hands, knees, or hips, mobility/flexibility exercises, muscular strengthening exercises, and aerobic exercises will slow arthritis' debilitating functional effects. The key is to find activities and exercises that you can perform painlessly. For example, non-weight-bearing cardiovascular exercise on a stationary bike, elliptical, or swimming is excellent for those suffering from moderate to severe arthritis on the knees, hips, and back. If a person has arthritis of the neck, breaststroke or backstroke rather than the front crawl/freestyle would be indicated. Your personal doctor and trainer would be beneficial in helping to determine which exercises and the intensity of training would be best to accommodate any physical limitations you may have.

If you are suffering an acute/recent episode of arthritis pain and inflammation, you must curtail the amount and intensity of your exercise. Monitoring discomfort level is essential. Pain in a joint during exercise is an excellent barometer; it means that either you are doing the wrong exercise or doing the exercise too much or too hard. "Low and slow" is your guiding light to safe and effective exercising, especially when exercising arthritic joints.

PAIN MEASUREMENT SCALE

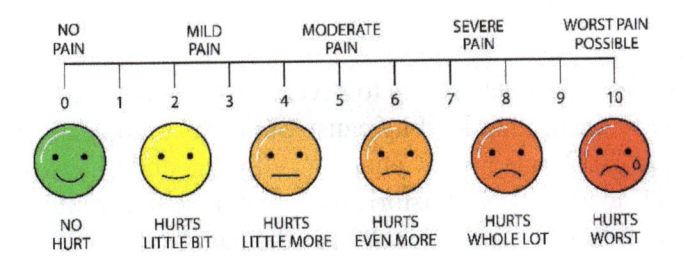

NO PAIN	MILD PAIN	MODERATE PAIN	SEVERE PAIN	WORST PAIN POSSIBLE
0 1	2 3	4 5 6	7 8	9 10
NO HURT	HURTS LITTLE BIT	HURTS LITTLE MORE	HURTS EVEN MORE	HURTS WHOLE LOT	HURTS WORST

Section 4, The Offense: The Older Adult Getting Active the Right Way, deals specifically with cardiovascular endurance, muscular strength, balance, agility, and coordination so you can implement a safe fitness program to help maintain mobility and function even if you are dealing with the debilitating effects of arthritis.

Conclusion

Arthritis in its many forms is a terrible disabling disease that can affect the quality of life for those it afflicts, young or old. However, through proper monitoring and management (medication, diet, and exercise), you can alleviate most symptoms to the point that, despite being an arthritic patient, you can lead a very regular, active, and functional life. If you have concerns, you should reach out for professional advice from your doctor, physiotherapist, chiropractor, personal trainer, and/or nutritionist. Remember, two, three, or four heads are always better than one when seeking advice about your health. Never be afraid to ask.

References

https://www.mayoclinic.org/

https://sunnybrook.ca/

https://www.medicalnewstoday.com/

https://www.healthline.com/health/arthritis

https://www.cdc.gov/arthritis/basics/types.html

https://www.webmd.com/arthritis/default.htm

https://www.mcmasteroptimalaging.org/e-learning/mobility

2.2. Heart Disease, Stroke and Hypertension

Introduction

Heart disease is a general term that refers to several illnesses of the heart and blood vessels. In Canada, heart disease is the second leading cause of death behind cancer, accounting for over 51,500 deaths in 2015. In 2012, one in 12 Canadians 20 years and older lived with some form of heart disease (Statistics Canada; 2018). Historically, men have had a higher incidence of heart disease than women, but this gap has narrowed over the past twenty years. One contributing factor for this is that women began to smoke more 30 to 50 years ago.

Heart disease is a condition in which the heart muscle is damaged or does not function properly. Plaque, which is composed of fat, cholesterol, calcium, and other substances, builds upon the inner walls of coronary (heart) arteries, and, over time, it hardens. This condition is known as atherosclerosis. As a result, there is narrowing of the inside of the coronary arteries which reduces blood flow to the heart muscle. If plaque ruptures from the arterial wall, a blood clot can form which can also block the flow of blood to the heart muscle.

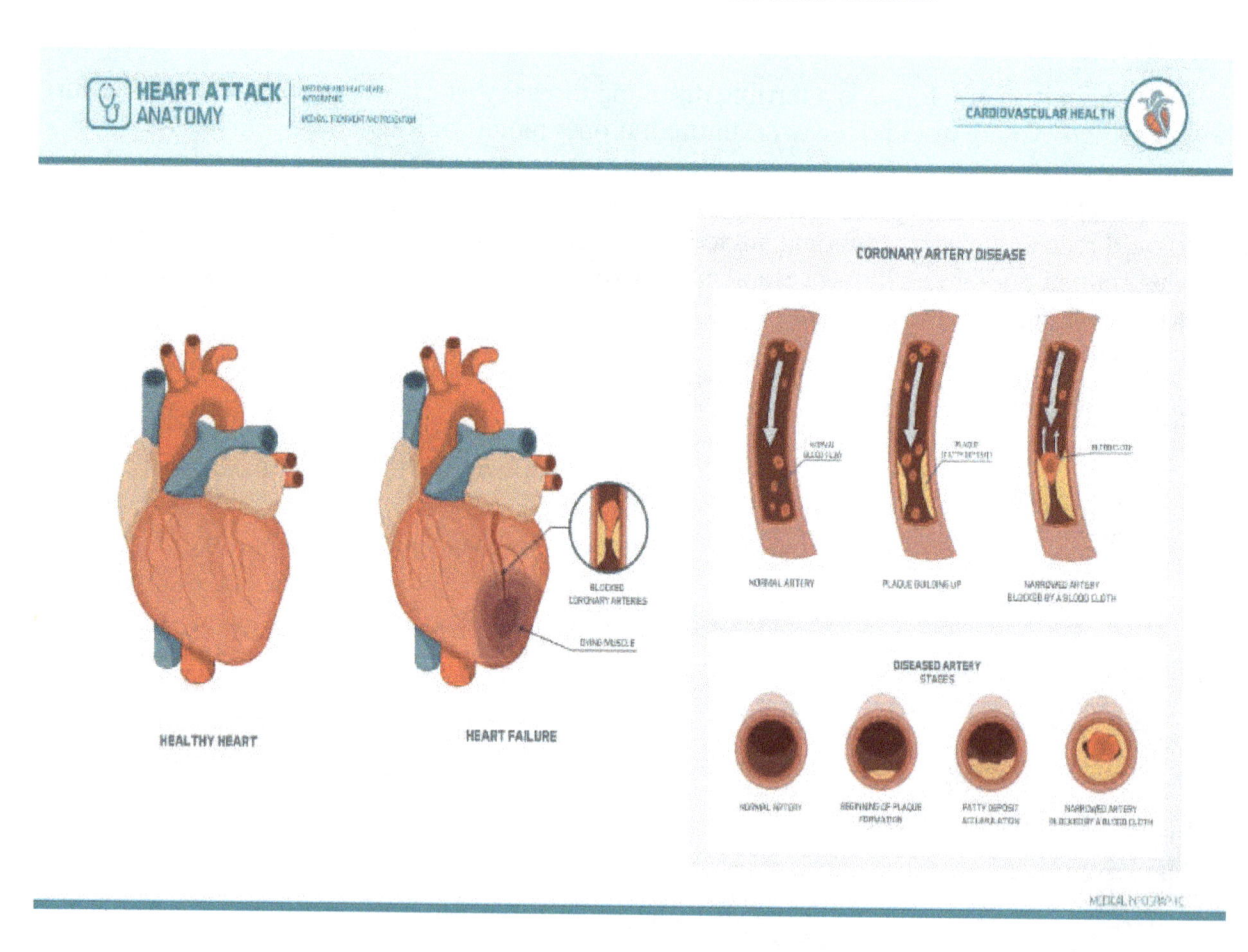

1. Heart Disease
Commonly known heart diseases include the following:

1. Ischemic Heart Disease
    Angina
    Cardiac Arrhythmias
    Acute Myocardial Infarction

2. Heart Failure

1. Ischemic Heart Disease (IHD)
Ischemic Heart Disease is the primary cause of heart disease and results from having reduced blood flow to the heart.

Risk Factors
There are unmodifiable and modifiable risk factors associated with IHD;

Unmodifiable Risk Factors;
1. **Age** – the older a person is, the greater their likelihood of developing atherosclerosis and IHD.
2. **Sex** – males have a higher prevalence than females.
3. **Family history** – genetic predisposition to IHD.
4. **Race** – people of African descent have a higher risk.

Modifiable Risk Factors;
1. **Obesity**
2. **High cholesterol and diets high in saturated (animal fats, meat) and trans fat (processed food)**
3. **Lack of exercise**
4. **Smoking**
5. **Chronic stress**
6. **Excessive alcohol consumption**

If Ischemic Heart Disease progresses to a moderate to severe blockage of a coronary artery, it can potentially lead to;

1. Angina
Angina is a primary symptom of IHD and presents as a heaviness, tightness, squeezing, pressure or pain in your chest. It is essential to differentiate between stable and unstable Angina.

Stable Angina:
- It usually happens during exertion and goes away with rest.
- Its onset can usually be predicted, and the pain is generally similar each time

- It will last five minutes or less.
- It disappears if you stop exerting yourself or use your angina medication.

Unstable Angina (Medical Emergency):
- Might signal a heart attack
- Occurs even at rest.
- It occurs unexpectedly and presents as a change in your usual pattern of angina.
- It lasts longer than stable angina, maybe 30 minutes or longer, and is usually more severe.
- Rest or angina medication may not be helpful in eliminating it.

2. Cardiac Arrhythmias (Irregular Heartbeats)

Cardiac Arrhythmias are a group of conditions that causes interruption to the electrical impulses that stimulate heart contraction, thereby causing the heart to beat too slowly, too quickly, or irregularly.

Categories of arrhythmia:
- **Bradycardia** – Slow heartbeat
- **Tachycardia** – Fast heartbeat
- **Irregular heartbeat** – Flutter or fibrillation
- **Early heartbeat** – Premature contraction

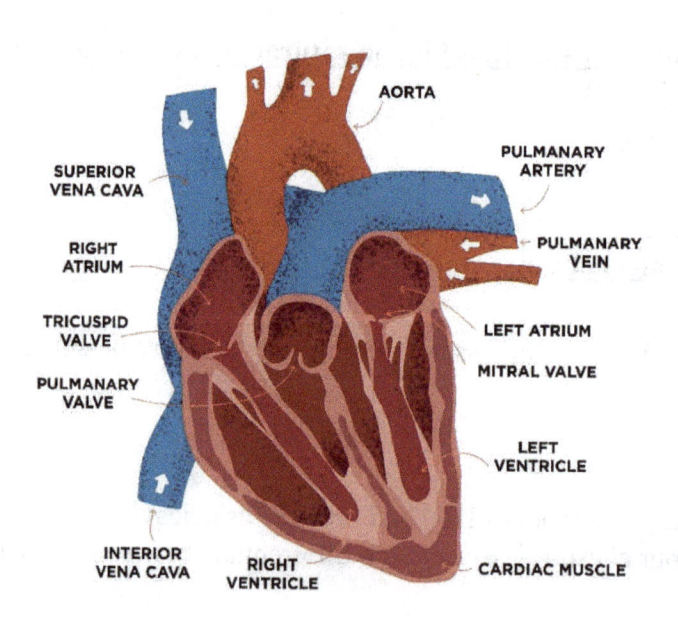

HEART ANATOMY

Heart Anatomy
- **Right and Left Atriums** – upper chambers of the heart
- **Right and left Ventricles** – lower chambers of the heart

Types of Arrhythmias:

I. Atrial Fibrillation (A-fib) – Irregular beating or quivering of the atrial chambers; and usually involves tachycardia (heart rate over 100 beats per minute). Atrial fibrillation (A-fib) is a common heart condition that most often develops in older adults over 65.

II. Atrial Flutter – Results from one area in the atrium not conducting electrical impulses correctly. Atrial flutter can lead to fibrillation without treatment.

III. Supraventricular Tachycardia – This is a regular but rapid and rhythmically heartbeat. These burst of accelerated heartbeats that can last only a few seconds or as long as a few hours.

IV. Ventricular Tachycardia – Results from abnormal electrical impulses that originate in the ventricles and causes an abnormally rapid heartbeat. A scar from a previous heart attack often predisposes the heart to this type of tachycardia.

V. Ventricular Fibrillation – The heart rhythm consists of rapid, uncoordinated, and fluttering contractions of the ventricles. The ventricles quiver and do not contract fully which restricts the heart from pumping out blood. Ventricular fibrillation is life-threatening and is often triggered by a heart attack.

VI. Long QT Syndrome – This heart rhythm disorder can cause uncoordinated, rapid, heartbeats which can result in fainting and can be life-threatening. Medications can make people vulnerable to this condition.

Causes of Arrhythmias:
- Smoking
- High blood pressure
- Heart disease, such as congestive heart failure
- Scarring or structural changes of the heart, often due to a heart attack
- Diabetes
- Certain medications
- Certain dietary and herbal supplements
- Drinking too much caffeine
- Alcohol abuse
- Stress
- Hyperthyroidism, or an overactive thyroid gland

Most arrhythmias are not severe or cause significant complications. Beta-blocker medication manages them well. However, arrhythmias can increase the risk of stroke or heart attack if not diagnosed and appropriately managed.

3. Acute Myocardial Infarction (Heart Attack)

It occurs when there is severe blockage of blood to the heart, and the heart muscle begins to die.

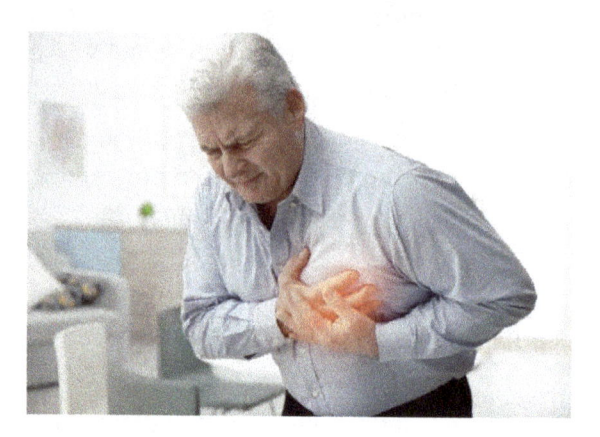

Warning Signs of a Heart Attack:

Warning signs of an impending heart attack can be subtle or very pronounced. A person should not ignore these signs and symptoms:

- Chest pain (if a person suffers from angina, this chest pain would occur unexpectedly and differs from a regular angina occurrence)
- Pain down the left arm
- Upper back pain
- Fatigue
- Shortness of breath
- Cold sweats
- Nausea (indigestion)
- Light-headedness and dizziness

HEART ATTACK
warning sign

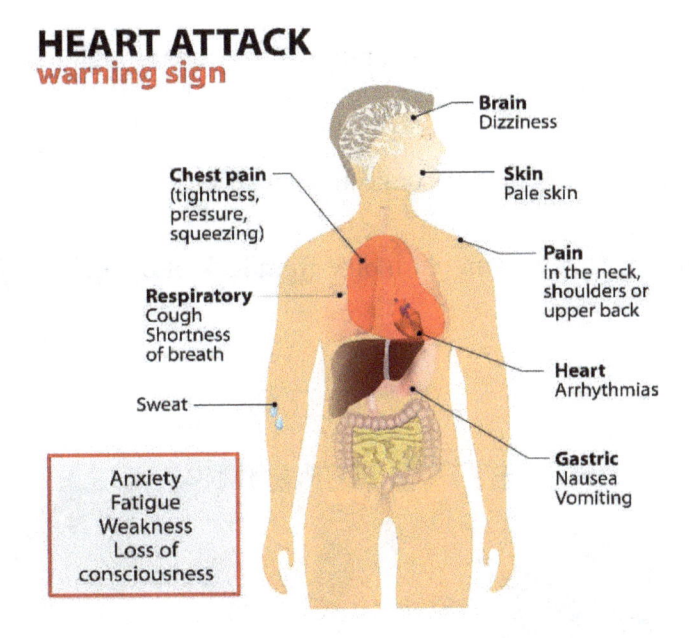

- Brain — Dizziness
- Chest pain (tightness, pressure, squeezing)
- Skin — Pale skin
- Respiratory — Cough, Shortness of breath
- Pain in the neck, shoulders or upper back
- Heart — Arrhythmias
- Sweat
- Gastric — Nausea, Vomiting
- Anxiety, Fatigue, Weakness, Loss of consciousness

Treatment

A heart attack is a medical emergency. Once the patient is stabilized, and out of life-threatening danger, the degree of IHD must be determined to initiate appropriate treatment.

Non-Invasive Treatment (Medications)
- Aspirin (blood thinner)
- Nitroglycerine
- Drugs to break up clots (thrombolytic therapy)
- Blood pressure medication
- Antiplatelet and anticoagulants (blood thinners)

Invasive Treatment
1. **Angioplasty** – Blocked artery are opened by removing the plaque buildup or using a balloon.
2. **Stent** – After angioplasty, a wire mesh tube (stent) is inserted into the artery to keep it open.
3. **Pacemaker** – Designed to help your heart maintain a normal electrical rhythm and is inserted beneath the skin close to the heart.
4. **Heart valve surgery** – Leaky valves are replaced to prevent the back flow of blood.
5. **Heart bypass surgery** – Rerouting of the blood around the blockage.
6. **Heart transplant** – This is performed when a heart attack has resulted in permanent tissue death to most of the heart.

2. Heart Failure

Heart failure occurs after other conditions, such as high blood pressure and heart attacks have damaged or weakened the heart muscle, resulting in the heart muscle not pumping blood as well as it should. The weakened heart muscle becomes too stiff and does not fill up properly between beats. As a result, there is less blood to be pumped out; alternatively, the heart muscle becomes so dilated (stretched) that it is not strong enough to pump blood out efficiently throughout the body.

When the heart muscle is not strong enough to pump blood through out the body, blood often backs up and causes fluid to build up in your:

Lungs – causing shortness of breath (Congestive Heart Failure)

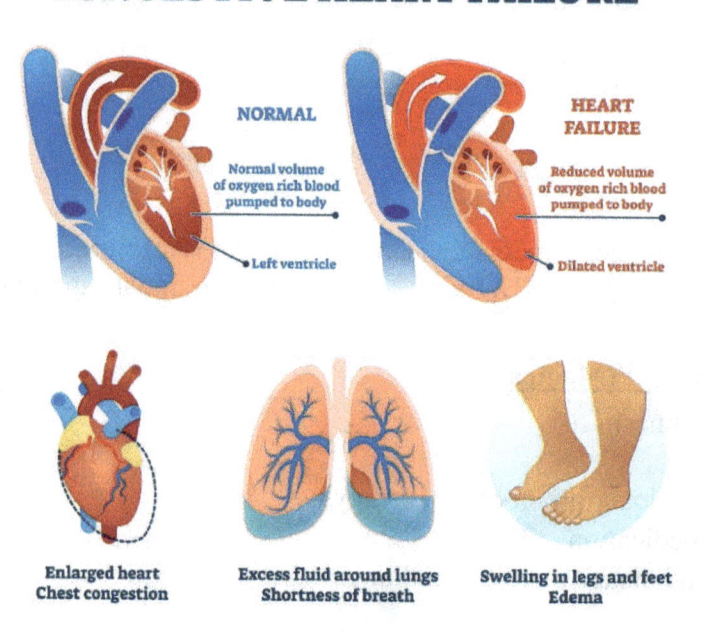

Legs – causing your legs to swell and turn blue from lack of oxygenated blood flow (Cyanotic Heart Failure).

The following conditions can damage the heart causing heart failure;
- Ischemic heart disease and heart attack
- Hypertension (high blood pressure)
- Faulty heart valves
- Myocarditis (inflammation of the heart muscle due to a virus including COVID-19)
- Heart arrhythmias
- Chronic diseases such as alcoholism, diabetes, kidney damage/failure, liver damage, hyper and hypo-thyroidism.

Symptoms of Heart Failure
- Shortness of breath
- Swelling in your ankles, feet and lower legs
- Fatigue and weakness,

- Reduced ability to exercise
- Heartbeat becomes rapid and/or irregular
- Lack of appetite
- Nausea
- Fluid retention and rapid weight gain
- Swelling or bloating of your abdomen

Heart failure is indicative of chronic severe heart disease. Some patients' symptoms will improve with proper treatment of the underlying cause (hypertension, heart valve failure, arrhythmias). Close medical monitoring of these patients is necessary since symptoms can worsen quickly with life-threatening consequences.

2. Stroke

By definition, stroke is not heart disease but can have a similar etiology and risk factors as ischemic heart disease and heart attacks. It can result from cardiac arrhythmias and is a vascular event with potentially life-altering and life-threatening consequences.

Strokes occur due to a disruption in the blood supply to the brain, resulting in the brain not getting sufficient oxygen and nutrients. The effects of a stroke depend on the area of the brain that has been damaged and the amount of damage.

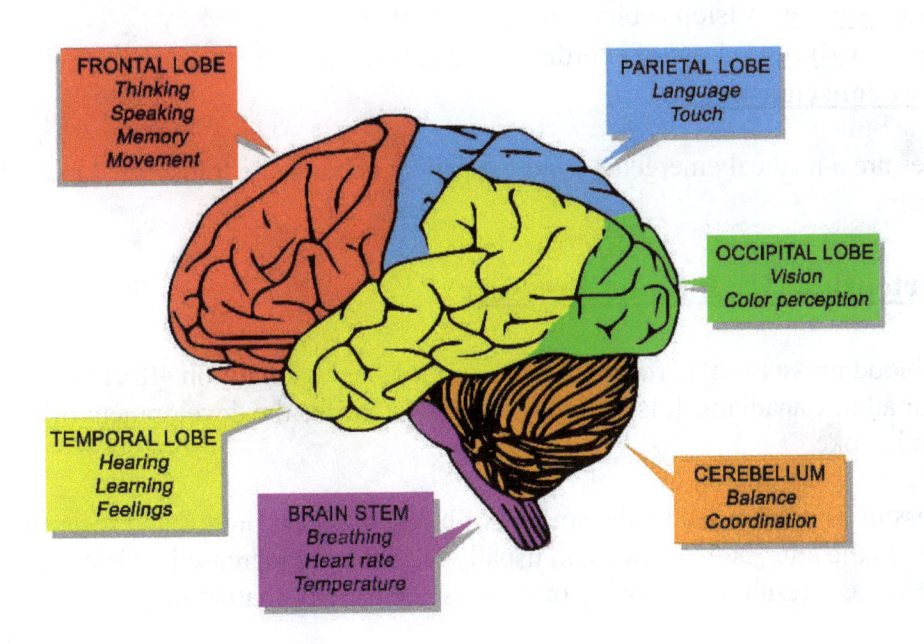

Types of Strokes

a. Ischemic Stroke – This is the most common cause of strokes. This type of stroke results from a blockage of the carotid artery (major blood vessels in the neck that supplies blood to the brain) or cerebral blood vessels due to atherosclerosis or a blood clot that travels from the heart. These blood clots primarily occur when the heartbeat is abnormal in some way (arrhythmias).

b. Hemorrhagic Stroke – This is caused when an artery/aneurysm (partial dilation of a blood vessel) in the brain ruptures.

c. Transient Ischemic Attack (TIA) – This is caused by an artery in the brain being briefly blocked by a small clot. It is often called a mini stroke. The TIA symptoms are usually transitory and last a few minutes and most often less than an hour. However, TIAs are a significant warning sign that a more severe stroke may occur soon. These are medical emergencies, and the person should be transported to the hospital immediately.

Risk Factors for Strokes

The risk factors for developing strokes resulting from atherosclerosis are the same as ischemic heart disease. Other causes of strokes, such as aneurysm, maybe congenital and be inherited.

Signs of a Stroke

Typically, signs of a stroke occur very suddenly;

- **Numbness, weakness, paralysis, physical distortion** – usually on one side of the body in the face, arm, or leg.
- **Slurred speech**
- **Severe headache** – Very severe with no identifiable cause.
- **Mental Confusion** – Difficulty following and understanding a conversation.
- **Trouble seeing** – Vision is blurry in one or both eyes.
- **Trouble walking** – Loss of coordination and balance
- **Loss of consciousness.**

Strokes are a medical emergency, and the patient needs to be transported to the hospital immediately.

3. Hypertension (High Blood Pressure)

High blood pressure (hypertension) is a common health condition affecting approximately one in four adult Canadians. It is a significant risk factor for the development of ischemic heart disease and stroke.

Blood pressure is determined by the amount of blood the heart pumps and resistance to this blood flow in the arteries. Hypertension usually results from increased resistance to blood flow in the arteries as a result of narrowing or decreased elasticity (hardening).

A blood pressure reading has two numbers and is given in millimeters of mercury (mm Hg).

Blood pressure measurement;

Systolic Pressure (Top Number) – This is the first or upper number and measures the pressure in the arteries when the heart beats blood from the left ventricle into the aorta and arteries of the body.

Diastolic Pressure (Bottom Number) – This is the second or lower number and measures the pressure in your arteries between beats.

Normal Blood Pressure – 120/80.
Hypertension – 140/90.

Symptoms of Hypertension
High blood pressure can be insidious since a person can have it for years without showing any symptoms. Some people with high blood pressure may experience signs and symptoms such as headaches, shortness of breath, or nosebleeds. However, these signs and symptoms aren't specific to high blood pressure and usually don't occur until a person's high blood pressure has reached a severe or life-threatening stage.

Two types of high blood pressure:
1. Primary (Essential) Hypertension – This type affects most adults. There's no identifiable cause for the person to have high blood pressure. This type tends to develop gradually and insidiously over many years.

2. Secondary Hypertension – This is high blood pressure caused by an underlying condition. This type typically appears suddenly and causes higher blood pressure than does primary essential hypertension. There are many conditions and medications that can lead to secondary hypertension, including:

- Certain over-the-counter and prescription medications, such as birth control pills, cold remedies, decongestants, pain relievers
- Kidney disease
- Adrenal gland tumors
- Adrenal gland tumors
- Obstructive sleep apnea
- Thyroid problems
- Illegal drugs, such as cocaine and amphetamines

High blood pressure not properly controlled increases the risk of severe health problems, including heart attack, stroke, and kidney failure. Fortunately, high blood pressure can be easily diagnosed, and once detected, can be controlled effectively by medication, diet, and exercise.

Please note, while doing muscle resistance type exercises, a person should never hold their breath because of the risk of elevating their blood pressure.

Conclusion

Heart disease is a significant and prevalent health problem in our society. Though a person cannot do anything about the genes they inherited (familial history) or getting older, they can take actions to minimize the risk of developing heart disease. These preventative measures include following a good diet with lots of fruits and vegetables, minimizing saturated and trans fats, participating in regular exercise, and reducing chronic stress.

It is important to understand heart disease, its risk factors, and its signs and symptoms. Then, as a person develops their health and fitness plan (refer to Section 4: The Offense, Section 5: The Defense, and Section 6: Special Teams), they must consider how heart disease compromises their present health status. The presence of risk factors or being diagnosed with heart disease, stroke, or high blood pressure will dictate modifications necessary in their health and fitness plan to accommodate these risks.

It is best practice for a person to consult with their medical doctor before starting any new exercise or nutritional plan. Safety comes first; this especially holds true when it comes to heart disease.

References

https://www.mayoclinic.org/diseases-conditions/heart-disease/symptoms-causes/syc-20353118
https://www.healthline.com/health/heart-disease
https://www.cdc.gov/heartdisease/facts.htm
https://www.webmd.com/heart-disease/ss/slideshow-visual-guide-to-heart-disease
https://www.nhlbi.nih.gov/health-topics/coronary-heart-disease

2.3. Cancer

Introduction

Cancer is devastating, period! It is the leading cause of death in Canada. Very few Canadians can say that their lives have not been adversely affected by cancer, directly or indirectly. It is estimated that there will be 225,800 new cases of cancer and 83,300 deaths attributed to cancer in Canada in 2020 (CMAJ March 02, 2020). Nearly half of all Canadians are expected to receive a cancer diagnosis in their lifetime. National health care cost for cancer is soaring, with an estimated price of over 10 billion dollars in 2020. Of course, the personal cost is priceless.

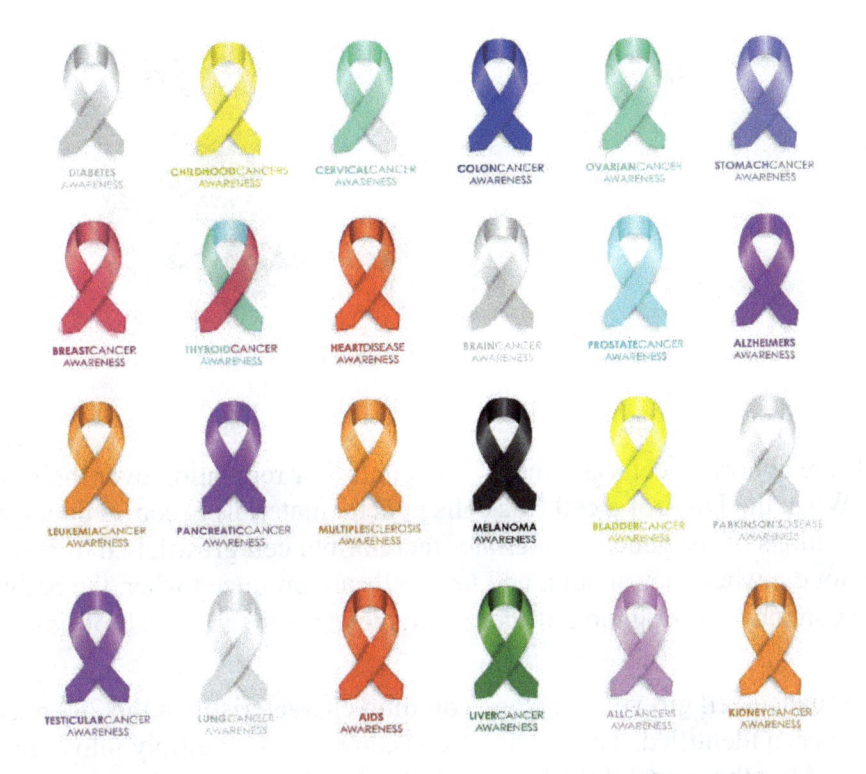

Lung cancer is the leading cause of death at 25.5%, followed by colorectal cancer at 11.6%, pancreatic cancer at 6.4%, and breast cancer at 6.1%. Unfortunately, due to the growing and aging population, the number of cases and deaths due to cancer is likely to increase.

What is Cancer?

To understand cancer better, it is helpful to understand the biology of a normal cell. A normal cell only divides when the body signals that more of those cells are needed to carry out its function.

Process of cancer development

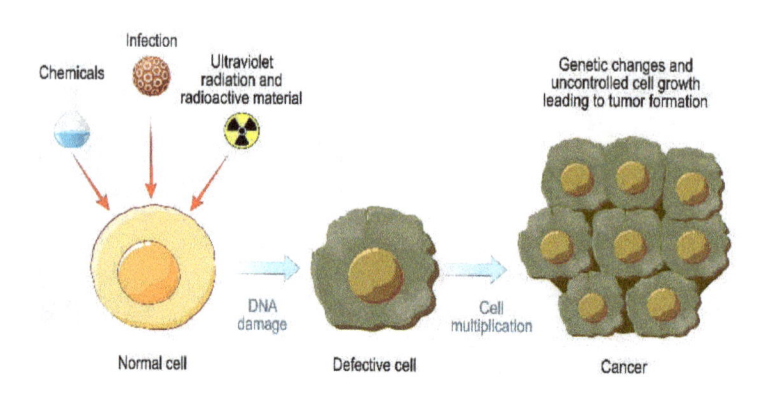

Cancer cells are abnormal cells and there is no control or regulation over their division and multiplication. When the DNA of a cell (the cells genetic material) becomes damaged or changed, the mutations of the genetic material affect normal cell growth and division. As a result, cells do not die when they should, and new cells are produced when the body does not need them. The continued propagation of these extra cells results in a mass of tissue or a tumor.

Unchecked mutated cell growth is the one common characteristic in the 200 plus types of cancers that have been identified. The mutated cells can not only multiply into a mass of tissue but they can spread to other parts of the body and invade other tissues. As a result, cancer is thought of as a genetic disease driven by gene mutations.

Typically, multiple mutations are required for an abnormal cell to develop into a tumor. The human body has many checks and balances to discover and destroy mutated cells to prevent cancer. However, under certain circumstances, even the healthiest person can develop cancer.

Possible causes for genetic mutation are:

    1. Genetics – Mutated genes are inherited from one or both parents. About 5% to 10% of breast cancer cases are hereditary. Angelina Jolie is probably the most famous person who has inherited the mutated genes for breast cancer and has had a double mastectomy and hysterectomy as a pre-emptive cancer-prevention procedure.

    2. Everyday environmental exposures and lifestyle factors – Diets high in fat (and red meat) have been associated with a high risk of colorectal cancer in several case-controlled studies, with saturated fats being specifically implicated.

    3. Cancer-causing substances exposure – Tobacco smoke, asbestos exposure and ultra-violet (UV) radiation from the sun, are three of the most commonly known cancer-causing substances.

    4. Certain viral infections –HIV, Hepatitis, and HPV are the best documented cancer-causing viruses.

There Is Hope

    As devastating as cancer is in our society, there is still hope. The survival rate for most cancers is rising due to earlier detection and new and improved treatments. The exception to this is pancreatic cancer, for which early detection is still challenging.

    Prevention and awareness programs focusing on smoking cessation and avoiding second-hand smoke, preventing sun exposure, and promoting proper nutrition such as reducing fat intake and an increase in fiber in our diet have significantly impacted the incidence and mortality rate of cancer.

    Interestingly, recent research has indicated that exercise can play a significant role in preventing certain types of cancer, especially colon and breast cancer. Exercise-induced changes in hormone levels, a reduction in the percentage of body fat, enhancement of the immune system, help in this regard.

    As well, exercise can be effective in the rehabilitation process of the cancer patient by reducing fatigue, nausea, and emotional stress.

Cancer Prevention by Lifestyle Choices

    It is well-accepted that a person's lifestyle choices influence their chances of developing cancer. Small and simple lifestyle changes can make a significant difference. The Mayo Clinic recommends the following cancer-prevention tips:

HOW TO REDUCE YOUR CANCER RISK

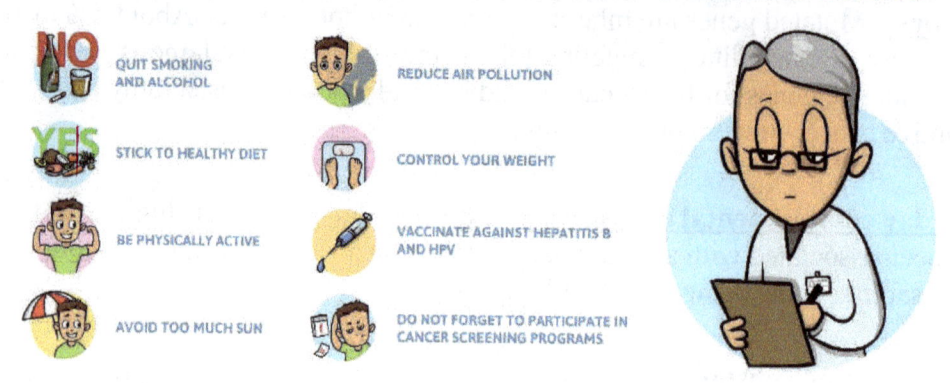

- QUIT SMOKING AND ALCOHOL
- STICK TO HEALTHY DIET
- BE PHYSICALLY ACTIVE
- AVOID TOO MUCH SUN
- REDUCE AIR POLLUTION
- CONTROL YOUR WEIGHT
- VACCINATE AGAINST HEPATITIS B AND HPV
- DO NOT FORGET TO PARTICIPATE IN CANCER SCREENING PROGRAMS

1. Avoid the Use of Tobacco

It has been very well documented that the use of tobacco substantially increases a person's cancer risk. Cancer of the mouth, throat, larynx, lung, pancreas, cervix, bladder, and kidney are just some of the cancers related to smoking tobacco. Chewing tobacco is associated with cancer of the oral cavity and pancreas. Research has shown that there is an increase your risk of lung cancer with exposure to second-hand smoke.

If you do not smoke or chew tobacco, it is better not to start. If you are a smoker or chew tobacco, ask your doctor about "stop-smoking and stop-chewing products" and other strategies for quitting. The lungs, in particular, have remarkable restorative abilities, so it is never too late to stop. The first line of prevention is not to start, or if you have started, stop smoking or chewing tobacco immediately.

2. Eat a Healthy Diet

Making good food choices at the grocery store and at mealtime might reduce a person's cancer risk.

Consider these healthy eating guidelines:

Consume vegetables and fruits for fiber – A diet heavy on vegetables, fruits, and foods from plant sources such as beans and whole grains helps increase dietary fiber intake which is important for the prevention colon cancer and helps manage a person's weight to avoid obesity.

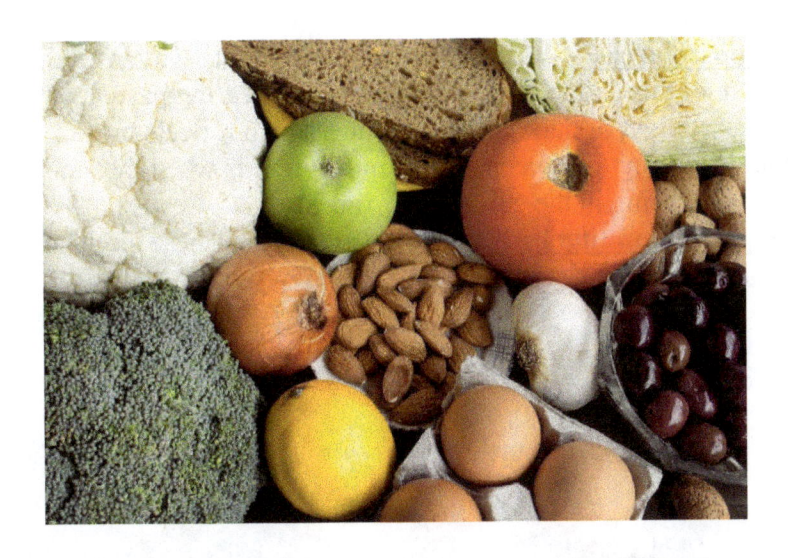

The Mediterranean diet (Chapter 5.2.10) has shown good cancer preventative prosperities by utilizing healthy mono and poly unsaturated fats found in fish, olive oil, and nuts.

Avoid obesity – Focus on serving smaller portions and leaner meals by choosing fewer foods, that are high in sugar, salt, saturated or trans fat, and calories.

Drink alcohol in moderation – The amount of alcohol you drink increases the risk of various types of cancer, including cancer of the liver, kidney, colon, and lung.

Limit processed meats – Several studies have concluded that the steady consumption of processed meat can increase the risk of certain types of cancer.

3. Maintain a Healthy Weight and Be Physically Active

Maintaining a healthy weight (good diet and exercise) might lower the risk of various types of cancer, including cancer of the colon, kidney, prostate, lung and breast.

Research has suggested that physical activity potentially lowers the risk of colon and breast cancer. The more exercise you do the better but it is recommended to include at least 30 minutes of physical activity in your daily routine. Refer to Section 4: The Offense: Getting Active the Right Way for specific exercise guidelines and Appendix 9.1.1 and 9.1.2 for cardiovascular and strengthening exercises.

4. Avoid direct Sun Exposure

Skin cancer is becoming one of the most common types of cancer diagnosed. Fortunately, it can be one of the most preventable.

1. **Find the shade** – Stay in the shade as much as possible and use sunglasses and a wide-brimmed hat when you are exposed to direct sun light.
2. **Use broad spectrum sunscreen** – Sunscreen with an SPF of at least 30 should be used daily, even on cloudy days. Apply sunscreen generously, and reapply often and at least every 2 hours if you're swimming or sweating.

3. **Cover exposed areas** – Wear loose-fitting but tightly woven clothing that covers as much of your arms and legs as possible. Avoid wearing pastels or bleached cotton, instead, wear bright or dark colour clothing which reflects more UV radiation.
4. **Avoid midday sun** – Between 10 a.m. and 4 p.m is when the sun rays are strongest so try to avoid being in the sun at these times.
5. **Sunlamps and Tanning beds are to be avoided** – These are just as toxic to your skin as natural sunlight.

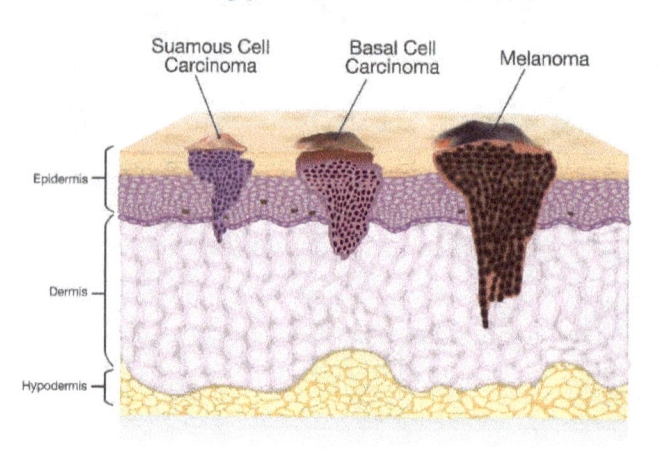

Early detection is important for all types of cancer. For skin cancer, be aware of the following:

a. Bump or Lesion

Basal cell carcinoma accounts for 8 out of 10 skin cancers. It may appear as a pink, white, or skin-colored bump or lesion on your neck, ears and face. The lesion may be flat, red, scaly or have a waxy appearance. Sometimes these lesions itch and become irritated, bleed, and then scab over. This type of skin cancer originates in the basal cells, which is the layer of the skin responsible for creating new skin cells after the old ones die. Basal cell carcinoma is clinically less severe than melanoma, and seldom spread to vital organs.

b. Open Sores and Growth

Squamous cell carcinoma often presents as a persistent red sore, nodule, or scaly patch. This form of skin carcinoma has a crusty exterior and often appear in areas that experience frequent sun exposure such as balding scalp, or the neck, hands, arms, face, rim of the ear or the lower lip. However, it can develop on any area of the body, including the genitals. Over the last 30 years, the number of squamous cell carcinoma diagnoses has increased by more than 200%.

c. Asymmetrical Moles

Melanoma often appears as asymmetrical mole with irregular borders. Melanoma is the most serious type of skin cancer. Men tend to see the development of Melanoma on their chest, back, head, and neck. Women, on the other hand, often develop melanomas on their lower legs. It is important to have any moles that change size (a normal mole is about ¼ - inch in diameter), color, shape, bleeds or itches evaluated by your medical doctor or dermatologist since these changes can indicate skin cancer. This form of skin cancer is becoming more prevalent in those younger than 40.

d. New Moles

The average adult has between 10 to 45 moles on their body, which usually develop before the age of 50. New moles that appear on an older adult skin are significant because there is a great likelihood to be cancerous or pre-cancerous. For the older adult or for anyone who is vulnerable to skin cancer (a person who has greater than a hundred moles or someone that works daily in the sun/outdoors) should have a yearly body scan examination by their doctor or dermatologist.

e. Pigmented Patch, a Dome, or Bump

A change in the skin is a very common sign of skin cancer. Be aware that the edges of a problematic skin patch will likely be less defined and appear more ragged, the coloring may be uneven, usually in varying shades of black, brown, white, tan, or blue. Skin cancer patches are asymmetrical while normal moles are mostly symmetrical.

5. Get Vaccinated

As mentioned previously under risk factors, certain viral infections have been well documented to cause cancer. It is important to discuss with your doctor about getting vaccinated against:

Hepatitis B – Hepatitis B has been documented to increase the risk of developing liver cancer. The hepatitis B vaccine can lower the risk of developing liver cancer in adults at high risk of contacting hepatitis B. Those who are at high risk include sexually active but not in a mutually monogamous relationship, people with sexually transmitted diseases, gay men, people who are regularly administered intravenous drugs, and health care and public safety workers who are exposed to infected blood or body fluids.

Human Papillomavirus (HPV) – HPV is a sexually transmitted virus that can result in cervical and other genital cancers and squamous cell cancers of the neck and head. The Gardasil 9 vaccine has been approved by the Canadian government for males between ages 9 to 26 and females between ages 9 to 45 to help protect against the HPV virus.

6. Get Regular Medical Care

Regular self-exams and screenings can help discover cancer early when treatment is most effective. Screenings and early detection are most effective for cancers of the skin, colon, cervix, and breast. Your doctor can help determine the best cancer screening schedule for you based on your risk factors.

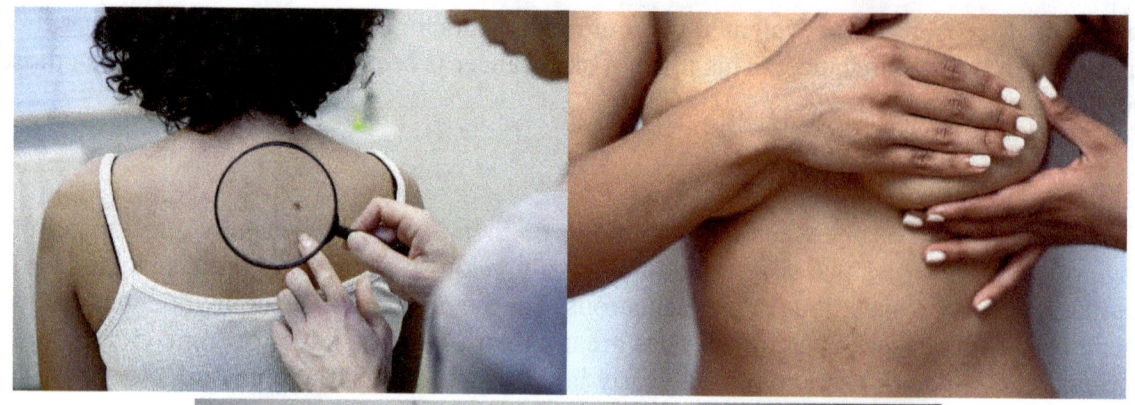

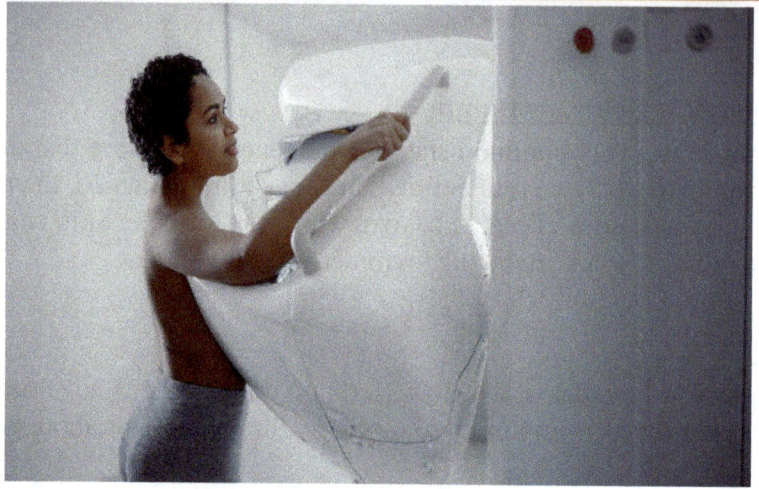

The Role of Exercise in Cancer

    The following are highlights from a review of medical articles by the Cancer Network studying the role exercise plays in cancer prevention and rehabilitation.

    To make a long story short, exercise has been shown to be beneficial in cancer prevention, recovery, and survival. Patients should be encouraged to exercise as vigorously as is safe in each of these oncologic setting,

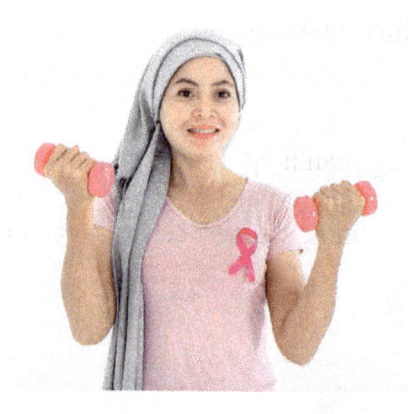

1. <u>During cancer treatment</u>, exercise helps counter the side effects of radiation and chemotherapy. The side effects of reduced fatigue and nausea has shown to occur with regular exercise. The current exercise guidelines listed in Section 4: The Offense – Getting Active the Right Way) should be followed. It is encouraged that for patients that are able, they should add some high intense exercise to complement their base of moderate intense activity.

2. <u>In the early survivorship setting</u>, exercise helps quicken the recovery from the effects of radiation and surgery. Exercise has been shown to help return the patient to as close to full function as possible which improves their quality of life.

3. <u>Exercise should be continued long -term</u> to improve a patients overall survival rate. Exercise decreases mortality rates so a vigorous physical activity program that is tailored to their limitations should be the goal for all cancer survivors.

Summary of the Study

It is recommended that a base of aerobic exercise of low-to-moderate intensity, such as walking, carried out 3 to 5 times a week for a total of at least 150 minutes per week be initiated. It is also recommended that when and where possible, resistance training be included to help restore muscle strength which was lost as a result of their treatment and covalence.

Mental/Emotional Health and Cancer

Whether you have been diagnosed with cancer or know a family or friend who has been, a wide range of feelings/emotions can develop that you may not use to dealing with. The intensity of these feelings can also be quite strong. The emotional and mental state of a person diagnosed with cancer or a family member or friend may change instantaneously with no apparent trigger. This is true before, during or after the cancer patient is done treatment. Feelings sad, overwhelmed, hopeless, fearful, anxious, angry, depressed, lonely, are all normal and should be expected.

The values a person grew up often affect how they think emotionally adapt to a diagnosis of cancer. For example, some people:
- Seek out help from counselors and other will not.
- Rely more strongly on their faith to help them cope while other will abandon their faith due to hopelessness and anger
- Rely on loved ones or other cancer survivors for support while others seek social isolation.
- Feel they have an obligation to their friends and families to be strong and protect them from the effects that their cancer diagnosis may have on them. This is especially true if they have small children.

What is important is to do what is right for you. Do not compare your feeling with how others are feeling. Your friends and family members probably share many of the same feelings you are experiencing but may express them in their own individualist way.

It is important to keep a hopeful attitude, seek social support because social isolation is emotionally detrimental, and seek professional support/help if needed. Don't hesitate, it is normal to need help after a life-changing diagnosis such as cancer.

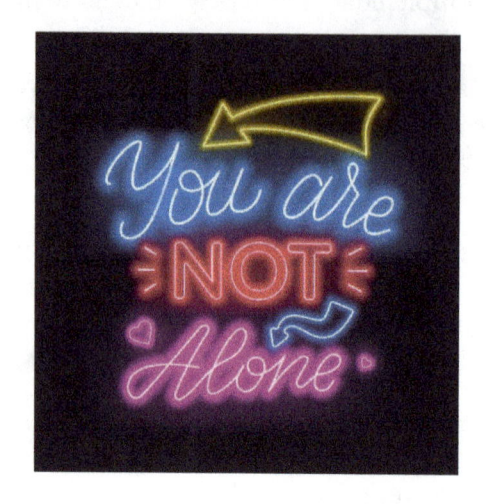

Conclusion

The current literature encourages people with cancer to be as active as possible before, during treatment and recovery. Being active may:
1. Improve your mood, reduce stress and help a person sleep
2. Boost a person's energy
3. Stimulate a person's appetite
4. Reduce side effects like nausea, fatigue, and constipation
5. Help a person regain their strength during recovery.

A person will need to check with their doctor before starting any health and exercise program. After the doctor has given the okay, the person should meet with an exercise specialist with experience in this area. They can help develop an exercise program that is safe, effective and fun. If a person is dealing with cancer, Section 4: The Offense – Getting Active the Right Way is meant only as a guideline for you. Each person's cancer and their treatment, rehabilitation and recovery are specific to them. As a result, their exercise and health plan must be tailored specifically to their needs. This can and should only be done under the personal supervision of a qualified health and exercise professional.

The war against cancer rages on, but the battle is being won. It is important to remember that a healthy lifestyle (proper diet and regular exercise) and early detection (regular physical examinations) are the most effective weapons against this dreaded disease.

References

https://www.cancernetwork.com/view/role-physical-activity-cancer-prevention-treatment-recovery-and-survivorship

https://www.cancerresearch.org/

https://www.cancer.gov/about-cancer/understanding/what-is-cancer

https://www.cancer.ca/

https://www.mayoclinic.org/diseases-conditions/cancer/symptoms-causes/syc-20370588

https://www.healthline.com/health/cancer

https://facty.com/conditions/cancer/10-signs-of-skin-cancer/1/

2.4. Diabetes

Introduction

Diabetes is a metabolic disease (a disease that disrupts normal metabolism, which is the process of converting food to energy on a cellular level) that causes high blood sugar. It is a significant health risk that is increasing in society as the population becomes more inactive, overweight, and obese. 10% of the Canadian population lives with either type 1 (an autoimmune disorder that results in insulin dependency) or type 2 diabetes (acquired and is insulin-resistant).

Research indicates that diabetes decreases a person's life span by 5 to 15 years and contributes to 30% of strokes, 40% of heart attacks, 50% of kidney failure requiring dialysis, and 70% of all nontraumatic leg and foot amputations. It is also the leading cause of blindness.

For the older adult, it is important to understand the causes, risk factors, signs and symptoms, and treatments for diabetes. If a person is diagnosed as pre-diabetic (high blood sugar levels that are not high enough to be classified as diabetic), that person can make lifestyle changes to prevent full diabetes. If a person has been diagnosed with type 1 or type 2 diabetes, it is important to monitor and manage the disease appropriately. Monitoring blood glucose levels is especially true when a person wants to make lifestyle changes concerning exercise and nutrition.

There are no contra-indications to exercising when a person has diabetes. Exercise is highly encouraged as an effective way to manage weight, high blood pressure, ischemic heart disease, and improve peripheral blood circulation in your legs. Many famous athletes who were diabetic have performed at the highest levels of their sport: Jackie Robinson (Baseball Hall of Fame), Bobby Clark (Hockey Hall of Fame), Author Ashe and Billy Jean King (Major Championship Tennis Winners) and Gary Hall (Five-Time Olympic Swimming Gold Medalist).

The secret to being diabetic and living a high quality of life is proper diagnosis, treatment, and continuous monitoring of blood glucose (sugar) levels. For the diabetic, monitoring blood glucose during exercise is especially important to avoid hyper or hypoglycemia, both of which can be life-threatening.

Understanding Diabetes

To understand diabetes, it is important to understand how glucose is normally processed in the body.

How Insulin Works
1. The pancreas produces the hormone insulin
2. Insulin is secreted into the bloodstream by the pancreas.
3. Insulin functions to enabling blood glucose (sugar) to enter your cells which lowers the amount of glucose in your bloodstream.
4. As your blood glucose level drops, a reduced amount of insulin is secreted from your pancreas.

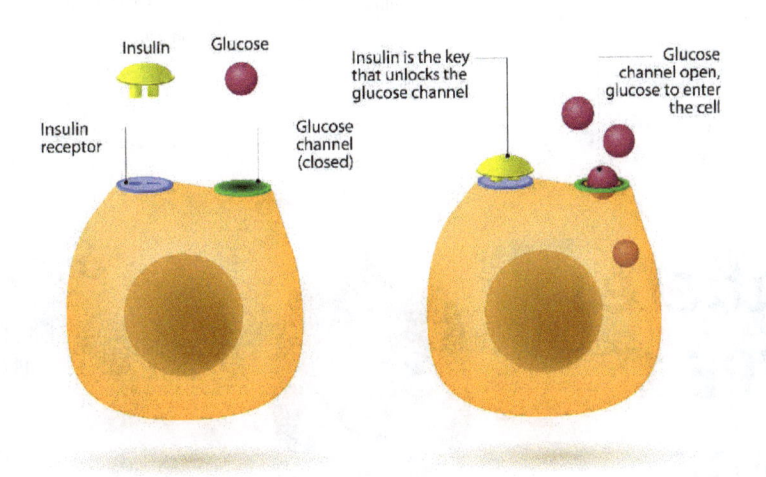

The Role of Glucose (Sugar)
- Glucose is the primary source of energy for the cells of the body's muscles, brain, and other tissues.
- The primary sources of blood glucose are from carbohydrates you eat and glucose stored in the skeletal muscles and liver as glycogen.
- Through the digestion of eaten food (carbohydrates) or the metabolic breakdown glycogen in the liver and skeletal muscles, glucose is absorbed into the bloodstream, where, with the help of insulin, it enters into the cells.
- Excess levels of glucose in the blood are converted into fatty acids and stored as fat in adipose tissue and the liver.
- When your blood glucose levels are low as the result of exercising or it has been a while since you have eaten, the liver breaks down stored glycogen into glucose to keep your blood glucose level within a normal range.

Types of Diabetes

DIABETES MELLITUS

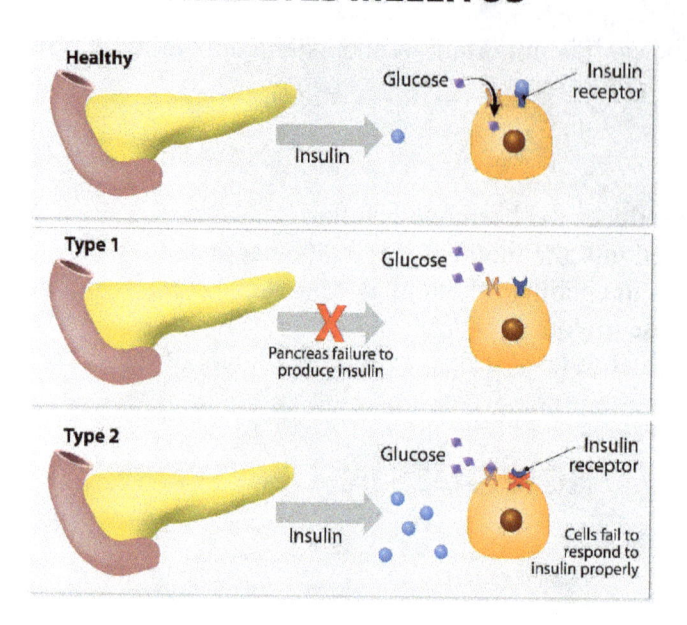

Healthy — Insulin → Glucose, Insulin receptor

Type 1 — Pancreas failure to produce insulin

Type 2 — Insulin → Glucose, Cells fail to respond to insulin properly

1. Type 1

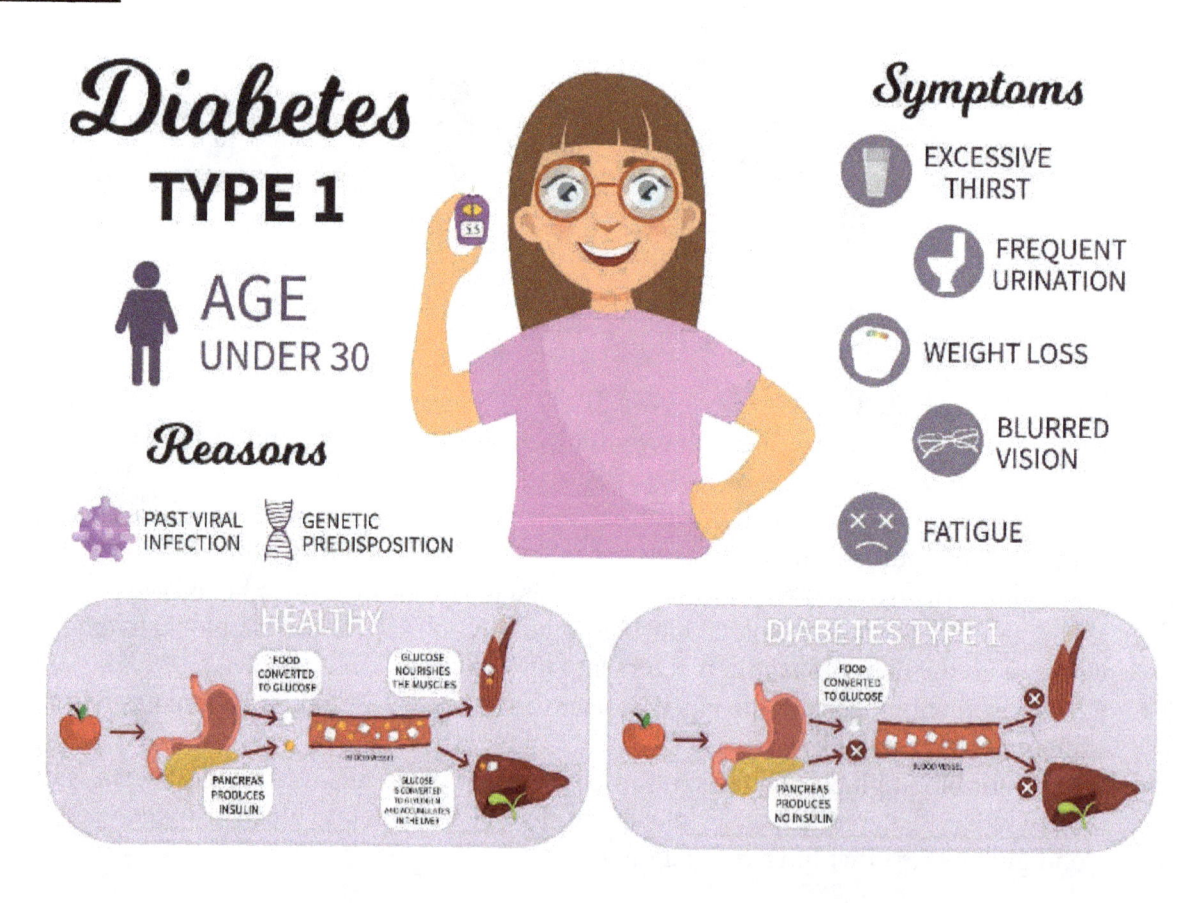

Diabetes TYPE 1

AGE UNDER 30

Reasons: Past viral infection, Genetic predisposition

Symptoms:
- Excessive thirst
- Frequent urination
- Weight loss
- Blurred vision
- Fatigue

HEALTHY: Food converted to glucose → Pancreas produces insulin → Glucose nourishes the muscles → Glucose is converted to glycogen and accumulates in the liver

DIABETES TYPE 1: Food converted to glucose → Pancreas produces no insulin

Type 1 diabetes, also known as insulin-dependent diabetes, is an autoimmune disease. The specific cause of type 1 diabetes is unknown; however, it is known is that with type 1 diabetes, the person's immune system, which typically fights harmful bacteria or viruses, attacks and destroys the insulin-producing cells in the pancreas. This results in type 1 diabetics being unable produce their own insulin and therefore they cannot regulate their blood sugar. Type 1 insulin-dependent diabetes accounts for approximately 10% of people living with diabetes.

To ensure their bodies have the right amount of insulin Type 1 diabetics inject insulin or use an insulin pump. This form of diabetes generally develops in childhood or adolescence but can also develop in adulthood.

2. Type 2

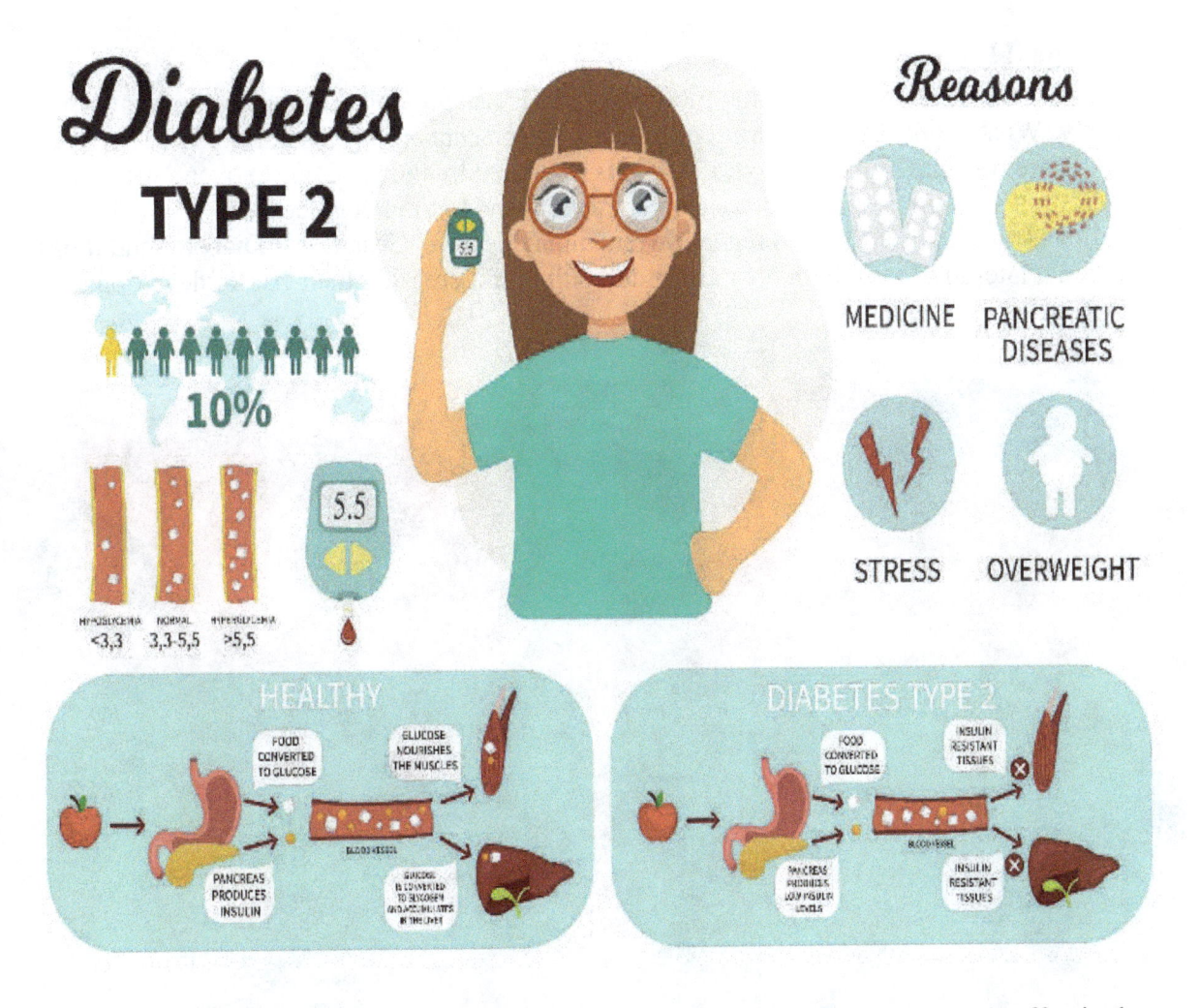

Type 2 diabetics cannot produce enough insulin or the cells of the body cannot effectively use the insulin that is produced. The exact cause is not known but it is believed that genetic and environmental factors play a significant role in developing type 2 diabetes. People who are overweight or obese have an increase likelihood to development of type 2 diabetes, however, not everyone with type 2 is overweight.

Type 2 diabetes can occur in childhood but most commonly develops in adults over the age of 40. Type 2 diabetes often requires insulin therapy but sometimes can be managed effectively with a good diet and regular exercise.

3. Prediabetes

A person is referred to as being Prediabetic when their blood sugar levels are slightly above normal but they are not high enough to be officially diagnosed as type 2 diabetes. Often, but not always, prediabetic's blood glucose levels will continue to rise and they will develop type 2 diabetes.

Corrective measures such as reducing weight can have significant preventative effectiveness against prediabetes developing into full-blown diabetes.

4. Gestational Diabetes

Gestational Diabetes occurs during pregnancy and is usually only last during the term of pregnancy. What happens is that during pregnancy, the placenta produces hormones that make the cells more resistant to insulin. Extra insulin is produced by the pancreas to overcome this resistance, but sometimes, the pancreas cannot keep up and too much glucose stays in your blood. It is estimated that 20% of pregnant women may develop Gestational Diabetes and it has the potential later in life, for both the mother and child, of increasing their risk of developing type 2 diabetes.

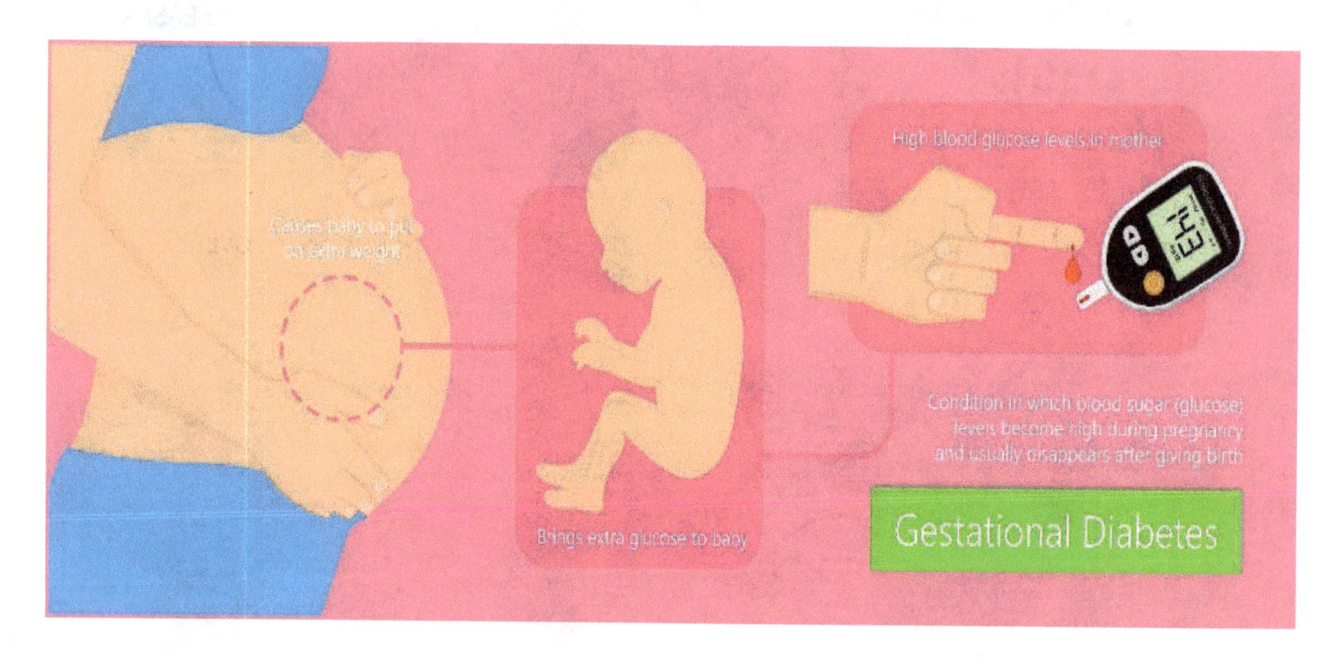

Signs and Symptoms of Diabetes

Depending on how much the blood sugar is elevated, the symptoms of diabetes may vary. It is not unusual for Prediabetic or Type 2 diabetics, usually adults, not to show symptoms. In type 1 diabetes, which usually affects children or adolescence, symptoms can occur quickly and be severe.

Be aware of the most common signs and symptoms of type 1 diabetes and type 2 diabetes:
- Frequent urination
- Dry mouth and increased thirst
- Unexplained weight loss
- Extreme hunger
- Urine smells like popcorn which means there is ketones in the urine. (Ketones are produced from the breakdown of muscle and fat when there is not enough glucose in the cells because of the insufficient availability or cell in-sensitivity to insulin.)
- Irritability
- Blurred vision
- Chronically tired and fatigue
- Frequent gum, skin and vaginal infections,
- Skin sores (cuts, blisters) heal slowly

Risk Factors of Diabetes

Risk factors differ for the various types of diabetes.

Type 1 Diabetes Risk Factors

It is unknown what exactly causes of type 1 diabetes but research has identified factors that may increase the risk:

- **Family history** – This is the number one risk factor if one sibling or parent has type 1 diabetes.
- **Environmental factors** – It is suspected that exposure to a viral illness increases the likely of developing in type 1 diabetes.
- **The presence of diabetic autoantibodies (immune system cells)** – If diabetic autoantibodies are present in parents, siblings or extended family members, there is an increased risk of developing type 1 diabetes.
- **Geography** – The reasons are unknown but certain Scandinavian countries, such as Finland and Sweden, have shown higher rates of type 1 diabetes.

Risk factors for Prediabetes and Type 2 Diabetes

Research clearly has identified that certain factors increase the risk for Prediabetes and Type 2 Diabetes but it is still unknow why some people with these risk factors develop these forms of diabetes and others don't:

- **Family history** – Once again genetics plays a significant role. The diabetic risk increases if a sibling or parent has type 2 diabetes.

- **Age** – The older a person gets, the increase risk of becoming diabetic. This is usually occurs because the older individual exercises less and as a result loses muscle mass and gains weight. It should be noted that type 2 diabetes is increasing among children, adolescents, and younger adults. This may be due to increased sugar intake and the increased incidence of obesity in this population.

- **Weight** – The higher percentage of fat tissue a person has, the more resistant their cells become to insulin.

- **Inactivity** – Physical activity helps control weight (less fat tissue), uses up blood glucose as energy rather than it being stored as glycogen in muscles and the liver, and makes your cells more sensitive to insulin.

- **Race or ethnicity** – The reasons are unknown but research indicates that certain ethnic groups, such as Black, Hispanic, Indigenous North Americans, and Asian American people, are at higher risk of developing diabetes. The reason for this is unknown but diet may play a significant role.

- **Gestational Diabetes** – This form of diabetes during pregnancy increases the risk of developing prediabetes and type 2 diabetes in both the mother and child later in life. Research also indicates that babies weighing more than 9 pounds (4 kilograms), have a higher risk of developing type 2 diabetes increases.

- **High blood pressure** – Having blood pressure over 140/90 millimeters of mercury (mm Hg) is linked to an increased risk of type 2 diabetes. This may be due to the fact that many people with high blood pressure are overweight and do not exercise, both of which are risk factors.

- **Polycystic ovarian syndrome** – This is a common condition characterized by irregular menstrual periods and obesity and has shown to increases the risk of diabetes.

Complications for Type 1 and Type 2 Diabetes

Complications of diabetes develop gradually. The risk of complications is higher the longer a person has diabetes and/or the less control they have over their blood sugar levels. Over a period of time the complications of diabetes may be disabling and life-threatening.

- **Cardiovascular disease** – The risk of various cardiovascular problems increases significantly in people with long standing diabetes. These cardiovascular problems include coronary artery disease (atherosclerosis), ischemic heart disease which includes angina (chest pain), heart attack, and stroke.

- **Nerve damage (neuropathy)** – This is a common complication with individuals who have had diabetes for an extended period of time. High blood sugar can cause injury to the walls of the tiny blood capillaries that nourish the nerves, especially in the legs. Symptoms of nerve damage are tingling, burning, pain and numbness that usually begins at the tips of the toes or fingers and eventually spreads upward. Damage to the nerves for digestion can result in the symptoms of nausea, vomiting, diarrhea, or constipation. Erectile dysfunction can occur in men.

- **Foot damage** – Nerve damage or poor blood flow involving the feet compromises healing and can result in cuts and blisters developing serious infections if not properly treated. Often with someone who has had long-standing diabetes, these lesions never heal resulting ultimately amputation of the toe, foot, or leg.

- **Kidney damage (nephropathy)** – The kidneys have a very delicate blood waste filtration system. Diabetes can damage the blood vessels of this filtering system and if severe enough, kidney failure can occur which may require dialysis or a kidney transplant.

- **Eye damage (retinopathy)** – The retina's blood vessels (diabetic retinopathy) can be damaged which can potentially lead to blindness. Cataracts and glaucoma are other vision problems that diabetics have an increase the risk of developing.

- **Skin conditions** – Bacterial and fungal infections of the skin are more likely to occur in diabetics.

- **Hearing impairment** – People with diabetes are more likely to have hearing impairments.

- **Alzheimer's disease** – There is an increase the risk of dementia, such as Alzheimer's disease in people with long-standing diabetes.

Treatment of Diabetes

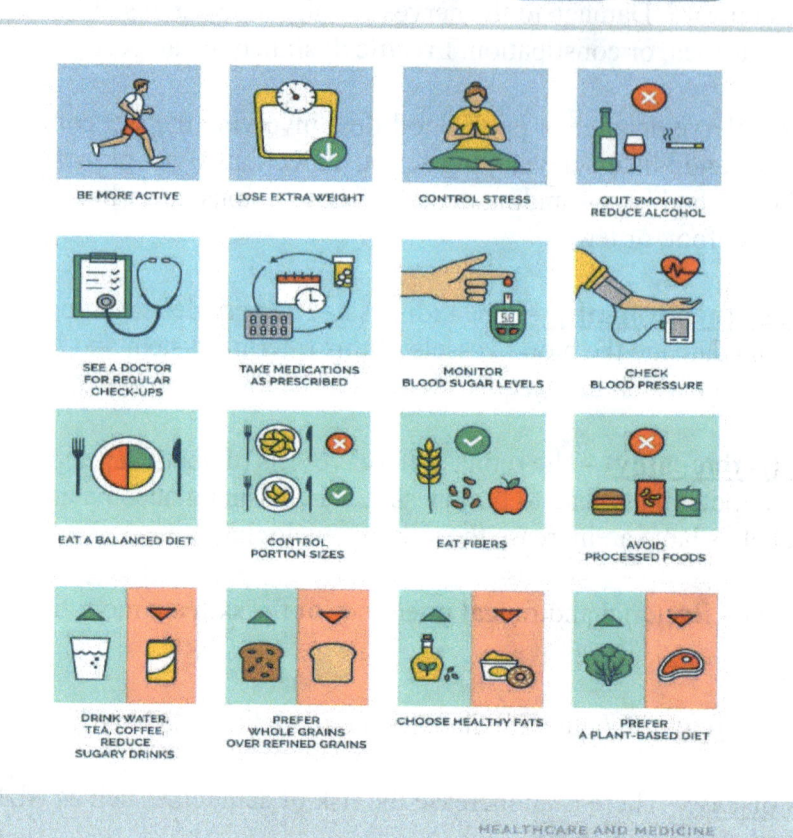

Type 1 Diabetes

The administration of insulin by injection or pump to replace the hormone the diabetics body can not produce is the main treatment for type 1 diabetes.

Insulin treatment varies by how quickly the insulin starts to work, and how long their effects last:

1. **Rapid-acting insulin** – begins to work within 15 minutes, and is effective for 3 to 4 hours.
2. **Short-acting insulin** – begins to work within 30 minutes and is effective for 6 to 8 hours.
3. **Intermediate-acting insulin** – begins to work within 1 to 2 hours and is effective for 12 to 18 hours.
4. **Long-acting insulin** – begins to work a few hours after injection and will be effective for 24 hours or longer.

Type 2 Diabetes
For some people type 2 diabetes can be managed by diet and exercise. If these lifestyle changes do not produce sufficient lowering of blood sugar levels, medication or insulin administration is necessary.

Diabetes Prevention

Type 1 Diabetes
Type 1 diabetes is an autoimmune disease therefore it is not preventable.

Type 2 Diabetes
Some risk factors for type 2 diabetes, such as your familial history (a person's genes) or advancing age, are not controllable. However, adhering to basic health principles such as eating a balanced diet, managing good weight control, getting regular exercise, and reducing chronic stress, can have significant preventative effects against the development of diabetes as a person gets older.

These preventive measures are discussed in detail under Sections 4: The Offense and Section 5: The Defense. However, it is necessary to discuss diet and exercise in more specific terms related to diabetes.

Diet and Diabetes
A good diet may or may not be enough to control Prediabetes or Type 2 Diabetes. However, a good diet is just good health practice.

Type 1 Diabetes
Blood sugar levels are sensitive to the types of foods you eat. Blood sugar levels rise rapidly with the ingestion of starchy or sugary foods (carbohydrates). Protein and fat, on the other hand cause a more gradual blood sugar increase. It is often recommended to limit the number of carbohydrates eaten each day and coordinate carbohydrate intake with insulin doses.

Working with a dietitian is advisable to get the expertise to help design an effective diabetes meal plan. It is important to get the right balance of carbohydrates, protein, and fat, to help control blood sugar and maintain healthy cognitive and bodily functions.

Type 2 Diabetes
To control your blood sugar and help you lose any excess weight it is important to eat the correct types of food. To manage type 2 diabetes carbohydrate counting is essential. With the help of a dietitian, you can figure out the correct amount of carbohydrates to eat at each meal and balance out your diet.

It is important keep your blood sugar levels steady by trying to eat small meals throughout the day and emphasize healthy foods such as:

- vegetables
- fruits
- lean protein such as poultry and fish
- healthy mono and ploy-unsaturated fats found in olive oil and nuts
- whole grains

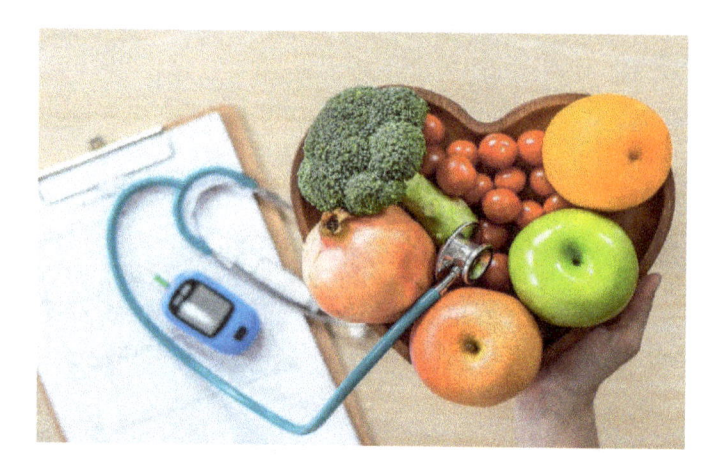

Everyone, but especially someone who has been diagnosed as prediabetic or having type 2 diabetic should avoid foods containing added sugar, salt, or is high in saturated fat (red meats and dairy) and trans-fat (processed foods).

Exercise and Diabetes

Word of Caution

It is strongly recommended to have a complete medical checkup before starting a new exercise program. For someone has been living with diabetes for several years this is especially relevant since over the years they may have developed mild to moderate chronic diabetes complications such as ischemic heart disease, peripheral neuropathy, or renal (kidney) neuropathy.

Your doctor will also recommend the best time to do physical activity based on the type of medication you are taking and when you are taking it. Insulin dosages can often be adjusted based on your physical activity schedule

Some General Tips when Doing Physical Activity as a Diabetic:
- Check blood glucose levels regularly.
- Stop exercising if feeling unwell.
- Drinking regularly and stay hydrated.
- Carry diabetic identification (e.g., neck medallion, wrist bracelet, or wallet card).
- Wear appropriate shoes and socks. As a diabetic, peripheral neuropathy is a significant concern, so bruises and blisters on the feet must be prevented.
- Be on the look out for any blisters or other wounds before and after exercise.

- If any of the following symptoms occur when exercising: severe fatigue, nausea, fainting, blurred vision, headache, dizziness, shortness of breath consult with your doctor immediately.
- Seek professional advice from a kinesiologist or personal trainer with experience with diabetic clients. They can advise on the intensity and what type of exercise to do.

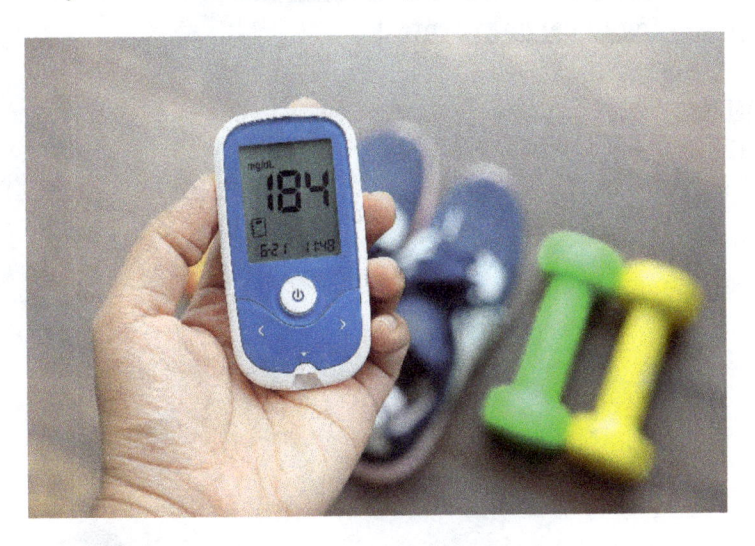

Physical Activity and Hypoglycemia (Low Blood Sugar)

Exercise increases muscle and cell sensitivity to insulin and this results in lower blood glucose levels. Consequently, there is an increased risk of hypoglycemia during and after exercise (up to 48 hours). This risk is even greater for people with type 1 diabetes or type 2 who take insulin or a drug that increases insulin secretion from the pancreas.

To Prevent Hypoglycemia:

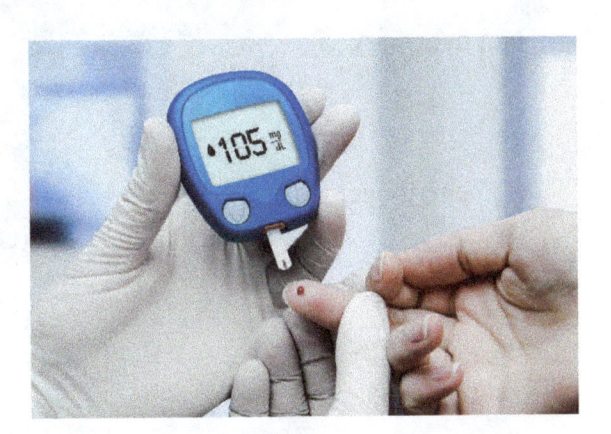

- It is important to anticipate a potential hypoglycemic episode, therefore regular monitoring of blood glucose (sugar) levels before and after exercising is necessary. If the activity lasts 60 minutes or more another reading midway through the session should be done.
- For up to 48 hours after the activity it is important to continue to monitor blood glucose (sugar) levels and essential if the activity was longer than 60 minutes.
- It should be standard practice to always carry a supply of concentrated sugar such as energy gels, glucose tablets or drink a regular soft drink, if there is potential for hypoglycemia.

To plan your meals, snacks and medication correctly based on the intensity and type of physical activity you are doing you should consult with your medical doctor and dietitian. A good rule to follow is to treat your hypoglycemia before starting to exercise if your blood glucose reading is less than 4 mmol/L

Guide to Supplemental Carbohydrates During Exercise
(1 energy gel package = 25g of carbohydrates)

Type of Physical Activity	Blood Sugar (Mmol/L)	Supplemental Carbohydrates
Short duration (less than 30 minutes) at low intensity	< or = 5.5	10 to 15g (.5 energy gel pkg)
	> 5.5	Not necessary
Medium duration (30 to 60 minutes) at moderate intensity	< or = 5.5	30 to 45g (1.5 energy gel pkg)
	5.5 to 9.9	15g per 30 to 45 minutes of exercise (.5 energy gel pkg)
	10.0 to 13.9	Not necessary
Long duration (More than 60 minutes) at high intensity	< or = 5.5	45g (1.5 energy gel pkg)
	5.5 to 9.9	30 to 45g (1.5 energy gel pkg)
	> 9.9	15g per hour (.5 energy gel pkg)

Reference: CHUM Hotel-Dieu Metabolic Medecin Day-Care Centre, 2013, Understand Your Diabetes and Live a Healthy Life, page 194.

Extra Strategies for Type 1 or Type 2 on Insulin
- Avoid delaying meals and avoid exercising on an empty stomach (fasting)
- Aerobic exercises should follow your weight resistance exercise routine.
- To avoid accelerating insulin absorption that could cause hypoglycemia don't inject insulin in an area of the body that will be worked during the activity (for example, do not inject into your dominate arm if you intend to play tennis).

Physical Activity and Hyperglycemia (High Blood Glucose Levels)

Blood sugar levels tend to drop since the cells become more sensitive to insulin during and after nearly all types of exercise. However, the body will produce more blood glucose than it uses due to the activation of stress hormones during short-duration high-intensity physical activity such as playing hockey (shifts), (shoveling snow), or basketball (stopping and starting). In these instances, transient hyperglycemia can result.

As well, stay well hydrated before, during and after physical activity because dehydration from vigorous exercise can also increase the concentration of glucose in the blood. This is especially true during the summer when the weather is hot and humid.

Blood sugar level	Symptoms
Hypoglycemia	sweating confusion hunger fast heartbeat shaking headache irritability trouble concentrating fatigue
Hyperglycemia	weakness headache extreme thirst dry mouth nausea confusion shortness of breath frequent urination blurry vision

Conclusion

Significant long-term and acute health risks can result from diabetes, and these must be considered when developing a new comprehensive health and fitness plan. Long-term health risks can result from complications of having diabetes for years and include chronic conditions such as ischemic heart disease, peripheral neuropathy and renal (kidney) failure. Acute health risks occur from a person suffering from hypoglycemia or hyperglycemia and can be life-threatening.

If diagnosed early and managed correctly, diabetes poses no contraindications to exercise, and in fact, exercise is highly recommended for those who have diabetes.

All diabetic patients must seek medical and professional health care advice before starting any new health and fitness program to ensure they follow proper nutrition and exercise guidelines.

References

https://www.mayoclinic.org/diseases-conditions/diabetes/symptoms-causes/syc-20371444
https://www.diabete.qc.ca/en/living-with-diabetes/physical-activity/advices/physical-activity-warnings-and-safeguards/
https://www.diabetes.ca/about-diabetes/what-is-diabetes
https://www.webmd.com/diabetes
https://www.medicinenet.com/diabetes_mellitus/article.htm
https://www.diabetes.org/diabetes/type-1/symptoms

2.5. Obesity

Introduction

Obesity is a progressive chronic disease characterised by excessive fat accumulation. Diabetes, osteoarthritis, heart disease, high blood pressure, and certain cancers are just some of the health conditions that obesity contributes to.

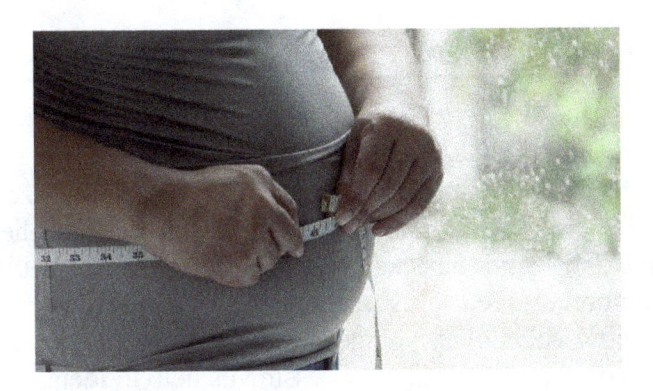

According to Stats Canada, Canadians are at epidemic proportions when it comes to being overweight or obese. They report that 67% of men and 54% of women are either overweight or obese. Sadly, 31.5% of Canadian children and youth between the ages of five and 17 are the same. According to the Canadian Heart and Stroke Foundation, among those aged 40 to 69 the prevalence of obesity has doubled, and it has tripled among those aged 20 to 39 over the past 30 years. It is estimated that in 2021 the annual economic cost of obesity in Canada will be over 9 billion dollars.

Losing weight is the number one "self-help" activity for most adult Canadians. In North America, the market for weight loss programs is estimated to be worth 104 billion dollars. Unfortunately, most of these dollars are spent on ill-advised "quick fix or fad diets," and most weight loss efforts fail.

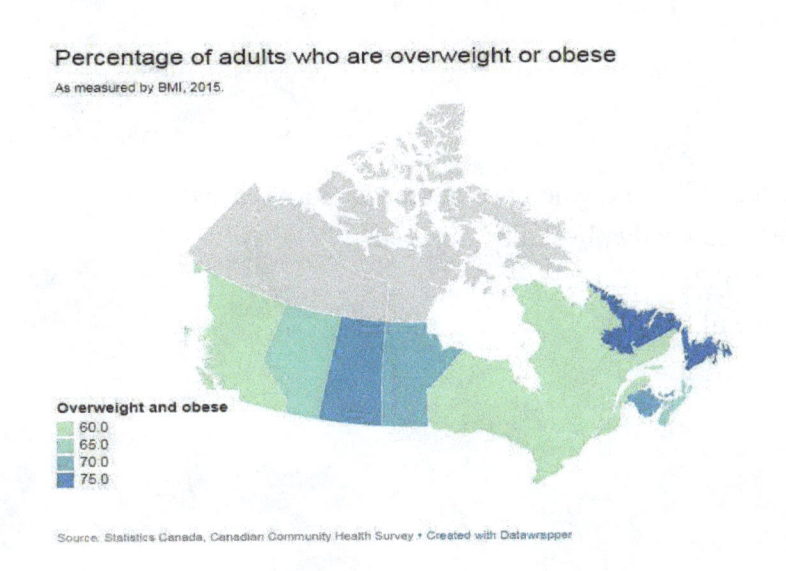

There are many risk factors for the development of obesity. Most often it is a combination of genetic factors (our genes), economic status, social environment, a lack of exercise, and diet that contribute to a person becoming excessively overweight or obese.

Health problems associated with obesity can be improved with even modest weight loss. Healthy dietary changes (no fad diets), more physical activity, social and behavior changes such as reducing chronic stress can help a person lose weight. Prescription medications and surgical procedures for weight loss are medical options for treating obesity.

Are You Over-Weight or Obese? - Guidelines for Body Weight Classifications in Adults

Body Mass Index (BMI) and Waist Circumference (WC) are recognized methods to help classify obesity as an indicator of health risk. It is important to note that these classifications are only guidelines. Weight classifications associated with BMI and WC should only be used as one component of a more comprehensive health assessment which would include an evaluation of your diet, the amount of physical activity you get, skinfold thickness measurements, and a review of your family history. Together, these assessments help to identify your health risk associated with obesity.

The BMI and WC classification systems are not intended for use with:
1. Those under 18 years of age
2. Pregnant and lactating women

1. Body Mass Index (BMI)
BMI is not a direct measure of body fat, but is moderately correlated with the skin fold thickness test which is a more direct measures of body fat. As well, research indicates that BMI appears to be as strongly correlated with the development of diabetes and heart disease in a person as are more direct measures of body fatness.

Limitations to BMI:
These body weight classification systems may over or underestimate health risks in specific groups such as:

1. Young adults (under 18 years) who have not reached full growth
2. Adults with a very lean body physique
3. Highly muscular athletes
4. Adults over the age of 65

BMI Calculation

1. Kilograms and Metres

BMI = Weight (kg)/Height (m)²

Example: Weight = 68 kg, Height = 165 cm (1.65 m)

Calculation: $68 \div (1.65)^2 = 24.98$

2. Pounds and Inches

BMI = weight (lb) / [height (in)]² x 703

Example: Weight = 150 lbs, Height = 5'5" (65")

Calculation: $[150 \div (65)^2] \times 703 = 24.96$

BMI Classification

BMI	Weight Status
Below 18.5	Underweight
18.5-24.9	Normal or Healthy Weight
25.0-29.9	Overweight
30.0 – 39.	Obese
> 40	Morbidly Obese

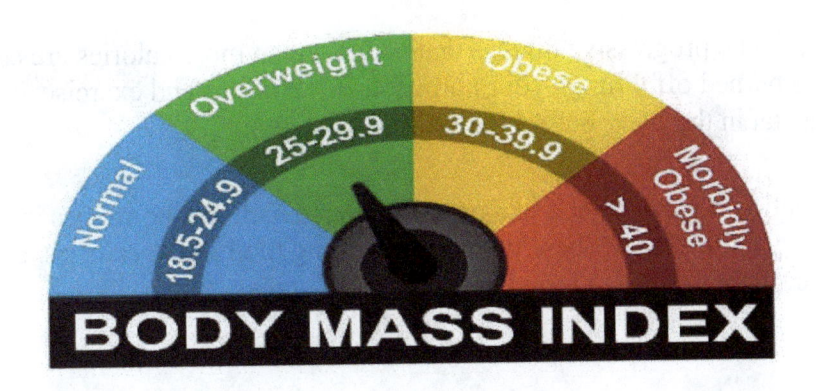

2. Waist Circumference (WC)

This measurement helps identify health risks associated with abdominal fat.

Measurement Technique:

Measure the circumference of the belly midway between the lowest rib and the top of the pelvis bone on the side. The tape measure should not compress any underlying soft tissues.

WC Cut Off Points	Risk of Developing Health Problems such as; coronary heart disease, high blood pressure and type 2 diabetes
Men - > 102 cm (40 inches)	Increased
Women - > 88 cm (35 inches)	Increased

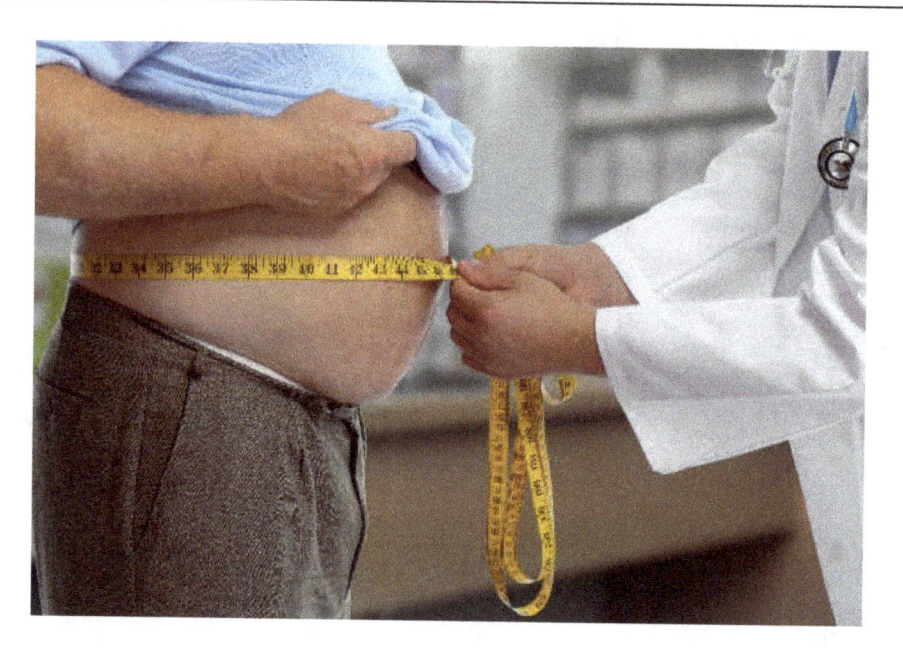

Causes of Obesity

Obesity is a chronic progressive disease that occurs when more calories are consumed from your diet than are burned off through your normal daily activities and exercise. The body stores excess calories as fat in the liver, but primarily in adipose tissue.

Although genetics, behavior (lack of exercise), metabolism and hormones influence body weight, the primary culprit is the obese person's diet being too high in calories, generally from nutritionally poor, highly processed food and sugary beverages.

Causes of Obesity

- Cultural
- Medications
- Genetics
- Environmental
- Endocrine Disorders
- Psychiatric Disorders
- Psychological

→ Obesity

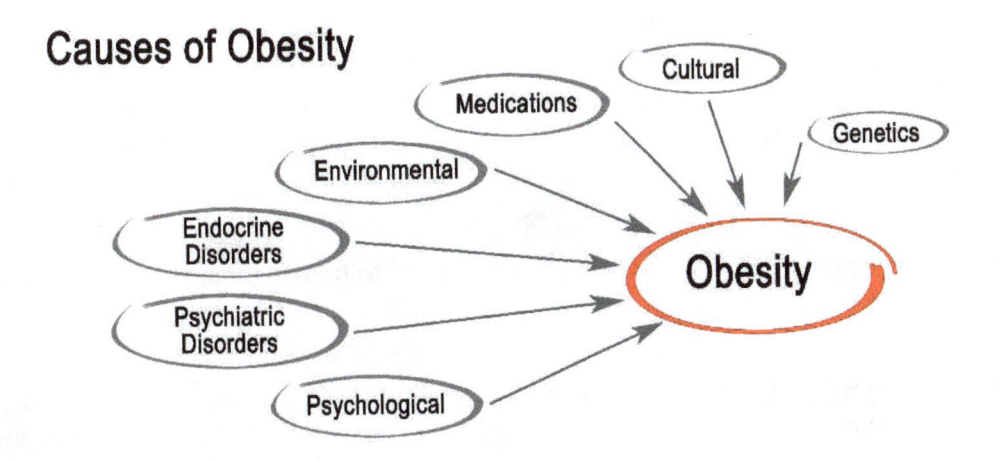

Risk Factors for Obesity

There are a number risk factors that combine and contribute to a person becoming obese:

1. Family (Genetics)

A person's genetic make-up affects:

- Metabolism – how efficient the body is at converting the food you eat into energy.
- How your appetite is regulated.
- How the calories are burned during exercise.
- Amount of fat stored in the liver and adipose tissue.
- How fat is distributed in the body.

The tendency for obesity to be prevalent in some families is not just the result of sharing common genes, but also because families share similar economic status, social environments, as well as eating, and activity habits.

2. Lifestyle Choices

- **Inactivity** – Watching television and looking at your computer, tablet, and smartphone are very common modern day sedentary activities that result a person burning fewer calories that they consume in a day.
- **Unhealthy diet** – A diet that is lacking in fruits and vegetables, full of fast food, and high in calories due to oversized portions contribute to weight gain.
- **Liquid calories** – Calories from alcohol and high-calorie beverages, such as sugared soft drinks often go unnoticed.

3. Certain Diseases and Medications
Medical causes that can contribute to obesity are:

a. Hypothyroidism – Results in a lower body metabolism due to inadequate production of thyroid hormone.

b. Steroid treatment – Corticosteroids are often used to treat asthma and arthritis and may increase the patient's appetite.

c. Cushing's Syndrome – Caused by high levels of cortisol. When cortisol levels increase, the body's cells can become resistant to insulin. This may lead to sustained high blood sugar levels and consequent weight gain.

d. Chronic stress and depression – Cortisol (stress hormone) stimulates the metabolism of fat and carbohydrates for glucose production for fast energy. Increase in blood glucose levels stimulates insulin release to control these elevated glucose levels. An increase in your metabolism can result in an increase in your appetite and can cause cravings for sweet, salty and high-fat foods.

e. Polycystic Ovary Syndrome – Thought to cause hormone-related issues, including consistently high levels of insulin, leading to weight gain.

f. Pre-existing medical conditions - Arthritis, heart disease, and diabetes, can also lead to decreased physical activity, resulting in weight gain.

g. Medications – Medications for diabetes, depression, beta-blockers as well as anti-seizure and antipsychotic medications, can lead to weight gain.

4. Social and Economic Issues
Having a safe place to walk and exercise, having access to healthier foods and being taught good cooking and eating habits are often unavailable for the socially and economically depressed. Your social group may also influence weight because if your friends or relatives are obese there is an increase likelihood you will become obese.

5. Age
Obesity is thought of as an adult problem but unfortunately obesity can occur at any age and is becoming more prevalent in children and adolescents as a result of poor diet and inactivity. In adults, hormonal changes and a sedentary lifestyle increase their risk of obesity. As well, the percentage of muscle mass a person has decreases at a rate of .5 to 1% after the age of twenty-five. Lower muscle mass contributes to a slower metabolism, resulting in reduced calorie needs. If dietary intake is not modified, you can expect to gain weight.

As we age, we must eat nutritiously and with appropriate portion sizes as well as become more physically active, or weight gain will result.

6. Pregnancy

Weight gain is required for a healthy pregnancy, but weight loss after pregnancy is often difficult. This post-partum weight gain often contributes to the development of obesity in women.

7. Quitting Smoking

A person often uses food to cope with smoking withdrawal. Quitting smoking is necessary for your health so consultation with your doctor or a dietitian can help prevent or minimise weight gain as you go through the process of withdrawing from smoking.

8. Lack of Sleep

A person's appetite can increase as the result of getting too little or getting an excessive amount of sleep. Weight gain occurs because you begin to crave easily accessible, highly processed foods that are high in calories and carbohydrates.

9. Previous Attempts To Lose Weight

Dieting to lose weight followed by rapid weight regain, the yo-yo affect of unsuccessful weight management, may contribute to further weight gain. "Yo-yo dieting" upsets your metabolism and results in a slower basal metabolic rate.

Having a few of these risk factors does not mean that you will develop obesity. Fortunately, you can counteract most risk factors through increasing your physical activity, practising good dietary habits and controlling chronic stress.

Complications of Obesity

People who suffer from obesity are at a higher rick of developing serious health problems, including:

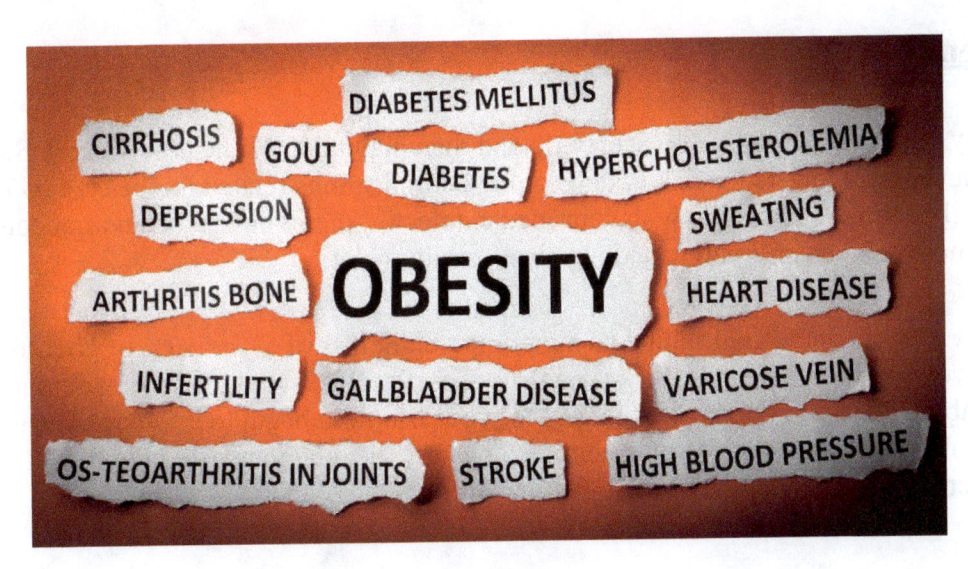

a. Type 2 diabetes – Obesity increases the risk of diabetes by increasing cellular resistance to insulin which affects how insulin is utilized to control blood sugar levels.

b. Heart disease and stroke – Obesity contributes to high cholesterol levels and high blood pressure which are major risk factors for developing heart disease and causing a stroke.

c. Osteoarthritis – Obesity promotes inflammation within the body and increases physical stress on weight-bearing joints, both of which increases the risk of developing osteoarthritis.

d. Certain cancers – Research suggests that obesity may increase your risk of cancer of the breast, liver, kidney, endometrium, uterus, cervix, ovary, oesophagus, gallbladder, pancreas, colon, rectum, and prostate.

e. Sleep apnea – Sleep apnea, a disorder in which breathing stops and starts during sleep, is more prevalent in people who are obese.

f. Digestive problems – There is an increase likelihood of developing heartburn, gallbladder disease, and liver problems if a person is obese.

g. Gynecological and sexual problems – In men obesity has been associated with erectile dysfunction and in women, irregular periods and infertility.

h. Discrimination – Significant inequities often exist for someone obese when they are trying to find employment and access healthcare and education.

i. Low self-esteem and depression – Developing low self-esteem and depression is common in an obese person because of having a poor body image and a diminished quality of life due to an inability to be physically active and carry out everyday activities comfortably.

Treatment

Obesity treatment is focused on achieving and then maintaining a healthy weight. Successful weight management lowers the risk of developing complications related to obesity and improves your overall health. Consultation with your medical doctor, dietitian, and behavioral counsellor can help improve a person's eating and physical activity habits.

Initially, the treatment goal should be a modest weight loss of 5% to 10% of your total weight. If you weigh 200 pounds (91 kg) and are obese by BMI standards, you would need to lose only about 10 to 20 pounds (4.5 to 9 kg) for your health to begin to improve. The more weight an obese person loses by implementing a healthy diet and increasing their level of physical activity, the greater the health benefits will be.

Behavioural changes are challenging and a successful treatment method for someone obese depend on their level of obesity, overall health, and motivation to participate in a weight reduction plan.

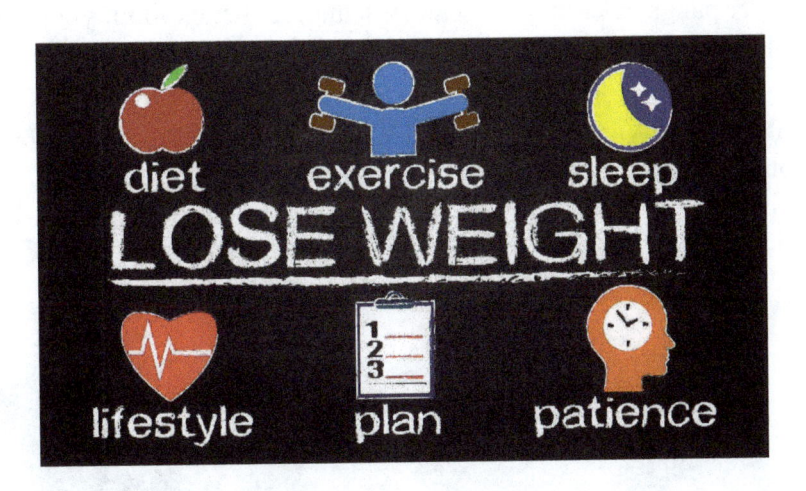

1. Dietary Changes

Reducing calories by reducing portion sizes and practising healthier eating habits by choosing higher quality whole foods (less processed food) are essential to overcoming obesity. When following a weight loss program, weight may fall off quickly initially, but ideally, the goal is to lose weight slow and steady over the long term.

Losing one pound a week is considered the safest and best way to keep weight off permanently.

It is important to avoid drastic and unsustainable fad diets. Empirical results show that these types of diet are unlikely to help you manage your weight long-term. To be successful, the goal should be to participate in a proven weight-loss program for at least six months and in their maintenance phase for at least a year.

There is no silver bullet or magic formula to achieve and maintain weight loss. The key is motivation, self-discipline and to chose a weight-loss programs that focuses on healthy foods and appropriate portion sizes.

Treating obesity through dietary changes include the following guidelines:

a. Cutting calories – One key to weight loss is reducing how many calories you consume. People need to review their typical eating and drinking habits to see how many calories they typically consume and where they need to cut back.

Controlling your portion size is very important. A dietitian can decide how many calories a person is limited to consume each day to lose weight. For women, the typical amount is around 1,500 calories, and for men 1,500 to 1,800 calories.

b. Feeling full on less – Some foods such as desserts, candies, fats, and processed foods contain a large number of calories for a small portion. In contrast, fruits and vegetables provide a larger portion size with fewer calories. By eating larger portions of foods with fewer calories, you can reduce hunger pangs, take in fewer calories and feel better about your meal, contributing to how satisfied you feel overall.

c. Drink lots of water – Water has no calories, but it can increase satiety (feeling full) and boost your metabolic rate. Timing when you drink water is significant too; drinking water half an hour before meals is the most effective practice. It will make you feel fuller so that you eat fewer calories.

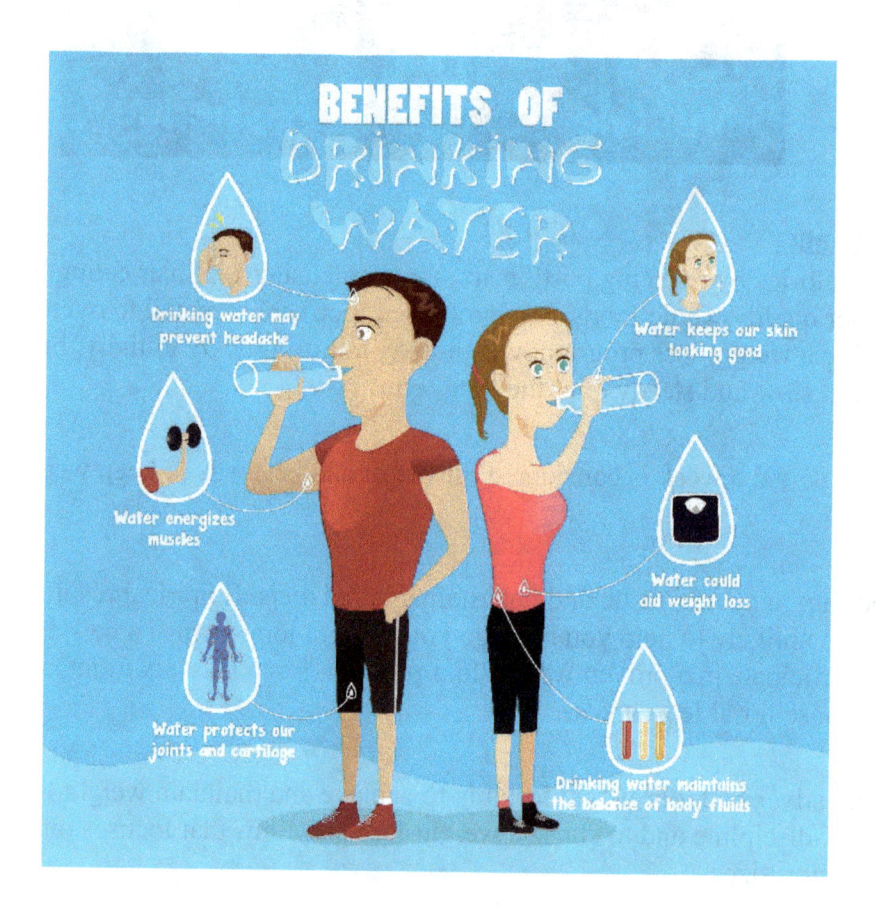

d. Making healthier choices – To make your overall diet healthier, eat more plant-based foods, such as fruits, vegetables, and whole-grain carbohydrates. Also, emphasise lean sources of protein such as beans, lentils, soy, and lean meats. Try to include fish twice a week. Limit salt and added sugar. Eat small amounts of fats, and make sure they come from heart-healthy sources, such as olive, canola, and nut oils. The Mediterranean diet (Chapter 5.2.10) meets most of these requirements.

e. Be careful of meal replacement strategies – These plans suggest that you eat only their "special foods," or replace one or two meals with their products such as low-calorie shakes or meal bars and eat healthy snacks and a healthy, balanced third meal that is low in fat and calories. This type of diet may help you lose weight in the short term. However, these diets likely won't teach you how to change your overall lifestyle and learn the long-term dietary changes needed for sustained weight loss and control.

Quick fixes/fad diets do not work long-term. To lose weight and keep it off, you have to adopt a healthy lifestyle which includes exercise and healthy eating habits that you can maintain over time.

Refer to Section 5: Defense – Protecting Your Health and Fitness, to learn more about developing healthy, sustainable nutritional habits.

2. Exercise and Activity

An essential part of a person's weight loss program should be increasing their level of physical activity and exercise. Research indicates that getting regular exercise; even simply walking helps a person lose and maintain their weight loss for more than a year.

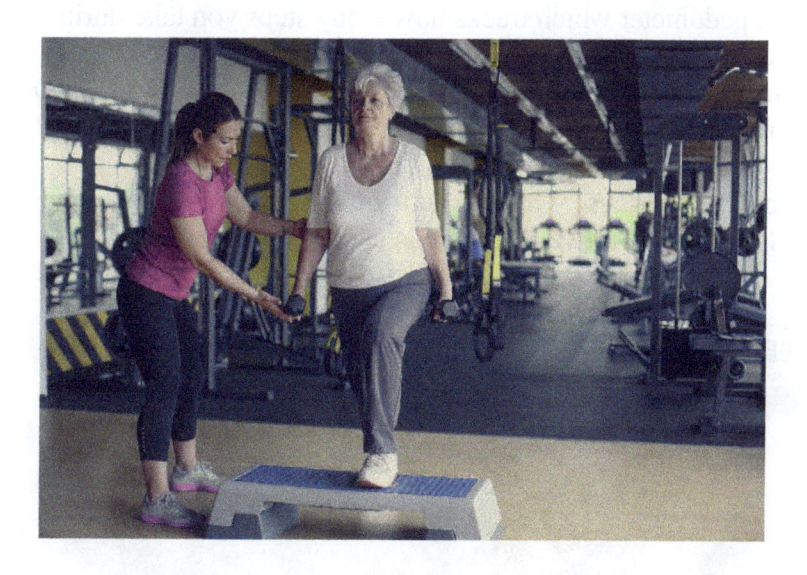

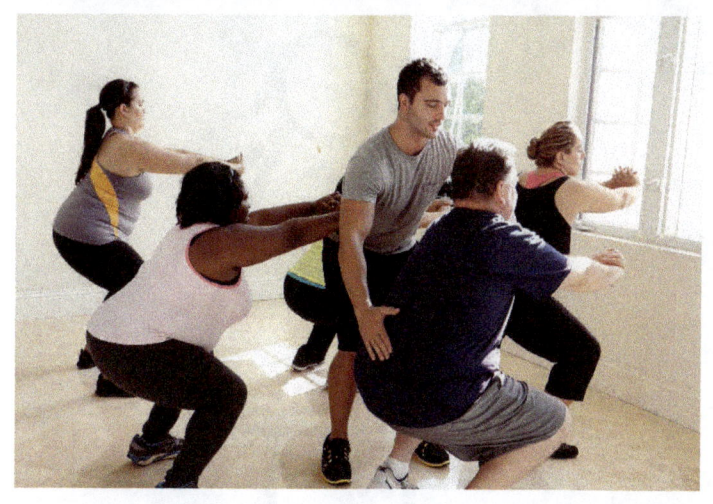

Keys to increasing activity level:

I. Exercise –From a cardiovascular fitness perspective, it is recommended that adults get at least 150 minutes a week (30 minutes five times per week) of moderately-intense physical activity. This level of exercise can help prevent further weight gain or maintain the loss of a modest amount of weight. At a certain point, a person may need to exercise longer each week to achieve greater weight loss. A person will need to gradually increase the amount of exercise they do, as their endurance and fitness level improve, to avoid weight loss plateauing.

II. Keep moving –The most efficient way to burn calories and shed excess weight is by exercising regularly but any physical activity burns calories and should be encouraged. Simple changes in your level of physical activity throughout the day can make a significant difference. Good examples of these are parking farther from store entrances, increasing the frequency of doing household chores, climbing stairs, and doing some gardening or other outdoor work.

The secret is to get up and move around regularly. Sitting for more than 30 minutes at a time is contraindicated. A pedometer which tracks how many steps you take during the day is an excellent way of recording effort and staying motivated. Reaching 10,000 steps every day is a common and recommended goal. Start slowly; don't feel pressured to do 10,000 steps initially. The number of steps can be gradually increased each week to achieve that goal.

Refer to Section 4: The Offense: Getting Active the Right Way for a comprehensive discussion on developing an effective, sustainable exercise program.

3. Behavior Changes

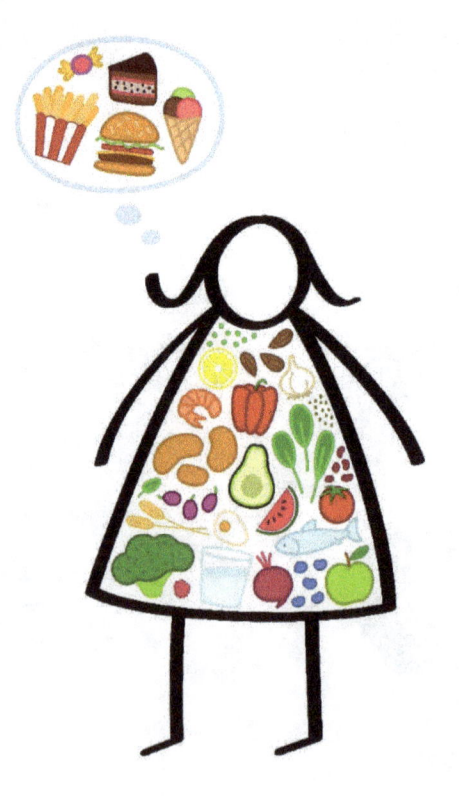

Making lifestyle changes to lose weight and to keep it off is difficult Developing a behavioural modification program with the help of a professional can be a great first step. To lose weight you must examining your current behavioral habits and determine what situations, factors and stressors are contributing to you being over weight.

Everyone experiences different obstacles in managing their managing weight, such as late-night eating to relax before bed to having a lack of time to exercise. The key is to identify your individual concerns and tailor behavior changes to address them.

Behavior modification/behavior therapy can include:

a. Individual Counselling –Poor behavioral issues related to over eating can be effectively addressed with professional counselling. It is vitally important to understand why you overeat, for example, feeling anxious. Professional therapy can help identify what these issues are and develop healthy ways to deal with them. Therapy can also teach you how to monitor your diet and physical activity levels, understand eating triggers, and cope with food cravings. When seeking professional counselling, considered it to be a long-term strategy and not a "one and done" thing. Change takes time.

b. Support groups – Group counselling is effective and often more cost effective if that is a concern. Support groups provide camaraderie and understanding and provides a safe environment where people can share their similar challenges with obesity.

4. Prescription Weight-Loss Medication

A healthy diet and regular exercise are necessary to effectively lose weight over a sustained period of time. However, in certain situations, weight-loss medication may be needed to augment behavioural changes related to diet and exercise. The primary purpose of weight-loss medications is to supress hunger signals that appear when trying to lose weight.

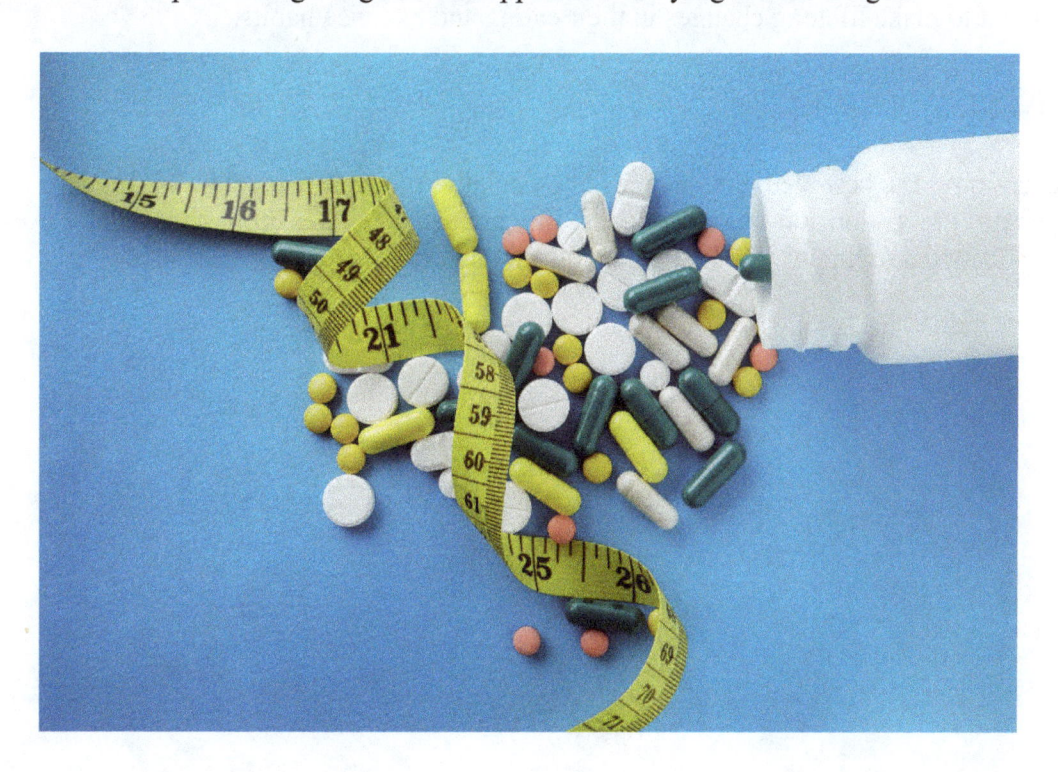

When taking a prescription weight-loss medication, close medical monitoring is necessary. Unfortunately, weight-loss medications have not been found to be 100% effective, and with long-term use, their effectiveness may become less.

A cautionary note, when a person is no longer taking weight-loss medication, they may regain the weight they had previously lost. This is why it is vitally important that proper dietary habits and physical activity/exercise have been ingrained into their daily routine.

5. Endoscopic Procedures for Weight Loss

Endoscopic procedures used for weight loss take many different forms. One procedure involves making the size of the stomach smaller so the amount of food that can be comfortably consumed is reduced. This can be done by stitching up a portion of the stomach or inserting a small water filled balloon into the stomach. Each of these procedures helps a person feel fuller faster.

Invasive endoscopic procedures are usually only considered when diet, exercise, and medication have not been successful.

6. Weight-Loss Surgery

Weight-loss surgery (bariatric surgery/gastric by-pass surgery) limits the amount of food a person can comfortably eat by decreasing the size of the stomach or decreases the absorption of food and calories by decreasing the size of the small intestine, or it does both. This type of procedure can pose serious risks and should be considered as a last resort to lose weight.

Weight-loss surgery is effective and can help a person lose as much as 35% or more of their excess body weight. However, there is no guarantee that you will keep the lost weight off long term. Even after successful weight-loss surgery, permanent weight loss depends on a person's commitment to make lifelong changes in their eating and exercise habits.

Prevention

Prevention is the best medicine and this is especially true with respect to weight management. Prevention and treatment for obesity are the same: a healthy diet, regular exercise, and a life- long commitment to watch what you eat and drink.

WEIGHT LOSS

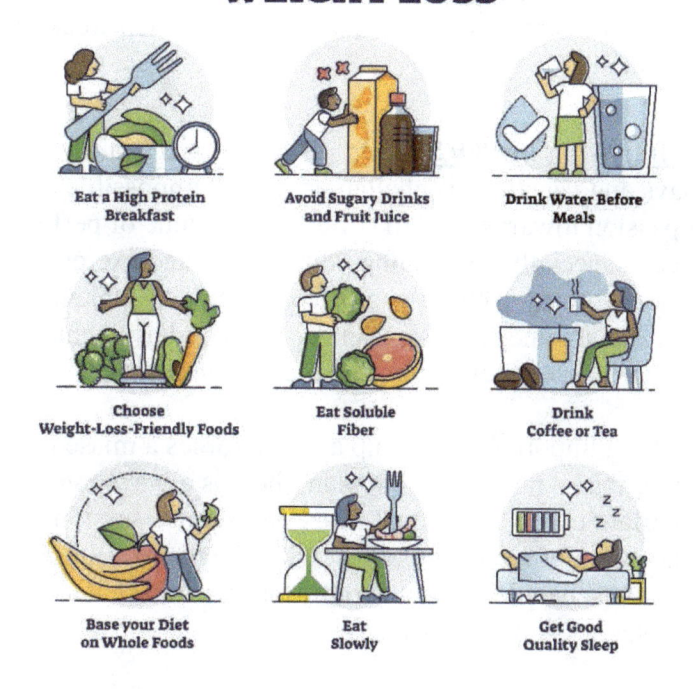

1. Exercise regularly – To prevent weight gain it is recommended that a person should try to get a minimum of 150 minutes and preferably closer to 300 minutes of light to moderate intense activity a week. Refer to Section 4: Offense – Getting Active the Right Way for a detailed discussion on developing an effective, sustainable exercise program.

2. Follow a healthy eating plan – For sustainable weight management, you should limit calorie consumption to between 1800 (adult female) and 2200 (adult male) calories per day. This is of course dependent on your activity level. Increase in activity allows you to consume more calories. Your diet should include large amounts of nutrient-dense foods, such as vegetables, fruits, and whole grains. As well, your diet should have only limited amounts of sweets, alcohol and saturated fats. It is recommended to eat three regular meals a day with limited snacking or five smaller meals through the day. Refer to Section 5: Defense – Protecting Your Health and Fitness for a detailed discussion on developing strong, sustainable dietary and nutritional habits.

3. Implement behavioral modification into your daily routine – Avoid food traps by identifying and avoiding situations that trigger out-of-control eating. Stress is a common food trigger that needs to be identified and managed effectively. Journaling is an effective way of tracking eating habits. Knowing when, what, and how much you eat, and how hungry you are when you eat is valuable information. Often unhealthy patterns emerge that can be modified. Developing strategies to handle situations that trigger unhealthy eating is a key element for effective weight management.

4. Monitor weight regularly – Research as shown that if you weigh yourself weekly you will be more successful with weight management. Monitoring weight regularly has two key purposes. First, it is a motivational tool that will reinforce to you that your dietary and exercise habits are working. Second, weighing yourself regularly will help detect small gains in weight before they become big gains. A person's weight is impacted by hydration status, hormone levels, exercise and time of day, so small fluctuations are normal. It is recommended that a person weigh themselves at the same time and on the same day each week to help minimise daily fluctuations.

5. Be consistent by following the 80/20 Rule – Sticking to a healthy-weight plan 24/7 and especially during holidays and vacations is challenging if not impossible. It is important and necessary to show compassion towards oneself. Life is not a game of perfect, so why should you even attempt to be perfect, especially concerning your dietary and exercise routine? Life is challenging enough without forcing 100% compliance. If you can achieve 80% compliance with respect to following your dietary and exercise routine, you will have achieved the consistency and sustainability necessary to see great results and meet your goals.

Don't worry if something important comes up and life forces a missed workout or consumption of something that is not part of the plan; there is always tomorrow's workout or the next meal. It is also important not to "make up" a missed exercise session or a "binged" night at your favourite restaurant. Attempting to "make-up" will take the joy out of life and mess up your planned dietary and exercise schedule. Forget about what you have eaten that you should not have or the missed exercises session and move on.

A good rule to follow is to "do your best and forget the rest." Losing weight by embracing behavioral lifestyle changes involving exercise and healthy eating should be considered a marathon, not a sprint. If you are compliant 80% of the time, you are doing great and should expect no more of yourself.

Conclusion

Obesity is fast becoming the number one health issue in our society. As we become more dependent on technology and are more sedentary, obesity is likely to become an increasingly important risk factor to our quality of life. But it does not have to be this way. Behavioral modification regarding the way we eat and the amount of exercise we get can minimise obesity. Small steps/missteps can add up to significant permanent changes. Weight loss and weight control are all about math: how many calories you consume minus how many you expend. If the answer to this equation is a negative number, you will lose weight and if it is a positive number, you will gain weight.
One pound is equal to 3500 calories. If you burn off only 115 calories a day more than you ingest, you will lose one pound a month or 12 pounds over a year. That may not sound like a lot, but that is better than gaining 12 pounds over the year. Plus, 115 calories a day is not a huge goal to aspire to. In real terms, that is the equivalent of 2 tablespoons of white sugar or a glass of wine a day.
Losing weight, especially when you are obese, is not easy. Effective weight management is necessary to improve the quality of your life and increase your life expectancy. The alternative should be unacceptable. If you need to, seek professional help from your medical doctor, a dietitian, and a behavioral specialist. Control your weight and your heart, joints, and mind will love you for it.

References

https://www.mayoclinic.org/diseases-conditions/obesity/
https://www.cdc.gov/obesity/adult/defining.html
https://www.webmd.com/diet/obesity/features/am-i-obese#1
https://www.healthline.com/health/obesity
https://obesitycanada.ca/
https://www.hsph.harvard.edu/obesity-prevention-source/obesity-causes/
https://www.canada.ca/en/health-canada/services/healthy-living/your-health/lifestyles/obesity.html

2.6. Dementia

Introduction

"Am I losing my mind?" is the quote most older adults, 50+ years, fear the most. Like cancer, most people have been affected in some way by the devastating consequences of a friend or loved one suffering from cognitive impairment or dementia as the result of aging. Dementia is a catch-all term used to describe the loss of memory, language, problem-solving, reasoning or other thinking abilities, as well as significant changes in mood and behavior that interfere with daily life. The most commonly known cause of dementia is Alzheimer's which accounts for 60 to 80% of dementia cases.

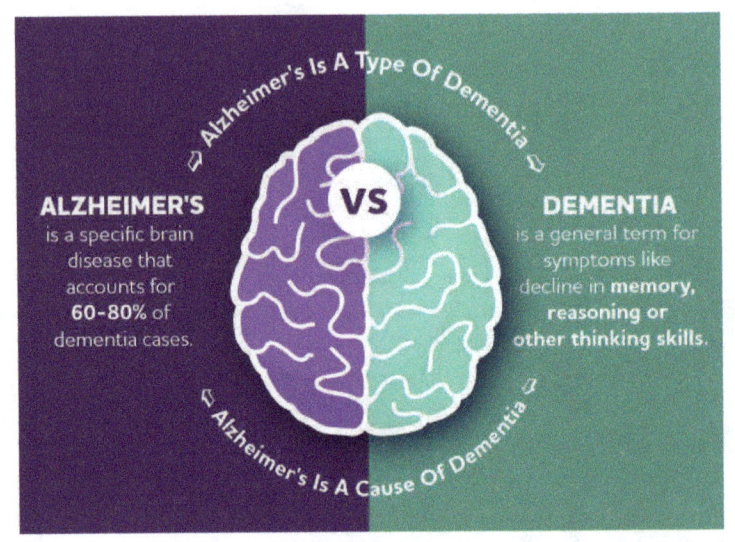

Image Source: alz.org

In 2016, over 500,000 Canadians were living with dementia. It is estimated that this number will almost double over the following ten years due to our growing aging population. Sixty five percent of people diagnosed with dementia over the age of 65 are women. Twenty percent of Canadians have experienced caring for someone suffering with dementia. The annual cost for Canadians to care for those living with dementia is greater than 12 billion dollars (Alzheimer's Society, Prevalence and Monetary Costs of Dementia in Canada, 2016).

It should be emphasised that dementia is an umbrella term and not a specific disease. It is a term that describes a group of symptoms affecting social abilities, memory and thinking. Several specific diseases may cause dementia.

DEMENTIA

Umbrella term for loss of memory and other thinking abilities severe enough to interfere with daily life.

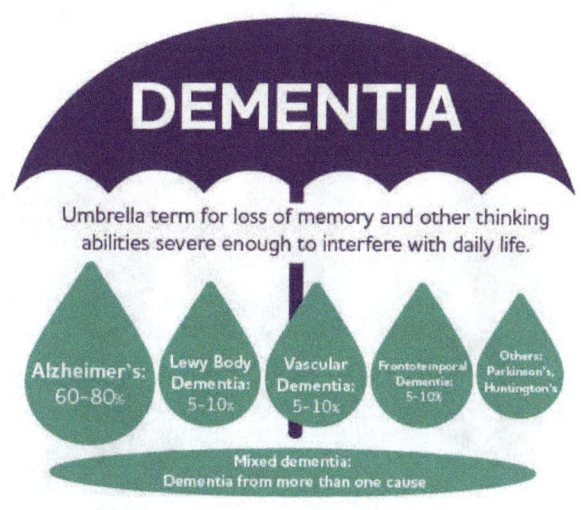

- Alzheimer's: 60-80%
- Lewy Body Dementia: 5-10%
- Vascular Dementia: 5-10%
- Frontotemporal Dementia: 5-10%
- Others: Parkinson's, Huntington's

Mixed dementia: Dementia from more than one cause

Image Source: alz.org

Difference between Normal Aging Memory Loss and Dementia

1. Age-Associated Memory Loss

Most people's memories will not decline rapidly or substantively as they age. However, after the age of 65, some form of memory loss will be experienced by almost 40% of the population. But this does not mean that they have dementia. For the majority of older adults, their memory loss is usually mild enough that it does not interrupt their ability to live their daily lives productively. The following list presents normal age-related memory changes:

- Daily life is not disrupted by memory loss.
- Details of a conversation or an event are sometimes difficult to remember.
- Occasionally forget events and things.
- Finding the right words to say becomes more difficult.
- Learning and remembering new things is not affected.
- Occasionally forgetting the name of an extended family member or acquaintance.
- The ability to complete tasks as they usually would get done is not affected.
- No medical condition is causing the occasional memory problems.

Age-associated memory impairment is characterised by self-perception of memory loss, and is considered a normal part of aging. Even though you may have difficulties remembering things on occasion, like where you left your keys, your computer password, or the name of a former classmate, this does not mean you have dementia. Unfortunately, with advancing age, you may not remember things as quickly as you used to, which can be an annoyance, but there is usually no cause for concern. Only 1% of those who suffer from age-related memory loss, will progress to dementia.

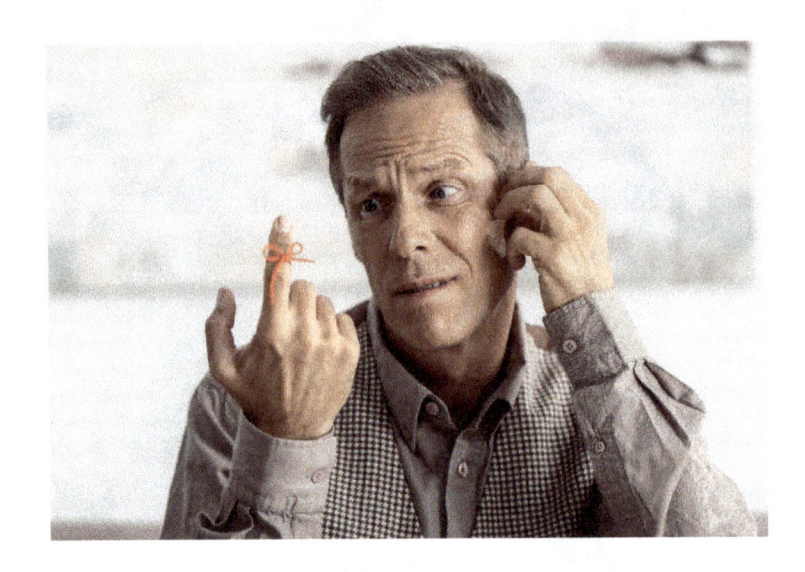

2. Mild Cognitive Impairment
This is a condition in between age-associated memory impairment and dementia. The symptoms, such as memory loss and disorientation, are mild. The symptoms are not severe enough to interfere with your normal routines and daily functions. A person with mild cognitive impairment has a 15% higher risk of developing dementia or Alzheimer's disease than if they just had age-associated memory impairment.

3. Dementia
The World Health Organization (WHO) estimates that, 5 to 8% of people over 60 years of age, will develop and live with dementia at some point as they continue to age. With dementia, your cognitive abilities seriously weaken and you are no longer able to take care of yourself.

Dementia is diagnosed when the memory loss so severe that:
- You are unable to remember details of recent conversations or events.
- You cannot recognise or remember the names of members of the family.
- You forget things more frequently.
- A person has frequent pauses when finding words (word loss).
- Memory loss is affecting a person's ability to stick to their regular routine and function normally
- You find it challenging to learn new things.
- you find it increasingly difficult to complete familiar tasks.
- Other people are starting to notice changes in a person's cognitive abilities

Dementia

Causes
Dementia is not a disease but a group of symptoms caused by other conditions. The symptoms of dementia are caused by loss or damage of nerve cells and their connections in specific areas of the brain. Dementia affects people differently and cause different symptoms such as memory loss, and difficulty with learning, decision-making, and language, depending on the damaged location in the brain.

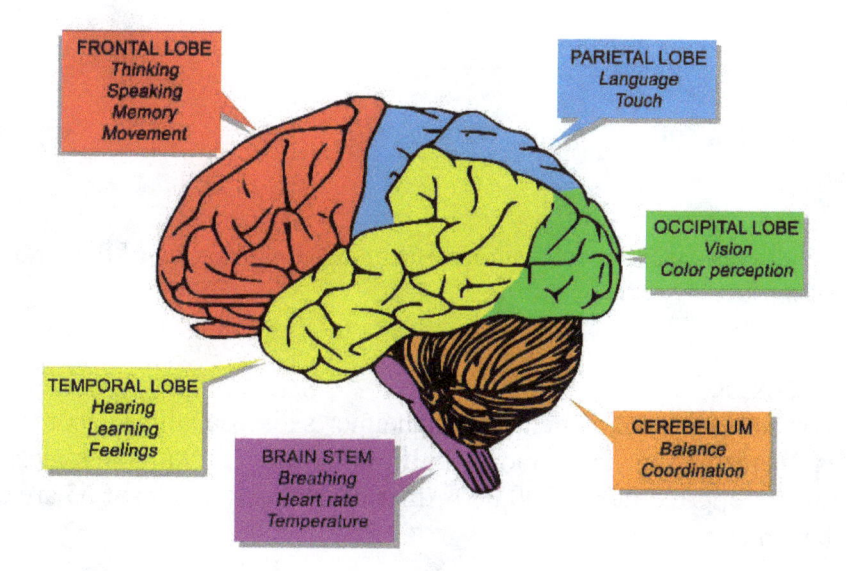

Symptoms

Most people associate dementia with memory loss, but many cognitive, psychological, and motor changes are also symptoms of dementia:

1. Cognitive changes
- Confusion and disorientation
- Difficulty with planning and organizing
- Memory loss, that is noticed by others
- Difficulty handling complex tasks
- Difficulty finding words and communicating effectively
- Difficulty with visual and spatial abilities. An increase feeling of disorientation such as getting lost while driving or loss in a grocery store.
- Difficulty with motor functions such as agility, balance and coordination.
- Difficulty reasoning or problem-solving

2. Psychological changes
- Hallucinations
- Paranoia
- Anxiety
- Agitation
- Personality changes
- Inappropriate behavior
- Depression

3. Motor Changes
- Reduced agility, balance, and coordination
- Reduced gait/walking speed

Progressive Dementias
1. Alzheimer's Disease
2. Vascular Dementia
3. Lewy Body Dementia
4. Frontotemporal Dementia
5. Mixed Dementia

Unfortunately, many causes of the symptoms under the umbrella of dementia are progressive and non-reversible:

1. Alzheimer's disease

The most common cause of dementia is Alzheimer's disease which accounts for 60-80% of dementia cases. Increasing age is the most significant risk factor with the majority of people 65 and older. However, approximately 200,000 Americans under the age of 65 are diagnosed with early-onset Alzheimer's.

Not all causes of Alzheimer's disease are known, but research has identified that a small percentage of Alzheimer's cases can be passed down from generation to generation due to the mutations of genes. It is suspected that many genes are probably involved in Alzheimer's disease but one important gene that has been identified to increases the risk of Alzheimer's is apolipoprotein E4 (APOE).

Pathology studies of patients with Alzheimer's disease have shown plaques and tangles in their brains. Healthy neurons and the fibers connecting them are thought to be damaged by these plaques and tangles.

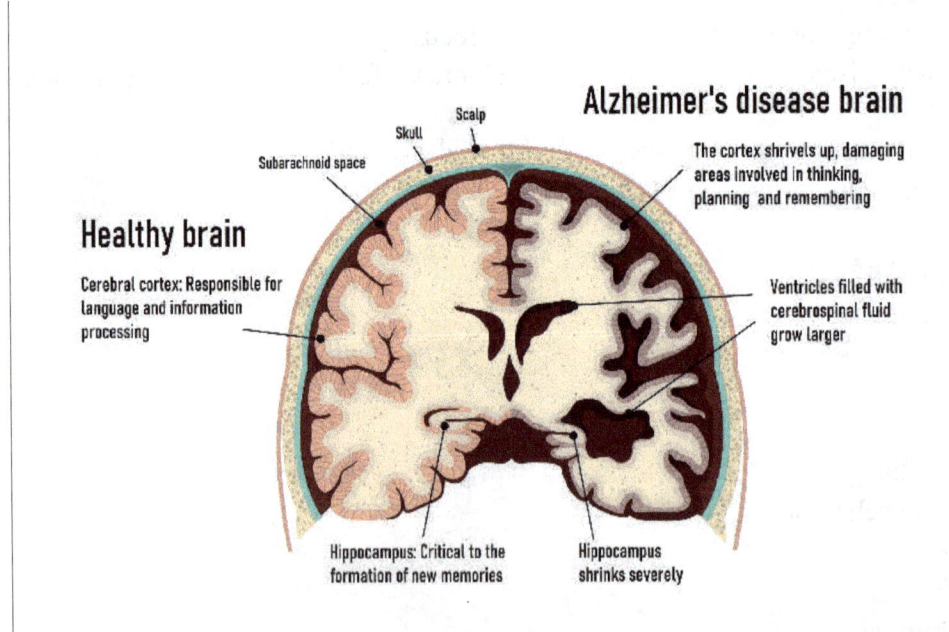

Alzheimer's disease is a progressive form of dementia affecting a person's cognitive, emotional, behavioral, and physical abilities at a severe level and is eventually fatal.

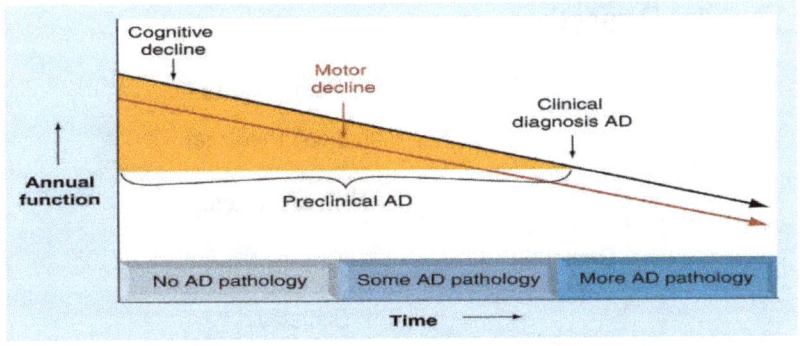

Image Source: https://www.ncbi.nlm.nih.gov/pmc/articles/PMC3121966/

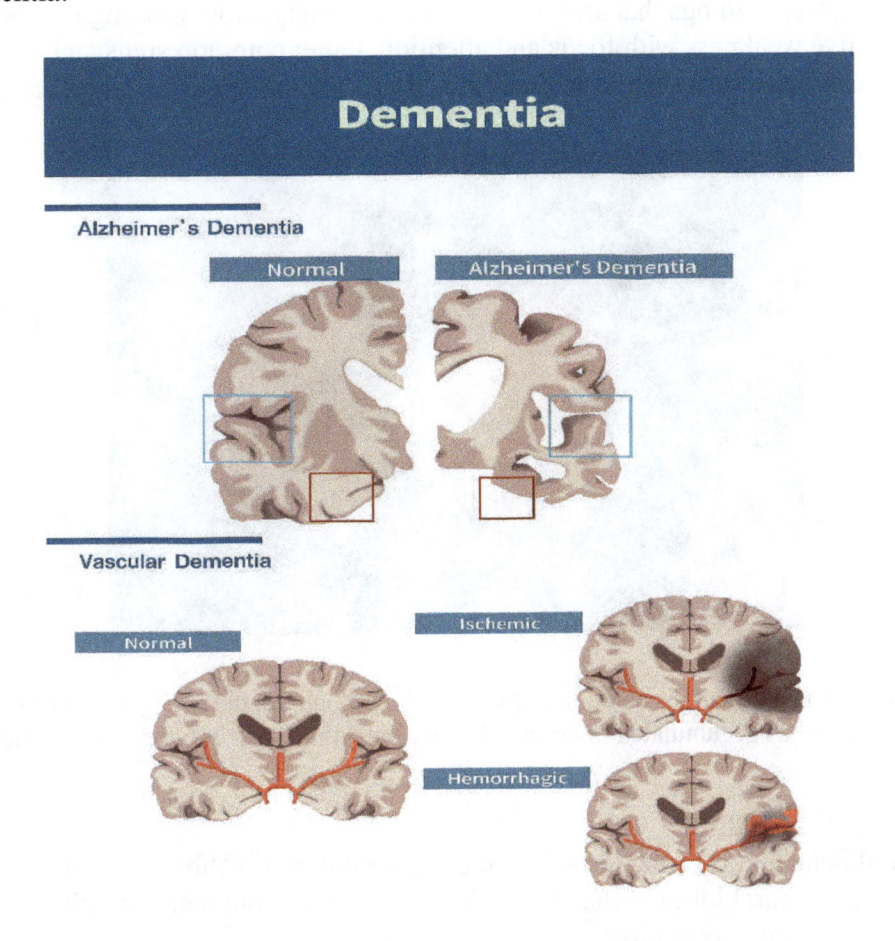

AD = Alzheimer's Disease

2. Vascular Dementia

This is the second most common type of dementia and is caused by damage to the blood vessels that supply blood to your brain. Difficulties with focus, organizing, problem-solving, and slowed thinking, are the most common symptoms. Memory loss is not as noticeable with this form of dementia.

Risk Factors for Vascular Dementia

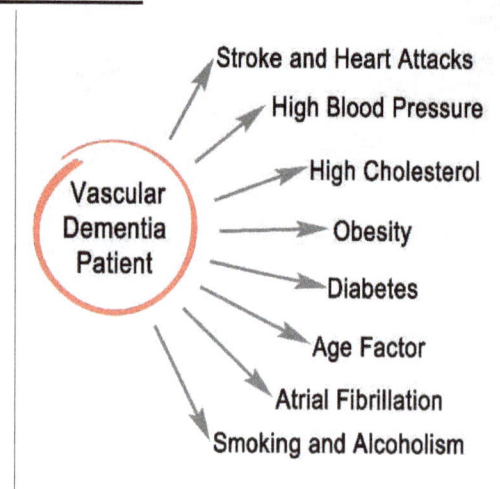

Vascular Dementia Patient:
- Stroke and Heart Attacks
- High Blood Pressure
- High Cholesterol
- Obesity
- Diabetes
- Age Factor
- Atrial Fibrillation
- Smoking and Alcoholism

3. Lewy Body Dementia

Lewy Body Dementia is a common progressive dementia. Lewy bodies are abnormal clumps of protein found in the neurons of people not only with Lewy body dementia but also with Alzheimer's disease, and Parkinson's disease. Distinguishing signs and symptoms of Lewy Body Dementia include seeing things that aren't there (visual hallucinations), acting out dreams in sleep, and cognitive weakness with focus and attention. Other common signs and symptoms are similar to Parkinson's disease such as uncoordinated or slow movement, tremors, and rigidity.

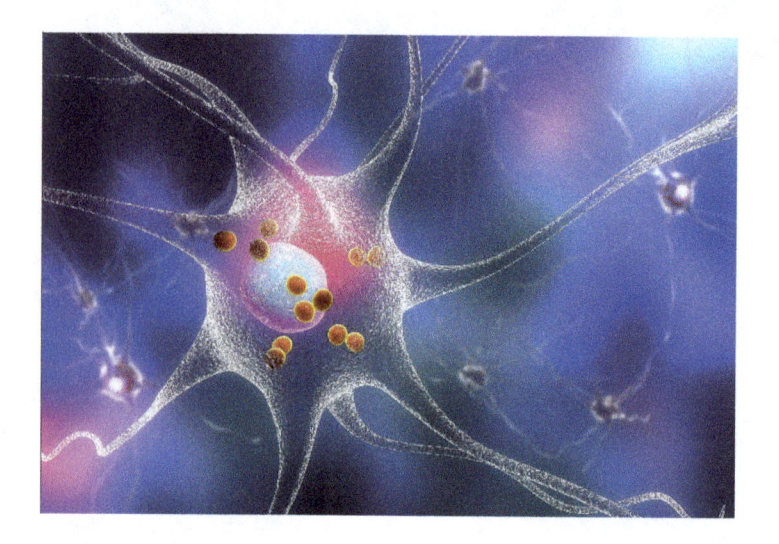

3D illustration showing neurons containing Lewy bodies which are the small red spheres. They are deposits of proteins accumulated in brain cells (neurons) that cause progressive degeneration.

4. Frontotemporal Dementia.

This form of dementia is characterised by the degeneration of neurons and their connections in the frontal and temporal lobes of the brain. These areas in the brain are associated with language, behaviour and personality.

MRI of Frontotemporal Dementia

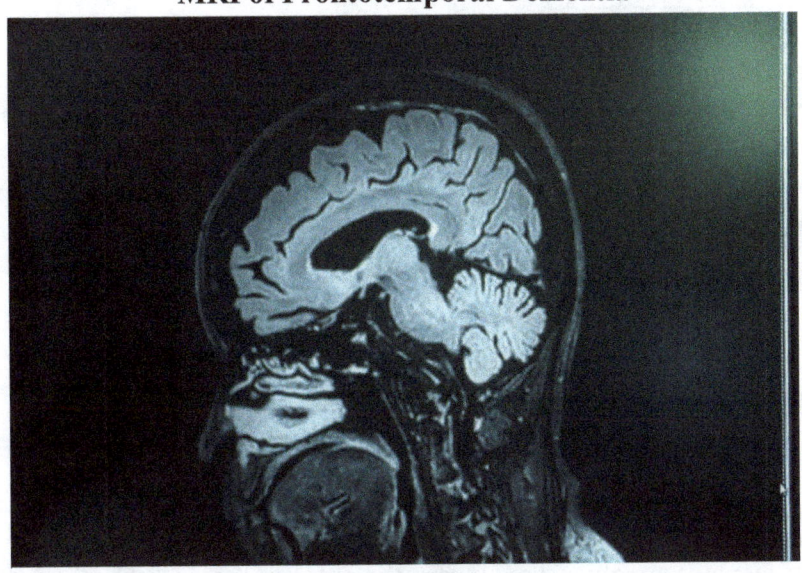

5. Mixed Dementia

Autopsy studies of dementia patients indicate that many had a combination of Alzheimer's disease, vascular dementia, and Lewy body dementia. Making an accurate diagnosis between Alzheimer's disease and vascular dementia is difficult because they are the most common and have similar symptoms.

Other Disorders Linked to Dementia

1. Huntington's Disease

Genetic mutation is the cause of this disease and results in nerve cells in the brain and spinal cord to deteriorate. Signs and symptoms usually appear around age 30 or 40 and include a severe decline in thinking (cognitive) skills.

2. Traumatic brain injury (TBI)/Chronic Traumatic Encephalopathy (CTE)

This cause of dementia is getting a lot of press coverage and caused by repetitive head trauma. Football players, hockey players, boxers and combat soldiers are vulnerable to this.

The symptoms of dementia might not appear until years after a player retires and include depression, memory loss, impaired speech, and explosiveness. This form of brain injury may also cause Parkinsonism. Unfortunately, Mohammad Ali is a good example of this.

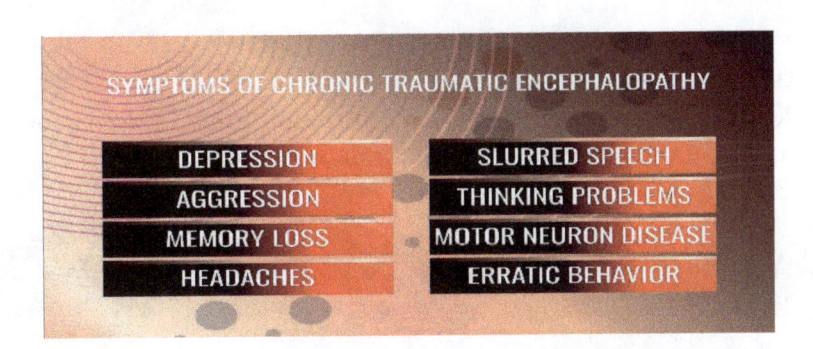

SYMPTOMS OF CHRONIC TRAUMATIC ENCEPHALOPATHY

DEPRESSION	SLURRED SPEECH
AGGRESSION	THINKING PROBLEMS
MEMORY LOSS	MOTOR NEURON DISEASE
HEADACHES	ERRATIC BEHAVIOR

3. Creutzfeldt-Jakob Disease (CJD)

Creutzfeldt-Jakob disease is rare and occurs in people without known risk factors. CJD can occur sporadically (no known reason), by inheritance (mutated genes) or by contamination (exposed to infected human tissue during a medical procedure, such as a cornea or skin transplant) Signs and symptoms usually appear after age 60.

4. Parkinson's disease

Parkinson's disease dementia occurs when patients suffering from Parkinson's develop dementia.

Dementia-Like Conditions that Can be Reversed

Some causes of dementia or dementia-like symptoms can be reversed with treatment:

1. Nutritional deficiencies

Nutritional deficiencies are always a concern for older adults. Dehydration, deficiencies in thiamin (vitamin B-1), which is common with alcoholism, and not enough vitamins B-6 and B-12 in your diet (vegetarians) can all cause dementia-like symptoms.

2. Medication side effects

This is very common in older adults who are often on many medications. The adverse reactions to a particular medication or due to several drugs adversely interacting can cause dementia-like symptoms.

3. Subdural Hematomas

Falls are common with older adults and if the head is injured it could result in bleeding between the surface of the brain and the covering over the brain and this can result in significant cognitive changes.

4. Poisoning

Exposure to heavy metals, such as lead (often used in paints years ago), poisons, such as pesticides, and recreational drug or heavy alcohol use, can lead to symptoms of dementia.

5. Infections and immune disorders

High fever can be a side effect of your body's attempt to fight off an infection and can result in dementia-like symptoms.

6. Metabolic problems and endocrine abnormalities

Dementia-like symptoms can result in people suffering from Thyroid problems, low blood sugar (hypoglycemia), too little or too much sodium or calcium.

Risk Factors for Dementia

Many factors can contribute to a person developing dementia. Risk factors, such as age and genetics, cannot be changed but others such as improving your diet and increasing the amount of exercise you get can be implemented to reduce your risk.

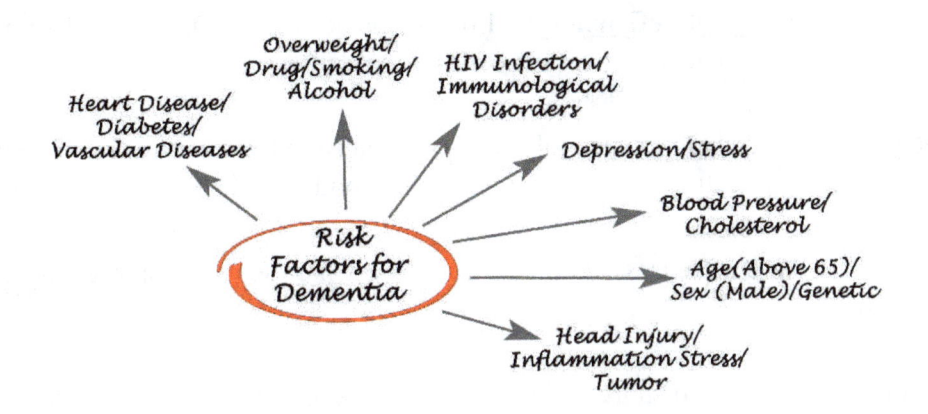

Risk Factors that you Can't Modify

1. Age – Even though dementia can occur in younger people, advancing age, especially after 65, is the number one risk factor for developing dementia

2. Genetics – Research indicates that a strong familial history for developing dementia increases a person's risk. Genetic testing can be used to determine if a person has specific genetic mutations that increase risk of developing dementia.

3. Down's Syndrome – By middle-age, people born with Down's Syndrome are more vulnerable to develop early-onset Alzheimer's disease.

Risk Factors You Can Modify

There are factors for Dementia that a person can control to help reduce the risk:

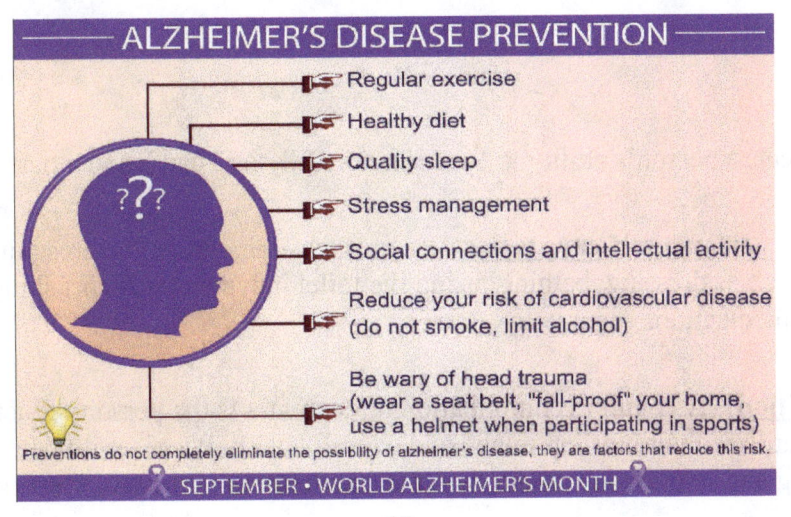

1. Diet and exercise – Research indicates that increasing your level of physical activity and exercise decreases the risk of dementia. No specific diet has been identified or established to reduce the risk of dementia. However, research indicates that people who follow a Mediterranean-style diet rich in vegetables, fruits, nuts, seeds and whole grains have a decreased incidence of dementia.

2. Vitamin and nutritional deficiencies – Low levels of vitamin D, vitamin B-6, vitamin B-12, and folate have been indicated to increase your risk of dementia.

3. Diabetes – Having diabetes, especially if poorly controlled, may increase a person's risk of dementia, since a complication of chronic diabetes is blood vessel and nerve disease.

4. Smoking – Smoking increases blood vessel disease which would increase a person's risk of developing dementia.

5. Sleep apnea – People who snore and have episodes where they frequently stop breathing while asleep (apnea) have been identified as having increase incidence of memory loss.

6. Chronic Sleep Deprivation – Researchers report that people in their 50s and 60s who regularly got less than 6 hours of sleep per night were 30% more vulnerable to develop dementia than those who averaged more than 7 hours of sleep per night.

7. Reduce Heavy alcohol use – Drinking alcohol excessively has been shown to increase the risk of dementia. As a general rule, less is better.

8. Depression – The onset of depression in an older adult might indicate the development of dementia. Avoiding social isolation, having hobbies and keeping mentally and physically active are important ways of minimizing the risk of developing late life depression.

9. Minimize Cardiovascular risk factors – Reducing high cholesterol, high blood pressure (hypertension), and saturated fats in your diet helps reduce the risk of atherosclerosis (hardening of the arteries) which has been associated with the development of dementia.

Complications

Dementia affects a person's ability to function normally and can leave a person vulnerable to:

1. Inability to perform self-care tasks – Progressive dementia interferes with your daily living activities such as dressing, bathing, using the toilet independently, brushing your hair and teeth, and taking medications accurately.

2. Poor nutrition – A common complication of dementia is the person reducing or stopping eating. This jeopardizes their nutrient intake and overall health. People with dementia often have difficulty chewing and swallowing which complicates their ability to eat independently.

3. Personal safety challenges – Walking, cooking and driving alone can present safety issues for people with dementia.

4. Pneumonia – Because dementia patients often have difficulty swallowing there is an increase risk of choking or aspirating food into the lungs which could result in pneumonia, coma and death.

Prevention

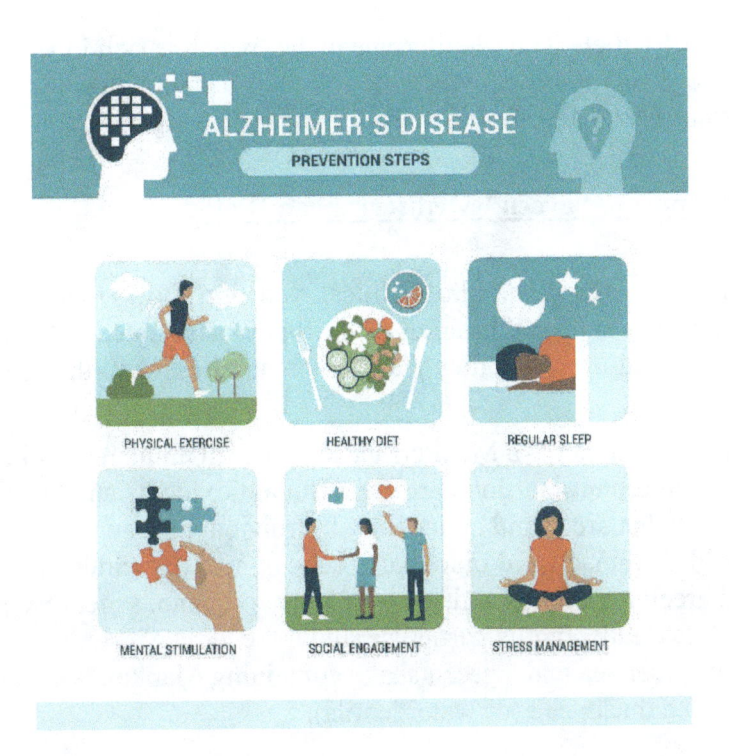

Actively preventing dementia is difficult since advancing age and genetics are unmodifiable risk factors. However, research indicates that living a healthy lifestyle does reduce the risk:

1. Quit smoking – Quitting smoking might reduce a person's risk of developing dementia by reducing blood vessel disease, but it will definitely improve your overall health.

2. Be physically and socially active – Research definitely supports increasing your physical activity levels and social interaction to help delay the onset of dementia. Achieving 150 minutes of exercise a week should be your minimum standard. Social isolation is a common problem with older adults and needs to be avoided.

3. Manage cardiovascular risk factors – Effectively treating diabetes, high cholesterol and blood pressure, and maintaining a healthy body weigh are good health recommendations and can be help reduce the risk of developing dementia by reducing blood vessel disease.

4. Keep your mind active –Reading, word games, puzzles are mentally stimulating activities, which research suggest may delay the onset of dementia and decrease its symptoms.

5. Get enough vitamins – Research studies have suggested that low levels of vitamin D may contribute to a person developing dementia but specifically Alzheimer's disease. Dietary vitamin D is plentiful in fish (salmon), red meats, eggs, milk. Vitamin D is activated with sun exposure and in the winter time or for those confined to living indoors, vitamin D supplementation is available. Nutritional supplementation of B-complex vitamins and vitamin C has also been suggested.

6. Maintain a healthy diet –The Mediterranean diet which is rich in vegetables, fruits, whole grains, and omega-3 fatty acids, which are found in fish and nuts, promotes health and potentially lowers your risk of developing dementia by improving cardiovascular health.

New Research in Support of "green" Mediterranean Diet:

Just published research in the Journal of Clinical Nutrition shows that following a Mediterranean diet slowed the loss of brain tissue (atrophy) associated with advancing age, but significantly, a "green" Mediterranean diet had even greater brain-health benefits.

A "green" Mediterranean diet is a Mediterranean diet with an increased intake of polyphenols which are micronutrients and are powerful antioxidants and have strong anti-inflammatory properties that are found abundantly in fruits (apples and berries – blue, black and strawberries), vegetables (spinach, red onion, artichokes), nuts (hazelnuts, pecans, almonds, walnuts), coffee and green teas, herbs and spices (cloves, oregano, sage, rosemary, thyme) and whole-grains such as flaxseeds. In this particular study, the "green" Mediterranean diet included 7 walnuts, 4-5 cups of green tea and a green shake containing Mankai, which is a branded strain of an aquatic plant called duckweed (or water lentils).

7. Get quality sleep – Practice good sleep hygiene (Chapter 5.3: Sleep: Don't Ignore It), and treat sleep apnea (periods where you stop breathing) with a CPAP machine.

Conclusion

Dementia is primarily an older adult issue and a general term that describes a group of symptoms affecting social abilities, memory and thinking. It is important to differentiate between age-associated memory loss and dementia. Not all memory loss means you are suffering from dementia. It depends on whether the severity of the symptoms affects your ability to carry out everyday activities.

Research indicates no real preventative measures for dementia, however, good health practices such as following the Mediterranean diet (diet high in vegetables, fruits, nuts and fish), getting regular exercise, and reducing chronic stress are best practices to follow.

Dementia, and the diseases associated with it, such as Alzheimer's Disease, can be devastating for the patient and their family. It is recommended that if someone has concerns, they should seek medical consultation for an accurate diagnosis so appropriate medical treatment and social support can be initiated and to rule out potential secondary medical causes that can be effectively treated.

References

https://alzheimer.ca/en/about-dementia/do-i-have-dementia/differences-between-normal-aging-dementia
https://www.mayoclinic.org/diseases-conditions/dementia
https://www.ncbi.nlm.nih.gov/pmc/articles/PMC3121966/
https://alzheimer.ca

2.7. Oral and Dental Health and Decay

Introduction

An essential part of our overall health and well-being is dental and oral health. Unfortunately, for many older adults, a lifetime of poor oral hygiene has led to tooth decay, cavities, gum disease, and a loss of teeth. Poor oral health has also been linked to cancer, diabetes, heart disease, dementia, and Alzheimer's disease.

It is a lifelong commitment to maintaining healthy teeth and gums, and regular dental checkups are essential. When oral/dental problems do arise, they must be addressed immediately to prevent complications, such as pain, headaches, and infections from occurring.

Nutrition is a significant part of an older adult's fitness and health plan. If you have difficulty with your teeth, gums, and bite (due to a loss of teeth), you will not be able to chew your food correctly. This can lead to malnutrition and other secondary health issues for older adults.

From a mental health perspective, an older adult's mouth and smile play a big part in how the feel about themselves. If you do not feel good about your teeth, you will smile and laugh less, which can reflect a depressed personality. As Dr. Dana Colson states in her book, Your Mouth: The Gateway to a Healthier You, "It is impossible to smile on the outside without feeling better on the inside."

For older adults, oral and dental health is an essential component of their physical and mental health.

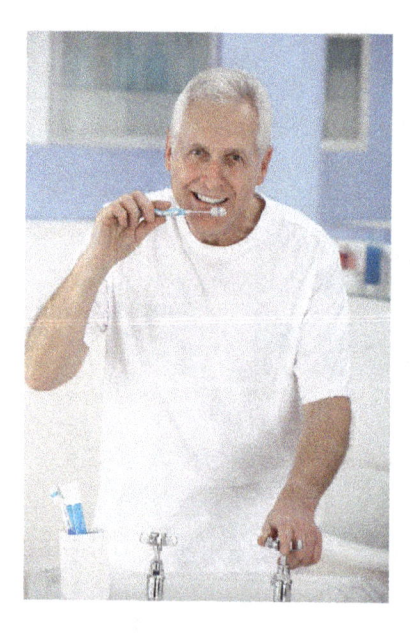

Connection Between Oral Health and a Person's Overall Health

Similar to other body areas, the mouth is full of primarily harmless bacteria, however under certain circumstances some of these bacteria can cause disease. Usually, the body's natural defenses/immune system and practising good oral health care, such as daily brushing and flossing, keep bacteria under control. Poor oral hygiene and acidic saliva from sugars and a lack of green vegetables in the diet, and dry mouth, are conditions which many older adults suffer from and which can allow these bacteria to reach high levels that lead to tooth decay, oral infections and gum disease.

Older adults often are prescribed medications, such as antihistamines, decongestants, diuretics, antidepressants, and pain killers that can leave the older adult to be vulnerable to reduced level of saliva. A good amount of salvia production is essential to wash away food and neutralize acids in the mouth that are produced by bacteria. Less salvia means less oral protection.

Oral health problems can become more severe by certain diseases such as diabetes, cancers, hepatitis, and malnutrition that lower the body's resistance to infection by weakening the immune system.

Health Conditions that can Result from Poor Oral Health

Poor oral health can contribute to the following diseases common among older adults:

1. Endocarditis – This infectious condition occurs when bacteria from the mouth, or other parts of the body, spread through the bloodstream and attach to the inner lining of the heart chambers or the heart valves (endocardium).

2. Cardiovascular Disease – Some research suggests that oral bacteria can cause inflammation and infections that may contribute to clogged arteries, heart disease, and stroke.

3. Pneumonia – Pneumonia and other respiratory diseases may result when certain bacteria in the mouth are pulled into the lungs.

Medical Conditions/Diseases That Influence Oral Health

1. Diabetes, cancers, hepatitis, malnutrition – These conditions affect and suppress the immune system and as a result the body's resistance to infection is lowered. Patients with these conditions have a higher incidence and severity of gum disease such as gingivitis and peritonitis.

2. Osteoporosis – Osteoporosis causes de-calcification and weakening of the periodontal bone resulting in tooth loss.

3. Alzheimer's disease – People with mental health condition often have poor oral hygiene that contributes to malnutrition which in turn results in worsening oral health.

Oral Health Hygiene

Good oral hygiene needs to be practiced daily to protect your oral health.

1. Brush teeth at least twice a day with a soft-bristled brush using fluoride toothpaste or electric toothbrush

Using a manual toothbrush to brush your teeth is standard practice, however, an electric tooth brush can be an effective alternative. An electric tooth brush does not require toothpaste and for older adults, who may suffer from arthritis of the hands, it can make brushing your teeth much easier.

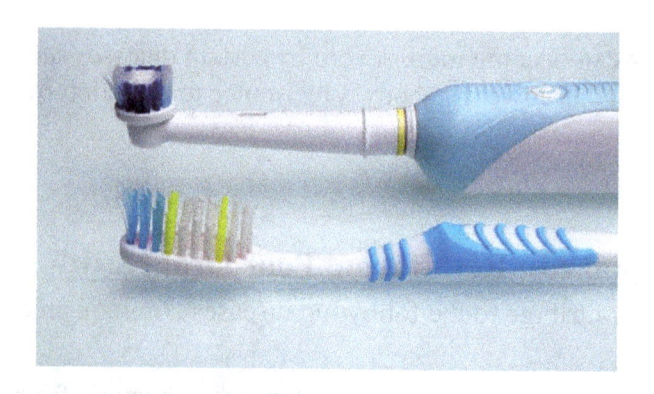

To operate it effectively, hold the electric toothbrush in one position and let the moving bristles do the work. There are two major models of electric tooth brushes.

1. <u>Rotating oscillating head</u> - one where the brush head rotates in both directions

2. <u>Sonic</u> – these have very fast vibrating bristles (bristles vibrate at a frequency over 50,000 times per minute and make a humming sound).

Most dentist feel that for superior cleaning and plaque removal, electric tooth brushes are preferred over manual tooth brushes.

2. Floss daily

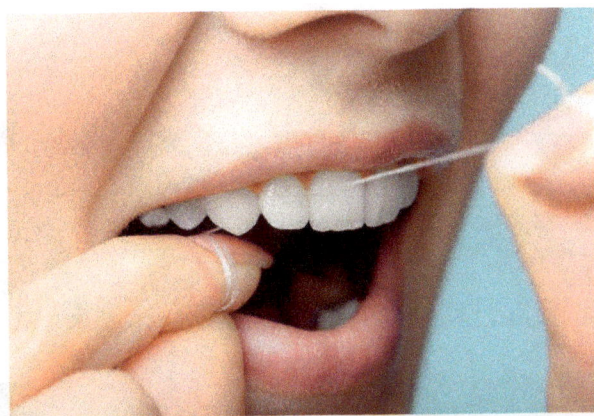

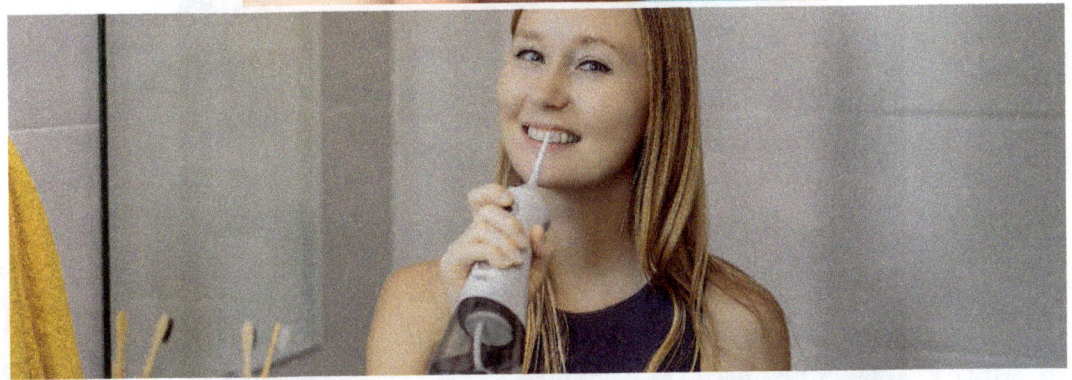

    To cleaning the tight spaces between the teeth standard dental floss is recommended. To use dental floss properly, you scrape up and down the sides of each tooth. A common mistake is people move the floss in and out or back and forth rather than up and down.

    A Waterpik®, is a device that shoots a stream of water at the teeth. This devise is effective at removing food particles from teeth as well as reduce bleeding from the gums and potential gum disease. An advantage of using a Waterpik® is that it can reduce bacteria even below the gumline but it should not be a substitute for brushing and flossing because it doesn't remove visible film and plaque on teeth.

    If you find that plain dental floss gets stuck in between your teeth, use waxed covered floss which allows the floss to move more easily or a floss wand, picks or picks with brushes.

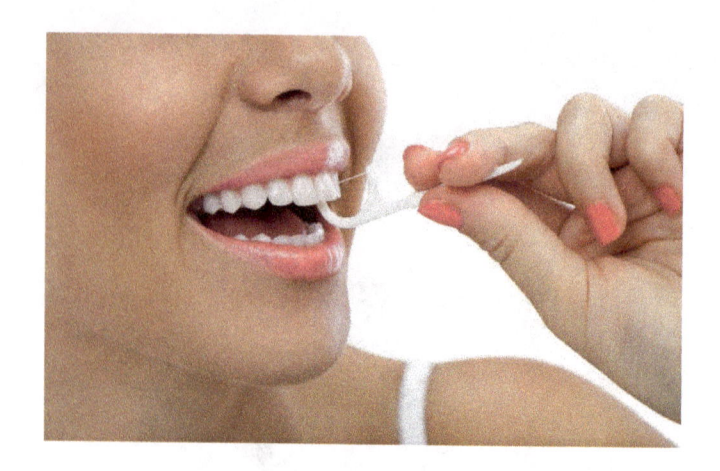

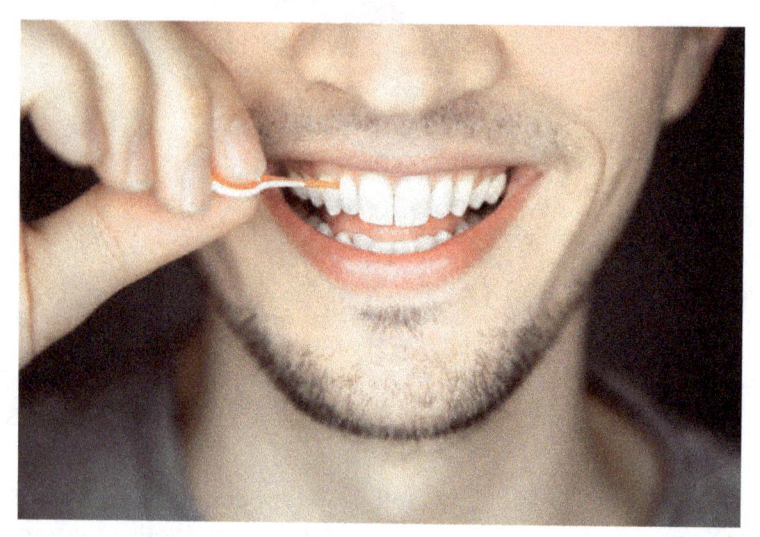

3. Use mouthwash to remove food particles left after brushing and flossing

Using mouthwash should not be considered a substitute for brushing and flossing. Mouthwashes may reduce the risk of cavities, gum disease, bad breath, or pain from oral sores.

There is a debate about the use of mouthwashes. Generally speaking, mouthwash is good, but not just any mouthwash. It is best to choose an alcohol-free mouthwash. Alcohol eliminates bad (and good) bacteria, but it dries out a person's mouth in the process. That dryness can irritate the oral tissues and exacerbate the very problems the person is trying to treat. Be aware that mouthwashes with chlorhexidine, cetyl pyridinium chloride, and zinc are likely to stain teeth. It has also been reported that chlorhexidine has caused anaphylactic (allergic) reactions. It is best to shop for mouthwashes that are PH balanced vs. the highly acidic alcohol-based mouthwashes.

4. Eat a healthy diet and limit food with added sugars

Sugar, natural (found in food) or artificial, is terrible for a person's health in many ways including facilitating tooth decay. Once sugar enters the mouth it combines with saliva and bacteria to develop plaque on teeth. This plaque produces acid that dissolves tooth enamel and ultimately leading to cavities.

5. Replace a splayed or worn toothbrush or at least every three months.

Brushing is only as effective as the quality of the toothbrush (manual or electric). A good toothbrush is a good investment.

6. Brush well

Brushing, to be effective, should be for two minutes and requires a concentrated/focused effort.

7. Schedule regular dental checkups and cleanings

Prevention is the best medicine to promote good oral and dental health. It is recommended to have a checkup, oral cancer screening, and cleaning every six months unless the dentist or hygienist recommends otherwise.

8. Avoid tobacco use

Research indicates that smokers are more likely to develop gum/periodontal disease, which can lead to a loss of teeth. Any type of tobacco product can irritate the gum tissue, and this makes it easier for bacteria to develop decay.
Smoking also discolours the teeth, causes dry mouth, and leaves the smoker more vulnerable to oral cancers.

Common Dental and Oral Health Conditions

1. Tooth Decay

Tooth decay/cavities are permanently damaged openings or holes on the hard surface of the teeth. It results from a combination of factors; not cleaning the teeth well, frequent snacking with sugary foods, sipping sugary drink and bacteria in the mouth.

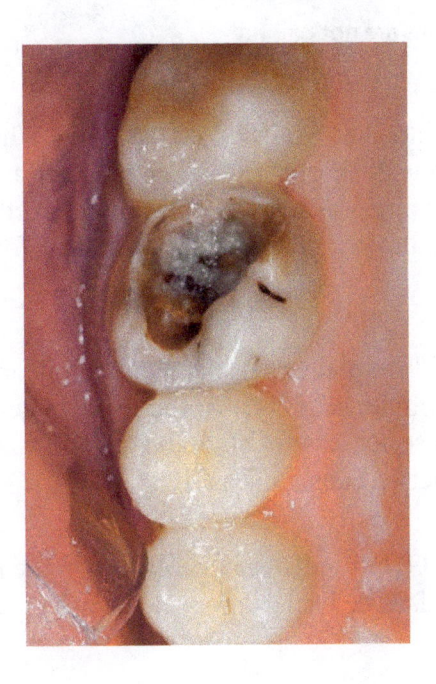

Tooth decay is a common health problem for the older adult. If cavities are not treated early, the decay progresses and affects deeper layers of the teeth. This can result in severe toothache, infection, abscess, and tooth loss.

Symptoms of Tooth Decay

The size and location of the tooth decay determines the signs and symptoms that a person will experience. When a cavity is small, it may not result in any symptoms, however as the decay progresses, it may produce the following signs and symptoms:

- Tooth sensitivity such as mild to sharp pain when eating or drinking something sweet, hot or cold
- Toothache
- Pain when biting down
- Pits in the teeth or visible holes
- Brown, black staining on the surface of a tooth

Causes of tooth Decay

Tooth decay is a process and progresses slowly:

The Stages of Tooth Decay

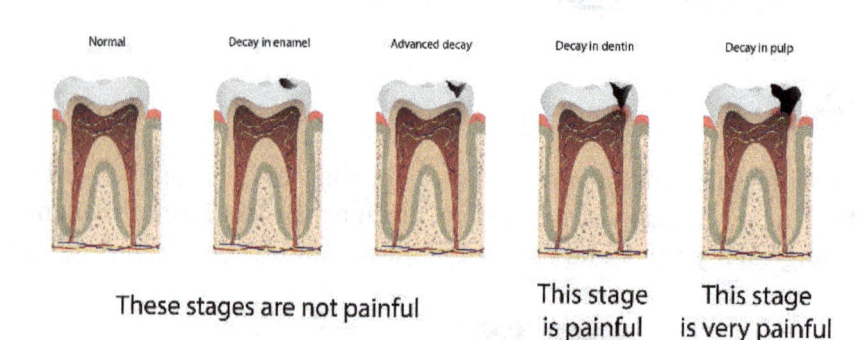

| Normal | Decay in enamel | Advanced decay | Decay in dentin | Decay in pulp |

These stages are not painful | This stage is painful | This stage is very painful

1. Plaque forms – Dental plaque naturally coats the teeth. When you eat starchy or sugary foods and do not clean the teeth well shortly after eating, bacteria begins to feed on them and acid is formed. If plaque is not brushed away and stays on the teeth, it will harden above and below the gum line into tartar (calculus). Tartar creates a shield for bacteria and makes removing plaque more difficult.

2. Plaque attacks – The acids in plaque attacks the minerals in the hard outer enamel of the tooth. Bacteria and acid can reach the next layer of the teeth, called dentin, once the other tooth enamel is worn away. Dentin is softer less resistant to acid and has tiny tubes that directly communicate with the tooth's nerve, causing sensitivity.

3. Destruction continues – Over time, decay continues to the inner tooth material (pulp) that contains nerves and blood vessels. The bacteria causes the pulp to become swollen and irritated.

Because there is no room for expansion inside a tooth, irritation of the nerve occurs producing pain.

Risk factors for Tooth Decay

Everyone is at risk of getting cavities based on the following risk factors:

1. Tooth location –The molars and premolars, teeth at the back of the mouth, are the most vulnerable to decay. The structure of these teeth with grooves, pits, and crannies leaves these teeth vulnerable. As well, compared to the easy to reach front teeth, they are harder to keep clean.

2. Certain foods and drinks – Sugary foods such as milk, pop, pastries, cereals, energy bars and drinks, tend to cling to the teeth for a long time. As a result, they are more likely to cause decay than foods that are easily washed away by saliva.

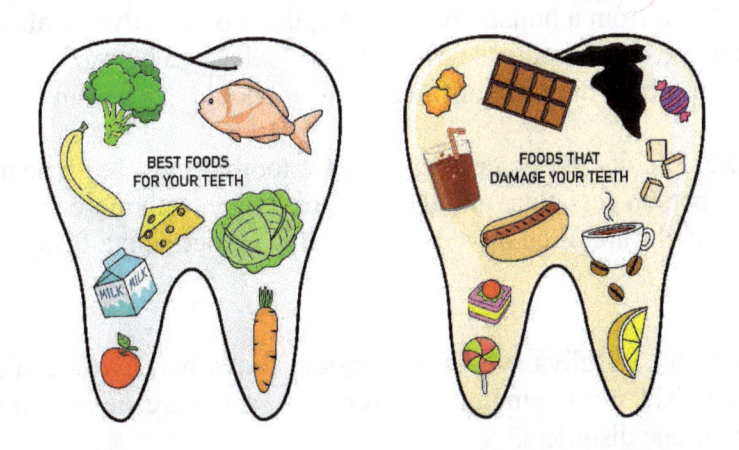

3. Frequent snacking or sipping - Mouth bacteria needs fuel to produce acids that attack the teeth and wear them down. Snacking, sipping pop, lemon water or other acidic drinks continually throughout the day creates a prefect environment for the bacteria to produce an acid bath over the teeth.

4. Inadequate brushing – The sooner a person cleans their teeth after a meal, the better to prevent plaque development. Studies have shown that as quickly as ten minutes after eating, the destructive process of tooth decay begins.

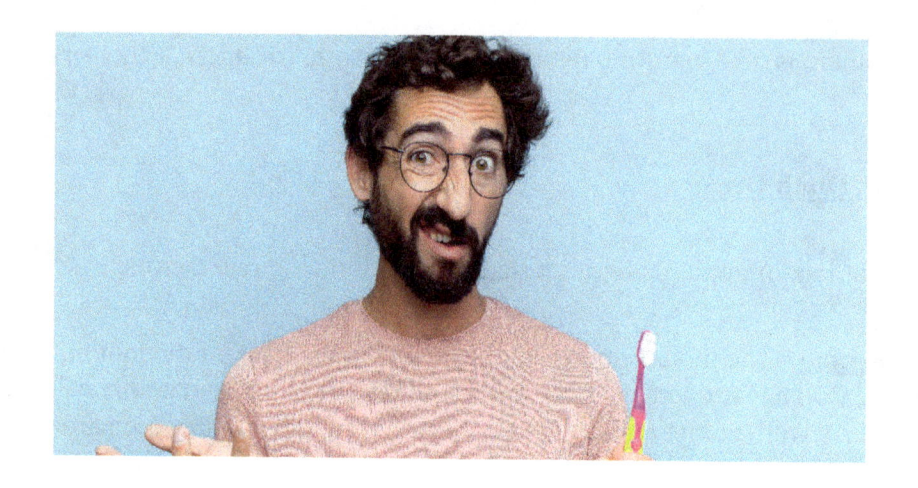

5. Not getting enough fluoride – Fluoride is a mineral that helps prevent cavities and can reverse the early stage of tooth decay. Fluoride is usually found in toothpaste and mouth rinses and is added to many public water supplies.

It should be noted that from a holistic perspective, there is controversy about the use of fluoride and that there are other products besides fluoride that can be used for cavity prevention. If a person has concerns about their use of fluoride, they should discuss this with their dentist.

6. Older age –Older adults are at very high risk for tooth decay. Teeth begin to wear down, and gums recede as a person gets older and these factors leave teeth more vulnerable to root decay. As well, older adults are often on medications that reduce saliva flow, which increases the risk of tooth decay.

7. Dry mouth – A lack of saliva, which is necessary to wash away food and plaque from teeth, causes dry mouth The most common causes of dry mouth are snoring, medication, mouth breathing, and autoimmune disorders.

8. Worn fillings or dental devices –Dental fillings weaken and break down over the years and these worn fillings allows plaque to build up more easily. Dental devices, such as dental bridges, can stop fitting well because of changes in the guns and jaw bones, and this allows decay to begin underneath them.

9. Heartburn – Wearing away the enamel of the teeth resulting in significant tooth damage can occur from heartburn (gastroesophageal reflux disease (GERD)) which causes stomach acid to flow into the mouth (reflux). Enamel erosion exposes more of the dentin to attack by bacteria, creating tooth decay.

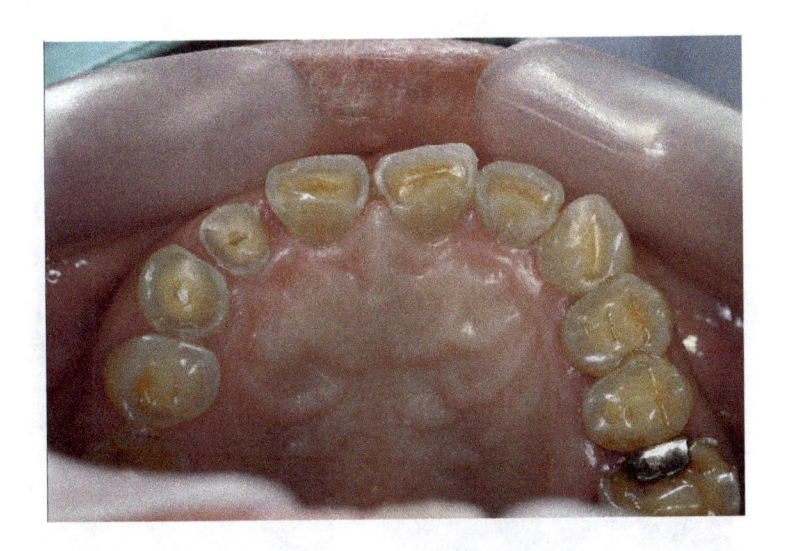

10. Eating disorders – Eating disorders such as anorexia and bulimia, interfere with saliva production. As well, repeated vomiting (purging) from these conditions can lead to significant tooth erosion and cavities because of the dissolving of enamel from stomach acid washing over the teeth.

Complications of Tooth Decay

Early cavity complications may include:

- Chewing problems
- Pain
- Swelling or pus around a tooth
- Tooth abscess
- Damaged or broken teeth
- Positioning shifts of teeth after tooth loss

Over time severe decay and large cavities may result and cause the following longer-term complications that affect your quality of life:

- Pain and difficult eating or chewing resulting in weight loss or nutrition problems.
- The quality of you daily living compromised because of chronic tooth pain.
- Endocarditis and pneumonia can result from a tooth abscess which is a pocket of pus caused by bacterial infection.
- A person's appearance, confidence and self-esteem may be affected by tooth loss.

Prevention of Tooth Decay

Older adults can minimize the occurrence and severity of tooth decay by practising good oral hygiene.

a. Use a fluoride toothpaste when you brush after eating, snacking or drinking –At least twice a day and, ideally after every meal or snack, brush your teeth using fluoride-containing toothpaste. Floss regularly to clean between your teeth. If you are used to drinking lemon water, it is best practice to brush your teeth before drinking it.

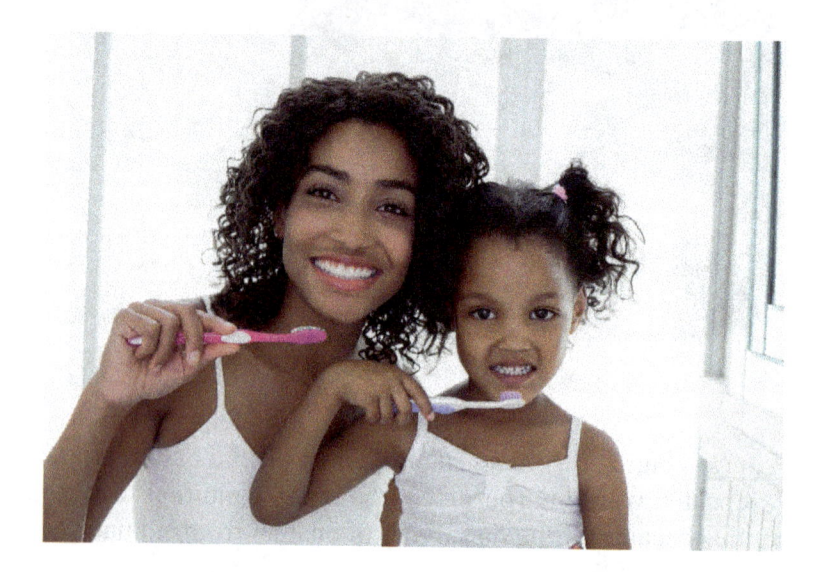

b. Rinse the mouth – Mouth rinse with fluoride is another layer of protection that helps minimize the risk of developing cavities.

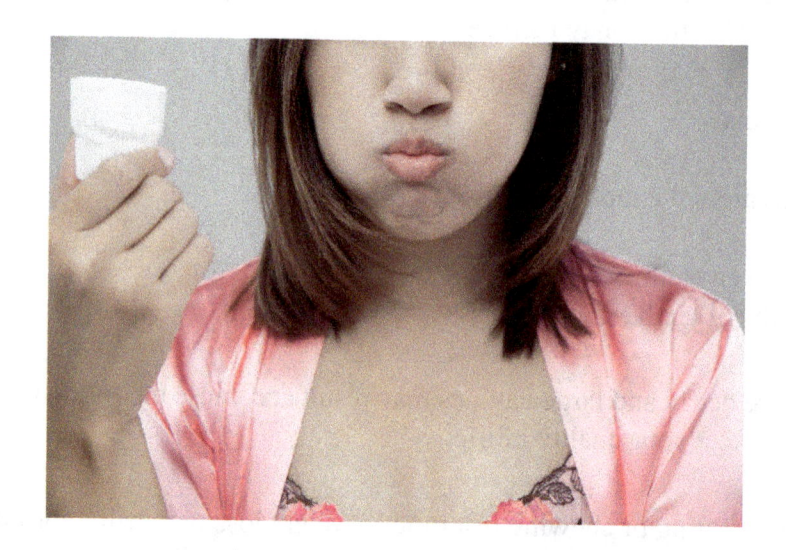

c. Regularly Dental Visits – Prevention is the best medicine. Regular oral exams and dental cleaning every six months or as recommended by the dentist and hygienist.

d. Dental sealants – A protective plastic sealant to the back teeth to seal off grooves and crannies that tend to collect food, and thus protecting tooth enamel from acid and plaque. Sealants need to be checked regularly but they usually last for several years before they need to be replaced.

e. Choose tap water or bottled water –Fluoride, which can help reduce tooth decay significantly, has been added to most public water supplies. The disadvantage of drinking only bottled water is that it doesn't contain fluoride.

f. Frequent snacking and sipping should be avoided – Whenever you eat sugary and starchy foods or drink sugary beverages your teeth are under constant attack from bacteria causing acid and plaque build-up.

g. Tooth friendly foods – The best way to prevent tooth decay is brushing and flossing soon after eating or drinking. It is important to avoid foods that get stuck in grooves and pits of the teeth for long periods. There are some foods and beverages that are better for oral hygiene than others. The foods include, fresh fruits (even though they contain natural sugars) and vegetables which increase saliva flow. The beverages include unsweetened coffee, tea, and 100% Xylitol sugar-free gum, which help wash away food particles.

h. Fluoride treatments – Your dentist may recommend fluoride treatments if they feel you are prone to demineralization of the enamel and decay of the tooth structure.

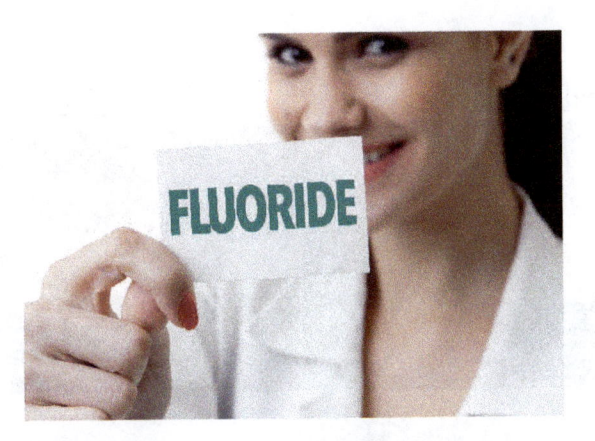

i. Antibacterial treatments – Antibacterial mouth rinses may be needed if your medical condition (immune suppressant diseases like some cancers) leave you vulnerable to tooth decay.

2. Gum Disease

1. Gingivitis

Gingivitis is a common and mild form of gum disease (periodontal disease). It causes irritation, swelling (inflammation) and redness of the gingiva which is the part of the gum at the base of the teeth. Gingivitis can lead to periodontitis, a much more severe gum disease, and tooth loss if it is not treated promptly.

The most common cause of gingivitis is poor oral hygiene. This condition can be reversed with regular brushing, flossing, and dental checkups.

Gingivitis

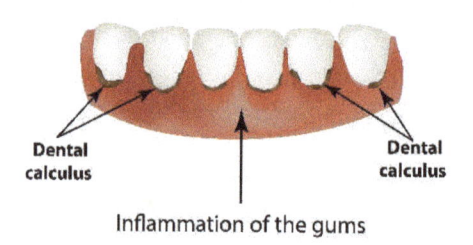

Symptoms of Gingivitis

Healthy gums appear as firm, pale pink and are fitted tightly around the teeth. You can suspect Gingivitis if you observe the following signs and symptoms:

- Swollen or puffy gums
- Dusky red or dark red gums
- Tender gums
- Gums that bleed easily during brushing or flossing
- Receding gums
- Bad breath

Causes of Gingivitis

Poor oral hygiene that allows plaque to form on teeth and over time results in inflammation of the surrounding gum tissues is the most common cause of gingivitis. Dry mouth from mouth breathing is also a common cause of gingivitis.

The progression of plaque to gingivitis:

1. Plaque forms on the teeth –When sugars in food interact with the bacteria typically found in the mouth plaque forms. Daily removal of plaque is necessary because it re-forms quickly.

With poor hygiene plaque builds up and the bacteria become more aggressive and damages the tooth and gum tissues.

2. Plaque turns into tartar – With poor brushing, long standing plaque on the teeth hardens under the gumline into tartar (calculus, very hard like stone), and this collects bacteria. Plaque becomes more difficult to remove because of the tartar. As a result, a protective shield develops for bacteria, which results in irritation along the gumline. Removal of the tartar can only be done by a professional dental cleaning.

3. Gingiva becomes inflamed (gingivitis) – If the plaque and tartar is allowed to remain on the teeth, increased irritation of the gingiva around the base of the teeth occurs. This causes inflammation of the gums and they become swollen and begin to bleed easily.

Gingivitis will progress to periodontitis and eventual tooth loss if not treated properly.

Risk Factors for Developing Gingivitis

Gingivitis is common, in people with poor oral hygiene. Other risk factors for the development of gingivitis include:

- Older age and the increase likelihood of poor oral hygiene
- Vitamin C deficiency as the result of poor nutrition. Again, often found with older adults
- Smoking or chewing tobacco
- Crooked teeth that are difficult to clean or poorly fitting dental restorations (Bridge work)
- Conditions such diabetes, hepatitis, and cancer treatment that decrease a person's immunity
- Mouth breathing and dry mouth
- Certain drugs, such as some beta-blockers, used for angina and high blood pressure and epileptic seizure medications.

Complications of Gingivitis

Gingivitis, can progress to periodontitis, which is a much more serious gun condition that can lead to tooth loss.

Systemic diseases such as respiratory disease, diabetes, coronary artery disease, stroke, and rheumatoid arthritis are often compromising the older adult health and affecting their ability to do the activities of daily living. This may increase the likelihood of poor oral hygiene and the development of chronic gingiva inflammation. Likewise, chronic gingivitis may exacerbate these conditions.

Prevention of Gingivitis

Prevention is similar to the prevention of tooth decay:

a. Practice Good Oral Hygiene – Ideally this means brushing your teeth after every meal or snack for at least two minutes. At minimum you should brush twice daily, in the morning and before going to bed, and flossing at least once a day. It is recommended that you flossing before brushing because it allows the cleaning away of loosened food particles and bacteria.

b. See Your Dentist Regularly –Dental check-ups and cleaning should be part of everyone oral hygienic routine. You may need professional cleaning more often if you have any of the risk factors listed previously.

c. Implement Good Nutritional Practices into Your Daily Routine – Eating lots of fruits and vegetables and minimizing sugar and starches is a good way to improve your oral health

d. The Order In Which You Eat Your Foods Makes a Difference–Eat foods containing sugar first and then follow with foods, such as raw vegetables and apples. that will help wash away or rinse the sugar from the teeth

2. Periodontitis

Periodontitis is a severe and advanced gum disease. Without treatment, it can destroy the bone that supports the teeth, resulting in loosened teeth and eventually tooth loss.

PERIODONTITIS
INFLAMMATION OF THE GUMS

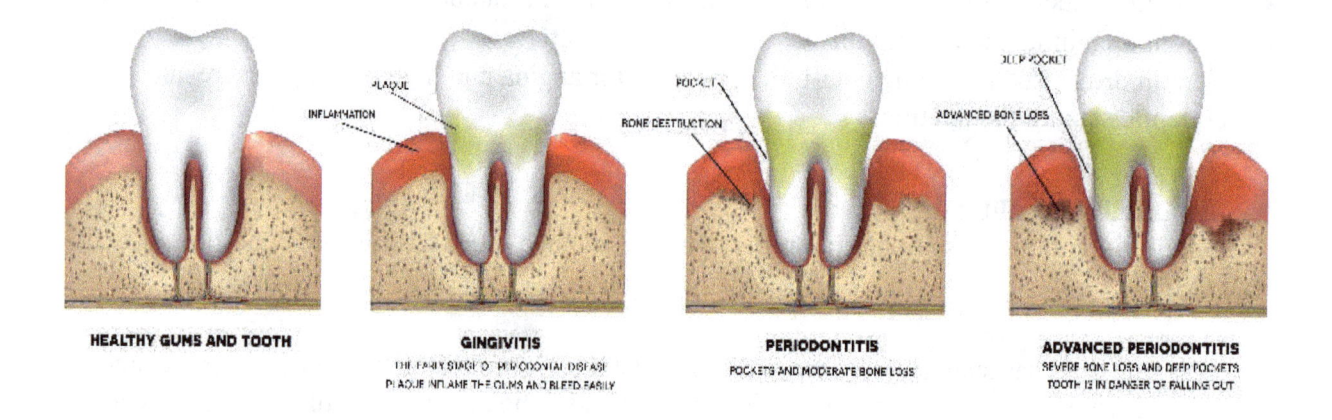

HEALTHY GUMS AND TOOTH	GINGIVITIS	PERIODONTITIS	ADVANCED PERIODONTITIS
	THE EARLY STAGE OF PERIODONTAL DISEASE PLAQUE INFLAME THE GUMS AND BLEED EASILY	POCKETS AND MODERATE BONE LOSS	SEVERE BONE LOSS AND DEEP POCKETS TOOTH IS IN DANGER OF FALLING OUT

Symptoms of Periodontitis

Symptoms of Periodontitis are similar to gingivitis, but are more advanced/severe.

Remember, healthy gums are firm, pale pink and snugly fit around teeth. Periodontitis will present as:

- Gums will appear as bright red, dusky red or purplish
- The gums will be swollen or puffy
- Gums, when touched, will feel tender

- Gums are bleeding easily
- (<u>Note</u> – there is no healthy reason why gums should bleed. Bleeding gums acts as a portal for bacteria to enter the body)
- After brushing or flossing the teeth, you will spit out blood
- Chewing food is painful
- Pus appears between the teeth and gums
- Gums are pull away from the teeth (recede), making the teeth look longer than normal.
- The teeth will have increased sensitivity to hot and cold food or beverages and sweet foods
- There will be increase separation between the teeth
- The teeth become loose increasing the likelihood of losing teeth
- The person's bite has changed because the way the teeth fit together when chewing has changed
- Bad breath

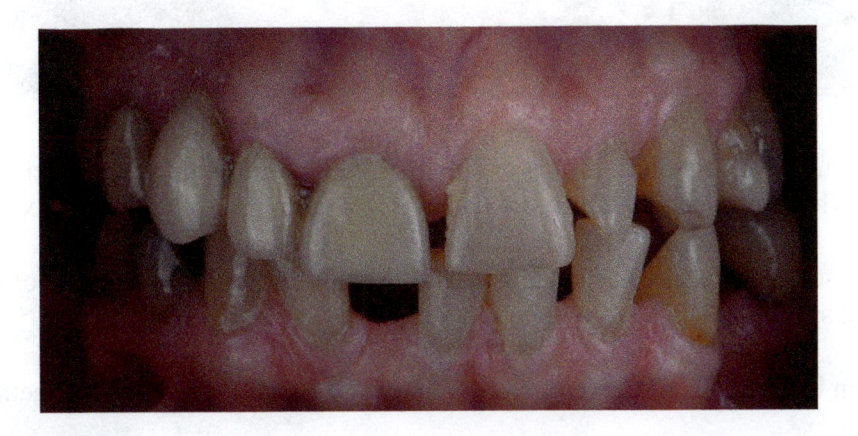

Causes of Periodontitis

In most cases, periodontitis is an advanced form of gingivitis and starts the same way, with plaque build-up.

- Plaque forms on the teeth
- Plaque, if not removed by brushing, hardens under the gumline into tartar (calculus)
- Plaque causes gingivitis (inflammation of the gums)
- Periodontitis results from chronic gum inflammation –the chronic inflammation causes pockets to develop between the gums and teeth. These pockets fill up with plaque, tartar, and bacteria. Over time these infected pockets increase in size and fill with more bacteria. These deep infections will eventually cause a loss of gum and bone, and ultimately the loss of teeth.

Complications of Periodontitis

Chronic inflammation of the gums stresses the immune system, resulting in the older adult becoming more vulnerable to disabling systemic health issues such as rheumatoid arthritis, coronary artery disease respiratory disease, diabetes, dementia and Alzheimer's Disease.

Prevention of Periodontitis

Preventing periodontitis is similar to that of tooth decay and Gingivitis, follow a good oral hygiene program that includes regular visits (2 to 4 times per year) with the dentist and hygienists.

3. Bruxism (Teeth Grinding)

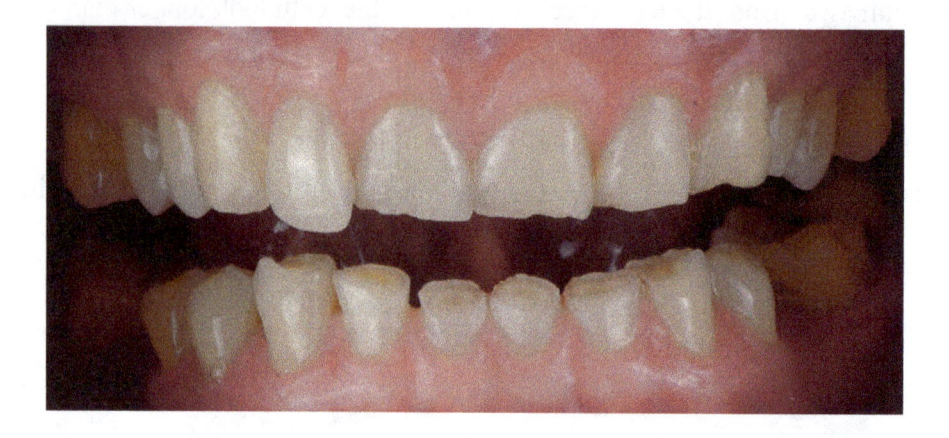

Bruxism occurs when a person grinds or clenches their teeth. A person may clench their teeth unconsciously when awake (awake bruxism) or clench or during sleep (sleep bruxism).

People who suffer from sleep bruxism are more likely to have other sleep disorders, such as sleep apnea and snoring.

Bruxism can be frequent and severe enough to lead to headaches, damaged teeth and jaw disorders.

Unfortunately, many people are unaware that they suffer from bruxism until complications develop. Be aware of the signs and symptoms of bruxism and seek regular dental care if you suspect that you suffer from this condition.

Signs and Symptoms of Bruxism
- Loud enough grinding or clenching of your teeth to wake up your sleep partner
- The tooth enamel is worn to the extent that the deeper layers of the tooth are exposed
- Flattened, fractured, chipped or loose teeth
- Increased pain or sensitivity of teeth
- Soreness of the temporomandibular joint (jaw joint), face or neck
- Jaw muscles are sore and tight resulting is a restricted range of motion of the jaw or a locked jaw that won't open or close completely
- Pain that feels like an earache, though it's not a problem with the ear
- Headaches in the temple region
- Disruption of sleep

Causes of Bruxism

Causes of bruxism is not fully understood, but is probably the result of a combination of genetic, physical, and psychological factors.

Awake bruxism – May result as a coping strategy or a habit during deep concentration or dealing with emotions such as stress, frustration, anxiety, and anger.

Sleep bruxism – Is associated with arousals during sleep causing sleep-related chewing activity.

Risk factors for Developing Bruxism

- **Type A Personality** – An aggressive, competitive, or hyperactive personality type can increase a person's risk of bruxism.
- **Familial History of Bruxism** – Genetics could play role since sleep bruxism has been found to occur in families.
- **Emotional Stress** – Physical response to emotional stress and anxiety can lead to clenching of the jaw and teeth grinding.
- **Medications** – Psychiatric medications, such as certain antidepressants have bruxism as a side effect. Smoking tobacco, drinking caffeinated beverages or alcohol, or using recreational drugs may increase the risk of bruxism.
- **Medical Disorders** – Mental health disorders such as depression, and medical conditions, such as dementia, gastroesophageal reflux disorder (GERD), Parkinson's disease, epilepsy, and sleep apnea increases the risk of bruxism.

Complications of Bruxism

Bruxism usually does not cause serious complications, but if the condition is severe enough it result in:

- Tension headaches
- Severe jaw or facial pain
- Flattening and damaging of teeth
- Movement disorders in the temporomandibular joints (TMJs), jaw joint
- Clicking sounds from the TMJ when the mouth is opened and closed

Bruxism is not normal under any circumstances even if grinding your teeth is a habit when stressed or doing certain mental or physical activities.

Treatment of Bruxism

1. Treat the underlying cause

a. Chronic emotional stress and anxiety management – Learning strategies that promote relaxation, such as mindful meditation. (Chapter 6.9: Mindful Mediation). Consulting your medical doctor or mental health professional is recommended if self management of your stress and anxiety is not successful.

b. Dental approaches

I. Splints and mouth guards – Their purpose is to create a physical barrier between the upper and lower teeth which will prevent them from grinding upon each other. The splints can either fit over the upper or lower teeth.

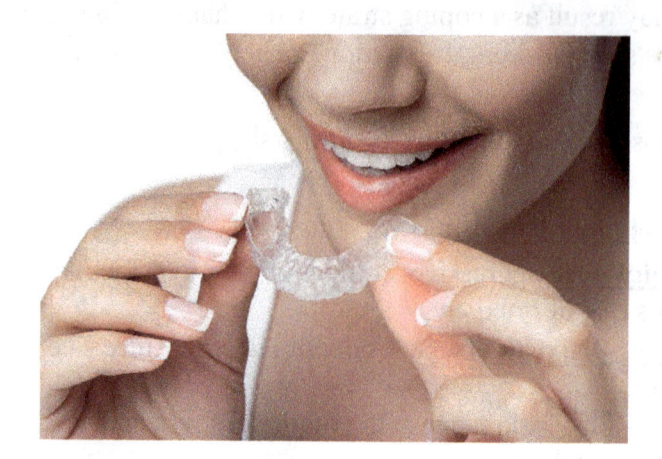

II. Dental correction – In situations when there is significant tooth wear and this has led to sensitivity or chewing problems, reshaping the chewing surfaces or the use crowns to repair the damage may become necessary.

2. Adjunct Treatments for Bruxism

In her book, "Your Mouth: The Gateway to a Healthier You," Dr. Dana Colson D.D.S. states the following as a practical approach and treatment for grinding and clenching the teeth:

"Pay attention to proper jaw alignment and doing facial exercises and massage to encourage proper positioning."

Some of Dr. Colson's recommendations are listed below;

1. Be aware of your jaw position – The ideal jaw position is one in which the teeth are a few millimetres apart, the tongue rests lightly at the junction of the upper teeth and gum tissue, and the lips rest lightly together.

Repeat the following phrase as a mantra to increase your awareness of the ideal position for the mouth to rest;

"Lips Together, Teeth Apart, Tongue in Place"

2. Facial Scan – Using a "facial scan" will help you become more aware of the tension you may hold in your jaws and face. You can perform a scan by having your eyes closed and asking yourselves the following questions:

1. Is there tension in my facial skin and muscles are or are they relaxed?
2. Do my teeth touch together lightly or tightly?

3. Are my lips together, teeth apart and jaw hanging loosely?

4. What is my tongue position? It should be positioned behind my front teeth with the tip lightly touching my upper palate at the junction of the teeth and gum tissue.

3. Facial Massage – Massaging muscles of the face, neck, and jaws provides relaxation.

4. Deep breathing – "Breath therapy" helps a person to relax physically and emotionally.

5. Downward jaw exercise – With the use your index fingers and thumbs position them just above the angle of the jawline and secure both borders of your lower jaw and, with your teeth apart, gently pull the jaw down and forward. Hold this position for 30 seconds to feel a gentle release.

6. Smile therapy – Smiling helps control emotions by reducing anxiety and stress. Research shows that when a person smiles, the brain receives a signal that they are happy, resulting in a release of endorphins. Endorphins are powerful hormones that make a person feel and look better by reducing pain and enhancing the immune system.

For further information on this topic and oral health, please refer to Dr. Colon's book, "Your Mouth: The Gateway to a Healthier You," referenced at the end of this chapter.

Tooth Loss and its Treatments: Implants and Dentures

If you are an older adult, losing your teeth due to decay or periodontitis can have significant physical and mental consequences. Physical, because it affects the structure of the jaw and its ability to chew. As a result, you may not be able to eat properly and suffer malnutrition. Mentally, losing teeth, especially the front teeth, affects your speech, smile, and appearance. Noticeable tooth loss could result in depression, social withdrawal, and isolation. These are things that an older adult must avoid.

Losing teeth due to decay or periodontitis, both chronic conditions, means that the older adult has not been practising good oral hygiene for an extended period. Tooth loss may indicate poor overall health care by the older adult and signify that other potential health concerns may exist.

Consequences of Losing One or More Teeth

Time is the enemy when one or more teeth are missing. If this situation is left untreated, the adjacent teeth attempt to close the gap by gradually shifting towards the open space. These shifting movements occur naturally by the body to compensate for the loss of a one or more teeth. Unfortunately, this shifting can result in a series of problems that make the initial lost tooth situation worse.

1. New spaces between other teeth are created when the shifting occurs. These new spaces create a great place for food to get caught and build up. These spaces are difficult to clean and

maintain and as a result become susceptible to tooth decay and gum disease. Both of these conditions can result in bone loss and over the long-term further loss of teeth.

2. The antagonist, which is the tooth in the opposing jaw (upper jaw if a lower jaw tooth is lost), starts to move in an attempt to find its former point of contact. The gum, around this now moving and loose tooth, begins to recede, and this increases its sensitivity. The tooth will continue to move and the gum will continue to rede until the tooth finds another point of contact or falls out if bone loss occurs.

3. Chewing by fewer teeth increases the stress on these teeth and can lead to premature wear.

4. The appearance of premature facial aging can occur as the result of sagging of the facial support tissues due to loss of bone structure in the jaw.

Treatments for Tooth Loss

1. Dental implants

One of the most common methods of tooth replacement is dental implants. They look and feel like an actual tooth, and are sturdy. Dental implants can be used to replace a single tooth or multiple teeth in different areas. Dental implants can last a lifetime if properly taken care of.

The process of placing a dental implant begins with replacing the tooth's root with titanium or Zirconia screws, which act as the foundation to place the false tooth placed on. Sufficient jaw bone is necessary for the screws to be put in place securely. Once the implant becomes securely fused to the jawbone a dental crown will be placed on top.

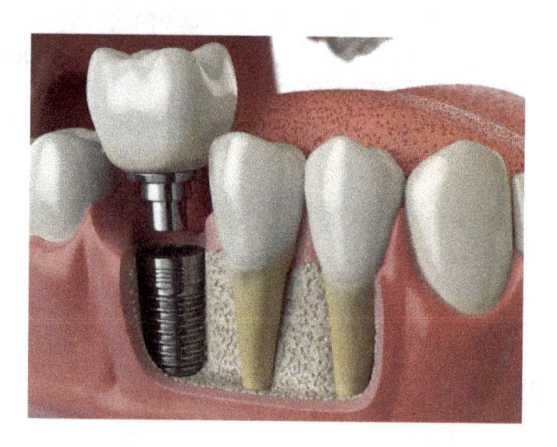

2. Implant-Supported Bridge

An ideal solution for multiple missing teeth in a row is an implant-supported bridge is. Replacing teeth with multiple dental implants can be very lengthy and expensive. Implanted-supported bridge, only requires the teeth at the two ends be secured in place with implants while the teeth in the middle do not require any screwing.

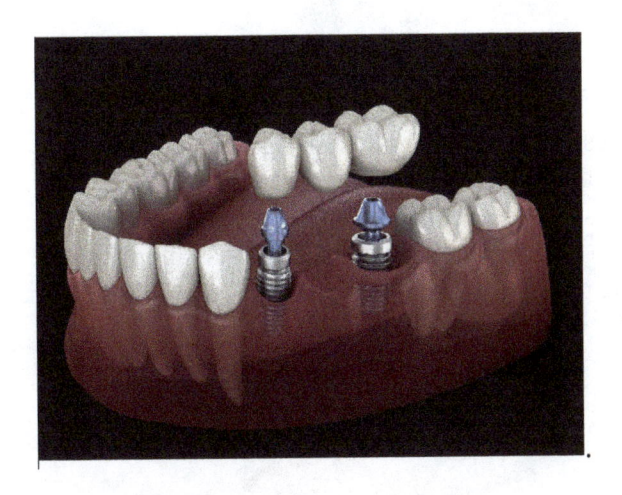

3. Traditional Tooth-Supported Bridge
With this type of bridge, existing teeth act as the anchors for the placement of the bridge.

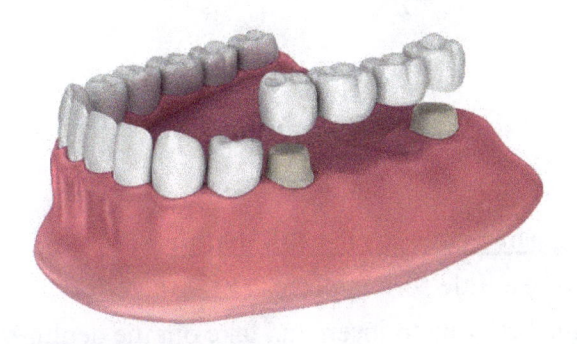

4. Removable Partial Dentures
A simple option to replace a few missing teeth is a removable partial denture. This is a very economical option when compared to the cost of multiple dental implants This type of denture is clasped into the correct place, so the false teeth are held in the appropriate spots.

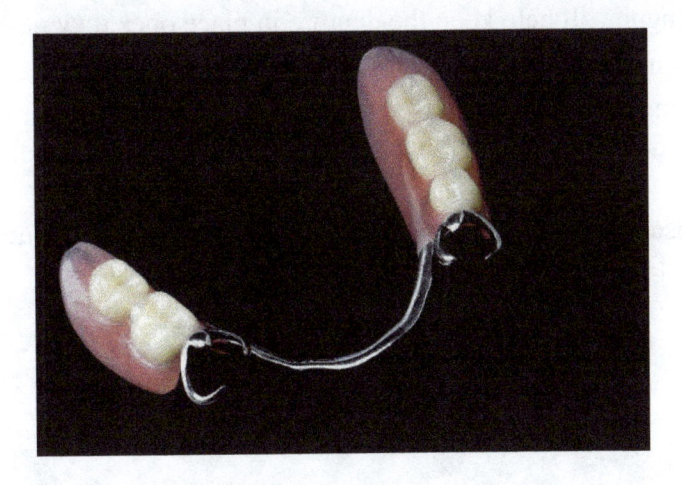

5. Full Dentures

Full Dentures are necessary when a person is missing the majority of their teeth and a partial bridge or implants are not an option. Full Dentures are effective at restoring the appearance and oral functions that were lost as a result of multiple missing teeth. Full dentures are made to replicate gum tissue and the teeth are made of either porcelain or plastic. A layer of saliva between the gums and the denture facilitates the suction that keeps the full dentures in place.

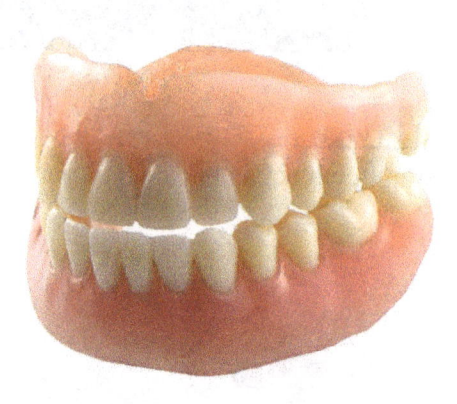

Be aware of the following when considering full dentures:

- The gums will initially be a little sore in places.
- Be patient in finding the best way to insert and take out the dentures.
- It is often necessary to return to the dentist often in the first few weeks to adjust the parts of the denture that are irritating the oral tissues.
- It takes some practice to learn to eat with the dentures in place. It is usually best to start with soft foods, and chew food equally on both sides of the mouth. Sticky or chewy foods should be avoided.
- The cheeks and tongue will help keep the denture in place once they get used to the denture.
- Speaking will become easier with repetition but will require practice.
- Yawning or laughing, exaggerated movements of the mouth may result in the dentures becoming dislodged at first. The denture may need to be adjusted or refit if this becomes a chronic problem.
- Initially, an increased production of saliva will occur, but normal production will return back to normal within a few weeks.

Oral Thrush

Oral thrush occurs when Candida Albicans, a fungus and a normal organism in the mouth, accumulates excessively on the lining of the mouth.

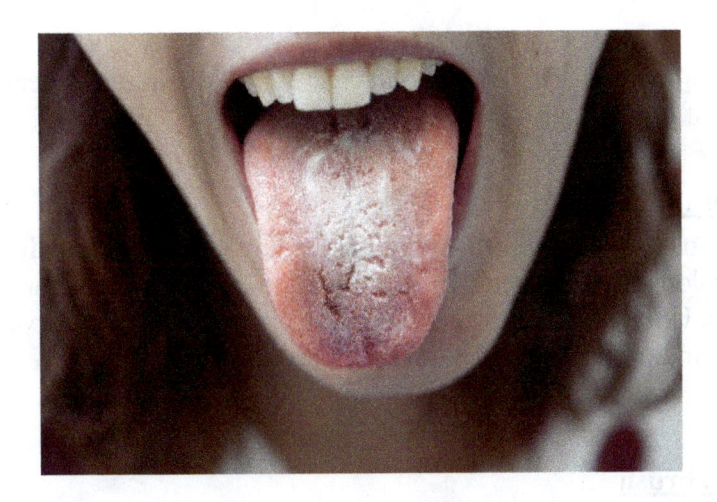

Oral thrush often occurs in older adults because of reduced immunity due to a pre-existing medical condition or the type of medication they are on. Oral thrush can be severe and difficult to control for someone who has a weakened immune system.

Symptoms of Oral Thrush
- Creamy white lesions on the tongue, inner cheeks, and sometimes on the roof of the mouth, gums, and tonsils. These lesions can have a cottage cheese-like appearance.
- Slight bleeding if the lesions are rubbed or scraped.
- Corners of the mouth may be red and cracked.
- Difficulty eating or swallowing as a result of redness, burning, or soreness in the mouth
- Ability to taste is diminished.
- A cottony dryness feeling in the mouth.

If the Oral Thrush is severe, the creamy white lesions may spread downward into the oesophagus and the patient may experience pain, difficulty swallowing and feel like food is getting stuck in their throat.

Causes of Oral Thrush
The primary cause is a weakened immune system that is unable to repel or maintaining a balance between "good" and "bad" microbes that naturally inhabit the body. When this occurs, the number of candida fungi grows exponentially allowing the oral thrush infection to take hold.

Risk factors for Oral Thrush
- **Weakened immunity** – This is the number one risk factor for the development of Oral Thrush. Some medical conditions such as cancer, and organ transplantation and HIV/AIDS, and their treatments can suppress the immune system.

- **Diabetes** – When diabetes is not diagnosed or not well controlled, the saliva will contain larger than normal amounts of sugar which encourages the growth of candida.
- **Medications** – Drugs such as the steroid prednisone, corticosteroid inhalants for asthma, or antibiotics can increase the risk of oral thrush by disturbing the natural balance of microorganisms in the body.

- **Other oral conditions** – Dry Mouth and wearing full dentures, especially upper dentures, can increase the risk of oral thrush.

Complications of Oral Thrush

Oral thrush is seldom a problem for healthy adults; however, in older adults with lowered immunity, or on a prolonged administration of steroidal medication for arthritis, thrush can become more serious. Untreated oral thrush can lead to more serious invasive systemic candida infections. Invasive candidiasis can affect the brain, bones, blood, heart, eyes, and other parts of the body.

Prevention of Oral Thrush

- **Rinse the mouth** – Brush your teeth or at least rinse your mouth with water if you use a corticosteroid inhaler.
- **Good oral hygiene** – Brushing teeth at a minimum of twice a day and flossing regularly.
- **Check dentures** – Partial or full dentures need to be removed at night and cleaned. Dentures need to fit correctly. Any irritation needs to be addressed immediately.
- **Regular dental checkups** – This is especially important if you suffer from diabetes or wear dentures.
- **Watch the diet** –Limit sugar-containing foods in your diet. Sugar, natural or artificial, encourages the growth of candida.
- **Maintain good blood sugar control with diabetes** – Controlling blood sugar reduces the amount of sugar in the saliva which discouraging the growth of candida.
- **Avoid dry mouth**

Dry Mouth (Xerostomia)

When, over a period of time, the salivary glands in the mouth do not make enough saliva to keep the mouth wet a condition called Dry Mouth develops. It is often due to aging issues, the side effect of certain medications, or radiation therapy for cancer.

For teeth to remain healthy, saliva is necessary because it washing away food particles and neutralizes acids produced by bacteria, as a result it limits bacterial growth and slows tooth decay. Saliva helps a person chew and swallow and the enzymes in saliva help the digestion of food.

Decreased saliva and dry mouth can be just a nuisance or can have a significant impact not only on your teeth and gum health but your general health as well.

Symptoms of Dry Mouth

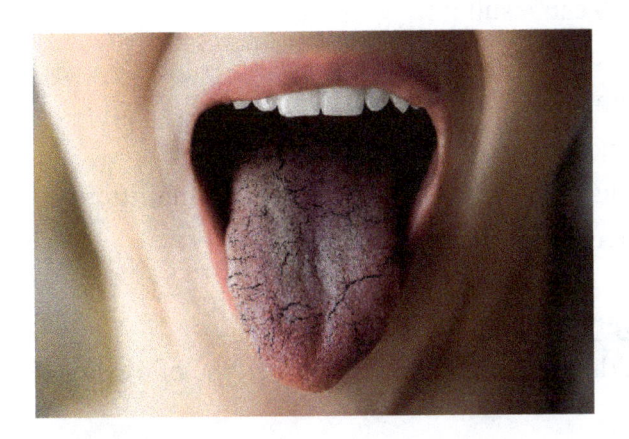

- Bad breath
- Dry or sore throat and hoarseness
- Dryness or a feeling of stickiness in the mouth, when awaking in the morning
- Dry or grooved tongue
- Your sense of taste changes. "Nothing tastes the same."
- Thick and stringy saliva
- Chewing, speaking, and swallowing become difficult
- Dentures become uncomfortable.

Causes of Dry Mouth (not enough saliva)

- **Aging** –Dry mouth is more prevalent in older adults because they are vulnerable to more risk factors such as the use of certain medications (see below), the body's decrease ability to process medications, inadequate nutrition, and having pre-existing long-term health problems such as diabetes, arthritis, obesity and dementia.
- **Medications** –Many prescription and over-the-counter drugs, produce, as a side effect, dry mouth. The most likely medications to cause problems for older adults are those used for depression, anxiety, high blood pressure, allergies (antihistamines), colds (decongestants), arthritis (muscle relaxants and pain medications).
- **Tobacco and alcohol use** – A person is more vulnerable to dry mouth symptoms if they are heavy drinkers or smokers or chew tobacco.
- **Cancer therapy** – The chemistry of the saliva and the amount produced can change as the result of chemotherapy drugs and radiation. Depending on the dosage and area treated the changes in saliva may be temporary or permanent.
- **Nerve damage** – Any trauma or neurologic injury to a person's head and neck area can result in dry mouth.
- **Open mouth sleeping** - Sleeping and breathing with the mouth open can also contribute to dry mouth. This often happens if the person is using a retainer to avoid grinding of their teeth (bruxism).

Complications from Dry Mouth

Developing dry mouth can result in:
- Increased plaque, gun disease and tooth decay
- Sores in the mouth
- Corners of your mouth or lips become red and cracked
- Difficulty chewing and swallowing leading to poor nutrition.
- Thrush (yeast infection)

Treatment for Dry Mouth

The underlying cause of dry mouth will determine the type of treatment necessary. These treatments could include:
- Use recommended products to moisturise the mouth
- Use prescribed medication that stimulates saliva
- Change medications that cause dry mouth

Home remedies include:
- Use a room humidifier to add moisture to the air at night. This is especially effective during the winter months when the furnace is on and the air is at its driest.
- Use skin and lip moisturizer to help heal dry or cracked areas
- Throughout the day moisten the mouth by sipping water or sucking on ice chips.
- To encourage saliva production use Xylitol lozenges, chew 100% Xylitol sugar-free gum or suck on sugar-free hard candies
- Non prescription saliva substitutes are available
- Breathe through the nose. Taping of mouth with surgical tape will encourage breathing through the nose
- Avoid products which can make dry mouth symptoms worse such as caffeine and alcohol (avoid using a mouthwash that contains alcohol), tobacco and over-the-counter antihistamines and decongestants

Conclusion

Oral and dental health are essential components to an older adult's physical and mental well being. Besides the primary health problems associated with tooth decay, gingivitis, periodontitis, teeth grinding, oral thrush, and dry mouth, secondary complications also arise, such as malnutrition, depression, and social isolation. All of these must be avoided to enhance the older adult's quality of life.

Fortunately, by having regular appointments with the dentist and dental hygienist, most oral and dental conditions are easily diagnosed and treated effectively. Prevention of most oral and dental problems can be accomplished through by practicing of good oral hygiene which includes frequent brushing of your teeth, especially after meals and snacks, and a diet that minimizes sugary foods.

As Dr. Dana Colson says in her book, Your Mouth: The Gateway to a Healthier You, "Our smile is our best vitamin," so the older adult needs to protect their smile the best they can. Dr. Colson also gives another valuable but straightforward piece of advice regarding the importance of proper mouth, teeth, and tongue position: to ensure that the tongue and teeth are always in proper oral alignment, remember and repeat the mantra, "Lips together, teeth apart, tongue in place." She explains that in the ideal oral position, the lips rest lightly together, the teeth are a few millimetres apart, and the tongue rests lightly at the junction of the upper teeth and gum tissue. Following this mantra is an excellent start to good oral and dental health.

Start taking care of your dental health today, your smile depends upon it, and as Dr. Colson says, "It's almost impossible to smile on the outside without feeling better on the inside." Is that not exactly what you want from your fitness and health plan?

References

Colson, Dana G., D.D.S. (2011) *"Your Mouth: The Gateway to a Healthier You,"* DJC Corp.
www.myoclinic.org
www.webMD.com
www.bloorwestsmile.com
www.medicinnet.com

2.8. Visual Challenges and Impairments

Introduction

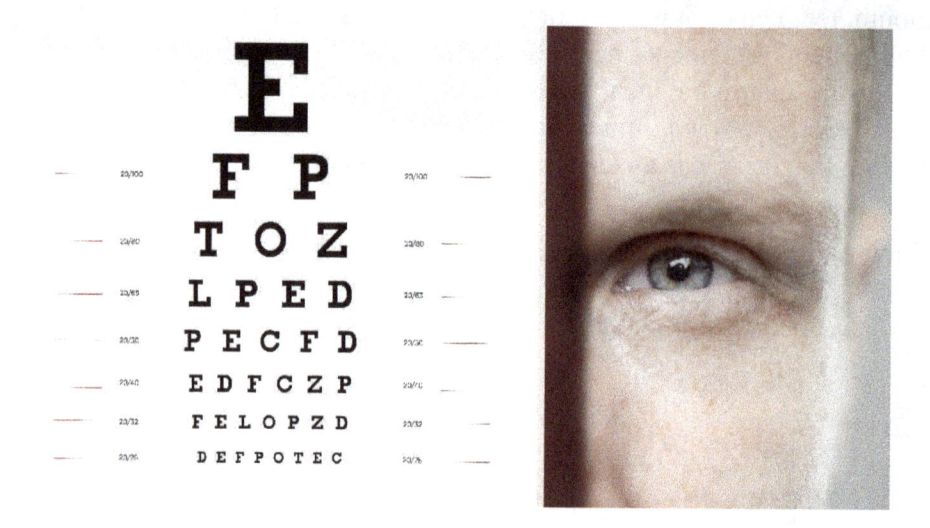

As an older adult, you face many physical and mental challenges and impairments. One of the most common is declining eyesight and other various eye/ocular conditions that can significantly affect your quality of life because four fifths of all information that the brain receives comes from the eyes.

Early in life, even if corrective eyeglasses are necessary to improve someone's vision, there is a tendency to take vision for granted. Wearing eyeglasses is commonplace; people nowadays wear non-prescription eyewear as a fashion statement.

Many older adults have not had their vision checked regularly because of declining mental health, finances, and challenges getting to the optometrists. As a result, many older adults are not even aware that there may be an issue with their vision. Conditions such as near and farsightedness, cataracts, and glaucoma could develop and progress insidiously. These conditions can significantly affect your visual acuity and ability to participate in your favourite hobbies such as golf, playing cards, riding a bike, and even carrying out your normal daily activities such as walking, climbing stairs, and cooking.

An additional challenge to the older adult is an increased risk of falling as the result of impaired vision. Proprioceptive reflexes help correct your position in space to prevent a loss of balance and reduce the risk of falling. Proprioceptive reflexes come from three sources in the body: our joints (postural or somatosensory reflexes), our ears (vestibular reflexes) and our eyes (ocular reflexes).

Arthritis in weight-bearing joints such as the knees and hips compromise the joint/postural/somatosensory proprioceptive reflexes ability to prevent falls. The vestibule-ocular reflex in the ears helps stabilize your vision when you move their head rapidly. Research indicates that the function of this reflex declines with age, which will affect your ability to determine whether it is your surroundings or your own body that is moving in certain situations. Combine this with decreased visual acuity, and the risk of falling becomes very high.

Understanding visual impairment is important. Most of the visual/ocular conditions that afflict the older adult can be treated effectively if detected early enough. Maintaining visual acuity is crucial for helping you maintain an active lifestyle and a high quality of life into your golden years.

What is presented in this chapter are the most common visual/ocular conditions that affect older adults. There are many other conditions, some of which could have life-threatening consequences. It is recommended that everyone visits their optometrist regularly. For those of you who are younger than 50 years of age, once every two years should be sufficient. For adults over 50 years of age a yearly visit to the optometrists is recommended.

Anatomy of the Eye

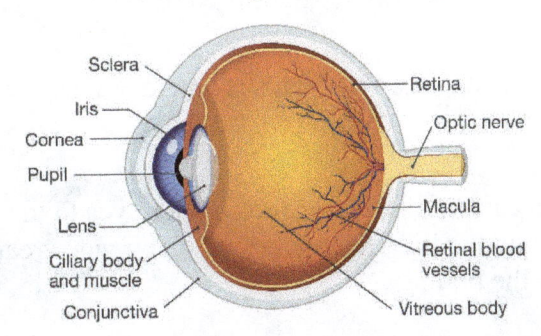

Without making things complicated, it is a valuable lesson to review the anatomy of the eye:

Cornea – The transparent part that covers the front of the eye. The iris, pupil, and anterior chamber (the fluid-filled inside front of the eye) are covered. The primary function of the cornea's is to bend or refract light.

Pupil – This is the opening in the center of the iris. It allows light to enter the eye. The pupils appear black in color, equal in size and perfectly round.

Iris – This is the part of the eye that is coloured. It functions to regulate the amount of light entering the eye. The iris closes the pupil to let in less light when it is bright and opens the pupil when the light is low to let in more light.

Lens –This focuses the light on to the retina. When healthy it is clear. It becomes cloudy when a person suffers from cataracts. The shape of the lens changes by using small ciliary muscles. By changing shapes, the lens can better focus on objects at different distances. The focusing of the lens is a reflex response.

Conjunctiva – This is a membrane that covers the eyelid and folds back to cover the sclera right up to the edge of the cornea.

Sclera –This is the outer white layer that protects everything inside the eye.

Vitreous Body (Humour) –The space between the lens and the retina is filled with this clear gel.

Choroid – It is positioned between the retina and the sclera and is made up of layers of blood vessels that nourishes the back of the eye.

Retina – Is made up of millions of light-sensitive cells called rods and cones, and other nerve cells that receive, organize and transmit visual information to the optic nerve.

Macula – This is the central area and functional center of the retina. It is about 5mm across and is responsible for your visible acuity (ability to see "20/20"), and color vision.

Optic Disc – This is the optic nerve head. This is where the nerve cells leave the eye and form the optic nerve.

Optic Nerve – Communicates visual images from your eyes to the brain. When a visual image is focused on the retina, energy in the light that makes up that image creates an electrical signal/impulse that the optic nerve sends to the brain

Refractive Eye Disorders

If the eye becomes irregularly shaped it makes it difficult for the cornea and lens of the eyes to take images and focus them clearly onto the retina and this results in vision becoming blurred and impaired.

1. Near and Far Sightedness

When light is focused directly on the retina, rather than in front or behind it, a person can see objects that are near and far clearly.

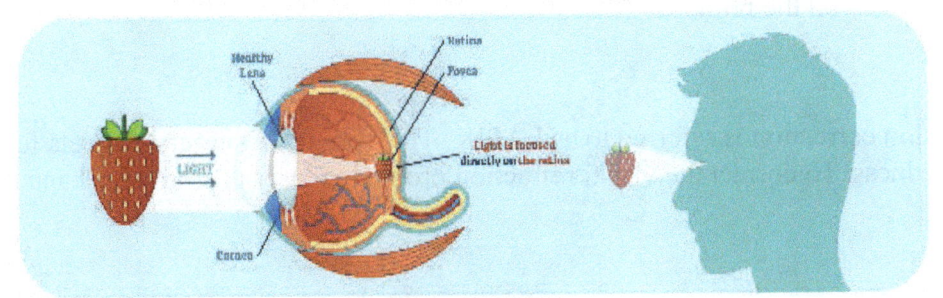

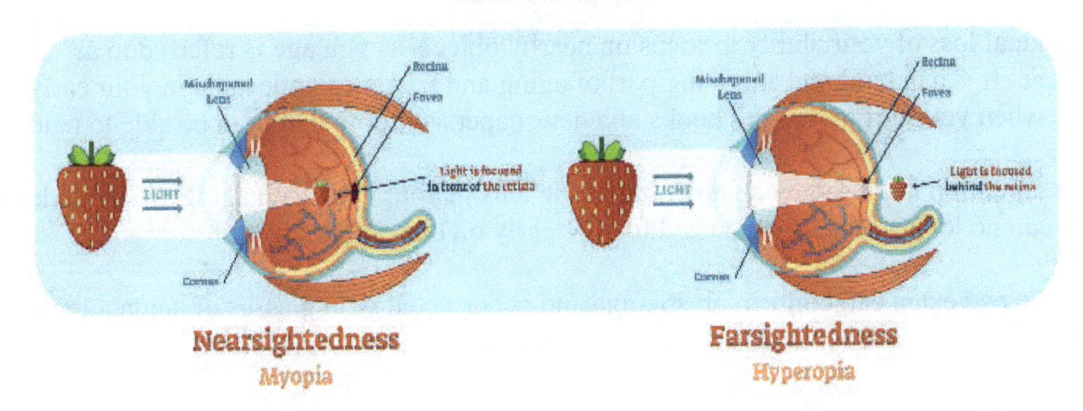

a. Nearsightedness (Myopia)

When a person can only clearly see objects close to them, they are referred to as being nearsighted. Objects in the distance are out of focused and blurry. Nearsightedness occurs when of the physical length of the eye is longer than the optical length. This results in the visual image not being focused directly on the retina but in front of it. This condition frequently develops in the rapidly growing children and adolescents and requires frequent changes in corrective eye wear.

b. Farsightedness (Hyperopia)

A farsighted person can see objects that are far away clearly but objects near to them are blurred. With farsightedness, the visual image is focused behind the retina rather than directly on it. It may be caused by the eyeball being too small at birth or the focusing power of the eye being too weak. This condition is often present from birth but often the child outgrows the condition.

Corrections for Refractive Eye Disorders

a. Eye Glasses or Contact Lens

Both of these conditions can be correct effectively by an optometrist prescription.

Nearsightedness –the focusing power of the lens in the eye is too strong because visual image is being focused in front of the retina. As a result, a diverging lens is needed to reduce focusing power so the image will be focused directly on the retina.

Farsightedness – this condition requires stronger focusing power because the visual image is focused behind the retina. A converging lens is necessary to increase focusing power and bring the images directly on the retina.

b. LASIK

Laser vision correction is referred to as LASIK. This refractive surgery corrects for both near and farsightedness. To correct the visual refraction problem a laser is used to reshape the cornea in the eye.

2. Presbyopia

A gradual loss of your ability to focus on nearby objects as you age is referred to as Presbyopia. It is a natural and annoying part of aging and becomes noticeable in your early to mid-40s when you start to holding books and newspapers at arm's length to be able to read them.

This condition is caused by a hardening of the lens in your eyes with aging. With hardening, the lens can no longer change shape and focus clearly on close-up images.

A basic eye exam can confirm presbyopia and is corrected with glasses or contact lenses. LASIK may or may not be indicated for this condition.

3. Astigmatism

Astigmatism is a refractive disorder caused by the eyes not focusing the light evenly on the retina resulting in blurred or distorted vision at any distance. Symptoms of astigmatism can also include eyestrain, headaches, squinting, and trouble driving at night.

No definitive reason why astigmatism occurs but genetics may be a reason. Amblyopia ("lazy eye") is a complication if Astigmatism develops early in life.

This condition results from an irregular curvature of the lens or cornea. Both of these two structures have curved surfaces that function to bend (refract) light onto the retina, to make the image. If the shape of either of these structures' changes, for example, one becomes egg-shaped, the light rays will not be bent the same way onto the retina, and two different images will develop resulting in blurred vision.

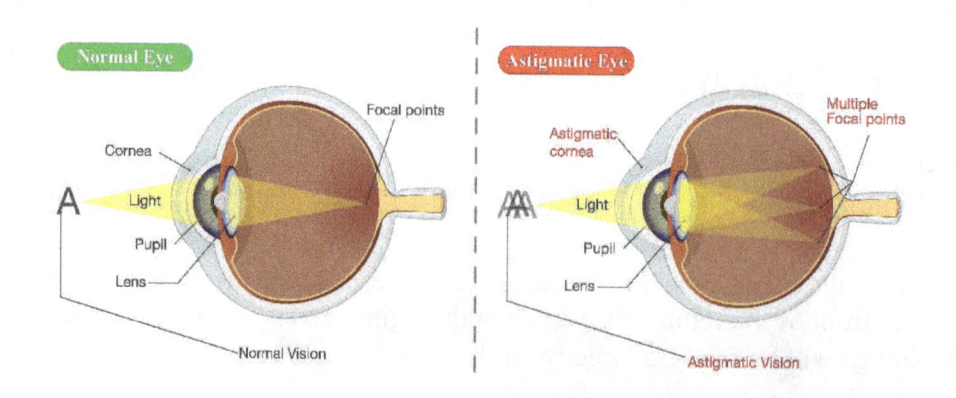

An eye examination will diagnosis this condition and there are three types of treatment: glasses, contact lenses, and refractive surgery, which permanently changes the shape of the eye.

4. Amblyopia (Lazy Eye)

When, early in life, vision is reduced in one eye, this abnormal visual development is called Amblyopia or what is more commonly known as Lazy Eye. The weaker/ lazy eye often wanders outward or inward.

This condition usually develops between birth to age seven and is the leading cause of decreased vision among children. Lazy eye rarely affects both eyes.

Treatment usually involves prescription glasses, contact lenses, or patching therapy.

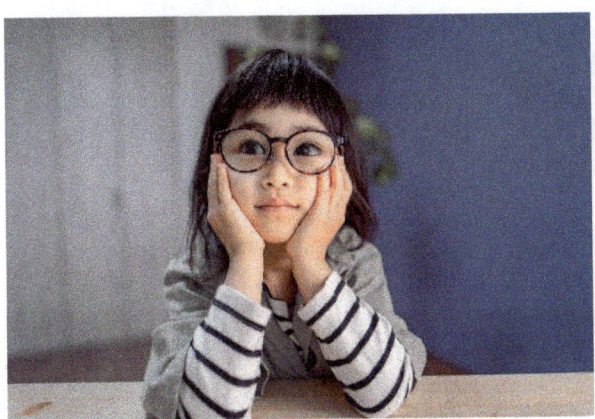

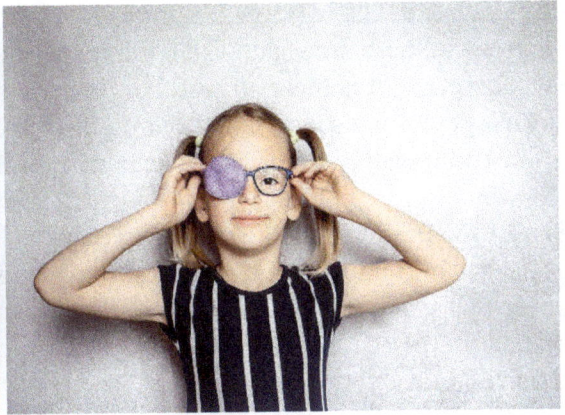

Vitreous Detachment

This is a common condition that primarily affects older adults. It appears more frequently in those who are nearsighted. If vitreous detachment occurs in one eye, the other eye is also likely to have it, or develop it in later years. Serious complications are rare.

How Vitreous Detachment Occurs

Vitreous gel is a jelly-like substance that helps maintain the eyes round shape. The vitreous gel contains millions of fine fibers attached to the retinal surface. With advancing age, the vitreous gel slowly shrinks away from the retina, and the fibers will often become detached from the retina.

Floaters and Flashes

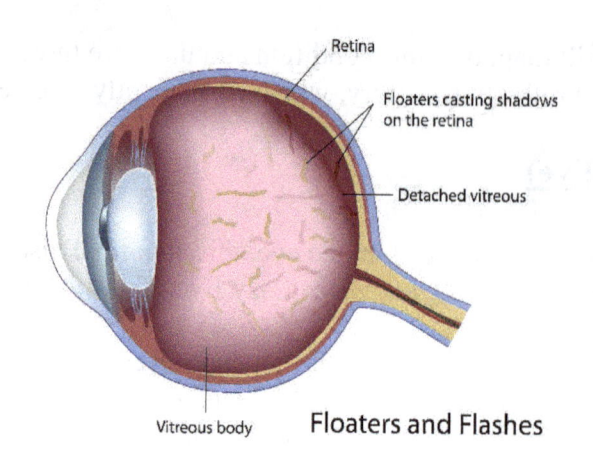

Symptoms of Vitreous Detachment

Floaters – These are shadows on the retina due to the vitreous shrinking and becoming somewhat stringy. It is these strings that produce shadows on the retina. It is best to think of floaters as specks that seem to be floating in your field of vision. If you look at the sky or into bright-lit while reading floaters will become more noticeable.

Bright flashes of light (lightning streaks) – If the number of floaters suddenly increases, bright flashes of light (lightning streaks) may suddenly appear off to the side of your vision whenever you move your eyes. These are most noticeable when the light is low or you move into a darkened room. The light flashes occur when the detached vitreous, bumps lightly against the retina as you move your eyes.

Floaters and light flashes never disappear completely but usually they will decrease during the weeks or months after the vitreous detaches.

Complications of Vitreous Detachment

Usually, vitreous detachment and its floaters and flashes are just annoying however, if the vitreous fibers pull very hard on the retina as they detach, retinal tears can be created, and these can lead to retinal detachment, which can potentially threaten your vision.

Age-Related Macular Degeneration

As the name suggest, Age-related Macular Degeneration is an eye disease that most often progresses over time. In people over age 60, it is the leading cause of severe, permanent vision loss. It results when the macula, the small central portion of the retina, wears down. It might cause severe vision problems but usually doesn't cause blindness.

Wet vs. Dry Macular Degeneration

1. Dry form –In our macula there are normally a few small yellow deposits, called drusen. Usually, drusen will not cause changes in vision, but they could distort your vision, especially when reading, if they get bigger and more numerous, If the condition worsens, the light-sensitive cells in the macula get thinner and die. A person may start to have blind spots in the center of their vision, and if the condition progresses, a person will lose central vision. This is the most common form of macular degeneration, making up 80- 90% of the cases. The dry form can lead to the wet form.

2. Wet form – This form of macular degeneration always occurs from the dry form. Abnormal blood vessels grow from underneath the macula, and leak blood and fluid into the retina. Initially, your vision becomes distorted so that straight lines look wavy. With progression, you may develop blind spots and loss of central vision. If the blood vessels and bleeding eventually form a scar, permanent loss of central vision will result.

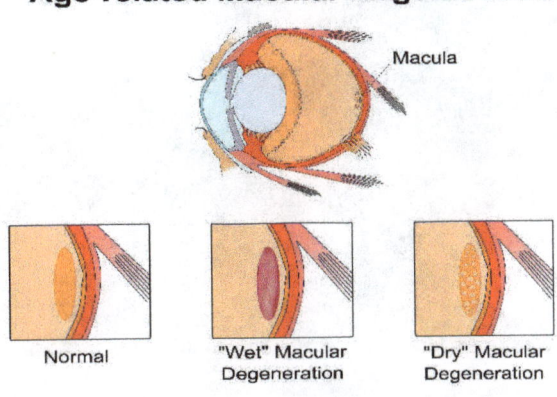

Age-related Macular Degeneration

Wet Macular Degeneration

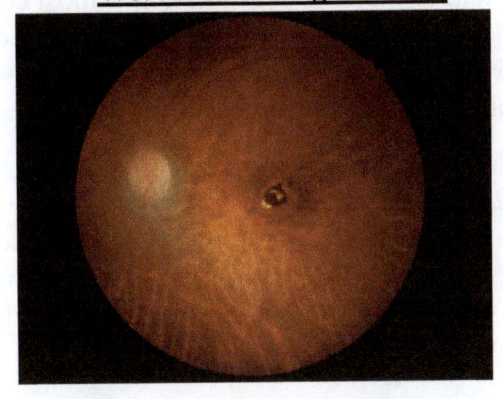

Dry Macular Degeneration

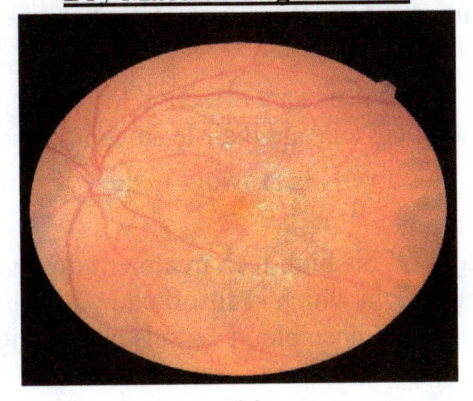

Symptoms of Macular Degeneration
Unfortunately, macular degeneration often does not get diagnosed until its later stages when both eyes are affected.

It is important to see your optometrist immediately if the following symptoms present themselves:
- Blurry and diminished vision making it hard to drive or read fine print.
- Your central vision becomes blurry and dark.

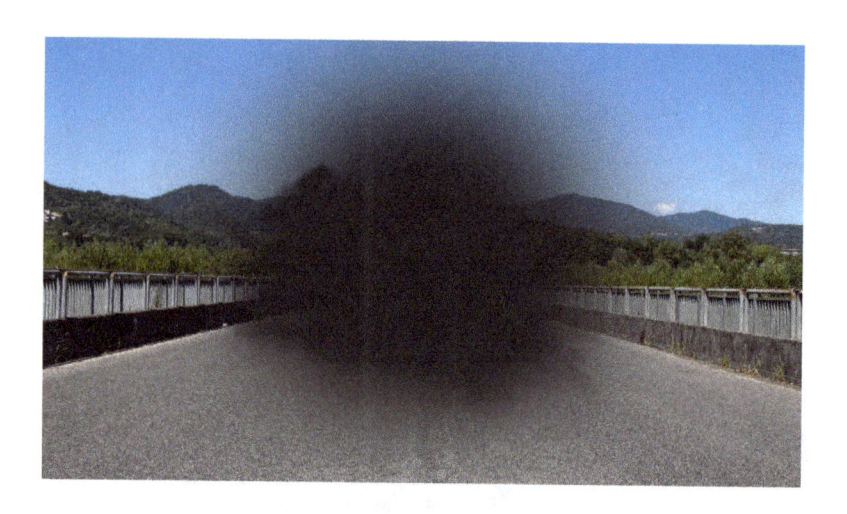

Causes of Macular Degeneration
As the name implies, age-related macular degeneration is most common in older people. Genetics may be a risk factor since there appears to be a familial history associated with it. Other risk factors include gender, being female, poor diet by eating lots of saturated fat, having high cholesterol, being obese, smoking, and having a light eye color.

How Is Macular Degeneration Diagnosed?
Macular degeneration can be detected by a routine eye examination. Increase accumulation of drusen is one of its most common early signs. The use of an Amsler grid is a commonly used diagnostic tool. This grid has a pattern of straight lines and macular degeneration can be suspected if some of the straight lines appear wavy, or are missing.

What Treatments Are Available for Macular Degeneration?
Macular degeneration has no cure but effective treatment can help prevent you from losing too much of your vision.
- **Anti-angiogenesis drugs** – These drugs are effective for wet macular degeneration by inhibiting the creation of blood vessels and their leakage into the eye.
- **Laser therapy** –Abnormal blood vessels growing in the eye can be destroyed by high-energy laser light.
- **Photodynamic laser therapy** – This high-tech treatment involves the injection of a light-sensitive drug into the blood stream which is absorbed by the abnormal blood vessels. The medication is triggered to damage those blood vessels by shining a laser into the eyes.

- **Low vision aids** –Devises such as special lenses or electronic systems can help people who have vision loss from macular degeneration by magnifying larger images.

Macular Degeneration Prevention

There is no definitive way preventing macular degeneration however, research does suggest that taking vitamins C and E, lutein, zeaxanthin, zinc, and copper supplements may help slow the disease.

Prognosis for People with Macular Degeneration?

The dry form, which causes the vast majority age related macular degeneration, is slow progressing so complete vision loss is rare. Vision loss is primarily is restricted to the central visionary field. In most cases, your central vision may be poor, but you are still able to perform most normal daily activities.

However, the wet form, which develops from the dry form, progresses much faster and is a leading cause of permanent vision loss from macular degeneration. Regular/yearly optometrist appointments and early detection for age related macular degeneration is important so appropriate treatment can begin to help maintain the quality of life of the older adult.

Glaucoma

Glaucoma damages the optic nerve, the health of which is vital for good vision. Abnormally high pressure in a person's eye is the cause this damage. Glaucoma is one of the leading causes of blindness for people over 60, but it can occur at any age.

Often a person will not notice a change in their vision as a result of Glaucoma until the condition is at an advanced stage because Glaucoma can progress very slowly. It is essential for the older adult to have regular eye exams that include measurements of their eye pressure so a diagnosis of Glaucoma can be made in its early stages and treated appropriately. Unfortunately, a person can not recover vision loss due to glaucoma. Fortunately, vision loss can be slowed or prevented if Glaucoma is diagnosed early. Once diagnosed, treatment is on going for the rest of your life.

Causes of Glaucoma

There is a familial history with Glaucoma. Research has indicated that Glaucoma tends to run in families and genes have been identified that are related to high eye pressure and optic nerve damage.

The Optic nerve damage is usually related to increased pressure in the eye. Increase in eye pressure results from a buildup of a fluid (aqueous humor) that flows throughout the inside of the eye. Normally, tissue called the trabecular meshwork, which is located at the angle where the iris and cornea meet, allows the internal fluid to drains out. When the fluid can't flow out at its regular rate, the eye pressure increases.

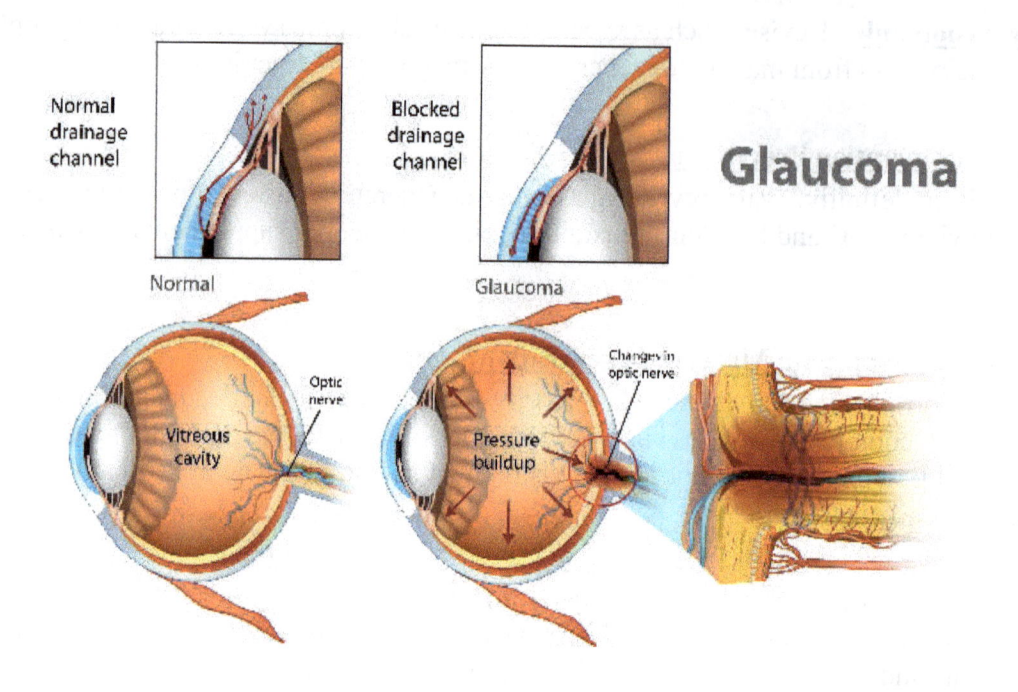

Types of Glaucoma:
1. Open-angle Glaucoma
The most common form Glaucoma is referred to as being open-angled. With this type of Glaucoma, the drainage angle formed by the cornea and iris remains open, but the trabecular meshwork is partially blocked. Eye pressure gradually increases because of this partial blockage and the optic nerve becomes damaged. The increase in eye pressure and the subsequent optic nerve damage and loss of vision is slow and often occurs before an older adult suspects that there is a problem.

2. Angle-closure Glaucoma
Angle-closure glaucoma, refers to the condition where the iris bulges forward to narrow or block the drainage angle formed by the cornea and iris. This blockage restricts fluid circulation through the eye, and pressure increases. People born with narrow drainage angles are at higher risk of developing angle-closure glaucoma.

Unlike Open-angle glaucoma, Angle-closure glaucoma may occur suddenly creating a medical emergency.

TYPES OF GLAUCOMA

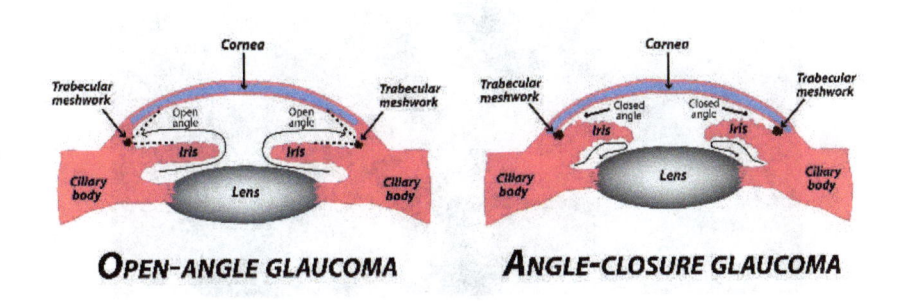

OPEN-ANGLE GLAUCOMA   **ANGLE-CLOSURE GLAUCOMA**

3. Normal-tension Glaucoma

In this form of Glaucoma, the optic nerve becomes damaged even though the eye pressure is within the normal range. The etiology for this is unknown however it is suspected that the person may have less blood supplied to their optic nerve or a sensitive optic nerve. Atherosclerosis/heart disease or diabetes, that impair circulation, could contribute to this form of Glaucoma.

4. Pigmentary Glaucoma

This type of glaucoma is caused by a build up of pigment granules from your iris in the drainage channels resulting in blocking the aqueous fluid from exiting the eye. Rapid movement of the head or vigorous activities such as jogging can stir up the pigment granules, which could ultimately lead to this condition if these accumulate in the drainage channels.

Symptoms of Glaucoma

Open-angle glaucoma
- Frequently occurs in both eyes
- Patchy blind spots in your central or side (peripheral) vision
- Tunnel vision in the advanced stages (only seeing central vision)

Acute angle-closure glaucoma
- Pain in the eyes
- Vision becomes blurred
- Redness of the eye(s)
- Severe headache
- Nausea and vomiting
- See halos around lights

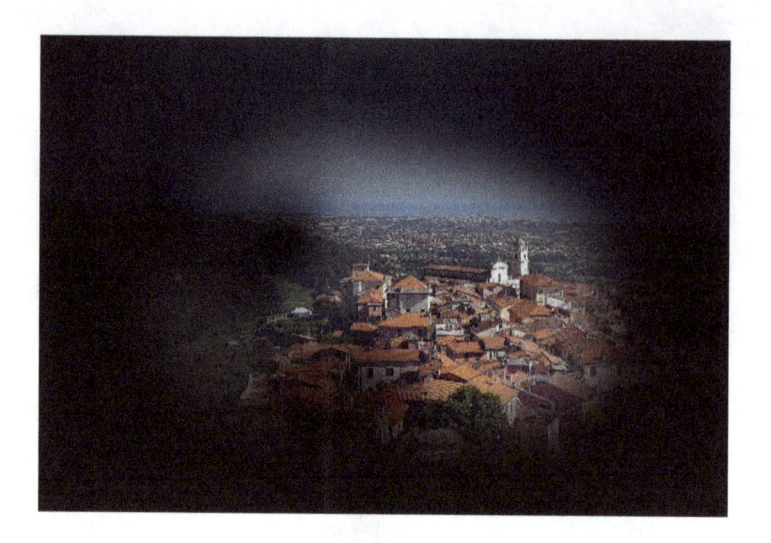

Glaucoma is a serious condition and if left untreated will eventually cause blindness. Even with treatment, within 20 years, approximately 15 percent of people with glaucoma will become blind.

Risk factors of Glaucoma

For the older adult, being aware of these risk factors is important because chronic forms of glaucoma can destroy vision before any signs or symptoms (listed previously) are apparent:

- **Age** - Being over age 60
- **Genetics** - Having a family history of glaucoma
- **Intraocular pressure** - Having high internal eye pressure
- **Heritage** - Being Black, Asian or Hispanic
- **Pre-existing certain medical conditions** - Diabetes, heart disease, high blood pressure, and sickle cell anemia
- **Structural issues** - Having corneas that are thin in the center
- **Refractory Vision** - Being extremely nearsighted or farsighted
- **Trauma** - Having had an eye injury or certain types of eye surgery
- **Steroidal medication** - Taking corticosteroid medications for arthritis or other inflammatory condition, (ie – eyedrops) for a long time

Prevention for Developing Glaucoma

Prevention is essential to slow or preventing vision loss.

- **Get regular dilated eye examinations** – If you have any risk factors and especially if you are over 60, regular comprehensive eye exams will help detect early-stage glaucoma before significant damage can occur.
- **Be aware of your family's eye health history** – Familial history of glaucoma is a significant risk factor.
- **Exercise safely** – Regular exercise my reducing the major risk factors of heart disease, obesity, and diabetes. As well, exercise may help prevent glaucoma by reducing eye pressure.

- **Prescription eye drops need to be taken regularly** – Specifically prescribed Glaucoma eye drops can reduce high eye pressure; however, they need to be used regularly even if no symptoms are present.
- **Wear eye protection** – Eye protection is essential when using power tools or playing high-speed racket sports in enclosed courts. Traumatic eye injuries can lead to glaucoma.

Cataracts

Clouding of the usually clear lens of your eye is referred to as Cataracts. Seeing through cloudy lens of the eye is similar to looking through a frosty or fogged-up window. The clouded vision due to cataracts can make reading, drive a car (especially at night) or seeing a family member of friend's face more challenging.

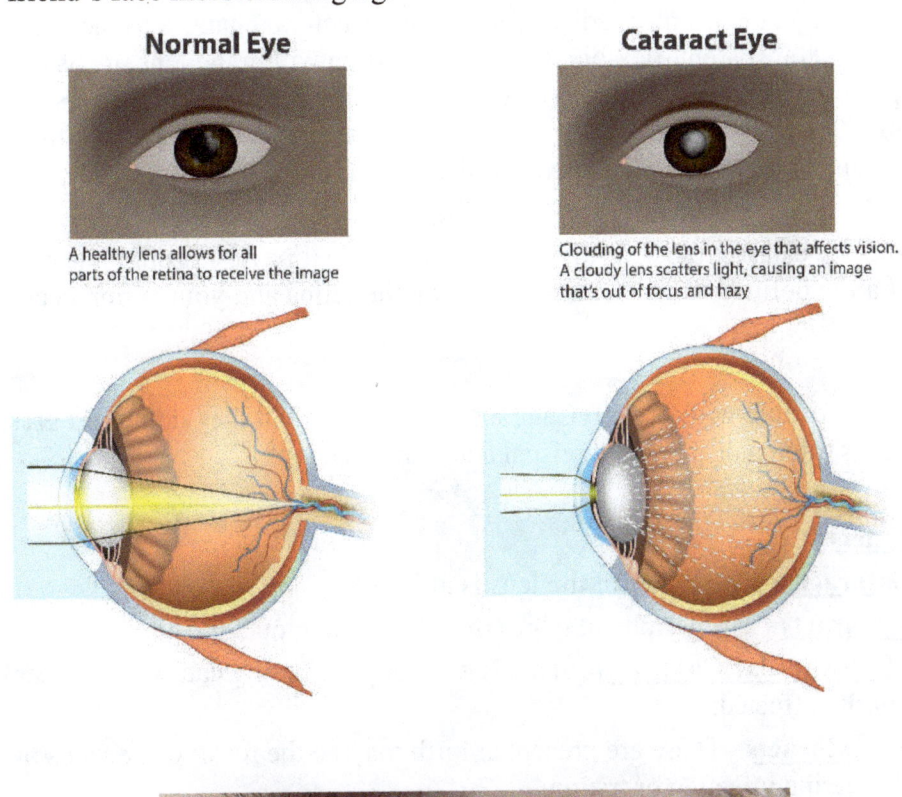

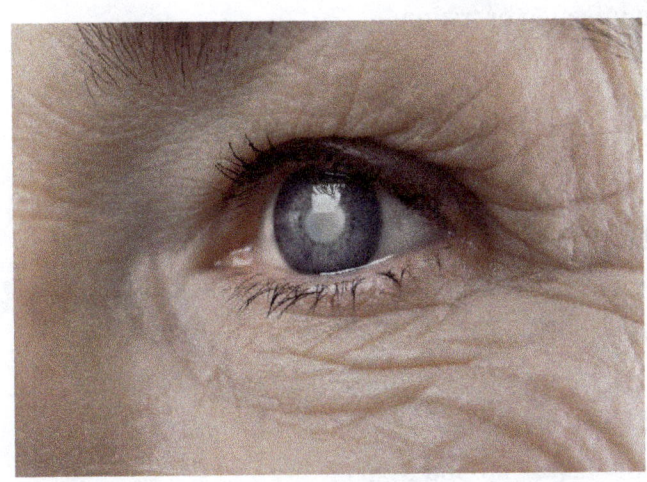

Normal Eye

A healthy lens allows for all parts of the retina to receive the image

Cataract Eye

Clouding of the lens in the eye that affects vision. A cloudy lens scatters light, causing an image that's out of focus and hazy

Cataracts are usually slow developing and eyesight is not affected early on. Unfortunately, cataracts will progress and eventually interfere with your vision. Initially, eyeglasses and stronger lighting will help a person vision, however with progression, cataracts will diminish vision and interfere with a person's usual daily activities. At this stage, cataract surgery may be necessary. Fortunately, Cataract surgery is an effective procedure and generally safe.

Causes of Cataracts
- Advancing age or injury can changes the tissue that makes up the eye's lens.
- Previous eye surgery or pre-existing chronic medical conditions, such as diabetes.
- Long-term use of steroid medications for arthritis or other inflammatory conditions.

How a Cataract Develops

With advancing age, or chronic medical conditions, structural changes to the lens occurs and the lens become less transparent, flexible, and thicker. Often within the lens, its tissue breaks down and the pieces clump together and create small clouded areas within the lens. With time, the lens continues to stiffen and the cataract continues to develop, creating a clouding effect that is denser and involving a more extensive part of the lens.

Once formed, the cataract blocks and scatters the light as it passes through the clouded lens. As a result, a sharply defined image is unable to reach the retina and your vision becomes blurred.

Generally, most people will develop Cataracts in both eyes but they do not progress evenly. As a result, there is often a difference in visual acuity between eyes.

Types of Cataracts
Neutral Cataracts – The center of the lens is affected.
Cortical Cataracts – The peripheral edges of the lens are clouded.
Posterior Subscapular Cataracts – This is a faster progressing cataract. The back of the lens is primarily affected.
Congenital Cataracts – These are present at birth may be the result of genetics or associated with an intrauterine infection or trauma.

Symptoms of Cataracts
- Vision becomes clouded, blurred, or dim.
- Reading or other activities require a brighter lighting
- Vision at night becomes more difficult.
- Eyeglass or contact lens prescription needs frequent changing.
- Increase sensitivity to light and glare
- A single eye may develop double vision
- Colours become yellowish or fading in brightness
- The appearance of "halos" around lights

Symptoms of a Cataract become more noticeable as the Cataract grows and more of the light that passes through the lens gets increasingly distorted.

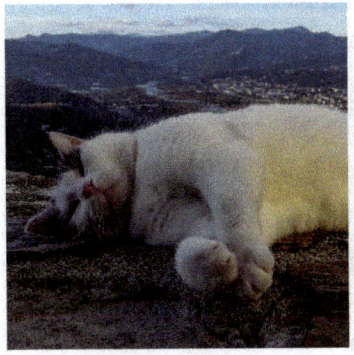

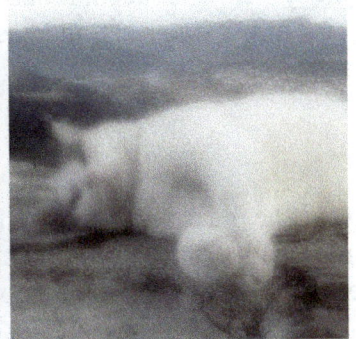

NORMAL VISION   **VISION WITH CATARACT**

Risk factors for Developing Cataracts
- Increasing age
- Excessive exposure to sunlight
- High blood pressure
- Diabetes
- Obesity
- Smoking
- Drinking excessive amounts of alcohol
- Previous eye inflammation or injury
- Lon-term use of corticosteroid medications
- Previous eye surgery

Prevention from the Development of Cataracts
How to prevent cataracts or slow the progression of cataracts is unknown but research suggest several potential prevention strategies:

- **Having regular eye examinations** – Early detection of cataracts is important before vision becomes significantly affected.
- **Quitting smoking** – This is always a good idea to minimize health risks.
- **Managing other health problems** – Good management of existing chronic health problems such as diabetes and arthritis. Long-term corticosteroid use for arthritis must be monitored for side effects
- **Choosing a healthy diet that includes plenty of fruits and vegetables** – Adding a variety of colorful fruits and vegetables to a person's diet ensures that they are getting the necessary amounts of vitamins and nutrients. Fruits and vegetables have many antioxidants, which help maintain a person's eyes. The Mediterranean diet (Chapter 5.2.10) is an excellent choice to follow.

- **Wearing sunglasses** –The suns ultraviolet light from may contribute to cataract development. Minimize eye exposure to ultraviolet B (UVB) rays is strongly recommended by wearing ultraviolet protective sunglasses.
- **Reducing alcohol use** – Like tobacco, reducing alcohol is always a good idea. Research indicates that the risk of Cataracts can increase with excessive alcohol consumption.

Conclusion

Vison care for you as the older adult is extremely important. Impaired or lost vision will significantly affect your quality of life. Fortunately, for most visual/ocular conditions, early detection facilitates effective treatment and a good prognosis.

Regular optometrist appointments are necessary and should become part of every older adult's health plan. You only have two eyes and diminished, or vision loss in one is a big thing. Open your eyes and don't diminish the importance of good eye care.

References

National Eye Institute, *"Facts About Astigmatism"*. October 2010
Rose, D. J. (2010) *Fallproof!:A Comprehensive Balance and Training Program*. Human Kinetics, 2nd edition
Ng., David. O.D., *Vitreous Detachment*, October, 2020
www.bochner.com
www.medlineplus.gov
www.healthline.com
www.sightsavers.com
www.webMD.com
www.mayoclinic.org

2.9. Hearing Impairments and Disorders of the Ear

Introduction

For older adults, hearing loss is a common disability that can significantly affect their functionality and quality of life. Approximately one in three people between the ages of 65 and 74 have hearing loss, and over 50% over 75 years of age have difficulty hearing. Hearing loss is more common in men than women. Fortunately, with the continuing developments in hearing aids, most hearing loss problems can be effectively managed, and the older adult's quality of life can be maintained.

Unfortunately, ear disorders are not limited to just diminished hearing. They can also affect your balance, create dizziness (vertigo) and chronic ringing in your ear (Tinnitus). Each of these can significantly affect your functionality. The cause/etiology of these conditions determines how effectively they are treated.

Ear health is extremely important. Not only does hearing loss have the potential to diminish your communication skills, which contributes to social isolation, but a loss of balance and dizziness leaves you vulnerable to falls. Chronic ringing in your ears can affect your mental health.

Older adults should have their hearing acuity checked yearly. If symptoms of loss of balance, dizziness, or ringing in the ear develops, they should seek medical attention immediately.

Anatomy of the Ear

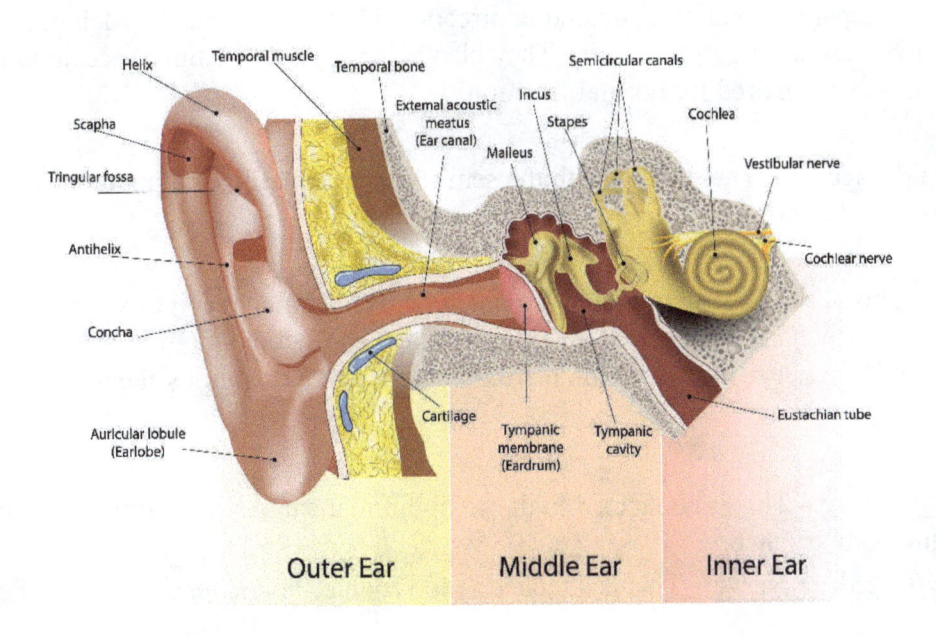

To better understand hearing loss and ear disorders, it is good to have a basic understanding of the ear's anatomy.

Outer Ear
External Ear (Pinna) - Collects and channels sound waves into the ear canal.

Ear Canal (Auditory Canal) – It is the passage way for sound waves, which are amplified and propelled toward the eardrum (tympanic membrane).

Middle Ear
Ear Drum (Tympanic Membrane) – This vibrates to transmit sound waves from the outer ear (ear canal) to the three ossicles inside the middle ear.

Auditory Ossicles (Malleus, Incus, Staples) – These are the smallest three bones the human body. Their function is to transmit sounds from the air to the fluid-filled labyrinth (cochlea) in the inner ear.

Eustachian Tube (Auditory Tube) – This links the nasopharynx, which lies behind the nose in the upper part of the throat, to the middle ear. It is approximately 35 mm (1.4 in) long and has three functions;

1. Equalize pressure - between the nasopharynx to the middle ear.
2. Protection - of the middle ear from loud sounds and nasopharyngeal secretions.
3. Drainage and ventilation of the middle ear.

Inner Ear
Semi-Circular Canals – Their function is related to maintaining balance in space. They are filled with liquid and cilia (microscopic hairs) line the canals. When the head moves, the fluid moves the cilia which acts as a motion sensor for the brain so the brain knows how to keep the body balanced, regardless of its position in space.

There are three parts to the semi-circular canals, the anterior, posterior, and horizontal canals. Each canal has a separate function in detecting directional balance (vertical nodding, lateral head tilting, and horizontal turning right to left). They also help measure rotational acceleration. The left and right canals are paired for normal function.

Utricle and Saccule – These work with the semi-circular canals to maintain balance. They measure linear acceleration.

Cochlea – This is fluid-filled and lined with stereocilia. Cochlea receives vibrational sound from the ossicles, which results in the stereocilia moving. The stereocilia movement converts the vibrational sound into nerve impulses which are transmitted to the brain by the auditory nerve.

Nerves
Vestibular Nerve – This is connected to the semi-circular canals; it is primarily responsible for maintaining body balance.

Auditory/Cochlear Nerve – This is attached to the cochlea and is responsible for hearing.

1. Hearing Impairment

1. Presbycusis

Presbycusis is hearing loss associated with aging and is the most frequent cause of hearing impairment in the older adult.

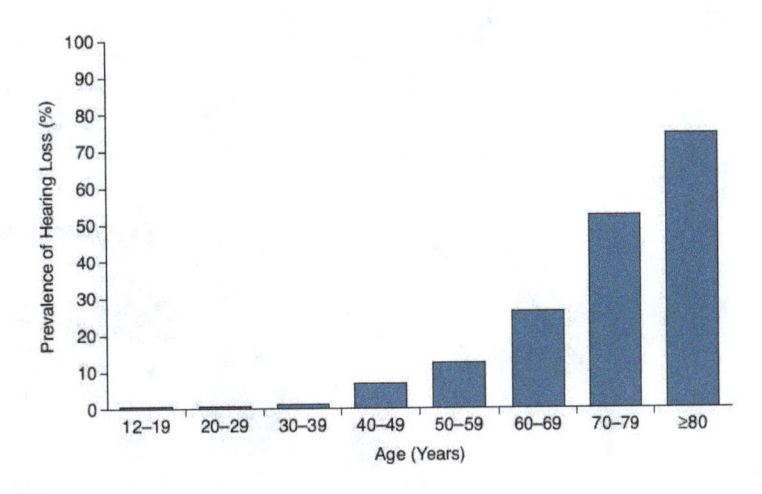

Image Source: nap.edu

Measuring Hearing Loss

Your level of hearing is measured as the minimum loudness in decibels (dB) that they can detect, also called the hearing threshold. A typical hearing test will measure the thresholds at multiple different frequencies, or pitches. An audiogram is a chart that is used to plot the thresholds (dBs), the minimum loudness a person can hear on the vertical axis and the different frequencies on the horizontal axis.

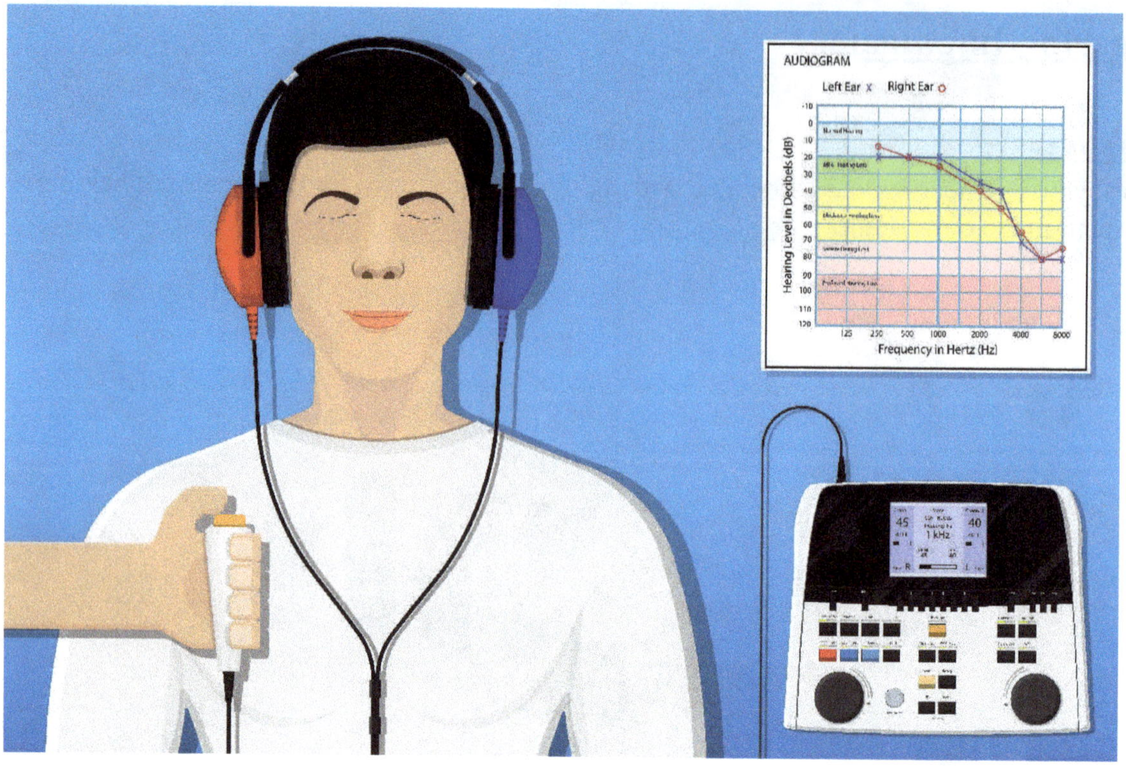
AUDIOGRAM
Left Ear x Right Ear o
Hearing Level in Decibels (dB)
Frequency in Hertz (Hz)
1 kHz

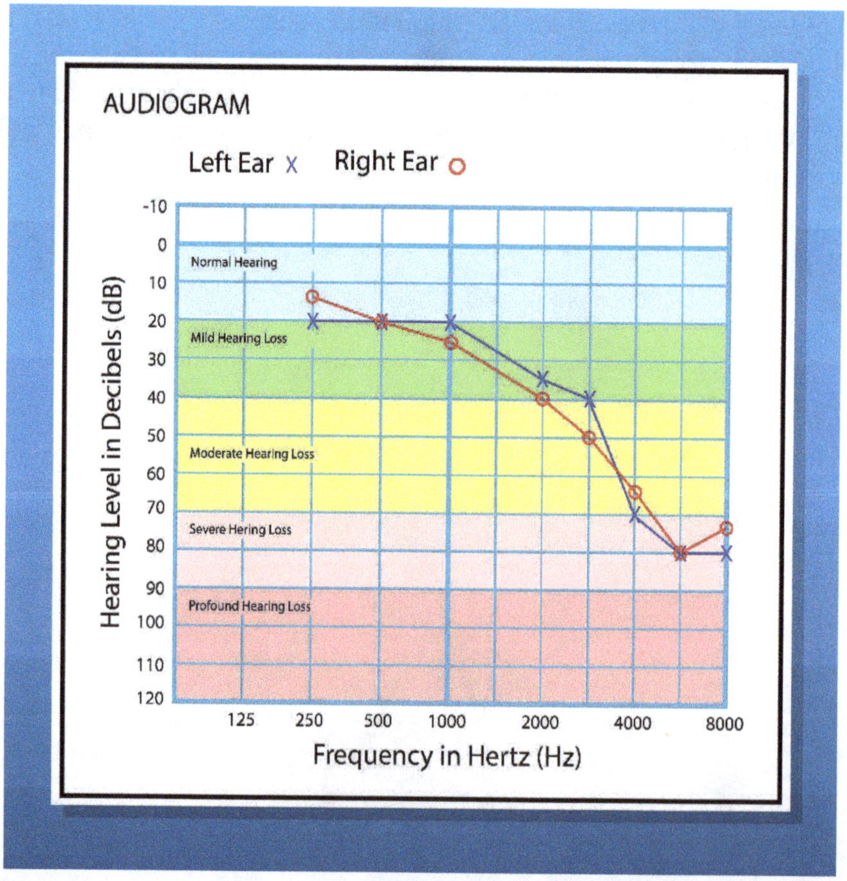
AUDIOGRAM
Left Ear x Right Ear o
Hearing Level in Decibels (dB)
-10
0
10
20
30
40
50
60
70
80
90
100
110
120
Normal Hearing
Mild Hearing Loss
Moderate Hearing Loss
Severe Hering Loss
Profound Hearing Loss
125
250
500
1000
2000
4000
8000
Frequency in Hertz (Hz)

A person's hearing acuity is measured by detecting air conduction with the use of earphones. A small vibrator is placed on the top of a person's head so the vibrated sound waves can largely bypass the eardrum and middle ear and be measured, by the earphones, as they pass directly to the cochlea in the inner ear.

Testing is done one ear at a time, and involves hearing low to high frequencies of tones. The intensity of each frequency of tone is varied with the aim of finding the lowest level of vibrational sounds that you can hear. For example, with a threshold of 55 dB, a person cannot hear any sounds below 55 dB, which is then used as the threshold for that tone's frequency. A person with normal hearing will have a flat line across the top of the audiogram in the normal range. Age-related hearing loss typically affects the higher frequencies first (the graph dips at high frequencies).

Most age-related hearing loss is symmetric. If there is asymmetric hearing loss, this can be a sign of trauma, infection, benign tumor (vestibular schwannoma), eustachian tube dysfunction, Meniere's disease, etc. and require further investigation.

Five Hearing Loss Thresholds Categories:
(Note – Any sound below the threshold cannot be heard)
(Example – Whispering – 30 dB, normal conversation – 60 dB, heavy traffic – 85 dB)

1. **Normal Hearing (0-25 dB)** – A person can hear the softest of sounds.
2. **Mild hearing loss (26-40 dB)** – More difficult to hear soft sounds if there is noise in the background.
3. **Moderate hearing loss (41-55 dB)** – It is more difficult to follow a conversation, especially if background noise is present.
4. **Moderate-Severe hearing loss (71-90 dB)** – Very difficult to follow conversations even in a quite room. A person may start to have difficulty with speech.
5. **Profound hearing loss (above 90 dB)** – Speech and language deteriorate. Hearing gets impossible without hearing aids.

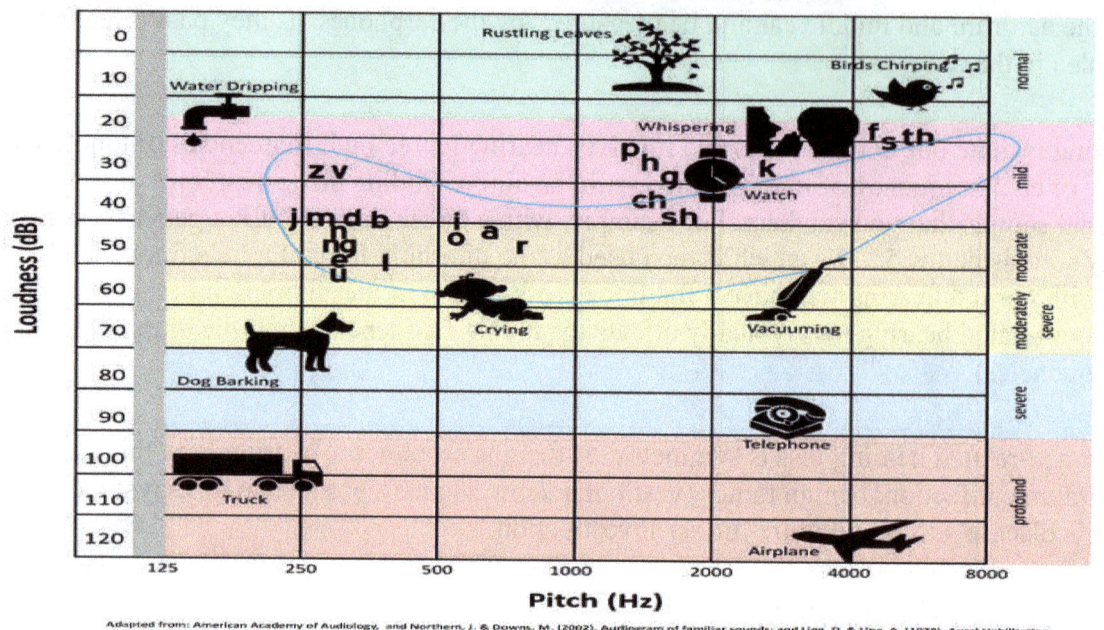

Types of Hearing Loss

    1. Sensorineural (involves inner ear)
    2. Conductive (involves outer or middle ear)
    3. Mixed (combination of the two)

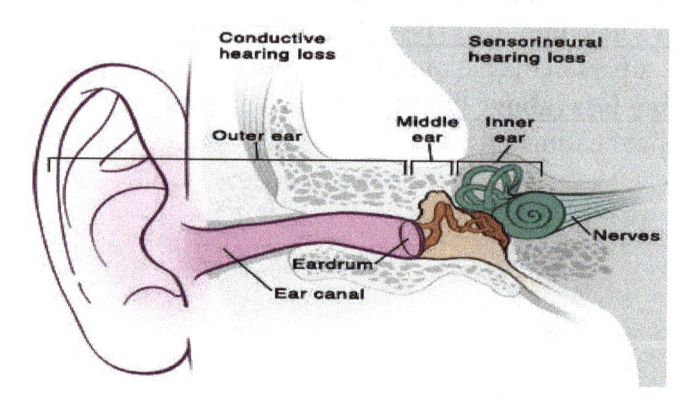

Image Source: saintlukeskc.org

1. Sensorineural Hearing Loss

Sensorineural hearing loss involves damage to the inner ear and is the most frequent age-related cause of the three types of hearing loss.

Specifically, wear and tear on the nerve cells or hairs (stereocilia) in the cochlea (inner ear) that send sound signals to the brain, results from acute or chronic exposure to loud noises and aging. When damage to these structures occurs, the electrical signals become diminished and hearing loss occurs. One of the earliest signs of hearing loss is the difficulty hearing higher-pitched tones (normal conversation) making it difficult to pick out words (they become muffled) against background noise.

Signs and Symptoms of Sensorineural Hearing Loss
1. **Difficulty following personal conversations** – Especially when there's background noise you have to continually asking people to repeat themselves.
2. **Public address announcements become difficulty to understanding**– Especially when spoke from a microphone or loudspeaker.
3. **Phone conversations become difficult to understand** – Sounds seem unclear and mumbled. You have to concentrate much harder to understand the other person.
4. **Difficulty hearing high-pitched sounds** – Such as fingernails scratching, bells ringing, whistles blowing, squeaky sounds.
5. **Ringing or buzzing in the ears (Tinnitus)** – This condition is common with sensorineural hearing loss.

Risk factors
These risk factors may damage or lead to loss of the hairs and nerve cells in your inner ear:

- **Aging** – Results in the inner ear structures (stereocilia) degenerating and becoming less sensitive to the vibrating sounds being transmitted from the ossicles.
- **Loud noise** – Exposure to loud sounds can damage the nerve cells (stereocilia) of your inner ear. This exposure can be from occupational or recreational activities. Damage can be from chronic long-term exposure to loud noises (farming, factory or construction sites or race cars) or an acute short blast of noise, (gunshot, rock concert) (See chart below: Comparing Loudness of Common Sounds).;
- **Heredity** – Familial history of hearing loss (mother, father, sibling) makes other family members more likely to suffer ear damage as they age.
- **Prescription medications** – Certain pain-relieving drugs (high doses of aspirin), antibiotics (gentamicin), certain chemotherapy drugs and the erectile dysfunction drug sildenafil (Viagra), can have the side-effect of damaging the inner ear.
- **High Fever** –Illnesses that can cause high fever, such as meningitis increase the risk of damage to the cochlea stereocilia.

Comparing the Loudness of Common Sounds [1]

Safe noise level is considered to be 70 dB., Less exposure time is necessary for loud noises to cause permanent hearing damage.

Sound levels of common noises

Decibels	Noise source
Safe range	
30	Whisper
40	Refrigerator
60	Normal conversation
75	Dishwasher
Risk range	
85	Heavy city traffic, school cafeteria
95	Motorcycle
100	Snowmobile
110	Chain saw, jackhammer, rock concert, symphony
120	Ambulance siren, thunder
140-165	Firecracker, firearms

Prevention Against Sensorineural Hearing Loss

1. Limit exposure time and use ears plugs – The best prevention is limiting the duration and intensity of your exposure to loud noise. Protect your ears from damaging noise in the workplace or recreational activities by using glycerin-filled earmuffs or plastic earplugs.

2. Regular hearing tests – This is especially important if you are constantly exposed a noisy environment.

3. Avoid high noise recreational risks – Wearing hearing protectors helps but minimizing high noise activities such as riding a snowmobile, hunting, using power tools, or listening to rock concerts is best.

Treatment for Sensorineural Hearing Loss

The only treatment for sensorineural hearing loss is hearing aids. Many shapes and sizes of hearing aids are available. It is important to find a type of hearing aid that fits your needs and type of hearing loss.

Types of Hearing Aids

1. Hearing Aids that Fit in Your Ear

These hearing aids are positioned directly in the ear and are custom-fitted, so they are the right shape and fit for optimum comfort and sound quality. There are no external wires or tubes, so they are very discreet.

Disadvantages include an increased susceptibility to wind noise and damage from ear wax and moisture in the ear. Depending on the level of hearing loss, they may not be appropriate for all patients.

Invisible-In-Canal (IIC)	Completely-In-Canal (CIC)	In-The-Canal (ITC) / Half Shell (HS)	Full Shell (FS)
Mild to Moderately Severe Hearing Loss	Mild to Severe Hearing Loss	Mild to Severe Hearing Loss	Mild to Severe Hearing Loss

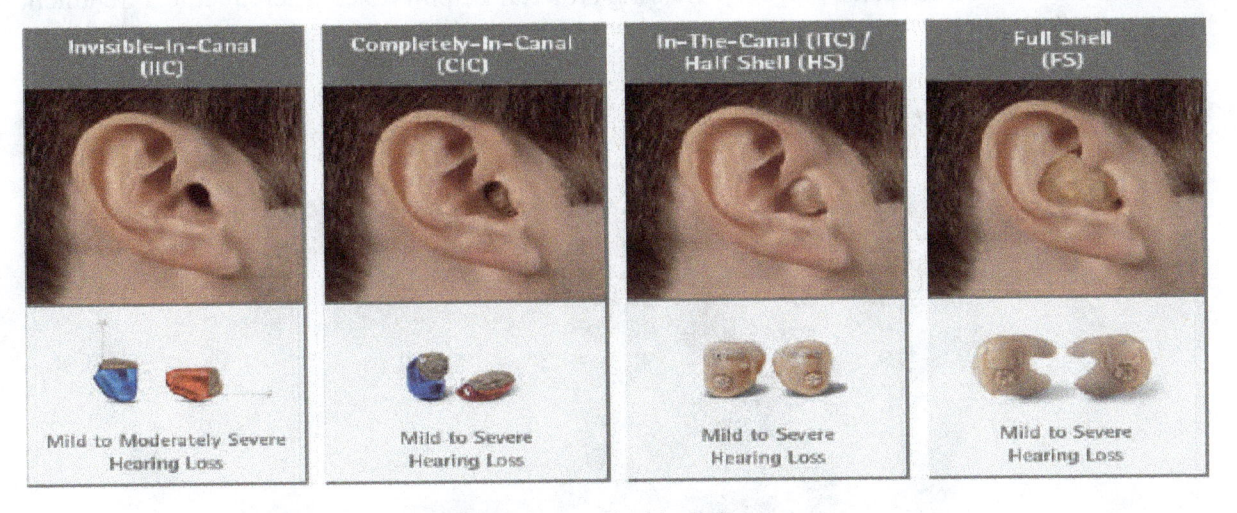

Image Source: harbinclinic.com

2. Behind-the-Ear Hearing Aids

These hearing aids are very powerful, have a longer battery life than the in-ear models, and are best used in cases of more severe hearing loss or smaller ear canals. All the hearing aid components are positioned behind the ear and there is a tube that connects the hearing aid to an earpiece in the ear canal. They are often found to be more comfortable since they do not fit deep into the ear canal.

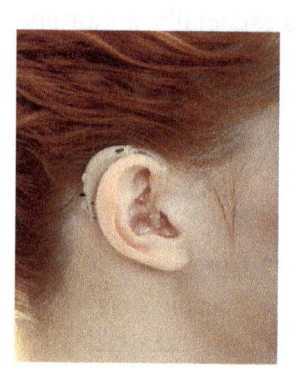

2. Conductive Hearing Loss

This occurs when sounds cannot be transmitted to the inner ear because there is blockage or damage in the outer or middle part of the ear, where sound is converted to vibrations and sent to the inner ear. This type of hearing loss is easily identifiable with causes such as wax build-up in the ear canal, damage/trauma/rupture to the eardrum due to poking, or a loud blast of noise, fluid, and infections in the middle ear, and osteoporosis. The latter occurs because the bones around the ear transmit vibrations to the middle ear. If there is less bone (osteoporosis), there is a diminished ability to transmit these vibrations.

Conductive hearing loss is usually medically treatable (removal of the ear wax in the ear canal, antibiotics for infections, surgery). Hearing aids can help in cases where medical treatment does not work.

3. Tinnitus (Ringing in the Ear)

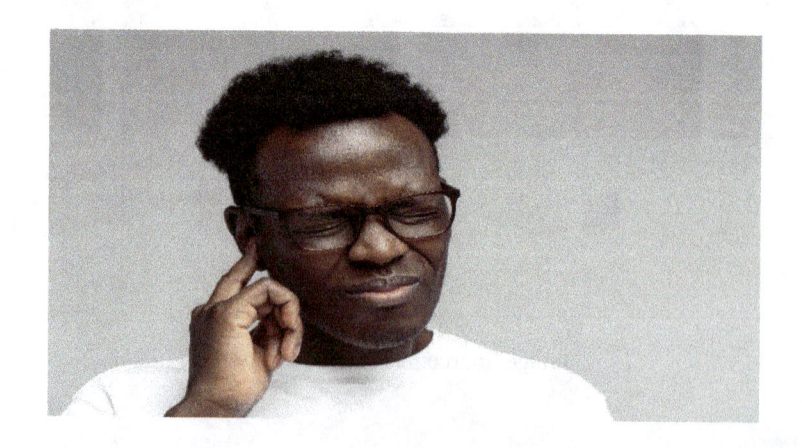

Hearing noises or ringing in one or both of your ears is referred to as Tinnitus. The noise is not caused by an external sound, and only the affected person can hear it. Tinnitus affects about 20% of the population and is very common and troublesome in aging adults. If not treated properly, it can significantly affect the older adults mental health and quality of life.

Usually an underlying condition causes Tinnitus, and can include, age-related hearing loss (Presbycusis), broken or damaged hair cells (stereocilia) in the cochlea, compromising of how blood moves through nearby blood vessels such as the carotid artery due to atherosclerosis, injury to the jaw joint (temporomandibular joint) or how the brain processes sound. Treatment focuses on identifying and eliminating the underlying cause or reducing the noise so the tinnitus less bothersome.

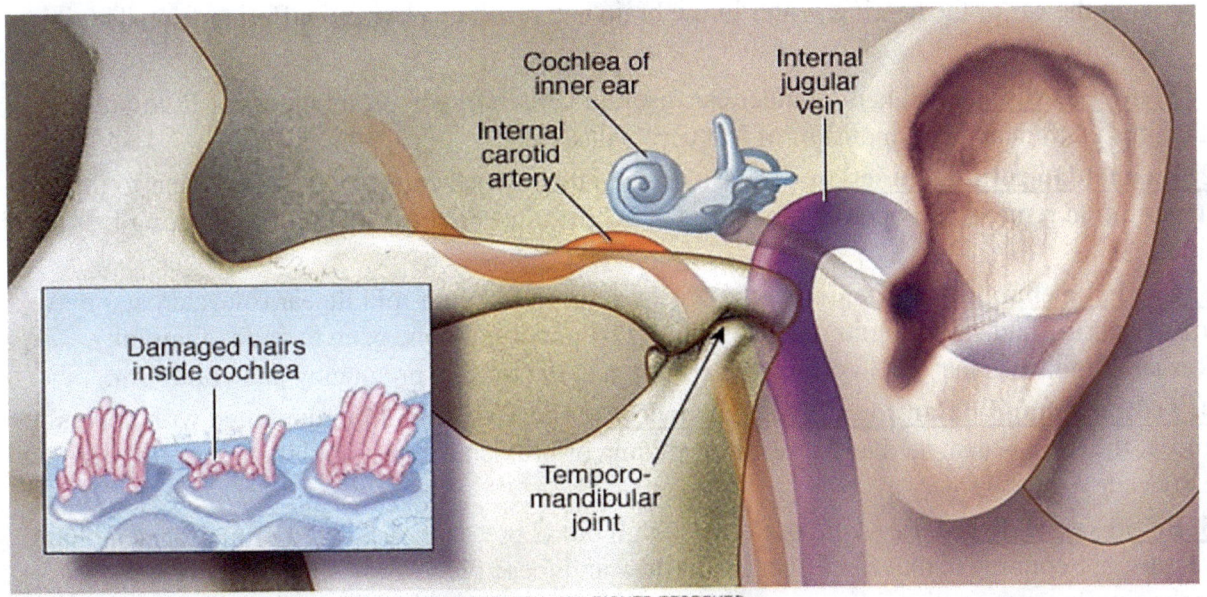

Symptoms of Tinnitus
Ringing in the ears is how Tinnitus is usually described but the noise has been reported to buzzing, clicking, hissing, and humming. The noises can be heard in one or both ears and will vary in pitch from a low roar to a high squeal. The Tinnitus can be so disruptive that it interferes with your ability to hear external sound or to concentrate. Tinnitus can occur intermittently or be present all the time.

Common Causes of Tinnitus
1. Ear infection or ear canal blockage – The outer ear canal becomes blocked as a result of a build-up of earwax, dirt, fluid (ear infection), or a foreign material. This blockage results in an increase in inner ear pressure and reducing hearing, which makes the tinnitus more noticeable.

2. Hearing loss – If the nerve hairs inside the inner ear (stereocilia in the cochlea) are damaged as a result of age or chronic exposure to loud sounds, they can produce random electrical impulses to the brain, causing tinnitus.

3. Head or neck injuries – Head or neck trauma usually causes tinnitus in only one ear. The stereocilia of the cochlea can be damaged, or the brain function linked to hearing becomes impaired.

4. Medications –Nonsteroidal anti-inflammatory drugs (NSAIDs), antibiotics, cancer drugs, diuretics, and antidepressants, may cause or worsen tinnitus. The higher and longer the dose of these medications, the worse tinnitus becomes. If a person stops using these drugs, Tinnitus often disappears.

Less Common Causes of Tinnitus
Other ear problems, chronic health conditions, and injuries or conditions that affect the nerves in the ear or the hearing center in the brain can result in a person suffering from Tinnitus.

1. Meniere's disease –This is an inner ear disorder caused by abnormal inner ear fluid pressure. Tinnitus is often an early indicator of Meniere's disease

2. Eustachian tube dysfunction –The Eustachian tube which connects the middle ear to the upper throat remains too open or too closed which results in the ear feeling full, hearing loss or tinnitus.

3. Ear bone changes – Stiffening of the bones (ossicles) in your middle ear (otosclerosis) may affect hearing and cause tinnitus. This is caused by abnormal bone growth and is familial. Research indicates that it will often affect women at the time of pregnancy and childbirth.

4. Temporomandibular Joint (TMJ) disorders – The TMJ is highly innervated with nerves and, if the joint is damaged as the result of trauma or bruxism (grinding/clenching teeth), tinnitus can occur.

5. Blood vessel disorders –Atherosclerosis, high blood pressure, or kinked or malformed blood vessels, are conditions that can affect blood flow and these blood flow changes can cause or make tinnitus more noticeable.

6. Other medical conditions –Diabetes, thyroid problems, migraines, anemia, and autoimmune disorders such as rheumatoid arthritis and lupus have all been associated with tinnitus.

Risk factors for Developing Tinnitus

1. Exposure to loud noise –Heavy equipment, chainsaws, and firearms, MP3 players are common sources of loud noise-related hearing loss. Noisy environments such as factories and construction work, musicians, and soldiers are particularly at risk.

2. Age – With advancing age, the number of functioning nerve fibers in your ears declines, potentially causing hearing problems often associated with tinnitus.

3. Sex – Men are more prone to experience tinnitus than women.

4. Tobacco and alcohol use – Long standing smoking and chronic alcohol use compromises your cardiovascular system resulting in high blood pressure and deterioration of your overall health.

Complications

The severity of Tinnitus varies from person to person but the complications associated with Tinnitus can affect the persons quality of life. The older adults, is especially vulnerable to these secondary symptoms.

- Trouble concentrating
- Memory problems
- Anxiety and irritability
- Headaches
- Depression
- Fatigue
- Stress
- Sleep problems

Treating these secondary conditions does not affect Tinnitus directly, but can significantly improve the quality of life of the person suffering from Tinnitus.

Prevention of Tinnitus

Precautions, similar to those for hearing loss, have been found to can help prevent certain kinds of tinnitus.

1. **Use hearing protection** – As with hearing loss, it is good practice to limit exposure to loud sounds and wear protective hearing devices that will help protect the nerve cells (stereocilia) in the inner ear.
2. **Turn down the volume** – Long-term exposure to amplified music can cause hearing loss and tinnitus.
3. **Take care of your cardiovascular health** – Tinnitus has been linked to obesity, high blood pressure and atherosclerosis so regular exercise, eating a healthy diet, and managing chronic stress are good preventative steps.
4. **Limit alcohol, caffeine, and nicotine** – These substances used over a long time can affect blood vessel health and blood flow in the carotid artery which can contribute to tinnitus.

3. Vertigo/Dizziness

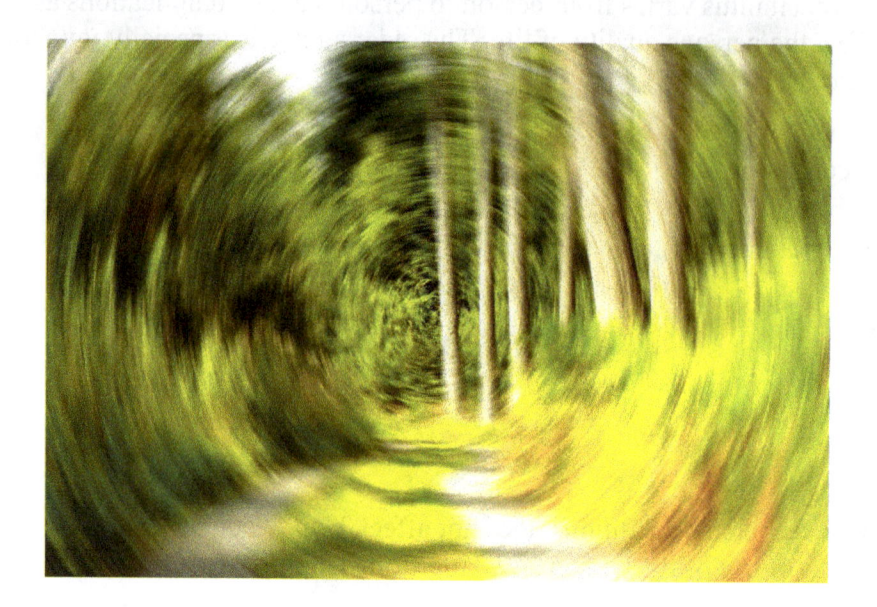

Vertigo is a symptom, not an illness. It is characterized by a sensation of spinning, as if a person's surrounding environment is spinning in circles around them. Vertigo/dizziness is a common complaint in older adults, affecting 70% of individuals who are 65 or older. Vertigo/dizziness is significant because it creates dynamic postural imbalances, which significantly increases the risk of falling.

There are many causes of vertigo/dizziness in older adults but Peripheral Vestibular Dysfunction (PVD) is the most frequent cause. PVD results from pathology of the ear's vestibular structures and of the eighth cranial nerve resulting in diminished sensory information to the brain regarding head position and movement. The most frequent form of Peripheral Vestibular Dysfunction in the elderly is Benign Paroxysmal Positional Vertigo (BPPV) followed by Meniere's disease.

Causes of Vertigo
1. Benign Paroxysmal Positional Vertigo (BPPV)

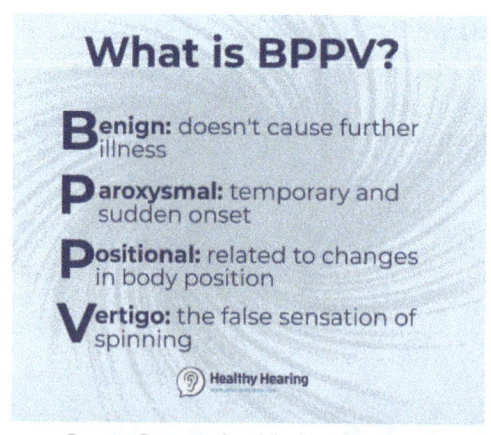

What is BPPV?
- **B**enign: doesn't cause further illness
- **P**aroxysmal: temporary and sudden onset
- **P**ositional: related to changes in body position
- **V**ertigo: the false sensation of spinning

Image Source: healthyhearing.com

As mentioned, the most frequent cause of vestibular dysfunction and vertigo/dizziness is Benign paroxysmal positional vertigo (BPPV). Women are affected more frequently than men.

BPPV presents as brief episodes of mild to intense dizziness that is triggered by changes in a person's head's position, such as when they move their head vertically up or down, when they lie down, or turn or sit up in bed.

BPPV is troublesome but rarely a serious problem, however, it significantly increases the chance of falls for older adults.

The Ear's Role in BPPV
The inner ear contains the vestibular labyrinth, which includes the three loop-shaped semi-circular canals that contain fluid and cilia (hairlike sensors) that monitor rotational head movement and the utricle and saccule which contain crystals that monitor linear head movement.

Unfortunately, these crystals in the utricle and saccule can become dislodged and when they do, they usually move into the posterior canal of the semi-circular canals. This new position of the crystals causes the semi-circular canal to become increasingly sensitive to head movements and results in you feeling dizzy.

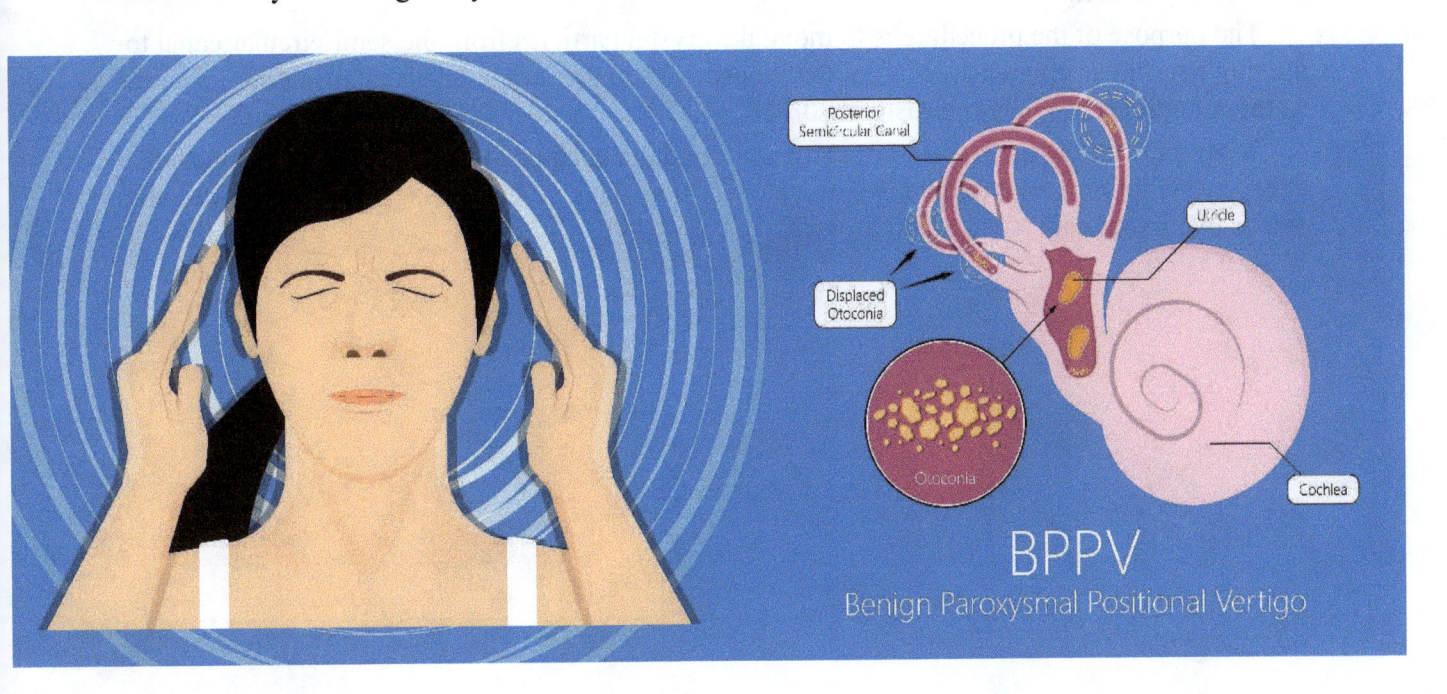

Symptoms of BPPV
- Dizziness and spinning (vertigo). You feel as if your surroundings are moving.
- Your balance is lost and you feel an increase sense of unsteadiness
- Nausea
- Vomiting

The symptoms of BPPV are transitory, usually last less than one minute, but often are recurrent.

The cause of BPPV varies but is almost always initiated by a change in head position.

Complications of Suffering from BPPV

Benign Proximal Positional Vertigo is uncomfortable because the spinning sensation results in a loss of balance and nausea but the most significant complication, especially for the older adult is the increased risk of falling.

Treatment for BPPV

Benign paroxysmal positional vertigo typically goes away on its own, usually within a few weeks or months. However, the "Canalith Repositioning Procedure", which is self administered, has been developed to help relieve BPPV sooner.

Canalith Repositioning Procedure

This procedure, which consists of several simple and slow maneuvers of the head, can be taught to you by your health care practitioner, physiotherapist and audiologist, so you can perform it yourself.

The purpose of the procedure is to move the crystal particles from the semi-circular canal to the tiny bag-like open area (vestibule) that houses one of the utricle or saccules in your inner ear so these particles can be more easily resorbed.

When performing the re-positioning procedure, hold each position for about 30 seconds or after any symptoms, or abnormal eye movements stop. This procedure is usually successful after one or two treatments.

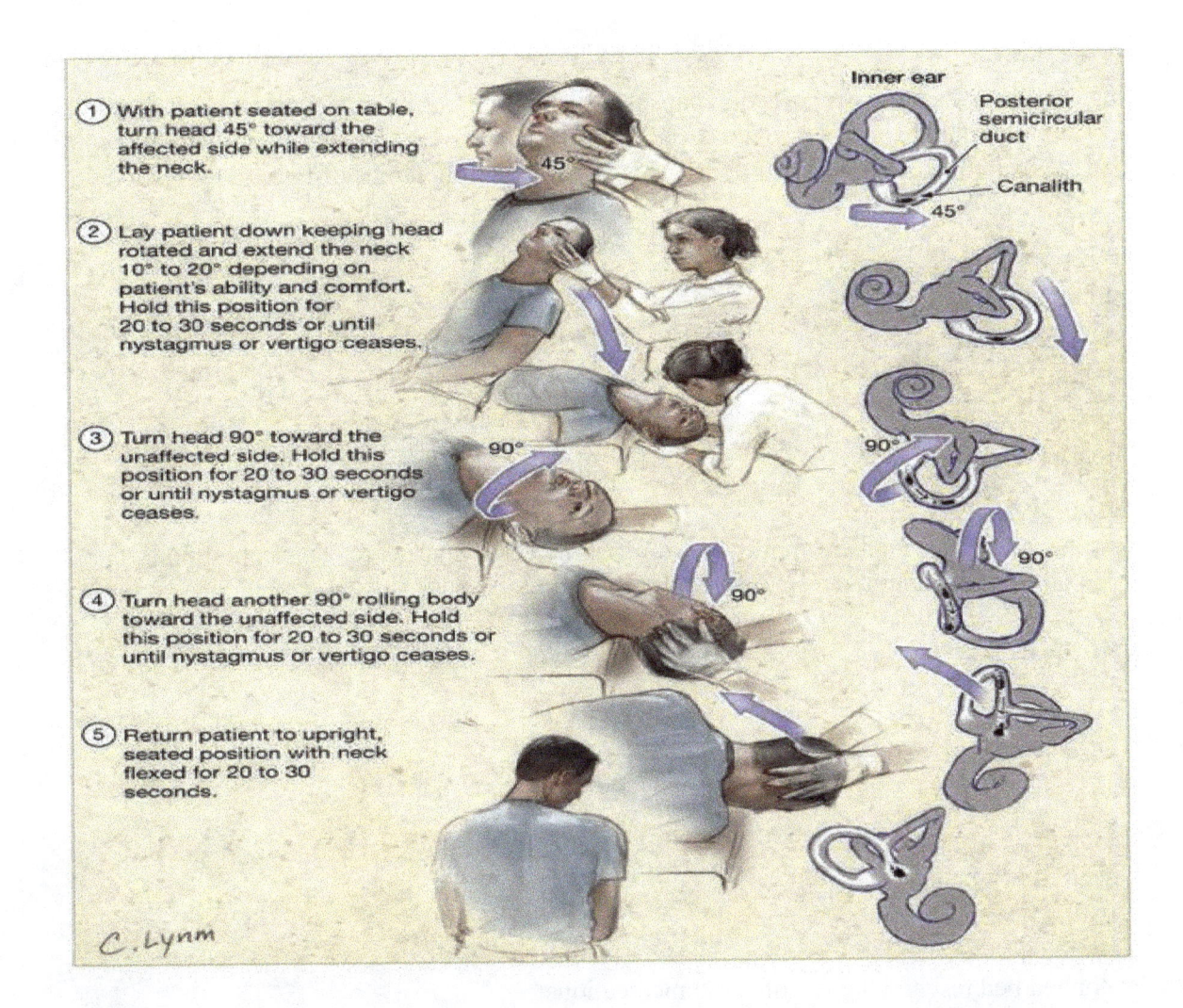

Surgical Alternative in the Treatment of BPPV

Rarely a surgical procedure may be recommended if the Canalith Repositioning Procedure doesn't work. With this surgical procedure, a bone plug is used in the inner ear to prevent the semi-circular canal from responding to general head or crystal movements. This surgical alternative is considered a treatment of last resort because of risk of hearing loss with this procedure.

Other Medical Conditions that can lead to vertigo include the following:

1. Meniere's Disease

This is the second leading cause of vertigo/dizziness in older adults. Meniere's Disease is characterized by vertigo, ringing in the ears (tinnitus), and hearing loss due to a build-up of fluid in the inner ear. It usually occurs in people between the ages of 40 and 60.

Viral infection, blood vessel constriction, or an autoimmune reaction are possible causes but the exact cause is unknown. Research indicates that a genetic familial component may also exist.

2. Labyrinthitis

This condition occurs when infection causes inflammation of the inner ear's semi-circular canals. The inflammation affects vestibulocochlear nerve ability to send information to the brain about head position, motion, and sound. Besides vertigo, complications of Labyrinthitis include;

- Hearing loss
- Tinnitus
- Headaches
- Ear pain
- Vision changes

3. Vestibular neuritis

Vestibular neuritis results from inflammation of the vestibular nerve. This condition is similar to labyrinthitis, but it does not affect your hearing. Besides vertigo, common symptoms are;

- blurred vision
- severe nausea
- feeling of being off-balance

Other Factors that Can Cause Vertigo

- A head injury
- Ear surgery
- Migraine headaches
- Prolonged bed rest and the use of some medications
- A stroke or a transient ischemic attack (TIA or mini-stroke)
- Shingles in or around the ear
- Otosclerosis, when a middle ear bone growth problem leads to hearing loss
- Cerebellar or brain stem disease

A Warning

Besides the increase risk of falling, it is unusual for dizziness/vertigo to signal a serious illness. However, if any of the following symptoms are present with vertigo a person should consult with their medical doctor immediately:

- A fever
- Hearing loss
- Trouble speaking
- Double vision or loss of vision
- A new, different, or severe headache
- Numbness or tingling
- Leg or arm weakness
- Falling or difficulty walking
- Loss of consciousness

Conclusion

Hearing loss/impairment and ear disorders such as tinnitus and Begin Proximal Postural Vertigo/Dizziness are significant conditions that can significantly affect the quality of life of the older adult if they go undetected and untreated. For the most part, diagnosis for these conditions is relatively straightforward and treatment successful.

The risk of social isolation due to communication problems resulting from hearing loss increases mental health challenges for older adults. As well, the increased risk of falling due to vertigo/dizziness cannot be underestimated.

The ideal situation is for older adults to have their hearing and ear health checked every year. The older adult's ability to communicate effectively and function and move safely without the threat of falling is greatly dependent on their hearing and ear health.

Early detection of hearing loss and the use of hearing aids ensures the auditory cortex in the brain remains active and makes hearing loss easier to rehabilitate as time goes on. Unfortunately, older adults often wait years to get hearing aids. By then, the auditory cortex has partially shut down and newly fitted hearing aids can do nothing.

Exercise and the maintenance of core strength (Chapter 4.2.2) is crucial to helping you compensate for imbalance that can occur as inner ear function declines. As discussed in Chapter 4.3, Fall Prevention: Agility, Balance and Coordination Training, the brain uses three main sets of reflex signals to maintain balance/orientation; 1. Vestibular (inner ear), 2. Visual (eyes), 3. Proprioceptive (joints, tendons and muscles). If one of these signals weakens (vestibular (inner ear)) the other two will compensate to a certain degree. Maintaining good leg and hip strength and core stability is significant for the older adult to maintain balance and prevent falls.

Those funny-looking structures on the side of your head are important. It is an excellent idea to make sure they are working correctly.

References

www.ncbi.nlm.nib.gov
www.healthline.com
www.myoclinic.org
www.hearinglife.ca

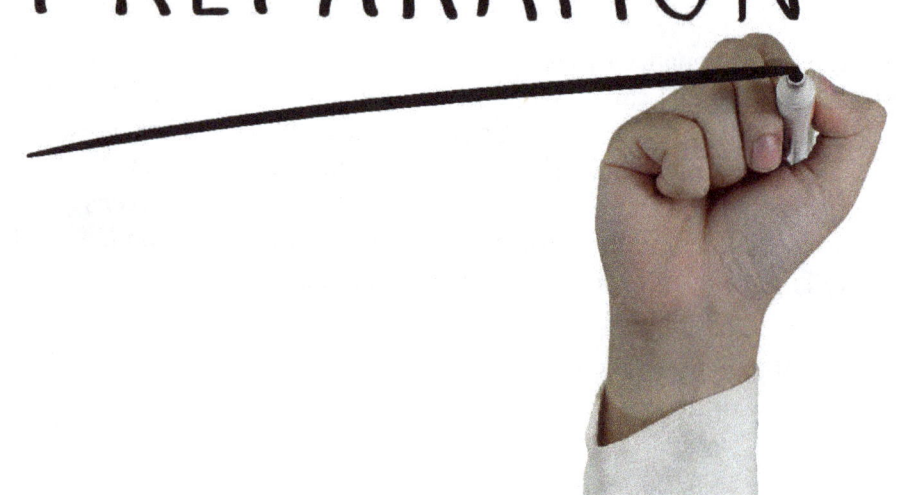

Section 3

Pre-Season – Preparation Time so You Can Perform at Your Best

SUCCESS NEEDS PREPARATION

3.0. Introduction: The Preseason: Preparation Time

In football or in any sport, the Preseason is a time for preparation. In the preceding section, the Off-Season, we studied the clinical conditions that pose opposition to a person's, and specifically an older adult's, health and quality of life. The clinical conditions presented were; arthritis, heart disease, cancer, diabetes, obesity, dementia, oral and dental decay, visual and hearing impairments. Understanding the clinical significance of these potential health challenges allows you to better prepare yourself for prevention and management.

The Preseason is the time to learn new skills, so the health and fitness lifestyle plan that you develop later (Section 4: The Offense, Section 5: The Defense, and Section 6: The Special Teams) will be successful in meeting these health and quality of life challenges. The new skills developed from reading this section are specific and invaluable. They will help guide you through challenging times as you implement your fitness and health plan.

You can refer back to this section often to help refresh your memory on how to proceed successfully. If you are not motivated and prepared properly before the season starts, before you begin to implement your fitness and health plan, you are destined for failure when the going gets tough. Preparation is essential because there will be many turbulent times when it will feel easier to quit than continue.

Success starts with good preseason preparation.

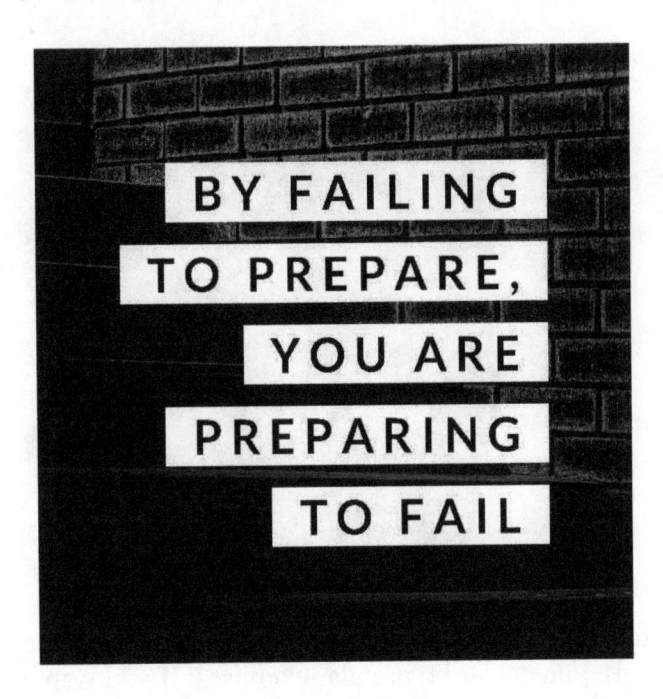

BY FAILING TO PREPARE, YOU ARE PREPARING TO FAIL

3.1. The Eight Golden Rules of Training

Introduction

As a personal physical trainer, I often get asked the secret of achieving a lifetime of improved health and fitness. Unfortunately, there is no "magic bullet," but there are "Golden Rules" that everyone can easily follow to increase the probability of long-term success.

I stress "long term" because that is this book's goal, and it should be everyone's goal. People often have great intentions of improving their health and fitness levels but don't follow through. At one time or another, most of us have set New Year's resolutions to improve our health and fitness. Unfortunately, after one, two, or six months, those well-intentioned goals/resolutions are long gone. A multitude of excuses are given, such as "I am too busy," "It's no fun," or "I got sick/injured and couldn't get started again." Whatever the excuse may be, the bottom line is that you are not improving your health, which is not a good thing.

Most people do not adhere to a long-term fitness and health plan because they start all wrong despite their good intentions. This chapter covers the eight most important rules of training. Close adherence to these rules is necessary if you are to have long-term success with your training.

1. Be Specific

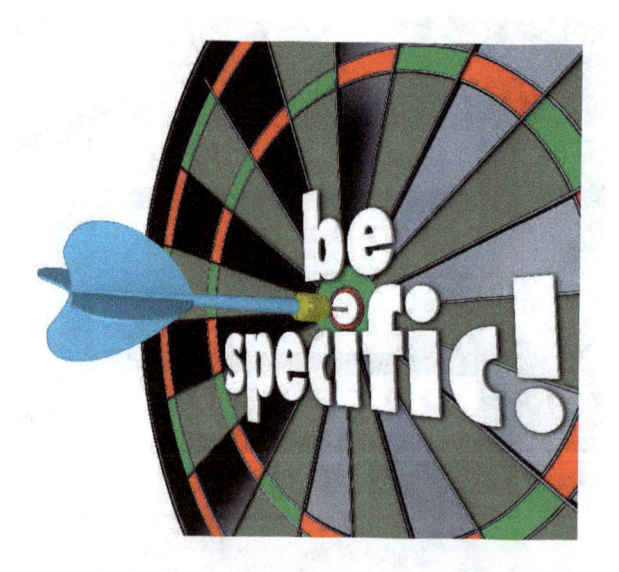

The best way to exercise is to be as specific as possible. Exercising the right way means that if you want a stronger heart, you do cardiovascular exercises; if you want stronger arms, focus your muscle resistance training of the arms. The same is true for each muscle group or region (chest, upper and lower back, hips, legs, and core) in the body.

Many exercises do have a cross-over effect. For example, doing a proper bicep curl requires you to engage your core for stabilization. However, if you really want to strengthen your core, there are specific exercises to do for each part of your core. The same goes for improving flexibility fitness. If you want to improve your ability to bend over and touch your toes, you must do stretches that will improve the flexibility of your lower back and hamstrings.

When you establish fitness goals, you must specify what you want to achieve. For example, if you set the goal that you are going to be a strong walker, you need to walk and walk at a specific pace to raise your heart rate enough to have a training effect. Once again, the same holds true for flexibility. A person stretching their legs does not improve their shoulder range of motion. To achieve maximum training results, you need to be as specific as possible concerning your cardiovascular, muscle strengthening, and flexibility exercises.

2. Start Low and Progress Slowly

small steps every day

Begin exercising at a low intensity and progress slowly when adding intensity is one of the most critical and misunderstood points concerning exercise. Not adhering to this principle far exceeds all other reasons people fail to reach their fitness and health goals.

Typically, when you start an exercise program, you are highly motivated and are "pumped" to get in the best physical condition possible, but that does not mean you should start too aggressively with an exercise routine. Your body is consistently, physically and emotionally, adapting to stress that it is subject to. If your body and mind are subject to the physical and emotional stress of exercise too quickly, injury and exhaustion develops. It takes time for positive physical and mental adaptations to exercise to occur.

People start their physical training at different fitness levels, so you should be starting at the level of intensity and frequency of exercising that is right for you. If you have not been training regularly for the past few months, starting by doing three cardio and three strength training sessions a week is too much. After two or three weeks, you will typically hit the "wall" physically and emotionally. Physically, when you are not giving your body sufficient recovery time, it starts to become achy and stiff, which exponentially increases your chance of injury.

Mentally and emotionally, when starting too aggressively, you are not giving yourself enough time to make regular exercise a habit. It takes doing something regularly about 21 times before it becomes ingrained as a habit. If you go from zero to six exercise sessions per week all at once, you have not created a habit, you have created a nightmare.

Over a few short weeks, you will not only become physically tired and achy, but you will also become emotionally tired. This is because you have added so much new activity into your already busy schedule. As a result, after about three weeks, you will not be looking forward to your training sessions and will be looking for ways to avoid them. You will start to accept the simplest of excuses for not exercising.

The failure of people to adhere to a regular exercise schedule is why fitness clubs are constantly looking for new clients. Fitness and health clubs do a terrible job of educating their new and existing clients on how best to introduce an exercise routine into their daily schedule. Consequently, after a couple of months, the best-intentioned client stops going. At first, they miss one scheduled exercise session per week, then it is two, then three, and so on. Failure is inevitable.

It is very discouraging to start enthusiastically and see this enthusiasm diminish over a few weeks because of injury or exhaustion. As Lao Tzu, the Chinese philosopher said, "The flame that burns twice as bright burns half as long." The key is to start slowly. For anyone who is beginning to exercise after a long layoff, their weekly exercise frequency should be no more than twice or three sessions per week. Equally important is to start with low intensity, which means low weights/resistance and short cardio exercise. You can learn more on how to start properly in Chapter 4.1.1: Cardiovascular Fitness Training and Chapter 4.2.2: Muscular Resistance Training: Developing Muscular Strength and Endurance.

The goal is for you to build upon this conservative start every couple of weeks. In a short period, you will be surprised at how well you are doing, and how much you are enjoying exercising. Most importantly, you will stay motivated and injury-free.

3. Consistency and Sustainability

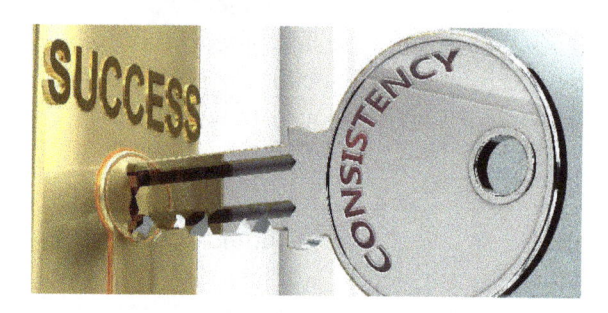

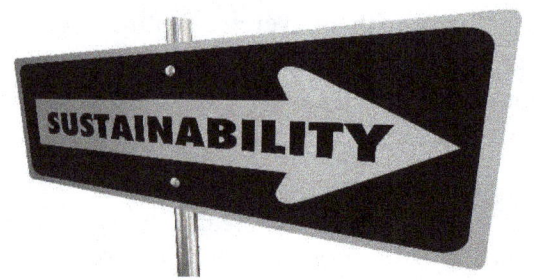

This rule is almost as important as the previous one. This is the key to training success. The Low and Slow rule focused on starting the right way so you can begin a successful routine and are less likely to lose motivation or get injured and stop. The consistency and sustainability principle focuses on getting the best results from your exercise routine.

As mentioned previously, the body responds very favorably to physical stress if introduced conservatively. However, to receive maximal benefit from exercise, it must be done consistently and sustained over a long period. Doing two strength training sessions and two cardio sessions one week and only one of each the next week will not allow you to achieve the result you want. The body needs consistent and sustained stress to build strength and endurance. Consistency and sustainability are the keys to successful exercising, but are often the overlooked components of the "overload" principle in training.

The lack of consistency and sustainability is also true concerning nutrition and why most diets fail. The changes that most diet programs introduce to a person occur too quickly and are too severe compared to what one is used to. The change is too drastic and, as a consequence, is not sustainable. You may lose weight initially, but once you veer off the recommended program, you will lack consistency, and the weight quickly returns.

It is a generally accepted principle in physical training that you will lose what new level of fitness you have gained twice as quickly as it took for you to attain it. As a result, start low and slow, be consistent, and do it over a sustained period to achieve your health and fitness goals.

4. Recovery Time

> **REST & RECOVERY DAYS:**
>
> 1. Rebuild & Repair Muscle Tissue
> 2. Strengthen Joints and Ligaments
> 3. Replenish Fluids & Energy Stores
> 4. Refresh Our Mental Energy
> 6. Reduce Risk of Injury
> 7. Avoid Overtraining

Image Source: theresidentbrainnerd-wordpress.com

Allowing sufficient recovery time is also an often overlooked but crucial aspect in developing a training schedule. Recovery time is an important indicator of your fitness level as well. Generally speaking, the more physically and emotionally conditioned you are, the less time you need to recover from a specific exercise session. The more intense your exercise session, the more recovery time is necessary. Time is your friend when it comes to building fitness, getting sufficient recovery, staying injury-free and motivated.

It is important to understand that all of your training sessions should not be of the same level of intensity. If you are doing three cardio sessions per week, one of your cardio sessions may be intense such as a spin class or interval (HIIT) training. The other two sessions should be more of mild or moderate intensity. The mild to moderate intense sessions may be a long, moderately paced walk or an easily manageable bike ride. These mild to moderately intense sessions are active recovery sessions. After an intense spin session or a hill walk, you will need to give yourself more recovery time (for example, two days) than you will need after a long slow walk or an easy bike ride (possibly one day).

Experience goes a long way to understanding how much recovery time you need. It is essential to listen to your body. Eight signs of overtraining and not giving yourself sufficient recovery time are:

1. Feeling consistently achy and sore between exercise sessions.
2. Restless sleep and not waking up feeling refreshed.
3. Your energy level is generally low. You do not feel like doing anything outside of work and exercise.
4. Mood swings. You feel more agitated and have less patience than usual.
5. Not looking forward to your workouts. You find it becoming increasingly laborious to do them.
6. You find that you are becoming prone to injury.
7. You find yourself suffering more head colds and chest infections because your immune system has become weaker.
8. Your resting heart rate is elevated. To monitor this, develop the habit of checking your heart rate before you get out of bed each morning.

The body's adaptation to exercise and its ability to develop strength and endurance occur while in recovery mode. It is essential that the body has sufficient time to recover to allow physical improvements to occur. Over time, you will see improvements and leave yourself less vulnerable to acute and overuse injuries.

5. Change Up Your Routine

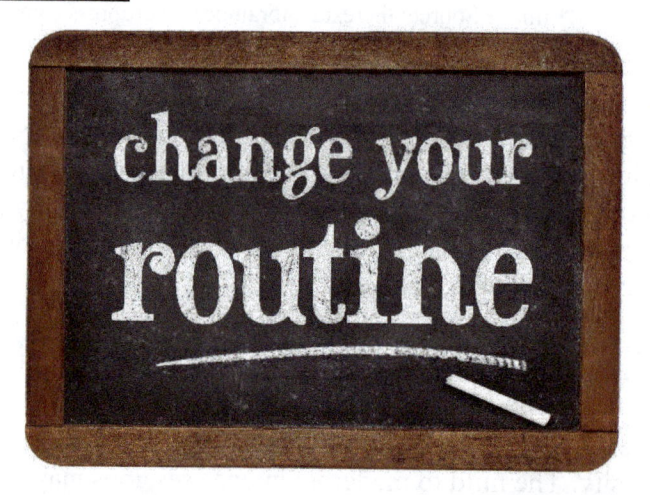

Variety is the spice of life, and for exercise, it is the key to avoiding hitting the dreaded plateau wall. As mentioned previously, the body has a remarkable ability to adapt to physical stress. However, if you don't consistently change how the physical stress of exercise is applied, the body will only adapt so much until growth slows and plateaus. The changes in your training routine don't have to be drastic, but they are needed relatively frequently. A good rule is to make changes in the exercise routine every five weeks or after every ten exercise sessions. For example, if you are doing upper body strength training twice a week, change the exercises in the routine after five weeks.

To illustrate: to strengthen the chest, you decide to do a certain number and types of push ups. That is a great exercise to do to achieve a stronger chest. A "regular" push up is done with the hands about shoulder-width apart. You may do them in a full plank position (on your toes) or, if that is beyond your fitness level at this time, you can do them in a modified position (knees touching the mat). The key to a good "regular" push up is to do them rhythmically on a count of one, two down, one, two up. Keep the body in a straight plank position with the core (stomach) tight, and lower to just before the nose touches the ground.

There are many variations to the "regular" push up so that a person can "confuse" the neuropathways to the muscles and avoid muscle memory and plateauing. For example, rather than the hands being shoulder-width apart, they can be positioned inward toward your ribs (Military) or outward so they are much wider than shoulder-width. Rather than going straight down, you can move your upper body forward and backward like pretending you are going back and forth under a fence. You can also vary the speed of the push up by doing them faster (down on one and up on two) or slower (down 1, 2, 3, 4, and up 1, 2, 3, 4) on each repetition. Varying how you exercise a particular muscle group is limited only by your imagination and what you can find on the internet. Just Google, "Various ways of doing a bicep curl, triceps extension or chest press," etc.

For cardio exercise, you can vary your exercise sessions between high-intensity spin classes or aerobic classes, long slow walks, hill walking, swimming, stair climbing, stair climber, running/jogging, etc.

The secret, however, is to keep varying the strength and cardio routines. By doing so, you will get better and quicker results, avoid plateauing in strength and endurance gains, and enjoy more variety in your workouts.

6. Prioritize Exercise in Your Daily and Weekly Schedule

SELF CARE IS A PRIORITY AND NECESSITY —NOT A LUXURY—

Prioritizing your exercise and health routine into your daily and weekly schedule is necessary to achieve successful training results. Unless a person emphasizes and embraces the importance of having consistent and sustainable workouts by prioritizing them as essential, life will get in the way. As a result, excuses will set in as to why you can't exercise on any particular day.

The first step in prioritizing is recognizing the importance of what you are trying to accomplish. There is a saying, "If you understand the whys, you can overcome the how's." Take the time to identify the "why" to exercise; if the purpose of exercising means a lot to you, then the "how" becomes more easily identifiable because it has become prioritized as an essential part of the daily and weekly schedule.

To prioritize the correct way, the person must be as specific as possible for the day, the time of day, and what they are specifically doing to exercise on that day. You should never say, "I will get to it when I can," or "I will see how I feel," or "I will decide later to do cardio or strength training."

When prioritizing a schedule, it is best to pick the same type of exercise on the same day and time each week. The more consistent you are in scheduling your training into your daily routine, the quicker exercising becomes a habit. The negative forces then will have less influence to divert you from exercising.

7. Gold Medal Performance

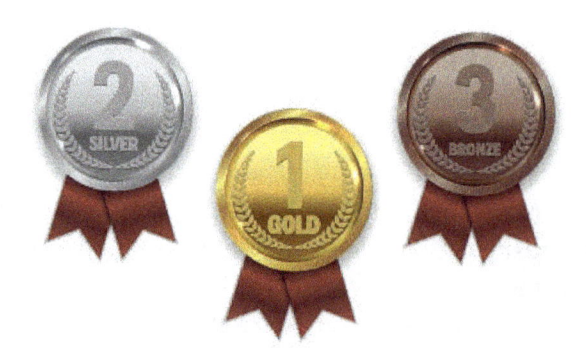

It is unrealistic for a person to expect a gold medal performance each time they exercise. This rule is essential to embrace. Even experienced, professional, and Olympic athletes know that they will not and cannot have a great exercise session every time they hit the gym or go for a cardio workout. Your body and mind are not built that way; but for many with less experience and, especially those type-A personality types, this rule is tough to accept. It is essential to show a little self-compassion (Chapter 6.6: Self-Compassion: The Proven Power of Being Kind to Yourself) and realize that it is sometimes a victory to show up and complete the exercise routine regardless of how well it was done.

A good rule of thumb to follow when you know you are not at your best when starting your scheduled exercise routine that day is if, after ten minutes of exercising, it just doesn't feel right and the exercise session is just too much of a struggle, stop, clean up, go home, have a nice meal, and a good sleep. Tomorrow is another day. Everyone has these days, but if you adhere to the 10-minute rule, you will be surprised how often you will get in the zone and complete your workout. It may not be a gold medal workout, but you will have done it and maintained consistency and sustainability.

8. 80/20 Rule

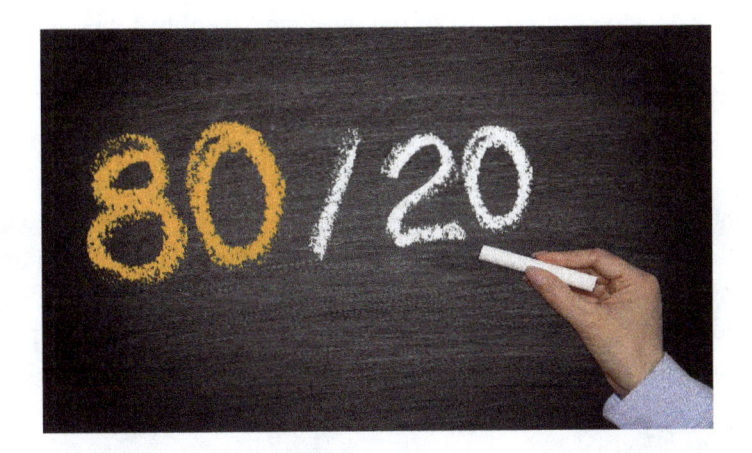

The 80/20 rule is my favourite rule and it is the "best" rule because it permits you to miss a scheduled workout. That is right; one has permission to skip a workout. Life is not a game of perfect, so why should anyone even attempt to be perfect, especially concerning their exercise routine. Life is challenging enough without forcing 100% compliance. If you can achieve 80% compliance in following your scheduled exercise or nutrition routine, you will have achieved the consistency and sustainability necessary to see great results and meet your goals.

Life will force you to miss a workout or eat something you usually would not. Don't sweat the small stuff; there is always tomorrow's workout coming or the next meal to eat properly again. It is also important not to "make up" a missed exercise session or a "binged" night at your favorite restaurant. "Make-ups" will mess up your finely planned schedule. Forget about it and move on. A good rule to follow is to "do your best and forget the rest." Successfully exercising and following a healthy diet is a marathon (remember consistency and sustainability), not a sprint, so being compliant 80% of the time is excellent.

Conclusion

This chapter has covered a lot of material; however, just like building a house, the structure crumbles down if there is not an excellent foundation to build upon. Without following the eight rules discussed, reaching your health and fitness goals becomes much harder. Adhering to these essential rules will ensure that your foundation is strong and increase the likelihood of you successfully following your health and fitness program. The results you desire will follow, so here's a review:

1. Make the program's exercises as specific as possible to the established goal.
2. Start low and slow. Give the body and mind time to adapt to the new stress of exercising regularly.
3. Be consistent and strive for sustainability. These are the key to developing strength and endurance.
4. Build into the program sufficient recovery time so the body can repair and become stronger. Look for signs of physical and emotional fatigue.

5. Modify the exercise routines every ten sessions to introduce muscle/neurologic confusion to avoid strength and endurance plateaus.
6. Prioritize exercise as an essential part of the daily and weekly schedule.
7. Don't expect a gold medal performance with every workout. Life is not a game of perfect, so your workouts will not be either.
8. Follow the 80/20 rule. It permits you to miss a workout.

By following these eight "golden" rules, you will instinctively look forward to your time exercising. Interestingly, you will probably feel out of sorts when life does get in the way, and you miss an exercise session. When this occurs, you will know that you have physically and emotionally adapted to your new fitness routine and are craving for it. Exercising has now become a positive addictive force in your life.

3.2. Learning to Overcome the Five Internally Generated Obstacles to Exercise

Introduction

Chapter 3.1. The Eight Golden Rules of Training discussed the importance of consistency and sustainability to achieve fitness and health goals. However, being aware of this golden rule is much easier than accomplishing it. Many obstacles get in the way of achieving the most well-intentioned and well-planned health and fitness goals. Barriers to achievement are especially true when it comes to exercising.

For as many people who exercise, there are excuses not to continue exercising. Some of these excuses are legitimate. There are times when exercise just does not fit into your schedule, and it would cause too much stress and increase the risk of injury to take the time to exercise. However, these "legitimate excuses" are rare. In most cases, people can modify their busy life, work schedule, or the intensity of their exercise to get it done.

External vs. Internal Generated Obstacles/Excuses to Your Fitness and Health Plan

External Obstacles/Excuses

External obstacles range from "the gym is too far away," "it is too hot/cold/wet," "I have no one to work out with," "my favorite instructor/personal trainer is away," "work is too busy," "my gym clothes are dirty," etc. Most of these external excuses are managed well with careful planning and adjusting of your schedule and staying motivated to exercise. Exercising should be fun, and most people agree that once they begin an exercise session, they enjoy it and are glad they made an effort to do it, even if it meant changing or reprioritizing their schedule.

Internal Obstacles/Excuses

Internally generated obstacles are not as easily identified as external obstacles and often a little harder to manage. They are developed mentally and often reflect your personality type. To overcome them requires a change in one's thought process, and often people are not willing to make an effort to do so. Consequently, over time, people succumb to their old habits and stop exercising. To complicate the matter further, these internally generated obstacles to exercise often pose a much more significant barrier to re-engage in an exercise routine at a later date than external excuses do.

The following are five common internally generated excuses that you need to be aware of and strategies to help overcome them so you can enjoy all the benefits that regular exercise can give.

1. Seeking Perfection

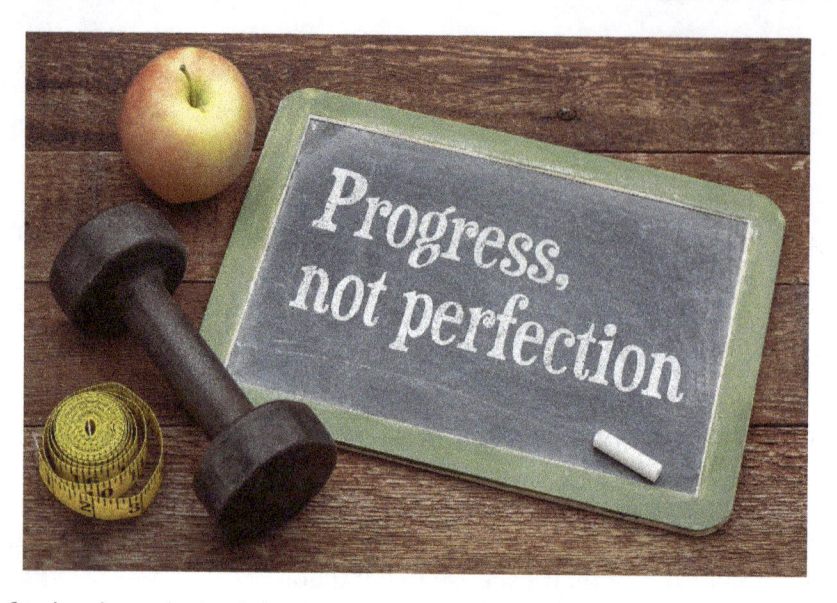

Seeking perfection is typical of the Type-A personality. It is unreasonable to expect every workout to be perfect, that you will be able to give it your best effort every time. Life gets in the way. Work, family, hormones, nutrition, stress, and lack of sleep are just some things that can and will affect your ability to perform optimally every time. When a workout is not going as well as hoped, don't sweat it, just do the best you can. Accept a less than perfect exercise session for what it is, an opportunity to still improve your health, both physically and mentally.

A less-than-stellar workout is better than no workout, and usually, what you perceive as an inferior workout is not all that bad. Often, your expectations are too high. If a person has an off day in their training, they need to accept it as a learning process. It is important to identify what may have been the cause of the "off day." Sometimes there are no apparent reasons; accept that too if it occurs. Remember, everyone has off days.

2. Don't Take It Too Seriously

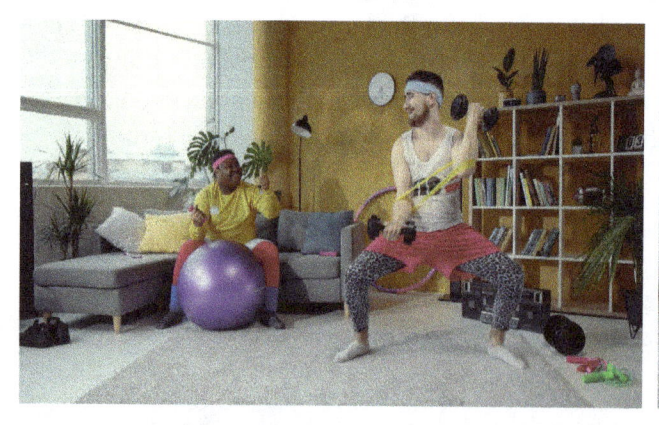

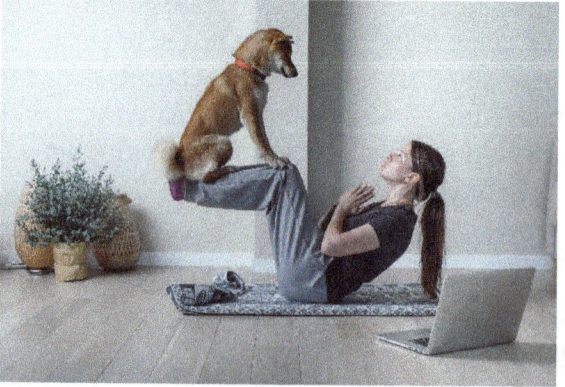

If you are not a professional athlete, why would you approach your exercise session as if you were? Exercising is fun, so allow it to be fun. You need to enjoy the time you have to exercise.

Mentally, think of it as a privilege to be healthy enough to exercise. The time a person has to exercise is special, but don't get hung up on it being more than it is – an opportunity to take care of your health. Whether you have had a great spin, yoga, aerobic, or weight lifting class, won or lost a tennis match or played well or not in a hockey game doesn't matter when considering the broader scope of things. What is important is that you made the time to participate, you enjoyed doing it and you are healthier for doing so. Remember that exercise is something that you do and not who you are. You need to identify yourself for what you are, a recreational exerciser, and not identify yourself to the specific results that occur from the activity. What this means is that you embrace the process or exercising regularly and not the results.

3. Don't Sweat the Small Stuff

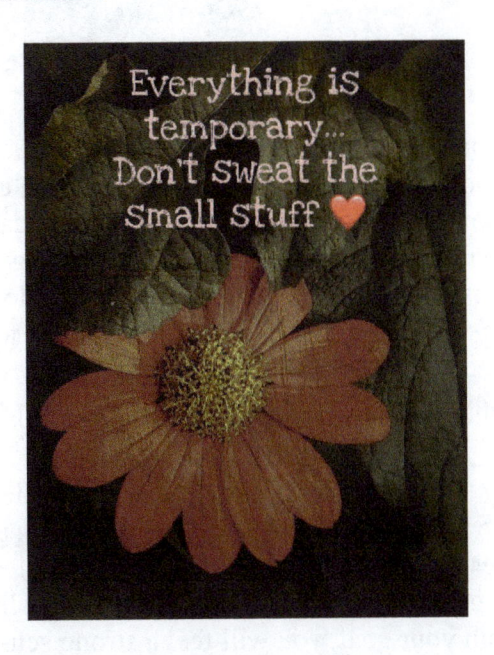

People need not stress over the small stuff they can't control. If it is raining or very hot and humid, don't get upset; just modify the intensity of the exercise and dress and hydrate accordingly. If a person cannot find their favorite hockey stick, tennis or squash racket, running/walking shorts, or shoes, they should use or wear their second favorite.

It is important to be physically and mentally prepared for the unexpected. You should lay out or pack sporting equipment and workout clothes the night before the exercise session and watch the weather channel so a warm, wet, or frigid day does not catch you unexpectedly.

You need to mentally prepare yourself and understand that the unexpected does and will occur from time. By being mentally and emotionally prepared, you are ready to deal with any situation. Remember, the quality of your fitness results is based on you training consistently, and giving your best effort, and not on external things that you can't control.

A good example is the 2012 Boston marathon that was held under very hot and adverse conditions. The experienced runners understood that they could not control the temperature and accepted that it would be an extremely challenging and an uncomfortable race. They adjusted their performance expectations accordingly. They understood that they would not be achieving a personal best time that day.

The lesson learned is don't let the small stuff ruin your exercise experience.

4. Don't Underestimate What Your Goals Should Be

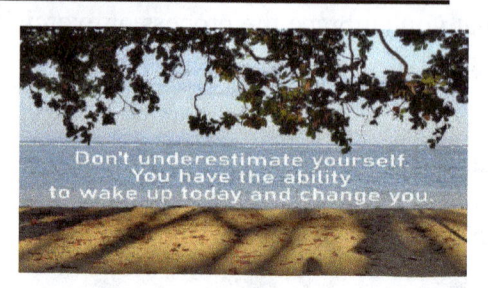

One of the great things about exercise and training is that the body responds favorably to an appropriate level of overload so that you can become strong, faster, and more skilled. When you set goals, it is essential that they are not set unrealistic high, but equally importantly is that they are not set too low. Setting goals can be very motivating, but setting expectations that are too high can be demoralizing. Conversely, setting goals that don't push you and are not challenging enough is frustrating. Set long-term goals, for example, six months to a year out, and set short-term goals of three months, one month, one week, or even one day. The great thing about short-term goals is that you can easily modify them if they are too easy or too hard to attain.

It is essential to be willing to change the exercise routine to achieve established short-term goals, which, in turn, will help ensure you will meet your long-term goals. You should not be afraid to "push" yourself. Over time and with experience, you will learn how hard or high you can set your expectations and goals. You need not go crazy, but pushing yourself can be motivating. When you do attain your goal, you will feel a strong sense of accomplishment and a natural high.

5. Be Mentally Engaged

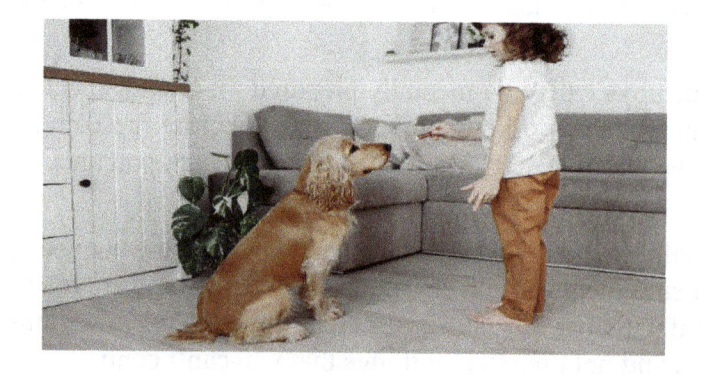

You only get the full benefit from your exercise session if you are mentally engaged in what you are doing. That does not mean that you should feel mentally exhausted at the end of your exercise session, but neither should you exercise with a laissez-faire attitude. You need to focus on the activity you are doing to perform it well and get the most out of it.

You cannot play golf or tennis well if you are not concentrating. If you are in an aerobic or yoga class, you will not achieve the full benefits from the class if you are not focusing on what the instructor is saying and doing. Even when you are out for a run or a walk, it is important that you focus on your gait and breathing to make sure you will not exercise too hard and hurt yourself. You will appreciate the extra effort you make in staying engaged in the activity you are doing. It is safer, and you are more likely to achieve your goals, making it more satisfying and enjoyable.

Conclusion

Internal obstacles can be deceiving. Often, you are unaware of them and how significantly they compromise your willingness to participate in a sport or to exercise. You need to be aware of these obstacles, and if they pop up, develop strategies to combat their harmful effects and turn them into positives.

Exercise should be fun, and the natural high you get from exercising and achieving your sporting goals is unparalleled. You need to find ways to make it as easy as possible to achieve your goals.

HINT

Find a friend or group to exercise with. Companionship increases accountability and can help you overcome many of the obstacles to exercise.

3.3. The Importance and Art of Goal Setting

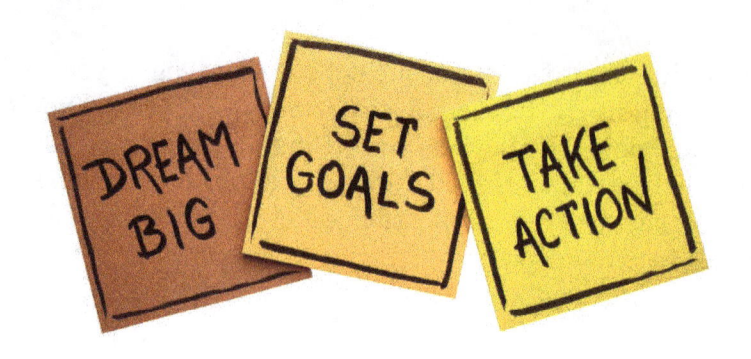

Introduction

The importance of goal setting cannot be overstated. Consciously and unconsciously, we all set goals every day. "I've got to get to the grocery store or get the laundry done today" are short-term goals that you may not even think of as goals. But if you did not think of them, they would not get done. Planning for a year-end vacation or striving for a job promotion would be considered long-term goals. Research has shown that the practice of writing down goals results in greater success in achieving them.

Goal setting only takes a few minutes of thought and effort and can effectively redirect your thoughts and actions into achieving something special. Remember, if you do not think it, you can't do it, and if you can't do it, it doesn't get done. Writing thoughts and goals down in a structured way brings them one step closer to reality.

The Structure of Successful Goal Setting

The secret to goal setting is to be **S.M.A.R.T.**
S – Specific
M – Measurable
A – Action-oriented
R – Realistic
T – Time lined

S.M.A.R.T. Goals

(S) Specific
– Be as specific and as clear as possible. The more detailed the description of the goal, the better you can visualize them and work toward making them a reality.

Examples:
- I want to be able to walk for one hour non-stop in 6 months (write the date down).
- I want to complete a 5-kilometer race for charity in three months (write the date down).
- I want to lose 10 pounds in 12 weeks (write the date down) and stay at that weight for the following year.

(M) Measurable
– If you can't measure it, you can't do it. You must identify specific metrics to measure your progress and achievements.

Examples:
1. Each month for the next six months, I will increase my ability to walk non-stop by 10 minutes.
2. After one month, I will be able to run two kilometers; after two months, I will be able to run four kilometers.
3. After one month, I will have lost four pounds, and after two months, eight pounds.
4. After I have lost 10 pounds, I will weigh myself every two weeks to ensure my weight stays stable.

(A) Action-Oriented
– List specific actions/steps that will be taken to achieve the goals. Be as straightforward as possible.

Examples:
1. I will walk three times per week. Monday (6 pm), Wednesday (6 pm), and Saturday (10 am). Each week I will increase the time I walk each day by 2.5 minutes.

2. I will run three times each week. Tuesday (5 pm), Thursday (5 pm), and Sunday (8 am). Each week I will increase the distance I run by 250 meters.

3. I will follow a balanced diet based on the recommendations of the Canadian Health Food Guide. I will record my nutrition and aim for a daily caloric intake of 2000 calories. I will also increase my exercise level to 30 minutes five days a weekday by implementing a moderately paced walking program. Monday, Tuesday, Thursday, and Friday at 6 pm and Sunday at noon.

(R) Realistic
– Setting goals must have a real chance of being accomplished based on the resources, time, and effort you can commit. If not, frustration, disillusionment, and failure will result. List how the goal is realistic/achievable.

Example:
1. I will review my activity schedule/nutrition diet weekly to make sure I am compliant with my action plans. If I cannot accomplish my action plan, I will modify my goals and action plan.

(T) Time lined
– Set a specific time (a week, a month, a year) to accomplish the goal. Set a long-term and short-term time line so progress can be measured.

Example:
1. Time lines have been listed previously. See the examples set out in the "Measurable" section above.

Setting Your Goals

The following table is to help direct your thoughts. Do not be limited by what is listed. Take your time; think carefully about motivating factors and the results that are expected.

Once the goals are identified, make them S.M.A.R.T. (as explained previously). It is not unusual to have difficulty organizing thoughts concerning SMART Goals. Useful goal setting takes practice.

Identifying Your Health and Fitness Goals:
Over the next months, I want to achieve the following (choose 3);

Exercise More (commit to a regular exercise routine)	
Increase Muscle Strength/Endurance	
Increase Cardiovascular Endurance	
Increase Flexibility	
Reduce Muscle/Joint Stiffness	
Lose Weight	
Reduce Blood Pressure	
Improve my Eating Habits (follow 80/20 rule)	
Drink 8 Glasses of Water Per Day	
Reduce the Amount of Alcohol I drink	

Reduce and Better Manage Stress	
Have a Happier and Healthier Outlook on Life	
Live an Active Lifestyle	
Have More Energy Feel Healthier	

First Goal:

Specific	
Measurable	
Action	
Realistic	
Time lined	

Second Goal:

Specific	
Measurable	
Action	
Realistic	
Time lined	

Third Goal:

Specific	
Measurable	
Action	
Realistic	
Time lined	

3.4. Visualization for Motivation to Promote Change

Introduction

Forever Active Older Adult Health and Fitness Playbook aims to inform and motivate everyone, and specifically the older adult, to begin a successful transformation of their fitness and overall health. The purpose of the preceding chapters; Chapter 3.1: The Eight Golden Rules of Training, Chapter 3.2: How to Overcome the Five Internal Obstacles to Exercise, and Chapter 3.3: The Importance and Art of Goal Setting were to help your health and fitness transformation become more attainable. The information presented in these chapters is valuable and practical, but unless you have the motivation to change your lifestyle and to improve your level of health, nothing else matters.

Understanding Motivation

For you to find the motivation to change and take care of your health can be elusive. Surprisingly, the fear of premature death due to a heart attack, stroke or diabetes, or the threat of premature physical disability due to being overweight, having osteoarthritis of the knees, hips, and lower back, or generalized muscle weakness is often not enough to motivate someone to exercise every day.

Fear can motivate but only for short periods. Humans are creatures of habit. Changing your daily living habits requires a change in the attitude about who you are and how you want to live your life. For most people, this is an uncomfortable thing to do.

Health starts with a motivational attitude that says, "How I think, how I handle stress, how I eat, and how active I am makes a difference in who I am, how I will interact with others, and how I will enjoy my life."

Your attitude will motivate you to make healthy choices in your life. If you are sedentary, overweight, or suffer from muscle stiffness and pain, then it is essential that you change your attitude and become motivated toward exercising, nutrition and mental health if you are to successfully change the habits that will change your life.

"A healthy body starts with a healthy attitude."

Use Visualization to Change Your Attitude and Develop Lasting Motivation

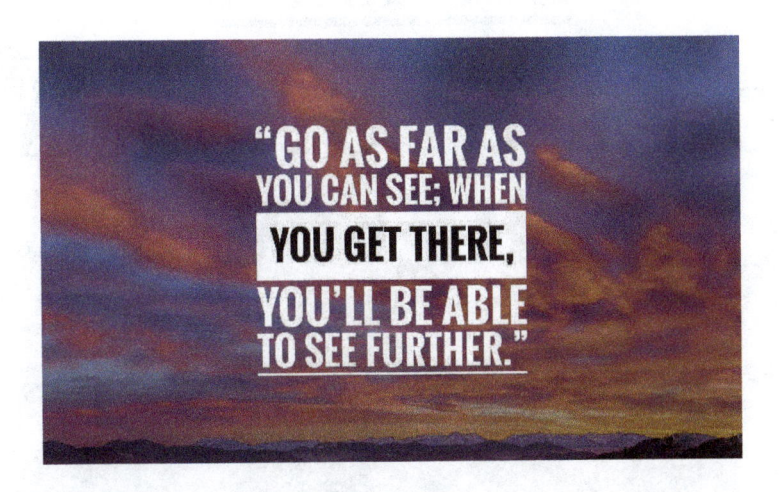

"GO AS FAR AS YOU CAN SEE; WHEN YOU GET THERE, YOU'LL BE ABLE TO SEE FURTHER."

The best way a person can change their attitude and stay motivated is by visualizing themselves as they would like to be. This means continually thinking about the benefits and rewards of being an active, fit, healthy, and focused person.

An excellent way to start on this visualization path is to identify someone you admire. It could be a friend, relative, or celebrity. It could be someone you know intimately and admire or someone you don't know at all, but most importantly, it needs to be someone who has the healthy lifestyle you crave.

Once you have identified your role model, you need to create a mental picture of yourself being like that person. You need to visualize yourself as who you intend to be in the future. It is important to be realistic and practice self-compassion (Chapter 6.6: Self-Compassion – The Proven Power of Being Kind to Yourself) when you do this. It's best to not hold yourself up to unrealistic ideals. You should strive to become the best you can be and use the example and experience of others to help guide the way.

Your self-image, the way you inwardly perceive yourself, is powerful, and largely determines your performance on the outside. Improvements in your outer life begin with improvements in on the inside, with your attitude. A healthy attitude is where the motivation for a transformational, physically fit, and healthy lifestyle must come. Once you have visualized and are motivated on how you want to live your life, being successful in this pursuit becomes just a matter of following the eight golden rules, understanding how to overcome their internal obstacles, and pursuing S.M.A.R.T. goals.

Conclusion

The Preseason preparation is over, and it's time to play the game. To be successful requires a strong offense, defense and special teams. The following sections will detail how to improve cardiovascular fitness, muscle strength, agility, balance and coordination, flexibility, nutritional balance, and build a strong, positive attitude, and a mindful approach to life.

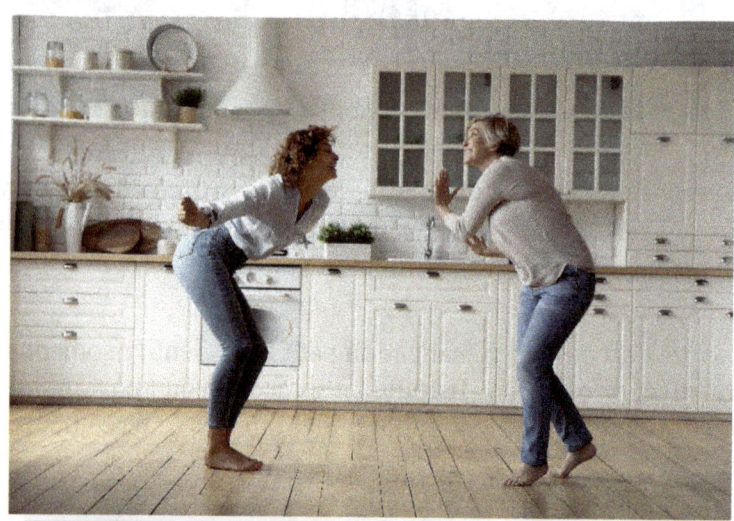

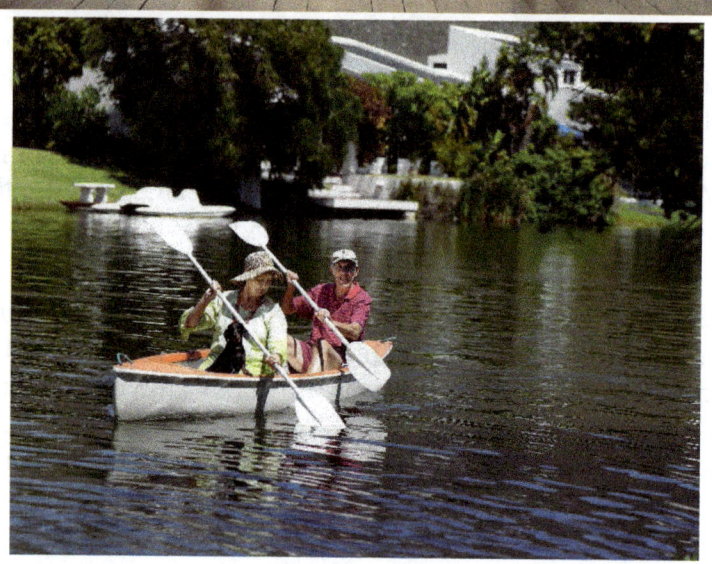

Section 4
The Offense – Getting Active the Right Way

4.0. Introduction: The Offense – Getting Active The Right Way

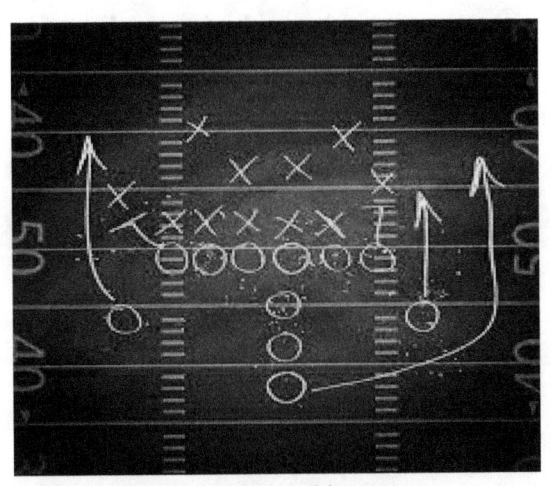

Image Source: mckinsey.com

In football, the glamour positions are all on offense. These positions include the quarterback, running backs, and wide receivers. Similarly, in fitness and health, cardiovascular activities and muscle strengthening exercises get most of the attention. However, for the older adult, another vitally important component of fitness and health are exercises and drills to improve agility, balance, and coordination.

Cardiovascular exercise strengthens the heart, lowers blood pressure, and helps control weight. These are important to fight off heart disease, obesity, and type 2 diabetes. There is also an added cognitive benefit. Research has established that cardiovascular exercise helps manage and alleviate chronic stress and fights off or slows down the disabling effects of dementia.

Muscular resistance exercises improve strength and mobility and help the older adult engage more effortlessly in the activities of daily living. After the age of 25, muscles begin to atrophy (waste away) at a rate of .5 - 1% each year. The older adult needs strong muscles to climb stairs, lift objects and participate in sports and hobbies that they enjoy. These activities all contribute to an enhanced quality of life for older adults. Resistance exercises slows muscular atrophy and the weakening process.

Agility, balance, and coordination exercises are not as well-known but are equally important for older adults. As you age, the number one risk factor for injury and disability increases. The reason for this is two-fold. First, as mentioned previously, muscles weaken with age. Weakened legs provide less mobility and support. Second, and less well known, the neurological connections that help control movement and maintain balance weaken. These neurological connections are called proprioceptor reflexes and originate from your eyes, ears, and joints. As a result, it is important and necessary that the older adult do specific exercises or drills to sharpen these proprioceptive reflexes. The better the proprioceptive reflex's function, the better protected the older adult is from falling and seriously hurting themselves.

A well-functioning offense is a vital component for a winning football team. The same is true for the older adult's health and fitness. A strong heart, strong muscles, and good agility, balance, and coordination are keys to a more enjoyable and higher quality of life.

4.1.0. Introduction: Cardiovascular Health, Fitness and Training

Cardiovascular fitness, muscular strength and endurance, and flexibility are the three major components to physical fitness. Each of these components is equally important for optimal health and well-being; however, cardiovascular fitness is the most important from a life-or-death perspective.

Heart disease and stroke are the second and third leading causes of death in Canada (Stats Canada). One in twelve Canadians (2.4 million) over the age of 20 have been diagnosed with heart disease. Men are twice as likely to be diagnosed with heart disease as women, and on average, males are diagnosed 10 years younger (55-64 years old) than females (65-74 years old). Approximately every seven minutes in Canada, someone dies from heart disease or stroke. The Conference Board of Canada estimates that heart disease and stroke cost the Canadian economy more than 20.9 billion dollars per year. (For a more in-depth study of heart disease, refer to Chapter 2.2: Heart Disease, Stroke and Hypertension).

As a preventative measure, cardiovascular training is of paramount importance. The following chapters will examine cardiovascular training and how to do it effectively and safely to gain maximal health benefits.

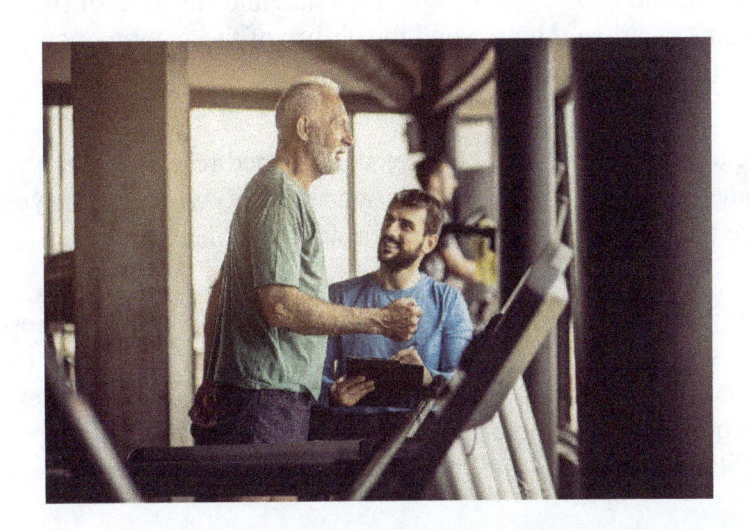

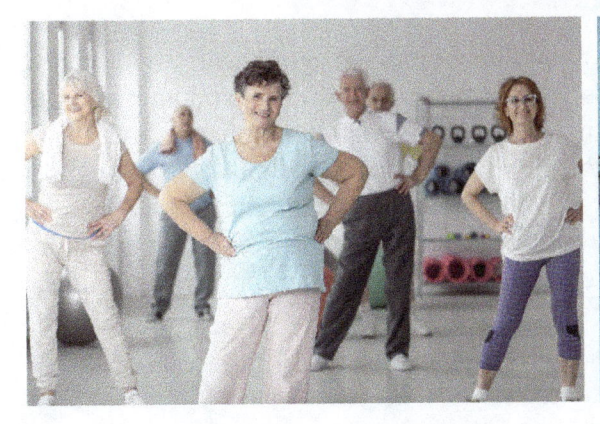

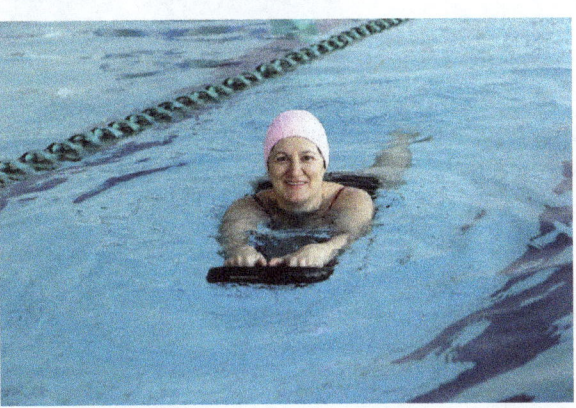

4.1.1. Cardiovascular Fitness Training

Introduction

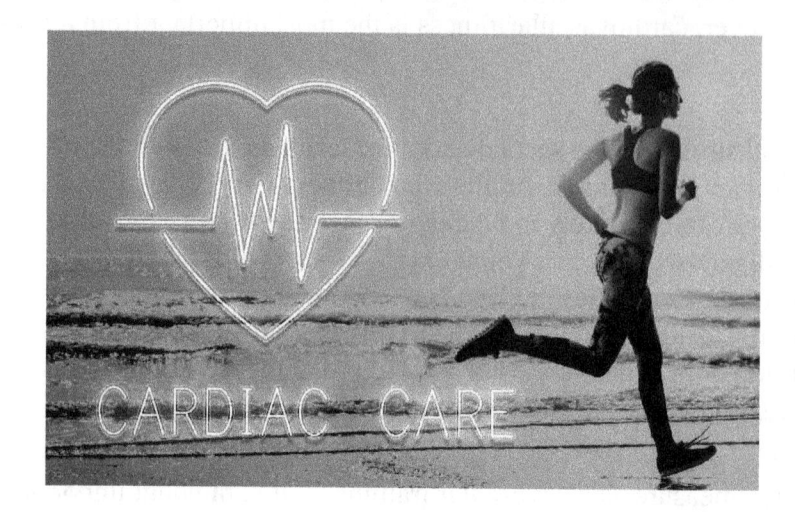

Of the three major components of fitness, the cardiovascular system is probably the most important. If you do not have a strong functioning heart, it doesn't matter how strong or flexible your muscles, tendons, and ligaments are. The structure and function of the cardiovascular system (arteries, veins, heart, and lungs) and the ability of these components to work together is critical for healthy, functional, and independent living.

Unfortunately, for the older adult, activities that seemed relatively easy to perform just a few years earlier become more challenging as their heart's ability to deliver oxygen to the working muscles to produce the needed energy to perform work declines.

The ventricular wall, the chamber of the heart that pumps blood to the rest of the body, increases in thickness by about 30% beginning at around age 25. This wall thickness, in part, is in response to an age-related increase in blood pressure as the aorta and arterial tree (the arteries that deliver blood to the muscles and organs) become thicker and less compliant with age. Physiologically, with age, the heart and blood vessels become less sensitive to neurological stimulation.

This decrease in neurologic sensitivity means two things. First, the aging heart can't achieve the maximum heart rate possible during a person's younger years. A lower maximum heart rate limits how hard a person can physically exert themselves. Second, blood pressure reflexes that accommodate changes in blood pressure as a person changes postural positions from sitting to standing do not respond as quickly. The slowness in blood pressure accommodation to changing postural positions often results in dizziness, confusion, weakness, or fainting as the older adult changes postures (increases the risk of falling) or during the initial stages of physical exertion (increases the risk of heart attack).

Fortunately, regular cardiovascular exercise can slow down these anatomical and physiological changes that occur with aging. The benefits of cardiovascular training (exercise that involves increasing the heart rate for a sustained period) are:

- Reduces the risk of cardiovascular disease or hardening of the arteries.
- Decreases resting heart rate, so the heart is not working as hard during times of non-exertion.
- Keeps resting blood pressure normal by improving arterial elasticity.
- Improves heart efficiency, so the heart works less forcefully during exertion.
- Helps control weight gain.
- Increases metabolism and energy and build stamina, so you do not experience fatigue as quickly when exerting yourself.

Older adults need to engage in cardiovascular fitness training on a consistent and sustained basis. Having a strong heart that can respond to changes in physical exertion goes a long way to enhance their quality of life.

Decreasing vs. Increasing MVPA (Moderate to Vigorous Physical Activity)

Decrease in Frequency of MVPA
1-2, 3-4, and ≥5 times of MVPA/week to decreased frequency or physically inactive

Up to 27% Increased Risk of Cardiovascular Disease

Coronary Heart Disease   Stroke

Increase in Frequency of MVPA
Physically Inactive to 1-2, 3-4, and ≥5 times of MVPA/week

Up to 11% Reduced Risk of Cardiovascular Disease

Coronary Heart Disease   Stroke

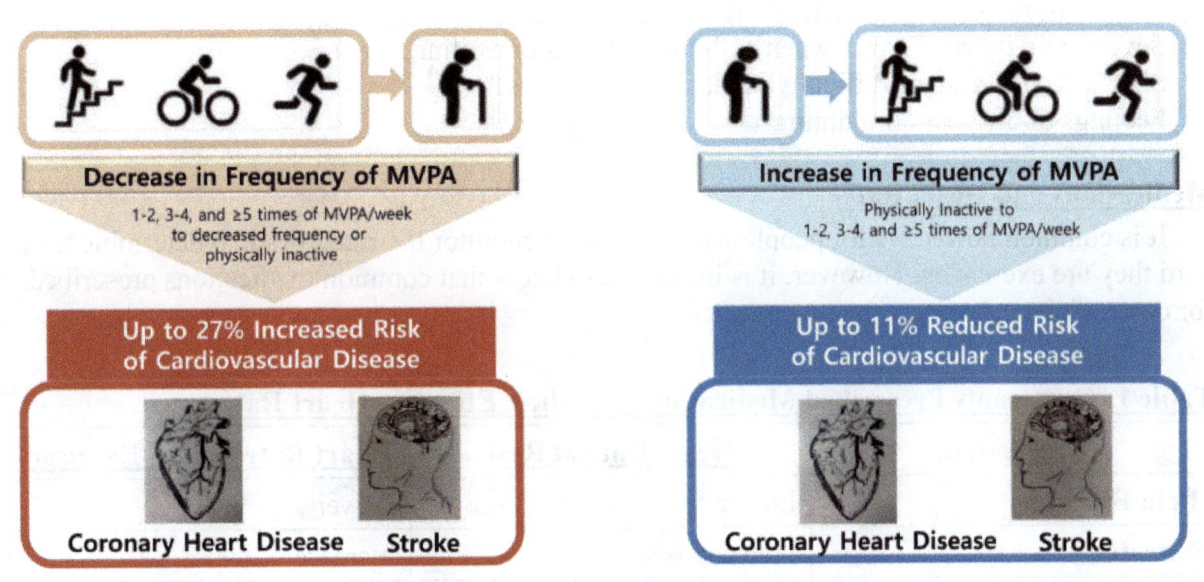

Image Source: bicyclenetwork.co.au

Safety First

Cardiac Risk Factors

It is important for safety reasons for everyone to have a medical examination before they start a regular exercise program. A medical examination is even more important for the older adult or anyone who has experienced anatomical and physiological changes with their cardiovascular system as they have aged.

The following are a list of conditions that increase the older adult's risk of cardiovascular disease:

1. Age
2. Family history of heart disease
3. Smoking
4. High blood pressure (Hypertension) – Systolic pressure greater than 140 or diastolic pressure greater than 90)
5. High cholesterol levels- (total cholesterol over 200 milligrams per decilitre)
6. Diabetes
7. Sedentary life style;
    – less than 60 minutes of light effort performed daily,
    – less than 30 minutes of moderate-intensity activity four times a week,
    – less than 20 minutes of vigorous activity four times a week.

Signs and Symptoms of Cardiovascular Distress

If you are exercising and experiences any of the following symptoms, you should stop exercising immediately, consult your doctor, or go to the hospital:

1. Pain and discomfort in the chest, lower jaw or left shoulder
2. Feeling of rapid, throbbing heart rate
3. Severe pain in leg muscles when walking, running or cycling
4. Shortness of breath or difficulty breathing
5. Feelings of dizziness or fainting.

Medications and Heart Rate

It is common nowadays for people who exercise to monitor their heart rate to determine how hard they are exercising. However, it is important to know that common medications prescribed for older adults may affect their heart rates.

Table 1: Commonly Prescribed Medications and their Effect on Heart Rate

Medication	Heart Rate at Rest	Heart Rate during Exercise
Beta Blockers	Lower	Lower
Nitrates	Increase	Increase
Calcium Channel Blockers	Increase	Increase
Digitalis	Neutral affect	Neutral affect
Antiarrhythmic Agents Class 1	Neutral or increase	Neutral or increase
Diuretics	Neutral affect	Neutral affect
ACE Inhibitors	Neutral affect	Neutral affect
Antidepressants	Neutral or increase	Neutral or increase
Nicotine	Neutral or increase	Neutral or increase
Thyroid Medication	Increase	Increase

Bronchodilators (Methylxanthines)	Neutral or increase	Neutral or increase
Bronchodilators (Sympathomimetic)	Neutral or increase	Neutral or increase
Bronchodilators (Cromolyn Sodium)	Neutral	Neutral
Bronchodilators (Corticosteroids)	Neutral	Neutral

Predicting Cardiovascular Fitness (MVO$_2$Max)

Most adults, especially older adults, are unconditioned and many have a compromised cardiovascular system due to high blood pressure and/or being overweight. As a result, before starting a regular cardiovascular exercise program, it is a good idea to determine, or generally estimate, your level of cardiovascular fitness.

Determining your cardiovascular fitness has two purposes. First, it will indicate how conditioned your cardiovascular system is. The level of cardiovascular conditioning helps determine the level of intensity with which you can do your cardiovascular exercises. Second, it can act as a motivational tool. If you follow cardiovascular guidelines and your exercise routine regularly, your cardiovascular fitness level will improve. This improvement will be reflected in a higher score on your cardiovascular fitness test.

Measuring aerobic (living with oxygen) capacity is the best way of predicting cardiovascular fitness. Aerobic capacity is determined by measuring VO$_2$MAX. This measurement represents the maximum volume of oxygen one uses when exercising at a sustained, maximal workload.

VO$_2$MAX measurement varies by sport due to, how much muscle is being used, the effects of gravity and drag (water when swimming, wind resistance when biking or running) on the effort, and is closely related to age. After age 25 VO$_2$MAX decreases by 1% per year. This decline is primarily due to a reduction in maximal heart rate with age. Research has shown that genetics (genes) can have a 20-30% effect on your VO$_2$MAX value. Your fitness level, sedentary vs. athletic, also has a significant effect and can influence your VO$_2$MAX value by 20%.

VO$_2$Max measures as milliliters of oxygen per kilogram of body weight per minute, MVO$_2$/Kg/min. Charts 1 and 2 illustrate VO$_2$MAX values for both men and women with advancing age. Women generally have VO$_2$MAX values 15-30% lower than men. Much of this difference is attributed to body size and composition. VO$_2$Max decreases as body fat percentage increases. Typically, women have a larger percentage of body fat than men.

Chart 1: Men's VO$_2$MAX values with age

Men's VO$_2$Max Rating	**20-29**	**30-39**	**40-49**	**50-59**	**60+**
Superior	>52.4	>49	>48	>45.3	>44.2
Excellent	46.5-52.4	45-49.4	43.8-48	41-45.3	36.5-44.2
Good	42.5-46.4	41-44.91	39-43.7	35.8-40.9	32.3-36.4
Fair	36.5-42.4	35.5-40.9	33.6-38.9	31-35.7	26.1-32.2
Poor	33-36.4	31-35.4	30.2-33.5	26.1-30.9	20.5-26
Very Poor	<33	<33.5	<30.2	<26.1	<20.5

Chart 2: Women's VO$_2$ MAX values with age

Women's MVO$_2$MAX Ratings	**20-29**	**30-39**	**40-49**	**50-59**	**60+**
Superior	>41	>40	>36.9	>35.7	>31.4
Excellent	37-41	35.7-40	32.9-36.	31.5-35.7	30.3-31.4
Good	33-36.9	31.5-35.6	29-32.8	27-31.4	24.5-30.2
Fair	29-32.9	27-31.4	24.5-28.	22.8-26.9	20.2-24.4
Poor	23.6-28.9	22.8-26.9	21-24.4	20.2-22.7	17.5-20.1
Very Poor	<23.6	<22.8	<21	<20.2	<17.5

Table 2 – VO$_2$MAX values for Sedentary Females and Males and Various Elite Athletes

	Female (mlO$_2$/kg/min)	**Male** (mlO$_2$/kg/min)
Sedentary Female/Male	38	43
Elite Athletes by Sport		
1. Cross Country Skiers	65	80
2. Middle Distance Runners	59	80
3. Swimmers	56	77
4. Speed Skaters	54	76
5. Cyclist	56	75
6. Rowers	42	61

Measuring MVO₂MAX

1. Lab Test

The most accurate and expensive way of testing for MVO₂MAX is to do a sophisticated lab test requiring a face mask to directly capture and measure the volume and gas concentrations of inspired and expired air. The lab test involves exercising on a treadmill or a bike at an intensity that increases every few minutes until exhaustion and is designed to achieve a maximal effort. The individual's maximal heart rate from this test and their resting heart rate can be used to develop a precise target heart rate range that is necessary for effective cardiovascular training.

2. Maximal and Submaximal Predictor Tests

Fortunately, there are less expensive and intrusive ways of predicting your MVO₂MAX. The first test requires maximal effort while running. The second test is a submaximal test performed by walking. These tests are less accurate than the lab test, but they give a relatively good idea of your MVO₂MAX value and cardiovascular fitness from which target heart rate ranges for training can be determined.

1. Maximal Running MVO₂MAX Predictor Test

Test Procedures:

— A 1.5-mile level running surface is used.

— The 1.5 miles are covered in as fast a time as possible. It is best to run at an even pace until near the end, just as in a race.

—Time the run, in minutes and seconds, and measure the heart rate at the end of the test.

VO2MAX is computed with the following equation:

$$\text{VO2MAX (ml. kg}^{-1}.\text{min}^{-1}) = 88.02 \times (3.716 \times \text{gender (0-female, 1-male)})$$
$$- (0.0753 \times \text{body weight in pounds})$$
$$- (2.767 \times \text{time for 1.5 miles in minutes and fractions of minutes})$$

Prediction value – 90%

Reference: George, J. D. et al. *VO2MAX estimation from a submaximal 1-mile track jog for fit college-age individuals*. Medicine and Science in Sports and Exercise, 25, 401-406, 1993.

2. Submaximal Rockport Walking MVO₂MAX Predictor Test

This test was developed and validated on subjects 30-69 years old.

The test was shown not to be valid in college-aged subjects but a correction factor can be applied for this group (see below).

Test Procedures:

— One mile is walked (no jogging) as fast as possible on a level surface.

— It is important that that the pace be as fast as possible.

– Record heart rate immediately at the end of the walk. If checking the heart rate by palpating, find the pulse as soon as the walk is finished and count for 15 seconds. If using a heart monitor, take the heart rate five seconds after finishing the test.

– Record the time for walking the one mile in minutes and fractions of minutes.

VO₂MAX is computed using the formula:

VO₂MAX (ml. kg.min) = 132.853 - (0.0769 x weight in pounds)
- (0.3877 x age)
+ (6.315 x gender (0-female, 1-male))
- (3.2649 x mile walk time (round to nearest minute)
- (0.1565 x ending heart rate)

Note – For individuals between 18-24 years old, subtract 6 ml. kg.min from the value obtained above.

Prediction value – 88%

References:
1. Kline, G. M. et al. *Estimation of VO₂MAX from a one-mile track walk, gender, age, and body weight.* Medicine and Science in Sports and Exercise, 19, 253-259, 1989.
2. Dolgener, F.A. et al. *Validation of the Rockport Fitness Walking Test in College Males and Females.* Research Quarterly for Exercise and Sport, 65, 1994, 152-158., 1994.

Once you have determined your general MVO₂MAX score and determined what level of fitness you are at (Chart #1 above) you can follow recommended cardiovascular training guidelines to determine the level of intensity (target heart rate zone based on % of MVO₂MAX) that your cardiovascular training needs to be at to produce a training effect and stronger heart.

Cardiovascular Training Guidelines

To exercise the cardiovascular system and improve MVO₂MAX value safely, efficiently, and effectively, a person needs to follow well-established training guidelines. Table 3 breaks these guidelines into three categories:

1. Beginner/sedentary (Not active)
2. Intermediate (mild to moderately active)
3. Advanced (highly active)

It is essential for a person to follow the golden rule of training and always start conservatively, low and slow (Chapter 3.1: The Eight Golden Rules of Training). Following the low and slow rule is important when a person begins their cardiovascular training because they are starting to stress the heart and this is stress that the heart has not had time to adapted to. Consequently, a person needs to pick a category that best describes their current level of fitness (MVO₂MAX) and activity.

It is important for a person not to choose a level based on their previous fitness level two, five, or ten years ago. If you are unsure whether you are a "couch potato" or "weekend warrior" or somewhere in between, it is best to be conservative and start in the beginner/sedentary category. Determining your MVO$_2$MAX will help in this regard.

From a physical, mental and emotional perspective it is always smart to start low and slow and build cardiovascular strength and endurance from that point. The last thing anyone wants is to injure themself or become mentally or emotionally fatigued due to exercising regularly. Injury or fatigue can cause a person to start to miss scheduled workouts. Consistency and sustainability are the keys to successful training (Chapter 3.1: The Eight Golden Rules of Training).

Please Note – The guidelines in Table 3 are established for reference only and do not substitute for a thorough medical examination and clearance from the doctor.

Table 3: Cardiovascular Training Guidelines (FITT) for Older Adult

Level of Cardiovascular Fitness	Beginner/Sedentary "Couch potato" (Very low to Low Fitness)	Intermediate (Mild to Moderately Active) "Weekend warrior" (Average Fitness)	Advanced (Highly Active) "Athlete" (Above-Average to High Fitness)
Goals	1. Improved health 2. Increased energy 3. Daily activities made easier 4. Weight reduction	1. Improved health 2. Weight Reduction 3. Participate in activities of greater intensity compared to those of daily living (i.e.- participation in sporting activities such as golf & bowling, gardening)	1. Improved health 2. Weight maintenance 3. Sports training for competition.
Frequency (F)	1-3 times/week	3-5 times/week	4-6 times/week
Intensity (I) (See Note 1 & 2)	1. Max HR - 55%-64% 2. RPE -3-4 3. Talk Test - carry on a conversation	1. Max HR - 65%-74% 2. RPE – 4-6 3. Talk Test – challenging to carry on a conversation	1. Max HR -75%-90% 2. RPE – 6-8 3. Talk Test – unable to carry on a conversation

Time (T)/Duration	15-30 minutes/session (Initially this does not have to be continuous)	30-60 minutes/session (Ideally continuous)	60+ minutes/session (Continuous)
Type (T) of Exercising (See Table 6)	1. Walking 2. Stationary bike 3. Swimming 4. Water aerobics 5. Basic fitness classes	1. Stair climbing 2. Treadmill 3. Fitness Classes 4. Cycling (spin) classes 5. Lower intensity sports	1. Complex movements 2. High intensity/activity sports 3. Interval training (HIIT) 4. Cross-training

Note 1: There is a high correlation between MVO_2MAX and Heart Rate. Therefore, heart rate is used as a substitute for MVO_2MAX when determining cardiovascular exercise intensity. (Reference - https://health.ucdavis.edu/sportsmedicine/resources/vo2description.html)

Note 2: Three Ways Determine Exercise Intensity.

1. Target Heart Rate (% of Max HR)	2. Rate of Perceived Exertion (RPE)	3. Talk Test
Step 1: Determine maximum heart rate; **Formula:** HRmax = 207 - (.7 x age) Example – 55 year old HRmax = 207 - (.7 x 55 yrs of age) = 169 bpm	This method to monitor exertion uses the Modified Borg Scale of exertion between 0 and 10.	Best and simplest method used for a beginner/sedentary person to measure intensity of their exercise
Step 2: Determine Target Heart rate range: (Based on intensity guidelines in Table 1); **Formula** – Max HR x lower % Example – Beginner (55-64% intensity) 169 x 55% = 93bpm 169 x 64% = 108 bpm Target HR range – 93-108 bpm	**Modified Borg Scale of Perceived Exertion** <table><tr><th>Rating</th><th>Perceived Exertion</th></tr><tr><td>0</td><td>Nothing at all</td></tr><tr><td>1</td><td>Very Light</td></tr><tr><td>2</td><td>Light</td></tr><tr><td>3</td><td>Moderate</td></tr><tr><td>4</td><td>Somewhat Hard</td></tr><tr><td>5-6</td><td>Hard</td></tr><tr><td>7-8</td><td>Very Hard</td></tr><tr><td>9</td><td>Very, Very Hard (Almost maximal)</td></tr><tr><td>10</td><td>Maximal</td></tr></table>	**1. Low Intensity – For beginner:** - Able to talk in complete sentences. **2. Moderate Intensity – best for cardiovascular training:** – Talk in broken sentences. **3. High Intensity & Interval training:** Shortness of breath makes it difficult to talk
Summary – for a 55-year-old who is a beginner (very low to low fitness level) they would try to raise their heart rate to between 93 and 108 bpm for 15-30 minutes Perceived exertion – 3-4 (Initially activity doesn't have to be continuous).	**Summary** – An intermediate (average fitness) older adult should do cardiovascular exercise at a perceived exertion level between 4-6 for 20 to 45 minutes 3 to 5 times per week.	**Summary** – If a beginner is breathless and unable to talk, the intensity is too high and they should slow down immediately.

High Intensity Interval Training vs. Moderate vs. Low Intensity Cardiovascular Training

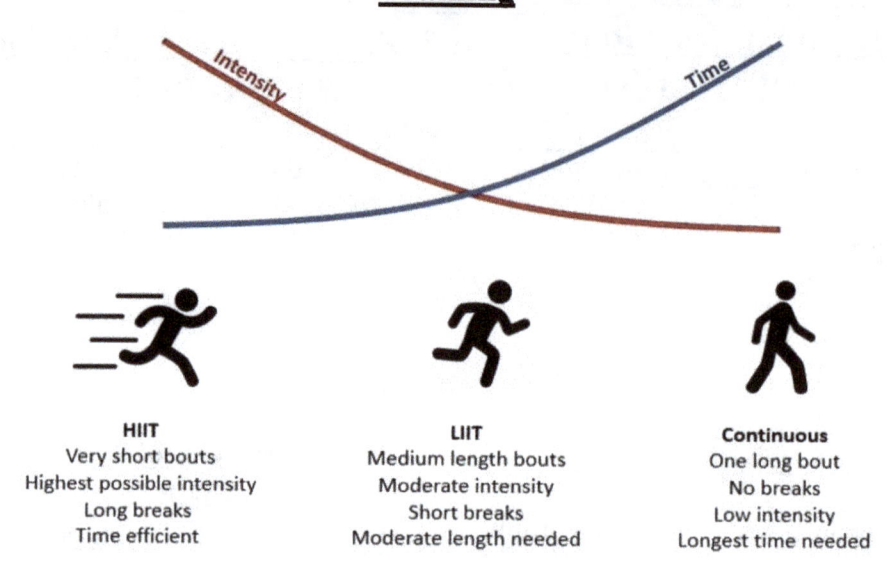

Image Source: theconversation.com

1. High Intensity Interval Training: Taking Cardiovascular Training to the Next Level (HIIT)

The guidelines for cardiovascular training listed in Table 3 (FITT Guidelines) should be followed. Please note that the three critical variables for each level of fitness for cardiovascular training are duration, frequency, and intensity. For the beginner/sedentary person, the most important of these is frequency. As mentioned previously, consistency and sustainability are the keys to effective training for beginners.

Once a strong baseline of cardiovascular fitness is established, intensity becomes the driving force for effective cardiovascular training. As Note 2 details, intensity is most easily be measured by heart rate (High correlation with MVO_2Max), perceived exertion, or the talk test. Measuring pace with a GPS device during walking or running or determining power with a power meter while riding are more sophisticated ways of monitoring intensity.

Research has shown that even though the guidelines listed above effectively slow the aging of the cardiovascular system, higher intensity exercise (HIIT) that involves achieving 80 - 95% max heart rate, or perceived effort of 8 - 10 or more is the most effective way to enhance and maintain cardiovascular fitness. The caveat is that a person MUST have a strong baseline of fitness before working at these high-intensity levels. It is important to note that it is unnecessary or advisable to work at these high-intensity levels for each cardiovascular workout.

There are two types of high-intensity workouts to enhance cardiovascular training;
1. **Aerobic-Capacity Interval Workouts** – short intervals, 30 seconds to three minutes, and performed at a very high intensity.
2. **Lactate-Threshold Workouts** – longer intervals, five to 12 minutes, and slightly less intense intervals.

The guidelines for each of these workouts are described in Table 4.

Table 4: Guidelines for the Two Types of High Intensity Interval Workouts

	Aerobic-Capacity Interval Workouts (HIIT)	**Lactate-Threshold Workout**
Duration	30 seconds-3 minutes	5-12 minutes
Recovery: Duration between Intervals	Same to 50% of the workout interval	25% length of interval
Intensity	**HR** – 90-95% max heart rate **RPE** – 85-90% (-9 - 10 on Borg Scale) **Talk Test** – breathless	**HR** – 85-90% max heart rate **RPE** – 70-80% (8-9 Borg Scale) **Talk Test** – breathless
Frequency	Based on recovery rate usually at least 2-3 days rest between sessions, but for older adults, one time/week to avoid overtraining Note – Cross training between running, cycling and swimming is effective to help avoid injury and makes training density more manageable	Based on recovery rate usually at least 2-3 days rest between sessions but for older adults, one time/week to avoid overtraining Note – Cross training between running, cycling and swimming is effective to help avoid injury and makes training density more manageable

2. Low-Intensity Cardiovascular Training

High-Intensity Interval Training (HIIT) is essential for elite and master athletes to improve their MVO_2MAX levels to compete successfully. However, an essential part of their cardiovascular training and the bedrock for the sedentary/couch potato and the average/weekend warrior is long-slow aerobic training. Even for the elite, well-trained person, it is recommended that they only do high-intensity training 20% of the time. The remaining 80% is reserved for low-intensity training.

Low-intensity training is much less intense, and as a consequence, it must be done for a more extended period to stimulate and improve the cardiovascular system. Duration and not intensity are the key to this type of workout. Table 5 details the guidelines for this form of aerobic cardiovascular training.

Table 5: Guidelines for Low Intensity Long-slow Aerobic Training

Duration	30 minutes to over 3 hrs
Intensity	60-70% max heart rate RPE – 4-6
Frequency	2-4 times/week Can be done frequently but if not given sufficient recovery time, it will result in a significant amount of fatigue

LOW INTENSITY CARDIO

VERSUS

HIGH INTENSITY INTERVAL TRAINING

COMPARING THE TWO MAIN TYPES OF CARDIO

Low intensity cardio is aerobic exercise that is performed at 60 to 80 % of your maximum heart rate or your target heart rate.

BENEFITS
Perfect for beginners
Increasing Endurance
Calories burned are fat at a greater degree

DRAWBACKS
Time consuming
Can get boring
Catabolic if overdone

EXAMPLES
Run at a moderate pace
Dancing
Cycling
Elliptical

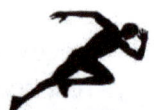

High-intensity interval training (HIIT), is a form of an exercise alternating short periods of intense anaerobic exercise with less-intense recovery periods.

BENEFITS
Accelerate fat loss
Break plateaus
Time efficient
Faster results

DRAWBACKS
More difficult
Injuries can occur
Easy to overtrain

EXAMPLES
30sec walk/ 30sec sprint
5 set of 10 burpees
Skipping rope
Box jumps
Tabata HIIT

Image Source: pinterest.co.uk

Types of Cardiovascular Activities

Table 6: Types of Cardiovascular Activities

Exercise	Advantage	Disadvantage	Skill Level
1. Walking and Running (Appendix 9.1.1.1 & 9.1.1.2)	– easy to do – convenient – walking is low impact – low cost	– some find it boring	– low
2. Riding **- Road Bike** **- Stationary Bike (Up-right or Recumbent)** **- Spin Classes** (Appendix 9.1.1.3)	– easy to learn – relatively inexpensive home equipment – can do when weather is poor – classes are in a social setting – non-weight bearing	– some find stationary bikes boring	– low
Running/Walking Treadmill and Elliptical (Appendix 9.1.1.2)	– usually easy to learn – low to moderate impact on joints.	– Can be expensive for home use – requires more balance and coordination	– low to moderate
Swimming and Aquatics (Appendix 9.1.1.4)	– usually, inexpensive – non-weight bearing	– higher level skill – can't do in comfort of home	– moderate to high

Conclusion

Cardiovascular fitness for the older adult is the most important fitness component to improved health, functional independence, and quality of life. With proper medical screening and following specific training guidelines (FITT), cardiovascular fitness training can be performed safely and effectively. Increased endurance, loss of weight, increased self-esteem, and self-image are just some of the many benefits of engaging in this form of exercise.

"Success is in the Doing," and if you don't enjoy what you are doing, you won't do it for long. The key is to pick cardiovascular activities that the individual will enjoy and look forward to doing. That does not mean that all exercise sessions will be easy, but overall, they should and need to be enjoyable.

Get started today, the heart depends on it.

4.1.2. Walking with an Activity Tracking Device: A Great Way to Get Started on the Road to Improved Health

Introduction

Exercising does not have to be intimidating. However, for many people, especially older adults, knowing how, when, and where to start exercising can be challenging. It is a common belief that a person needs sophisticated equipment or be a member of an expensive fitness facility to start exercising. This is just not the case.

Fitness starts at home. Most people exercise every day just by walking, but many don't consider this "actual exercise." Maybe that is because it is easy to do and is taken for granted because a person can do it anytime, anywhere. But walking is an excellent form of cardiovascular exercise and has many other health benefits for the older adult such as:

- Boost's energy
- Reduces stress and improves mood
- Helps reduce the risk of chronic disease, heart disease, and stroke
- Helps in weight control and helps prevent and control type 2 diabetes
- Strengthens bones and helps prevent or control osteoporosis
- Improves joint mobility.

With the development of pedometers, smartwatches, and smartphones, it is now easy to measure how much exercise a person gets from walking each day. Counting walking steps is a great way to kick-start a cardiovascular fitness program, measure progress, and stay motivated.

How Many Steps is Enough?

Because we are so accustomed to walking, it is taken for granted as a form of exercise. Just because it is easy to do does not mean it is not valuable. However, just like other types of exercise, there are guidelines for walking to have a significantly positive health effect.

The following table lists guidelines to determine when you are walking enough to get health benefits:

Number of Steps/days	Health Effect
< 5,000	**"Below Average".** Not enough physical activity
5,000 to 7500	**"Average"** What most people do daily but not enough to provide all the health benefits of walking
7,500 to 10,000	**"Above Average"** Somewhat active"
10,000 to 12,500	**"Active".** A good target to aim for
> 12,500	**"Highly active"** At this level a walker is receiving significant health benefits

How to Measure How Many Steps are Taken

At first glance, a person may think that 10,000 or more steps per day are a lot, but when you consider that it only takes about 5 minutes at average walking speed to do 500 steps, then to do 10,000 steps does not seem too daunting a task. If a person adds up the number of minutes that they walk throughout the day, it usually amounts to well over an hour and a half. But rather than count the number of minutes walked, a more precise, effective, and inexpensive way to monitor the number of steps taken in a day is to use a pedometer, smartwatch, or smartphone.

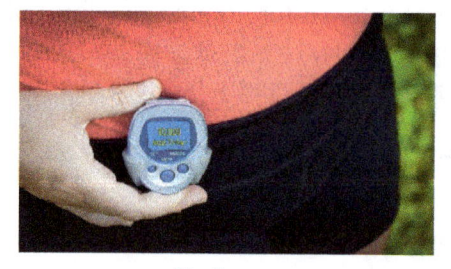

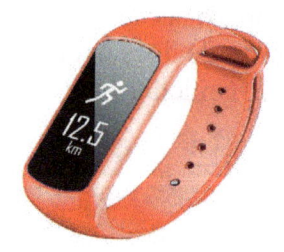

Pedometer   **Fitbit**

Smartwatch   **Smartphone**

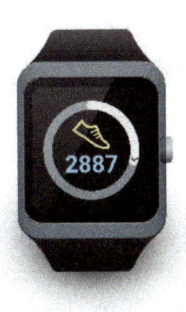

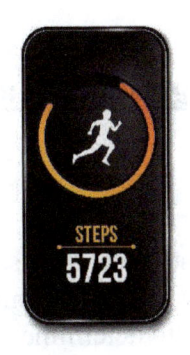

    A pedometer is a battery-powered, pager-size devise worn on a belt. It records and displays the number of steps taken based on the body's hip movements. Some pedometers only count steps, while others also track the distance walked and the calories burned. The average cost of a pedometer is between $17 to $30 depending on the device's sophistication. It is an excellent device for older adults if they are not too tech-savvy or don't possess a smartwatch or smartphone.

    One of the significant advantages of wearing a pedometer or using smart devices is that they give you accurate feedback about their activity level. For example, suppose you had a day requiring a lot of sitting and noticed at lunch or before dinner that the number of steps taken is below your average. In that case, you can make it a point to take an extra 5, 10, or 15 minutes during the day or evening to get the recommended number of steps. Therefore, these step/activity tracking devices are great tools to help you become more aware of their activity level; and help you become more accountable in keeping as active as you need to be.

Conclusion

    Counting the number of steps taken in a day is an excellent way for you to start on the road to improved fitness and health. With time you can begin to consider the intensity or speed at which you are walking to enhance the health benefits of the activity.

    People may discover that they begin to think of ways to get more "steps" throughout their busy days. Strategies such as walking upstairs rather than using the escalator or parking the car a little farther from work or grocery/retail stores are great ways of forcing the legs to walk a little more.

    Good fitness starts in modest ways. The first step is often the hardest step to take, and utilizing a pedometer or smart device to track your steps/activity is an excellent way of counting those first steps towards better health.

    You should make it a habit to monitor your daily activity; it is invaluable feedback (refer to Chapter 8.0: Evaluation of Effort – Measuring Progress and Success).

4.1.3. Monitoring Heart Rate for Effective Cardiovascular Training

Introduction

The older adult must do cardiovascular training safely and without over-exerting themselves. The talk test (the ability to talk in complete sentences) and rating perceived effort on a scale of one to ten are two ways to determine the intensity of your effort. However, heart rate monitoring is the most accurate way for older adults to evaluate their exercise intensity and to ensure that they don't endanger themselves by overdoing it.

Self Monitoring   **Smart Watch on the wrist**

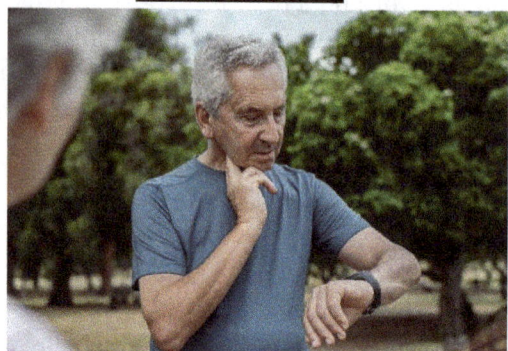

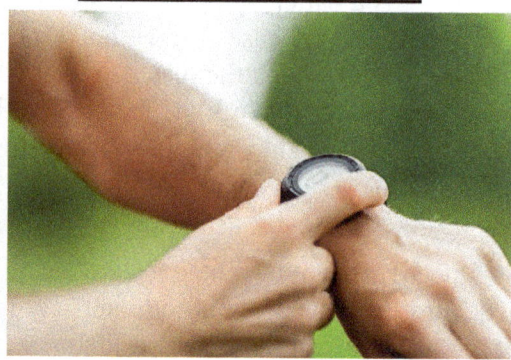

Chest Strap Monitoring

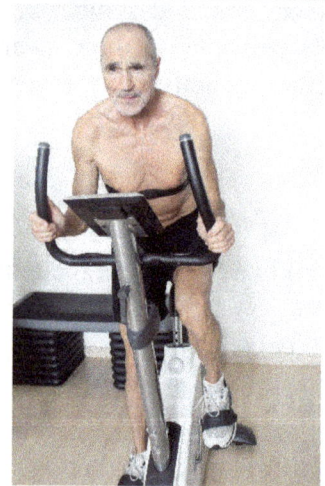

Key Points to Remember

1. Effective cardiovascular training requires you to train at different cardiovascular training intensities. Following the 80/20 rule, 20% of the training sessions will be at high intensity, and 80% will be at a low to moderate level of intensity.

212

2. Monitoring heart rate is the best and most accurate method for determining training intensity. Unlike subjectively monitoring perceived effort or the ability to hold a conversation (talk test) while exercising, heart rate monitoring is objective.

3. Though heart rate monitoring is an objective measure of how hard the heart is working to deliver oxygen to the working muscles, it can be affected by factors other than exercise effort. Medications, physical fatigue, illness, overtraining, and hot, humid weather can profoundly affect heart rate and must be considered when determining and monitoring the intensity of a particular exercise session.

4. Avoid becoming addicted to the heart rate monitor. Monitoring heart rate during exercise is important, but it does not have to be monitored every minute. While exercising, determine perceived effort and use the talk test (see table below) as convenient ways of monitoring exercise intensity and then monitor heart rate every 10 minutes to confirm that work is staying in the correct training zone.

Subjective Ways to Monitor Exercise Intensity

1. Modified Borg Scale of Perceived Exertion		**2. Talk Test**
Rating	**Perceived Exertion**	**1. Low Intensity – For beginner:** – Able to talk in complete sentences. **2. Moderate Intensity- best for cardiovascular training:** – Talk in broken sentences. **3. High Intensity & Interval training:** – Shortness of breath makes it difficult to talk
0	Nothing at all	
1	Very Light	
2	Light	
3	Moderate	
4	Somewhat Hard	
5-6	Hard	
7-8	Very Hard	
9	Extremely Hard (Almost maximal)	
10	Maximal	

Advantages of Monitoring Heart Rate Objectively

1. Adjustments to exercise intensity can be made immediately to meet the training goals for that particular workout.

   (<u>Example</u> – if the exercise intensity goal is between 125 & 130 bpm and after 10-15 minutes, heart rate is only at 120, the walking pace needs to be increased. Conversely, if the heart rate is 135, the person is exercising too hard, and the pace needs to be slowed).

2. Heart rate monitoring is an excellent way of monitoring improvements in your fitness level. Lowering the resting heart rate is one of the first physiological signs of improved fitness. As your fitness level improves, you will exercise at a greater intensity (walk faster) at a lower heart rate. The lower heart rate for the same amount of effort means the heart has become more efficient. The lower heart rate is excellent motivational feedback that your training is working and provides you confidence and incentive to continue training.

General Cardiovascular Training Guidelines

To receive the most benefit from cardiovascular exercise the American College of Sports Medicine recommends;

<u>Intensity (Target Heart Rate Zone)</u> – 60-80% of maximum heart rate
<u>Duration</u> – At least 20 – 60 minutes per workout
<u>Frequency</u> – three to five times a week.
<u>Type of Exercise</u> – Anything that you will enjoy and that will elevate your heart rate for a sustained period of time (examples: walking, running, swimming, biking).

Specific Cardiovascular Training by Monitoring Heart Rate

1. <u>Maximum Heart Rate Calculation</u>

HR_{Max} = the maximum attainable heart rate the body can reach before total exhaustion
<u>Determination;</u>

      a. <u>Most Accurate</u> – Exercise lab stress test
      b. <u>Two Estimation Formulas (variability range of 10 bpm)</u>;

         1. HR_{Max} = 220 – age
            <u>Males</u> - 220-age
            <u>Females</u> - 226-age

<u>Reference</u> – Stanton, John. (2010). *Running: The Complete Guide to Building Your Running Program.* Penguin Canada

2. $HR_{Max} = 207 - (age \times .7)$

<u>Reference</u> – Pfitzner, Peter., Douglas, Scott. (2009). *Advanced Marathoning*, Human Kinetics

2. <u>Calculating Target Heart Rate Training Zone</u>
    <u>Formula</u>:
        1. HR_{Max} x <u>Lower %</u> Heart Rate Training Zone
        2. HR_{Max} x <u>Upper %</u> Heart Rate Training Zone

<u>Key Point</u> – Staying within the "target zone" or the "intensity" with which it is recommended to exercise is critical to meeting cardiovascular exercise goals.

Three Common Heart Rate Training Zones (Intensities)

<u>Training Zone</u>	**<u>% of Maximum Heart Rate</u>**	**<u>Purpose</u>**
1. Beginner & Intermediate: Base Training (Endurance) -Active Walking (Long Slow Distance)	60-70%	Conditioning of muscles, ligaments and heart for more intense exercise
2. Advanced: Strength & Endurance Training – Hill Training/Tempo (fast)	70-80%	Work on proper form, strength and endurance
3. Advanced: Speed Training – Speed (interval) training on the track	> 80 %	Improve fitness, technique

Example- Heart Rate Training Zone Calculation:

Female, age 55

Step 1 – Calculate – Max heart rate:
> Two formulas:
> 1. Max HR – age = 226-55 = 171
> 2. 207 – (age x 70%) = 207-(55 x .7) = 169

Step 2 – Calculate – Heart Rate Training Zone:

> Formula – Max Hr x Target Zone Percentage

> 1. Base Training (Sunday walks – Average/Intermediate Fit Person)- Intensity between 60 & 70%)
> Lower Training HR – 169 x .6 = 102 bpm
> Higher Training HR – 169 x .7 = 119 bpm

> 2. Strength Training (Hills – Intensity between 70-80%)
> Lower Training HR – 169 x .7 = 119 bpm
> Higher Training HR – 169 x .8 = 136 bpm

> 3. Speed Training (Track – intensity greater than 80%)
> Training Zone – 169 x >.8 = >136 bpm

Use this Chart for Calculating Heart Rate Training Zone for the Various Training Intensities

Age	Max Heart Rate (220-age)	1. Base Training (Long Slow Distance -Sunday Walks) 60%	70%	2. Strength Training (Hills) 70%	80%	3. Speed Training (Track) > 80%
30	190	114	133	133	152	> 152
31	189	113	132	132	151	> 152
32	188	113	132	132	150	> 150
33	187	112	131	131	150	> 150
34	186	112	130	130	149	> 149
35	185	111	130	130	148	> 148
36	184	110	129	129	147	> 147
37	183	110	128	128	146	> 146
38	182	109	127	127	146	> 146
39	181	109	127	127	145	> 145
40	180	108	126	126	144	> 144
41	179	107	125	125	143	> 143

(Males)

42	178	107	125	125	142	> 142
43	177	106	124	124	142	> 142
44	176	106	123	123	141	> 141
45	175	105	123	123	140	> 140
46	174	104	122	122	139	> 139
47	173	104	121	121	138	> 138
48	172	103	120	120	138	> 138
49	171	103	120	120	137	> 137
50	170	102	119	119	136	> 136
51	169	101	118	118	135	> 135
52	168	101	118	118	134	> 134
53	167	100	117	117	134	> 134
54	166	100	116	116	133	> 133
55	165	99	116	116	132	> 132
56	164	98	115	115	131	> 131
57	163	98	114	114	130	> 130
58	162	97	113	113	130	> 130
59	161	97	113	113	129	> 129
60	160	96	112	112	128	> 128
61	159	95	111	111	127	> 127
62	158	95	111	111	126	> 126
63	157	94	110	110	126	> 126
64	156	94	109	109	125	> 125
65	155	93	109	109	124	> 124
66	154	92	108	108	123	> 123
67	153	92	107	107	122	> 122
68	152	91	106	106	122	> 122
69	151	91	106	106	121	> 121
70	150	90	105	105	120	> 120
71	149	89	104	104	119	> 119
72	148	89	104	104	118	> 118
73	147	88	103	103	118	> 118
74	146	88	102	102	117	> 117
75	145	87	102	102	116	> 116
76	144	86	101	101	115	> 115
77	143	86	100	100	114	> 114
78	142	85	99	99	114	> 114
79	141	85	99	99	113	> 113
80	140	84	98	98	112	> 112

Age	Max Heart Rate (226-age)	Base Training (Long Slow Distance - Sunday Walks) 60%	70%	Strength Training (Hills) 70%	80%	Speed Training (Track) > 80%
30	196	118	137	137	157	> 157
31	195	117	137	137	156	> 156
32	194	116	136	136	155	> 155
33	193	116	135	135	154	> 154
34	192	115	134	134	154	> 154
35	191	115	134	134	153	> 153
36	190	114	133	133	152	> 152
37	189	113	132	132	151	> 151
38	188	113	132	132	150	> 150
39	187	112	131	131	150	> 150
40	186	112	130	130	149	> 149
41	185	111	130	130	148	> 148
42	184	110	129	129	147	> 147
43	183	110	128	128	146	> 146
44	182	109	127	127	146	> 146
45	181	109	127	127	145	> 145
46	180	108	126	126	144	> 144
47	179	107	125	125	143	> 143
48	178	107	125	125	142	> 142
49	177	106	124	124	142	> 142
50	176	106	123	123	141	> 141
51	175	105	123	123	140	> 140
52	174	104	122	122	139	> 139
53	173	104	121	121	138	> 138
54	172	103	120	120	138	> 138
55	171	103	120	120	137	> 137
56	170	102	119	119	136	> 136
57	169	101	118	118	135	> 135
58	168	101	118	118	134	> 134
59	167	100	117	117	134	> 134
60	166	100	116	116	133	> 133
61	165	99	116	116	132	> 132
62	164	98	115	115	131	> 131
63	163	98	114	114	130	> 130
64	162	97	113	113	130	> 130
65	161	97	113	113	129	> 129
66	160	96	112	112	128	> 128
67	159	95	111	111	127	> 127

68	158	95	111	111	126	> 126
69	157	94	110	110	126	> 126
70	156	94	109	109	125	> 125
71	155	93	109	109	124	> 124
72	154	92	108	108	123	> 123
73	153	92	107	107	122	> 122
74	152	91	106	106	122	> 122
75	151	91	106	106	121	> 121
76	150	90	105	105	120	> 120
77	149	89	104	104	119	> 119
78	148	89	104	104	118	> 118
79	147	88	103	103	118	> 118
80	146	88	102	102	117	> 117

Conclusion

Cardiovascular training challenges the heart to work harder. For the older adult who is often unfit and may have a compromised cardiovascular system due to high blood pressure, obesity, diabetes, etc., monitoring their heart rate as they exercise is very important from a safety perspective. By monitoring heart rate, a person can accurately determine their training intensity and if they are training within their prescribed training zone.

Purchasing a heart rate monitor is an excellent investment to ensure the safety and effectiveness of training. As you become more fit and the intensity of your cardiovascular training increases, the need for accurate monitoring of your heart effort becomes even more important.

4.2.0. Introduction: Muscular Resistance Training

There are three major components to a comprehensive fitness plan; cardiovascular fitness, muscular strength, and flexibility. Developing and maintaining muscular strength as a person gets older is often the most elusive of the three fitness components because it usually involves buying a gym membership and leaving home to go to the gym or, if there is space, buying a set of weight, rubber resistance bands and working out at home. As well, it is often more inconvenient and usually less enjoyable for someone to do muscular resistance exercises than taking a walk, going for a run, riding their bike, or stretching in their living room in front of their TV.

People are creatures of habit, and older adults are especially like that. We like "our" daily or weekly routine, and anything that we find inconvenient or stretches us out of this routine or comfort zone often is discarded and forgotten. In other words, it just does not get done. However, maintaining your muscular strength and endurance as you age is vitally important to remain active and enjoy a high quality of life into your golden years.

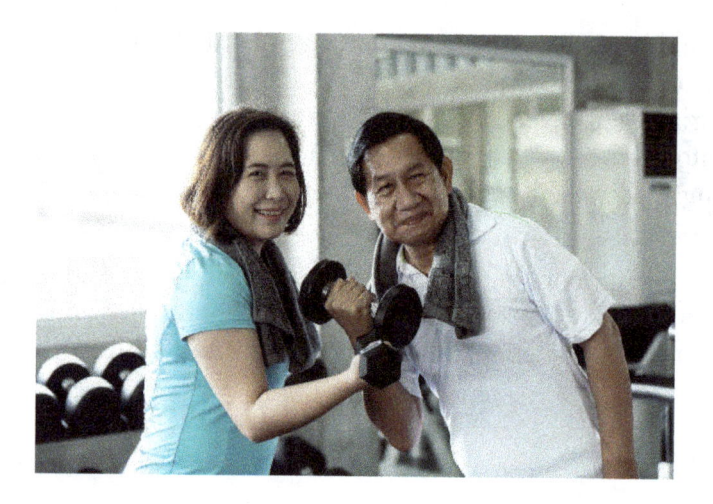

Starting and maintaining a muscular strengthening and endurance program does not have to be a daunting task. There are benefits to joining and going to the gym. It promotes social interaction, and there are usually professional trainers there who are trained to help develop a muscle resistance program tailored to a person's specific needs. As well, the gym can be a very motivating place to exercise. There is a particular energy at the gym that is hard to replicate at home.

If exercising at home is your only option, a good muscle-resistant exercise program can be developed using minimal equipment (One or two resistant bands of varying strength) and your body weight.

Maintaining muscle strength for the older adult cannot be emphasized enough. A person must find a convenient, affordable, sustainable way of introducing muscular resistant exercises into their daily and weekly routine. A person's ability to walk, climb stairs, lift objects and participate in their favourite physical activities depends upon it.

4.2.1. Muscular Resistance Training: Developing Muscle Strength and Endurance

Introduction

There are three dimensions of human frailty; time, disease, and disuse.

The passage of time is inevitable, so it is important to enjoy each moment the best you can.

The onset of disease is the result of internal system fatigue or external exposures that damage the body tissues (Chapter 1.2: Introducing the Older Adult: The Science of Aging). Medical technology has helped make the impact of disease significantly less.

Disuse – Sedentary living or lack of activity – is devastating to functional capabilities and is the number one cause of human frailty. To maintain or improve your quality of life, you must embrace physical activity.

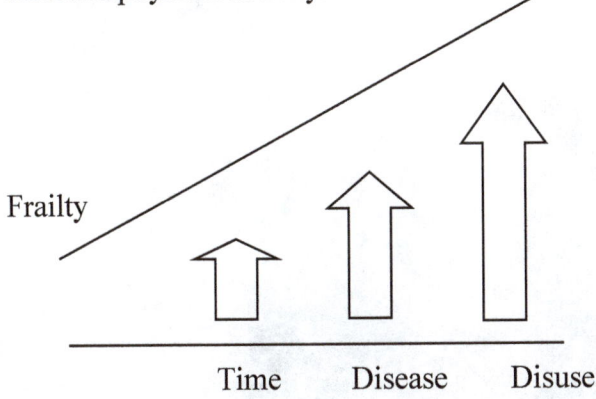

For the older adult, one of the most significant signs of aging and physical dysfunction is the loss of muscle mass (sarcopenia). By the age of 25, most men and women's muscle tissue begin to atrophy or waste away. On average, men lose about 5% and women 3% of their muscle mass each decade. The majority of the muscle mass loss is related to inactivity, but a decline in the hormones testosterone and growth hormone contribute to this loss.

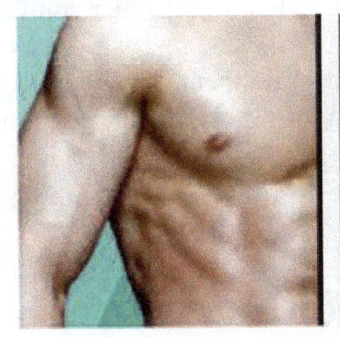

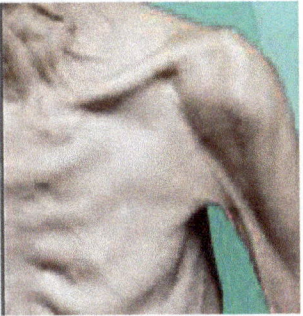

Image Source: healthjade.net

The loss of muscle mass has a significant effect on the older adult's ability to function physically. Most activities of daily living such as lifting and carrying items, climbing stairs, getting in and out of chairs and cars, gardening, house cleaning, and involvement in recreational activities require moderate levels of muscle strength. The loss of muscle mass and strength impact the older adult's agility, balance, coordination, and, consequently, their ability to walk and increases their risk of falling.

Fortunately, muscle resistance or strength training can significantly reduce muscle mass loss that occurs with age. The benefits of muscle resistance training include:

- Increased muscle and bone strength
- Increased muscle mass and decreased body fat
- Increased resting metabolism
- Improved core strength and posture
- Promotion of joint stability
- Improved body image and self-esteem.

All of these benefits are essential to enhance the older adult's quality of life.

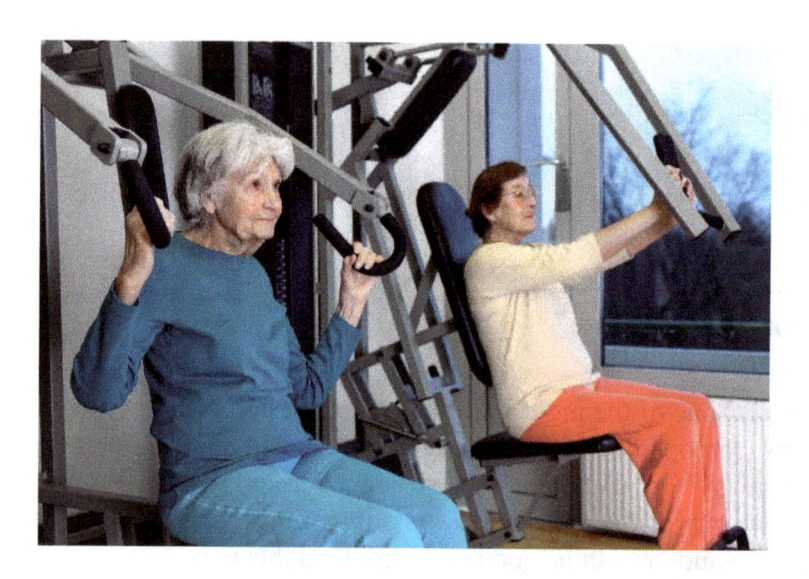

Muscle resistance training must be a key component to the older adult's fitness and health program. There are risks involved when performing muscle resistant type of exercises, and safety guidelines must be strictly adhered to when performing them. This is especially true for older adults who are usually de-conditioned when they start their fitness program.

1. Safety for Resistance Training

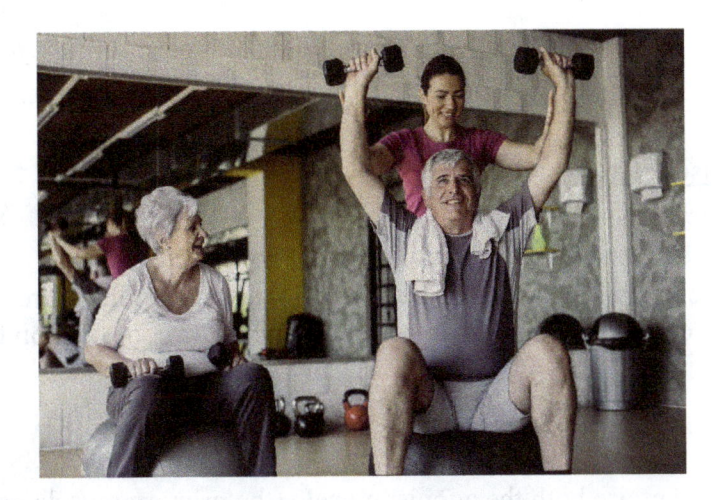

Safety has to be the number one priority for older adults when they exercise. The following safety rules must be adhered to when strength training;

1. **Medical clearance** – You must ensure that you have no medical reasons for not participating in a strength training program by having medical clearance by their doctor.
2. **Adhere to medical recommendations** – If there are modifications that your doctor recommends, these must be adhered to rigorously and completely.
3. **Warm-up is necessary** – You must ensure that you are thoroughly warmed up before beginning your resistance training. A good warm-up would include 5-10 minutes of dynamic stretching (Appendix 9.1.4.1) and light cardiovascular exercise.
4. **Perform each exercise biomechanically correct** – You must completely understand each resistance exercise and perform them correctly (Appendix 9.1.2.2.1).
5. **Be under control** – All movements of the exercise must be performed with perfect technique, under control and with no jerky movements. Good technique is especially relevant when you start to feel fatigued during the last few repetitions of a set.
6. **NEVER hold your breath** – This is rule number one when performing resistance exercises or any time you are lifting an object.
7. **Know your lifting limit** – Always use a weight that can be controlled, performed through a complete range of motion, and pain-free. To determine how much weight you should be lifting, you can calculate your one max repetition from the chart and formula below and lift a safe percentage of this weight (refer to the Intensity section in the FITT chart below for the correct percentage of one max rep to lift).

2. Key Principles to Resistance Training

The following should be considered when developing and performing a muscle resistance exercise program:

1. The type of exercise selected
- What is its specific purpose?
- Is it the most effective exercise to accomplish what you want it to do?
- Is it safe? Does the exercise produce or require too much instability? Are you physically capable with respect to your flexibility, agility, balance, and coordination to perform this type of exercise?

2. Muscle balance
A person needs to exercise both the agonist muscle (the primary muscle you are targeting) and antagonist (the counter or paired muscle). For example, you must exercise both the bicep and triceps muscles but not with the same amount of resistance. Also, it is necessary to exercised both the right and left sides of the body to prevent dominance of one side.

3. Exercise order
You should first exercise the larger muscle groups, such as the chest and back muscles, before exercising the smaller muscles such as the biceps and triceps of the arm.

4. Rest between sets
You can modify the intensity of the exercise by increasing or decreasing the amount of rest between sets. Typically, 1 to 3 minutes between sets is recommended for the older adult.

5. Breathing
You should <u>never hold your breath</u> when you are doing resistance-type exercises. Proper breathing is essential for older adults who may have high blood pressure. As you perform a resistance exercise, you should breathe out (exhale) and, during the return to the original position, breathe in (inhale).

6. Technique
Proper technique is vitally important to maximize the exercise's effectiveness and prevent serious injury.

7. Speed of movement
Most resistance training should be performed slowly and under total control. The rule of thumb is two beats to push or pull the resistance and two or four beats to return to the original position.

8. Loading
Always start with a light load to ensure proper technique and avoid injury.

9. Avoid pushing to fatigue

Perform all exercises to the last point of success rather than the first point of failure. In other words, it is best to stop one rep early than a half a rep late (safety first).

3. Establishing Your One Repetition Maximum Calculation (One Rep Max)

One repetition maximum (one rep max) calculation means determining the maximum amount of weight you can lift once. To avoid injury by experimenting with heavy weights, a formula has been established to calculate your one rep max number. Determining your one rep max for each exercise/muscle group is essential because you will lift a percentage of this one rep max for each exercise.

The percentage of the one rep max that is used varies depending on the individual's fitness level and purpose for their exercise. For example, a 30-year-old well-fit football player may want to increase their leg power. They will do fewer repetitions per set (5 to 8 reps) but a higher percentage (90-95%) of their one-repetition maximum to accomplish their goal. However, a 60-year-old non-conditioned female whose goal is to slow the loss of muscle mass in their legs as they age will do a higher number of reps per set to start (10, 12, 15) and lift only 50-60% of their one-repetition maximum.

These percentages are listed under the heading Intensity in the FITT Prescription chart which follows.

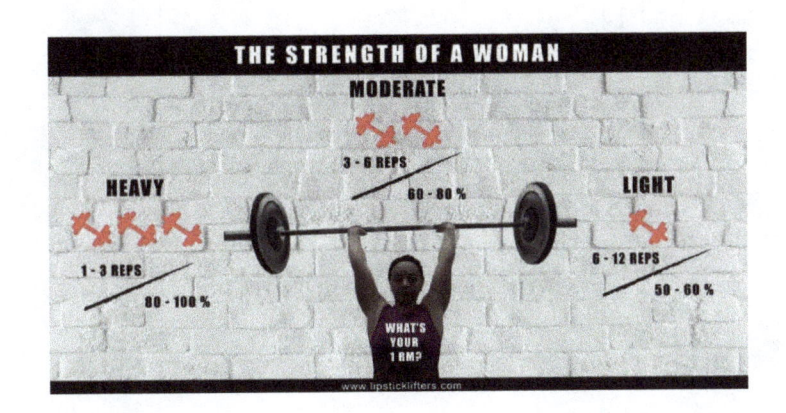

One Repetition Maximum Calculation
One Rep Max Calculation Chart

Repetition Completed	Coefficient
1	1.00
2	.943
3	.906
4	.881
5	.856
6	.831
7	.807
8	.786
9	.765
10	.744
11	.723
12	.703
13	.688
14	,675
15	.662
16	.650
17	.638
18	.627
19	.616
20	.606

Calculation Formula

One Rep Max (1RM) = Load (wt. lifted)/Coefficient (Based on the number of repetitions completed with the weight lifted)

(Example – a person lifted 50 lbs 8 times – 1RM = 50lbs /.786 (coefficient for number of times lifted) = 65 lbs.)

Calculating one max rep is especially relevant and important for the older adult whose muscles, tendons, and ligaments are not as pliable and do not recover from the stresses of exercise as quickly as they would for a younger person. Lower intensity strength training (60% one rep max vs. 90% one rep max) will promote endurance and mild to moderate increases in strength, which is usually more applicable to the older adult needs.

Prior to beginning a resistance training program, you must establish realistic goals (Chapter 3.3: The Importance and Art of Goal Setting) so that the correct muscle resistance program can be developed to achieve them.

4. Progression in Resistance Training

The key to achieving good results from a muscular resistance training program is consistency and sustainability. Over time you will get stronger, and you will have to change and increase the amount of weight you lift to see progress. This is called the "overload" principle. No matter the age, muscles will adapt positively to strength/resistance training because muscles are very sensitive to the stimulus/weight applied. As you get stronger and add more resistance into your routine, additional strength development will occur. However, with increased resistance, there is an increased risk of injury.

It is essential to implement progression (making the exercise harder) properly in resistance training programs. The following is a list of progressions that can be implemented safely to increase the level of difficulty of the program when you are ready to do so;

1. **Increase the amount of weight lifted gradually and change the way the weights are lifted**

    This is the most commonly abused principle for progression in a muscular resistance program. The usual thought process when you want to make your program harder and the simplest way for you to do that is to increase the amount of weight. Unfortunately, there are multiple problems with this line of thinking.

    First, most people increase the amount of weight they push or pull too quickly. It is vitally important that you are physically well adapted to the weight you are using before increasing the lifted weight. Usually, 8 to 10 sessions at a particular weight is necessary before physical adaption occurs. Even if you find it easy to get through a set at a specific weight in fewer sessions, it is best to adhere to the 8-10 session guideline. On the other hand, if you find it challenging to complete your reps/sets before getting exhausted, it is best to extend the number of sessions before progressing to more weight.

    Second, the amount of weight a person adds is usually too much, and they don't make accommodations for the significant increase in weight. This situation often occurs when the weights available are few and/or increase in increments by 5 or 10 lbs rather than 2.5 pounds. The safest rule of thumb is never to increase the amount of weight used by more than 2.5 pounds at a time. If 2.5-pound increments are not available and you must increase by 5 pounds, you must decrease the number of reps or sets. Once you accommodate to the new reduced reps/sets, you can increase the number of reps or sets to what they were before.

    Third, most people do the same type of exercise for a particular muscle group repeatedly. It is essential to change the type of exercise you are doing for a specific muscle group every ten sessions. This process is called "muscle confusion." By increasing the amount of resistance you are using, but not changing the type of exercise for a particular muscle group, you are not stimulating the muscles and neurologic system optimally. You are just "patterning" your exercises which means you are using the same biomechanics or "pattern" to lift more weight.

This "patterning" leads to a faster rate of plateauing and significantly slows the rate of progress you will see for the effort expended.

For most muscle groups, you can do multiple types of exercises to achieve strength gains. Appendix 9.1.2.1.1 lists various core exercises, Appendix 9.1.2.2.1 lists a variety of whole-body strengthening exercises and Appendix 9.1.2.3.1 list body-weight strengthening exercises that are available for the different muscle groups. Workout sheets 9.2.0 are available that presents core, whole-body and body-weight muscular strengthening routines. You can modify these routines to address your particular goals and needs.

2. Reduced rest time between sets

A very effective way of introducing progression and increasing the intensity of a muscular resistance workout session is decreasing the time between sets. Because reducing recovery time between sets increases the intensity of the exercise session, you must be careful because it also increases the chance for injury since fatigue sets in earlier than usual.

This way to introducing progression should only be used when you are well-conditioned and used intermittently (every fourth exercise session) to change the dynamics of the exercise session. Introducing this type of variety into your muscular resistance exercise routine is excellent and helps your exercise routine produce the most effective results.

How to Progress Your Resistance Training Program...

Increase... Sets/Reps Resistance/Weight

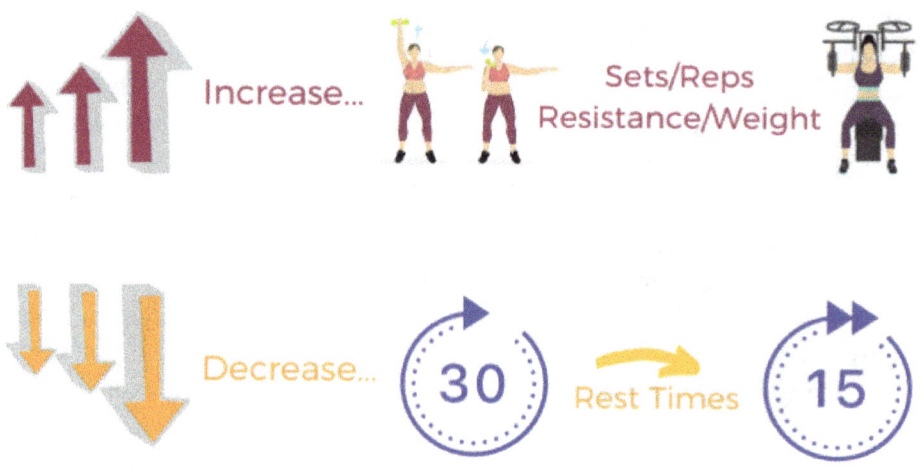

Decrease... 30 Rest Times 15

Image Source: weightlossresources.co.uk

3. Single joint to multi-joint movements

If your fitness level is average or poor when you start your fitness program, all exercises you do should be single-joint exercises. This means, only one joint is moving and being exercised at a time. For example, you could do machine leg extension exercise to strengthen the quadriceps (front thigh muscle). During this exercise, only the knee moves. As you get stronger, you can introduce multi-joint exercises to strengthen the quads, such as a squat or lunge. With these exercises, the hip and knee are involved. These exercises involve not only two joints but also multiple muscle groups and increase the need for good balance. Squats and lunges are advanced and progressive exercises.

4. Stability to instability

Adding instability (stability ball, BOSU) adds significantly to the challenge/difficulty of an exercise. You need good strength, agility, and balance before you progress to this level of difficulty. A good example is standing lateral shoulder raises (exercising the Deltoids and Upper Trapezius muscles) versus sitting lateral raises on a stability ball. When standing, you can stabilize yourself through your feet, but when sitting on a stability ball, you lose this stability, and the difficulty of the exercise increases considerably.

5. Slow to fast movements

It is recommended that a consistent 2:2 beat ratio (2 beats to contract and 2 beats to lengthen the muscle) or 2:4 beat ratio (2 beats to contract the muscle and 4 beats to lengthen the muscle) be used when doing resistance exercises. Doing resistance exercises at this pace allows the muscle/joint proprioceptor reflexes to have time to help control the movement. Faster movement (1:1 or 1:2) requires a more immediate neurologic reaction for muscular recruitment and coordination to control the movement. Introducing faster movements is a significant progression in intensity of the exercise. It is important to be aware that if you are not well conditioned, you will not be able to neurologically recruit the muscle fibers necessary in a shorter/faster period. As a result, there is a greater likelihood of injury if you introduce this type of progression too early into your exercise routine.

The most discouraging thing when exercising is having to stop because of injury. By following the five principles listed above, the likelihood of injury dramatically diminishes. Regaining your health and fitness and then maintaining it is a marathon, not a sprint. Introduce progression slowly. Your body will greatly appreciate it.

5. Exercise Guidelines

Chapter 3.1: The Eight Golden Rules of Training reviews the major guidelines for safely and effectively implementing an exercise program. Three of these guidelines need to be emphasized concerning muscle resistance exercising.

1. Progress low and slow

The first consideration must always be safety. The older adult's body can adapt to the stresses placed upon it, but it needs time to make this adaptation. For the older adult, the time for this physical adaption to occur is a little longer than for someone in their 20's and 30's.

As well, for exercise to be consistent and sustainable (two keys to effective training), mental adaptation must also occur. If you progress too hard and too fast, you have not had time to mentally adapt, resulting in mental/emotional fatigue and a lack of motivation to continue.

2. Have sufficient recovery time

The need for recovery between exercise sessions takes on a particular significant purpose for the training and re-conditioning of the older adult. Physical adaptations/strength gains occur during periods of recovery. The metabolism of the older adult, especially if you are unfit, is slower, so you need more time to recover/adapt physically to the new stresses of exercise.

If the older adult becomes physically injured, tired, or sore, this will affect their mental/emotional adaptation and motivation. Recovery time between exercise sessions is as important as the exercise sessions themselves.

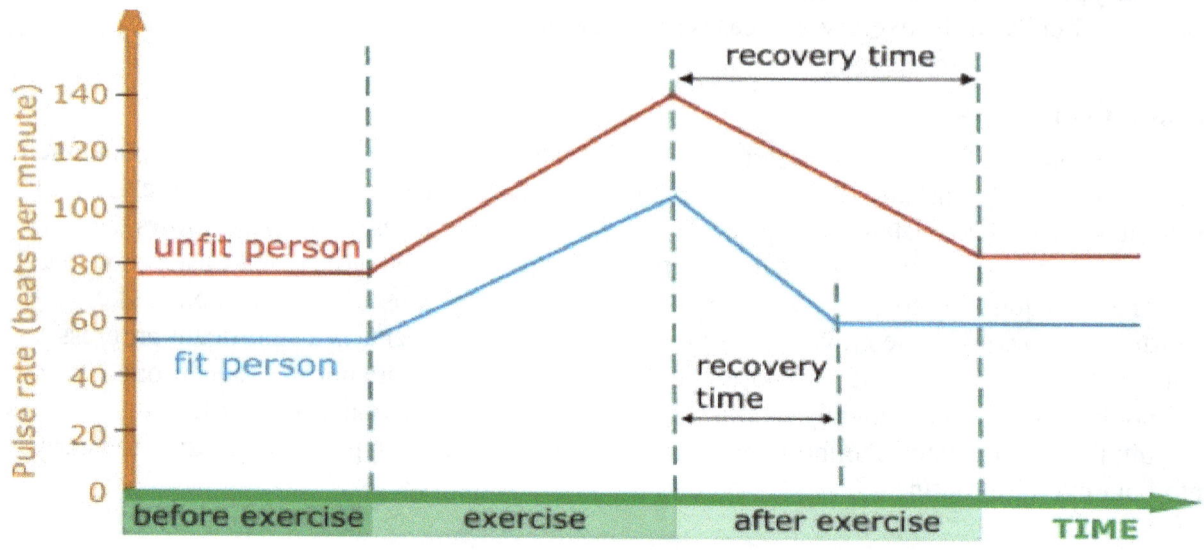

Image Source: ironcompany.com

3. Consider physical and cognitive limitations

Section 2: The Off-Season: Studying the Opposition and Section 6: Special Teams: Mental Health discuss the various physical and cognitive challenges that the older adult faces. These physical and cognitive challenges need consideration when developing an effective muscular resistance exercise program. For example, suppose arthritis of the knee is present. In that case, the goal should be to strengthen the upper leg muscles (quadriceps and hamstrings) without weight-bearing activities that may aggravate the arthritic knees. As a result, non-weight-bearing leg extensions and leg curls on an exercise machine are indicated, and weight-bearing exercises such as squats and lunges are contra-indicated.

Knee Pain

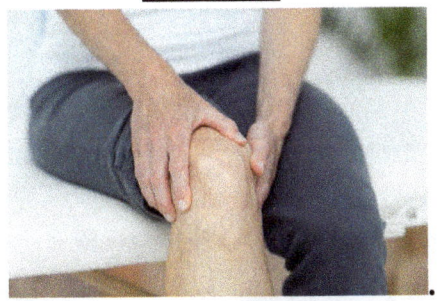

Machine Leg Extensions (Indicated)   **Squats (Contra-indicated)**

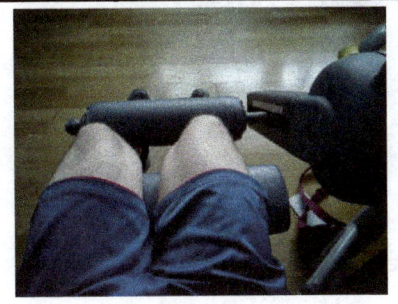

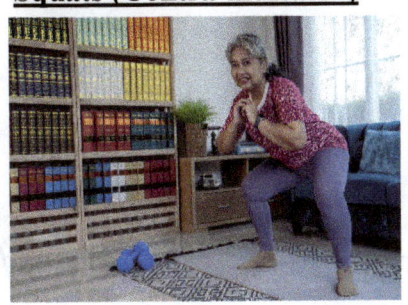

6. The FITT Template

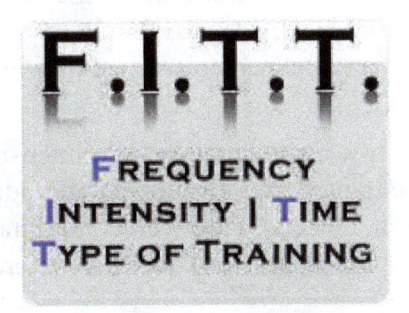

Image Source: sites.google.com

The FITT template (Frequency, Intensity, Time, Type) is the framework used to structure a person's muscular resistance exercise program.

Steps:
1. Establish your muscular strengthening goals (Section 3.3: The importance and Art of Goal Setting)
2. Follow the FITT template;

   a. Frequency (F) – This indicates how often per week you will do muscular resistance exercises. For the older adult, 2x/week is sufficient to develop and maintain strength gains. These exercise sessions should occur on non-consecutive days. Ideally, there should be two or three days for recovery between each exercise session.

Older adults who train 2x's/week develop as much or more lean muscle mass weight as those who train 3x's/week.

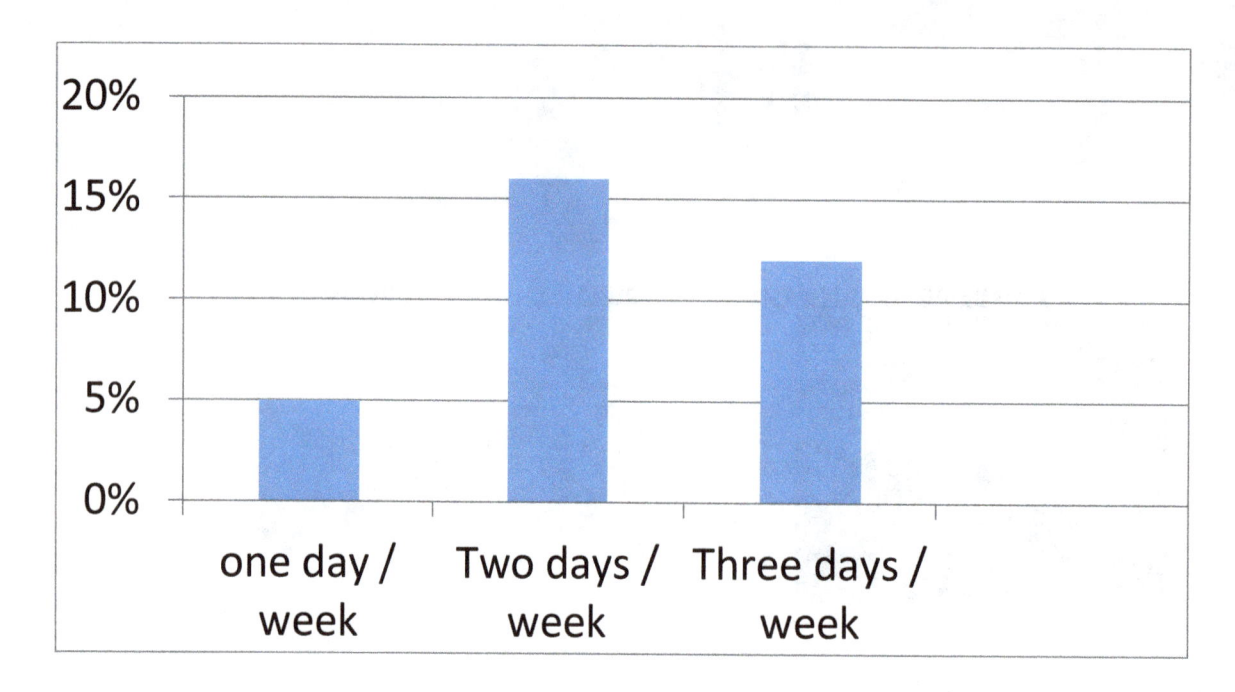

[Bar chart showing: one day/week ≈ 5%, Two days/week ≈ 16%, Three days/week ≈ 12%]

    b. Intensity (I) – The intensity of the workout for the older adult is significant. Too intense, and the person will find it too hard, fatigue quickly, need more recovery time, all without enjoying the experience. Too easy, and the person will get discouraged from a lack of progress.

    It is always best to start with a low or moderately light intensity (Rating 4) (refer to the chart below). The intensity can increase to moderate (Rating 5) or moderately hard (Rating 6) after initial physical and mental adaption. Once you are well conditioned, intense workouts (Rating 7) can occur sporadically (once every fourth session) over a 10-exercise session set.

Rating of Perceived Exertion

Rating	Perceived Exertion
1	Very, very light
2	Very light
3	Moderately light
4	Light (safe)
5	Moderate (safe)
6	Moderately hard (safe)
7	Hard (safe)
8	Very hard
9	Very, very hard
10	Extremely hard

The intensity that you experience in an exercise session is influenced by your level of fitness. The golden rule of starting slow must be followed. This may mean doing only one set or doing only 3, 5, 8, or 10 reps per set to start (a set is the number of repetitions of a particular exercise you do in a row). As a person's physical conditioning improves, the number of reps per set and the number of sets for a particular exercise may increase.

The Rule of Thumb for the number of reps and sets is as follows:
To develope:
1. Power – 4 to 6 sets of 3-8 reps at 90% one rep max
2. Strength – 2- 3 sets of 8-12 reps at 70-80% one rep max
3. Strength and endurance (Recommended for older adult) – 3 sets 12-15 reps at 50-70% one rep max

Note – for the person who is severely de-conditioned an intensity of 40-50% one rep max is recommended to start.

c. Time (T)/Duration – The duration that you work out will be dependent on your fitness level and whether you are doing 1, 2, 3 sets or 8, 12, 15 reps, and whether you are doing a whole-body workout (chest, back, arms, core, hips and legs) or doing just a few selected muscle groups (chest and back or legs). It is best to limit the workout duration to 60 minutes, which includes a 5-minute dynamic stretch at the beginning and a 5-minute static stretch at the end.

d. Type (T) of Exercise – There is an endless variety of ways to exercise the various muscle groups in the body. Appendix 9.1.2.1.1 illustrates multiple core exercises and Appendix 9.1.2.2.1 illustrates the various whole-body exercises that you can do with dumbbells or on a weight machine.

Most of these exercises can also be done using your body weight as resistance (Appendix 9.1.2.3) or with various weight resistance apparatuses such as Resistance Bands (Appendix 9.1.5), Stability Ball (Appendix 9.1.6), BOSU (Appendix 9.1.7), TRX (Appendix (9.1.8), Medicine Ball (Appendix (9.1.9), Floor sliders (Appendix 9.1.10). The use of different exercise equipment over time helps maintain motivation in two ways; first, by introducing variety into your resistance program to prevent boredom; second, by stimulating "muscle confusion" to prevent plateauing of strength gains.

The most popular weight resistance apparatuses are listed and illustrated below.

Refer to the appropriate appendices for a description of exercises associated with these apparatuses.

Various weight resistance and instability apparatuses

1. Weight machine
(Appendix 9.1.2.2. Whole Body Weight Strengthening)

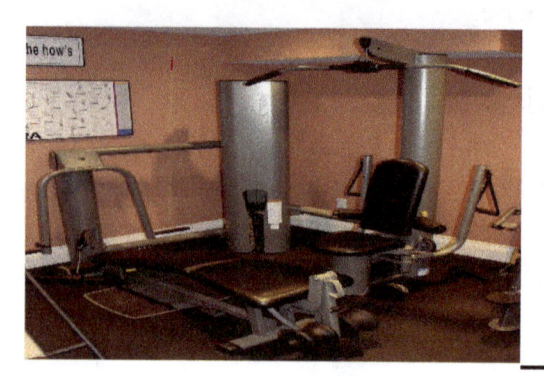

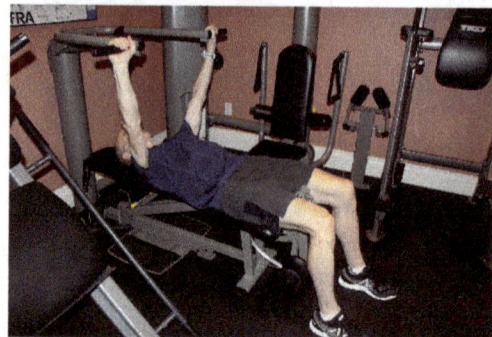

2. Dumbbells
(Appendix 9.1.2.2. Whole Body Weight Strengthening)

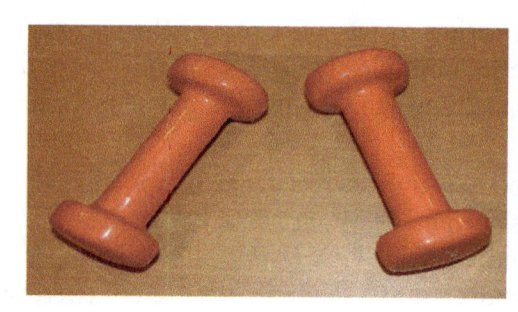

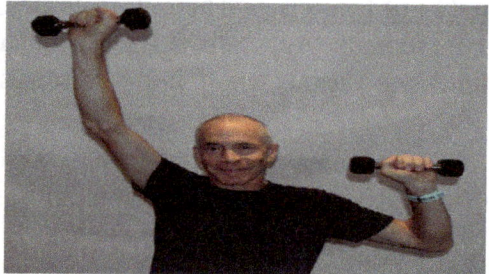

3. Resistance bands
(Appendix 9.1.5.)

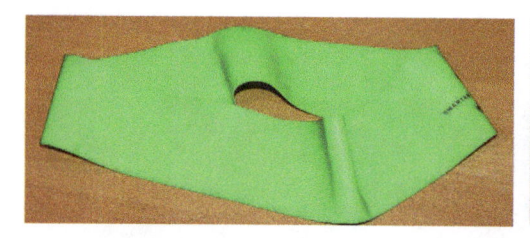

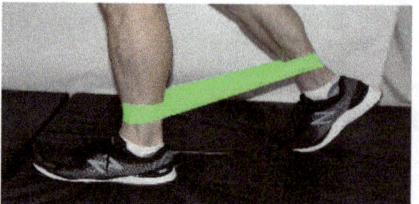

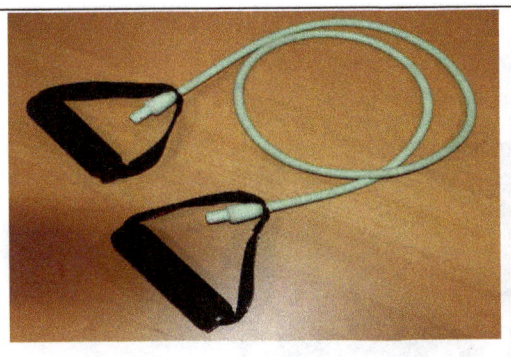

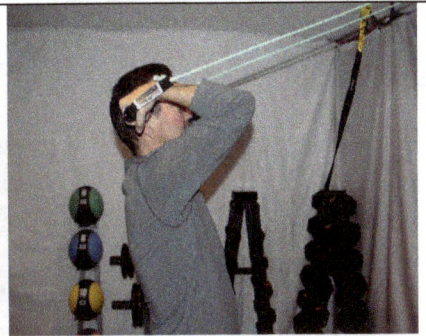

4. Stability Ball
(Appendix 9.1.6.)

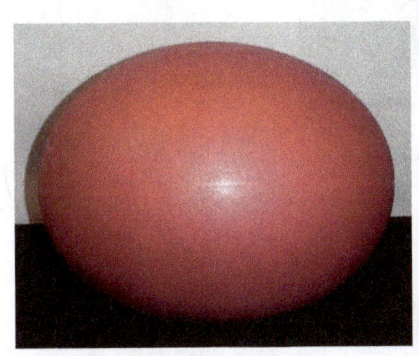

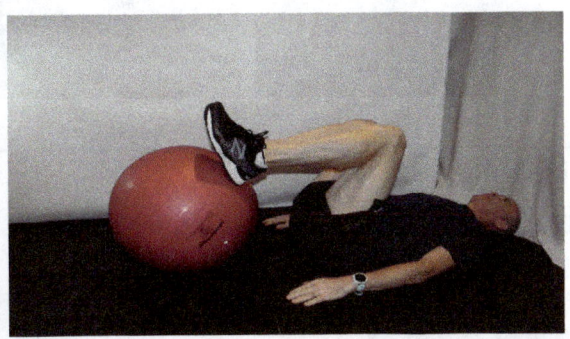

5. BOSU
(Appendix 9.1.7.)

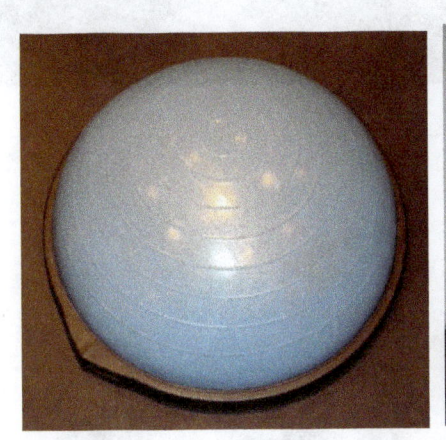

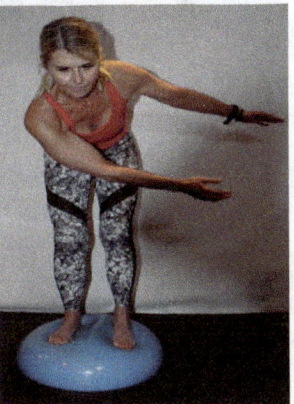

6. TRX
(Appendix 9.1.8.)

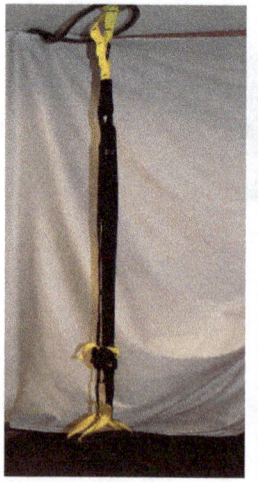

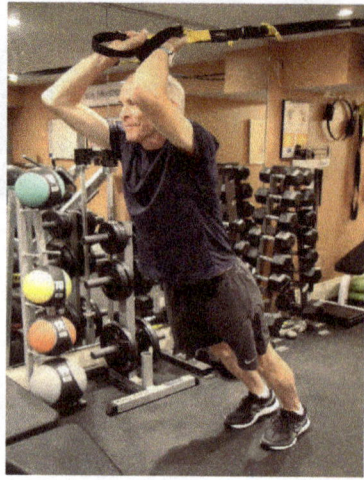

7. Medicine balls
(Appendix 9.1.9.)

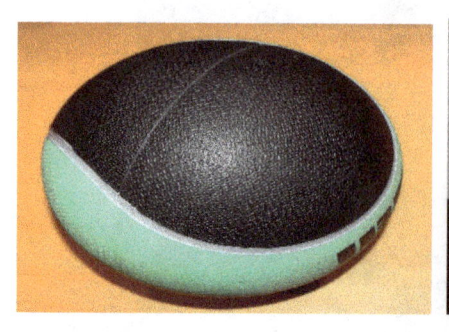

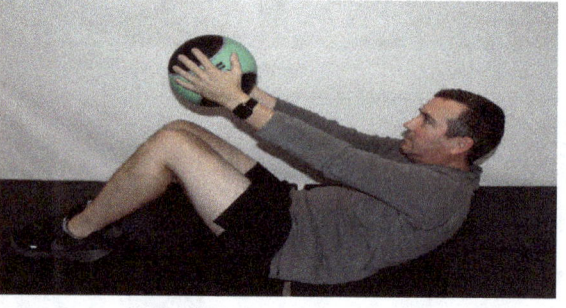

8. Floor Slider
(Appendix 9.1.10.)

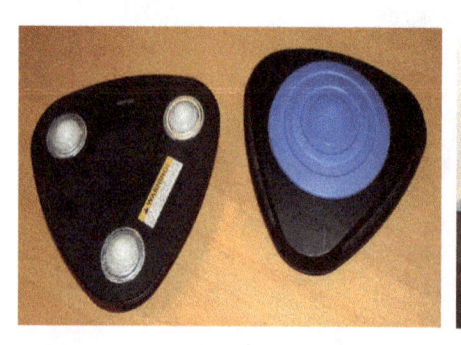

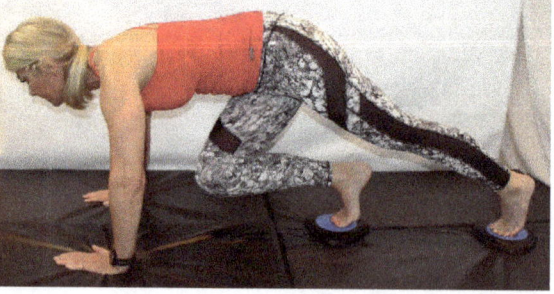

7. FITT Template: Resistance Training Guidelines

Description	Beginner (Minimal Experience)	Intermediate (Regular Exerciser)	Advanced (Serious lifter)
Goals	1. Learning proper technique 2. Learning correct exercises 3. Developing core strength 4. Gaining muscular endurance	1. Refining proper technique 2. Learning new exercises 3. Developing core strength 4. Gaining muscular strength 5. Exercise variety	1. Exercise variety 2. Increasing muscular size 3. Maximizing core strength 4. Maximizing training time
Frequency	1-2 x's/week	2-3 x's/week	3-5 x's/week
Intensity (% 1 rep max)	< 40-60% 1RM	60-70% 1 RM	80-90% 1RM
Result	Muscular endurance	Muscular strength and endurance	Maximum strength and power
Reps	12-15, no muscle failure (May feel a mild burn)	8-15 (May feel fatigue last 3 reps)	3-8, reaching failure
Sets	1-3	2-3	3-5
Rest Between sets	30sec.-1 min	30sec.-2 min	2+ min
Type (Equipment Choice)	1. Weight training machines 2. Body weight exercises 3. Stability ball	1. Weight training machines 2. Pulleys 3. Dumbbels/barbells 4. Body weight exercises 5. Instability equipment	1. Weight training machines 2. Pulleys 3. Free weights 4. Body weight exercises 5. Stability ball 6. Medicine ball, etc.
Time (Routine Choice)	1. Total body – Balanced workout (6-8 exercises)	1. Total body 2. Split programs Example: – chest and back – arms and shoulders – hips, quads and hamstrings	1. Split programs Example: – chest and back – arms and shoulders – hips, quads and hamstrings

		(2-3 exercises per muscle group)	2. Advanced designs (eg. circuit training, splits, pyramids) – 2 muscle groups per workout (2-3 exercises per muscle group)

8. Paired Muscle Groups

To achieve proper muscle balance, you must make sure that the right and left sides of the body are exercised with equal weight resistance. If one side is significantly weaker than the other side, the weak side needs special attention (increase the number of reps and sets but not increase weight resistance) to ensure proper strength balance is regained.

The muscle resistance program must also be structured so that the muscle pairs (the muscles that oppose each other) are exercised equally, even though the weight resistance for the paired muscle groups will not be the same.

The chart below lists the paired muscle groups in the body.

Muscle	**Opposing/Paired muscle**
Quadriceps (Quads are worked at approximately 3:2 ratio to the hamstrings. Example – quads at 15 lbs and hamstring at 10 lbs)	**Hamstrings**
Hip Abductors (Lateral buttocks muscles – Gluteus Medius, Gluteus Minimus, Tensor Fasciae Latae)	**Hip Adductors** (Groin muscles)
Ankle Extensors Gastrocnemius	**Ankle Flexors** Tibialis Anterior
Chest and Shoulders Pectoralis Major, Deltoids	**Upper Back** Trapezius Rhomboids Latissimus Dorsi Rotator Cuff Muscles
Front of the Upper Arms Biceps (Biceps are worked at a 2:1 ratio to triceps. Example – Biceps at 20 lbs and Triceps at 10 lbs.)	**Back of the Upper Arms** Triceps

Wrist Extensors	**Wrist flexors**
Forearm extensors	Forearm flexors

Core
(All muscle groups that make up the core must be exercised for proper muscle balance)
Lower back extensors,
Rectus Abdominus (six-pack muscle)
Abdominal obliques

Conclusion

It is vitally important that older adults maintain their muscular strength and endurance to perform routine daily activities and participate in their favourite recreational sports/activities. Muscle resistance exercises are the way to accomplish this goal.

Fortunately, because the older adult is often faced with many health challenges, the frequency, intensity, time/duration, and type of specific exercises can be changed/modified to accommodate almost any special need or condition that the older adult presents with. However, when performing these exercises, safety is paramount, and the specific safety guidelines listed must be strictly adhered to.

When muscular resistance exercise programs are done safely, consistently, and sustained over a period of time, muscle strength gains will occur and this will allow the older adult to maintain a high quality of life well into their golden years.

References

www.forever-active.com
Can-Fit-Pro, (2007) *Foundations of Professional Personal Training*, Human Kinetics,
Rose, Debra J. (2010), *Fall Proof: A Comprehensive Balance and Mobility Training Program*, Human Kinetics.
Baechle, Thomas., Westcott, Wayne.(2010), *Strength Training Older Adults*, Human Kinetics.

4.2.2. Core Strengthening

Introduction

Attempts to identify "The Core", its functional importance, and what exercises are best to help condition and strengthen it have been confusing and often misleading. "The Core" is the front and back torso. Specifically, these muscles include;

Front and sides:
- Erectus abdominis (what you think of when you think "abs")
- Transverse abdominis (the deepest internal core muscle that wraps around your sides and spine)
- The internal and external obliques (the muscles on the sides of your abdomen)

Back and hips:
- Erector spinae (a set of muscles in your lower back)
- Gluteal muscles (hip musculature).

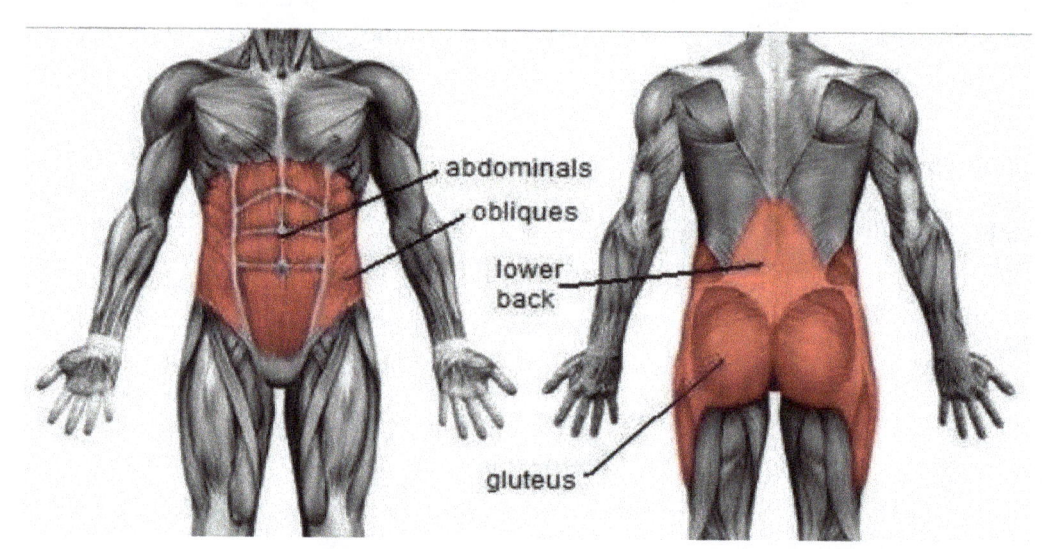

Image Source: physiofitness.org.uk

"The Core" is critical to the older adult in maintaining good posture and helping stabilize the spine during functional movements such as walking, bending, twisting, reaching, and lifting.

Any activity that involves stabilizing the trunk and maintaining good posture (abdominal bracing) will engage the core muscles and help condition these muscles.

Having a well-conditioned core is essential to help prevent lower back injuries and maintain good functional capacity and high quality of life.

Core Exercises

Specific core exercises are described and illustrated in Appendix 9.1.2.1.1

Key Points to remember when doing Core Exercises;
1. **Abdominal Bracing** – Basic technique used during whole-body core exercise training.
   – Pull the navel into the spine
2. **NEVER** hold your breath
3. **Go Slow** – The slower a core or whole-body exercise is done and the longer each repetition is held, the more effective and beneficial the exercise will be.

4.2.3. Whole Body Muscular Strengthening

Introduction

As you age, you lose muscle mass. Medically, this is called sarcopenia. The rate of loss accelerates as we age. After age 25, the rate of loss is approximately .5 - 1% per year. After the age of 50, the rate of loss is greater than 1% per year, and after age 70, the rate of loss doubles to greater than 2% per year. This muscle loss with age results from a gradual decrease in production of the hormones testosterone and growth hormone, and a lack of exercise.

Muscle Loss with Age (Sarcopenia)

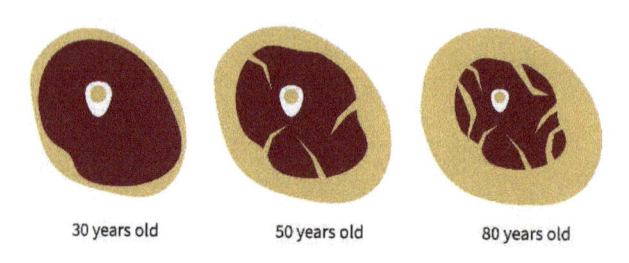

30 years old   50 years old   80 years old

SARCOPENIA

The loss of muscle mass and strength in the older adult affects their ability to be functionally active and leaves them vulnerable to falling.

Strength training is necessary to slow the rate of muscle loss in older adults. However, unlike core strength training, strength training of the chest, shoulders, arms, hips, and legs needs to be very specific. To maximize safety and the effectiveness of any strength training exercise, you need to isolate the target muscle in the most specific way possible. As a result, proper positioning to start the exercise and correct biomechanics while performing the exercise is of the utmost importance.

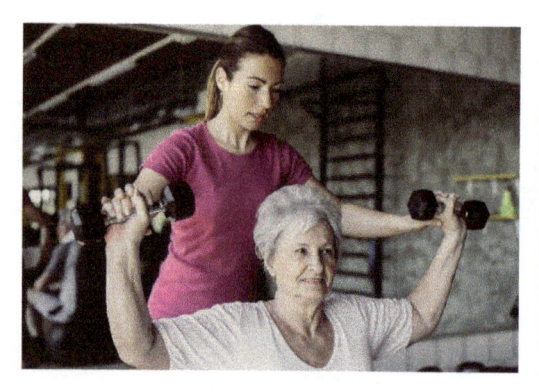

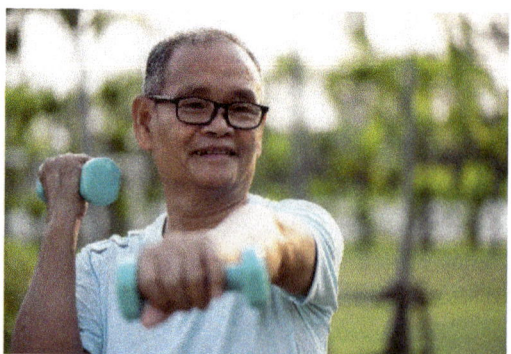

Muscles get stronger based on the overload principle. However, doing too much too soon leaves the person vulnerable to injury. It is important to remember that time is on your side.

Everyone should start with light resistance and progressively increase the resistance slowly. Reconditioning muscles, tendons, and ligaments takes time.

The best advice is to:
1. Start with low resistance.
2. Add additional resistance and the number of repetitions and sets slowly.
3. Be as consistent as possible in doing your exercise routine.
4. Make strength training a lifelong commitment. People will lose it if they don't do it so do it!

"Success is in the doing."

Muscle Strengthening Exercises

Muscle strengthening exercises are illustrated and described in Appendix 9.1.2.2.1.

4.2.4. Bodyweight Strength/Resistance Training

Introduction

One of the most common excuses used by people who do not exercise is that they cannot afford a gym membership or buy home exercise equipment. Fortunately, one does not need to spend money on either of these to get a good muscle strengthening and endurance workout. The solution is simple and not fancy; you just need to use your body weight as resistance.

By utilizing the "overload" principle of strength training (a greater than typical stress or load on the body is required for training adaptation) and one's body weight as the load, you can develop an effective muscle strengthening program. Push-ups and sit-ups are the most commonly known and used bodyweight strength training exercises. This form of resistance training is excellent at developing tone and endurance in the muscles. Most importantly, it can be easily and safely used by the older adult.

Bodyweight Exercises

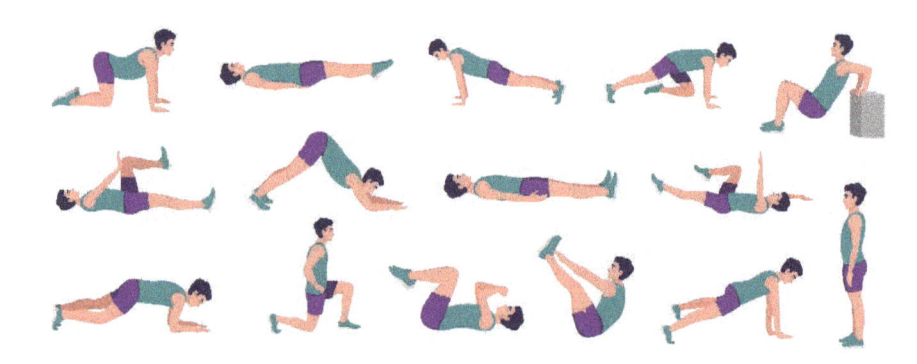

Advantages

1. **No need for external resistance equipment** – You do not require weights, dumbbells, barbells, rubber bands or machines. Making use of bodyweight exercises are ideal for those who do not have access to a gym or various types of resistance apparatuses.
2. **External weights may be incorporated** – This is for the sake of increasing the difficulty or intensity of most bodyweight exercises.
3. **These exercises are excellent at "toning" the body and developing strength endurance** - You can accomplish this by increasing the number of repetitions and sets (increasing the load) of a particular exercise.
4. **The intensity of body resistance exercises can be increased or decrease** – You can modify the intensity of the exercise by using different body positions to do the same exercise. For example, doing push-ups on your knees (easier) vs. on your toes, one-arm push-ups (harder) vs. two-arm push-ups or doing wide-arm push-ups (easier) vs. narrow-positioned (military) type push-ups.

1. **Improves agility, balance, and coordination** – Most bodyweight resistance exercises will result in improved agility balance and coordination.
2. **Core is engaged** – Bodyweight exercises require core engagement; further strengthening of these muscles can occur with the use of unstable surfaces such as stability ball or BOSU.

Disadvantages

1. **The intensity of the exercise is limited** – This is because bodyweight exercises only use your own weight to provide the resistance for the movement. Since the resistance load (bodyweight) is always fairly consistent, it makes it challenging to develop increased muscle strength (compared to muscle endurance) through muscle hypertrophy (increase size of the muscle).

However, as mentioned previously, the intensity of bodyweight exercises can be increased by including additional weights (such as wearing a weighted vest or holding a barbell, kettlebell, or a weight plate) or by altering the exercise position to put the body at a leverage disadvantage (such as elevating the feet on a stability ball, bench or the feet hanging from straps (TRX) during a push-up) or by using only one limb or incorporating isometrics into the exercise (holding a position for a period like 30 seconds). One well known and fantastic bodyweight isometric exercise is planks.

2. **Plateauing** – The body adapts to the stresses you put on it. To avoid plateaus in strength gains, you must constantly change the type of exercise and resistance you are using. Even though you can modify body resistance exercises to a certain degree, you are more limited than if you had access to free weights and weight machines.

3. **Boredom** – Once again, the limitation in the type and routine of exercises that you can do with bodyweight resistance exercises lends itself to repetition and possible boredom.

Bodyweight Resistance Exercises

Most body weight resistance exercises have several variations/modifications that can be performed to make them more or less challenging.

Bodyweight resistance exercises are described and illustrated in Appendix 9.1.2.3.1

Conclusion

Bodyweight resistance training is a convenient and effective way to tone and develop muscle endurance. An older adult can easily perform these to maintain muscle strength and endurance. It is cheap; compared to buying a gym membership or home weight equipment, and portable since the resistance you use (body weight) goes wherever you go.

Professional athletes utilize body resistance exercises to complement their weight resistance routines. These routines are used extensively in physical rehabilitation programs. They can be used safely at any age and can be easily modified to meet the fitness levels and physical compromises that the older adult may present with.

Bodyweight resistance exercises have the added advantage that they help develop flexibility, balance, agility and coordination. This advantage makes this form of exercise ideally suited for the older adult in their fall prevention program.

4.3. Fall Prevention: Agility, Balance and Coordination Training

Introduction

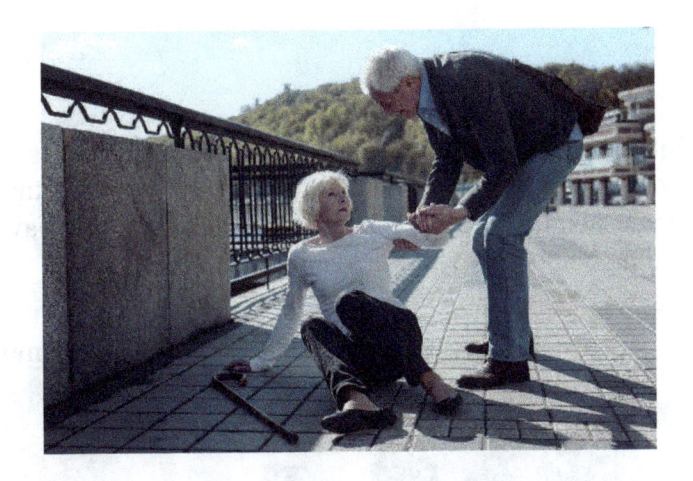

Falling is the number one risk factor for injury and disability for older adults. The frequency of falls increases with age and frailty level. Research shows that among people over 64 years of age, 28-35% fall each year. For older adults over 70, approximately 32%-42% fall each year. Older people living in retirement and nursing homes fall more often than those living in the community. Approximately 30-50% of people living in long-term care institutions fall each year, and 40% of them experience recurrent falls.

The impact of falls on the quality of life for older adults is significant. The chart below illustrates the type of injuries that result from falls by older adults.

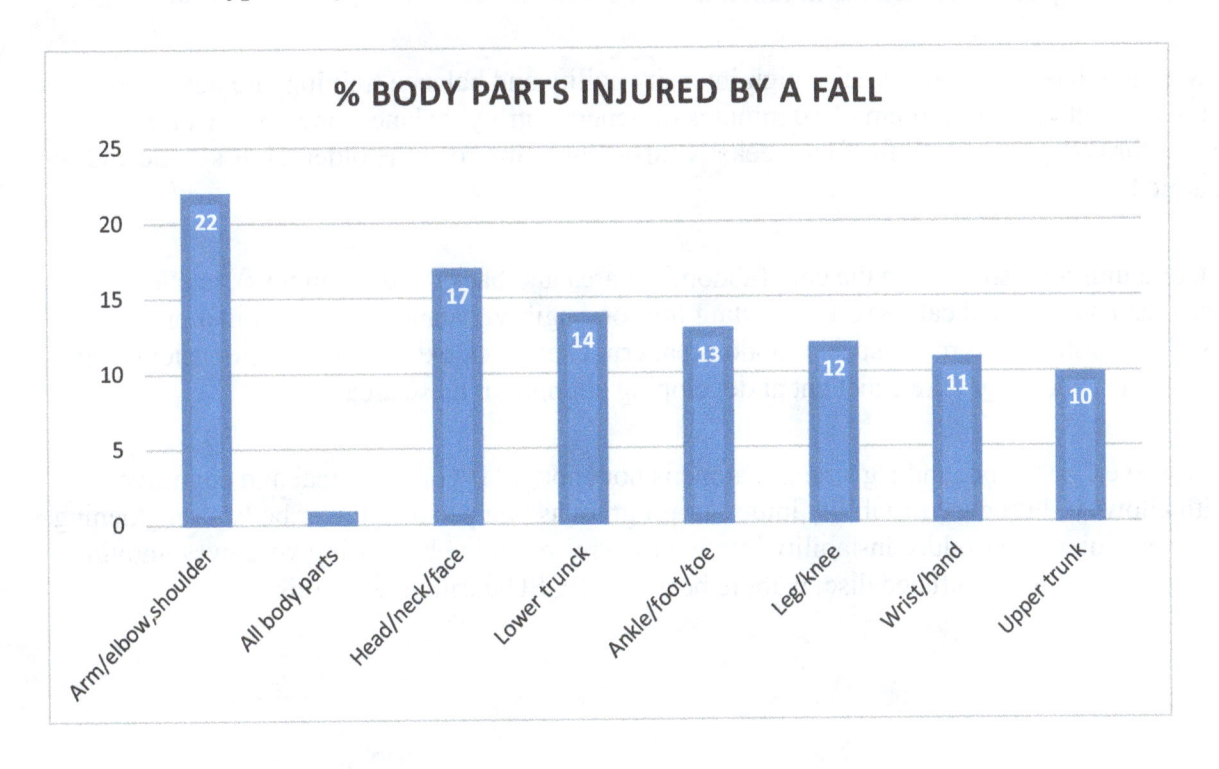

% BODY PARTS INJURED BY A FALL

Body Part	%
Arm/elbow/shoulder	22
All body parts	1
Head/neck/face	17
Lower trunk	14
Ankle/foot/toe	13
Leg/knee	12
Wrist/hand	11
Upper trunk	10

Physical frailty and immobility (muscle weakness, poor cardiovascular endurance, lack of flexibility), and cognitive impairment (dementia and depression) reduce functional capacity and balance, leaving the older adult increasingly vulnerable to falling. Older adults who are socially isolated have a higher incidence of falling than those socially active and engaged.

Prevention

Given the risk of falling and the potentially severe impact of a fall, it is essential that agility, balance, and coordination training is implemented into the older adult's fitness and health plan. Recent research indicates that agility, balance, and coordination training have positive benefits for all age groups, including competitive and recreational athletes.

Agility training   **Balance Training**   **Coordination Training**

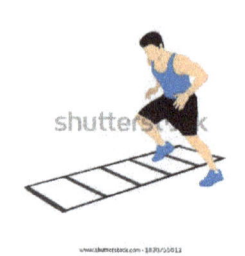

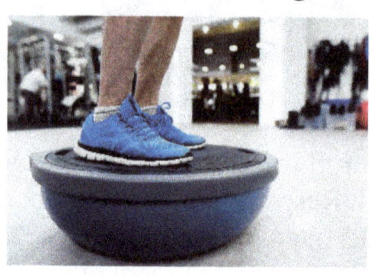

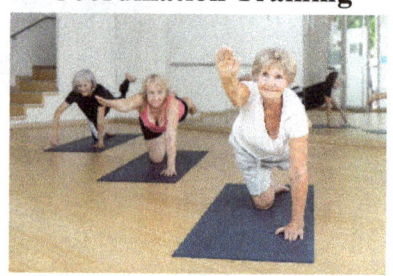

As discussed in Section 2: Studying the Opposition, with advancing age, the older adult suffers a gradual decline in sensory (eyes and ears), motor (muscles, tendons and joints), and cognitive (reasoning, memory) functions, all of which affect their ability to maintain good agility, balance and coordination as they move and change position. Physical and cognitive training can help slow this decline in function.

Research has shown that precise high intensity agility and balance training, are not necessary for fall prevention. A minimum of 10 minutes of general agility, balance, and coordination training three days per week for four weeks is sufficient to improve the older adult's static and dynamic balance.

Good muscular strength in the core (abdominal area and back), hips (buttocks), and legs (quads, hamstrings, and calves) are important for good agility, balance, and coordination. Muscular resistance exercises such as abdominal crunches, back extensions, leg extensions, leg curls, squats, and lunges are excellent at developing strength in these areas.

However, good core and leg strength alone is not enough. If your physical and cognitive health allows it, introduce instability into your program as you perform lower body strengthening exercises. You can introduce instability into your exercise routine by closing your eyes, moving your head, or using an inflated disc, wobble board, or BOSU during the exercise.

Inflated Balance Disc   **Wobble Board**   **BOSU**

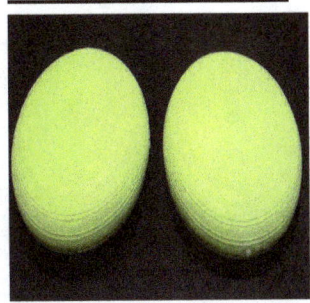

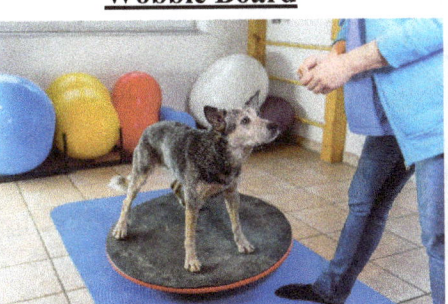

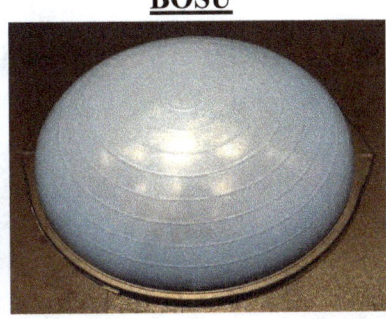

Instability exercises stimulates proprioceptive reflexes vital in maintaining good balance and preventing falls. Agility exercises using an agility ladder is also an excellent way to improve balance.

Agility Ladder

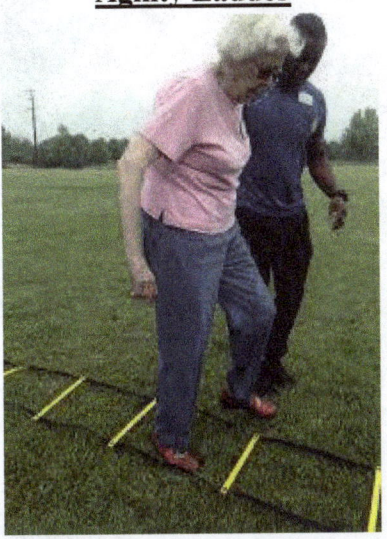

Image Source: countrymeadows.com

Good agility, balance, and coordination are necessary for people of all ages but are essential for older adults. This type of training improves their fitness levels and functional performance but most importantly, it helps prevent falls and injury.

For older adults, agility, balance, and coordination training improves their quality of life. It allows them to effectively carry out activities of daily living such as stair climbing, bending, lifting, carrying, and participating in physical activities such as golf, bike riding, skating, gardening, and walking.

Agility, Balance and Coordination Training

Two key factors that contribute to improved agility, balance, and coordination are;

1. Core and Lower body muscle strength

Exercises that strengthen the core and legs will improve posture, agility, balance, and coordination by giving the older adult the strength to move with more rhythm and coordination and maintain balance and make corrections when they fall off balance.

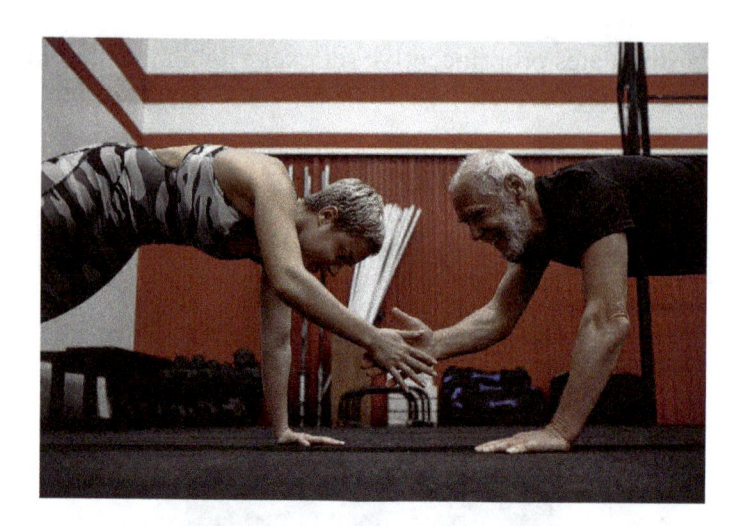

2. Improved timeliness of neurological signals from the eyes, ears and muscles/joints to the brain and then back to the muscles (proprioceptive reflexes)

Agility drills can help train the brain to signal the muscles to move more quickly and make balance corrections, to avoid falling.

Proprioception

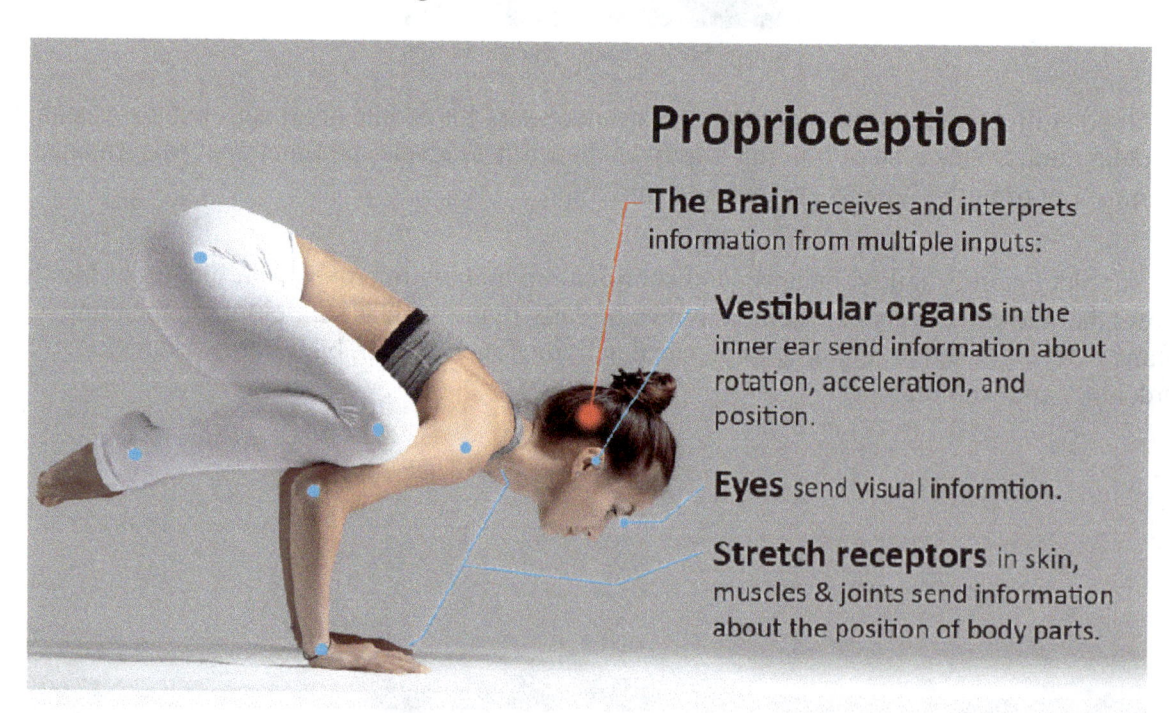

The Brain receives and interprets information from multiple inputs:

Vestibular organs in the inner ear send information about rotation, acceleration, and position.

Eyes send visual informtion.

Stretch receptors in skin, muscles & joints send information about the position of body parts.

Image Source: shamimkhanphysio.co.za

Agility Ladder Drills

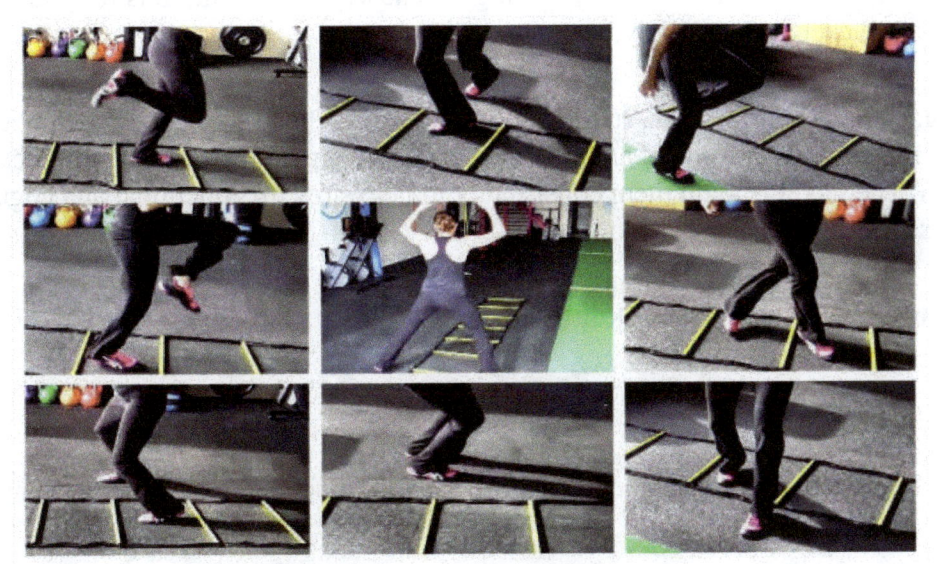

Image Source: redefiningstrength.com

Fall prevention training is about developing good core and lower body muscle strength, along with improving proprioceptive reflex reaction time.

Tables 1, 2, and 3 in Appendix 9.1.3.1 illustrate muscular strengthening, balance, and agility/coordination exercises that can easily be implemented at home to improve the older adult's defense against falling.

When performing these exercises, just like any new exercise routine, it is important to start slowly (Section 3: Chapter 3.1: The Eight Golden Rules of Training). It is necessary to focus on doing the exercises biomechanically correct and increasing the number of repetitions or length of the exercise only after they are performed without significant fatigue or muscle soreness.

These exercises should become part of everyone's, but especially the older adult's, fitness and health routine.

Workout sheets 9.2.4 presents these exercises again, but in a table format to be copied and used to record and track daily, weekly, and monthly accomplishments. Tracking the date and which exercises have been done allows monitoring of progress. By accurately monitoring progress, you will know when to add progressively more challenging exercises to your routine, so fall prevention is enhanced.

Conclusion

Falling is a huge risk for older adults and can significantly affect their quality of life if they injure themselves. Leg strengthening exercises, and specific agility, balance, and coordination exercises are preventative measures and should become part of the older adult's exercise routine.

Doing these exercises frequently, at least twice a week at low intensity, is more effective than doing them sporadically at high intensity to fatigue. The key to prevention is for you as older adults to do these exercises regularly.

Walking, riding a bike, skating, running, bowling, yoga, Pilates, tai chi, or any other physical activity that requires leg movement and coordination will help improve your agility, balance and coordination. The secret is to do them consistently to help slow the functional and cognitive aging process and minimize the risk of falling.

Remember, "Success is in the Doing."

References

www.forever-active.com

www.findingbalancealberta.ca

Canfitpro (2003) Older Adult Specialist Certification Manual

Canfitpro Foundations of Personal Training Certification Manual

Rose, D. J. (2010) Fallproof!:*A Comprehensive Balance and Training Program.* Human Kinetics, 2nd edition

Baechle, Thomas R., Westcott, Wayne L. (2010) *Fitness Professional's Guide to Strength Training the Older Adult.* Human Kinetics, 2nd edition

4.4. The Value of Cross-Training

Introduction

One of the common complaints people make about exercising is that they get bored of doing the same routine, the same exercises, over and over again. Section 3.1. The Eight Golden Rules of Training explains that it is important to "change up your exercise routine" every five weeks to avoid a plateauing of gains made with cardiovascular fitness and muscle strength. Changing up your exercise routine regularly has the added benefit of helping prevent you from becoming bored, which can destroy motivation. Cross-training is an excellent way of changing things up and introducing variety into one's fitness program.

Cross-training is fitness conditioning that incorporates several different methods, types of movement, exercises, and equipment into a person's training routine. The great advantage of cross-training is that by exercising in different ways, more muscle groups are worked and conditioned than if a person was only doing one type of exercise/movement.

For example, rather than just running or walking all the time, include bicycling, which works the same muscle groups but differently because it is a non-weight-bearing exercise. Or you could include another great cardiovascular exercise, swimming, into your routine, which will work the upper body much more than running, walking, or biking.

Another benefit of cross-training is that by introducing different forms of exercise, the neuro-muscular system is stimulated in a variety of ways so your agility, balance and coordination improve compared to just doing the same type of exercise and movement patterns repeatedly.

Injury prevention is another excellent benefit of cross-training. Because the muscles, ligaments, and tendons are not stressed the same way all the time there is less chance that these tissues will break down and get injured. The body responds to overload stimulation, and the more ways it can be stimulated and challenged, the better it will respond.

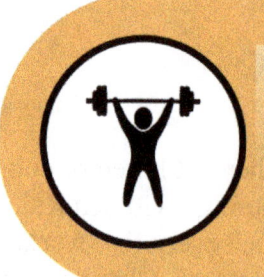

What is Cross Training?
Cross training involves a fitness routine that includes several different forms of exercise to help "everyday" exercisers and athletes achieve and maintain a high level of overall fitness.

Benefits of Cross Training
- Improves overall fitness
- Reduces the risk of overuse injuries
- Limits stress on the same muscle groups
- Conditions different muscle groups
- Helps you develop new strength and skills
- Alleviates boredom from doing the same workout

Why Cross Training Works
When you do the same movements and workouts on a regular basis your, body becomes more efficient at doing them. Unless you challenge your body, your fitness level can stagnate or even decline. Cross training allows you to break through "muscle memory" and push through to the next level of fitness.

What are Ideal Cross Training Exercises?
- Running
- Swimming
- Cycling
- Rowing
- Stair Climbing
- Rope Jumping
- Dance
- Calisthenics
- Basketball
- Plyometrics
- Free Weights
- Yoga
- Pilates

Image Source: grow.rootworks.com

Benefits of Cross-Training

The benefits of cross-training are many because of the use of a variety of exercises, movements, and equipment:

1. **Opportunity to condition the entire body** – More muscles can be exercised because of the variety of activities introduced into the exercise routine.
2. **Reduces the risk of injury** – This is because you are not stressing the bones, joints, and soft tissues the same way all the time.

3. **Promotes recovery** – When a variety of exercises and methods are used, specific muscles are recovering/resting when others are being exercised and stressed.
4. **Increases flexibility of choosing what exercises to do and when** – For example, when the pools are closed on weekends, you can do land training or muscle resistance training.
5. **Produces a higher level of all-around conditioning vs. just doing cardiovascular or muscle strength conditioning** – Higher level of conditioning can be yielded because you can work your muscles at a higher intensity more frequently because the muscles are not being stressed the same way all the time.
6. **Training can continue when injured** – For example, swimming or biking with a foot injury or running or walking through a shoulder injury.
7. **Improves agility, balance, and coordination** – This occurs because with cross-training you are not regularly performing a single movement pattern during exercise. For example, running is a forward linear cardiovascular exercise, whereas an aerobic exercise class introduces various movement patterns.
8. **Reduces exercise boredom** – You reduce boredom thanks to eliminating repetition in your exercise routine.

Examples of Cross-Training

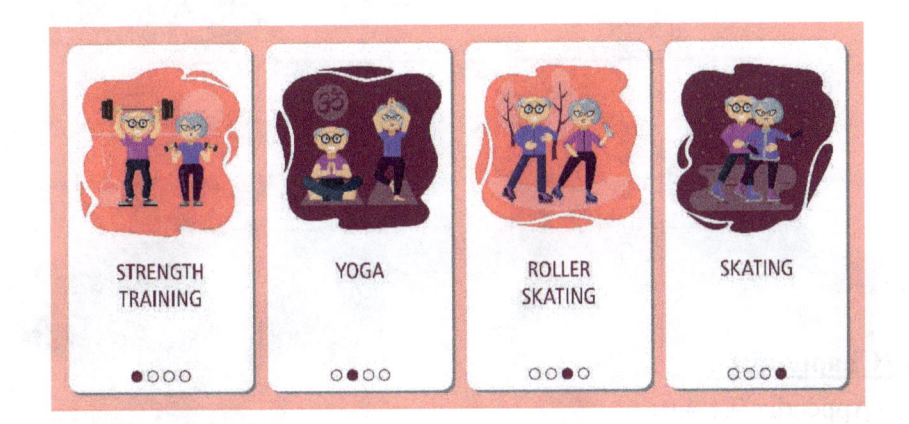

1. Cardiovascular training (Chapter 4.1.1):
- Walking (road or treadmill) (Appendix 9.1.1.1)
- Running (road or treadmill) (Appendix 9.1.1.2)
- Biking (stationary biking, road biking, spin classes) (Appendix 9.1.1.3)
- Swimming (pools or open water swimming (lakes)) (Appendix 9.1.1.4)
- Rowing
- Stair climbing
- Rope jumping
- Skating
- Cross country skiing
- Racquet sports (tennis, squash, badminton)
- Elliptical training
- Aerobic and aquatic classes

2. Muscular Resistance Training (Chapter 4.2.1):
- Dumbbell training (Appendix 9.1.2.2.1)
- Weight machines (Appendix 9.1.2.2.1)
- Barbells
- TRX (Appendix 9.1.8)
- Rubber tubes and bands (Appendix 9.1.5)
- Body resistance exercises (push-ups, sit-ups, burpees) (Appendix 9.1.2.3.)
- Pilates
- Boot camp
- Yoga (Appendix 9.1.4.3)
- Circuit training – doing a variety of exercises in sequence and each performed for a specific time period (ie – 30 to 60 seconds)

Circuit Training

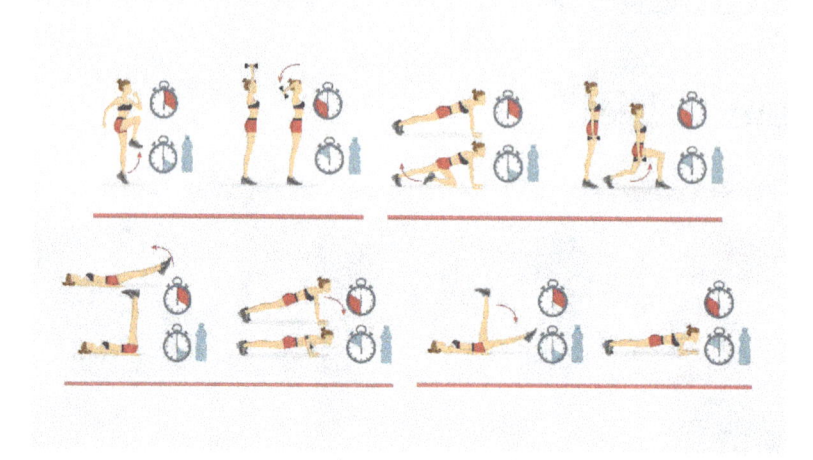

3. Flexibility (Chapter 5.1):
- Stretching (Appendix 9.1.4.0)
- Yin Yoga (Appendix 9.1.4.3)

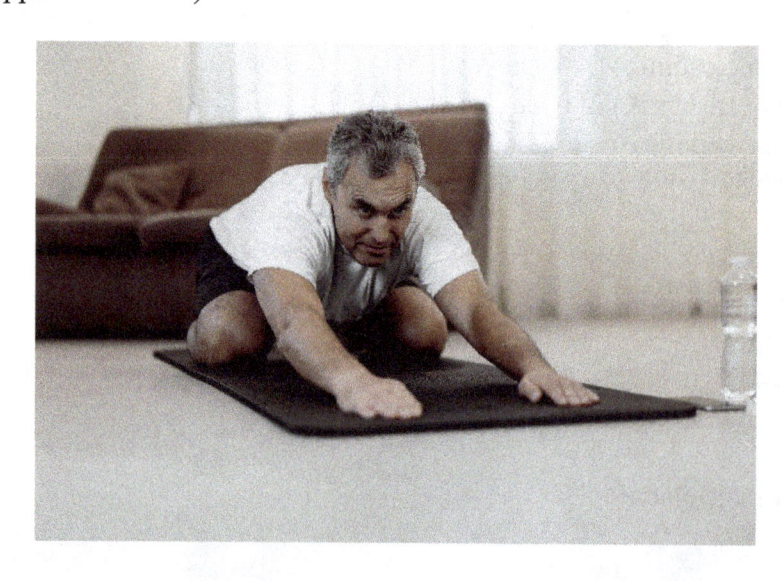

4. Agility, Balance and Coordination Drills (Chapter 4.3):

- Agility ladder (Appendix 9.1.3.1)
- BOSU (Appendix 9.1.7)
- Stability ball (Appendix 9.1.6)
- Inflated discs
- Pylons
- Obstacle course
- Floor Sliders (Appendix 9.1.10)

Agility Ladder

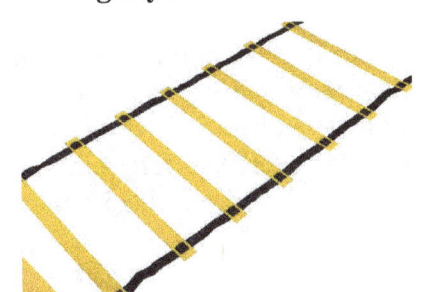

BOSU for Balance

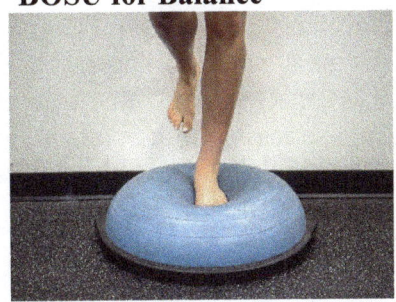

Yoga or Dance for Coordination

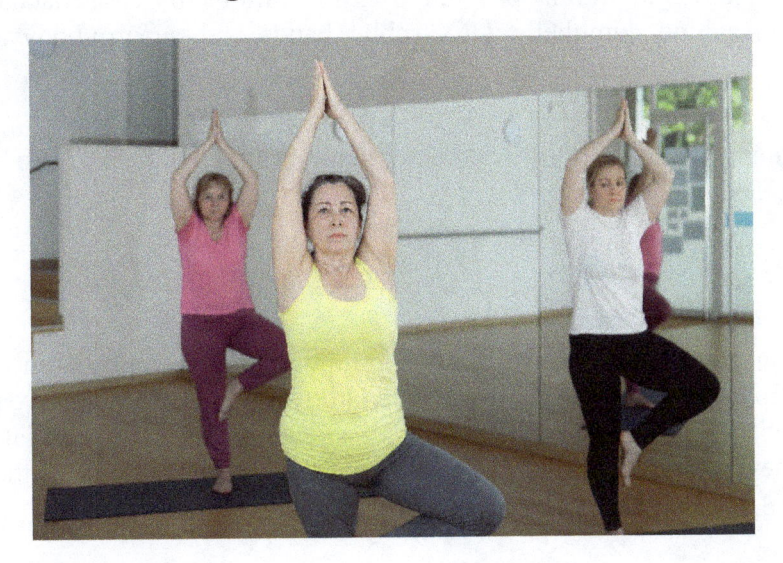

5. Speed and Power

- Sprinting
- Plyometrics (sudden explosive exercises)

Plyometrics

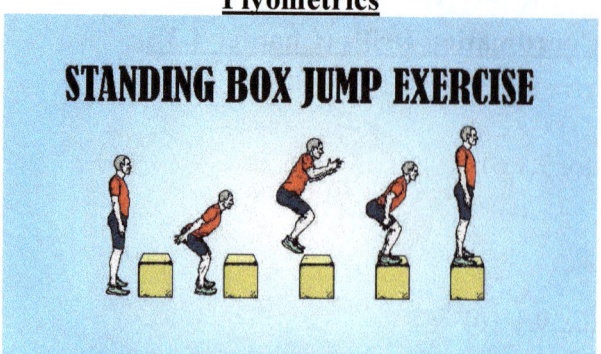

STANDING BOX JUMP EXERCISE

Implementation

One of the great benefits of cross-training is the ease of its flexible application. You can introduce different activities to challenge the same muscle groups daily, or even during one particular exercise session. For example, instead of devoting an entire workout to a specific exercise like running, you could blend in several cardiovascular exercises during the session. You could devote 15 minutes to running on the treadmill, 15 on the elliptical, 15 minutes on the stationary bike, and 15 on stair climbing.

Another example is if you plan to do an hour of musculature resistance training, you should add variety into your strength training program by using various muscle resistance apparatus such as the weight machine, dumbbells, TRX, rubber bands, and perform bodyweight resistance exercises.

With cross-training, the possibilities and combinations are endless. You are limited only by your imagination.

Risks

One of the advantages of implementing cross-training into a training routine is the variety of physical stress introduced to the body. However, adding variety (different movement patterns by the body) also produces increase risk. When adding a new activity, it is essential that the person not dive into the new activity too quickly. As we previously discussed, one of the golden rules of exercise (Chapter 3.1) is to introduce exercise "low and slow."

Even if the cardiovascular system is well-trained from regularly participating in spin classes, it does not mean your muscles, tendons, and ligaments are work-hardened to withstand the stress of running. The benefits of exercising are very specific. That is why cross-training is so beneficial because it expands the specificity of exercise. It exercises more muscles in more ways. Start a new exercise method slowly and let the body adapt to the new movement pattern.

When people cross-train and try a new activity/exercise, they tend to try to go too fast or lift too much weight. In other words, they start at too high an intensity before the body has had time to adapt. Unfortunately, often the result is that the person cannot maintain proper form throughout the exercise set, and they end up hurting themselves.

Conclusion

Cross-training should be part of everyone's training routine. It allows a higher intensity of training, as well as an opportunity to train a wider breadth of muscles while reducing physical stress and the possibility of injury to bones, joints, and soft tissues.

Mentally, this routine is excellent since it prevents boredom by introducing variety into a person's exercise routine and helps keep you motivated to keep exercising. Consistency and sustainability are the keys to a successful health and fitness program (Section 3.1: Eight Golden Rules of Training), and cross-training facilitates this.

Everyone should always consult their medical doctor before engaging in any new exercise/fitness program. For older adults, cross-training is an excellent way of starting an exercise program safely and enjoyably.

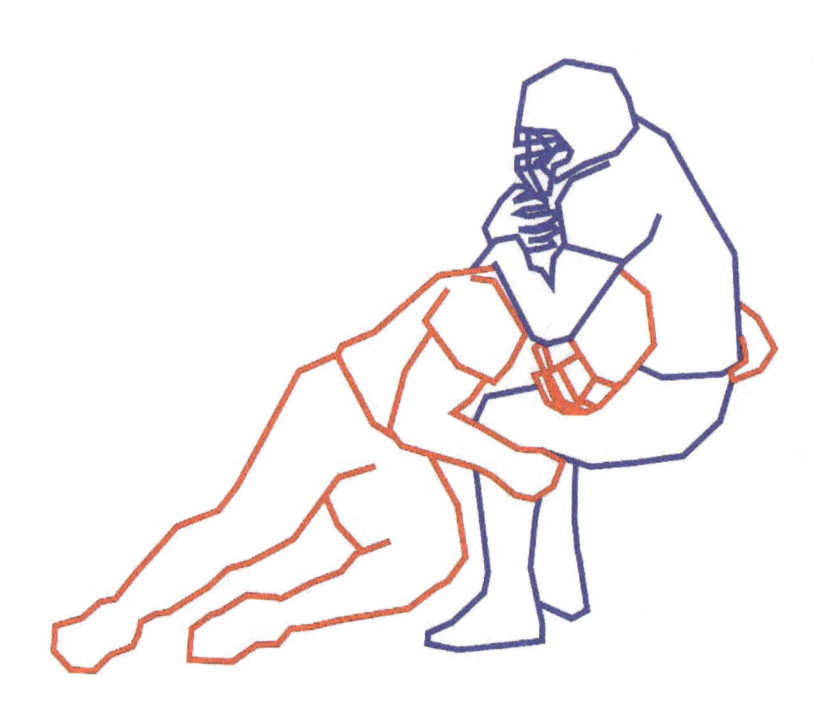

Section 5
The Defense – Protecting Your Health and Fitness

5.0. Introduction: The Defense – Protecting Your Health and Fitness

In football, your defense is as important as your offense. If your defense can't get the football back from the opposition, your offense can't score and win the game. For fitness and health, you must maintain your flexibility for mobility, have good nutrition for vitality and weight control, and get plenty of sleep for physical and mental recovery. Having a good defence in the name of flexibility, nutrition, and sleep, allows the older adult to take advantage of their offence plans for cardiovascular fitness, muscular strength, agility, balance and coordination.

Defense is not as glamorous as the offense. Everyone likes to score points, but not everyone wants to tackle. Likewise, everyone can find their preference and comfort zone to walk, run, bike, or swim and even do some resistance training to feel stronger. Still, not everyone loves to stretch or eat nutritiously (who loves to give up their sugary sweets and high-fat French fries?) or finds it easy to fall and stay asleep. If you are going to have a successful health and fitness plan, being flexibility and eating and sleeping well is necessary.

Embracing the information in this section will help you achieve your health and fitness and goals. If you ignore the importance of this section, and your health and fitness plan will not achieve optimal results, and you will be more vulnerable to injury and other health risks (Section 2: The Opposition).

The Defense

1. Flexibility

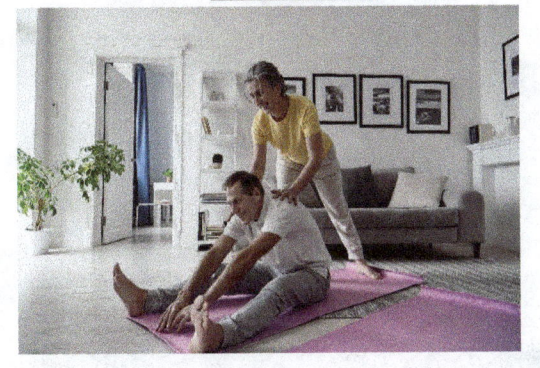

2. Nutrition

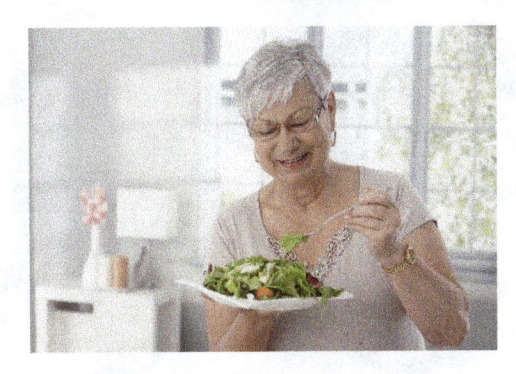

3. Sleep

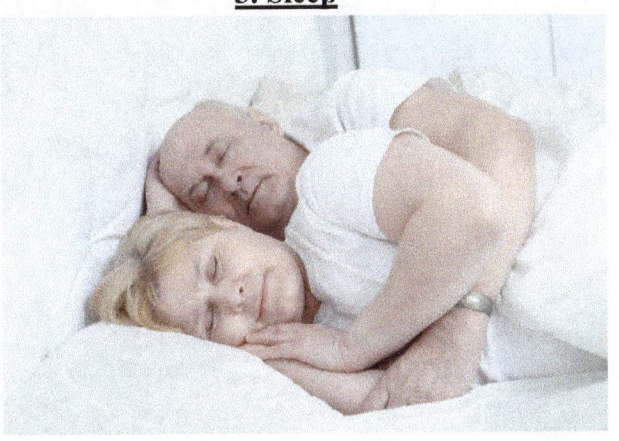

5.1.0. Introduction: Flexibility

One of the most overlooked components of fitness is flexibility. However, joint and muscle stiffness is one of the most common complaints of older adults. A lack of flexibility compromises your ability to perform daily living activities such as bending over to pick something off the floor, reaching above your shoulders into the kitchen cabinets, reaching behind your shoulders to put on your coat, and bending and twisting to get into and out of your car. A lack of flexibility also compromises performing recreational sports activities such as golf, curling, biking, bowling, skating, and hobbies such as gardening. Most significantly, a lack of flexibility leaves you vulnerable to muscle and joint injury in your upper and lower back, shoulders, and legs.

The good news is that stretching can improve your flexibility or, at the very least, help maintain what flexibility you do have. You can find many ways to stretch to avoid the boredom of repetition. The old saying, "Use it or lose it," is very true for stretching and flexibility. Stretching regularly will help you maintain your youthful flexibility. If you do not stretch, you will slowly stiffen up to the point that even the simplest of activities such as bending forward to put on and tie your shoes or lifting your arm to comb your hair becomes challenging.

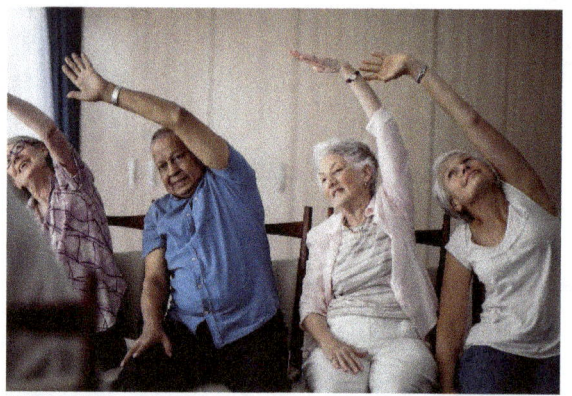

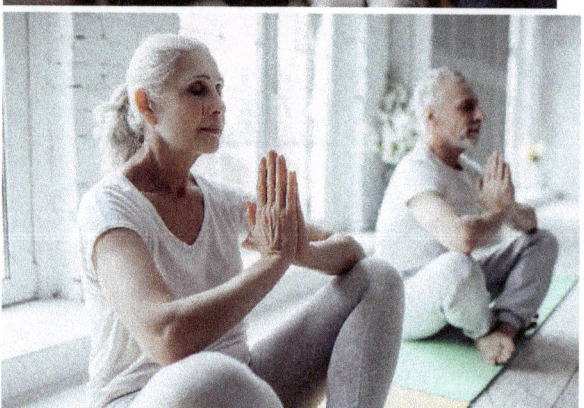

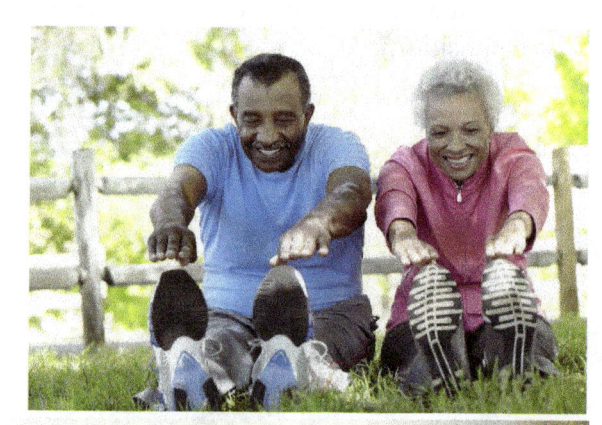

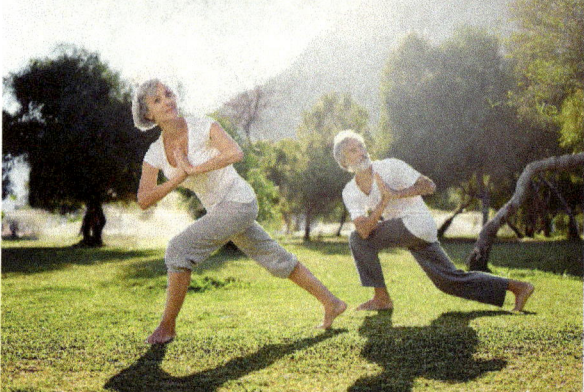

5.1.1. Flexibility Defined

Definition of Flexibility

Flexibility is the ability of a joint to move freely and pain-free through a complete range of motion. It is important to understand that every individual's "normal" range of motion for a particular joint is different. Some people are genetically more flexible than others. Extremely flexible individuals (hyper-mobile) have to be careful of joint instability that leaves them just as vulnerable to injury as someone who suffers from a lack of joint mobility (hypo-mobile).

Types of Flexibility

There are two types of flexibility: Static and Dynamic.

Static flexibility is a range of motion about a joint where there is no active movement involved by the musculature surrounding the joint. An example of this would be sitting for an extended period.

Dynamic flexibility involves the use of movement around the joint. An example of this type of flexibility would be bending over to put on your socks or walking up a flight of stairs. It is important to have good static and dynamic flexibility to prevent physical dysfunction.

Types of Stretching

It was previously thought that stiffness around a joint happened due to muscular tightness. However, it is now known that a lack of flexibility is due to connective tissue tightness. Connective tissue is composed primarily of non-elastic collagen fibers with some elastic fibers as well. Examples of connective tissues are ligaments, tendons, cartilage, and muscular fascia. The connective tissue will respond to various types of stretching.

Two main methods of flexibility training are static and dynamic stretching.

1. Static Stretching

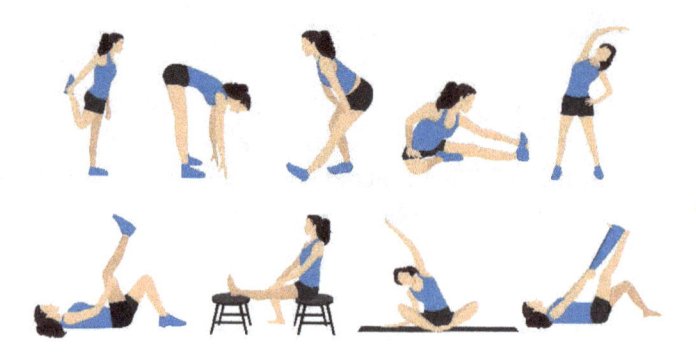

Static stretching is the most widely used stretching technique and involves slow, gradual, and controlled elongation of the muscle. The muscle is stretched to the point of mild tension and held for 10-30 seconds or longer. The continuous low-intensity stretch allows the muscle spindles and nervous system to adapt slowly to the new stretched position and causes the muscle to relax.

It is best to do this form of stretching at the end of a workout. Its advantage is that this is a simple, controlled type of movement. Its disadvantage is that it will improve flexibility only at the specific body position that the stretch is held. Therefore, it has limited effectiveness in increasing flexibility in multiple ranges of motion and is best used to complement the dynamic method of stretching.

2. Dynamic (Active) Stretching

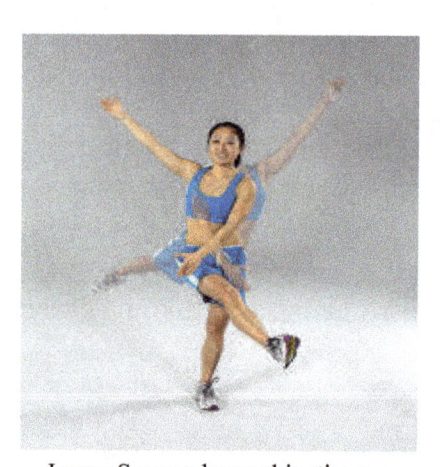

Image Source: humankinetics.me

This method of flexibility training uses increasingly dynamic movements through the full range of motion of a joint. Dynamic stretching is very important for maintaining the ability to perform dynamic functional activities of daily living, such as reaching and bending. When performed correctly, dynamic stretching warms up the joints and reduces muscle tension. The dynamic stretch begins at a slow pace and gradually increases in speed and intensity. You must always do dynamic movements under control which means no ballistic type movements such as high speed uncontrolled reaching, kicking or bouncing movements.

It is best to do dynamic stretching at the beginning of your exercise session but only after a mild cardo warm-up. It is a beneficial way to increase flexibility and prepare the body for activities that require a wide range of motion, especially when speed is involved, such as golf, tennis, and biking. Good examples of dynamic stretching are lateral arm or leg swings and torso twists.

FITT Guidelines for Flexibility Training

Frequency	– 4-7 x's/week (daily if possible) – Stretching should be done before activity to prevent injury and after activity to prevent stiffness and improve overall flexibility
Intensity	– Stretching should never be painful or produce significant discomfort – The goal is to bring the muscle to the point of slight tension – It is very important that you NEVER hold your breath and that you continue your breathing pattern throughout the stretch
Time	Static stretches should be held for 5-20 seconds or longer and repeated 2-4 times Dynamic stretches should be done initially for 5-20 seconds or 3-10 repetitions
Type	Static – Done at the end of activity after a cool down Dynamic – Done at the beginning of activity after a mild cardo warm-up

Rules for Effective Flexibility Training for the Older Adult

1. Don't overdo it. Always work within your limits.
2. NEVER hold your breath as you perform a stretch. Breathe normally and comfortably. On static stretching, exhale as the muscle lengthens to assist in relaxation.
3. Perform flexibility exercises for each muscle group for total-body improvements.
4. Always perform flexibility stretches after the body has warmed up. Warm muscles will lengthen more easily and with less discomfort.

Conclusion

Flexibility training is invaluable to prevent premature physical dysfunction in performing activities of daily living and injury during recreational activities.

When performed in a controlled manner, stretching activities are safe and can easily be implemented into your daily routine. Stretching exercises to improve flexibility are illustrated and explained in Appendix 9.1.4.1. As well, there are Workout Sheets, 9.2.5., that have various dynamic and static routines that can be used to record your daily stretching workouts. Recording stretching sessions is a good and effective way of keeping you accountable for stretching consistently.

5.1.2. The Biology of Stretching

Among the general public, there is much confusion about stretching. Common questions are, is it necessary, am I too old, which muscles need to be stretched, how long do I stretch for, is dynamic stretching better than static stretching? There is no such confusion in the professional world of physical fitness and athletics; stretching is necessary and should be an integral component of everyone's exercise routine.

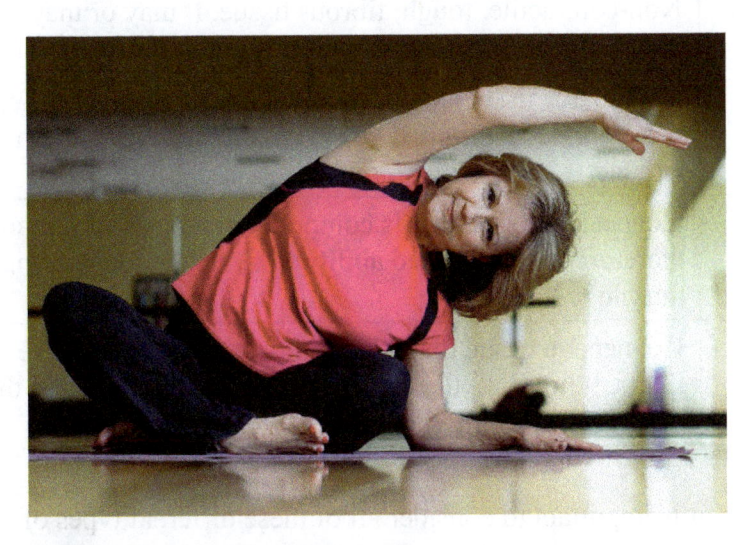

The benefits of stretching are far-reaching and vitally important for older adults. The most important benefit is injury prevention. Gentle dynamic stretching is needed before you begin exercising to ensure your muscles are warmed up and loose, and gentle static stretching after exercise is necessary to prevent soft tissue contracture and stiffness. Another important benefit of stretching is that it allows you to prepare for your exercise session mentally. This moment to mentally prepare is essential if you have had a busy day at work and had to rush to the gym, field, or arena to exercise. Stretching allows you a few moments to regroup and refocus on your upcoming exercise routine, run, bike ride, walk, or game. This way, you are physically and mentally prepared. After exercise, stretching allows you a few moments to relax and reflect on your training or game. It will enable you to cool down gently rather than abruptly.

Stretching improves the flexibility of the soft tissues of the body. The soft tissues include the muscles, tendons, ligaments, and fascia that hold the joints together.

Table 1: Description of the body's soft-tissues that surround the Joints

Tissue	Description
Muscles	Contractile tissue that moves and position the bones by their ability to lengthen and shorten.
Connective Tissue	Non-contractile, tough, fibrous tissue. It may or may not be flexible, depending on its function and its ratio of elastic to non-elastic fibers.
Ligaments	Connective tissue that is comprised primarily of non-elastic fibers and therefore have a limited ability to stretch before tearing. They join bone to bone.
Tendons	Connective tissue that is comprised primarily of non-elastic fibers and therefore have a limited ability to stretch before tearing. They join muscle to bone.
Fascia	Connective tissue that is quite flexible due to its large number of elastic fibers. It holds all the layers of the body together and therefore is present extensively throughout the body.

When you stretch, it is important to consider all of these different types of soft tissue because each has different needs and requirements.

1. **Muscle fibers** – These need to be stretched slowly and gently. You need to "relax" into the stretch regardless if you are performing a dynamic or static type stretch. If a muscle is aggressively stretched, it will initiate the "stretch reflex" and contract to guard itself against tearing. It is OK to feel some resistance and even mild discomfort, but never pain. Normal rhythmic breathing while stretching is essential. You should NEVER hold your breath while stretching.

   A good cue to effective stretching is to visualize the muscle lengthening as it is being stretched. For stretching to be effective, hold the stretch from 5-20 seconds or more.

2. **Ligaments and tendons** – They function to help stabilize the joints they cross. It is important not to stretch these structures past their normal limits and create a hypermobile joint. The hypermobility would leave the joint vulnerable to injury. If ligaments and tendons lack normal flexibility due to injury or disuse, you must stretch them very specifically and carefully.

3. **Fascia** – This is deeply entwined in the muscle structure at every level and requires you to hold the stretch for 90-120 seconds to effectively change its length. Yin Yoga is an excellent way of performing fascia stretching since each pose is held from 3-5 minutes. Because of each pose's length, it is important that Yin Yoga is performed very gently. If the stretch is painful, you will not be able to hold the stretch for the necessary length of time or practice the stretch regularly.

Fascia

Image Source: assignmentpoint.com

The real secret to improving flexibility is to repeat or practice stretching regularly. Performing a stretching routine once a week for 30 minutes is not as effective as performing the same stretches 6 times a week for 5 minutes at a time. It is important to get into the habit of stretching dynamically before engaging in exercise and performing static stretches after the exercise.

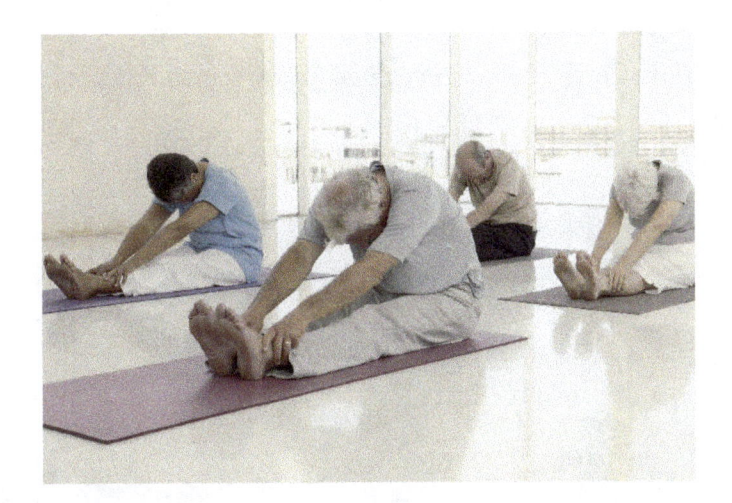

World-class athletes recognize the importance of good flexibility to enhance their athletic performance and prevent injury. They have taken the time to learn how to stretch properly. The great thing about stretching is that anyone can do it. The same stretches that a, world-class athlete does anyone can do. Fortunately, it does not take great physical conditioning or athletic prowess to stretch. It takes a bit of understanding on how to do it properly and the discipline to do it regularly.

Appendix 9.1.4.1. – Describes in detail and illustrates a comprehensive list of dynamic and static stretching exercises.

Workout sheets 9.2.5 – List a comprehensive 45-minute dynamic and static stretching routine and a stretching routine that can be completed in 10-minutes. Utilize the worksheets to record your daily accomplishments.

Conclusion

If you learn how to stretch properly and safely (Appendix 9.1.4.1), and take the time to stretch, you will enjoy your cardiovascular and muscle strengthening exercising much more. An older adult will find activities of daily living such as bending over, getting out of chairs, reaching behind to put your coat on, lifting your arms above your shoulders and head easier to do and this means more independence and enhanced quality of living.

You can listen to music or watch your favorite TV show while stretching. The key to successful stretching is to do it consistently, so you must make it as enjoyable as possible. Make it fun!

Begin to stretch regularly starting today, you will never regret the time you spend doing it.

References

Frederick, Ann., Frederick, Chris. (2006). *Stretch to Win*. Human Kinetics
www.forever-active.com

5.1.3. Yin Yoga: a Meditative Way to Improved Flexibility

Introduction

Yin Yoga is based on the Taoist concept of Yin and Yang, opposite and complementary principles in nature. Yin is the stable, unmoving, hidden aspect of an object, while Yang is changing, moving, and revealing aspect. These two objects always coexist, and everything in nature can describe in terms of its Yin and Yang.

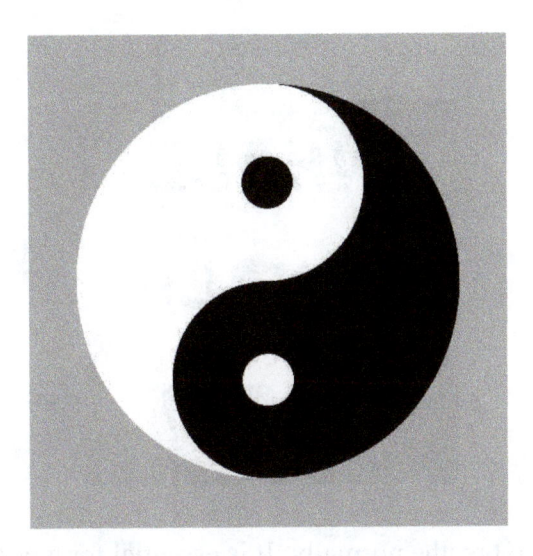

Yoga can be described as Yin or Yang based on which tissues of the body the yoga poses are targeting. A practice that focuses on gentle traction and the stretching of connective tissue (ligaments, tendons, and fascia) is Yin Yoga, and a practice that focuses on exercising and stressing the muscles is Yang Yoga.

How to Practice Yin Yoga

1. Be Relaxed, Be Patient

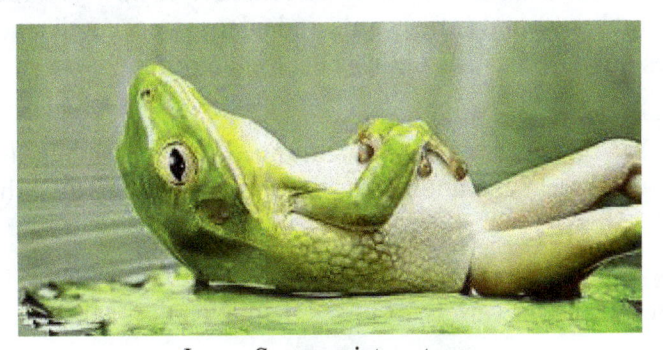

Image Source: pinterest.com

Dense connective tissues (ligaments, tendons, and fascia) do not respond to quick rhythmic and repetitive stresses the way muscles do. Connective tissues change and relax slowly after maintaining a constant stretch for two to five minutes. To correctly stress the connective tissue around a joint, the muscles in that area must be relaxed. As a result, when practicing Yin Yoga, it is important not to be anxious or aggressive and force the body into poses.

When you begin a pose, you should make a modest effort to approximate the pose as best as possible and then patiently wait. The power and effectiveness of Yin Yoga derives from time, not effort. Learning to relax as a pose is held is an important skill to acquire because it will allow you to release tension and get deeper into the pose.

2. Breathe Normally

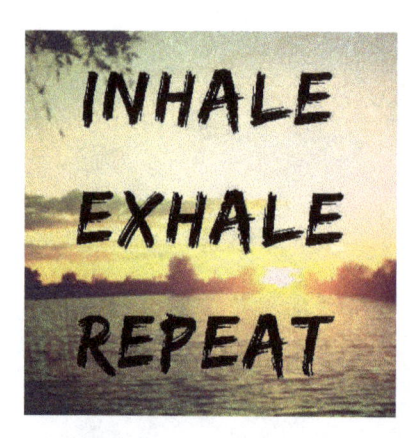

The key in Yin Yoga is to breathe normally. It is essential for a person not to hold their breath or artificially alter their breathing into a rhythmic cadence. Each Yin posture will affect your breathing differently, so it would be counterproductive to attempt to control it.

Guiding Principles

1. Every yoga pose is experienced by and affects each person differently. You should not become fixated on "mastering a pose." The poses are meant to be therapeutic, not to challenge your pride. Some poses may be uncomfortable but result in a healthy physiological response, while others may not. You need to be sensitive to how you feel while holding a pose and how your body responds afterwards and adapt your practice accordingly. If one particular pose does not agree with you, it's best to avoid it.

2. Forward bends are Yin and, as a result, are calming. They can be held for a more prolonged period. Backward bends are Yang and more stimulating to the body, which is why they do not need to be held as long.

3. Yin practice requires a smaller variety of poses than a Yang practice.

4. Use pillows, blankets, and bolsters to support yourself if you find poses strenuous. Yin yoga should never be stressful. If you find yourself unable to relax, you are being too aggressive.

5. For effective long-term Yin practice, it is essential to develop consistency and discipline. However, it is equally important to allow your practice to remain dynamic and to modify your practice routine to suit your needs.

Yin Postures

Yin postures and poses are also illustrated and explained in Appendix 9.1.4.3.

Key Points:

1. Start by holding each pose for two minutes and progress up to four or five minutes maximum.
2. Your practice should include four to eight poses depending on your available time and needs.
3. Over time, you may vary the poses to add variety and balance to your practice.

Utilize workout sheets in chapter 9.2.5. to record your weekly Yin Yoga practice.

Conclusion

Yin Yoga uses long (two to five minutes) relaxed and passive floor postures/poses to stretch and stimulate the body's deep connective tissues. This form of yoga is accessible to almost anyone regardless of age, fitness level, or health condition. Yin yoga is an ideal complement to dynamic aerobic and muscular resistance exercises and traditional stretching routines.

Try it; you will love it, and you will emotionally and physically benefit greatly from it.

References

www.forever-active.com

Grilley, Paul. (2012). *YinYoga Principles and Practice*. White Cloud Press. 10th Edition

5.1.4. Myofascial Self Massage: An Effective Way to Improve Flexibility

Introduction

Myofascia, like tendons and ligaments, is an essential element of the musculoskeletal system. It is not as well known or understood as muscle, tendons, and ligaments. Still, it is equally important when considering your ability to achieve and maintain good flexibility, especially as you age. That is why myofascia deserves a chapter of its own.

What Is It?

Fascia or myofascia is the dense, tough tissue that surrounds and covers all of your muscles and bones. This outer fascial covering is very strong and very flexible. It has a tensile strength of over 2000 pounds.

Under a microscope, myofascia resembles a spider web or fishnet. It is very organized and very flexible in a healthy state.

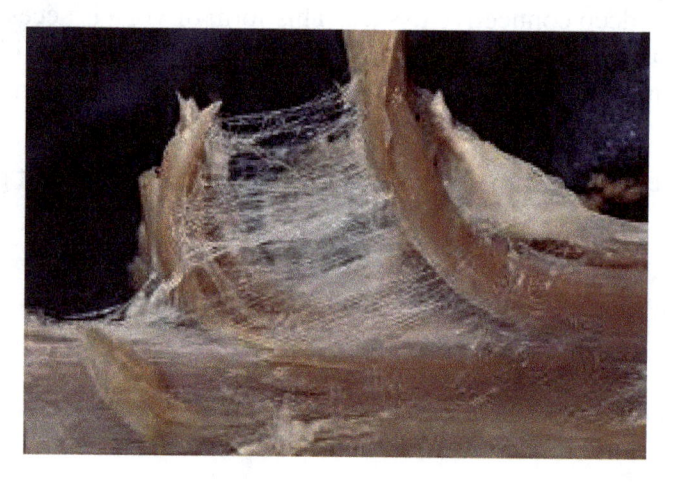

Image Source: healthyhabits.ca

Myofascia can best be described as a complete body suit which runs from the top of your head down to the bottom of your toes. It is continuous, has no beginning or end, and can be found almost everywhere in your body. Like yarn in a sweater, the entire body is connected to every other part of the body by the fascia. It is a continuous weave of material. And, like a pull in a sweater, damage to an area of fascia can affect other distant areas in your body even years later.

Why the Myofascia is Important for Your Health

In the normal healthy state, the fascia is relaxed and soft. It can stretch and move without restriction. When a person experiences physical trauma or inflammation, the fascia loses its pliability. It can become tight, restricted, and a source of tension throughout the rest of the body, and a number of health-related problems can result;

- Headaches
- Generalized muscle pain and spasms
- Chronic back and neck pain
- Re-aggravation of previous injuries
- Sciatica and the sensations such as numbness and pins and needles
- Restrictive Breathing
- Poor posture and reduced flexibility

Things that can cause the myofascia to become too tight are:

- Inflammation
- Traumas, such as falls, sport or work injuries, or car accident
- Poor posture
- Lack of stretching
- Prolonged sitting or standing
- Emotional/psychological stress
- Repetitive motions, such as factory work or keyboarding

Treating the Myofascia

Myofascial Release (Self-Massage)

Myofascial Release is an effective therapy that can effectively treat tough, tight myofascial tissue and improve its health by making it more relaxed, pliable, and soft.

Myofascial Release is applied directly to the body and uses slow deep pressure to restore the proper health of the fascia. The pressure should never be beyond tolerance. You may experience a slight tingling or burning sensation in the skin, which is perfectly normal and safe.

The purpose of myofascial release techniques is to help to relax and lengthen tight myofascial tissue. Myofascia is interconnected throughout the body, which means treating or relaxing one area of the body may positively affect another area. For example, relaxing the myofascia in the hips and low back may help reduce tension in the neck and shoulders, which may have been causing shoulder and neck restriction and headaches.

Utilizing a Roller for Self-Myofascial Release

Self-Myofascial Release is the process of using a roller to massage targeted muscles and fascia to improve soft tissue elasticity. Other benefits of self-myofascial release include;

- Removal of waste by-products (via blood) to facilitate tissue recovery and repair.
- Increase neural stimulation
- Increase range of motion
- Improve proper contraction of muscle tissue

Myofascial Rollers

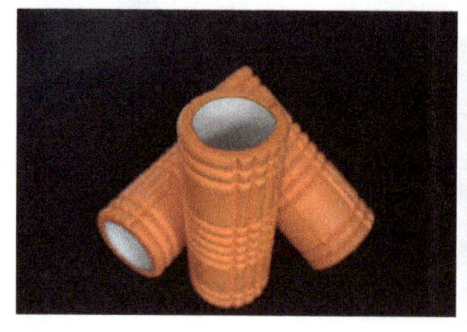

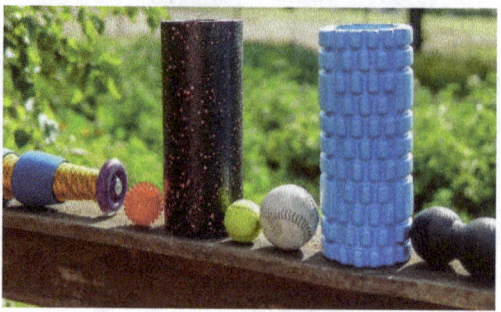

Guidelines for Safe and Effective Use of a Myofascial Roller

1. **Discomfort** – Mild to moderate discomfort is expected when beginning self-myofascial release. This discomfort will decrease over time as the normal length-tension relationship of the fascia is restored.
2. **Control of Grid** – It is important to maintain adequate pressure on the grid so it will not shift during the massage movement.
3. **Grid Placement** – AVOID grid placement on;
    a. bony structures such as the neck
    b. joints
    c. inside the upper arm
    d. any bruised areas of the body
4. **Breathing** – Connect the breath to each movement and focus on complete inhales and exhales
5. **Proper body positioning and technique** – For maximum effectiveness, the grid must be positioned as illustrated and movement must occur as described (Appendix 9.1.4.4).

Contraindications for the Use of the Grid

- Large bruises
- Phlebitis
- Severe varicose veins
- Open wounds
- Undiagnosed lumps
- Skin infections
- Diabetes
- Cancer of the bones
- Pregnancy – lower back and adductor regions
- General rule – never use the grid over joints or bony prominences or inside of the upper arms.

Myofascial Self Massage Release Positions

Myofascial release positions are illustrated in Appendix 9.1.4.4.

Utilize the workout sheet in Chapter 9.2.5. to record your myofascial massage routine

Key points:
- Never use the grid over joints or bony prominences or inside of the upper arms.
- All movements (rolling) are done slowly with gentle to deep pressure for a count of 10.
- Focus on deep, controlled breathing, which is in rhythm with your rolling.
- If you find a sensitive spot, you may apply pressure with the grid over this spot for 10 to 30 sec.
- Correct posture and positioning of the grid are necessary for effective results.
- It will take practice to learn how to perform each movement correctly.

Conclusion

Myofascial self-massage is an effective way to release tension in the muscles and fascia and help restore flexibility. Initially, the various positions may feel awkward, and the pressure may feel uncomfortable. However, with practice, the roller will become easier and more comfortable to use.

Myofascial self-massage is an excellent adjunct therapy to improve soft tissue pliability and flexibility and complements a regular stretching program.

People will move more freely and feel the difference in their muscles when they do this form of self-massage regularly.

Reference

www.forever-active.com
Phillips, Cassidy. *SMRT-Core Personal Training.* 5th Edition
Earls, James. Myers, Thomas. (2010) *Fascial Release for Structural Balance.* North Atlantic Books,

5.2.0. Nutrition: Introduction

"We are what we eat."

We hear that phrase all the time, and unlike many phrases we hear, there is truth in those five words. The carbohydrates, proteins, and fat that we ingest from our diet are the building blocks for our bodies (muscles, bones, and other tissues) and supply the energy for our movement and function.

It is never a good idea to have too much of a good thing, and this is especially true when it comes to eating. Our society today suffers from an epidemic of obesity as a result of eating the wrong foods too much, and too often. Stats Canada in 2018 reported that 26.8% (7.3 million) of adults 18 years and older were considered obese based on the Body Mass Index criteria (BMI). Another 36.3% (9.9 million) were deemed to be overweight. Based on these statistics, 63.1% of the Canadian population lives with increased health risk due to excess weight.

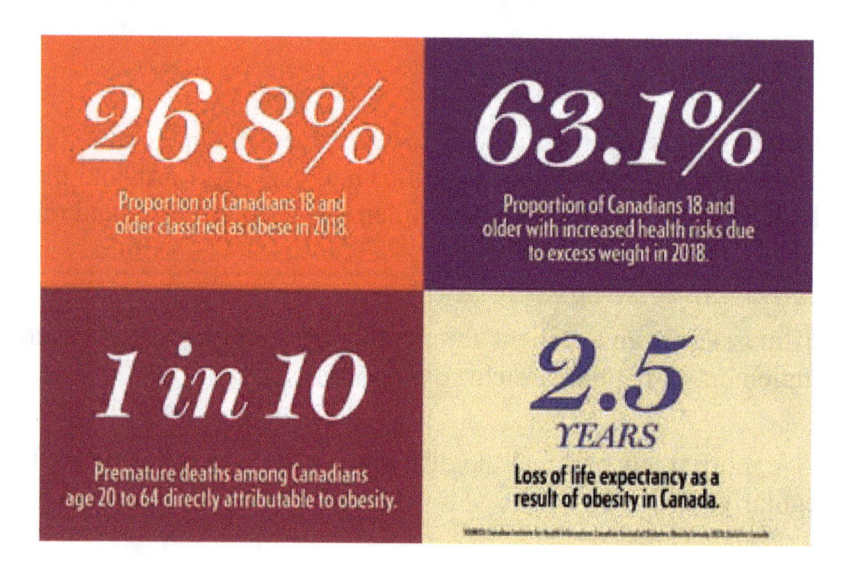

26.8% Proportion of Canadians 18 and older classified as obese in 2018.

63.1% Proportion of Canadians 18 and older with increased health risks due to excess weight in 2018.

1 in 10 Premature deaths among Canadians age 20 to 64 directly attributable to obesity.

2.5 YEARS Loss of life expectancy as a result of obesity in Canada.

To counteract this epidemic, a whole industry based on dieting and weight control has developed and is flourishing. In 2020, the Canadian weight loss industry was estimated to be worth 7 billion dollars and has been growing on average by 6% per year over the last ten years. The health care cost of obesity is also a staggering $7 billion per year and growing.

Research has established direct associations between obesity and the incidence of osteoarthritis, chronic back pain, asthma, gall bladder disease, type 2 diabetes, cardiovascular disease (hypertension, stroke, congestive heart failure, and coronary artery disease) and several types of cancers (colorectal, kidney, breast, endometrial, ovarian, and pancreatic cancers). Psychological conditions such as low self-esteem and depression have been linked to people being overweight and obese.

The human and economic cost of being overweight and obese is clearly defined. But what is the reason for this epidemic? Is it genetic, what and how much a person eats, or a lack of exercise? The answer is probably a combination of all of these.

The Genetic Factor

From a genetic perspective, research has identified over 400 different genes to be associated people being overweight or obese. However, only a few genes appear to significantly influence your predisposition to obesity. It is estimated that genes may contribute about 25% to the cause of obesity for most people. Genes can influence appetite, food cravings, metabolism, satiety (the sense of fullness), the tendency to use eating as a way to cope with stress, and body-fat distribution.

Environmental Factors

As significant as genetic influences may be for some people concerning obesity, environmental factors are the driving force behind obesity in most people and are the primary cause for the dramatic rise in the prevalence of obesity in our society. Environmental factors encompass anything in society that influences a person to overeat or exercise too little.

For a detailed investigation on obesity, read Chapter 2.5: Obesity.

Section 5.2: Nutrition will focus on helping the older adult understand the topic of nutrition more clearly. Unfortunately, we are bombarded daily with often misleading marketing advertisements and "informative" articles in the newspaper, magazines and on-line about what we should and should not be eating, what new revolutionary diet will solve our overweight problem, what vitamins and other supplements we need to take, etc.

The goal of this section is to correctly inform you about how to read nutrition labels, what the new Canadian Health Food Guide recommendations are, the truth about the effects of salt and sugar in your diets, the good and bad about cholesterol, the issue that revolves around Gluten, dietary supplementation and a review of the most popular diets. It is hoped that after a review of this section, you can make educated dietary decisions regarding what you buy and how to prepare the food you are planning to enjoy.

References

www.globalnews.ca
www.reportlink.com/weight_loss/reports
www.canada.ca

5.2.1. Nutrition Primer

Introduction

Nutrition is the study of food and how the body uses it. For older adults, nutrition presents particular challenges.

First, as a person ages, there is often a change in food fondness. Many older adults experience a loss of appetite due to sensory changes such as loss of smell and taste. Medication may also affect sensory stimulation to food. Second, the ability to digest and absorb food can be reduced, causing constipation and inadequate absorption of essential nutrients. Third, a lack of activity or an increasingly sedentary lifestyle can reduce appetite. If you are not burning as many calories as before, your appetite won't be as strong, leading to inadequate nutritional intake. Fourth, the loss of a spouse and having to prepare meals for only one could lead to a decreased motivation to shop and prepare good nutritious meals.

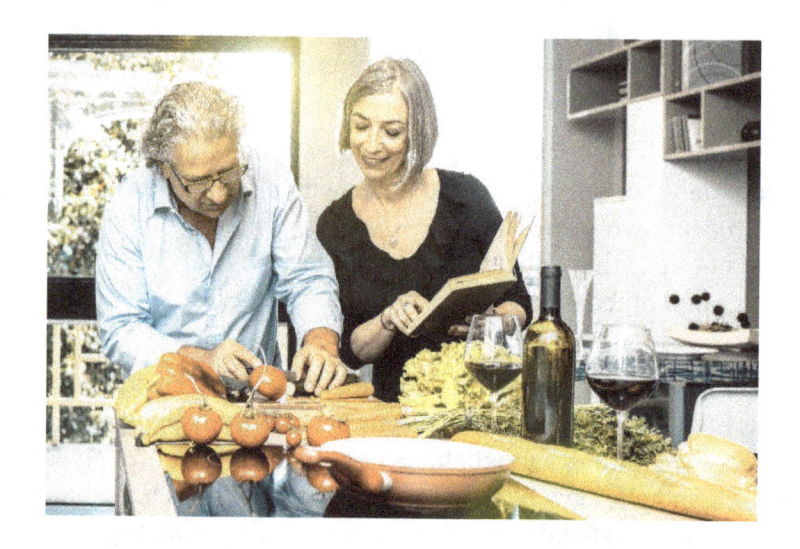

The average older adult should consume approximately 1,800 calories daily for women and 2,200 calories a day for men. An active older adult will need an even higher daily caloric intake to promote recovery and regeneration of muscle. You can add supplements to your diet if you cannot obtain these nutrients from the food you consume. However, taking vitamins and mineral supplements may interact with prescription medicine. Consultation with a medical doctor is necessary before taking any supplements.

Your diet has a profound effect on your health. A chronically poor diet facilitates the onset of physical ailments and disease. Proper nutrition can help slow the aging process, maintain healthy and vital cells, provide better cell replication and decrease disease associated with tissue breakdown. Reducing consumption of refined foods, sugar, salt, fast foods, and nutrient-deficient food is an excellent start to improving your diet and health.

No cell in the body escapes the influence of your food choices. Eating the wrong foods will compromise your body's long-term health. It is never too late to make changes in your dietary habits. As soon as your diet improved, you will feel its immediate effects, and it may even slow down the progression of a disease or prevent a new one from arising.

Important Benefits of Good Nutrition for the Older Adult

- Increased energy and stamina
- Decreased body fat and prevention of heart disease and certain types of cancer
- Better ability to regenerate tissue
- Stronger muscles and reduced loss of muscle mass.
- Stronger bones, ligaments, and tendons
- Better weight control
- Proper hormone and enzyme development for proper body function
- Healthier skin, hair, and nails.
- Decreased feelings of depression and a stronger, more positive mental outlook
- Increased ability to cope with stress.

Essential Nutrients

The body needs six essential nutrients or components of food to function properly. Three are referred to as macro-nutrients, and three are micro-nutrients.

1. Macro-Nutrients
Provide energy for body movement and function. Energy in food is measured in units called calories.

a. Carbohydrates
– Supply four calories per gram

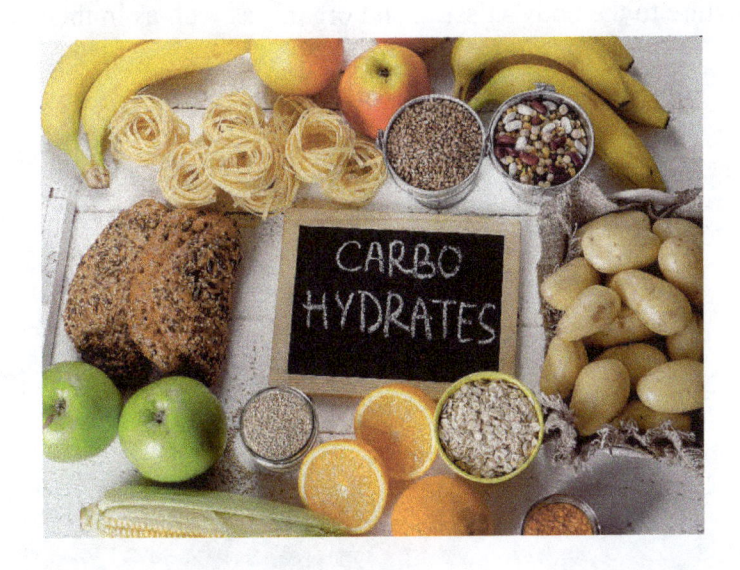

I. Simple carbohydrates – These are carbohydrates that contain one or two sugar molecules. They are digested and converted to glucose which results in a rise in blood sugar levels quickly. Unfortunately, they are abundant in all the things we love to eat such as ice cream, cheese, refined sugars, candies, beer, juice, pop, and white/refined grains Because these carbohydrates do not possess fiber, they are called empty calories and provide no significant nutritional value for the number of calories consumed.

II. Complex Carbohydrates – These carbohydrates have two or more sugar molecules, contain fibre and are most familiar to us as starchy foods. They are found abundantly potatoes, vegetables, fruit, whole-grain cereals and bread, lentils, beans, and nuts. Due to the presence of fibre, complex carbohydrates molecules are digested and converted to glucose slowly.

b. Protein
– Supplies four calories per gram

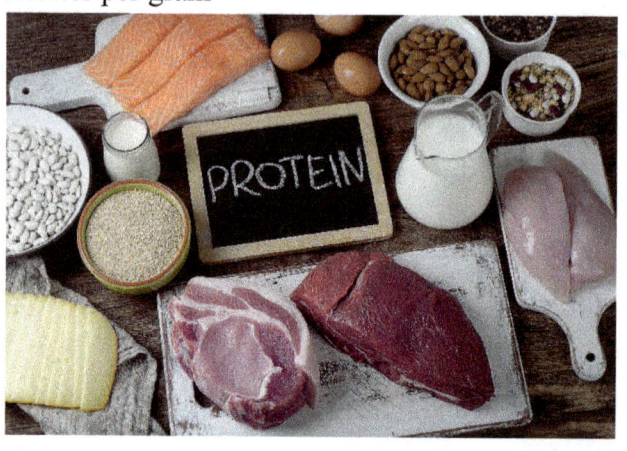

Proteins are macromolecules formed by 20 different types of amino acids. A protein is formed by the attachment of hundreds to thousands of these amino acids in long chains. Excellent sources of protein include fish, dairy products, meats and beans. Proteins are necessary to give physical structure to the body's tissues and organs, as well as in their functional regulation.

c. Fat
– Supplies nine calories per gram

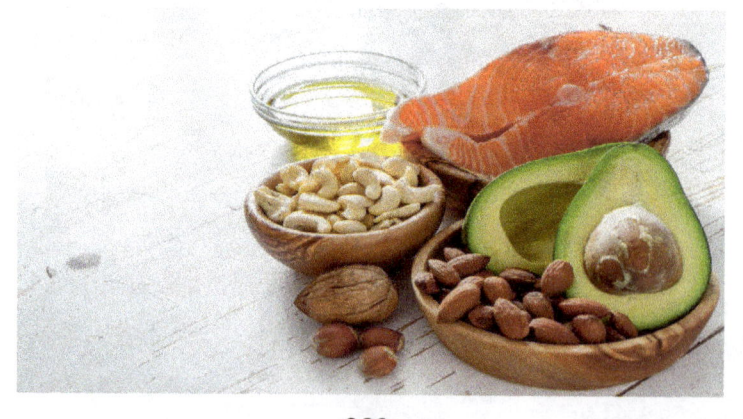

A glycerol backbone and three fatty acid tails make up a fat molecule. Fat provides energy and is necessary for the formation of cell membranes and the synthesis of essential hormones/chemicals in the body.

Three types of Fat:

1.Unsaturated fats (good fats) – These fats are liquefied at room temperature and are beneficial fats because they can ease inflammation, improve blood cholesterol levels, stabilize heart rhythms, and other beneficial roles. Unsaturated fats are predominantly from plants such as:

- Nuts and seeds
- Vegetable oils

"Good" unsaturated fats come in two forms:

    a. Mono-unsaturated fats – These are found in high concentrations in:
- Olive, canola and peanut oils
- Seeds such as sesame and pumpkin seeds
- Nuts such as pecans, hazelnuts and almonds
- Avocados

    b. Poly-unsaturated fats – These are found in high concentrations in:
- Flaxseed oils
- Flax seeds
- Fish
- Sunflower
- Walnuts
- Corn
- Soybean

An important type of polyunsaturated fat are Omega-3 fats. These are not manufactured by the body so they must come from food such as:
- Canola and soybean oil
- Walnuts
- Flax seeds
- Fish
- Supplementation

Research has indicated that high blood levels of omega-3 fats lower the risk of premature death from heart disease and improve mental health among older adults.

2.Saturated Fats –At room temperature these fats are in a solidified form and are found in animal products such as:
- Butter
- Cheese
- Meat and poultry

Traditionally, saturated fats were considered bad fats, but recent studies have indicated that this may not be the case. However, the overarching message continues to be that people should replace saturated fat with good fats, especially polyunsaturated fats to help lower "bad" LDL cholesterol, which will help reduce the risk of heart disease.

3. Trans Fat – This form of fat is "Bad Fat." It forms when unsaturated fats change from a liquid state to a solid state by a process called hydrogenation. This form of fat is commonly found in processed foods such as:
- Margarine
- Potato chips
- Frozen French fries
- Crackers
- Cookies

Trans fats raise blood levels of "bad" LDL cholesterol and lowers "good" HDL cholesterol, so trans fats are considered the worst type of fat for the heart, blood vessels, and rest of the body. Trans-fats are also associated with the creation of inflammation in the body which has been implicated in stroke, heart disease, and other chronic conditions such as osteoarthritis and diabetes, Trans fats need to be avoided in your diet.

2. Micro Nutrients

Micronutrients are vitamins and minerals which the body requires to function normally. Unfortunately, they are not produced in our bodies and are only derived from the food we eat or supplementation.

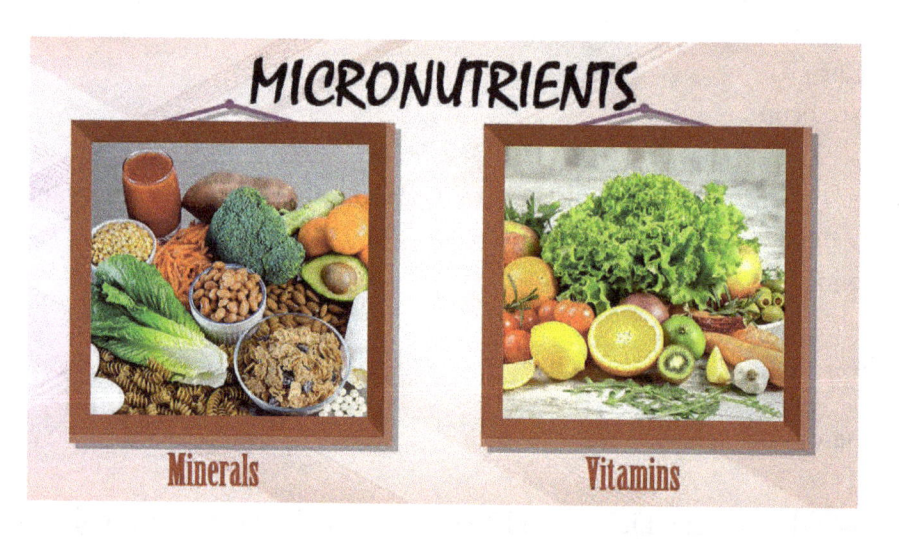

Image Source: steadfastnutrition.in

Vitamins – Vitamins are organic substances needed for the metabolism of carbohydrates and fats. There are two types; fat soluble or water soluble.

Fat-soluble vitamins (vitamin A, vitamin D, vitamin E, and vitamin K) – These dissolve and get stored in adipose (fat) tissue and therefore accumulate in the body. If a person/older adult is supplementing their diet with these vitamins, they must be careful of the dosage to avoid toxicity.

Water-soluble vitamins – (vitamin B1, B2, B3, B5, B6, B9 (Folate), B12, and C) – these can not be absorbed and stored by the body, because they get dissolve in water before they can be stored. Any unused water-soluble vitamins are excreted through the urine.

Minerals (calcium, iron, copper, fluoride, iodine, selenium, magnesium, zinc, and chromium) – These are essential inorganic substances necessary for the body to function normally. They regulate body fluids, involved in the transportation of oxygen in the blood, and are a necessary component for bone health, and hormone development. Each mineral is crucial for proper cell function even though the total amount of minerals in the body is small. Mineral deficiencies are rare since minerals are available in a wide variety of foods,

Nutrients needed for good health can be supplied by a healthy diet that includes plenty of vegetables, fruits, lean proteins, healthy (polyunsaturated) fats, and whole grains. Unfortunately, not everyone, especially the older adult who lives alone, eats a healthy diet. Supplementing a diet with multivitamins is necessary when nutritional requirements are not met through diet alone.

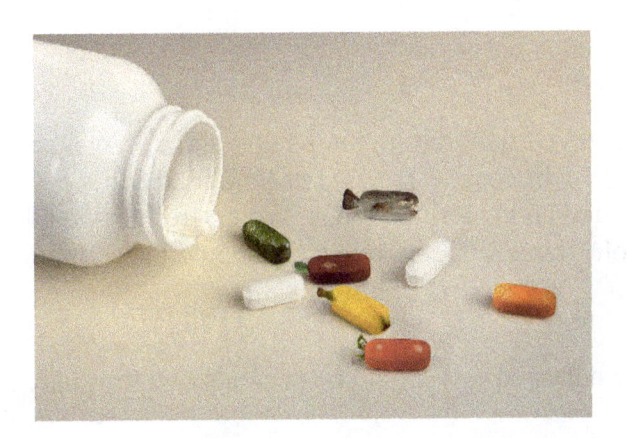

Water – The body is 60% water and it is necessary for body temperature regulation and metabolism, digestion, and lubrication of joints. Dehydration is a concern for older adults because their thirst mechanism and body composition change with age. Older adults have less water in their bodies than younger adults.

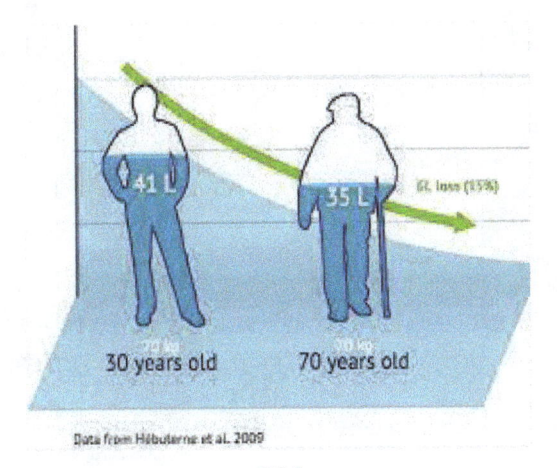

The body loses water during both regular daily activities and exercise. Thirst, the first sign of dehydration, often occurs after the body has become dehydrated, so it is essential to drink water even before feeling thirsty. If their urine is dark yellow, a person needs more water. Ideally, the urine should be pale yellow or clear.

Early signs of dehydration include:
- Fatigue
- Light headiness, dry mouth
- Loss of appetite
- Headache

Advanced signs of dehydration include:
- Difficulty swallowing
- Clumsiness
- Blurred vision
- Muscle spasms
- Delirium

Balanced Diet

Regardless of your age, you should limit your sugar and salt intake, refined carbohydrates, saturated fats, fried foods, hydrogenated (trans) fats, and food additives. Ensure that your meals are focused on whole natural and unrefined foods. Water, fresh fruit and vegetables, lean red meats, poultry, fish, whole grains, and unrefined oils should make up the bulk of your weekly diet.

Table 1 shows how a balanced diet should be presented on the plate.

Table 1: Balanced Diet

Nutrient	Percentage of your Diet/Plate	Food Choices
Carbohydrates	65%	Fruits Vegetables Whole Grains
Proteins	25%	Fish Seafood Lean red meats Poultry Eggs Low fat dairy products Beans & Legumes Nuts and seeds

Fats	10% Only 10% should be saturated fats (solid at room temperature such as butter and animal fat)	Eggs Cold water fish Oils (olive, flax, sunflower) Nuts and seeds (almonds, walnuts)

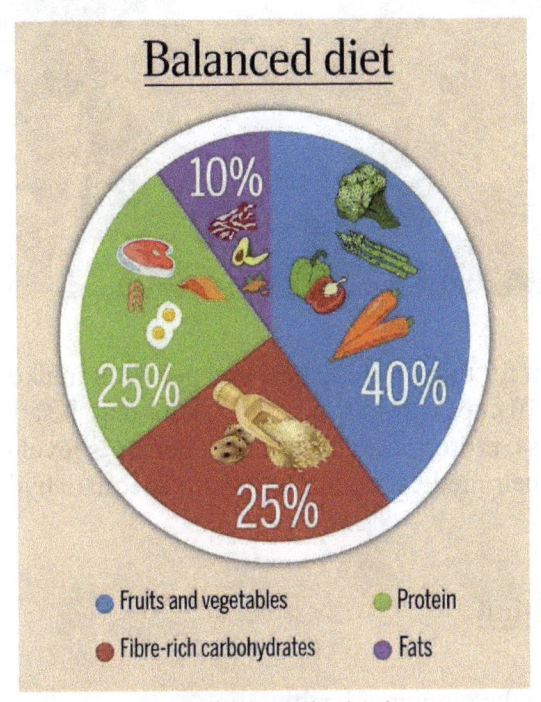

Image Source: femina.in

Eating and Physical Activity and Exercise

Physical activity and exercise put additional stress on muscles, ligaments, tendons, and bones. Maintaining a balanced diet is essential to ensure that muscle glycogen stores are available to fuel the activity/exercise and make sure proper tissue development and maintenance occurs following the activity.

Pre-exercise snacks are important to help avoid fatigue during and after the activity/exercise sessions. Pre-exercise healthy snacks include fruits and vegetables, yogurt, fruit smoothies, dates and raisins, nuts, and whole-grain cereal/crackers. After exercise, it is essential to replenish muscle glycogen stores to promote recovery. The post-exercise snack should be high in carbohydrates and include some protein. A 4:1 ratio of carbohydrate to protein is a rule of thumb for nutritional recovery after a workout of moderate to heavy intensity.

Hydration

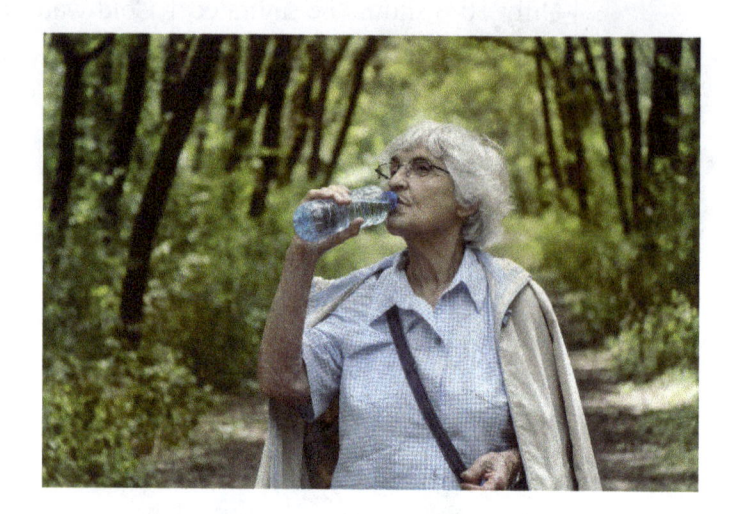

As we age, our sensation for thirst diminishes, and our fluid intake can suffer. A good rule of thumb is to consume six to 10 cups of water per day. There may be additional hydration requirements based on illness, prescription drugs and a person's level of physical activity. Older adults should consult with their medical doctor to ensure adequate hydration with physical activity and medication.

A Plan for Good Nutrition

Here are basic guidelines for developing a healthy diet:

1. Eat a variety of foods. Follow Canada's Health Food Guide recommendations (Chapter 5.2.3. The Canadian Health Food Guide) with respect to amounts from each food group (protein foods, dairy, whole grains, and fruits and vegetables).
2. Choose a diet low in fat and limit saturated and trans fats and cholesterol for heart disease prevention.
3. Eat plenty of vegetables, fruits, and whole grains.
4. Limit simple sugars.
5. Minimize salt intake.
6. Drink alcoholic beverages in moderation.
7. Balance food intake with physical activity.
8. Monitor caloric intake for weight control.

Be realistic with respect to diet. Follow the 80:20 rule (Chapter 3.1: The Eight Golden Rules of Training). This means that during the week, eat 80% healthy foods and you are allowed 20% or less of unhealthy foods. No one is perfect and realistically your diet will not be, so give yourself permission to indulge in less healthy foods but the key is to do this only 20% of the time.

Eat Well, Live Well for a Lifetime

The Dieticians of Canada have developed the LIFE program for older adults. It promotes:

L – Lifestyle – Being active and feeling good with family and friends and avoiding social isolation leads to a healthy lifestyle.

I – Independence – Healthy eating protects against illness and maintains daily life.

F – Food Choices – Be realistic, adventurous, flexible, and sensible with dietary choices.

E- Energy – Healthy eating and regular physical activity gives you the energy needed to get going and keep going.

Conclusion

Everyone, but especially the older adult, must, on a regular basis, eat well for health and vitality. The 80:20 rule is a realistic plan to follow. Eating well 80% or more of the time is excellent. Remember, you do not have to be perfect with your diet, but "you are what you eat," so it is important to make good food choices most of the time. It is best to combine regular exercise with a balanced diet for effective weight control.

Good nutrition is a crucial defense strategy for older adults to enhance their quality of life as they enter their golden years.

References

www.hsph.harvard.edu/nutritionsource/vitamins/
https://health.clevelandclinic.org/drink-up-dehydration-is-an-often-overlooked-health-risk-for-seniors/

Ogasawara, Sherry., Watters, Kyra., Sherk, Kerri., Sampson, Linda., Hutton, Janice. (2007). *Can-Fit-Pro: Nutritionist and Wellness Specialist: Certification Manual*. 4th Edition,

5.2.2. How to Read Nutritional Labels

Introduction

Since December 2005, companies selling food products in Canada have been required to have Nutritional Facts Labels on their food products. These labels were divided into two parts:

1. A nutritional fact table
2. A list of ingredients

In 2015, the Canadian government made amendments to improve the understanding of these labels so Canadians can make more informed choices.

The Changes to the Nutrition Facts Table

The following are changes/improvements to the Nutritional Facts Table:

1. **Changed the reporting of serving sizes** – The reporting sizes now reflect how much a Canadians typically eat in one sitting. This change will improve consistency on how serving sizes are listed which will make it easier to compare similar foods.
2. **Revised the % daily values** – This revision is based on new scientific data.
3. **3Total sugars are now listed with a new % daily value** – This is an important change since people are now encouraged to minimize their daily intake of sugar (Chapter 5.2.4: Sugar)
4. **Potassium is now listed** – This addition gives Potassium a much higher profile. Potassium is an essential mineral needed to maintain healthy blood pressure. High blood pressure is a significant cardiovascular risk factor for the older adult. Research indicates and many Canadians are getting an insufficient amount of this nutrient.
5. **Vitamins A and C were eliminated** – The typical Canadians diet supplies sufficient qualities of these nutrients so it was not as important to have them listed on the nutritional labels.
6. **Potassium, iron and calcium, are now listed by their amounts in milligrams (mg)** – These minerals needed a higher profile due to their nutritional importance, especially for older adults.
7. **The Percent daily value now has a footnote at the bottom of the table** – This footnote states that: 5% or less is a little and 15% or more is a lot. This is especially important to help the consumer understand how much is too much for nutrients like sugar and sodium/salt in the food they are buying.

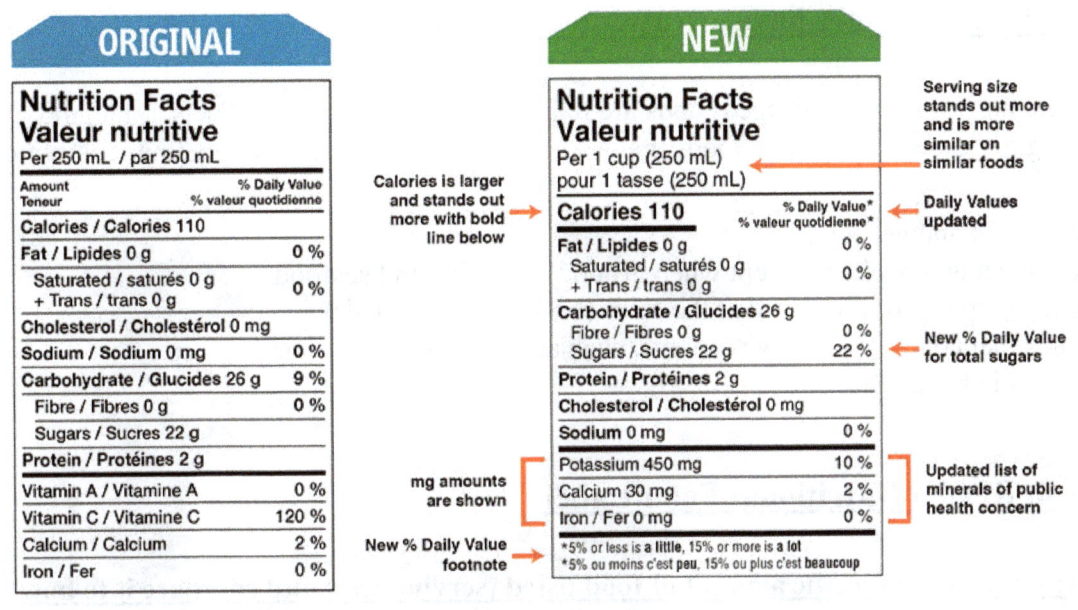

Image Source: Canada.ca

Changes to List of Ingredients label

The new changes will make the List of Ingredients easier to find, read and understand. These changes include:

1. **Sugar-based ingredients are now grouped in brackets after the name "sugars."** – All of the sources of sugar added to a food will now be more easily identified.
2. **Common names are now used to list food colours**
3. **Ingredients are now separated by bullets or commas** – This makes the ingredient list easier to read
4. **There is a 'Contains' statement** – which will indicate the presence or potential presence of:
    - Most common food allergens
    - Sources of gluten
    - any sulphites added

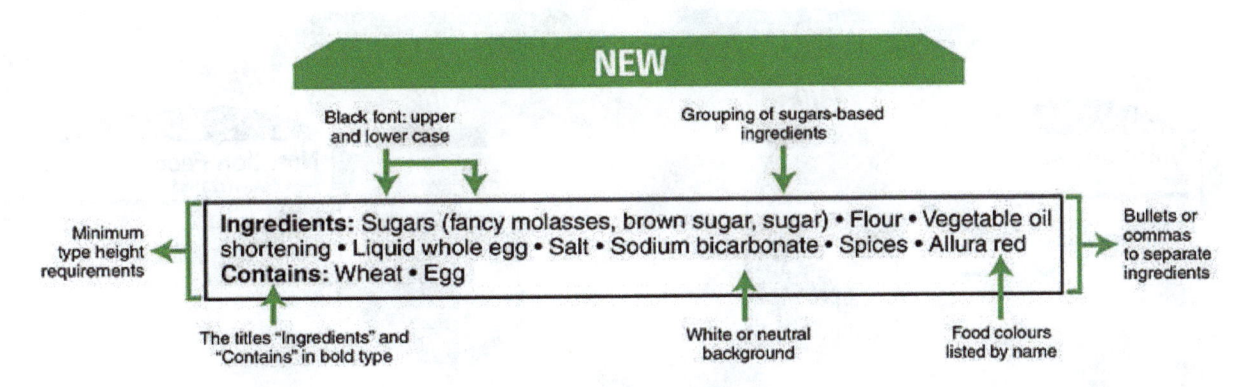

Image Source: Canada.ca

291

Not all food packages have a Nutrition Facts table

While almost all pre-packaged foods are required to have a Nutrition Facts Table, the following are examples of some foods that are exempt from the nutrition labeling requirements:

- Fresh fruit and vegetables
- Raw meat and poultry (except when ground), raw fish and seafood
- Foods prepared or processed at the store (bakery items, salads)
- Foods that contain very few nutrients, such as coffee, tea, herbs, and spices
- Alcoholic beverages

Steps to Read a Nutritional Food Label

Step 1: Look at the specific amount of food listed (serving size) and compare it to how much you would actually eat during a serving.

The serving sizes listed on the label are based on regulated reference amounts, and this may be different from what a person would typically eat. The serving sizes listed will make a difference concerning the number of calories and nutrients consumed.

Three key points to be aware of when looking at serving size:

1. Single Serving packaging – The serving size listed will be the amount in the whole container if the amount is within 200% of the reference amount.

Example –250 ml is the reference amount for milk, therefore the serving size shown on the container will be the amount of milk in the entire container if it is less than 500 ml (200% of 250 = 500 ml). The illustration below demonstrates that on a 473 mL carton of milk, the serving size will be shown as "Per 1 carton (473 mL)" since this is below the 200% threshold (500 ml) for the reference serving size for milk.

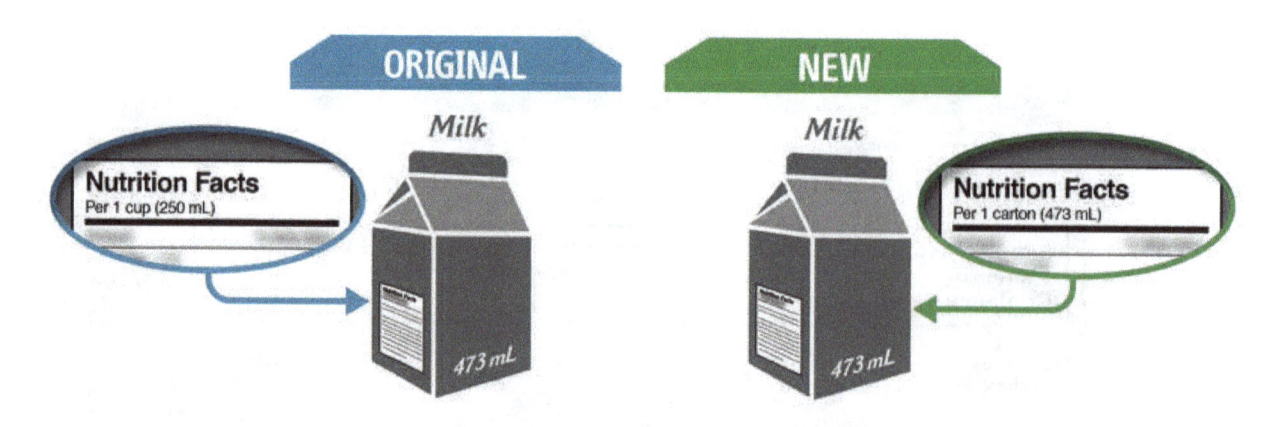

Image Source: Canada.ca

2. Multi-serving packages

The serving size referenced will be in an amount as close as possible to the food's reference amount.

Serving sizes are listed based on the type of food being looked at:
   a. Foods that can be measured
   b. Foods that come in pieces or are divided when served
   c. The amount of food typically eaten

a. Foods that can be measured (i.e. Yogurt (mL, tablespoon or teaspoon))

Yogurt, is a good example. The reference amount (what someone might typically eat at one sitting) is 175 g. Based on this reference amount, the serving size on all tubs of yogurt will listed as 175 g. It is much easier to compare nutrient content of different brands by listing consistent serving sizes.

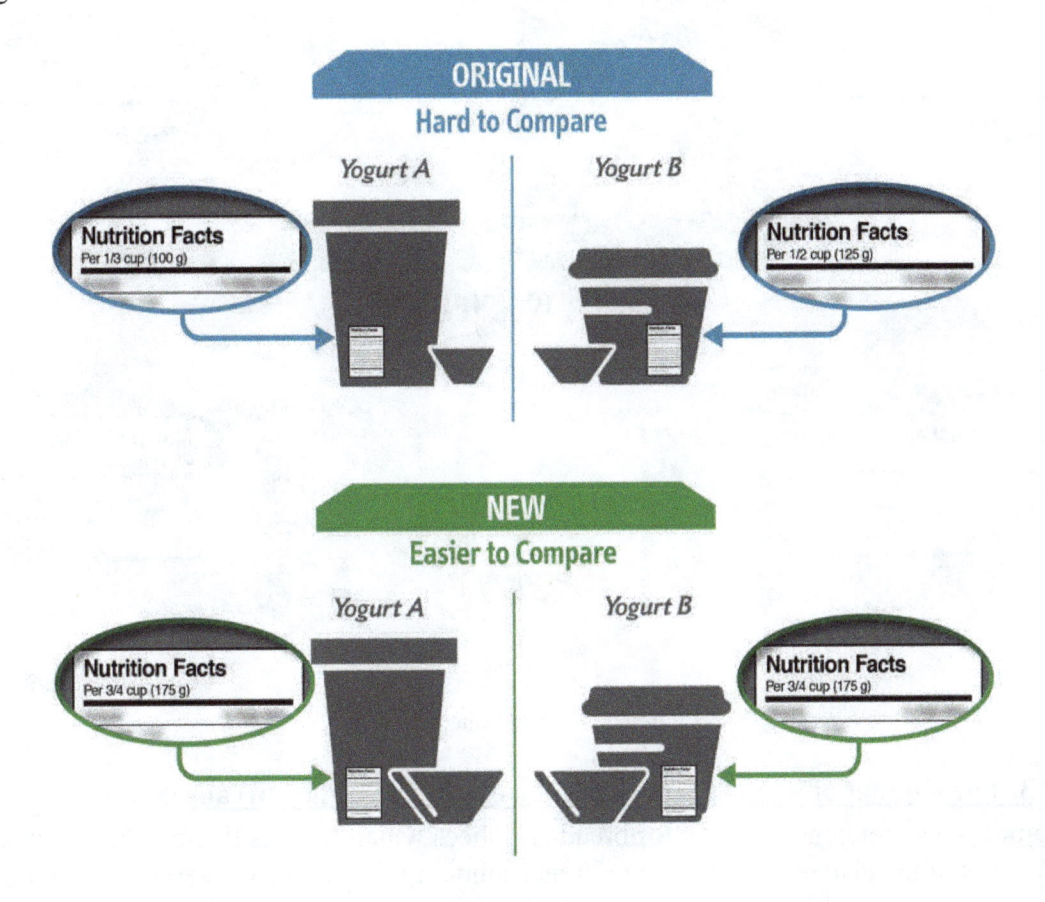

Image Source: Canada.ca

b. Foods that come in pieces (i.e. crackers (number of pieces) or are divided when served (i.e. lasagna (where a serving is a fraction of the food))

For example, on cracker boxes the serving size will be as close as possible to the reference amount of 20 g. The number of crackers from brand to brand may change but the serving size weights will be very similar so it is easier to compare different types of crackers.

ORIGINAL — Hard to Compare

Crackers A: Nutrition Facts Per 8 crackers (28 g)
Crackers B: Nutrition Facts Per 8 crackers (14 g)

NEW — Easier to Compare

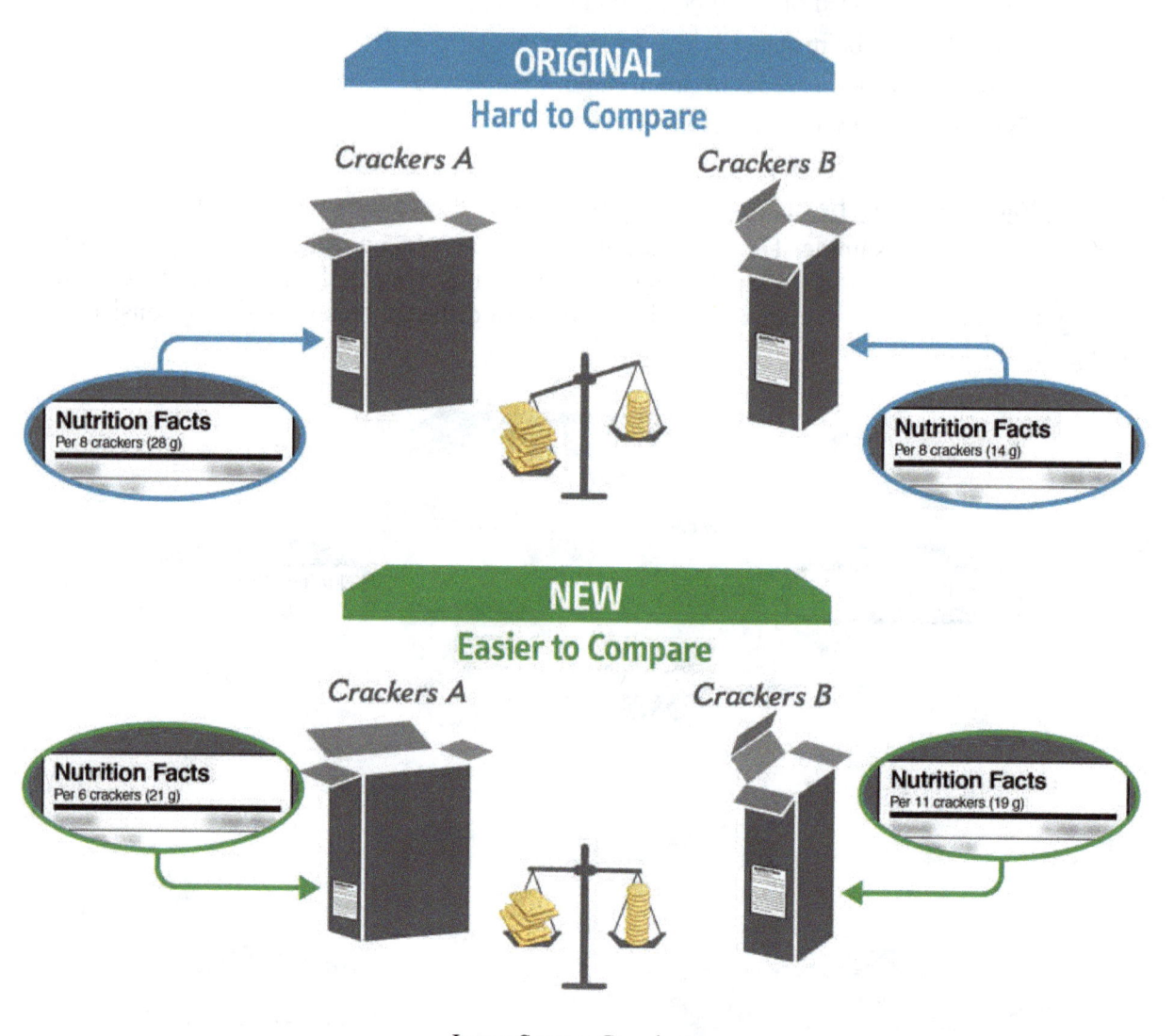

Crackers A: Nutrition Facts Per 6 crackers (21 g)
Crackers B: Nutrition Facts Per 11 crackers (19 g)

Image Source: Canada.ca

3. The amount of a food that is typically eaten (example – breads (slices))

<u>Example</u> –The reference amount for bread is 2 slices which reflects the fact that most people eat two slices of bread at one time. This reference amount is shown as the serving size on the nutrition label along with the 2 slices of bread weight in grams. Once again, being consistent by showing the reference amount of two slices of bread and the weight of these two slices of bread makes it easier for the consumer to compare different types of bread.

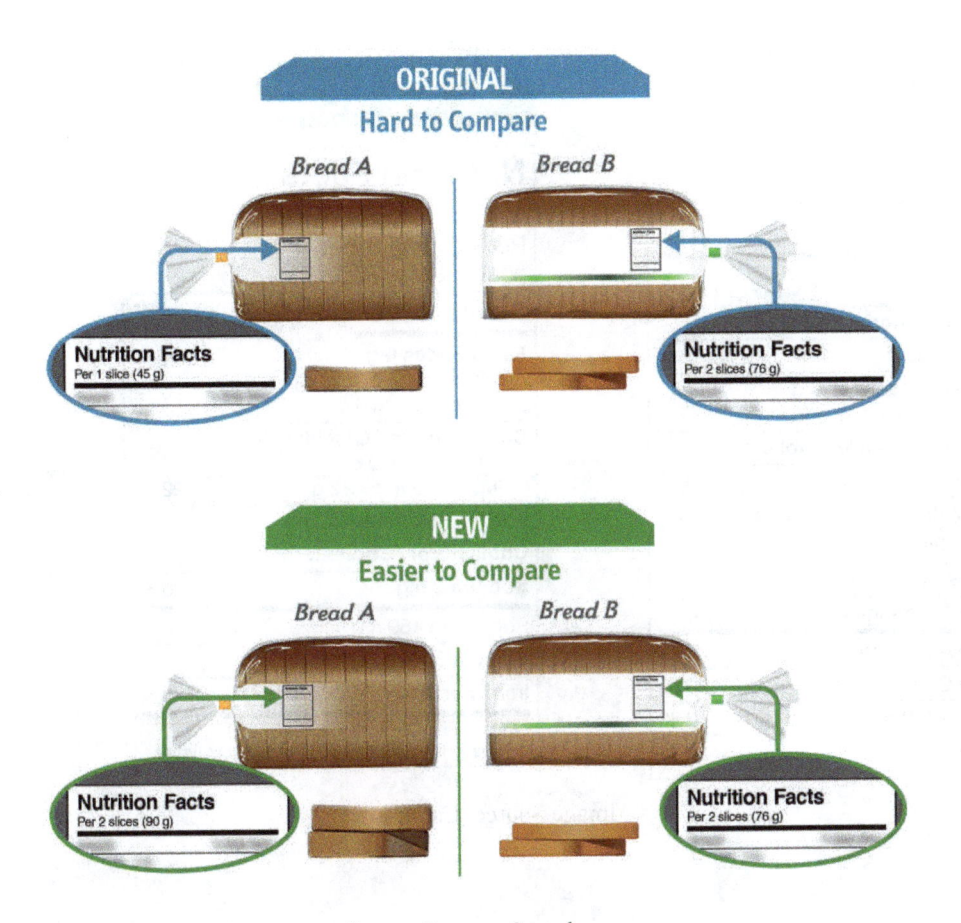

Image Source: Canada.ca

Step 2: Investigate if a food has a little or a lot of a nutrient by using the % Daily Value

The % Daily Value is a comparative benchmark when deciding the nutritional value between two food brands. It is best used to determine which food brand has a higher percentage of a nutrients that you want to limit in your diet (e.g., saturated and trans fats, cholesterol, sodium, sugar).

By using the recommendation in the footnote at the bottom of the nutritional label, (<5% is a little and >15% is a lot), it can be determined if a particular brand has less than or greater than the amount that is recommended for fats, carbohydrates/sugars, protein, cholesterol, sodium, potassium, calcium and iron.

Image Source: Canada.ca

Step 3:

1. Look at the number of calories per reference amount (serving size)

2. Look at the core nutrients (Fats, Carbohydrates, Proteins, Cholesterol, Sodium, Potassium, Calcium and Iron)

Image Source: Canada.ca

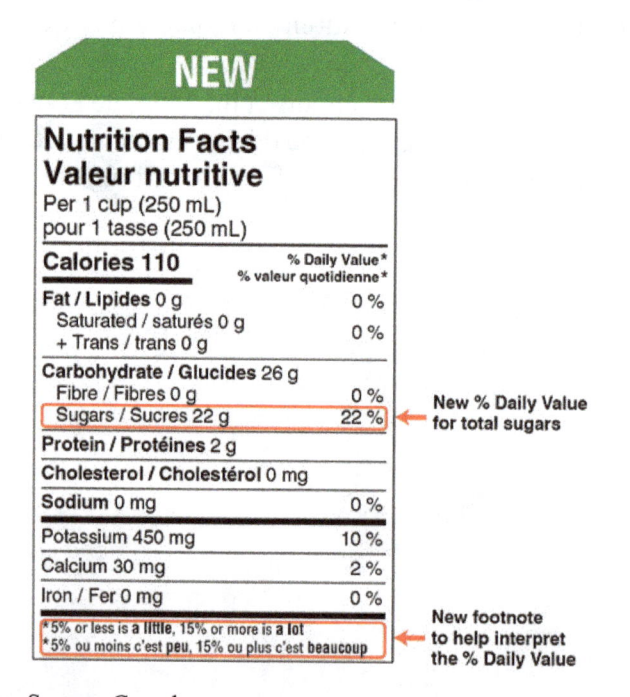

1. Calories
If you eat more than the reference amount, you will also be consuming more calories than what is listed. Portion sizes influence the number of calories consumed.

Example – If the Nutrition Facts table has information based on two slices of bread, eating four slices means doubling the calories and the amount of nutrients listed to calculate what the intake would be.

2. Fats
The fat listed in the Nutrition Facts table includes saturated fat, trans fat, and all other fatty acids present in the food.

Saturated Fat and Trans Fat have one combined % daily value in the nutrition facts table because both types of fat have negative effects on blood cholesterol levels. Therefore, choose a lower % Daily Value of fat type foods.

3. Carbohydrates
There are different types of carbohydrates:
- **a. Starch** – Such as in pasta and rice.
- **b. Fiber** – Such as whole grain products (like whole grain bread, high fiber cereals), legumes (e.g., dried peas, beans and lentils), vegetables and fruit.
- **c. Sugars** – Such as sucrose, glucose, fructose and dextrose.

In the Nutrition Facts table, the total amount of carbohydrates is listed in grams (no daily %) for the specified amount of food. This total amount includes starch, fiber, and sugars.

Pay particular attention to % daily amount of sugar. It is generally accepted that the less sugar, the better.

4. Protein
There is no % Daily Value for protein because protein intake is generally adequate for Canadians who consume a mixed diet.

5. Cholesterol
The % Daily Value for cholesterol is optional, so it may or may not be in the Nutrition Facts table. Whether or not the % Daily Value is displayed, the amount of cholesterol will be listed in milligrams.

6. Sodium
Salt is a common ingredient in processed and prepared foods, such as canned soups and processed meats. Most Canadians get more salt than they need, so a lower % Daily Value is preferred.

7. Potassium, Calcium, and Iron

These are based on a recommended daily intake. Having the % Daily Value makes it easier for consumers to understand the relative amount of this nutrient present in a food product.

Step 4: Be aware of nutritional claims and health claims on the packaging:

1. Nutrition Claims

The government has rules in place that must be met before a nutrition claim can be made on a label or advertisement. The regulations for nutrition claims apply to all foods pre-packaged and not pre-packaged.

A manufacturer can choose whether or not to include nutrition claims on the label or in the advertisement of a food. Many products will have nutrition claims as these claims highlight a feature of interest to consumers.

Examples of Nutritional Claims:

a. "Source of Fiber" – This means the food contains at least 2 grams of dietary fiber in the amount of food specified in the Nutrition Facts table under carbohydrates.

b. "Low fat" – This, means the food contains no more than 3 grams of fat in the amount of food specified in the Nutrition Facts table under fat.

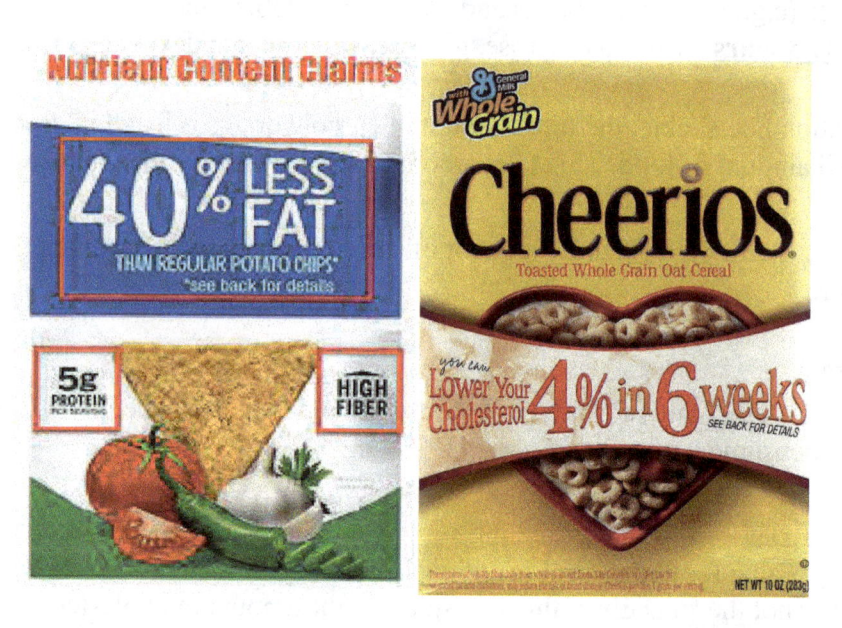

Image Source: fdareader.com   Image Source: twincities.com

c. "Fat Free" – This means that based on the serving size that the food has a negligible amount cholesterol (less than 2 mg) and it is also low in saturated fat and trans fat.

d. "Sodium-free" – "Free" means that the amount of a nutrient in the particular serving size of the food nutritionally insignificant. For example, "sodium-free" claim means the serving size of food specified contains less than 5 mg of sodium.

e. "Reduced in Calories" – This means at least 25% less energy (calories per serving) than the food it is being compared to.

f. "Light" – "Light" is allowed only on foods that are either "reduced in fat" or "reduced in energy" (Calories). "Light" can also be used to describe sensory characteristics of a food, provided that the characteristic is clearly identified with the claim (e.g., light tasting, light coloured).

2. Health Claims

Health claims are a type of nutrition claim. Health claims about the following diet/health relationship are permitted:

1. A healthy diet low in saturated and trans fats may reduce the risk of heart disease.
2. A healthy diet with adequate calcium and vitamin D, and regular physical activity, help to achieve strong bones and may reduce the risk of osteoporosis.
3. A healthy diet rich in a variety of vegetables and fruit may help reduce the risk of some types of cancer.
4. A healthy diet containing foods high in potassium and low in sodium may reduce the risk of high blood pressure, a risk factor for stroke and heart disease.

Step 5: Read the List of Ingredients

The List of Ingredients on food packaging is mandatory.
- The ingredients present in the greatest amount in a product are listed first.

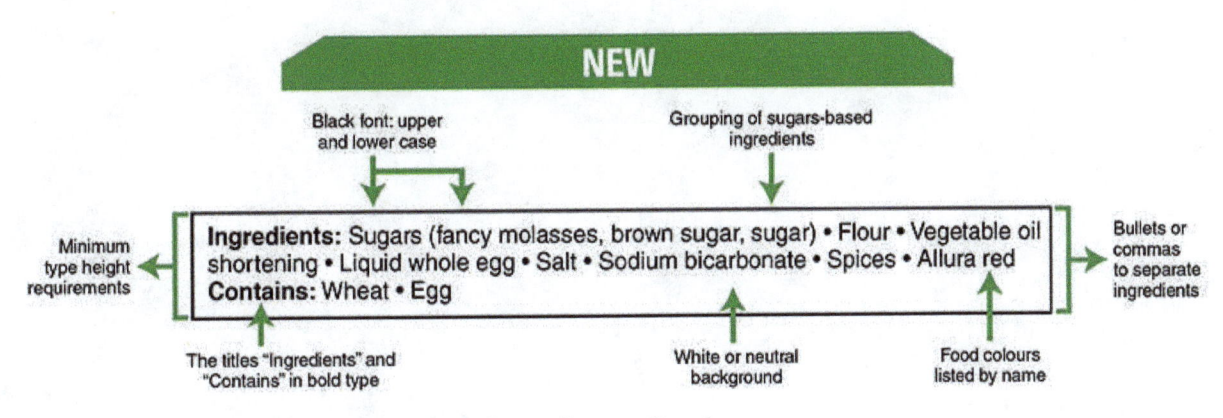

Image Source: Canada.ca

After the name "Sugars" - sugar-based ingredients are grouped in brackets and listed in descending order by weight. This improves the consumers ability to:

- see that sugars have been added to the food
- understand how much sugar has been added to the food compared to other ingredients.
- identifies the sources of sugars added to the food

"Contains" – This helps people, who are allergic or who want to avoid certain ingredients (i.e. – wheat or eggs), identify if those ingredients are in the food being considered.

Conclusion

The Nutrition Facts Label is an excellent source of information about the nutritional value of foods based on portion size. You can use it to monitor total caloric intake, fat, sodium, and cholesterol intake and help identify foods high in fiber, vitamins, and minerals.

Often, identical foods from two different manufacturers can have significantly different nutritional make-up (one can be high in sodium and the other low). It is well worth your time and effort to determine which one has the highest nutritional value. Good nutrition starts with reading the Nutrition Facts Label on the packages on food.

References

www.canada.ca/en/health-canada/services/food-labelling-changes.html
www.forever-active.com

5.2.3. Canadian Health Food Guide

Introduction

In January 2019, Health Canada unveiled the new Canadian Health Food Guide and an interactive, mobile-friendly website, https://food-guide.canada.ca. The new guide has been generally well-received by medical, nutritional health, and wellness professionals, with many calling it "relevant and evidence-based… and will help Canadians make healthy food choices."

Canada's has had a food guide since 1942. The first food guide, The Official Food Rules, recognized wartime food rationing and attempted to prevent nutritional deficiencies and improve Canadians' health during the second world war. Many times, since 1942, the food guide has been transformed, adopting new looks, new messages and new names. However, the focused has always been on improving the nutritional health of Canadians by promoting proper food selection.

The Canadian Health Food Guide is a valuable tool that older adults should consider as an educational tool designed to help them follow a healthy diet. Knowing what to eat and how much to eat starts with education, and the Canadian Health Food Guide fills this need.

The Health Food Guide was developed by merging national nutrition goals, data from food consumption surveys, utilizing sophisticated dietary analysis, and monitoring food supply and production. The food guide meets nutrient requirements while emphasizing variety and flexibility in food choices.

The new Canadian Health Food Guide reflects growing scientific literature that a diet that is plant-based is more in line with a healthy lifestyle than one based on meat and dairy.

Major Points Emphasised in the New Canadian Health Food Guide

1. Three Food Groups

The old four basic food groups, fruits and vegetables, meat and alternatives, grain products and milk and milk products have been reduced to three;

- proteins – a new umbrella category that combines dairy and meat and plant-based proteins such as tofu and chickpeas.
- whole grains.
- fruits and vegetables.

The key element to the New Canadian Health Food Guide is to eat less meat and dairy and more plants. The new guide clearly states, "Among protein foods, consume plant-based more often... The regular intake of plant-based foods – vegetables, fruit, whole grains, and plant-based proteins – can have positive effects on health." These positive effects include a lower risk of colon cancer, type 2 diabetes and cardiovascular disease.

2. "Half Your Plate" Method or "Half Fruit and Vegetable" Rule

Portion sizes, as described in the old food guide, such as two tablespoons of peanut butter, 2 ounces of cheese or 3.5 ounces of meat, and the number of servings per day, such as seven grain products or three meats, are out. There is a new simplified rule to follow: eat a diet made up of roughly half of two food groups; whole grains, and protein and half of the remaining food group; fruits and vegetables. The new guide is all about "proportions not portion," and this is accomplished by the "half fruits and vegetables" rule or also known as the "half your plate" method.

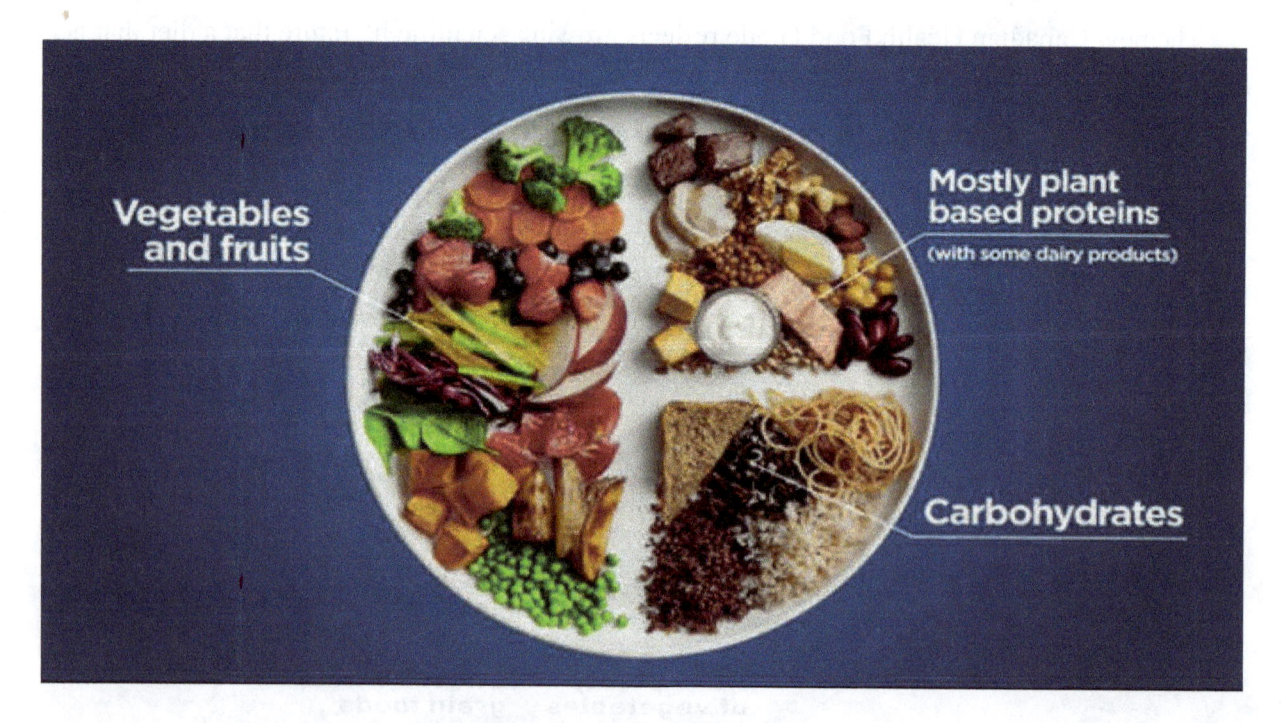

Image Source: globalnews.ca

3. Drink Water

The new guidelines encourage water to be Canadians "beverage of choice." Encouraging an increase in water consumption has two purposes. First, it promotes hydration, which is extremely important for older adults, and second, to reduce alcoholic beverages and sugary drink. In 2015, primary source of total sugars in Canadian diets was sugary drinks. Unfortunately, but not surprising, children and adolescents had the highest average daily intake of sugary drinks. Previously, the Canada's Food Guide stated that a healthy equivalent option to a serving of fruit was 100% fruit juice. The New Canadian Health Food Guide reverses this and states clearly that 100% fruit juice is a "sugary drink" associated with obesity, type 2 diabetes and dental decay.

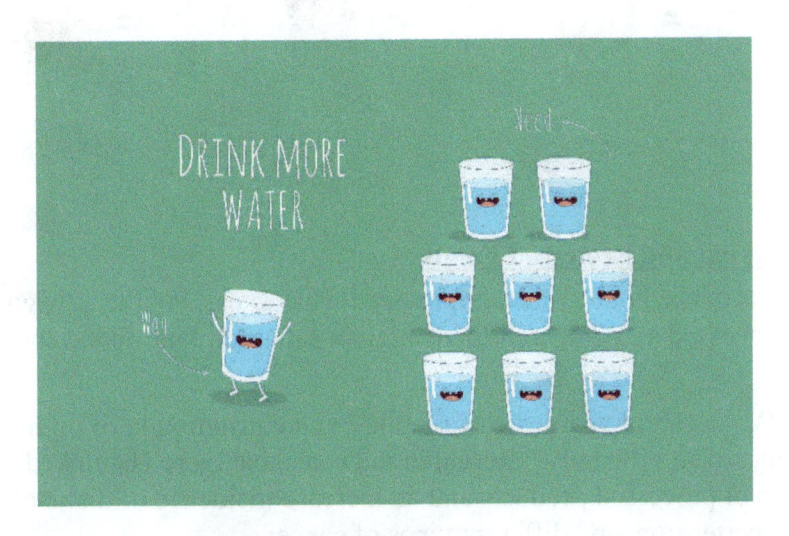

Alcohol consumption also has a new warning. The new guide states that alcohol, "contributes a lot of calories to the diet with little to no nutritive value."

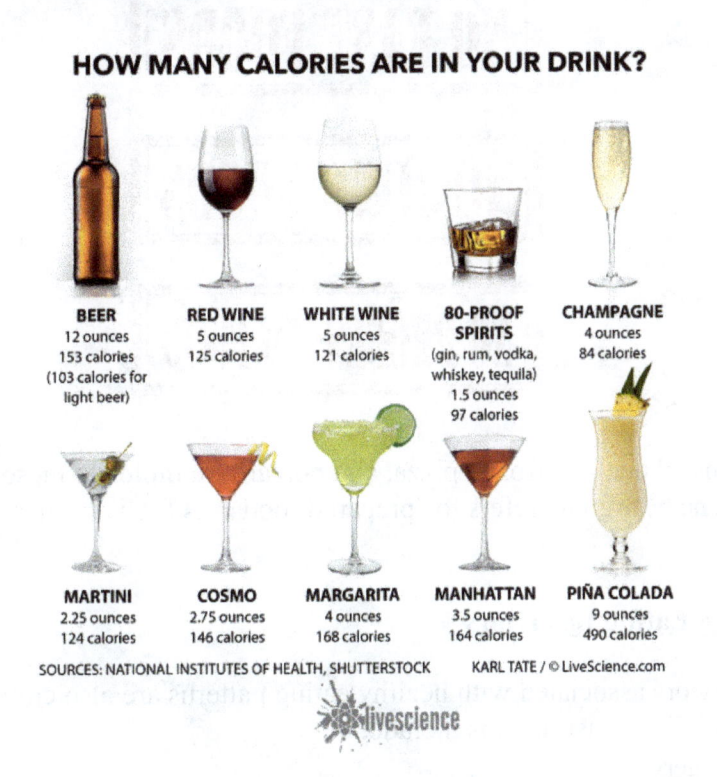

HOW MANY CALORIES ARE IN YOUR DRINK?

BEER — 12 ounces, 153 calories (103 calories for light beer)
RED WINE — 5 ounces, 125 calories
WHITE WINE — 5 ounces, 121 calories
80-PROOF SPIRITS (gin, rum, vodka, whiskey, tequila) — 1.5 ounces, 97 calories
CHAMPAGNE — 4 ounces, 84 calories
MARTINI — 2.25 ounces, 124 calories
COSMO — 2.75 ounces, 146 calories
MARGARITA — 4 ounces, 168 calories
MANHATTAN — 3.5 ounces, 164 calories
PIÑA COLADA — 9 ounces, 490 calories

SOURCES: NATIONAL INSTITUTES OF HEALTH, SHUTTERSTOCK   KARL TATE / © LiveScience.com

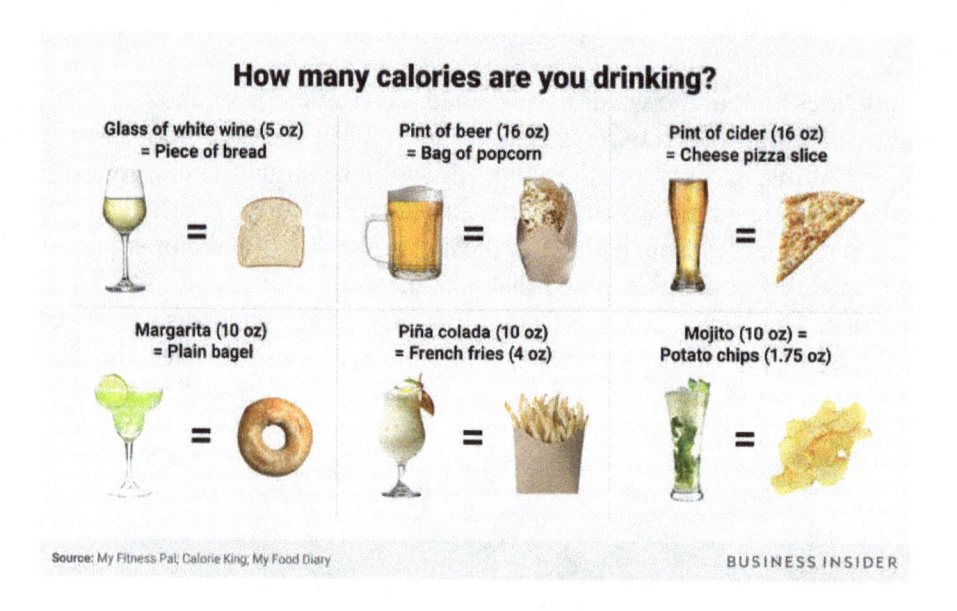

4. Eat Fewer Processed and Prepared Foods

Previous versions of the Food Guide emphasized what to eat, but the new guide emphasises what not to eat – processed and prepared foods high in saturated fats, added sugars and sodium.

The guide states, "In recent years, the availability and consumption of highly processed products have increased significantly." Research indicates that there is a linked between the higher consumption of processed products and an increase incidence of diabetes, cardiovascular disease, obesity, hypertension, and different types of cancer.

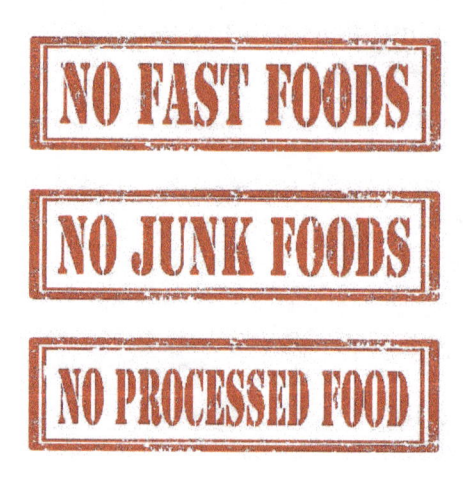

Hot dogs, muffins, chocolate, frozen pizza, and pop are examples of these processed foods listed in the guide. The new guide refers to "prepared foods" as foods from restaurants or similar ready-to-eat meals.

5. New Emphasis on Eating Behaviors

Instructions on behaviors associated with healthy eating patterns are also emphasized in the new Canadian food guide. These instructions include:
- Eat meals with others.

- Cook more often
- Be mindful of your eating habits
- Enjoy your food

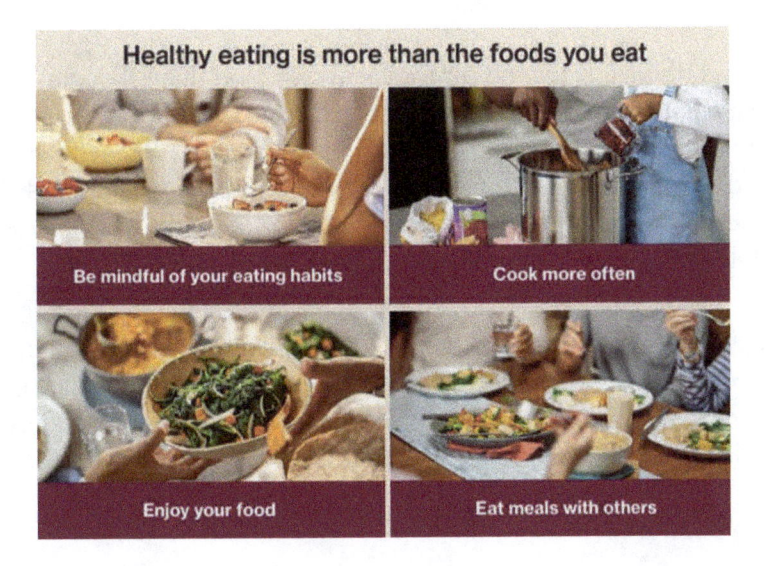

Image Source: wechu.org

Conclusion

The Canadian Health Food Guide is not without its detractors, namely that it is not specific enough with respect to what to eat and how much to eat. That was the "old" food guide, and this newer version's purpose is to be a guide and is purposely not meant to provide a meal plan for the perfect diet. The Canadian Health Food Guide is just that, a guide to help people develop the skills and behaviors important to having a healthy diet and a healthy relationship with food.

Being a "guide" is a good change and approach. The failure of diets that specify when to eat, how much to eat, and what to eat, shows that this approach to nutritional health does not work. The principles laid out in the new food guide are adequate and simple enough for everyone, including the older adult, to learn and follow. Old "bad" nutritional habits are challenging to break, and the first step to making positive change is to understand what needs to be done. The New Canadian Health Food Guide accomplishes this goal.

By following its recommendations, you will eat better and live a healthier life.

References

https://www.canada.ca/en/health-canada/services/canada-food-guide/about/history-food-guide.html

https://food-guide.canada.ca/en/

5.2.4. Sugar

Introduction

Besides weight loss, there are few hotter topics in nutrition than of sugar. Health scientists are now calling sugar the new smoking because of its potential ill health effects. Because older adults are vulnerable to developing type 2 diabetes, monitoring how much sugar they ingest and managing their blood sugar levels is of great importance. Refer to Chapter 2.4. for an in-depth discussion on diabetes and chapter 5.2.9. Glycemic Index: Its Usefulness in Controlling Blood Glucose Levels in Older Adults.

Canada's new Health Food Guide (Chapter 5.2.3.) states very clearly that a person must minimize their sugar intake. Unfortunately, this is easier said than done since sugar is added to many foods that we purchase at the grocery store. Hidden sugar in foods makes reading and understanding nutritional labels on food products more important (Chapter 5.2.2. How to Read Nutrition Labels).

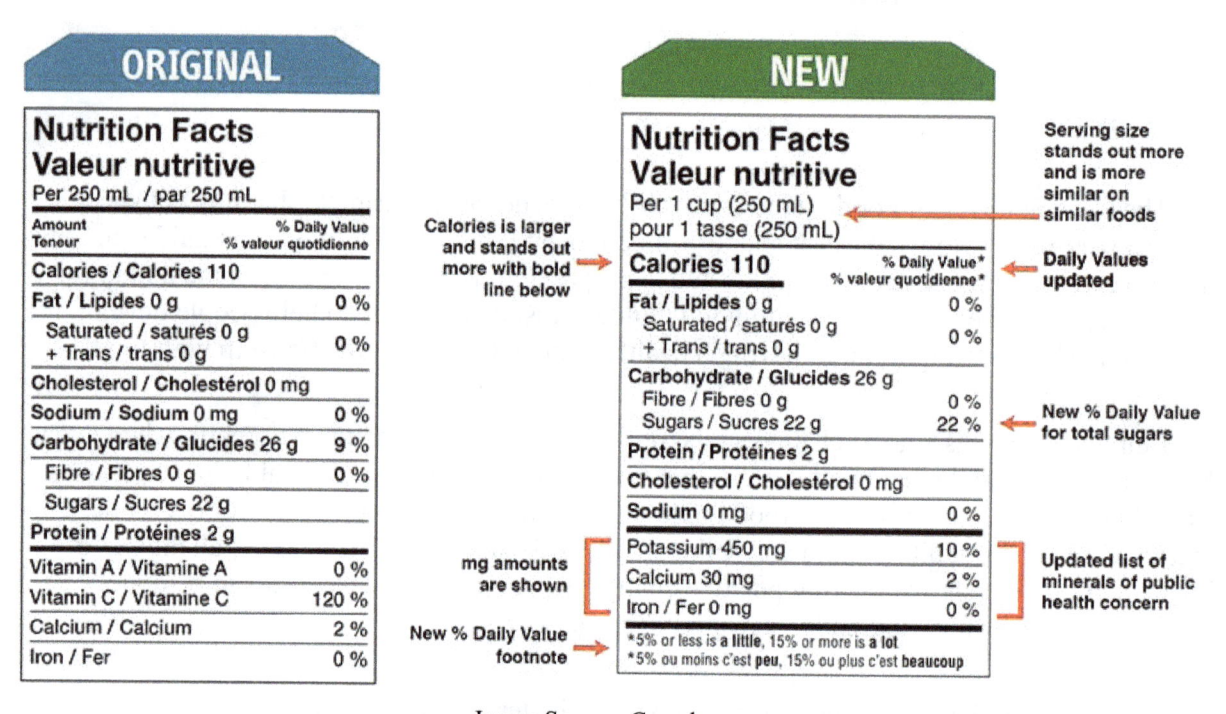

Image Source: Canada.ca

What is Sugar?

Sugars are a staple in the North American diet as they add flavor to food, but the old adage that it is never a good thing too have too much of a good thing, definitely applies to sugar.

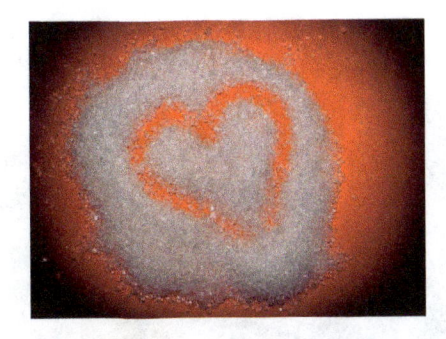

Sugar is the generic name for sweet-tasting, soluble carbohydrates, many of which are added to food.

1.Simple sugars (monosaccharides) : glucose, fructose, and galactose.
2.Compound sugars (disaccharides or double sugars) are two monosaccharides joined together.

Common examples of compound sugars are;

- Sucrose (table sugar) = Glucose + fructose
- Lactose (milk sugar) = Glucose + galactose
- Maltose (part of many foods and beverages such as bread, beer, cereals, and energy bars) = 2 glucose

In the body, compound sugars are hydrolyzed into simple sugars that enter the bloodstream.

Natural and Added Sugars

Key Point – You do not need to avoid all sugars

1. Natural Sugars

Fruits and vegetables, grains, and dairy are foods that contain carbohydrates so they naturally contain sugar. It is important to know that it is ok to consume whole foods that contain natural sugars. High amounts of fiber, essential minerals, antioxidants are contained in fruits and plant foods, while protein and calcium are present in dairy foods. These foods are digested slowly, so the sugar in them is released into the blood stream gradually, allowing a steady supply of energy to the cells. The risk of some chronic diseases, such as heart disease, diabetes, and some cancers have been shown to be reduced with a diet containing a significant number of fruits, vegetables, and whole grains.

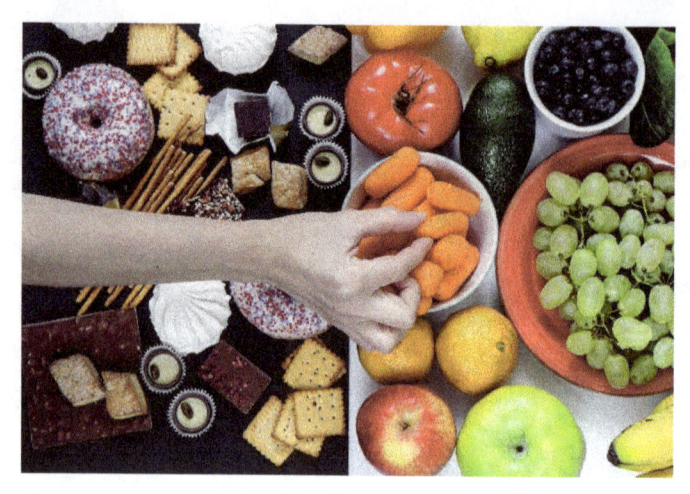

Image Source: health.com

2. Added Sugars

Sugars are added at home and by the food industry to add sweetness, thickening, and browning to the food. White and brown sugar, cane syrup, and honey are common sugars added in food preparation. **These types of sugars need to be avoided.**

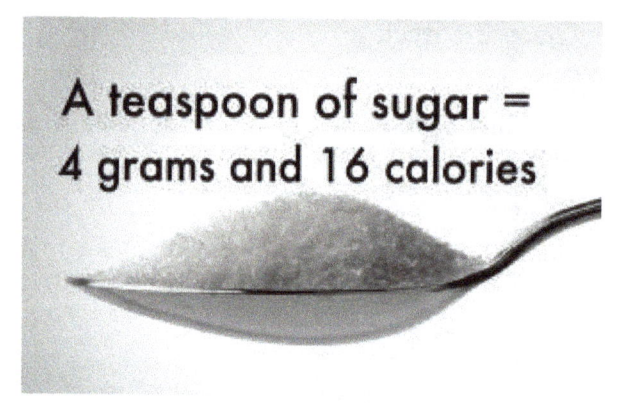

Image Source: 10tipsforhealth.com

Pop and fruit drinks, cereals, flavored yogurts, candy, cakes, cookies, and most processed foods are the top sources for added sugars. Many foods, not thought of as sweetened, like soups, bread, cured meats, and ketchup also have significant amounts of added sugar.

How Much Sugar is Too Much?

The average person's diet contains too much added sugar. Canadians consume on average 16 teaspoons of sugar/day, which is 30 kg/year or 15 bags of sugar.

Health Canada does not explicitly recommend an amount of sugar Canadians should consume daily. However, the World Health Organization (WHO) in 2015 suggested that adults and children reduce their intake of sugars to less than 10% and ideally 5% of daily calories. For the average adult who eats a 2,000-calorie diet, that amounts to 50 (10%) or 25 (5%) grams (4 calories = 1 gram of sugar) or approximately 10 or 5 teaspoons (5 grams ~ 1 teaspoon). However, WHO states very clearly that "less is best."

It is recommended by the American Heart Association that no more than 5- 6 teaspoons (25 grams) of sugar be added a day for women and 7- 9 teaspoons (36 grams) a day for men.

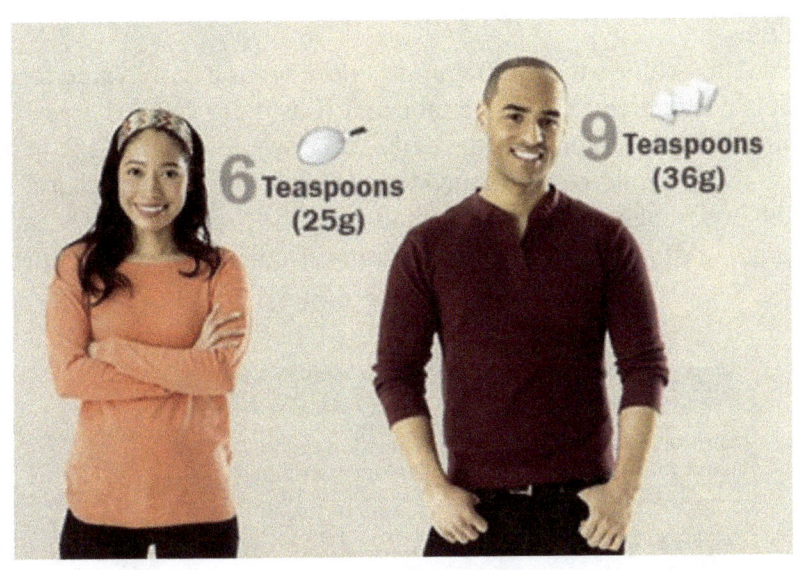

Image Source: webmd.com

Acute and Chronic Signs of Too Much Sugar

1. Acute signs a person is eating too much sugar
- Weight gain.
- Unexplained bloating.
- Low energy.
- Insomnia.
- Weakened immune system.
- Constant cravings.
- Premature aging of the skin – caused by long-term damage to the proteins, collagen and elastin of the skin which leads to premature wrinkles.

2. Chronic effects of consuming too much sugar
- Diabetes,
- Inflammation
- Heart disease
- Higher blood pressure
- Fatty liver disease
- Significant weight gain

Reading Nutritional Labels for Sugar Content

1. Nutrition Table

For a standard 2,000 calorie diet, 100 grams is now set as a daily value for total sugars. For a particular food, it is considered "a lot" of total sugar if its daily value is greater than 15% (15 grams). Added sugars is the reason why the daily value would exceed 15% in most foods. Examples of these foods would be sweetened yogurt, fruit juices and cookies. Unfortunately, it is still difficult to tell how much sugar has been added by the food industry because the nutrition label lumps the amount of added sugars and naturally occurring sugars together as total sugars in grams.

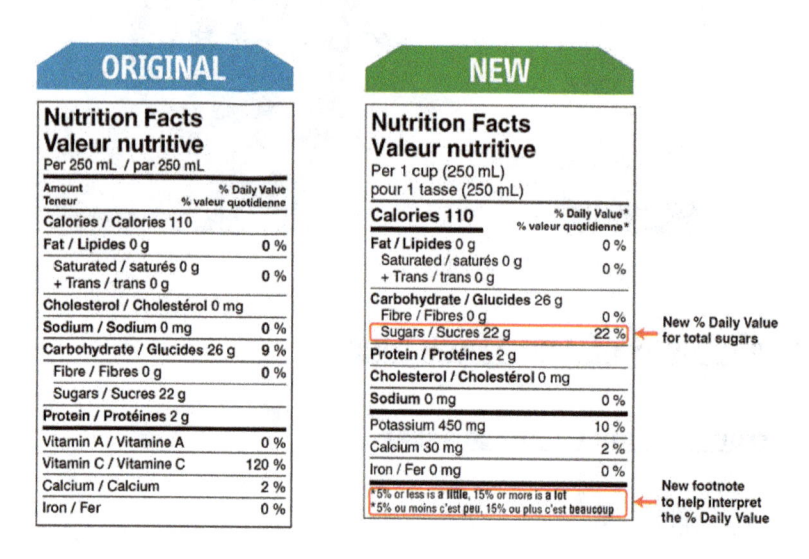

Image Source: Canada.ca

2. Ingredient List

Under the common name "Sugars" all sugar ingredients are listed. The combined weight of all the sugar ingredients determines where the common name "Sugars" is placed in the ingredient list. The different types of sugar on the list are listed in order by their weight, from most to least.

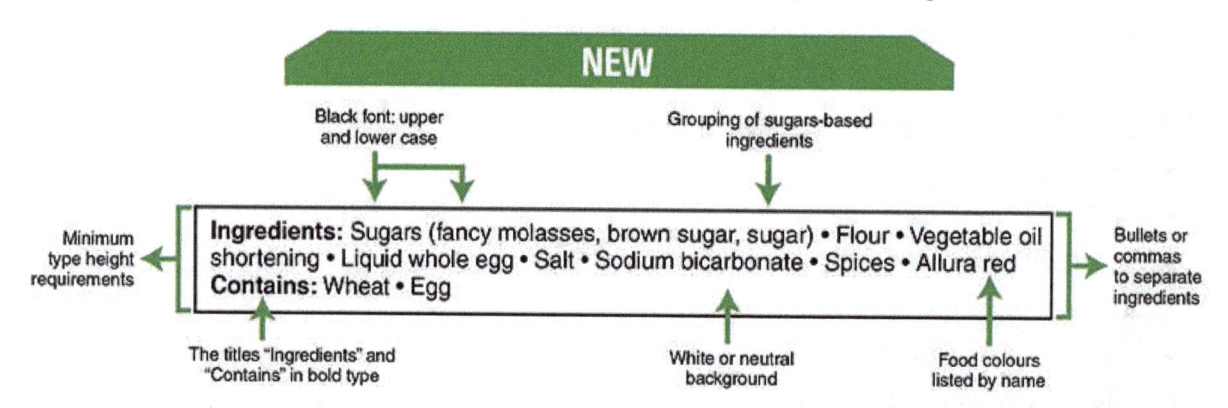

Image Source: Canada.ca

Understanding Sugar Content Claims on Packaging

There are five types of sugar-related claims on food packages;

1. **"No Added Sugar"** – No sugar has been added to this food. However, artificial sweeteners (i.e. aspartame) may have been added.
2. **"Unsweetened"** – No sugars are added nor are sugar alcohols (ie sorbitol) or artificial sweeteners (i.e. aspartame).
3. **"Sugar-Free" (a.k.a. zero sugar, sugarless)** – No more than five calories per serving is allowed. (i.e. sugarless gum and artificially sweetened drinks).
4. **"Reduced Sugar"** – These foods have been reformulated or processed to contain at least 25% less sugars than the regular version.
5. **"Lower in Sugar" or "less sugar"** – This product has not been reformulated but compared to other foods in the same food group, it contains 25% less sugar.

Sugar Addiction

Research suggests that sugar can be addictive. Signs that one may be addicted to sugar include:

- Headaches
- Lethargy and feeling tired
- Sugar cravings
- Muscle and joint pain
- Nausea
- Insomnia

Breaking Sugar Addiction

1. **Keep sugary foods away** – Avoid buying and stocking cookies, candy, cookies, and other high-sugar foods. It is recommended to consume fruit as a substitute.
2. **Sweeten foods at home** – Start by buying plain yogurt, unflavoured oatmeal, unsweetened iced tea, and then add sweetener at home. Slowly begin to reduce the amount of sugar you add so your taste buds have time to adapt to less sugary foods.
3. **Read food nutrition labels to become aware of hidden sugars in foods** – Become familiar with how to read nutrition labels (Section 5.2.2. How to Read Nutrition Labels) and avoid products that list sugar as the first ingredient.
4. **Eat breakfast** – A good strategy to avoid giving in to cravings is to start the day with a filling, nutritious meal. Excellent breakfast choices include unsweetened oatmeal, eggs, and fruit.

By following these four steps, your taste and cravings will change over time. and you will become increasingly satisfied with less sweet foods.

Conclusion

It is not unusual for a person to have a love-hate relationship with sugar; they love its taste but hate its health effect. For the older adult, it is necessary to balance this relationship because excessive sugar intake increases the risk of diabetes, heart disease and obesity.

Eating foods such as fruit and vegetables with naturally occurring sugars is good. This sugar is released slowly into the bloodstream, and these foods are full of necessary fiber, vitamins, and minerals. It is best for you to avoid foods with added sugars, such as processed foods.

Becoming familiar with and reading nutritional labels is an excellent first step to lowering daily sugar consumption. Being careful of how much sugar is added during meals and snacks and looking for whole food substitutes for sugary snacks are also excellent strategies to break that sugar habit/addiction.

References

www.canada.ca/en/health-canada/services/canada-food-guide/about/history-food-guide.html
www.webmd.com
www.mayoclinic.com

5.2.5. Salt/Sodium

Introduction

Salt/sodium is an essential mineral in the older adult's diet. But, just like sugar, too much of a good thing is not advisable. A person may use salt at their dinner table to add flavor to their meals, but that is not the primary source of salt/sodium in your diet. Salt is commonly added to foods by manufacturers for taste and food preservation, so reading nutritional labels should become a habit for consumers when they grocery shop. Different brands of the same food have different salt content.

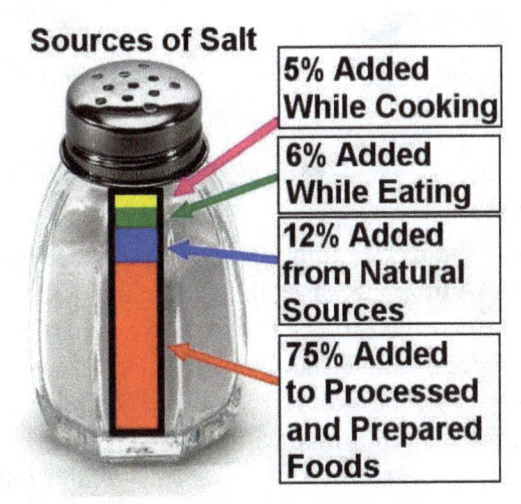

Image Source: pinterest.com

Table salt is 38% sodium. Sodium is necessary to regulate body fluid volumes, electrolyte balance, and the transmission of nerve impulses for muscle contraction and function. Unfortunately, high sodium content in diets has been associated with increased blood pressure, a major risk factor for cardiovascular diseases in older adults (Chapter 2.2. Heart Disease).

It is estimated that the average North American's sodium intake is 3.5 grams/day (1.5 teaspoons of salt). The World Health Organization recommends less than 1.5 grams of sodium per day which equals 2/3 teaspoons of salt . The Canadian Health Food Guide does not make a specific recommendation on the amount of salt/sodium to be consumed daily but strongly recommends reducing the consumption of processed foods because highly processed foods are the main source of sodium for Canadians.

1 tsp salt ≈ 2,300 mg sodium

Image source: lucaborghi.net

- American adult daily consumption (>3,400 mg)
- Adult upper level (2,300 mg)
- Adult recommended daily (1,500 mg)
- Adult needed daily (180 mg)

image source: drashchiheart.com

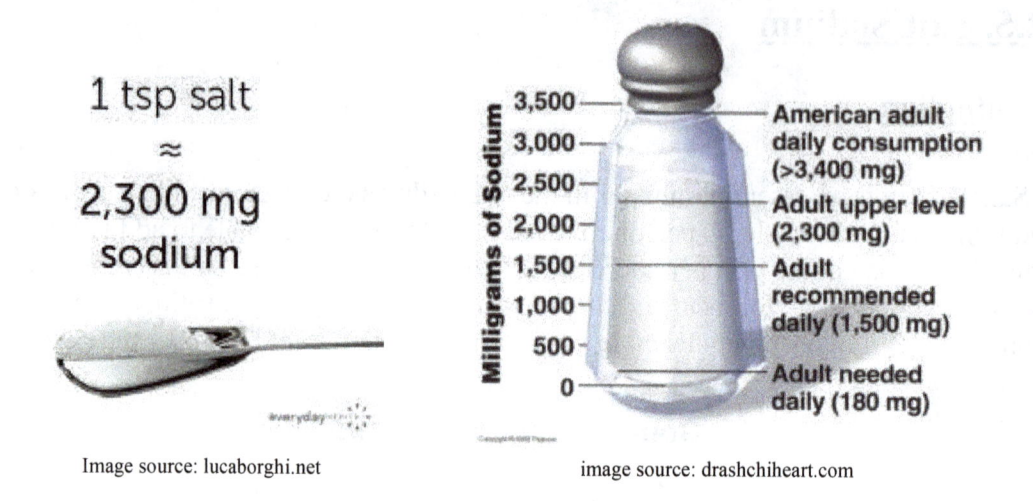

Harmful Effects of Salt

When the blood contains too much sodium, osmosis draws excess water from the cells into the bloodstream. As the blood volume increases inside the arteries, the pressure inside the arteries also increases, which means that the heart has to work harder because there is increase load (higher blood volume) and resistance (increase pressure) to overcome for it to pump blood around the body. As well, over time, the walls of the blood vessels can be stretched because of the increase in blood volume. This stretching or dilation makes the blood vessels more susceptible to damage, such as atherosclerosis, leading to a greater risk of heart disease and stroke.

An overstimulated immune system has also been linked to sodium. This suggests a link with various autoimmune diseases such as rheumatoid arthritis, psoriasis, celiac disease, alopecia (thinning of hair), multiple sclerosis, lupus, allergies, and other conditions.

It is recommended that you increase you consumption of potassium while reducing sodium intake. Potassium lessens the adverse effects of sodium on high blood pressure. Potassium is in various unrefined foods, especially fruits and vegetables.

Sources of Salt/Sodium

Salt/sodium occurs naturally in seafoods, meats, eggs, dairy products and some vegetables, however, the majority comes from processed and convenience foods in our diet.

The top salty foods in North America are processed foods:
- Cold cuts and cured meats
- Soup
- Sandwiches
- Pizza
- Bread and rolls

How much Sodium/Salt?

What does 1,500 mg of sodium (2/3 teaspoon of salt), the recommended daily intake, look like?

- 1 egg = 140 mg
- 1 cup fresh milk = 25 mg
- 1 serving of plain yogurt = 40 mg
- 1 serving of plain, low-fat yogurt = 76 mg
- 1 serving (1 cup) of raw celery = 180 mg
- 1 serving (1 cup) cooked spinach: = 150 mg

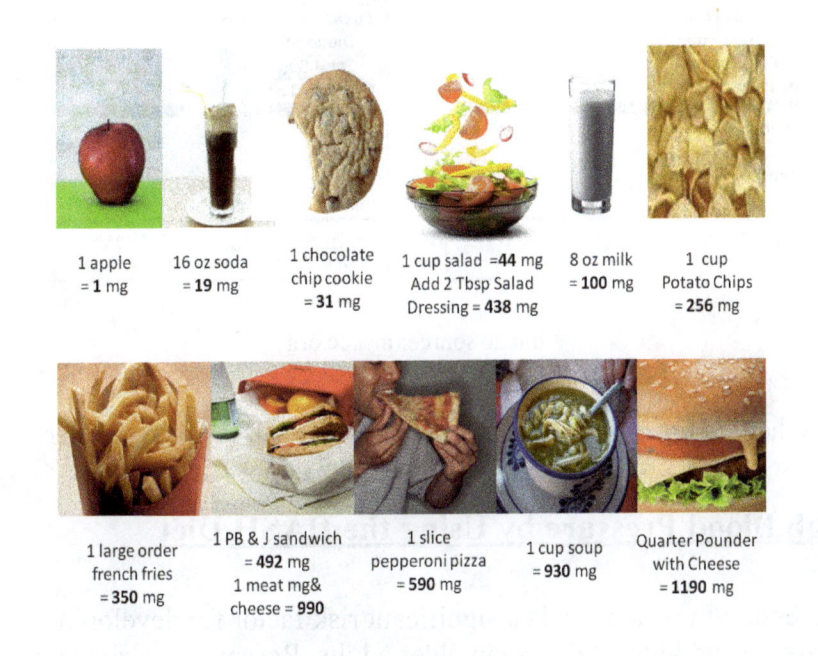

| 1 apple = 1 mg | 16 oz soda = 19 mg | 1 chocolate chip cookie = 31 mg | 1 cup salad = 44 mg Add 2 Tbsp Salad Dressing = 438 mg | 8 oz milk = 100 mg | 1 cup Potato Chips = 256 mg |

| 1 large order french fries = 350 mg | 1 PB & J sandwich = 492 mg 1 meat mg& cheese = 990 | 1 slice pepperoni pizza = 590 mg | 1 cup soup = 930 mg | Quarter Pounder with Cheese = 1190 mg |

Image source: thedietitiansdigest.com

How to Reduce Salt Intake

1. To help reduce added, unnecessary salt:
2. The consumption of processed and prepared foods should be reduced.
3. Purchase products with claims of no salt added, sodium-reduced or low sodium.
4. Eat more fresh vegetables and fruit.
5. Minimize the amount of salt added while baking, cooking or at the table,.
6. Be adventuresome when seasoning your food. Experiment with garlic, fresh or dried herbs and lemon juice.
7. Seek out nutrient information on menu items and make your preference toward meals lower in sodium.
8. Read nutritional food labels. Nutritional tables on food labels indicate how much sodium is in the food. It is listed in mg as well as % daily value. If the percentage is less than 5% it is considered "a little" and more than 15% is considered "a lot." (Chapter 5. 2.2: How to Read Nutritional Labels.

Regular chicken with noodles soup	Low-sodium chicken with noodles soup

Nutrition Facts
 1 serving per container
 Serving size 8 oz
 Amount per serving
 Calories 60
 % Daily Value*
 Total Fat 2g — 3%
   Saturated Fat 0.5g — 3%
   Trans Fat 0g
 Cholesterol 15mg — 5%
 Sodium 890mg — 37%
 Total Carbohydrate 8g — 3%
   Dietary Fiber 1g — 4%
   Total Sugars 1g
 Protein 3g
 Vitamin A — 4%
 Vitamin C — 0%
 Calcium — 0%
 Iron — 2%
	Nutrition Facts
	 1 serving per container
	 Serving size 10.75 oz
	 Amount per serving
	 Calories 160
	 % Daily Value*
	 Total Fat 4.5g — 7%
	   Saturated Fat 1.5g — 8%
	   Trans Fat 0g
	 Cholesterol 30mg — 10%
	 Sodium 140mg — 6%
	 Total Carbohydrate 17g — 6%
	   Dietary Fiber 2g — 8%
	   Total Sugars 4g
	 Protein 12g
	 Vitamin A — 30%
	 Vitamin C — 0%
	 Calcium — 2%
	 Iron — 6%

Image source: mskcc.org

Key Point - When it comes to your everyday diet, less salt is always better.

Lowering High Blood Pressure by Using the DASH Diet

    High blood pressure/hypertension is a significant risk factor for developing cardiovascular disease and kidney disease in older adults. Research has shown that a diet low in sodium effectively lowers your high blood pressure.

    The DASH Diet (Dietary Approaches to Stopping Hypertension) is based on two studies; the DASH and DASH-Sodium studies. These studies examined ways of using diet to reducing blood pressure.

    The <u>DASH study</u>, compared three eating plans:

1. A diet plan with nutrients comparable to a typical North Americans diet.
2. The same typical North American plan but included more fruits and vegetables.
3. The DASH diet, that is rich in fruits, vegetables, low-fat dairy foods and lower in cholesterol, saturated fat and total fat.

    The results of the study showed that the diet higher in vegetables and fruit and the DASH diet reduced blood pressure, but the DASH diet had the quickest and largest effect on lowering blood pressure. An added benefit of the DASH Diet was that low-density lipoprotein (LDL) or "bad cholesterol" and total cholesterol levels were reduced.

The <u>DASH-Sodium study,</u> involved the DASH Diet but involved three different sodium amount diet plans:
1. DASH diet that included 3,300 mg of sodium per day (a normal amount for many North Americans);
2. DASH diet that included 2,300 mg of sodium (1 teaspoon of salt);
3. DASH diet that included 1,500 mg of sodium (2/3 of a teaspoon of salt).

The results indicated that the less salt people consumed, the greater the decrease in blood pressure. People that already had high blood pressure saw the greatest decrease in blood pressure.

Difference Between the DASH Diet and the Canadian Health Food Guide Recommendations

The DASH diet and the new Canadian Health Food Guide are very similar. The consumption of fruits, vegetables, protein choices such as nuts, seeds, beans whole grains, poultry, fish, low-fat dairy products and lean meats, are heavily emphasised in both diets. However, the DASH diet is specifically focuses on a lower consumption of, sugar, and salt, and saturated fat.

In contrast to the new Canadian Health Food Guide, which has moved away from specific serving sizes to the ½ plate method (The guide recommends that a quarter of the plate with whole-grain foods, and a quarter of the plate with protein foods and the other half of the plate with vegetables and fruit), the DASH diet specifies serving sizes for each food group and the number of servings per day.

The DASH Eating Plan

DASH Food Groups and serving sizes (Daily servings except where indicated):

1. **<u>Vegetables (4-5 servings)</u>**
   1/2 cup cooked vegetables
   1 cup raw leafy vegetables

2. **<u>Fruit (4-5 servings)</u>**
   1 medium piece of fruit
   ¼ cup dried fruit
   ½ cup fresh, frozen or canned fruit

3. **Grains (mainly whole grains) (7-8 servings)**
   1 slice bread
   1 cup ready to eat cereal
   1/2 cup cooked rice, pasta or cereal

4. **Low Fat or No-Fat Dairy Foods (2-3 servings)**
   1 cup milk
   1 cup yogurt
   1½ oz cheese

5. **Lean Meats, Poultry and Fish (2 servings or less)**
   3 oz. cooked lean meats, skinless poultry, or fish

6. **Nuts, Seeds and Dry Beans (4-5 servings per week)**
   1/3 cup nuts
   2 tbsp peanut butter
   2 tbsp seeds
   1/2 cup cooked dry beans or peas

7. **Fats and Oils (2-3 servings)**
   1 tsp soft margarine
   1 tbsp low-fat mayonnaise
   2 tbsp light salad dressing
   1 tsp vegetable oil

DASH Diet
What To Eat?

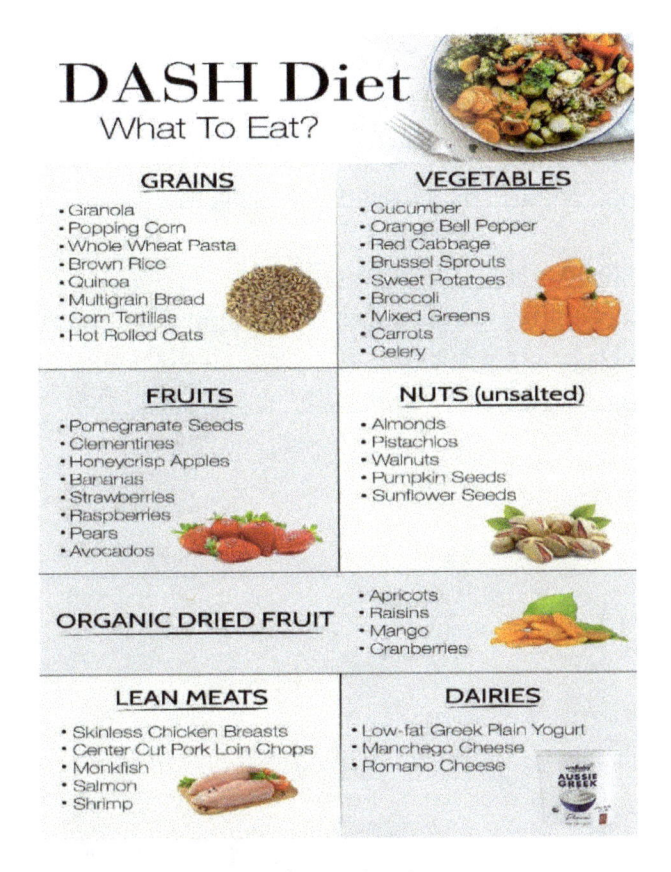

GRAINS
- Granola
- Popping Corn
- Whole Wheat Pasta
- Brown Rice
- Quinoa
- Multigrain Bread
- Corn Tortillas
- Hot Rolled Oats

VEGETABLES
- Cucumber
- Orange Bell Pepper
- Red Cabbage
- Brussel Sprouts
- Sweet Potatoes
- Broccoli
- Mixed Greens
- Carrots
- Celery

FRUITS
- Pomegranate Seeds
- Clementines
- Honeycrisp Apples
- Bananas
- Strawberries
- Raspberries
- Pears
- Avocados

NUTS (unsalted)
- Almonds
- Pistachios
- Walnuts
- Pumpkin Seeds
- Sunflower Seeds

ORGANIC DRIED FRUIT
- Apricots
- Raisins
- Mango
- Cranberries

LEAN MEATS
- Skinless Chicken Breasts
- Center Cut Pork Loin Chops
- Monkfish
- Salmon
- Shrimp

DAIRIES
- Low-fat Greek Plain Yogurt
- Manchego Cheese
- Romano Cheese

Image source: pinterest.com

Conclusion

For the older adult, salt is a paradox. On the one hand, it's easy to love the flavour it adds to food. This is important because as we age our taste buds' sensitivity and our appreciation of food diminishes. Anything that can add to the enjoyment of eating is important. On the other hand, salt, and specifically sodium, which makes up 38% of salt, has been established to contribute to high blood pressure and the development of cardiovascular disease.

75% of the sodium a person ingests has been added to the food by the manufacturer. This fact makes reading and understanding nutritional labels very important.

It is recommended that no more than 1,500 mg of sodium (just 2/3 of a teaspoon of salt) be ingested daily. The Canadian Health Food Guide recommends "less is best" for sodium. For those vulnerable to high blood pressure, following the DASH Diet is very effective in lowering your high pressure.

References

https://www.hsph.harvard.edu/nutritionsource/salt-and-sodium/

https://www.mayoclinic.org/healthy-lifestyle/nutrition-and-healthy-eating/expert-answers/sea-salt/faq-20058512

https://www.medicalnewstoday.com/articles/146677

https://www.canada.ca/en/health-canada/services/publications/food-nutrition/sodium-intake-canadians-2017.html

https://www.heartandstroke.ca/healthy-living/healthy-eating/dash-diet

5.2.6. Cholesterol

Introduction

There has been more controversy over cholesterol, its role in heart disease, and whether one's diet can control it than any other nutritional topic. Eat eggs, don't eat eggs, avoid butter, eat as much butter as you want, are just two examples of the flip flop that has occurred in the research related to cholesterol.

Research has established that high blood levels of a specific type of cholesterol called Low-Density Lipoprotein (LDL), high blood pressure, obesity, a sedentary lifestyle, and smoking contribute to the development of heart disease. Statistics Canada estimates that 27% of adults aged 20-39 and 43% of adults 40-59 have medically determined unhealthy LDL cholesterol levels (3.4 mmol/L or higher). Pertinent to the older adult, a recent study revealed that having elevated cholesterol levels for one to 10 years almost doubles the risk of heart disease. This risk of heart disease means that quickly lowering elevated blood cholesterol levels is essential.

Statins, are medications that effectively lower blood cholesterol levels However, the effect that diet has on blood cholesterol levels is still debatable. Low LDL cholesterol levels is a good thing. The question is, how does a person achieve and maintain low cholesterol levels when high-fat diets are popular in North American society?

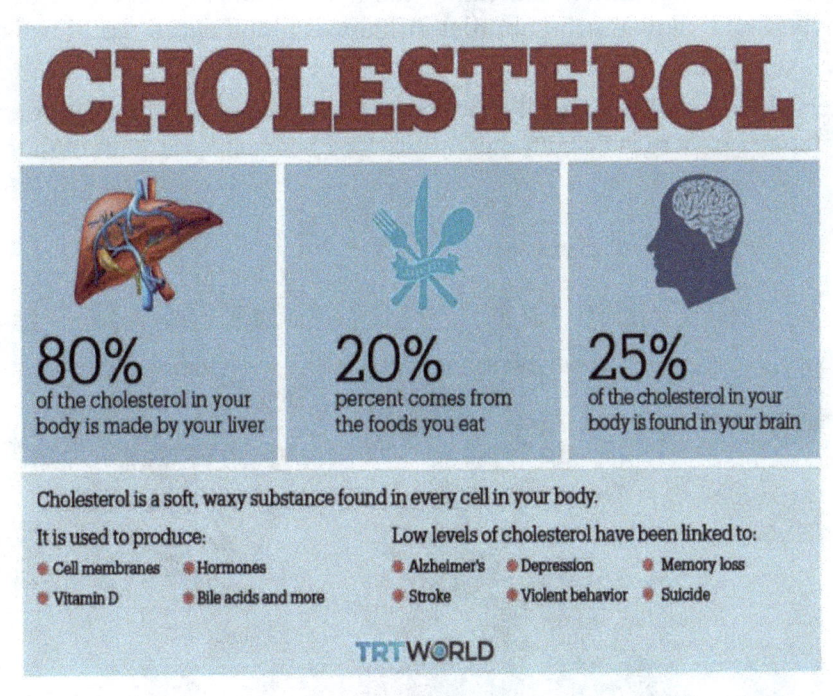

Image source: trtworld.com

Understanding Cholesterol

1. Cholesterol is a modified steroid lipid (fat) molecule and is important for the structural integrity of human cell membranes.
2. Cholesterol is necessary for brain function and the bio-synthesis of bile acids, vitamin D, steroid hormones.
3. Any food that contains animal fat has varying amounts of cholesterol.
4. Cholesterol only comes from food that comes from animals. Cheese, egg yolks, pork, beef, fish, shrimp, and poultry are major dietary sources of cholesterol.
5. Plant are not significant sources of cholesterol.
6. Cholesterol in the blood is carried by two types of lipoproteins:

    a. Low-density lipoprotein (LDL) – 'Bad' cholesterol.
     – High blood levels of LDL results in a build-up of cholesterol in the arteries and the development of atherosclerosis, which increases the risk of heart attacks.

    b. High-density lipoprotein (HDL) – 'Good' cholesterol
     – HDL helps remove cholesterol from the body by carrying it to the liver

7. LDL and HDL cholesterol balances are influenced genetically, but unhealthy lifestyle choices can contribute to high levels of LDL cholesterol in the blood. This means that a healthy diet, regular exercise, and sometimes medication can help reduce high cholesterol. There is scientific controversy as to how much your diet influences blood cholesterol levels, but even a little bit is better than nothing at all.

8. A cholesterol blood profile typically measures triglycerides, which is another type of fat in the blood. Unfortunately, there is also an increase risk of heart disease with high triglyceride levels.

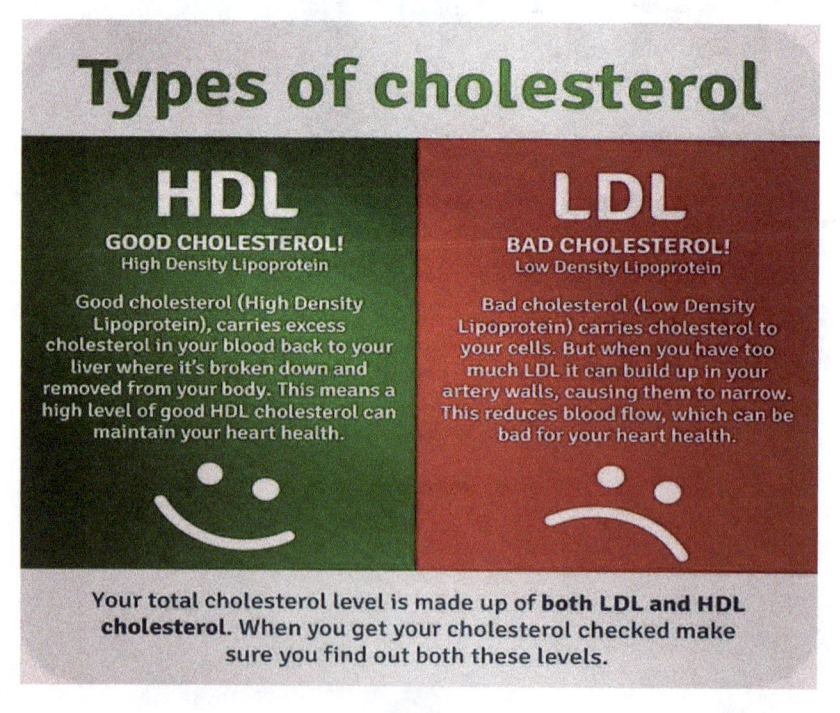

Types of cholesterol

HDL — GOOD CHOLESTEROL! High Density Lipoprotein

Good cholesterol (High Density Lipoprotein), carries excess cholesterol in your blood back to your liver where it's broken down and removed from your body. This means a high level of good HDL cholesterol can maintain your heart health.

LDL — BAD CHOLESTEROL! Low Density Lipoprotein

Bad cholesterol (Low Density Lipoprotein) carries cholesterol to your cells. But when you have too much LDL it can build up in your artery walls, causing them to narrow. This reduces blood flow, which can be bad for your heart health.

Your total cholesterol level is made up of **both LDL and HDL cholesterol**. When you get your cholesterol checked make sure you find out both these levels.

Image source: pinterest.com

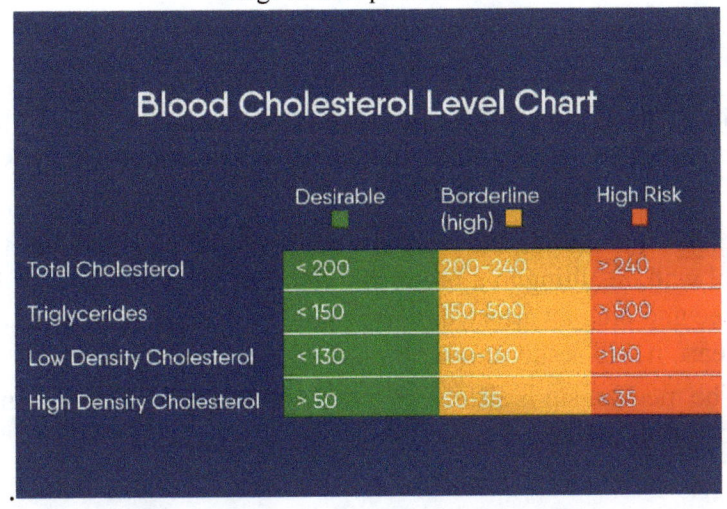

Blood Cholesterol Level Chart

	Desirable	Borderline (high)	High Risk
Total Cholesterol	< 200	200-240	> 240
Triglycerides	< 150	150-500	> 500
Low Density Cholesterol	< 130	130-160	>160
High Density Cholesterol	> 50	50-35	< 35

Note - Cholesterol is measured in mg/dl

Symptoms of High Cholesterol

A blood test is the only way to detect high cholesterol levels since it has no overt symptoms, just complications such as heart disease.

Risk factors

1. **Poor diet** – Research has shown that a diet high in the consumption of red animal meat, which has high levels of saturated fat, full-fat dairy products, and trans fats, found in some commercially baked pastries and processed foods can contribute to increase blood cholesterol levels.
2. **Obesity** – There is a greater risk of high cholesterol levels if your body mass index (BMI) is greater than 30.
3. **Lack of exercise** – Exercise increases the amount of HDL, or "good" cholesterol in the blood.
4. **Smoking** – The walls of the blood vessels can be damaged by smoking which makes them making them more prone to accumulate fatty deposits and the development of atherosclerosis. Levels of HDL, or "good" cholesterol may also be lowered as the result of smoking.
5. **Age** –The body's metabolism and chemical processes changes with age, and the liver becomes less able to remove LDL cholesterol.
6. **Diabetes** –Higher levels of a dangerous cholesterol called very-low-density lipoprotein (VLDL) and HDL cholesterol levels are lowered as the result of high blood sugar levels.

Complications from High Cholesterol

High cholesterol can cause cholesterol and other deposits to accumulate on the walls of the arteries (atherosclerosis) resulting in reduce blood flow through the arteries, which can lead to complications, such as:

1. Heart Disease:

a. Chest pain – This occurs if there is a restriction in blood supply to the heart as the result of cholesterol / fatty deposits accumulating in the arteries (atherosclerosis).

b. Heart attack – Plaques on the arterial wall can build up and restrict blood flow or tear or rupture the arterial wall, resulting in a blood clot that can block the flow of blood, or the plaques can break free and plug an artery downstream. If the blockage results in restricting blood flow to part of the heart. it will result in a heart attack.

c. Stroke –The mechanism is similar to a heart attack and occurs when a blood clot blocks blood flow to part of the brain.

2. Weight Gain

3. Achy joints

4. Stomach distention

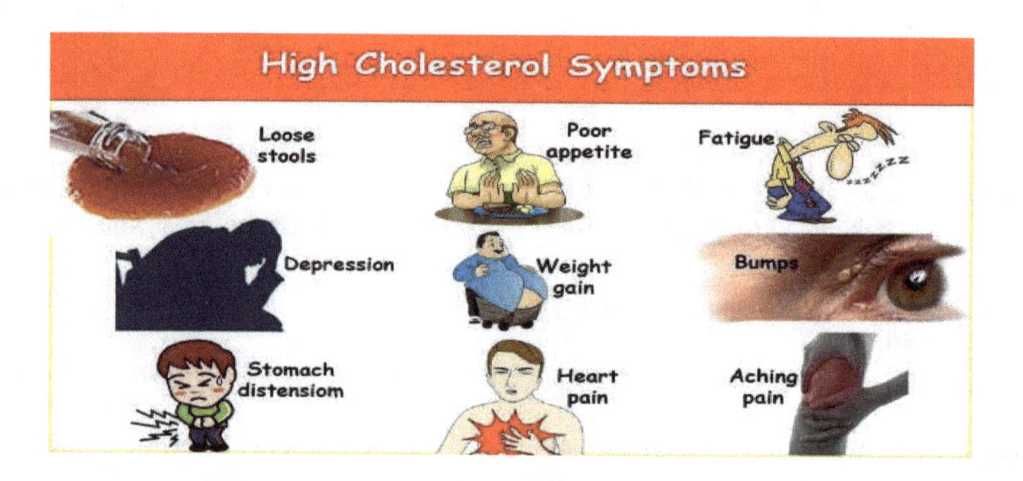

Image source: worldcreativities.com

Prevention

Depending on the influence that genetics has on the cholesterol level, a heart-healthy lifestyle can reduce the risk of developing high cholesterol.

Good preventative strategies include:
- Quit smoking
- Maintain a healthy weight
- Exercise on most days of the week for at least 30 minutes
- Limit the amount of cooked animal fats and use good fats (nuts) in moderation
- Eat a low-salt diet that emphasizes fruits, vegetables, and whole grains
- Drink alcohol in moderation, if at all

- Manage stress
- Read Nutritional Labels - Develop the habit of reading nutritional labels on all food purchases, including meats and dairy products. Sometimes the numbers and daily value percentages for cholesterol are surprising.

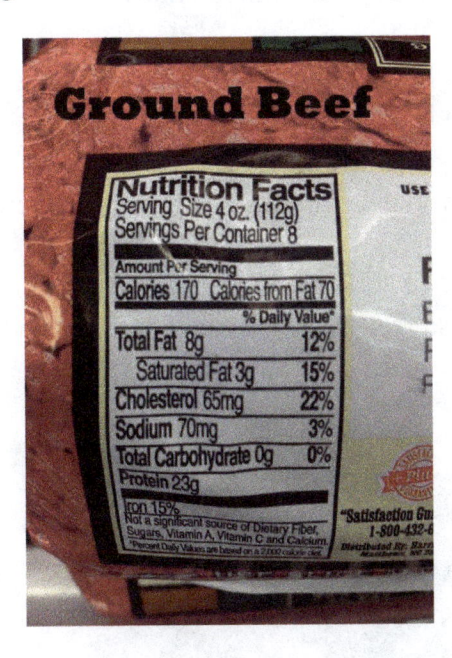

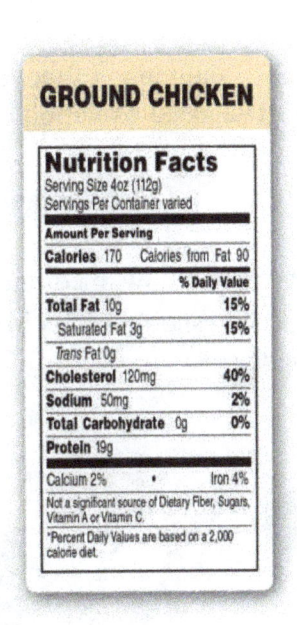

Image source: gnutritionco.com   Image source: catalog.prpaper.com

Remember, greater than 15% of daily value is too high and bad, and less than 5% is low, which is good.

Additional Preventative Measures

Three Other Preventative Measures have been advocated in the research recently:

1. Avoid Oxidized Cholesterol

Fried foods are a primary source of oxidized cholesterol. This oxidized cholesterol (not dietary cholesterol in and of itself) increases the risk of heart attacks by causing increases in free radical formation, which increases the risk of heart disease and cancer.

Key Point – The concern is not the LDL particles themselves but whether the cholesterol and fat residing in the LDL particles have been oxidized. This means that unoxidized cholesterol is good and has nothing to do with heart disease, and as long as natural cholesterol-rich foods such as red meats, eggs, and dairy products, are not fried or heated to high temperatures. It is oxidized cholesterol that you must avoid.

Tip – Because red meat is usually cooked at high temperatures (searing of the meat) it is best practice to eat it as rarely as possible because it is high in saturated fat.

2. The Stability (Oxidation) of Cooking Oils

It is important to cook with stable oils that don't oxidize easily at high temperatures. Fat in the oils undergo oxidation at high temperatures just like cholesterol in red meats.

The relative degree of saturation of the fatty acids in the oil is the most important factor in determining an oil's resistance to oxidation both at high and low heat is.

1. <u>Olive oil</u> – should be used for cooking only at low to medium heat. At high heat, it creates free radicals.
2. <u>Canola oil</u> – can be used at low, medium, and high heat.
3. <u>Butter and coconut oil</u> – should be avoided because they are high is saturated fats and will raise cholesterol levels.

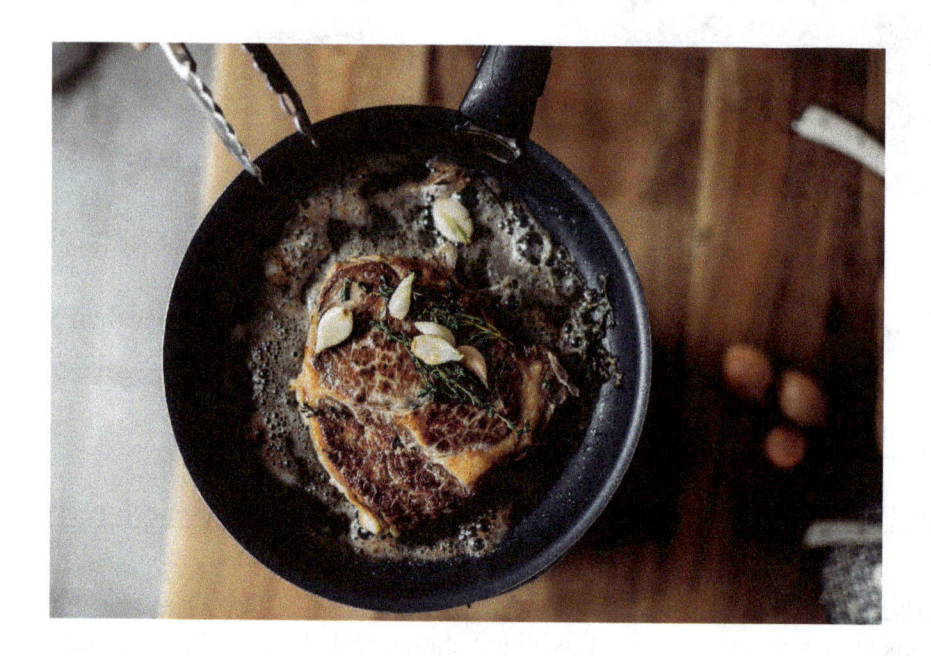

3. Limit Sugar Consumption

The majority of the body's cholesterol (80%) is produced by the liver, and influenced by insulin levels. High dietary sugar intake spikes blood sugar and insulin levels, resulting in the sugars being taken to the liver where it is used for fuel or converted to fat, some of which are stored. Over time, this increases body weight or the fat re-enters the blood and raises the level of small-density LDL.

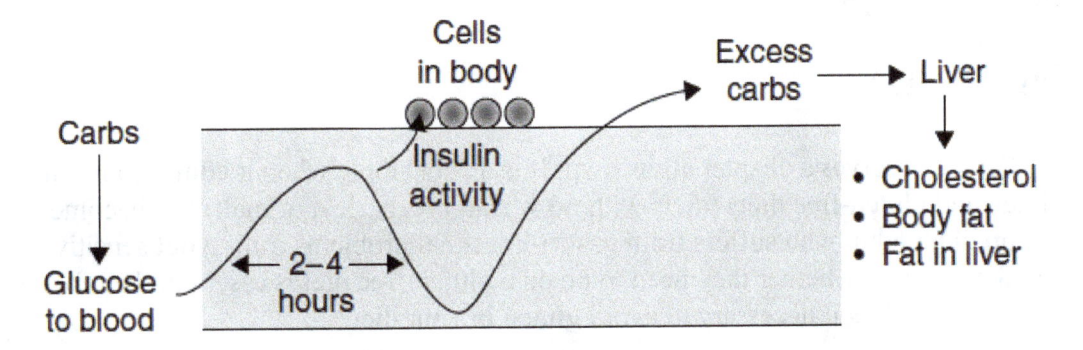

Carbohydrate metabolism: healthy versus imbalanced.

Image source: doctordoni.com

Optimize insulin levels by avoiding peaks in blood glucose levels by avoiding high sugar intake levels, which will automatically help optimize cholesterol levels.

Conclusion

For older adults, managing their blood LDL cholesterol level is as essential for good nutritional health as controlling their sugar and salt/sodium intake. A high LDL cholesterol level is a significant risk factor for developing heart disease, which the older adult is already susceptible to developing because of their vulnerability to conditions such as high blood pressure, obesity, and lack of exercise.

Good nutritional habits like increasing the consumption of fruits and vegetables while reducing the amount of saturated fat in their diet, modifying how they cook their meat and reading nutritional labels will help, as will getting regular exercise.

References

https://www.mayoclinic.org/diseases-conditions/high-blood-cholesterol/symptoms-causes/syc-20350800
https://www.health.harvard.edu/topics/cholesterol
https://www.healthline.com/health/cholesterol/effects-on-body
https://www.heartandstroke.ca/heart-disease/risk-and-prevention/condition-risk-factors/managing-cholesterol
www.forever-active.com

5.2.7. Gluten

Introduction

Gluten deserves a chapter all its own. It is a "hot" topic when it comes to nutrition. Avoiding gluten and gluten-free diets (diets with no wheat, rye, barley, or malt) has become very popular. For an older adult who suffers from gastro-intestinal problems, ruling out sensitivity to gluten and determining whether they need to be on a gluten-free diet is essential. But for a symptom-free individual, is it necessary to avoid gluten in your diet?

There is much controversy when it comes to gluten. This chapter will explain what gluten is and its role in nutrition. Hopefully, this will help you make an educated decision as to whether gluten should or should not be part of yourdiet.

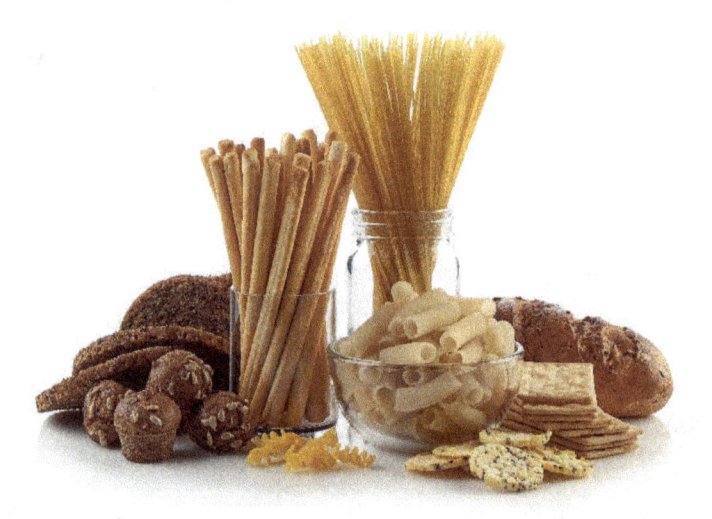

What Is Gluten and Its Usefulness

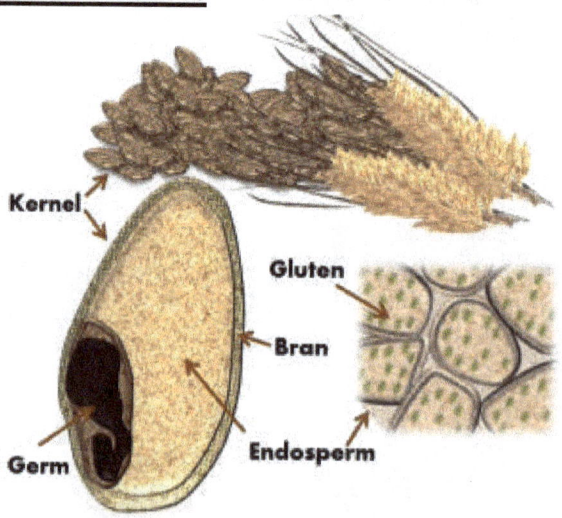

The Gluten protein is mainly found in the endosperm of grain Kernel (seed)

Image source: katiepinktolley.com

Gluten is a protein found in wheat, rye, barley and malt. Gluten helps dough rise, keep its shape, and gives it the chewy texture when baked. Gluten is used in dermatological, cosmetics, and hair products. It is estimated that 0.5 to 1% of people in North America have gluten sensitivity or intolerance to gluten (Celiac Disease). If gluten is present at a level greater than 10 ppm it must be identified on the food label.

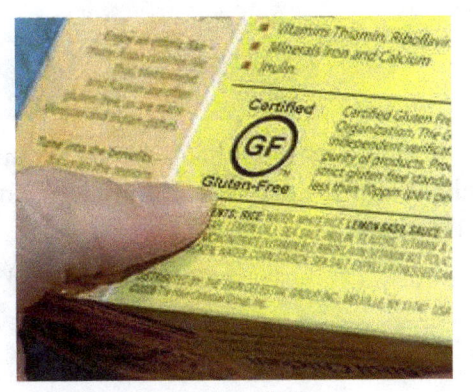

Image source: drweil.com

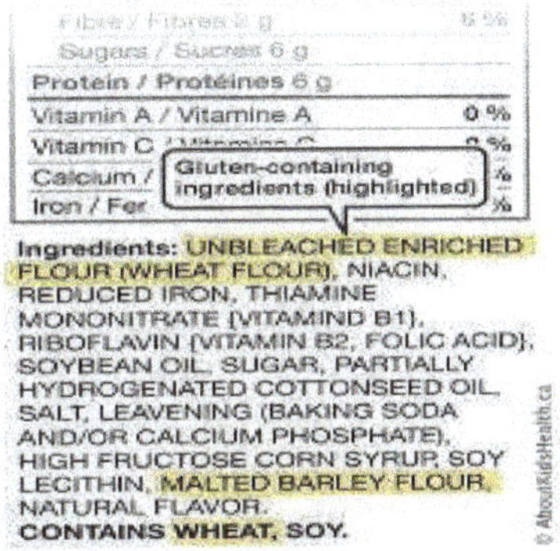

Image source: aboutkidshealth.ca

Celiac Disease

Celiac Disease results from eating gluten. It is an autoimmune condition (genetics) causing inflammatory damage to the small intestine's lining. The inflammatory response causes a flattening of the nutrient absorbing villi lining the small intestine which prevents essential micronutrients from being absorbed.

If not appropriately treated, chronic malabsorption may result, leading to bloating, diarrhea and weight loss. Eventually, the nervous system, skeletal system, and internal organs such as the liver can be adversely affected.

Diagnosis for Celiac Disease

1. **Blood Test** – A blood test for the IgA-tissue transglutaminase (TTG) antibody is necessary for screening. To make this test valid, you must be on a regular (gluten-containing) diet.

2. **Biopsy** – A small intestinal biopsy, where flattening of the small intestine villi is observed,
3. is needed for a definitive diagnosis of celiac disease.

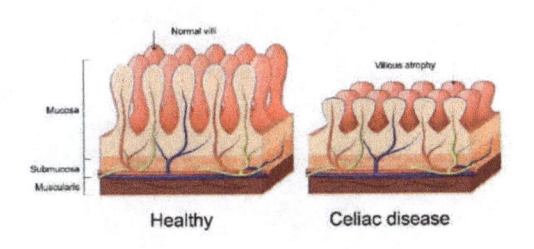

CELIAC DISEASE

Healthy   Celiac disease

Treatment for Celiac Disease

Celiac disease has no cure, but intestinal healing can occur and symptoms managed well by following a strict gluten-free diet.

Gluten-Free Diet

This diet is necessary to manage the signs and symptoms of Celiac Disease but many people who are not Celiac but follow a gluten-free diet claim improved health, weight loss, and increased energy. More research is needed to substantiate this claim.

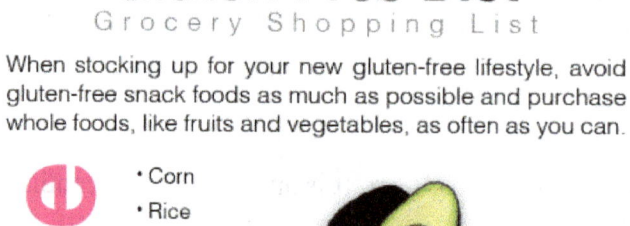

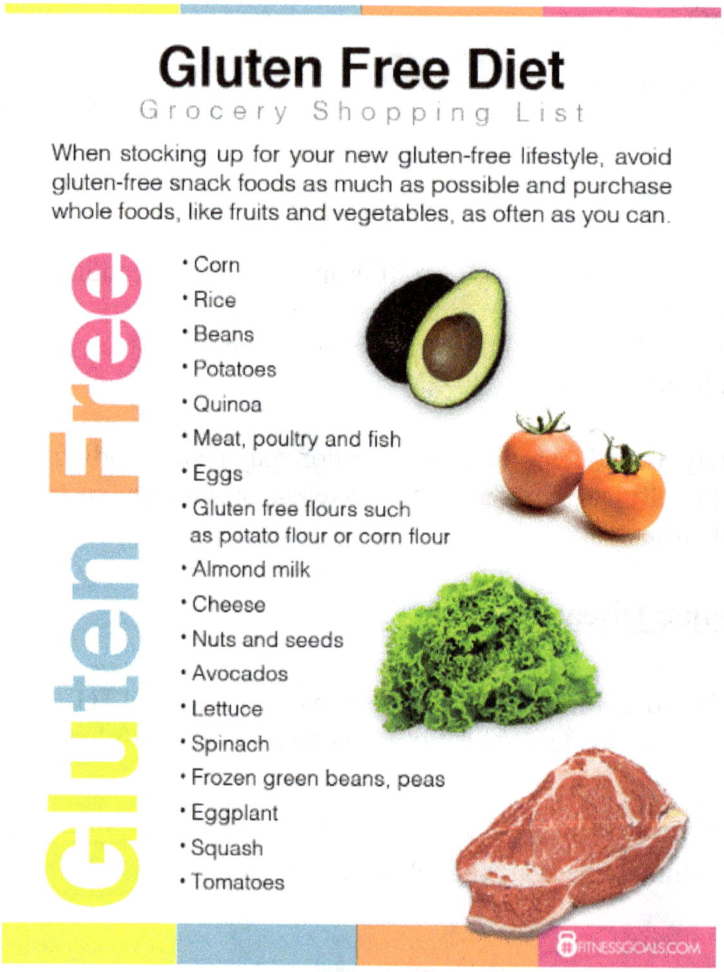

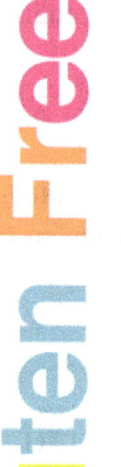

Gluten Free Diet
Grocery Shopping List

When stocking up for your new gluten-free lifestyle, avoid gluten-free snack foods as much as possible and purchase whole foods, like fruits and vegetables, as often as you can.

Gluten Free
- Corn
- Rice
- Beans
- Potatoes
- Quinoa
- Meat, poultry and fish
- Eggs
- Gluten free flours such as potato flour or corn flour
- Almond milk
- Cheese
- Nuts and seeds
- Avocados
- Lettuce
- Spinach
- Frozen green beans, peas
- Eggplant
- Squash
- Tomatoes

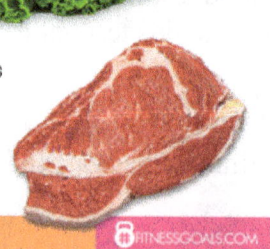

Following a gluten-free diet requires careful food selections:

1. Naturally gluten-free foods include:

- Lean, non-processed meats, fish, and poultry
- Eggs
- Most low-fat dairy products
- Fruits and vegetables
- Beans, seeds, legumes, and nuts in their natural, unprocessed forms

2. Grains, starches, or flours that can be part of a gluten-free diet include:

- Quinoa
- Corn – cornmeal, grits, and polenta labeled gluten-free
- Flax
- Rice, including wild rice
- Soy
- Gluten-free flours – rice, soy, corn, potato, and bean flours
- Arrowroot
- Buckwheat
- Millet

3. Avoid foods and drinks containing the following:

- Wheat
- Rye
- Malt
- Barley
- Triticale – a cross between wheat and rye

Oats – Oats are naturally gluten-free, but may get contaminated during production with wheat, barley, rye or other gluten containing grains. No cross-contamination has occurred if the oats are labeled gluten-free, however, some patients with celiac disease still cannot tolerate them.

Processed Foods that often Contain Gluten

Wheat or wheat gluten is often used to thicken and help bind dough, as well as improve taste and colour. Reading nutrition labels of processed foods is necessary to determine if wheat, barley, rye, and malt have been used in the product.

The following foods should be avoided unless they are labeled as gluten-free or made with corn, rice, soy or other gluten-free grain:

- Candies
- Cereals
- Beer, ale, porter, stout (usually contain barley)

- French fries
- Gravies
- Matzo
- Pastas
- Hot dogs and processed lunchmeats
- Soups, bouillon or soup mixes
- Vegetables in sauce
- Seasoned rice mixes
- Seasoned snack foods, such as potato and tortilla chips
- Breads
- Communion wafers
- Cookies and crackers
- Cakes and pies
- Croutons
- Malt, malt flavoring and other malt products (barley)
- Salad dressings
- Sauces, including soy sauce (wheat)

Conclusion to Gluten-free Diet

To avoid symptoms and complications of Celiac Disease, it is necessary to maintain a strict gluten-free diet for life.

Non-Celiac Gluten Sensitivity/Intolerance

Little research has been done on Non-celiac gluten sensitivity, but it is hypothesised that this condition involves the immune system reacting differently than it does with celiac disease.

With celiac disease, the immune system triggers an attack on its own tissues, specifically the small intestine.

In contrast, with Non-celiac gluten sensitivity/intolerance, there is a direct reaction to gluten. The gluten protein is directly recognized as an invader by the immune system which creates inflammation inside and outside the digestive tract to fight this perceived invader.

It's is not clear whether this immune response physically damages the organs or other tissues similar to what celiac disease does or simply causes symptoms.

Non-celiac gluten sensitivity may affect up to 6 percent to 7 percent of the population. It is estimated that 50 percent of the population may have some degree of gluten sensitivity.

Differentiating the Diseases

There is no direct test to diagnose non-celiac gluten sensitivity/intolerance. The first step is to use the antibody blood screening test rule out celiac disease. If that is negative, step 2 is to do a gluten challenge test which involves eliminating gluten from your diet and observe if symptoms clear up, and then "challenging" the system by reintroducing gluten into your diet, and observe if symptoms return.

Non-Celiac gluten sensitivity is diagnosed if the blood test for Celiac disease is negative but you are experiencing symptoms when gluten is part of your diet, but those symptoms clear up when gluten is removed from your diet.

Symptoms of Non-Celiac Sensitivity/Intolerance
Two categories of symptoms:

1. Gastrointestinal
- Nausea
- Diarrhea
- Bloating
- Abdominal pain

2. Extra-intestinal manifestations
Non gastrointestinal symptoms are far more common with gluten sensitivity cases than in celiac disease.

a. Neurologic
- Chronic headache
- Depression
- Anxiety – which may be due to anticipation of abdominal pain
- Brain fog –short-term memory lapses, confusion, disorientation and difficulty concentrating,

b. Systemic
- Fatigue
- Joint and muscle pain
- General feeling of being unwell
- Neuropathy – Numbness and pins and needles in the extremities

Key points;
1. Symptoms for non-celiac gluten sensitivity/intolerance are often similar to those of celiac disease and so accurate diagnosis is based on first ruling out celiac disease by blood test and biopsy if necessary.

2. Symptoms associated with non-celiac gluten sensitivity/intolerance develop quickly (within a few hours to a day) of ingesting gluten and disappear just as quickly once gluten is eliminated from the diet. As long as gluten is avoided the symptoms do not reappear.

It should be noted that a person with Non-Celiac gluten sensitivity may not have to suffer lifelong with this condition. Some research suggests that someone with non-celiac gluten sensitivity should retest their gluten sensitivity every couple of years.

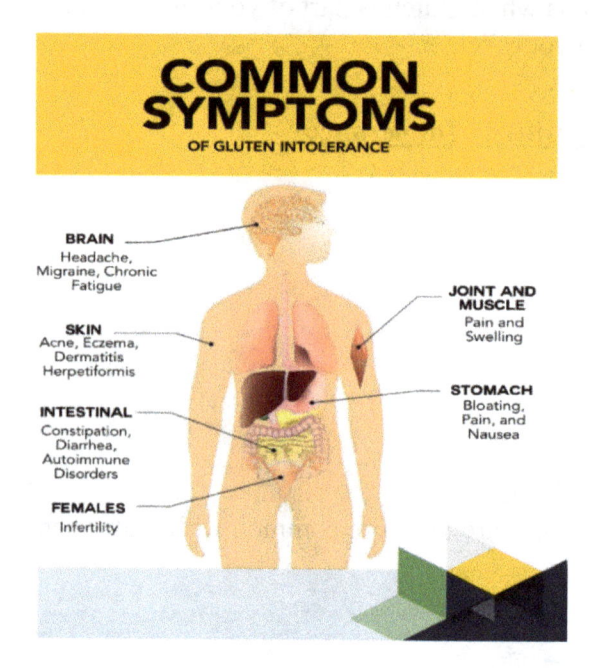

Image source: paleofoundation.com

Conclusion

If a person is eating wheat, rye, barley, or malt, then gluten is part of their diet. It is estimated that 90% of people who are either celiac or have gluten sensitivity/intolerance are never diagnosed. If an older adult has been suffering from chronic gastro-intestinal, neurologic and/or systematic symptoms and the cause has not been diagnosed, it is recommended that a celiac blood test and gluten challenge diet test be done. This would rule out gluten as a potential cause of these symptoms.

People in the general population and world-class athletes swear that they feel better and perform better when they follow a gluten-free diet. Whether this is a placebo effect is not known. The bottom line is, if a person subjectively feels better on a gluten-free diet, even if the reason cannot be medically explained, there is no reason to discontinue the diet.

From an orthodox medical perspective, if you have not been diagnosed with celiac disease or are not showing symptoms of non-celiac gluten sensitivity/intolerance, there should be no reason, except personal preference, to follow a gluten-free diet.

References

www.forever-active.com
https://www.mayoclinic.org/healthy-lifestyle/nutrition-and-healthy-eating/in-depth/gluten-free-diet/art-20048530
https://www.celiac.ca/gluten-related-disorders/celiac-disease/
https://www.verywellhealth.com/gluten-sensitivity-vs-celiac-disease-562964

5.2.8. Dietary Supplementation

Introduction

The quality of an older adult's diet is always a concern. Nutritional challenges that face the older adult include: living alone and being social isolated, a lack of motivation to cook well for only themselves, diminished appreciation of food because of a loss of taste, difficulty getting to the grocery store to shop and having to rely on others to pick out good whole foods rather than picking up easy-to-prepare processed food, and the cost of food.

As well, as you get older nutritional needs change:

- **Calcium and Vitamin D** – these mineral and vitamin become very important to help maintain bone health as the threat of developing osteoporosis grows with advancing age.

- **Vitamins B 6 and 12** – these vitamins are essential. They help make DNA, the genetic material in all cells, and help keep the body's blood cells and nerves healthy.

- **Dietary Fiber** – to help have regular bowel movements and reduce the risk of heart disease and Type 2 diabetes.

- **Increase potassium and limiting sodium intake** – to lower the risk of developing high blood pressure.

- **Good quality fats** – for preventing heart disease by consuming monounsaturated and polyunsaturated fats versus trans fats and saturated fats and found in processed foods.

If an older adult are not able to manage their diet properly and get the necessary calories, vitamins and minerals to maintain their health and slow down the aging process, then they need to consider dietary supplementation.

Vitamin and Mineral Dietary Supplementation

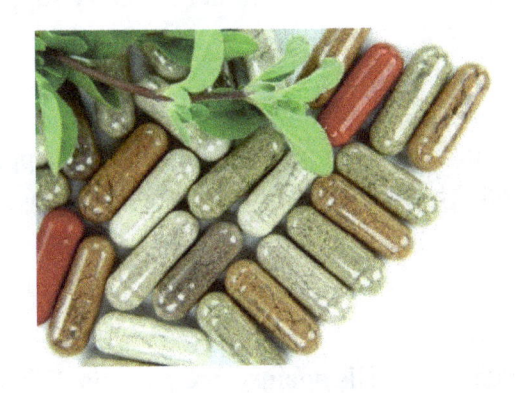

Vitamins

These organic substances that are essential, in varying small amounts, for proper body function. Vitamins are not produced by the body so they must obtain them from your diet or elsewhere. There are two types of Vitamins: water soluble and fat soluble.

1. Water-soluble vitamins (B-1, 2, 3, 5, 6, 7, 9, 12 and vitamin C) – These are transported in the bloodstream, the body uses what it needs and then excretes the excess through the urine. There is no storge of these water-soluble vitamins in the body so regular intake of these nutrients is necessary to prevent deficiencies.

2. Fat-soluble vitamins (A, D, E, K) – These are carried throughout the body and dissolved in fat. The body stores these vitamins in body fat; therefore, it is unnecessary to get a daily dose of fat-soluble vitamins every day. Over supplementation of vitamins E and K can create toxic levels within the body.

Minerals

Minerals are inorganic substances that are essential for life processes. There are only small amounts of minerals in the body but each mineral has an important role to play in cell function. Calcium and iron are the major minerals, but zinc, copper, magnesium, chromium, iodine, fluoride, and selenium are the other mineral that play important roles in body function. Minerals are plentiful in various foods, so mineral deficiencies are rare.

Advancing age can affect an older adult's eating habits and the quality of their diet. The following are risk factors that can affect how well an older adult eats:
- Mental capabilities/dementia
- Taste changes
- Oral health and hygiene
- Social isolation
- Dysphagia (difficulty swallowing)
- Medications (polypharmacy)
- Cultural/religious beliefs

The best way to determine if vitamin and mineral dietary supplementation is necessary is to have a dietary assessment done by a registered dietitian.

Dietary supplementation can change how medicines will work in your body so consultation with your doctor is necessary prior to taking any supplement. If dietary supplements are recommended by your doctor, it is important to get the doctor's recommended brand and take it as directed.

Antioxidants

Antioxidants help protect your cells against free radicals. When the body's breaks down food or when you are exposed to tobacco smoke or radiation free radicals are produced. Research indicates that free radicals can play a significant role in the development of cancer, heart disease, and diabetes, all of which commonly afflict the older adult.

Antioxidants, such as beta-carotene (fruits, sweet potatoes, dark green or orange vegetables (peppers, spinach, broccoli)), Vitamin C (tomatoes, berries (strawberries, raspberries, blackberries, blueberries), and citrus fruits), Vitamin E (nuts (walnuts, pecans), olive and peanut oil, wheat germ,) may help protect against free radicals damaging cells.

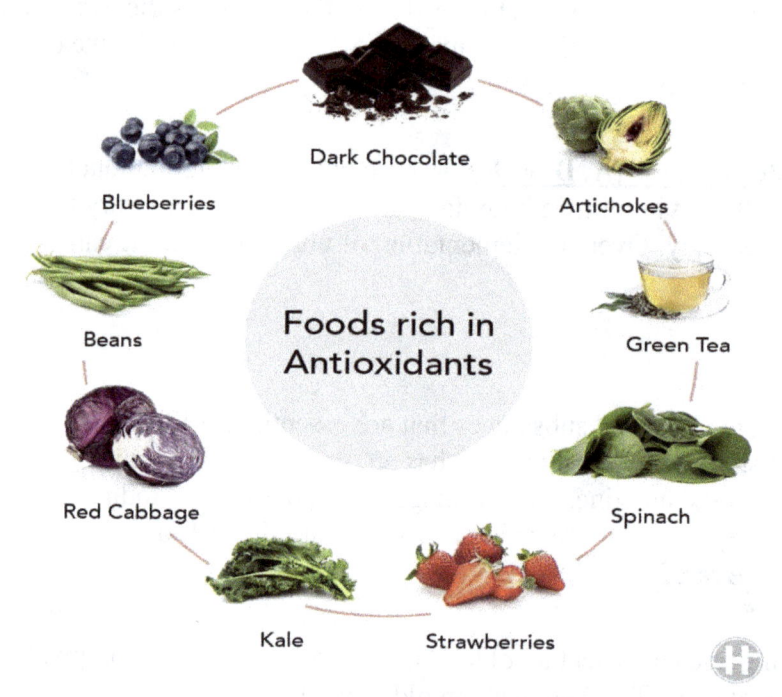

Image source: healthifyme.com

Antioxidants are plentiful, and it should not be a problem for you to get in sufficient amounts. Avoid one food group or a particular food from being your sole source. The key is having variety by incorporating different types of vegetables, nuts, fruits, and whole grains into your diet.

There is controversy in the science community about the effectiveness and safety of antioxidant supplementation. Recent research suggests that taking large doses of an antioxidant supplement has no preventative effect on chronic diseases such as diabetes and heart disease. As well, some studies have shown that the consumption of large doses of some antioxidants could potentially be harmful. Prior to taking a dietary supplement, the best practice is check with your doctor.

Herbal Supplements

Herbal supplements come from plants and their seeds, flowers, berries, oils, and roots. Herbal supplements have been used for many centuries and are believed to have healing qualities. These are a few that are most popular; gingko, ginseng, echinacea, garlic, St. John's Wort, flaxseed, and black cohosh.

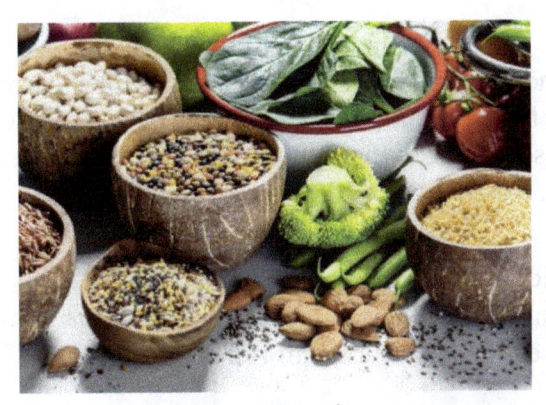

Image source: voice.ons.org

The scientific community is undecided about effectiveness of treating or preventing some health problems by using herbal supplements.

Two points you should keep in mind when considering using herbal supplements:

1. Dietary supplements may pose risks to people with some medical issues because they may harmfully interact with their medications.

2. Regulations for the manufacturing and distribution of prescription and over-the-counter drugs is much more stringent than they are for herbal supplements.

Prebiotics and Probiotics

Like every surface of the body, the digestive tract lining is covered in microscopic bacteria which creates a micro-ecosystem called the microbiome. What the microbiome is fed has a significant role in a person's health.

The healthier your microbiome is, the healthier you will be. Having a diet that nourishes a balance among the 1,000 different bacteria in the digestive tract is the key to a healthy microbiome.

There are two ways to maintain this balance:

- **Prebiotics** – foods that help existing microbes to grow
- **Probiotics** – adding living microbes directly to the digestive tract

1. Prebiotics

Prebiotics are fiber foods from plants. Like fertilizers, they stimulate healthy bacteria growth in the digestive tract.

Prebiotics are found in many foods that contain complex carbohydrates such as vegetables, fruits, berries, quinoa, barley, potatoes, sweet potatoes, and whole-wheat bread. The body does not digest these carbs so they pass through the digestive system and become food for the microbes and bacteria.

The list of prebiotic foods is long and plentiful, and usually, supplementation is unnecessary. However, supplementation should be considered if the diet is compromised and deficient in fiber containing fruits and vegetables, which unfortunately is the case for many older adults.

Prebiotic Rich Foods

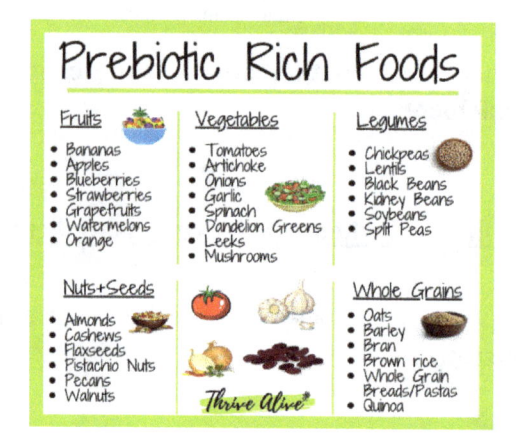

Fruits
- Bananas
- Apples
- Blueberries
- Strawberries
- Grapefruits
- Watermelons
- Orange

Vegetables
- Tomatoes
- Artichoke
- Onions
- Garlic
- Spinach
- Dandelion Greens
- Leeks
- Mushrooms

Legumes
- Chickpeas
- Lentils
- Black Beans
- Kidney Beans
- Soybeans
- Split Peas

Nuts+Seeds
- Almonds
- Cashews
- Flaxseeds
- Pistachio Nuts
- Pecans
- Walnuts

Whole Grains
- Oats
- Barley
- Bran
- Brown rice
- Whole Grain Breads/Pastas
- Quinoa

Image source: thrivealivee.com

2. Probiotics

Probiotics, unlike prebiotics, contain live organisms / bacteria that directly add to the number of healthy microbes in the digestive system.

Yogurt, sauerkraut, and pickles are probably the most common probiotic foods.

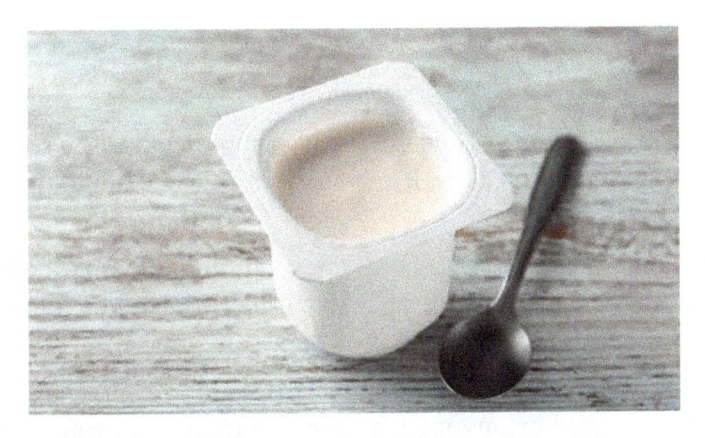

Image source: healthyeating.org

Probiotic supplements contain live organisms and a single dose may include a particular bacteria or microbe strain or blend of bacteria/microbes.

Is Probiotic Dietary Supplementation Necessary?

For the aging adult who often suffer from poor diets, suppressed immune systems and increased antibiotic use, studies have concluded that probiotics are beneficial. Research has also shown probiotics to be beneficial for those suffering from irritable bowel syndrome, infectious diarrhea, inflammatory bowel disease (Crohn's and ulcerative colitis), bloating, and gas. Other conditions reported to benefit from probiotic supplementation are yeast infections, urinary tract infections, eczema, and inflammation from rheumatoid arthritis.

Side effects can include allergic reactions, stomach upset, bloating, and diarrhea. However, the three latter side effects usually go away once the body has adapted to the ingestion of probiotic supplementation.

Probiotic supplementation is not recommended for older adults whose immune system is severely compromised due to chronic illness or inflection.

Adverse effects

- Probiotics side effects, if they occur, tend to be mild and digestive symptoms. (such as gas or bloating).

- May cause infections, especially in immuno-compromised patients.

- Diabetic patients should be doubly cautious about taking probiotic drinks available in the market as they contain high level of sugar.

- Probiotic products taken as a dietary supplement are manufactured and regulated as functional foods, not drugs.

Image source: slideshare.com

Caution

Probiotics are not drugs and are considered dietary supplements, as a result, the government does not monitor their manufacturing as well as they do for drug manufacturing.

It is best practice to only take probiotics after consolation with your doctor or pharmacist about how beneficial probiotics might be in your specific case and which brands are most well respected.

Probiotics should not be used by anyone who is being treated for cancer or suffers from an immune deficiency without a doctor's okay. Stop taking probiotics if there are any acute complications or long-lasting side effects.

Conclusion

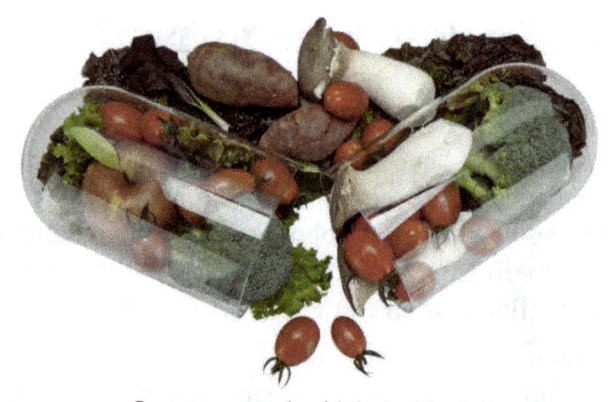

Image source: health.harvard.edu

Nutritional supplementation may appear to be a quick and easy way to improve an older adult's diet and allow them to get the nutrients necessary for healthy living and disease prevention. However, current research suggests that, if it is possible, it is best to stick to a healthy diet (follow the Canadian Health Food Guide, Chapter 5.2.3), be physically active (Section 4.0: The Offense: Getting Active the Right Way), keep an active mind (Section 6: Special Teams: Mental Health), don't smoke, see the doctor regularly, and, in most cases, only use dietary supplements when suggested by the doctor or pharmacist.

References

https://www.nia.nih.gov/health/dietary-supplements
https://www.eatright.org/health/wellness/healthy-aging/special-nutrient-needs-of-older-adults
https://www.mayoclinic.org/healthy-lifestyle/nutrition-and-healthy-eating/multimedia/antioxidants/sls-20076428?s=5
https://www.nccih.nih.gov/health/dietary-and-herbal-supplements
https://www.albertahealthservices.ca/assets/info/nutrition/if-nfs-ng-seniors-health-overview.pdf
https://www.todaysgeriatricmedicine.com/

5.2.9. Glycemic Index: What It Is and Its Nutritional Usefulness for Controlling Blood Glucose Levels

Introduction

The older adult experiences many physical and cognitive changes as they enter their golden years. Their hair turns grey, their skin becomes more wrinkled, and losing height and gaining weight are noticeable physical changes. The occasional loss in short-term memory is probably the most noticeable cognitive change. What is not quite apparent are the metabolic changes (the process of changing food into energy) occurring inside the older adult's body.

Body fat increases, muscle mass and intracellular body water is reduced, as you age. These changes leave the older adult vulnerable to developing insulin resistance and type 2 diabetes. Over 20% of people over 60 years have developed type 2 diabetes and impaired glucose tolerance is present in another 20%. (Refer to Section 2.4. Studying the Opposition: Diabetes for an in-depth study of diabetes).

Older adults who have type 2 diabetes often have near-normal glucose levels after fasting but are hyperglycemia after meals. Fortunately, research has shown that the incidence of type 2 diabetes can be reduced by 58% with healthy lifestyle interventions. Lifestyle changes have been proven to be even more successful at reducing the relative risk of diabetes in people over 60. Increasing exercise and improvement in diet are the key lifestyle changes needed for effective blood glucose management.

One focus of dietary modifications is on the quantity and type of carbohydrates a person is ingesting. Blood glucose levels are significantly affected by different carbohydrate foods. Using the glycemic index (GI), which ranks carbohydrates by their overall impact on blood glucose levels is a useful way of quantifying this. The more fiber or fat that is in a food (fruits, vegetables and nuts), the lower its GI, and the more a food has been processed (white bread), the higher its GI.

Research has shown that low GI foods slowly release glucose to the bloodstream, increasing cellular insulin sensitivity resulting in lower insulin release. In contrast, high GI foods (white sugar and processed foods) results in higher average insulin and blood glucose levels indicating cellular insulin insensitivity.

The research concludes that there is a clinically significant benefit on blood glucose levels with low GI foods. Understanding and minimizing which foods have a greater effect on raising blood glucose levels can have a significant preventative impact for you in your fight against developing type 2 diabetes.

The glycemic index is the best tool to identify which foods should be avoided for good blood glucose/diabetic control.

What is the Glycemic Index?

Some foods that contain simple carbohydrates (no fiber) can make blood sugar shoot up very fast. That's because simple carbohydrates found in pop and white bread for example, are easier for the body to metabolize and change into glucose, (the sugar the body uses for energy), than more slowly digested complex carbohydrates, (starchy fiber containing carbohydrates), like those in fruits, vegetables, and whole grains. It is much harder to controlling your blood sugar and you will increase the risk of developing type 2 diabetes by eating easily metabolized carbohydrates.

The glycemic index is a scale that helps identify "good carbs" that are metabolized/ digested slower from the faster metabolized/digested "bad carbs." The older adult can use the glycemic index as a tool to modify and improve their diet and help keep their blood sugar steadier without medication.

The glycemic index for a particular food is a number. It is a relative number that indicates the speed that the body metabolizes a specific foods carbohydrate into glucose and releases it into the bloodstream compared to the ingestion of pure glucose. The key point is that two foods can have different glycemic index numbers even though they have the same amount of carbohydrates because they contain different types of carbohydrates (simple vs complex carbohydrates). The GI can help manage blood glucose levels because it identifies foods that are metabolized differently and the speed that the glucose from the carbohydrate is released into the bloodstream.

The smaller the GI number for a particular food, the better because it impacts your blood sugar level more slowly.

- 70 or higher = High (bad)
- 56-69 = Medium
- 55 or less = Low (good)

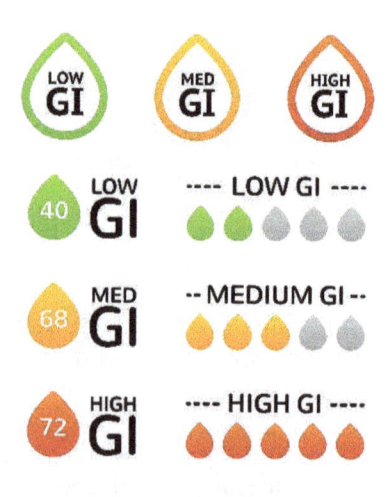

GI is often on packaged food labels. The internet is also a great source to find the GI lists for common foods.

Lower GI are more natural foods vs refined and processed foods which typically have a high GI value.

GI can Change

GI number for a food on paper could be quite different than the GI number, for that same food, that is on your plate. Be aware that there are several factors that influence a foods GI number when it is served:

1.Preparation – The longer a complex carbohydrate (pasta, vegetables) is cooked, the higher their GI.

2.Ripeness – A ripened fruit has a higher simple sugar content and GI number.

The GI of a meal is affected by combining a high-glycemic-index food with lower ones.

You Must Consider the Big Picture:

Generally speaking, the GI helps people control their blood glucose levels. Foods with a low GI are preferred, but the GI of a particular food should not be the only thing considered when making food choices.

A low GI doesn't mean that particular food is super healthy. A food with a low GI number only means that it is metabolized more slowly so its glucose is released into the bloodstream slower, which helps you control your blood glucose/sugar levels. However, that same food may be high in saturated fats which has a negative effect on your blood cholesterol level. AS well, calories, vitamins, and mineral content of food ingested are vitally important and must be considered. For example, GI for potato chips is lower than oatmeal and about the same as green peas but the nutrient value in potato chips is much lower than for oatmeal or peas.

Glycemic Load

The portion size of the carbohydrate ingested matters a great deal. Whatever kind of carbohydrate it is, if you eat it in excess, it will affect your blood sugar levels. That's what the glycemic load indicates. The GI only indicates how quickly a foods carbohydrate is metabolizes and enters in the blood stream, it doesn't tell you how high your blood sugar could go when you eat the food. Glycemic load will indicate this.

Glycemic load is a relative number that indicates how high your blood glucose level will go after eating a particular food. One unit of glycemic load approximates the effect of eating one gram of glucose. It's a number that may be seen along with the GI in lists. Glycemic load helps indicate how much glucose per serving a food can deliver. Remember that excess glucose (glucose that the body can't use for energy) is converted into fatty acids and stored as fat in adipose tissue and the liver, so the amount of glucose that a food delivers and how much you eat of that food is important for weight management. A glycemic load that is less than 10 is low; more than 20 is high.

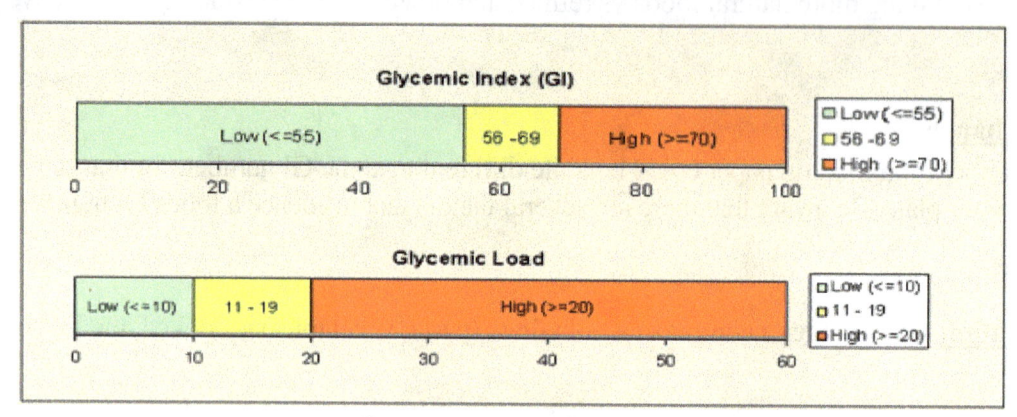

Image source: mendosa.com

Conclusion

For older adults, controlling blood sugar levels is a good and necessary defensive step to prevent the development of type 2 diabetes.

To help control blood sugar levels, a diet with a low GI and load is best:

Eat:

- More fruits, vegetables, whole grains, legumes, nuts, and other foods with a low GI Chart below)
- Fewer foods with a high GI, like white rice and bread, potatoes, ice cream.
- Less of sugary foods, such as pastries, candy, and sweet drinks (pop and fruit juices)

It is important to note that high GI foods can be part of your regular diet, but they need to be served in smaller portions along with nutritious, low-GI foods.

Glycemic Index

Low GI (<55), Medium GI (56-69) and High GI (70>)

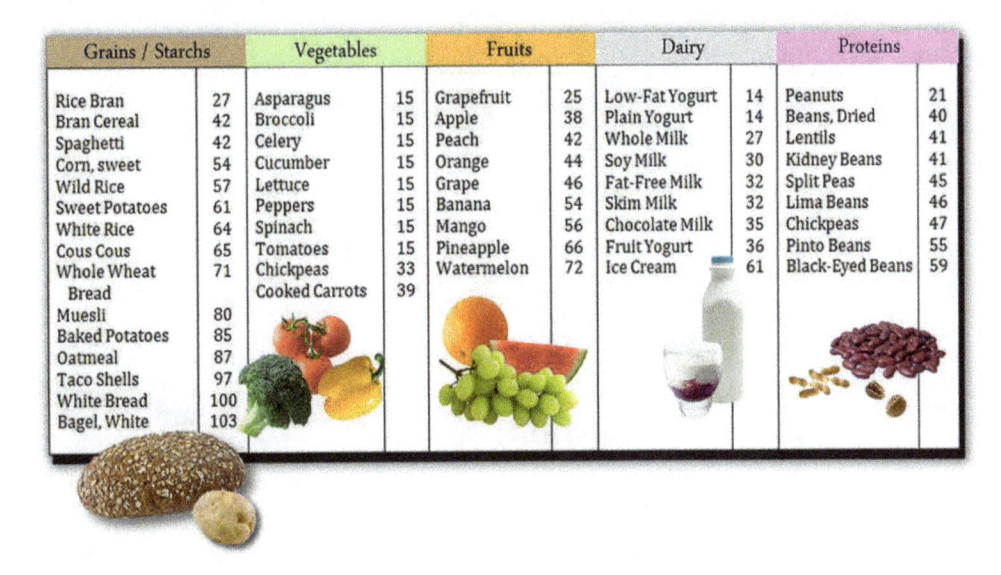

Grains / Starchs		Vegetables		Fruits		Dairy		Proteins	
Rice Bran	27	Asparagus	15	Grapefruit	25	Low-Fat Yogurt	14	Peanuts	21
Bran Cereal	42	Broccoli	15	Apple	38	Plain Yogurt	14	Beans, Dried	40
Spaghetti	42	Celery	15	Peach	42	Whole Milk	27	Lentils	41
Corn, sweet	54	Cucumber	15	Orange	44	Soy Milk	30	Kidney Beans	41
Wild Rice	57	Lettuce	15	Grape	46	Fat-Free Milk	32	Split Peas	45
Sweet Potatoes	61	Peppers	15	Banana	54	Skim Milk	32	Lima Beans	46
White Rice	64	Spinach	15	Mango	56	Chocolate Milk	35	Chickpeas	47
Cous Cous	65	Tomatoes	15	Pineapple	66	Fruit Yogurt	36	Pinto Beans	55
Whole Wheat Bread	71	Chickpeas	33	Watermelon	72	Ice Cream	61	Black-Eyed Beans	59
Muesli	80	Cooked Carrots	39						
Baked Potatoes	85								
Oatmeal	87								
Taco Shells	97								
White Bread	100								
Bagel, White	103								

Image source: narfa.com

Glycemic Index

70 - 100
- white wheat bread, donuts, baguette, crackers, waffles
- white rice, boiled potatoes and mash, french fries
- watermelon
- cornflakes

50 - 70
- rye & wholegrain bread
- muesli, corn, couscous, brown rice, spaghetti, popcorn, yams
- ice cream, sweet yogurt
- banana, grapes, kiwi

30 - 50
- coarse barley bread
- strawberries, apples, pears, oranges
- milk & soy milk
- natural yoghurt
- oatmeal, beans

10 - 30
- pearled barley, lentils
- greyfrut, cherry, apricot, plum
- dark chocolate 70% cocoa
- whole milk
- cashews, walnuts

0 - 10
- hummus, chickpeas
- garlic, onion, green pepper
- eggplant, broccoli, cabbage, tomatoes
- mushrooms
- lettuce

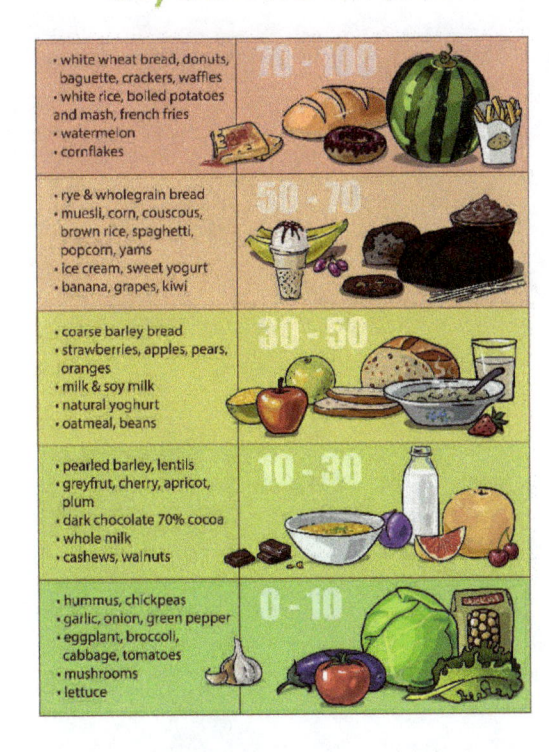

References

www.webmd.com

www.health.harvard.edu/diseases-and-conditions/the-lowdown-on-glycemic-index-and-glycemic-load

https://www.mayoclinic.org/

5.2.10. Weight Loss and a Review of the Most Popular Diets

Introduction to Weight Loss

Losing weight is almost a 300-million-dollar business in Canada. The reason: in 2019, Statistics Canada estimated that around 27.7 percent of Canadian adults were considered obese, so there is a big need for the average Canadian to lose weight. Unfortunately, most Canadians have found that setting a goal to lose weight is much easier than actually losing the weight. It is estimated that over 80% of people who attempt to lose weight fail to do so.

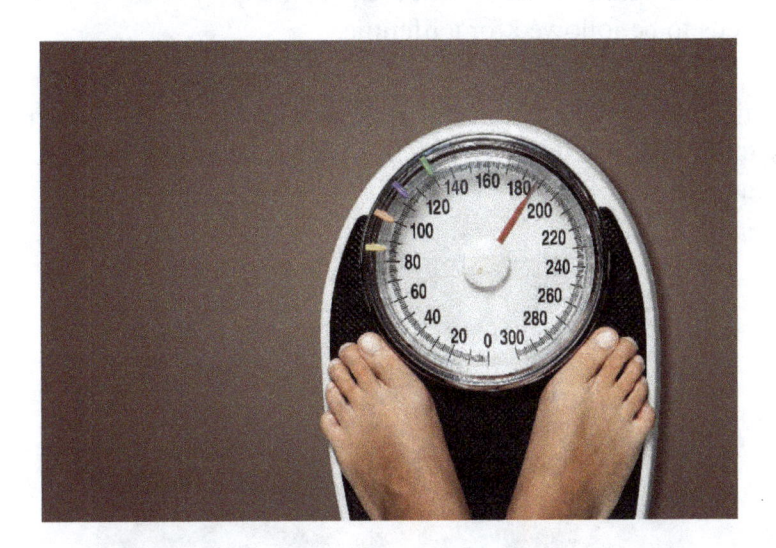

Despite the high rate of failure by their clients, the weight loss industry, like their clients' waistlines, continues to expand. Plant-based diets, intermittent fasting, low carbs, low fats, eating like a caveman, eating like the Italians, and eating within a daily set point system have all been advocated as "the way" to lose weight. Still, unfortunately, none have proven to be truly effective long-term for most of their clients.

What is at the root of the problem? Is it the structure of the diet that is at fault, or is it a lack of motivation by the clients? Perhaps it is the pressure by society for instant gratification, so people eat and drink too much and exercise too little. The answer is probably a combination of all three of these reasons.

It is hard to lose weight, and your motivation to lose weight must be high. To illustrate, pick up an iron; it feels heavy and probably weighs two or three pounds. Now think of the iron as fat, and it becomes clear that two to three pounds of fat is a lot of weight to lose. But when someone thinks about losing weight, they don't say, "I want to lose two or three pounds," they say they want to lose 10-20 pounds. That is over six times the weight of an iron. Is that a realistic goal? Even if a person loses 10-20 pounds, the real question is, can they keep the lost weight off?

What people must realize, and what most diets fail to educate their clients on, is that weight management is a life-long endeavor. It is about changing your eating and nutritional habits for a lifetime. Weight management must be thought of as a marathon, not a sprint. As difficult as it may be, most people can follow a restrictive caloric diet for a relatively short (one, three, or six months, or even a year) period (a sprint). However, over this time, the question is, can good eating habits be effectively ingrained to allow the person to keep the weight off (the marathon)? If a person can embrace good nutritional habits, the weight will stay off. If they can't, they become another failed statistic.

Weight loss and weight management is not about the mechanics of restricting caloric intake; most diets do this very well. It is also not about avoiding carbohydrates or fats, though in certain health situations when a person is vulnerable to type 2 diabetes and heart disease, these are good practices. Weight loss and weight management is about mentally accepting that whatever diet or method is used, it needs to be followed for a lifetime.

Following a particular diet or nutritional plan, long-term does not mean a person needs to be perfect, but if they follow the 80/20 rule (Chapter 3.1: The Eight Golden Rules of Training), they are more likely to succeed.

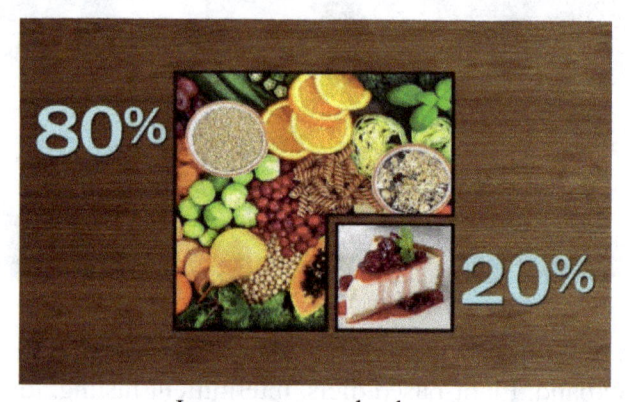

Image source: webmd.com

For older adults, weight management and good nutrition are important to enhance their quality of life through their golden years. This chapter will review the key points to consider when deciding on a diet. Ten of the most popular diets on the market today will also be reviewed. Each of these diets will help you lose weight, but the question is, which one is best structured for a particular individual to be successful long-term?

When people consider a particular diet, they must ask themselves how they can adapt this dietary program into good life-long nutritional habits based on their economic, social, and behavioral situation. This adaptation is the key to successful weight management.

Crunching the Numbers for Weight Loss

Crunching the numbers for weight loss is relatively simple:

Calories:
- The **energy** people get from consuming food and drink.
- The **energy** they use during physical activity.

3500 calories = 1 pound of body fat

Reduce caloric intake and/or increase exercise by 500 calories/day and a person will lose one pound a week (500 calories/day x 7 days = 3500 calories/week).

What 500 Calories Look Like

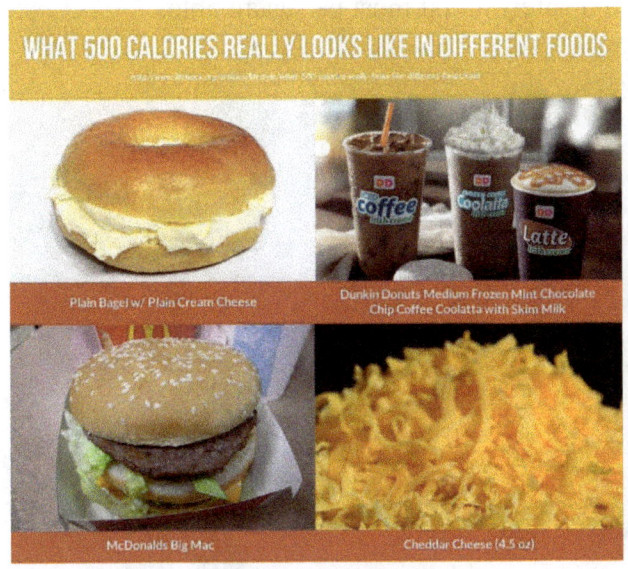

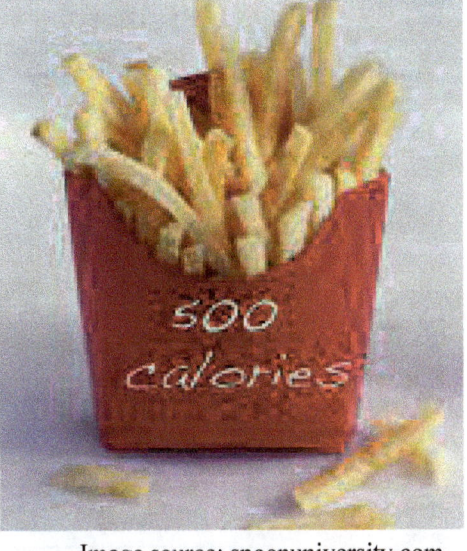

Image source: lifehack.org

Image source: spoonuniversity.com

Exercise

APPROXIMATE NUMBER OF MINUTES TO BURN 500 CALORIES

BODY WEIGHT:	120 lbs. 54.5 kilos.	140 lbs. 63.5 kilos.	160 lbs. 72.5 kilos.	180 lbs. 82 kilos.	200 lbs. 91 kilos.	220 lbs. 100 kilos.	240 lbs. 109 kilos.
Aquaerobics	131	113	99	88	79	72	66
Boot camp workout	78	63	52	45	39	35	31
Boxing - Heavy Bag	66	57	49	44	40	36	33
Cross country skiing	56	48	42	38	34	31	28
Cycling - outdoor	75	64	56	50	45	41	38
Cycling - spinning class	53	45	39	35	32	29	26
Ice skating	75	64	56	50	45	41	38
Jogging - 6.5 miles/hour	53	45	40	35	32	29	26
Martial Arts	53	45	39	35	32	29	26
Pilates	150	129	113	100	90	82	75
Racquetball	61	53	46	41	37	33	31
Rollerblading	75	64	56	50	45	41	38
Rowing	66	56	49	44	39	36	33
Running - interval sprints	24	21	18	16	14	13	12
Strength training - maximum rest	110	94	82	73	66	60	55
Strength training - minimal rest	64	55	48	43	38	35	32
Swimming laps	71	61	53	47	42	39	35
Walking - 3.5 miles/hour	107	92	80	71	64	58	53
Yoga	210	180	158	140	126	115	105
Zumba	67	57	50	44	40	36	33

Image source: breakingmuscle.com

It all sounds so simple, but unfortunately, the history of weight loss has shown that it is not.

What Diet That Is the Right One for You: An Introduction

When wanting to lose weight, it is easy to fall prey to quick loss gimmicks. Weight management is important, but you have to do it safely and it must be sustainable.

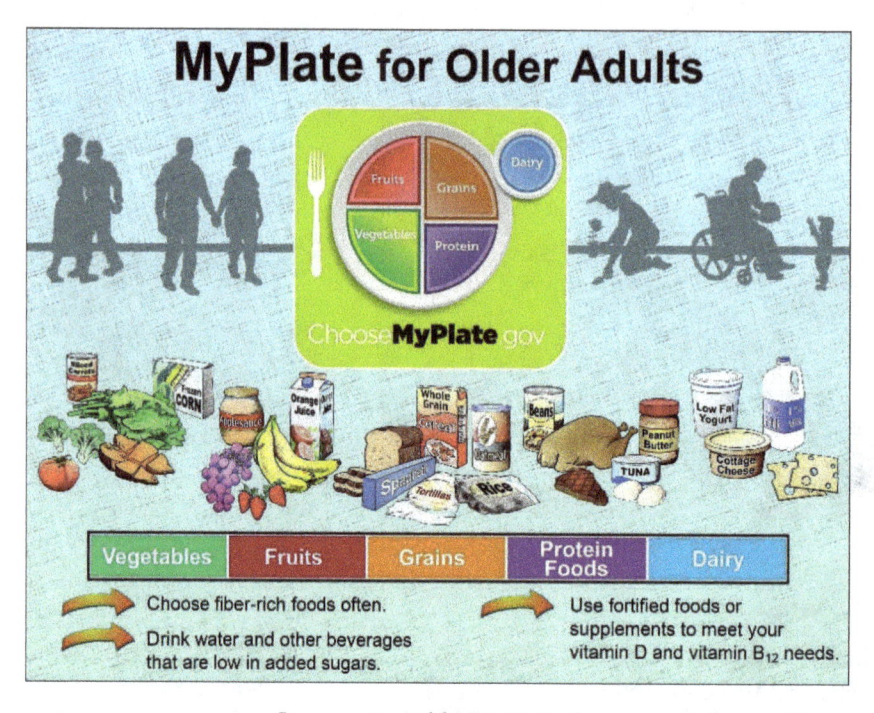

Image source: blogs.ext.vt.edu

Diets must be evaluated carefully to find one will work for you. A good first step is to consult your doctor and dietitian before starting any weight loss program. They will review your medications and any of your medical issues that might affect your ability to lose weight and provide guidance on an appropriate diet program. You can also discuss various exercise programs that you could safely begin. This discussion is especially important if you have physical or medical challenges which may require you to modify the way you exercise. Exercise is a key component to successfully losing weight and keeping it off.

When Choosing a Diet:

1. Consider Personal Needs

Unfortunately, no universally successful weight loss program or diet exist. It is essential to consider your weight loss goals, lifestyle and personal preferences. To be successful, you need to find a tailored and flexible diet plan to meet your individual needs.

Prior to jumping in and starting a new weight loss program, consider the following:

a. Re-evaluate the Diets you unsuccessfully tried before:
- How successful or unsuccessful were you in following the diet?
- While on the diet, how did you feel physically and emotionally?
- What did you enjoy or dislike?
- What worked or didn't work?

b. What are Your Preferences When it comes to Dieting:
- Do you prefer dieting on your own or would find being a part of a dieting support group more motivating?
- If using a support group is preferred, should this be done with in-person meetings or zooming on-line?

c. Do you have budget or logistic restrictions?
- Does your budget allow you to buy meals or supplements? Are there any restrictions for you to attend support meetings or visit weight loss clinics for weigh ins?

2. Look for a Safe, Effective Weight Loss/Diet Program

A slow and steady diet approach best. This type of program usually beats fast weight loss gimmicky diets and is easier to maintain long-term. The general medical recommendation is that one should not lose more than one to two pounds a week.

If a medical condition dictates the need for faster weight loss, you must do this safely under medical supervision.

As mentioned previously, a long-term commitment to eating healthy, exercising regularly, and modifying your social behavior is necessary to ensure successful weight loss. Behavior modification, which involves breaking old unhealthy eating habits is essential, and over the long-term could have the greatest impact on your weight loss efforts.

3. Pick a Plan You Will Enjoy and Stay With.

Key features to Consider:

1. Flexibility
A successful diet plan will include a variety of foods from all the major food groups while being flexible enough to allows the occasional indulgence (Chapter 3.1- 80:20 rule). The diet plan must feature foods that are readily available and that you enjoy eating. The consumption of sugary drinks, alcohol, and high in sugar treats will be limited because they have no nutrient value.

2. Balance

The diet plan must include essential nutrients and sufficient calories. Eating large quantities of certain foods while drastically cutting calories; or eliminating entire food groups, such as carbohydrates, can cause nutritional problems. Safe, healthy, and balanced diets do not require excessive vitamins and mineral supplements.

3. Likeability

Your diet needs to be sustainable, therefore it must include foods that you enjoy eating, not foods that you could only tolerate over the duration of the plan. You won't stick to the plan long-term and weight loss is unlikely, if you do not like the food or if the plan is overly restrictive, repetitive and boring.

4. Physical Activity

All diet plans should include physical activity. Burning calories by exercising helps avoid the need for moderate to severe caloric restriction from dieting. Exercise also helps counter muscle mass loss that occurs with weight loss and helps keep the weight off long-term. Exercise should be an important part of every weight loss and weight management plan.

The table below lists common diets on the market that will be reviewed in this chapter. Most diet plans fit into a few major categories, but there is overlap between elements of all these diets.

Most weight loss programs will help a person los weight, however the weight loss differences between diets will be generally small. The key to successful long-term weight management is picking which of these diets will facilitate and ingrain healthy long-term eating habits. That should be the barometer to judge the effectiveness of a diet.

Diet type and Examples	Flexible	Nutritionally Balanced	Sustainable for Long-Term
Balanced • DASH • Mayo Clinic • Mediterranean • Weight Watchers • Noom (DASH = Dietary Approaches	Yes. - No foods are off-limits.	Yes.	Yes. - Emphasis is on making permanent lifestyle changes.

Diet type and Examples	Flexible	Nutritionally Balanced	Sustainable for Long-Term
to Stop Hypertension)			
High protein • Paleo	No. - Emphasizes lean meats, dairy.	On very restrictive plans deficiencies are possible	Possibly. - Over time, the diet may be hard to stick to.
Low carb • Atkins • South Beach	No. - Carbs are limited; fats or proteins or both are emphasized.	Deficiencies are possible on very restrictive plans.	Possibly. - The diet may be hard to stick to over time.
High Fat • Keto	No. - High-fat, - adequate-protein - Low-carbohydrate.	No.	No. - The diet may be hard to stick to over time.
Meal replacement (Not reviewed)	No. - Replacement products take the	Possibly. - Balance is possible if you	Possibly. - Cost of products

Diet type and Examples	Flexible	Nutritionally Balanced	Sustainable for Long-Term
• Jenny Craig • Nutrisystem • SlimFast	place of one or two meals a day.	make healthy meal choices.	varies; some can be cost prohibitive.
Fasting • Intermittent Fasting	Somewhat. - Calories are limited/restricted at certain times of the day or on alternating days.	Yes.	Possibility. - If a person has existing health concerns such as diabetes this type of diet should be avoided.

Key Questions to Ask Before Starting a Diet Program

Knowledge is power when trying to determine the best diet for you. It does not mean a particular diet is right for you just because it is trendy or all your friends are doing.

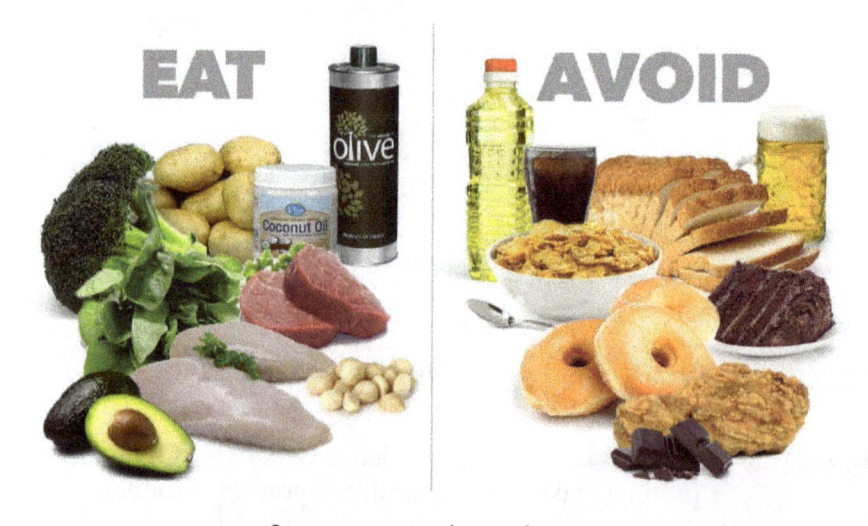

Image source: traineatgain.com

Key Questions to Ask:

1. What's involved?

- Are special meals or supplements required?
- Does it encourage and teach positive, healthy changes to help maintain weight loss?
- Can the plan be adapted to accommodate your needs?
- Does it offer in-person or online support?

2. Is the diet scientifically supported?

- Does science support the diets weight loss approach?
- If you go to a weight loss clinic what training and experience do the dietitians and doctors have and will they communicate with your regular doctor?

3. Are there short-term or long-term risks involved with the diet?

- If you have a health condition such as diabetes or heart disease, or take medications, are the dietary recommendations safe.
- Is the diet too calorie restrictive? Are all essential nutrients requirements being met?

4. Result Expectations?

- What is the expected timeline for weight loss?
- Does the diet promote before and after photos that seem too good to be true?
- Is the diet designed to maintain weight loss over time?
- Does the program claim that they can target specific areas of your body (no diet can do that)?

The Keys to Weight Loss Success

1. **Long-term changes in behavior** – Successful weight loss management requires changes in eating habits and physical activity. Long-term changes mean embracing these changes for life. If you revert to old unhealthy habits, any success you did have in losing weight will be lost.
2. **You can't feel deprived** – Diets that leave you feeling hungry are not sustainable and consequently ineffective. Successful diets must encourage healthy lifestyle changes, without leaving you feeling hungry all the time.
3. **A person must remain vigilant** – Weight control is a marathon, not a sprint. Combining more activity with a healthy diet is the best way to manage your weight. Don't expect perfection but when you do revert to old unhealthy eating or inactivity, make corrective changes quickly and more forward.

10 Popular Diets

Warning: Everyone, especially an older adult, needs to check with their doctor before starting a diet. This is especially necessary if you suffer from any chronic health condition, such as heart disease, diabetes, arthritis, cancer, or dementia (Section 2: The Off-Season- Studying the Opposition to Health).

1. Atkins Diet

Dr. Robert C. Atkins, cardiologist, developed this diet in the 1960s. This diet emphasizes consuming protein and fats while restricting carbohydrates. The theory behind the diet is that eating too many carbohydrates, especially refined carbohydrates like sugar and white flour contribute to weight gain, cardiovascular problems and blood sugar imbalances. The Atkins Diet has softened over time and eating more complex carbohydrates, such as high-fiber vegetables, is encouraged.

Calorie counting or portion control is not required, but the diet does require the person to track their carbohydrate intake. It uses a "net carbs system," which equates to the total carbohydrate content of an item minus its fiber content. For example, 4 ounces of raw broccoli, approximately ½ cup, has a total carb value of 2.3 grams of which 1.3 grams is fiber. This means it has a net carb value of 1 gram.

The Atkins Diet promotes its dietary plan by stating that by reducing carbohydrates in your diet, fat stores, rather than carbohydrates, will be used for energy, blood sugar levels will be managed more effectively, and the high consumption of protein and fat will not leave you feeling hungry or deprived. Once your goal weight is achieved, the Atkins Diet will help you identify the number of grams of net carbs you can eat each day without you gaining or losing weight (your carbohydrate tolerance)

The Atkins Diet, acknowledges that exercise can help manage your weight as well as offer other health benefits but states that exercise isn't a necessary component of a weight loss program.

Four Phase Atkins Diet
Based on your goals, you can start at any of the first three phases of this diet.

Phase 1: Induction
This is the strictest phase of the diet and lasts approximately two weeks. Most nutritional guidelines recommend getting 45 to 65% of your daily calories from carbohydrates, but in this first phase it restricts you to about 10 %. This equates to eating about 20 grams of net carbs a day, mainly from "Foundation" vegetables such as celery, broccoli, cucumber, asparagus, peppers and green beans.

During this phase, you must avoid sugary baked pastries, pasta, bread, nuts, grains, alcohol. As well, you are encouraged to drink at least eight glasses of water a day.

Phase 2: Balancing

In this phase, as you lose weight, you can slowly add back some nutrient-rich carbohydrates, such as berries, seeds and nuts. Once you are about 10 pounds from your goal weight you can move onto pre-maintenance phase 3.

Phase 3: Pre-maintenance

This phase lasts until you have reached your goal weight. This phase allows you to gradually increase the range of foods you can eat, including fruits, starchy vegetables, and whole grains. If you continue to lose weight, you can add about 10 grams of carbs to your diet each week. However, if your weight loss stops you must cut back again on the number of carbohydrates you are consuming.

Phase 4: Lifetime maintenance

Once you have reached your goal weight, this phase begins. You determine your "carbohydrate tolerance" in this phase and continue eating this way for life.

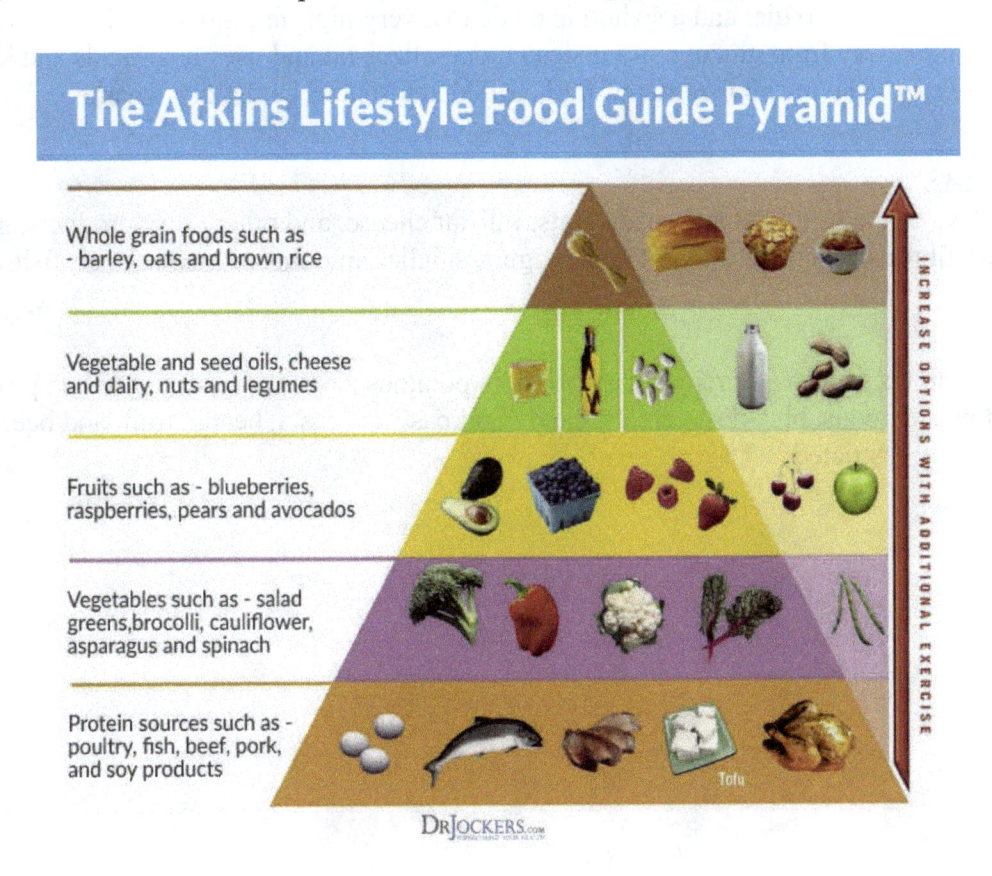

Results

The main reason for weight loss on the Atkins Diet is because of a lower overall calorie intake from eating fewer carbohydrates. The extra protein and fat consumed helps keep you feeling full longer which helps contribute to you lowering your overall calorie intake.

Risks

In the first phase, when you initially and significantly lower carbohydrate intake certain side effects may be felt:

- Weakness
- Fatigue
- Headache
- Dizziness
- Constipation

2. Keto (Ketogenic) Diet

This diet severely restricts carbohydrates to 50 grams per day, and emphasizes that 60 to 80% of your daily calories should come from fat with only moderate protein consumed.

The premise behind the diet is that because the North American diet is over 50% carbohydrates, glucose metabolized from carbohydrates is readily available for energy. But, when following the Keto diet and a switch is made to a very high-fat, low-carb diet, the body, by necessity, shifts away from glucose and instead metabolizes fat and uses fatty acids and ketone bodies for energy. The metabolization of fat is called ketosis, hence the diet's name.

Food Choices

Mainstays of the Keto diet are, seeds, nuts, full-fat cheese, and other dairy products, non-starchy and fibrous vegetables, plain Greek yogurt, smaller amounts of meats, eggs, fish, and oils.

Carbohydrates, such as, starchy vegetables like potatoes, sweet potatoes, corn and peas, bread and baked goods, breakfast cereals, candy and pastries, pasta, beans, fruit, and beer must be significantly restricted.

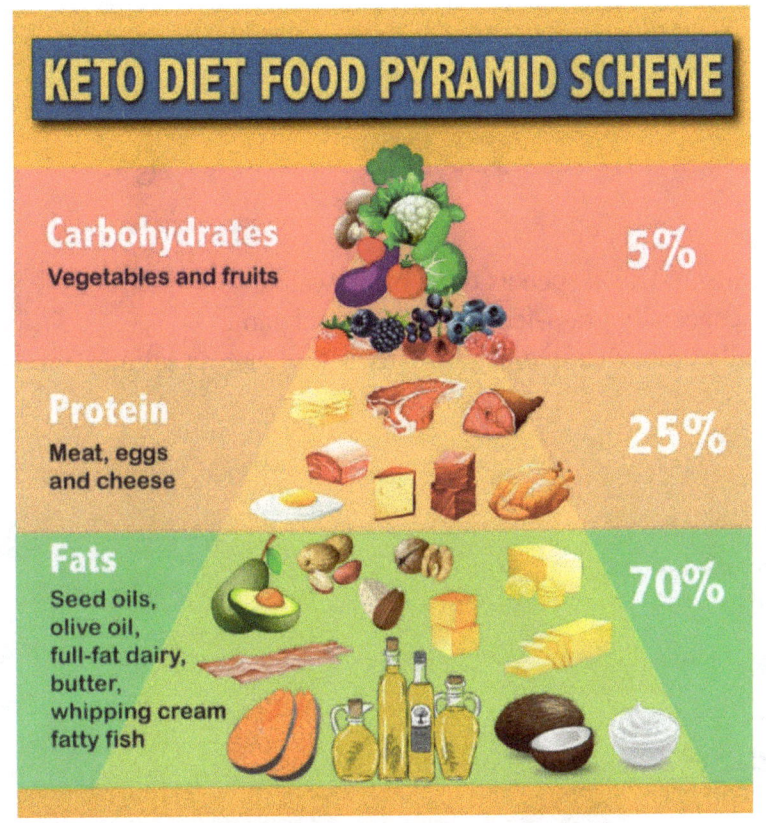

Image source: recoveryourgroove.com

Results
This diet does produce weight loss, but because it takes being on the diet two to three weeks before the body begins to burn fat vs carbohydrates, the results may be slower to occur than that seen with low carbohydrate diets.

Risk
Keto diet is tough to follow long-term because it is a very restrictive diet. As well, because the saturated fat content is high in this diet, and limits the amounts of vegetables, fruits, and whole grains that should be consumed, it is not optimal for a person's general overall health.

3. Paleo (Paleolithic) Diet

This dietary plan is based on what foods would have been obtained by hunting, gathering and eaten approximately 2.5 million to 10,000 years ago during the Paleolithic era. These foods include vegetables, fruits, lean meats, fish, seeds and nuts. Foods that became common when farming emerged about 10,000 years ago such as dairy products, legumes, and grains are limited.

The theory behind the diet is that there is a mismatched between the modern diet that emerged with farming practices and how the body is genetically manufactured. In other words, the rapid change in our diet has outpaced the body's ability to adapt, and this mismatch contributes to the prevalence of heart disease, diabetes and obesity, seen in our society today.

Food Choices

What to eat:
- Vegetables
- Fruits
- Nuts and seeds
- Oils from fruits and nuts, such as olive oil or walnut oil
- Lean meats, especially grass-fed animals or wild game
- Fish, especially those rich in omega-3 fatty acids, such as salmon, mackerel, and albacore tuna

What to avoid:
- Dairy products
- Highly processed foods
- Refined sugar
- Salt
- Potatoes
- Grains, such as wheat, oats, and barley
- Legumes, such as beans, lentils, peanuts, and peas

Being physically active and drinking water daily are encouraged.

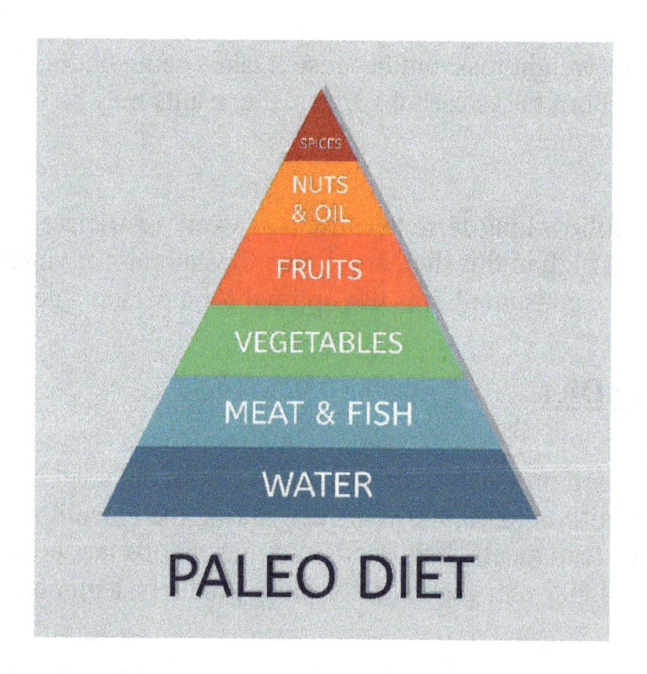

Results
Some clinical trials suggests that this restrictive diet may provide some benefits when compared with diets that emphasize vegetables, fruits, whole grains, lean meats, legumes, and low-fat dairy products. These benefits may include:

- Improved glucose tolerance
- Better blood pressure control
- Better appetite management
- More weight loss
- Lower triglycerides

Longer randomized trials needed to understand the overall health benefits and possible long-term risks of a paleo diet.

Risks

The paleo diet differs from other healthy diets primarily in the absence of whole grains which are considered good sources of fiber, vitamins, and other nutrients, and dairy products, which are good sources of protein and calcium.

4. Intermittent Fasting

This diet necessitates that you don't eat for a specific period of time each day or week.

There are different approached to carrying out intermittent fasting:

1.Alternate-day fasting –A regular diet is eaten every other day. On the other day you either completely fast or have one small meal (less than 500 calories).

2.5:2 fasting – You fast two non consecutive days a week. The other five days you consume your regular diet.

3.Daily time-restricted fasting – You eat a normal diet each day but only within an eight-hour window such as noon to 8 pm.

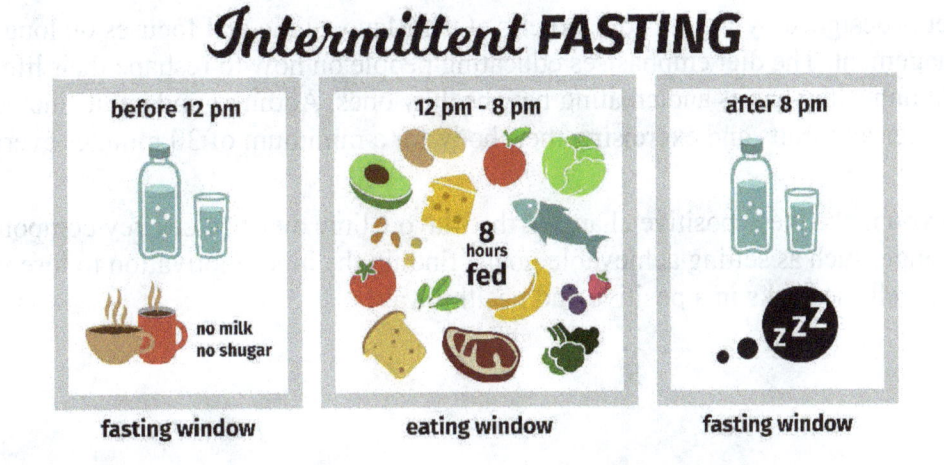

Intermittent FASTING

before 12 pm	12 pm - 8 pm	after 8 pm
no milk no shugar	8 hours fed	zzz
fasting window	eating window	fasting window

363

Potential Benefits

Some research suggests that compared to other diets, intermittent fasting may be superior in improving conditions associated with inflammation, such as:
- Arthritis
- Asthma
- Stroke
- Heart Disease
- Alzheimer's disease
- Multiple sclerosis

Results

Intermittent fasting may be as effective as a typical low-calorie diet for weight loss because it reduces over all calorie intake.

Risks

Unpleasant side effects have been reported with intermittent fasting but they tend to diminish in about a month.
- Headaches
- Fatigue
- Nausea
- Hunger
- Insomnia

If you are pregnant or breastfeeding it is not recommended that you skip meals to manage post-partum weight gain weight. Intermittent fasting is safe but everyone, especially an older adult who may have pre-existing medical issues, should consult with their doctor before starting this diet plan.

5. Mayo Clinic diet

This diet is designed by weight-loss experts at the Mayo Clinic and focuses on long-term weight management. The diet emphasises educating people on how to reshape their lifestyle by breaking old unhealthy habits and creating new healthy ones. Adding good habits include eating more vegetables and fruits and exercising their body for a minimum of 30 minutes every day.

To help you make these positive changes, the Mayo Clinic diet stresses key components of behavior change, such as setting achievable goals, finding the inner motivation to lose weight, and how to handle setbacks in a positive and healthy way.

Diet Details

- The a one-size-fits-all approach is not part of this diet. The diet is flexible and encourages you to design the diet to accommodate your own personal needs and health history.
- A large variety of foods are a key element of the diet. This includes an unlimited amount of fruits and vegetables.
- Learning and establishing establish healthy lifestyle habits and stop unhealthy ones
- Encouraging you to become more active to improve overall health and reduce health risks
- No precise counting calories is required or the need to eliminate groups of foods
- The diet is focused on the long-term not a quick fix and it is a diet most people can follow for life.

There are two main phases to the Mayo Diet:

1. Lose It

This is the "starting" phase and last approximately two weeks. Its goal is to have you lose 6 to 10 pounds safely which will jump-start your weight loss journey. In this phase, you focus on three key behaviours;

- Adding five healthy habits,
- Breaking five unhealthy habits
- Adopting another five bonus healthy habits.

The theory behind this quick start phase is that it gives you a psychological/motivational boost to "buy into" practicing essential healthy habits and to carry these forward into the second phase of the diet.

2. Live It

Establishing a lifelong diet and health approach is the emphasis of this phase. A main component of this phase is educating you about menu planning, portion sizes, food choices, and the need for increase physical activity. During this phase, you should continue to lose weight at a steady rate of about one to two pounds (0.5 to 1 kilogram) a week until you reach your goal weight which you should be able to maintain permanently if the behavioural changes taught are followed correctly.

Follow the Mayo Clinic Healthy Weight Pyramid

Precise calorie counting is not part of the Mayo Clinic diet. Instead, the diet presents a guide for a person to make smart eating choices.

The rule in using the weight pyramid is: eat more food (fruits and vegetables) from the food groups at the base of the pyramid base, less food sweets and fats) at the top, and to exercise more.

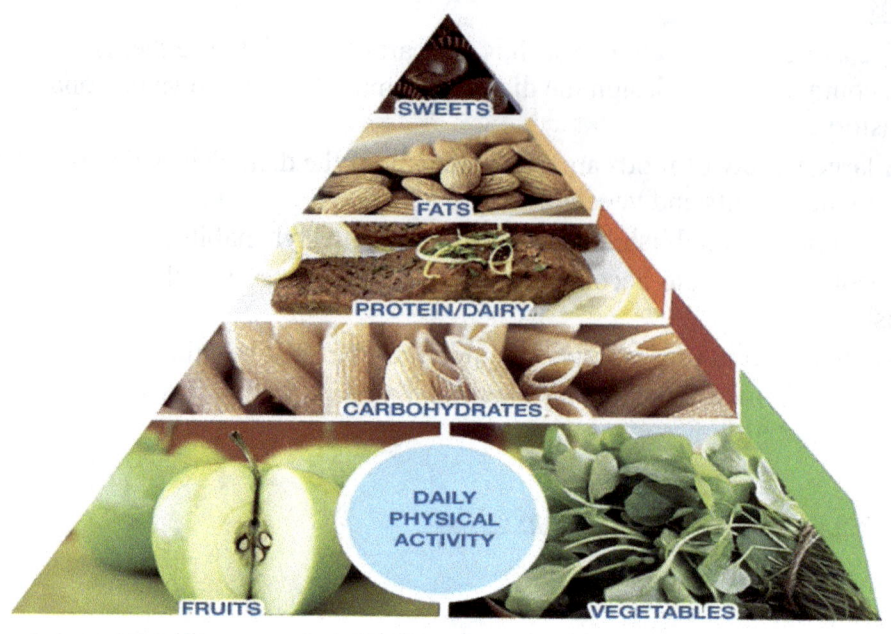

Control Portion Size and Eat Healthy Foods

The theory behind the healthy weight pyramid is that you focus your diet on large amounts of healthy foods (vegetables and fruit) at the base that contain a smaller number of calories per serving. As well, these foods will make you feel fuller faster so you will tend to eat less.

The rest of the diet pyramid focuses on making healthy choices and eating moderate amounts of carbohydrates (complex whole-grain carbohydrates), proteins (lean sources of protein such as legumes, fish and low-fat dairy), and fats (heart-healthy unsaturated fats).

The three key elements of The Mayo Clinic diet are:

- Educating you on how to estimate portion sizes and designing healthy meal plans.
- You are not require you to eliminate any foods.
- You can have sweets as long as you limit them to 75 calories a day.

Increase your Physical Activity

Increasing your level of physical activity is an important component to The Mayo Clinic diet. Practical and realistic suggestions for exercise and physical activity throughout your day are presented. An example would be using the stairs instead of an elevator or parking your car farther from work so you would have to walk a longer distance.

The diet recommends getting a minimum of 30 minutes of exercise but emphasises that even more exercise will lead to further health benefits and weight loss.

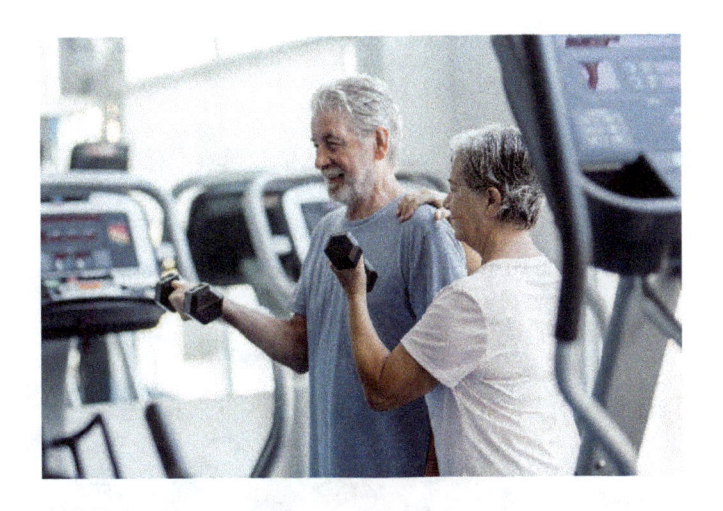

Results

Any diet plan that restricts calories in the short term will help a person lose weight. The Mayo Clinic Diet is no different. However, the goal of this diet is to help you keep the weight off permanently by learning to make smarter food choices and embracing behaviour modification techniques that will help substitute good habits for bad habits.

Risks

This is a relatively safe diet but consultation with your doctor and dietitian is always encouraged before starting a new diet program. Nutrient deficiencies are not usually a problem with The Mayo Diet because it encourages you to eat a lot's of vegetables and fruits which provide plenty of essential nutrients and fiber. It is important to note that you may experience minor, temporary digestive symptoms such as bloating and intestinal gas as you adjust to an increase amount of fiber in your diet.

Fruit does contain natural sugar which does affect carbohydrate intake, and this may temporarily raise blood sugar levels. If you are diabetic, you should aim for more vegetables than fruits in your diet. As well, it is recommended that rather than use fruit as your snack, you eat vegetables and add a source of protein such as a piece of chicken, Greek yogurt or low-fat cheese (cottage cheese).

6. Mediterranean Diet

The Mediterranean diet has become a very favourable diet in the science community and popular with the general population. Its name originates from the fact that the diet uses cooking methods and traditional flavors of the Mediterranean.

In the 1960s, interest grew in the Mediterranean regions diet and way of cooking with the observation that Mediterranean countries, such as Greece and Italy had fewer deaths resulting from coronary heart disease than in North America and western Europe.
The Mediterranean Diet is endorsed as a healthy and sustainable diet by the World Health Organization.

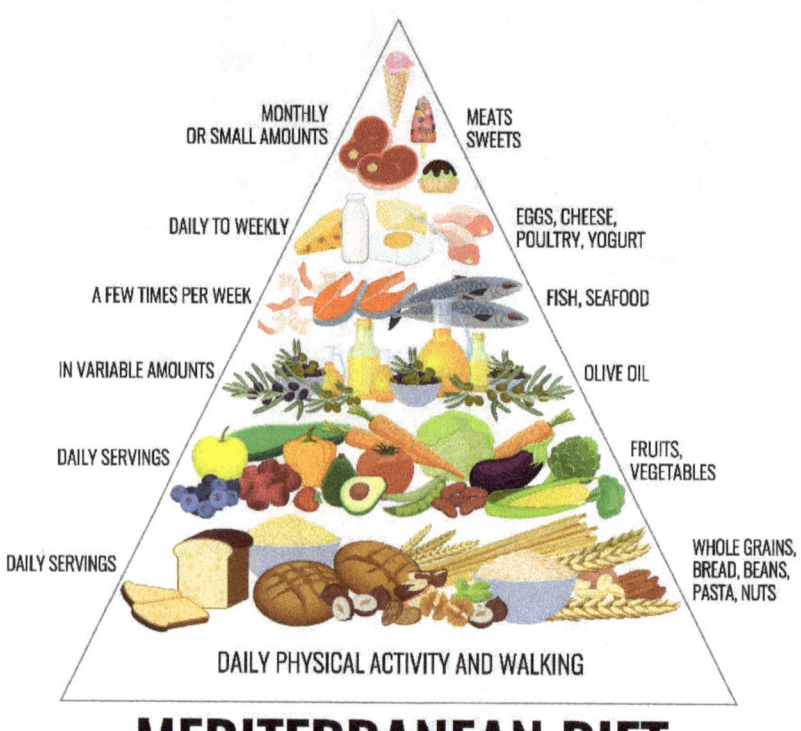

What is the Mediterranean diet?

Fruits, vegetables, whole grains, nuts, beans, herbs make up the foundation of the Mediterranean diet. Poultry, seafood, eggs and dairy, are also a significant part of the Mediterranean Diet. Only occasionally is red meat eaten.

The primary source of added fat in the Mediterranean diet is olive oil. This oil should only be heated to moderate temperatures. (Refer to chapter 5.2.6: Cholesterol for a more complete discussion on this subject). Olive oil, along with seeds and nuts contain monounsaturated fat, which lowers low-density lipoprotein (LDL or "bad") and total cholesterol levels which are major the risks factors for heart disease.

The Mediterranean diet is rich in omega-3 fatty acids, a polyunsaturated fat that helps reduce inflammation in the body because it encourages the consumption of fatty fish such as mackerel, herring, salmon, sardines, lake trout and tuna. High levels of Omega-3 fatty acids in the diet are important because it also helps decrease triglycerides, reduce blood clotting, and decreases the risk of stroke and heart failure.

The main components of the Mediterranean diet include:
- Limited intake of red meat
- Daily consumption of vegetables, fruits, whole grains, and healthy fats (olive oil, nuts and seeds)
- Weekly intake of fish, poultry, beans, and eggs
- Moderate portions of low-fat dairy products

Two other key elements of the Mediterranean diet are being physically active and sharing meals with family and friends. These elements are also emphasised in the New Canadian Health Food Guide.

The Mediterranean diet typically allows the consumption of a moderate amount of red wine.

Tips on Eating the Mediterranean way
- **Increase your consumption of fruits and vegetables** – the goal is for 7 to 10 servings a day.
- **Choose whole grain foods** – This includes pasta, cereal and bread.
- **Use healthy fats** – When cooking, replace butter with olive oil but only cook this oil at moderate heat. Substitute butter or margarine on bread by dipping bread in flavored olive oil.
- **Eat more seafood and reduce red meat consumption** – Have fish a minimum of twice a week but avoid deep-fried fish. Make sure red meat is lean and the portions small.
- **Low fat dairy is good** – Low-fat plain Greek yogurt is excellent. When serving cheese, make the portions small.
- **Reduce added salt** – Substitute salt with herbs and spices to boost flavor.

New Research in Support of "Green" Mediterranean Diet: Just published research in the Journal of Clinical Nutrition shows that eating a Mediterranean diet slowed the age-related loss of brain tissue (atrophy) but significantly, a "green" Mediterranean diet had even greater brain-health benefits.

A "green" Mediterranean diet is a Mediterranean diet with an increased intake of polyphenols which are micronutrients and are powerful antioxidants and have strong anti-inflammatory properties that are found abundantly in fruits (apples and berries (blueberries, blackberries and strawberries), vegetables (spinach, red onion, artichokes), nuts (hazelnuts, pecans, almonds, walnuts), coffee and green teas, herbs and spices (cloves, oregano, sage, rosemary, thyme) and whole-grains such as flaxseeds. In this particular study, the "green" Mediterranean diet included 7 walnuts, 4-5 cups of green tea and a green shake containing Mankai, which is a branded strain of an aquatic plant called duckweed (or water lentils).

7. South Beach Diet

The South Beach diet is a modified low-carbohydrate diet created in 2003 by cardiologist Arthur Agatston, M.D. This is not a strict low-carb diet such as the keto diet but compared to a typical eating plan, it is higher in protein and healthy fats. It should be noted that there is also a stricter keto (ketogenic diet) version of the South Beach diet (75% fat, 20% protein and 5% carbohydrates).

The goal of the South Beach diet, like all carbohydrate limiting diets, is to restrict carbohydrate intake, which then forces the body to use fat for energy instead of carbohydrates or protein.

Diet details

The South Beach diet is not a strict carbohydrate limiting diet. It attempts to introduce a diet that can be followed for a lifetime by developing a fiber-rich, nutrient-dense diet that balances complex carbs, lean protein, and healthy monounsaturated and polyunsaturated fats. Consumption of unhealthy fats such as saturated and trans-fats is discouraged.

Compared to a strict low-carb diet that restricts carbohydrate intake to 20 to 100 grams a day, the maintenance phase of the South Beach diet allows 28% or 140 grams of your daily calories to come from carbohydrates.

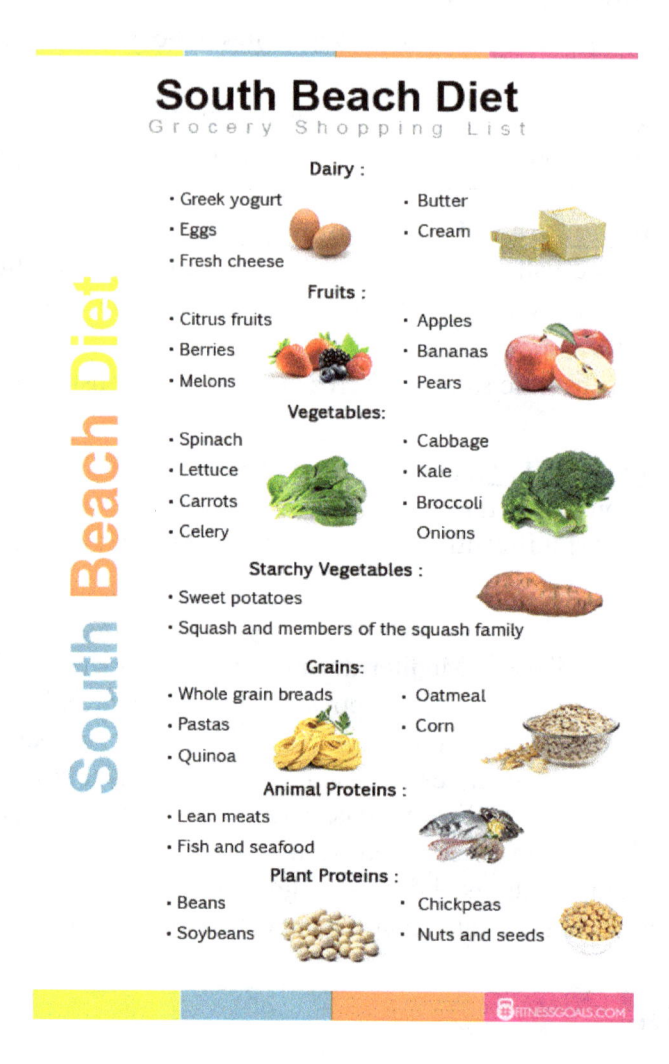

South Beach Diet
Grocery Shopping List

Dairy:
- Greek yogurt
- Eggs
- Fresh cheese
- Butter
- Cream

Fruits:
- Citrus fruits
- Berries
- Melons
- Apples
- Bananas
- Pears

Vegetables:
- Spinach
- Lettuce
- Carrots
- Celery
- Cabbage
- Kale
- Broccoli
- Onions

Starchy Vegetables:
- Sweet potatoes
- Squash and members of the squash family

Grains:
- Whole grain breads
- Pastas
- Quinoa
- Oatmeal
- Corn

Animal Proteins:
- Lean meats
- Fish and seafood

Plant Proteins:
- Beans
- Soybeans
- Chickpeas
- Nuts and seeds

Exercise

Exercise is recommended by the South Beach Diet to be an essential part of your daily life because it will boost your metabolism and help prevent weight loss plateaus.

Three Phases of the South Beach diet

Phase 1
This phase last two weeks. Its goal is to eliminate food cravings that are high in sugar and refined starches. The theory is by eliminating these simple carbohydrates, it will jump-start weight loss. This phase requires your diet to be almost free of carbohydrates (rice, bread, fruits, pasta, rice, bread, fruit juice and alcohol). In this phase, your diet should include lean protein, such as skinless poultry, lean beef, seafood, soy products, high-fiber vegetables, low-fat dairy, and foods with healthy, unsaturated fats, including avocados, nuts, and seeds.

Phase 2
This is a long-term weight loss phase and you stay in this phase until you reach your goal weight.

During this phase, the diet does allow you to add back complex carbohydrates such as vegetables, fruits, whole-wheat pasta, brown rice, whole-grain bread, brown rice, fruits, and more vegetables which were eliminated in phase 1.

Phase 3
This is the maintenance phase and is intended to be a healthy way to eat for life. The goal is that you follow the lifestyle principles that the first two phases introduced. You can eat all food types in moderation in this phase.

Results
The South Beach diet promotes that you will lose eight to 13 pounds in the first two weeks (Phase 1). It also makes the claim that most of the weight loss will be from your midsection. In Phase 2, the goal is to lose one to two pounds a week.

Risks
This diet is safe if followed as outlined. However, you may experience problems from ketosis (when you limit carbohydrate intake there is less glucose available for energy, so the body breaks down stored fat for energy. Ketones result from the metabolism of fat). Nausea, mental fatigue, headache, and bad breath, dizziness and dehydration are some of the side effects from ketosis.

8. Noom
Unlike most diets that focus creating weight loss by reducing calories by restricting the intake of carbohydrates, protein and fat, Noom uses a psychology-based approach to introduce healthy eating habits. According to its website, Noom uses technology, an app, to "help a person change not just how they eat, but how they think."

The convenience of the app is the key to this diet plan.

The Program

Noom's weight loss program is a comprehensive wellness plan that focuses on changing behaviours towards food, exercise, and mental health. The theory is that by changing your social behaviors you will loss weight and keep it off long-term.

1.Use their app – Enter your age, gender, weight, goal weight, general health and other aspects of your life such as your social circles.

2.Record daily your meals including any snacks– Based on this information the app provides feedback on food choices to help you reach your weight loss goals.

3.Record your daily exercise –Exercise recommendations are given to help motivate you to become more physically active. The app also has a pedometer to record how many steps you take each day.

4.Regular Feedback –A messaging feature is used by "your coach" to provide regular feedback and motivation to help over come any obstacles you may encounter. A virtual support group is also offered.

Over the initial 16-weeks of the program daily articles are provided about weight loss, nutrition, exercise, and advice to help prevent or manage chronic diseases like, diabetes, osteoarthritis, and high blood pressure. Interactive challenges to maintain motivation are also presented.

What You Can Eat and What You Can't

Nooms app encourages higher nutrition foods, smaller portions and fewer calories but no food is off limits. To simplify your nutrition plan, foods are colour coded (green, yellow, and red) based on their nutrient count to simplify eating. Fore example, Red doesn't mean bad and be avoided, but that these foods are higher in calories and should be eaten in smaller amounts.

Green foods – these should make up the bulk of your diet because they contain the most nutrients:
- Fruit: Bananas, strawberries, apples, oranges
- Vegetables: Greens and brightly coloured ones are recommended. Carrots, spinach, broccoli, bell peppers.
- Protein: Tofu.
- Dairy: Skim milk, non-fat Greek yogurt, non-fat cheese.
- Whole grains: Oatmeal, brown rice, quinoa, whole-grain bread

Yellow foods – these have fewer nutrients and more calories and eaten in moderate amount.
- Fish: Tuna, salmon
- Protein: Grilled chicken, turkey breast, lean ground beef, eggs
- Legumes: Black beans, chickpeas
- Dairy: Greek yogurt, low-fat cheese

- Grains: Whole-grain

Red foods – These need to be eaten less often and in smaller portions since they are low in nutrients and high in calories.
- Nuts: Almonds, cashews, walnuts
- Seeds: Flaxseed, sunflower seeds, chia seeds
- Nut butters: Peanut butter, almond butter.
- Oils: Olive oil, avocado oil, coconut oil

The color-coded ingredient lists and recipes available include a sufficient variety of foods so, weather you follow a specialized vegan or gluten free diet, you should have no problem accommodating to this diet recommendations.

THE NOOM DIET
WHAT CAN I EAT?

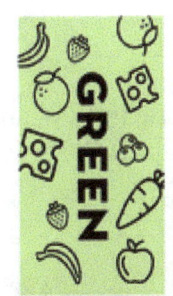

GREEN
- **HEARTY VEGGIES:** Carrots, sweet potatoes, spinach, broccoli, cucumbers
- **FRUITS:** Apples, strawberries, oranges, blueberries, apples, bananas, tomatoes
- **HEALTHY DAIRY:** Non-fat cheese and non-fat greek yogurt
- **WHOLE GRAINS:** Brown rice and oatmeal

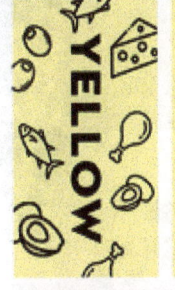

YELLOW
- **LEAN PROTEIN:** Tuna, salmon, turkey breast, and grilled chicken
- **BETTER DAIRY:** Yogurt and low-fat milk, plus eggs, and low-fat cheeses
- **HEALTHY FATS:** Avocado and olives
- **GRAINS AND LEGUME:** Black beans, chickpeas, quinoa, couscous, whole grain tortillas

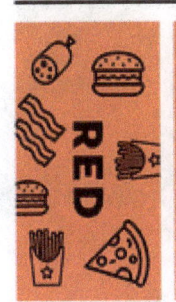

RED
- **PROCESSED MEAT:** Ham, bacon, salami
- **OILS AND CONDIMENTS:** Olive oil, coconut oil, avocado oil, mayonnaise, ranch
- **SUGAR:** Including sources like fruit juice
- **GUILTY PLEASURES:** Pizza, hamburgers, fries, chocolate

Image source: goodhousekeeping.com

Level of Effort

Daily recording of what you have eaten and how active you have been is necessary so the program to give you the right feedback and advise. Using the app could be a barrier for use for older adults who may not be too familiar in using this type of technology.

Virtual Coach/Support

The Noom's coaches can help with motivation and answer questions you may have but they aren't nutritionists and are more like behavior-change specialists that offer strategies and encouragement so you stay on track toward your weight loss goals.

Results

Research suggests that Noom does help people lose weight. The daily reminders and coaching tips for eating cooking, and exercise can be helpful, and may help you be more successful than doing it alone. As with all weight loss efforts, setting goals and changing unhealthy behaviors that could sabotage your actions are critical.

9. Weight-Watchers Diet

The company, Weight Watchers, has changed its name to WW and introduced its "myWW" program. In 2019 it was named the best weight loss diet in U.S. News & World Reports' annual Best Diets Assessment.

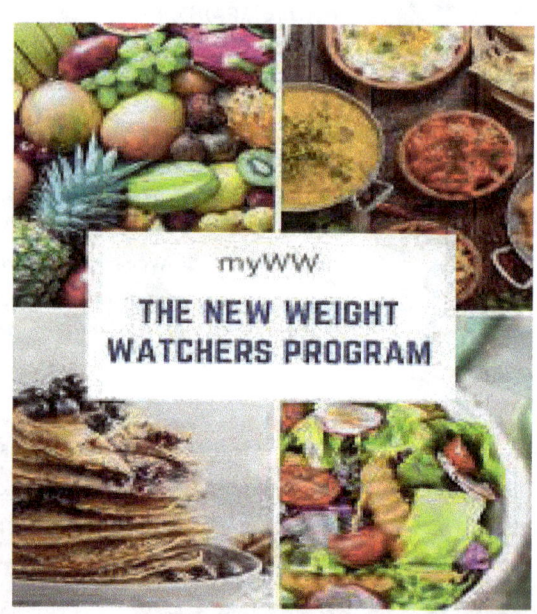

Image source: the pounddropper.com

Their motto is "eating what you love" remains and no food is off-limits but a colour-coding system is used to help move you towards healthier foods. The way it works is that you have a daily SmartPoints budget and some foods are designated as ZeroPoint. Based on the colour-coded plan you choose, you will either have a larger SmartPoints budget but fewer Zeropoint foods to choose from or, a smaller SmartPoint budget and a larger number of ZeroPoint foods to choose from.

MyWW Three Option Program

1. Green plan – This plan has over 100 ZeroPoint foods with the largest SmartPoints budget to spend on foods.
2. Blue plan – There are more (over 200) ZeroPoint foods but a smaller SmartPoints budget than the green plan.
3. Purple plan – This plan has the largest number (300) of ZeroPoint foods and the smallest SmartPoints budget.

The WWapp is used to track your SmartPoints budget, daily meals, exercises and help you build a virtual community.

Key Components to the MyWW Plan

1. Behaviour Modification

A big component of the MyWW plan is helping you improve behaviours like grocery shopping, healthy food preparation, cooking, dining out. The goal of modifying your behavour is to support your weight loss journey without sacrificing the enjoyment of eating.

2. Exercise

Exercise is encouraged and you will earn FitPoints for your activity. The more intensity the cardiovascular and strength training is, the more FitPoints are earned. The FitPoints are individualized to your sex, age, weight and height.

3. Personalized Coaching

MyWW plans are designed to be lifestyle-change program with regards to your nutrition, diet and activity level. The MyWW program provides an option of adding personal coaching to encourage and support these changes.

"Just-for-you recipes," exercise, life-style physical activity suggestions, and science-backed mindset/behavioural skills are included with the program and research has shown that personal coaching can help a person lock in these behavior and lifestyle changes.

What You Can Eat

Depending of which of the three MyWW plan (**Green**, **Blue**, **Purple**) you chose, will determine what foods you can eat. The different plans allow you to easy mix and match foods to suit your weight loss goals and taste preferences. Pre-packaged foods are available if that is your preference.

1. Smart Points

Every food is given a value (SmartPoints) based on calories, saturated fat, protein, and sugar.
These points are designed to help educate a person into healthier eating. The SmartPoint value of a food goes up the more calories, saturated fat, and sugar it has. As a result, your

SmartPoint budget will be used up quicker the more you consume foods with higher SmartPoints, therefore you are forced to eat less food to stay within your SmartPoint budget.

2. Personal SmartPoints budget –SmartPoints can be used any way you like, even on alcohol or dessert, as long as you stay within your daily SmartPoint budget target.

Your sex, age, height, weight, and height, used by the app to set your SmartPoint budget with the aim of helping you reach your goal weight.

MyWW plan is developed to be flexible with respect to the foods available to be eaten. As well, if your SmartPoints are not all used up on a particular day, you can bank up to four SmartPoints each day into your weekly SmartPoints budget.

3. ZeroPoint System

Each MyWW plan (Green, blue and purple) has its own list of ZeroPoint foods. These foods form the basis of a healthy eating pattern. A person can enjoy them without measuring or tracking.

Green Plan – The fewest amount of ZeroPoint foods allowed, all focused on fruits and veggies. But it has the largest SmartPoints budget to spend.

Blue Plan – SmartPoints budget shrinks but there are over 200 ZeroPoint foods, including fruits, vegetables, and lean proteins.

Purple Plan – Has the smallest SmartPoints budget but there are over 300 ZeroPoint choices including fruits, vegetables, lean proteins, and whole grains.

MyWW Plan Options

	Green	Blue	Purple
Min Daily Smart Points Allowance	30	23	16
Zero Smart Points Foods	About 100 Fruits Non-starchy Vegetables	About 200 Fruits vegetables Very Lean Proteins Eggs Legumes NonFat Dairy	About 300 Fruits Vegetables Very Lean Proteins Eggs Legumes Nonfat Dairy Whole Grains
Previous WW Program	Like Freestyle	Like Beyond the Scale	Like Simply Filling

Image source: pinterest.com

Level of Effort
Everything about the MyWW plan is focused on making it easier for a person to change their life-style and dietary habits for the long term. How much a person has to modify their eating and exercise habits and how willing they are to make those changes will dictate the amount of motivation, effort and determination necessary.

Results
The MyWWplan is a personalized weight loss program that focuses on wellness and building healthy habits. It has been well researched and these studies show that you can lose weight and keep it off by using this program.

The philosophy of the MyWW plan is that the process of losing weight is just a part of a comprehensive lifestyle plan. An added dimension of the WW program that it helps create a community of support to help you be successful.

WW is safe and suitable for anyone looking to improve their health. Its focuses on low-calorie foods that are nutritious which makes it great for people with high cholesterol, diabetes, high blood pressure, and heart disease.

This program is not cheap if you want to take advantage of all that is offered, however, if it helps you lose weight and keep it off, it is money well spent.

10. DASH Diet
(Also reviewed in Chapter 5.2.5. Salt)

Dietary Approaches to Stop Hypertension (DASH) is designed to help prevent and treat high blood pressure (hypertension). The diet is meant to be a life-long approach to healthy eating by encouraging a reduction of the sodium in your diet and to eat nutrient rich foods that help lower blood pressure. Foods's rich in as potassium, calcium, and magnesium help do this.

Helping to preventing osteoporosis, cancer, heart disease, stroke, and diabetes are other possible health benefits from following the DASH diet. Fruits, vegetables, fish, poultry, nuts, low-fat dairy foods, and moderate amounts of whole grains, are foods emphasized with the DASH diet

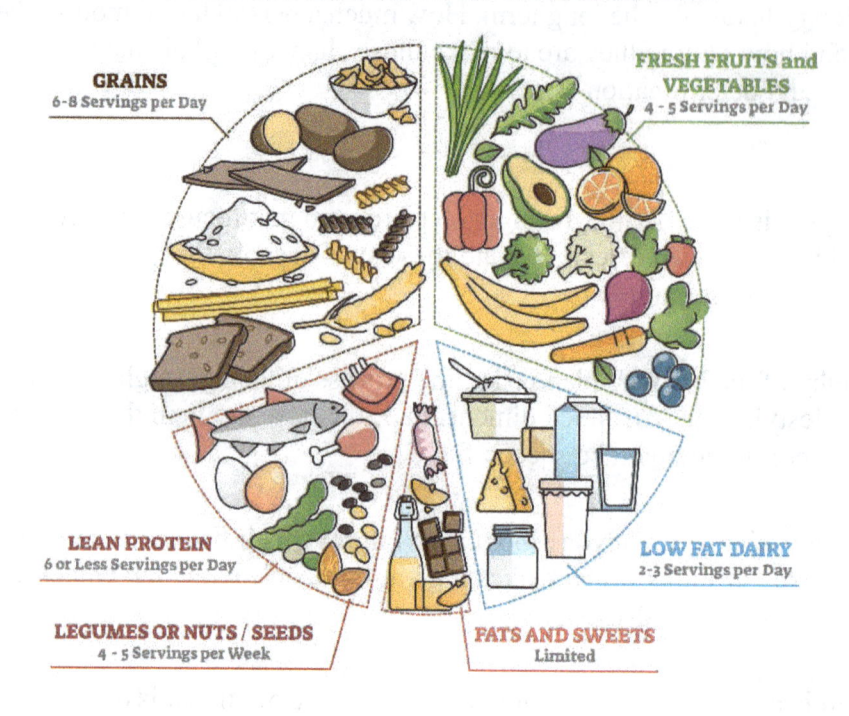

The DASH Diet
DIETARY APPROACHES TO STOP HYPERTENSION

GRAINS — 6-8 Servings per Day

FRESH FRUITS and VEGETABLES — 4 - 5 Servings per Day

LEAN PROTEIN — 6 or Less Servings per Day

LEGUMES OR NUTS / SEEDS — 4 - 5 Servings per Week

FATS AND SWEETS — Limited

LOW FAT DAIRY — 2-3 Servings per Day

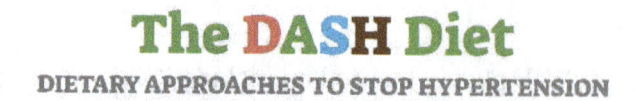

The typical daily sodium consumption in the North American diet is about 3,400 mg a day.

<u>**Standard DASH diet**</u> – No more than 2,300 milligrams (mg) of sodium a day.

<u>**Lower sodium DASH diet**</u> – limits the consumption of sodium to 1,500 mg day.

What You Can Eat

Whole grains, vegetables, fruits, vegetables, fish, poultry, legumes, low-fat dairy products, and a small amount of seeds, nuts, red meat, sweets, and healthy mono and poly-unsaturated fats are emphasized in the DASH diet. The diet is low in saturated fat, trans fat, and total fat.

Example: recommended servings from each food group for the 2,000-calorie-a-day DASH diet:

1. Grains: 6 to 8 servings / day	Bread, cereal, rice and pasta.
2. Vegetables: 4 to 5 servings / day	Carrots, tomatoes, sweet potatoes, broccoli, dark greens.
3. Fruits: 4 to 5 servings / day	Oranges, bananas, berries (strawberries, blue berries, raspberries) grapefruits.
4. Dairy: 2 to 3 servings / day	Milk, low-fat cheese, yogurt, eggs
5. Lean meat, poultry and fish: 6 one-ounce servings or fewer / day	Cutting back on meat portion will allow room for more vegetables.
6. Nuts, seeds and legumes: 4 to 5 servings / week	Walnuts, almonds, sunflower seeds, kidney beans, lentils, peas.
7. Fats and oils: 2 to 3 servings / day	Limit total daily fat to less than 30% of total calories. Mono and poly-unsaturated fats are emphasised.
8. Sweets: 5 servings or fewer / week	Sweets in moderation are allowed. Focus on cutting back on added sugar, (read nutrition labels, Chapter 5.2.2) which has no nutritional value but can pack on calories.
9. Caffeine	The DASH diet does not limit caffeine consumption but recognizes that caffeine can cause blood pressure to rise at least temporarily.

DASH Diet and Weight Loss

The DASH diet will help guide you toward healthier food choices and, in the process, help your loss weight but the real benefit of the DASH Diet, especially for the older adult, is that can effectively help manage or prevent high blood pressure.

Managing Sodium Dietary Intake

The foods emphasized in the DASH diet are naturally low in sodium by following the DASH diet, you will reduce your sodium intake. The following are suggestions to help you further reduce your daily sodium intake:

- Avoid adding salt when cooking. When flavouring food use sodium-free spices instead of salt. It can take weeks or months for your taste buds to get used to less salty foods so using spices helps with this transition.
- Buying foods labeled "no salt added," "sodium-free," "low sodium," or "very low sodium"
- Rinsing canned foods to remove some of the sodium

Exercise

You will have better success losing weight and lowering blood pressure if you combine the DASH diet with increase physical activity.

Conclusion

Losing weight and keeping it off is not easy. A person needs support from their doctor, dietitian, family and friends to succeeded long-term. If you are having trouble picking out a diet that is right for you or sticking to a particular diet, you need to talk to your doctor or dietitian rather than following gimmicky trends.

Healthy eating isn't an all-or-nothing proposition. Follow the 80/20 rule (Chapter 3.1. The Eight Golden Rules of Training) and show some self-compassion when things are not going well (Chapter 6.6: Self Compassion: The Proven Power of Being Kind to Yourself). Most importantly, you must make healthy life-long changes in the way in which you eat and how much exercise you get.

References

https://www.mayoclinic.org/healthy-lifestyle/weight loss/in-depth/weight loss/art-20048466
https://www.webmd.com/diet/a-z/noom-diet
https://www.webmd.com/diet/a-z/weight-watchers-diet

5.3. Sleep – Don't Ignore Its Importance for Recovery and Health

Introduction

Sleep, and its recuperative powers, are essential to living a healthy and productive life. Unfortunately, with the challenges of daily life, it is increasingly difficult to find the time and ability to get the necessary sleep. Older adults usually have more time to sleep, as most are retired and don't have the responsibility of raising children, but they generally find it increasingly hard to get a good quality of sleep. Insomnia, the inability to get adequate sleep, is common among older adults. Findings indicate that insomnia affects 31% to 38% of adults aged 18 to 64 years, and increases to 45% for those aged 65 to 79. Women tend to have a higher incidence of insomnia than men.

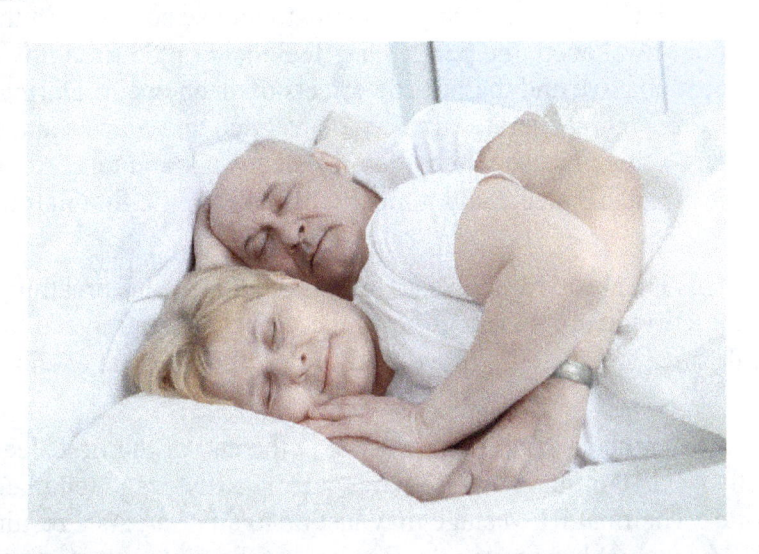

Eight hours of sleep a night is generally recommended to recover from the day's activities and prepare for the following day. Unfortunately, eight hours in bed does not correlate to eight hours of sleep. It is not uncommon for you to wake up in the morning after trying to get those eight hours of sleep and still feel tired.

The science of sleep is well researched, and sleep conditions that affect a person's sleep are now well understood. This chapter on sleep will try to bring clarity to the issue with the hope that a better understanding of sleep, the problems that affect sleep, and the techniques to improve it will lead you to have a better sleep.

What Happens When We Sleep?

During sleep, the body rests, and the brain gets "recharged," but the brain also stays active and controls many of the body's functions, including breathing.

Stages of Sleep

When you sleep, you typically drift between two sleep states, (1) Non-REM and (2) REM, in 90-minute cycles. (REM = rapid eye movement).

1. Non-REM Sleep – This sleep state has three stages, and each has distinct features.

Stage 1 – This is the "drowsiness sleep" stage, and occurs when you are first falling asleep. You can be easily awakened in this stage.

Stage 2 – In this stage, you are in "average sleep." It is not too deep, not too light, and it's where you typically spend about half the night.

Stage 3 – This is the "deep sleep" stage. Trying to arouse someone in this stage is more challenging, and once awakened, the person may feel disoriented for a few minutes. It is the stage where the most positive and therapeutic effects of sleep occur. During this stage of sleep, the body repairs and regenerates tissue such as bone and muscle and strengthens the immune system. Stage three is also when you may sleepwalk and talk. About 20% of the night is spent in deep Stage 3 sleep, and it mostly happens in the first half of the night.

2. REM sleep – This is the active sleep state where dreams occur, breathing and heart rate increase and become irregular, muscle groups relax or become paralyzed to keep you from acting out your dreams, and the eyes move back and forth under the eyelids.

REM sleep occurs 90 minutes after sleep onset or at the end of the first sleep cycle. The first REM period typically lasts 10 minutes, with each recurring REM stage lengthening as Stage 3 deep sleep gets shorter. The final REM stage may last up to an hour. As a result, most of your deep sleep (Non-REM Stage 3) happens in the first half of the night; most of your REM sleep occurs in the second half of the night.

Generally, as we get older, we sleep more lightly and get less restorative deep sleep (Non-REM Stage 3). As well, aging is associated with shorter periods of sleep, even though studies have shown that the amount of sleep needed doesn't appear to diminish with age.

WHY YOUR BODY LOVES SLEEP

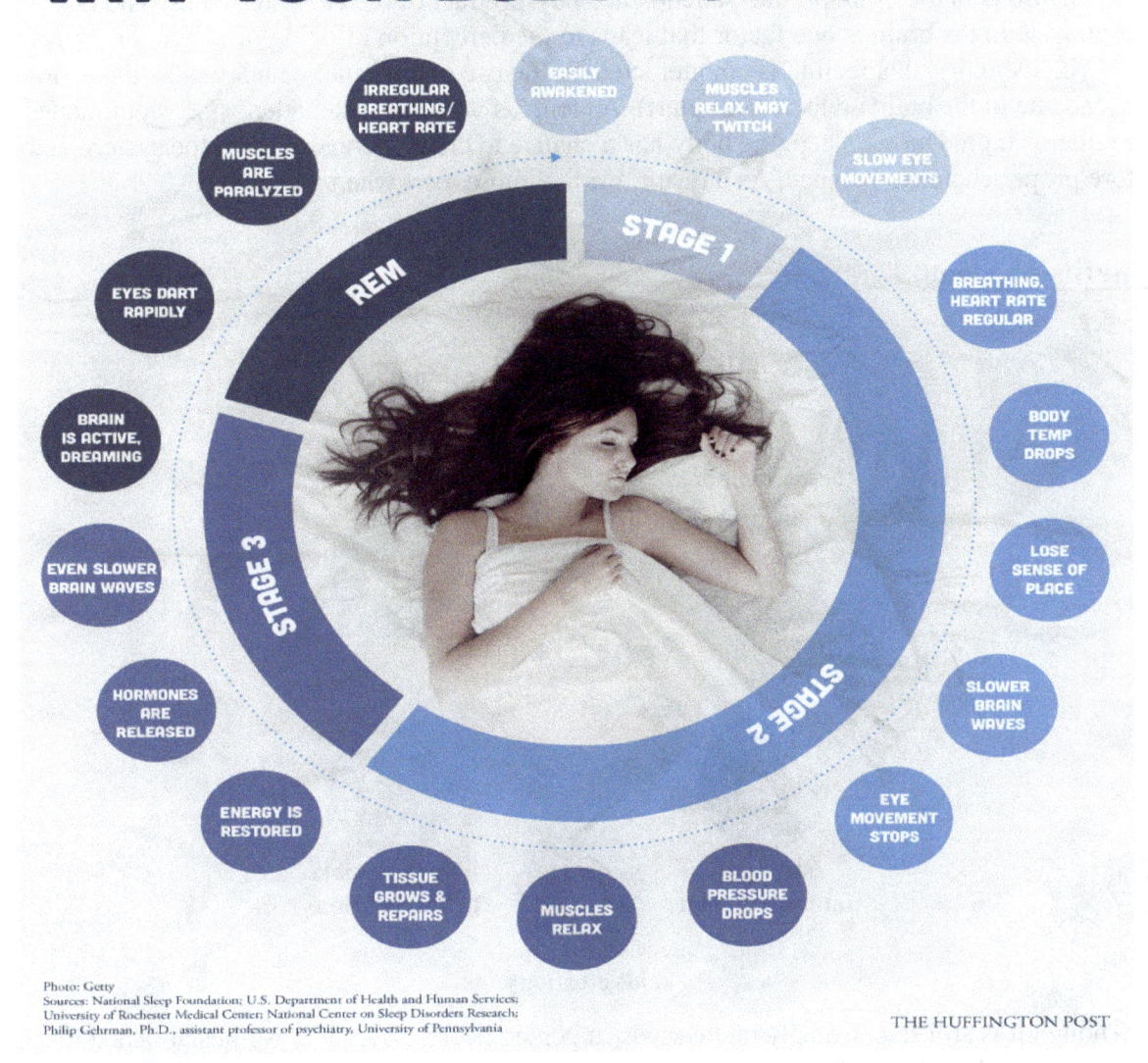

Photo: Getty
Sources: National Sleep Foundation; U.S. Department of Health and Human Services; University of Rochester Medical Center; National Center on Sleep Disorders Research; Philip Gehrman, Ph.D., assistant professor of psychiatry, University of Pennsylvania

THE HUFFINGTON POST

Why You Need Sleep

Over the years, many theories have been put forth on why we need sleep. One of the most respected is called the Restorative Theory.

This theory states that sleep serves to "restore" what is lost in the body while awake. In other words, sleep provides an opportunity for the body to repair and rejuvenate itself. This theory is supported by the fact that many of the primary restorative functions in the body like muscle growth, tissue repair, protein synthesis, and growth hormone release occur primarily, or in some cases only, during sleep. Interestingly, in a recent animal study, animals deprived entirely of sleep and not allowed "restorative time" lost all immune functions and died in just a matter of weeks.

To further support the restorative theory, it has been determined that other rejuvenating aspects of sleep are specific to the brain and cognitive function. For example, while a person is awake, neurons in the brain produce adenosine, a by-product of the cells' activities. The build-up of adenosine in the brain is one factor that leads to the perception of being tired and the "drive to sleep" (incidentally, this feeling is counteracted by the use of caffeine, which blocks the actions of adenosine in the brain and keeps us alert). As long as we are awake, adenosine accumulates and remains high. During sleep, the body has a chance to clear adenosine from the system and restore proper chemical balance. As a result, we feel more alert when we awake.

Benefits of Sleep

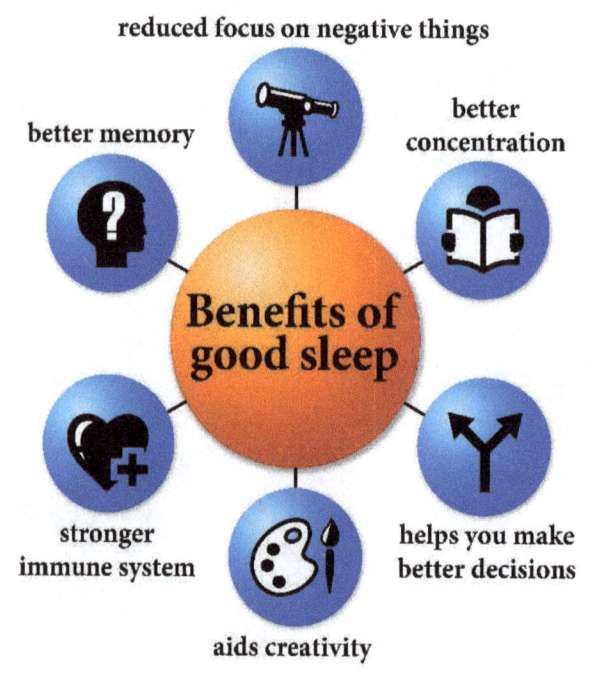

Though it is still scientifically unclear why a person needs sleep, it is well established that there are many health benefits of sleep.

1. Improved Memory – During sleep, mental memories are strengthened, and physical practice skills learned while a person is awake are ingrained. This mental ingraining process is called consolidation.

2. Longer life – Many long-term studies have shown that too little sleep is associated with a shorter lifespan due to sickness or disease due to a suppressed immune system.

3. Curb Inflammation – Inflammation is linked to heart disease, stroke, diabetes, arthritis, (Section 2: The Off-Season: Studying the Opposition) and premature aging. Research indicates that people who get less than six hours of sleep a night have higher blood levels of inflammatory proteins than those who get more sleep.

4.Creativity – Researchers have found that people seem to strengthen the emotional components of memory during sleep, which helps spur creativity.

5.Cognitive and Physical performance – Many studies have linked enhanced or deteriorating mental and physical performance to good or poor sleep patterns.

6.Weight control – Sleep and metabolism are controlled by the same brain sectors. When you are sleepy, Ghrelin, a hormone that increases appetite, goes up in the blood. Researchers found that dieters shed similar amounts of total weight regardless of sleep, but well-rested dieters lost more fat – 56% of their weight loss – while those who were sleep-deprived lost more muscle mass.

7.Avoiding Accidents – Sleeplessness affects physical agility, coordination, balance, cognitive reaction time, and decision-making. This is especially important to older adults because it means that sleep deprivation increases the risk of falling.

8.Managing Depression – Sleep has been found to reduce anxiety and impatience and stabilize mood. Sleep helps restore chemical balance in the brain to help those vulnerable to depression. For older adults, getting adequate sleep is very important for their mental health.

Chronic Medical Conditions Associated with Deprivation of Adequate Sleep

Complications of Insomnia

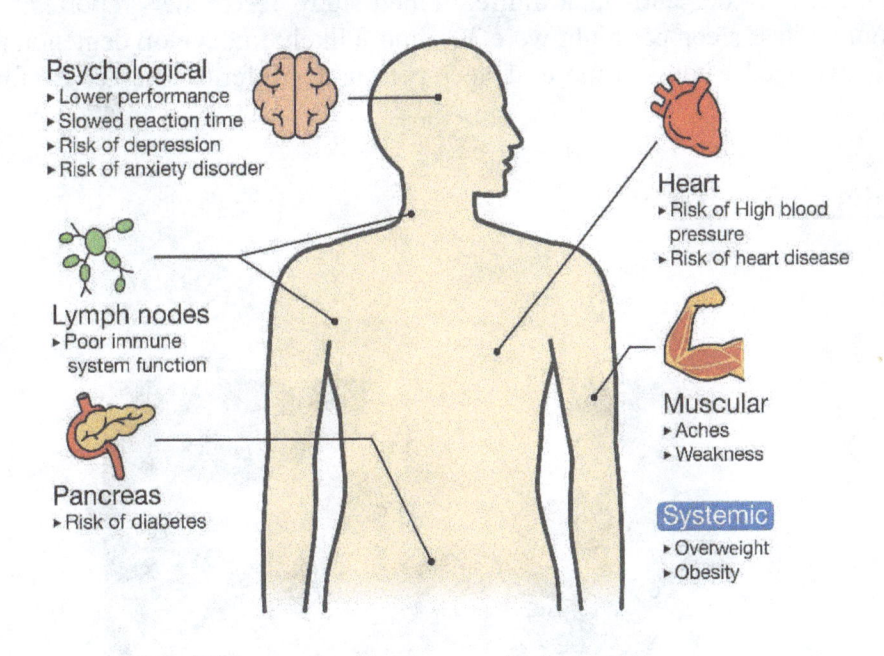

Psychological
- Lower performance
- Slowed reaction time
- Risk of depression
- Risk of anxiety disorder

Lymph nodes
- Poor immune system function

Pancreas
- Risk of diabetes

Heart
- Risk of High blood pressure
- Risk of heart disease

Muscular
- Aches
- Weakness

Systemic
- Overweight
- Obesity

1. Obesity – Several studies have linked insufficient sleep and weight gain. For example, studies have shown that people who habitually sleep less than six hours per night are much more likely to have a higher-than-average body mass index (BMI); people who sleep eight hours have the lowest BMI (refer to Chapter 2.5. for a comprehensive review of Obesity).

2. Diabetes – Researchers have found that insufficient sleep may lead to type 2 diabetes by influencing the way the body processes glucose (the high-energy carbohydrate that cells use for fuel). One sleep restriction study found that a group of healthy subjects who had their sleep cut back from eight to four hours per night processed glucose more slowly than they did when they were permitted to sleep 12 hours. If glucose is processed slowly between meals, any excess glucose is stored as fat (refer to Chapter 2.4. for a comprehensive review of Diabetes).

3. Heart Disease and Strokes – Studies have found that a single night of inadequate sleep for people who have existing hypertension can cause elevated blood pressure throughout the following day (refer to Chapter 2.2. for a review of Heart Disease).

4. Mood and Depression – In one study, subjects who slept four and a half hours per night reported feeling more stressed, sad, angry, and mentally exhausted than when well-rested. In another study, subjects who slept four hours per night showed declining optimism and sociability levels due to inadequate sleep. These self-reported symptoms dramatically improved when subjects returned to a standard 8-hour a night sleep schedule (refer to Chapter 6.3. for a comprehensive review of Depression).

5. Dementia – Researchers have found that getting chronic in-adequate sleep in your 50s and 60s can increase the risk for dementia later in life. In their study, researchers reported that people who got 6 hours or less sleep per night were 30% more likely to develop dementia than those who regularly averaged 7 hours or more of sleep per night. (Refer to Chapter 2.6 for a review of Dementia)

Sleep Disorders

1. Insomnia

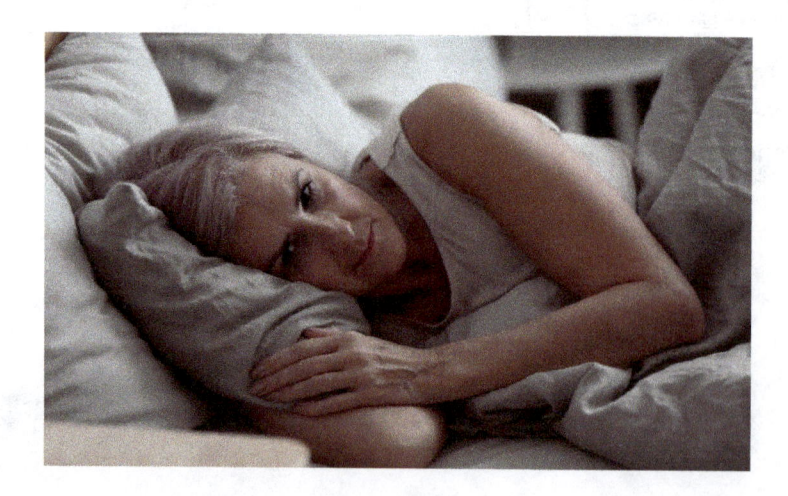

Insomnia is the most common sleep disorder in adults. Over one-third of the adult public report insomnia symptoms. For 10% of the population, insomnia is a persistent problem that impairs daytime functioning. Insomnia is common among older adults, women, shift workers, and people with medical or psychological disorders.

Insomnia is a condition that involves the following symptoms:
- Difficulty falling asleep
- Waking up frequently during the night
- Difficulty returning to sleep
- Waking up too early in the morning
- Un-refreshing sleep
- Daytime sleepiness
- Difficulty concentrating
- Irritability

<u>**Insomnia becomes a clinical problem when**</u>;
- You experience trouble falling asleep three or more nights per week
- Day time functioning is impaired
- Sleep difficulties have persisted for more than one month

Causes of Insomnia

- **<u>Emotional/Mental</u>** – stress, anxiety, and depression
- **<u>Physical</u>** – Chronic pain in joints from arthritis, frequent nighttime urination
- **<u>Medical</u>** – Respiratory, cardiovascular and digestive problems
- **<u>Medications</u>** – cold and allergies, heart, thyroid, pain, birth control, depression.

Treatment for Insomnia

> **PATIENT HANDOUT**
> ## A sleep hygiene checklist
>
> ☑ **Avoid naps.** Napping during the day can disturb the normal pattern of sleep and wakefulness.
>
> ☑ **Avoid stimulants,** such as caffeine and nicotine, and alcohol as bedtime approaches. While alcohol is well known to speed the onset of sleep, the process of the body metabolizing the alcohol can cause arousal, thus disrupting sleep.
>
> ☑ **Exercise.** All forms of exercise help to ensure sound sleep. Vigorous activities should be conducted in the morning or late afternoon, while a relaxing exercise, like yoga, can be done before bed to help initiate a restful night's sleep.
>
> ☑ **Avoid food too close to bedtime**—particularly large meals and chocolate (which contains caffeine). And try not to make any significant change to your diet. For example, if you're struggling with a sleep problem, it's not a good time to start experimenting with spicy dishes.
>
> ☑ **Soak up some natural light.** This is particularly important for older people who may not venture outside as frequently as children and younger adults. Light exposure helps maintain a healthy sleep-wake cycle.
>
> ☑ **Establish a regular bedtime routine.** Try to avoid emotionally upsetting conversations and activities before going to sleep.
>
> ☑ **Associate your bed with sleep.** It's not a good idea to watch television, use your computer or phone, listen to the radio, or read while in bed.
>
> ☑ **Ensure a pleasant, relaxing sleep environment.** The bed should be comfortable, and the room should not be too hot, cold, or bright.
>
> Adapted from: The National Sleep Foundation Web site. Available at: https://sleepfoundation.org/sleep-topics/sleep-hygiene. Accessed March 9, 2017.

1. Identify and treat the secondary cause – Secondary causes can be emotional (chronic stress), physical (joint pain), medical (indigestion, high blood pressure, asthma), medications (antidepressants, antihistamines for allergies).

2. Behavior Therapy

    a. Stimulus Control Therapy: This means creating a sleep environment that promotes sleep. This sleep environment involves a quiet and darkened room, comfortable bed, pillows, and sheets. Three hours before bedtime, no food, caffeine, alcohol is allowed.

    b. Cognitive Therapy: This involves learning to develop positive thoughts and beliefs about sleep. The goal is to think of going to bed and sleeping as a positive experience, not something to be labored through or dreaded. No reading or watching TV that is cognitively stimulating/arousing.

    c. Sleep Restriction: This involves following a program that limits the time in bed to get to sleep and stay asleep throughout the night.

3. Relaxation techniques – These include yoga, meditation, and guided imagery which may be especially helpful in preparing the body to sleep.

4. Exercise – Exercise fatigues the body and reduces mental stress, promoting deeper sleep. However, to reduce the effect of endorphins that are released during exercise, a person who has difficulty sleeping should exercise earlier in the day

5. Nutrition – It is important to follow a properly balanced diet by minimizing fat, sugar, nicotine, caffeine, and alcohol intake (alcohol is known to speed up the onset of sleep, but it disrupts sleep in the second half as the body begins to metabolize the alcohol, causing arousal). There should be no heavy meals close to bedtime (this is important for weight control as well).

6. Good sleep hygiene – Maintaining a regular wake and sleep pattern is important. Going to bed at the same time each evening helps get the mind and body in the routine of telling itself that it is "time to sleep."

7. Medications/sleep aids (hypnotics) – Sleep medications for the treatment of insomnia are called hypnotics. You should only take them when:

- The cause of insomnia has been evaluated by a medical doctor or a sleep specialist.
- The sleep problems are causing difficulties with your daily activities.
- Appropriate sleep-promoting behaviors are unsuccessful.

It is important to note that there are possible side effects of taking hypnotics such as morning sedation, memory problems, headaches, sleepwalking, and a night or two of poor sleep after stopping the medication. Women who are pregnant or nursing should not take hypnotics.

2. Sleep Apnea

Sleep Apnea is a type of sleep disorder characterized by pauses in breathing or instances of shallow or infrequent breathing during sleep. Each pause in breathing, called apnea, can last from at least ten seconds to several minutes and may occur five to thirty times or more in an hour.

An individual with sleep apnea is rarely aware of having difficulty breathing, even upon awakening. Usually, sleep apnea is recognized as a problem by others witnessing the individual having apnea episodes during sleep or suspected because of its effects on the body (increased appetite and weight gain, increased drowsiness during the day). Symptoms may be present for years (or even decades) without identification. During this time, the sufferer of sleep apnea may become conditioned to the daytime sleepiness and fatigue associated with significant levels of sleep disturbance.

The diagnosis of sleep apnea is confirmed with an overnight sleep test called a polysomnogram, or "sleep study."

Types of Sleep Apnea

1. Obstructive sleep apnea – (84%) – This occurs when the soft tissue in the back of a person's throat relaxes during sleep and blocks the airway. This often causes the person to snore loudly.

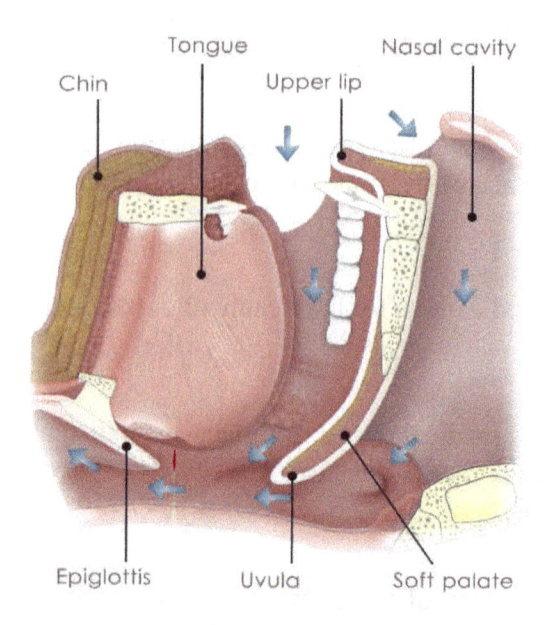

Open airway during sleep

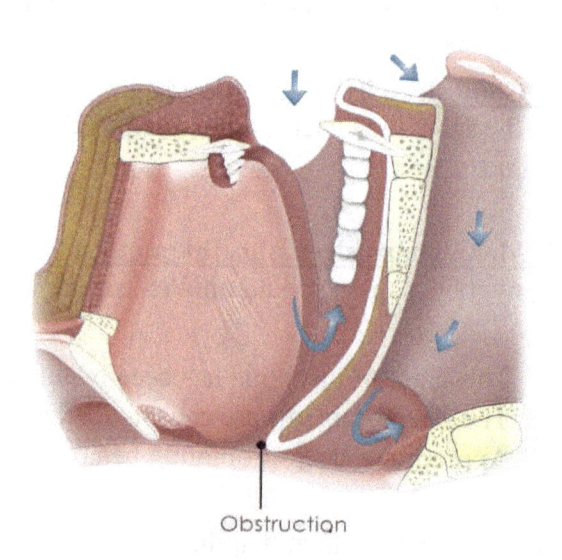

Sleep apnea present with obstruction

2. Central sleep apnea – (4%) – This involves the central nervous system and is due to the brain failing to signal the muscles that are controlling breathing. People with central sleep apnea seldom snore.

3. Complex sleep apnea – (12%) – This is a combination of obstructive sleep apnea and central sleep apnea.

What Happens During a Sleep Apnea Episode?

During each pause in breathing (apnea), the airflow to the lungs stops, as well as the oxygen level in the blood. The brain responds by briefly disturbing your sleep long enough to kick start breathing, which often resumes with a gasp or a choking sound.

1. Obstructive sleep apnea –You probably won't remember these awakenings. Most of the time, you will stir just enough to tighten your throat muscles and open your windpipe.

2. Central sleep apnea – You may be conscious of your awakenings.

Clinical Significance/Risk during an Apnea Episode

The breathing pauses (apnea) reduce blood oxygen levels, which puts additional strain on the heart and cardiovascular system by raising blood pressure, which increases the risk of stroke or heart attack. Reduces blood oxygen levels is potentially very serious for the older adult whose health may already be compromised due to high blood pressure, heart and lung disease.

Major signs and symptoms of sleep apnea

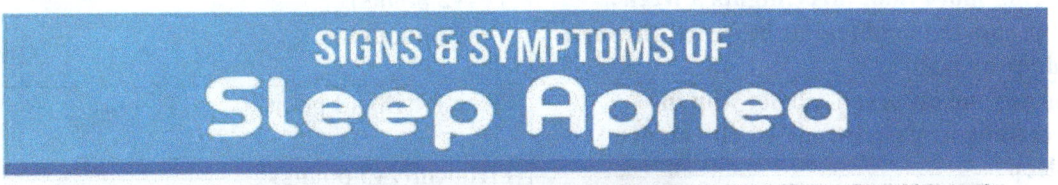

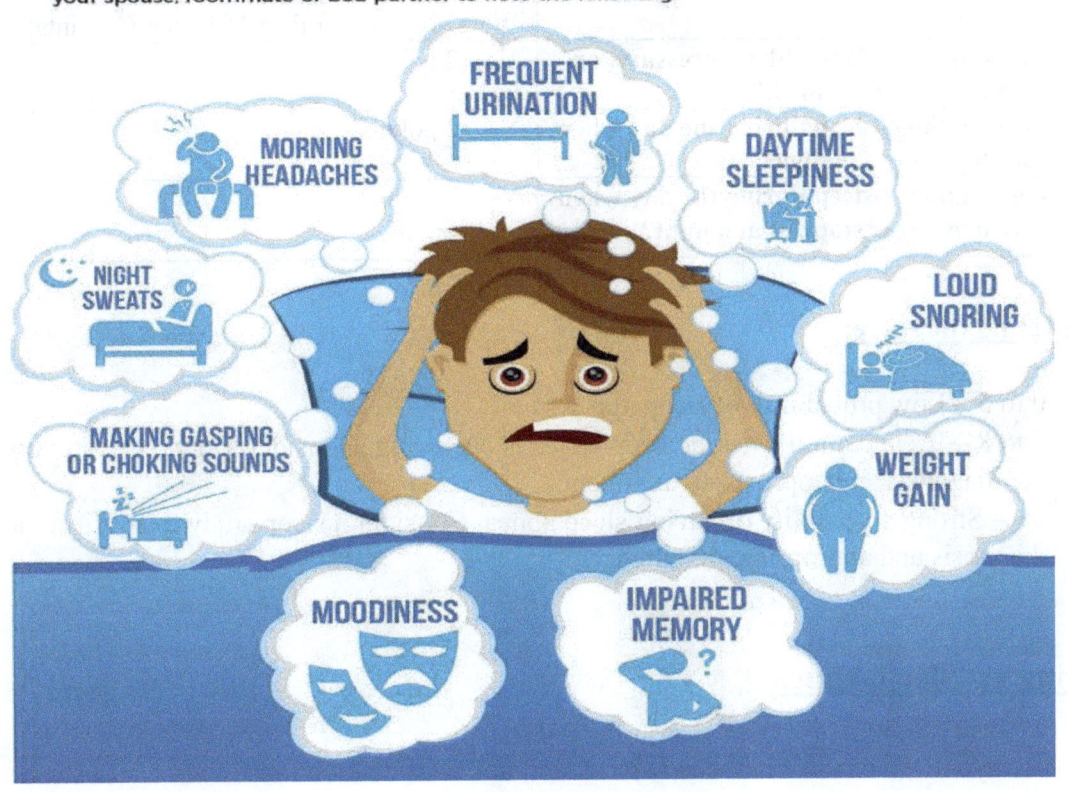

Image Source: gpsdentalsa.com

- Pauses in breathing occur while snoring and possibly choking or gasping following the pauses.
- Fighting sleepiness during the day, at work, or while driving. You may find yourself rapidly falling asleep during the quiet moments of the day when you are not active.

- Morning headaches.
- Memory or learning problems and not being able to concentrate.

- Feeling irritable, depressed, or having mood swings or personality changes.
- Waking up frequently to urinate.
- Dry mouth or sore throat on waking.

Do You Have Sleep Apnea?

These questions can help determine if you should be tested for sleep apnea.

Question	Score
1. Snoring more than three nights a week?	Yes (2 points)
2. Is the snoring loud (can it be heard through a door or wall)?	Yes (2 points)
3. Has anyone observed a brief stop in breathing or gasp for air when you are asleep?	Occasionally (3 points) Frequently (5 points)
4. Collar size?	Men – Greater than 17 inches (5 points) Women – Greater than 16 inches (5 points)
5. Is there a history of high blood pressure, or are you being treated for it?	Yes (2 points)
6. Dozing or falling asleep during the day when you are not busy or active?	Yes (2 points)
7. Dozing or falling asleep during the day when you are driving or stopped at a light?	Yes (2 points)

Interpreting the score:

- 0 to 5 – Low probability of sleep apnea.
- 6 to 8 – It's uncertain whether sleep apnea is occurring. Consider a sleep study to confirm the diagnosis and appropriate treatment.
- 9+ – Strong probability of having sleep apnea. Consider a sleep study to confirm the diagnosis and appropriate treatment.

Snoring vs. Sleep Apnea

Not everyone who snores has sleep apnea, and not everyone who has sleep apnea snores.

The most significant telltale sign is how you feel during the day. Typical snoring doesn't interfere with the quality of your sleep (though it may significantly affect your sleep partner's quality of sleep) as much as sleep apnea does. Therefore, you are less likely to suffer extreme fatigue and sleepiness during the day.

Risk Factors for Sleep Apnea

Risk Factors for Obstructive Sleep Apnea	Risk Factors for Central Sleep Apnea
<ul><li>Overweight</li><li>Male</li><li>Related to someone who has sleep apnea</li><li>Over the age of 65</li><li>Black, Hispanic, or a Pacific Islander</li><li>A smoker</li><li>Thick neck (>17")</li><li>Deviated septum</li><li>Receding chin</li><li>Enlarged tonsils or adenoids</li><li>Allergies or medical conditions that cause nasal congestion or blockage</li></ul>	<ul><li>Male</li><li>Over age 65</li><li>Heart disease</li><li>Stroke</li><li>Neurologic Disease</li><li>Spinal or brain stem injury</li></ul>

Treatment for Sleep Apnea

Self-Help Treatments (Very Similar to Insomnia)
Lifestyle modifications can go a long way in reducing sleep apnea symptoms.

1. Weight loss – Overweight people have extra tissue in the back of their throat, which can fall over the airway and block the airflow into the lungs while they sleep.

2. Quitting smoking – Smoking is believed to contribute to sleep apnea by increasing inflammation and fluid retention in the throat and upper airway.

3. Avoiding alcohol, sleeping pills, and sedatives – Observe this avoidance before bedtime as they relax the muscles in the throat and interfere with breathing.

4. Avoiding caffeine and heavy meals – Observe this avoidance within two hours of going to bed.

5. Maintaining regular sleep hours – Sticking to a steady sleep schedule will help with relaxation. Apnea episodes decrease when you get plenty of sleep and rested.

Bedtime Tips for Preventing Sleep Apnea

1. Sleep on the side – You should avoid sleeping on your back, as gravity makes it more likely for the tongue and soft tissues to drop and obstruct the airway.

2. The tennis ball trick – To keep from rolling onto your back while you sleep, you could sew a tennis ball into a pocket on the back of their pajama top or wedge a pillow stuffed with tennis balls behind your back.

3. Prop the head up – Elevate the head of the bed by four to six inches or elevate the body from the waist up by using a foam wedge. A special cervical pillow can also be used.

4. Open the nasal passages – Try to keep nasal passages open at night using a nasal dilator, saline sprays or breathing strips.

Medical Treatment Options

1. Continuous Positive Airflow Pressure (CPAP) Machine

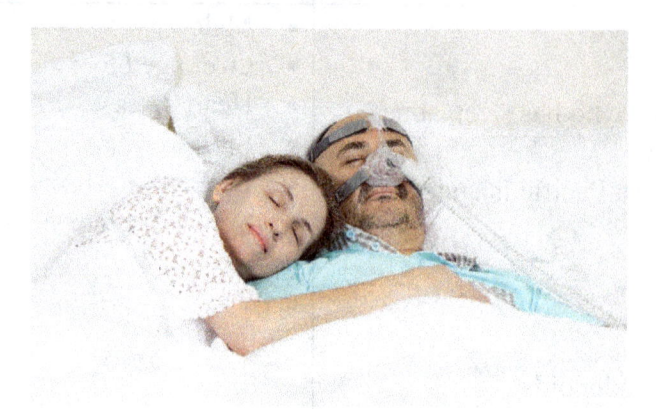

   The CPAP machine is the most common treatment for moderate to severe obstructive sleep apnea. The CPAP device is a mask-like machine that provides a constant stream of air that keeps the breathing passages open while a person sleeps. Most CPAP devices are the size of a tissue box.

   In many cases, the patient will experience immediate symptom relief and a huge boost in their mental and physical energy.

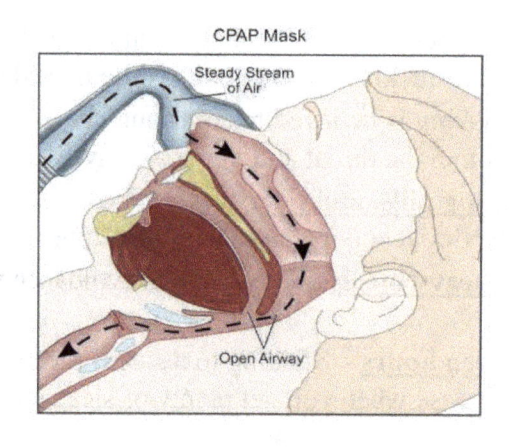

Image Source: cpapdepot.co.au

2. Dental Devices for Sleep Apnea
   Dental devices are usually only effective for mild to moderate sleep apnea. Most dental devices are acrylic and fit inside the mouth, much like an athletic mouth guard. Their purpose is to adjust the position of the lower jaw. Two common oral devices are the mandibular repositioning device and the tongue retaining device. These devices open the airway by bringing the lower jaw or tongue forward during sleep.

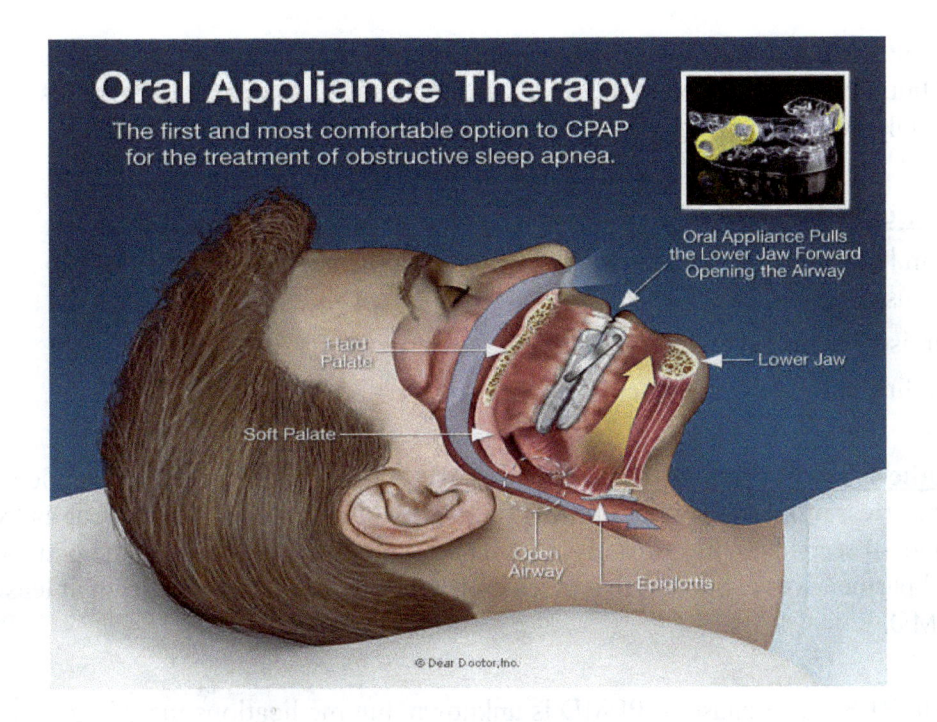

Image Source: midlandparkfamilydentistry.com

It is very important to get fitted by a dentist specializing in sleep apnea and see the dentist regularly for any potential dental/oral problems. It may also be necessary to have the dentist occasionally adjust the mouthpiece to fit better.

3. Surgery as a Treatment for Sleep Apnea

If a person has exhausted other apnea treatment options, they may want to discuss surgical options with their doctor or sleep specialist. Surgery can increase the size of your airway, thus reducing your episodes of sleep apnea.

The surgeon may remove tonsils, adenoids, or excess tissue at the back of the throat or inside the nose. The surgeon may alternatively reconstruct the jaw to enlarge the upper airway. Surgery carries risks of complications and infections, and in some rare cases, symptoms can worsen after surgery.

3. Leg Movement Disorders

There are two leg movement disorders that can lead to poor sleep and daytime drowsiness. Both of these conditions can occur in the same person.

1. Restless Legs Syndrome (RLS) —Older adults often are affected by this condition. It is estimated that more than 20% of people over 80 years old suffer from this condition. People with RLS experience uncomfortable tingling and crawling or pins and needles feelings in their legs. These uncomfortable feelings in the legs often make it hard for the older adult to fall asleep or stay asleep, resulting in day time drowsiness.

RLS, is not usually related to a serious underlying medical problem. Its cause is not fully understood but it has been linked to medical conditions such as nerve abnormalities, kidney failure and dialysis, and iron deficiency.

Treatment usually involves:
- Warm baths or packs and massaging of the legs (usually lower legs) to help relax lower leg muscles.
- Exercise – helps blood circulation in the lower legs.
- Avoiding caffeine.

2. Periodic Limb Movement Disorder (PLMD) – This condition causes people to jerk and kick their legs (less often in the upper limbs) frequently during sleep. It can occur as frequently as every 20 to 40 seconds. Unfortunately, PLMD not only disrupts sleep for the patient but also for their bed partner. It is estimated that at least 40% of older adults suffer from at least a mild form of PLMD.

Similar to RLS, exact cause of PLMD is unknown, but medications including antidepressants, antihistamines, and some antipsychotics are known to make the condition worse. Just like RLS, PLMD may be related to problems with limb nerve conduction due to diabetes or kidney disease or low iron levels

If symptoms are severe enough, treatment usually involves prescription medication to minimize limb movements.

Safe Sleeping Tips for Older Adults

As mentioned previously, insufficient sleep by older adults can lead to a higher risk of falls and deteriorating mental health.

Fall prevention safety tips include:

1. Keep a telephone and a list of important phone numbers by the bed – Receiving a phone call during the night can be both disturbing and startling. You do not want to have to "jump" out of bed, half-asleep, to get to the other side of the room for your phone. It is also important to have a phone close to the bed to call for help from bed in the event of an emergency. A list of significant phone numbers should be put by the phone on the nightstand beside your bed.

If you keep a cell phone beside your bed, turn it to mute so you are not disturbed when you receive notifications.

2. When in bed, a light switch should be is within easy reach – This will reduce stumbling in the dark if there is a need to get out of bed (night time urination). Motion sensor lights are effective in bedrooms, hallways and bathroom.

3. Reduce hazards in the bedroom – Rugs, stools, furniture and electrical cords, stools, should be removed from walking areas so they don't become trip hazards, especially in the dark.

Conclusion

The amount and quality of sleep a person gets is necessary and essential for living a healthy and productive life. For older adults, early detection of the signs and symptoms of sleep deprivation (insomnia) or sleep apnea is a vital component in managing potential physical and mental health challenges that they are already vulnerable to.

It is clinically important for you to get your "beauty" sleep. A good quality sleep, along with a solid nutritional plan/diet and maintaining flexibility, is necessary to defend the body against the health challenges (Section 2: Studying the Opposition to the Older Adults Health) and to assist the offense (Section 4: The Offense: Getting Active the Right Way) in promoting a healthy lifestyle. Managing sleep needs to be a significant part of everyone's fitness and health plan.

References

www.nia.nih.gov
www.sleepfoundation.org
www.webmd.com
www.betterhealthwhileaging.net
http://forever-active.com/sleep-insomnia-and-sleep-apnea/

Section 6

Special Teams – Mental Health: Supporting the Offense and Defense

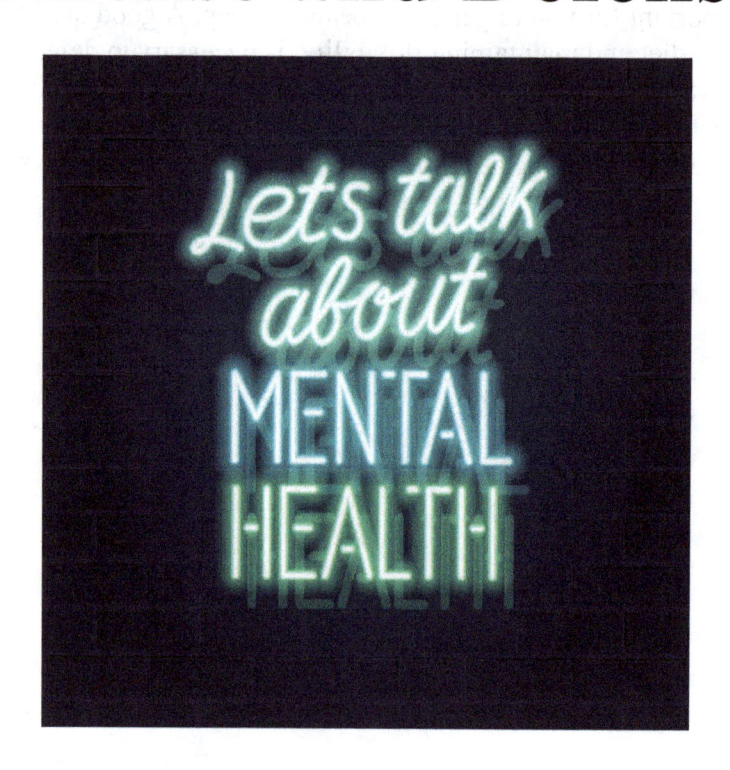

6.0. Introduction: Special Teams – Mental Health – Supporting the Offense and Defense

Special teams are essential to a football team. How well a team executes kickoffs, kick returns, punting, and punt returns often determine a win or a loss. Special teams may not get the hype and attention that the offense or defense gets, but they play a vital role in supporting the offense and defense.

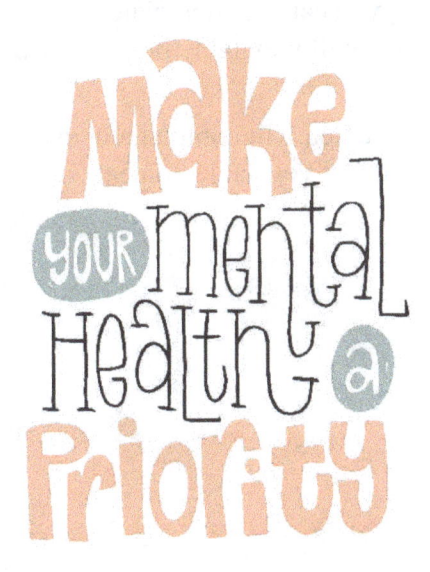

Make your mental health a priority

In Forever Active Older Adult Health and Fitness Playbook, the special teams focus is on mental health. Without being mentally healthy, you cannot successively implement the offense and defense health and fitness plans that you developed. The older adult faces many health challenges (Section 2 – The Off-Season: Studying the Opposition to Older Adults Health), functional mobility and social isolation challenges. The ability of older adults to mentally handle these challenges in a healthy and productive manner dramatically influences their quality of life.

This special team's section has 14 topics/chapters. Each topic has a significant role in influencing older adults' mental health and, in fact, all people's mental health, regardless of their age.

6.1. Understanding and Managing Cognitive Health
6.2. The Six Components of Wellness
6.3. Understanding Depression
6.4. Developing Mental Fitness
6.5. Finding Meaning/Purpose in Life
6.6. Self-Compression: The Proven Power of Being Kind to Yourself
6.7. Self-Leadership
6.8. Learning from Others Through Good Communication Techniques
6.9. Mindfulness and Mindfulness Meditation
6.10. Make Life a Joyful Journey

6.11. Dealing with Grief
6.12. Social Intimacy
6.13. Physical and Sexual Intimacy
6.14. Find Zen in Your Life

Each of these topics should be considered a building block used to become mentally stronger. No matter how physically strong, flexible, agile, and well-fed you may be, if you are not emotionally and mentally healthy, you cannot appreciate all that is good in your life nor manage the bad and sometimes the ugly that will inevitably present itself.

Embracing the information presented will complement every abdominal crunch, bicep curl, mile walked, ran or biked, and fruit and vegetable you eat.

6.1. Understanding and Managing Cognitive Health

By: Ann Fitzhenry Bedard, MSc. Occupational Therapy

Introduction

In Section 2, The Off-Season – Studying the Opposition, Dementia was discussed (Chapter 2.6.) as a potentially significant opponent to the older adult's mental health and quality of life. Dementia was defined as an umbrella term describing declining cognitive health symptoms to varying degrees. It stressed that minor declining cognitive health of older adults was expected, and this was referred to as "age-associated memory loss." The term "mild cognitive impairment" was a term used to describe individuals who fall between what is considered normal age-related cognitive changes and the early signs of dementia.

This chapter focuses on what is meant by cognitive health and how a person can optimize cognitive skills to improve their mental health so they can enjoy the highest quality of life possible.

Cognitive Health Defined

Good cognitive health means having good conscious intellectual skills (cognitive skills) such as thinking, speaking, reasoning, planning, problem-solving, and memory. Cognitive skills allow you to manage your daily life and personal affairs, maintain social relationships, enjoy meaningful connections with friends and family, complete hobbies, work or volunteer activities, and travel. As such, they are critical to your quality of life.

To perform these cognitive skills effectively requires a complex and highly sophisticated interplay of several neurological activities originating in the brain. Your overall cognitive ability depends not just on each cognitive skill individually but the interaction of several of these skills. As the brain begins to shrink (atrophy) in size as part of the normal aging process (.5-1% after the age of 60), the neurological activity necessary to perform these cognitive skills begins to be compromised. With progressive atrophy, the symptoms of dementia may begin to show themselves, and cognitive health declines.

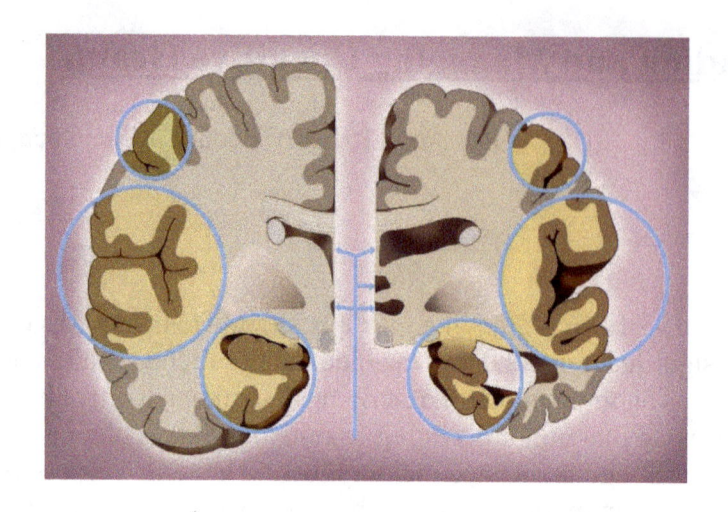

Key Cognitive Skills and their Interactions for Strong Cognitive Health

Key Cognitive Skills:
1. Attention
2. Memory
3. Language
4. Thinking, planning and problem solving

1. Attention – Attention is the ability to focus on the sensory (vision, hearing, touch) information being presented to you. This involves the following components:

Sustained attention – Not letting your mind wander from the task you are doing.
Filtering out background/unimportant information – Focusing on the key details and not being distracted by noises or activity in another part of the room.
Shifting your attention – Smoothly from one concept or activity to another, whether in a conversation, following directions or moving between two tasks such as answering the phone while cooking.

2. Memory – Memory is a complex skill dependent upon attention to ensure that appropriate/significant information is selected and encoded, is available to be stored, and can be retrieved as needed.

The major sub-categories of memory are:

Short term memory – It allows you to recall straightforward information needed for a short time only, such as a grocery list or why you went to the basement.
Working memory – It allows you to remember and hold multiple ideas or concepts in your mind to complete complex tasks such as organizing an event, writing a letter, or having a theoretical discussion with a group of friends.
Long-term memory – This is a broad term that includes remembering people and events that happened in your past. It is usually preserved even after short-term and working memories have diminished.
Types of Long-term Memory:
- **Declarative memory** – this is recalling facts of one's life. This includes people who have been in one's life, their names and where they have been.

Lapses in these kinds of memory are among the first signs of showing mild cognitive impairment or early dementia.
- **Procedural memory** – this frequently overlooked type of memory refers to your ability to complete activities that were previously learned very well, such as playing the piano, riding a bicycle, or cooking a favorite meal. Sometimes referred to as "muscle memory."

3. Language – This refers to the ability to understand and communicate verbal information, whether spoken or written. It requires two essential processes:

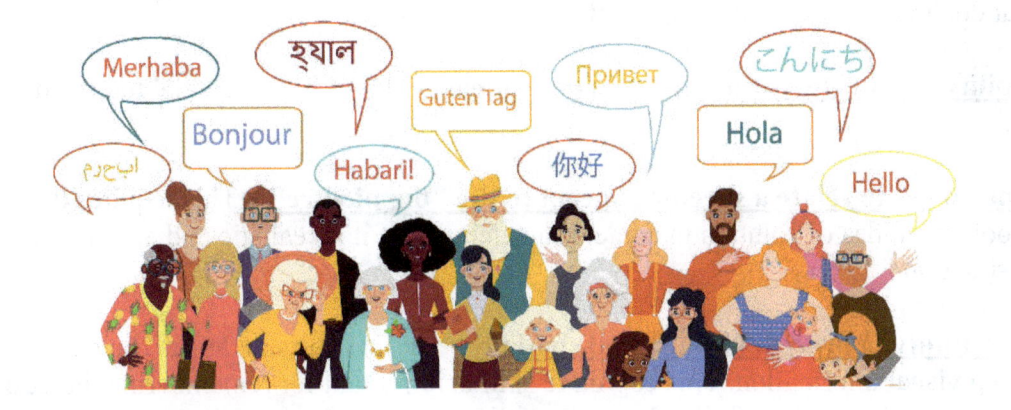

- **Receptive skills** – These are required to listen, read and understand the information presented. Attention and working memory both contribute to competency in receptive skills.
- **Expressive skills** – These allow you to communicate your ideas verbally or in writing. A good example of difficulty with expressive skills and a common issue for older adults is their challenge of finding the correct words to express themselves. "It's on the tip of my tongue" is a normal phenomenon, that with declining cognitive health, often becomes a significant cognitive/speech impairment, where an older adult frequently cannot find the correct words that they want to use.

4. Thinking, Planning and Problem Solving

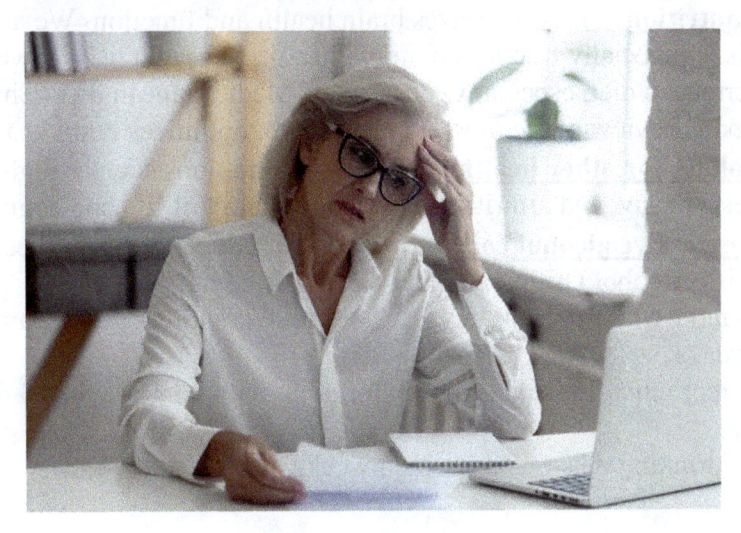

403

These cognitive skills are interrelated and depend significantly upon each of the cognitive abilities outlined above: attention, memory, and language. In order to solve a problem or plan an activity, you need to be able to pay attention to the relevant information, interpret visual input, understand any verbal communication, and hold key ideas in your head simultaneously.

Building on the four Key Cognitive Skills above, you need the following cognitive skills:

1. Ability to generate a wealth of ideas and discard those that are not helpful – Often called "brainstorming," this is the ability/skill to distinguish between those ideas that work and those that don't is an important component of this skill set.

2. Ability to sequence or organize steps or ideas – This skill is essential to effective planning.

3. The ability to relate a specific concept to the "big picture" – This requires the cognitive skill to look at an idea or solution in context to determine if it is realistic and appropriate to the specific situation.

4. The ability to process visually and spatially – This involves understanding and interpreting visual information. This cognitive skill is important for remembering directions, how to put things together such as fixing the coffee maker, organizing a garden layout and driving safely.

Maintaining Strong Cognitive Health

1. Follow the general health recommendations outlined throughout Forever Active Older Adult Health and Fitness Playbook.
These include:

- **Regular Exercise** – This has been shown repeatedly to have a strong protective effect on cognitive skills.
- **Adequate sleep** – This is essential for mental awareness.
- **Good nutrition** – This optimizes brain health and function. We are what we eat, and this is especially true for cognitive health. Research has shown that the Mediterranean diet, especially the "green" Mediterranean diet (Chapter 5.10 Weight Loss and a Review of the most popular diets), optimizes brain health and function.
- **Controlling for other health concerns** – Conditions such as high blood pressure, diabetes, obesity, and arthritis affects your quality of life and cognitive health.
- **Avoid excessive alcohol consumption** – To reduce long-term health risks, Canada's Low-Risk Alcohol Drinking Guidelines recommend:
  – No more than 10 drinks a week for women, with no more than 2 drinks a day most days.
  – No more than 15 drinks a week for men, with no more than 3 drinks a day most days.
  – Not drinking on some days each week.

Note – many health experts feel these guidelines are far too liberal and a person should significantly limit or eliminate their alcohol consumption.
- **Avoid abusive drug use** – This includes legal and illegal drugs. With older adults, excessive use of pain medication is a potential problem. It can contribute to marked difficulties in their cognitive abilities.

2. Meditation

Meditation has been found to be effective in enhancing concentration and focus while reducing chronic anxiety and stress, which can interfere with cognitive function.

3. Stay Mentally Active

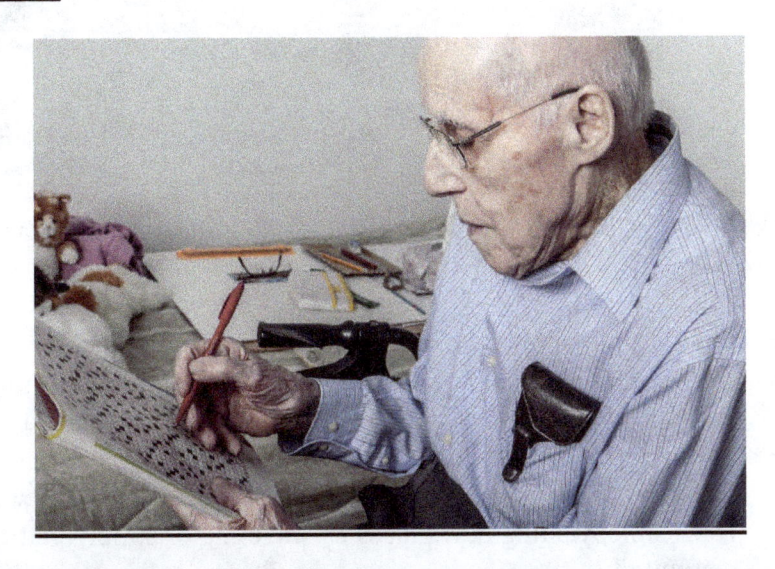

- **Stay engaged in hobbies and pastimes that keep you thinking** – This can be reading, writing, playing games, knitting, woodworking, stamp or coin collecting, etc.
- **Learn new skills** – Whether you take an art class or learn a new language, develop computer skills or follow through on another new interest, it all helps to keep you engaged. Research has shown that tackling activities that are more demanding and taking you out of your comfort zone can be especially helpful in protecting your cognitive abilities.

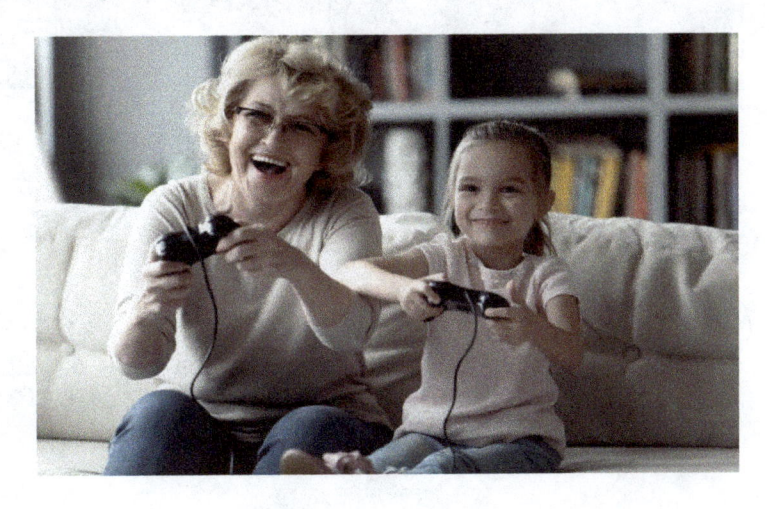

4. Stay Connected:

It is important to have both a sense of purpose and a sense of connection.

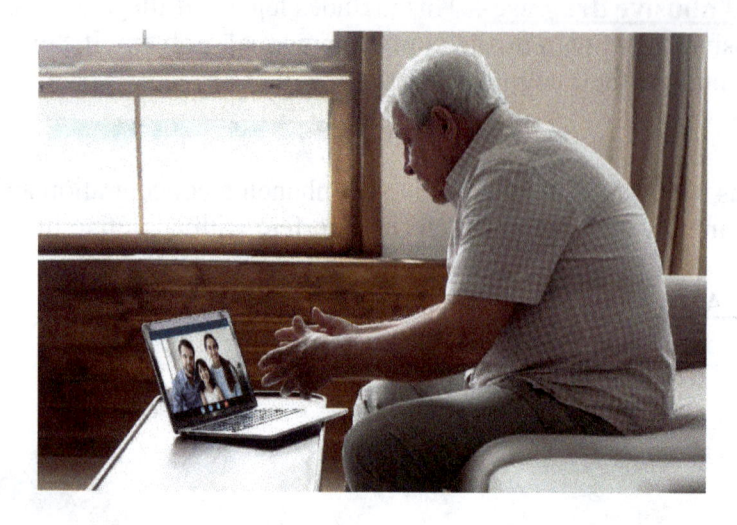

Research has shown the tremendous benefits of maintaining social interaction and relationships as you age. This includes:

- Regular interactions with family and friends.
- Volunteering, which is a terrific way to remain involved in your community and can provide a sense of purpose or meaning to your day.
- Participating in clubs and groups that allow you to exchange ideas and consider new perspectives on books, movies, political ideas, and more.
- If possible, visiting new places by traveling or simply getting out in your community

5. Manage Your Environment:

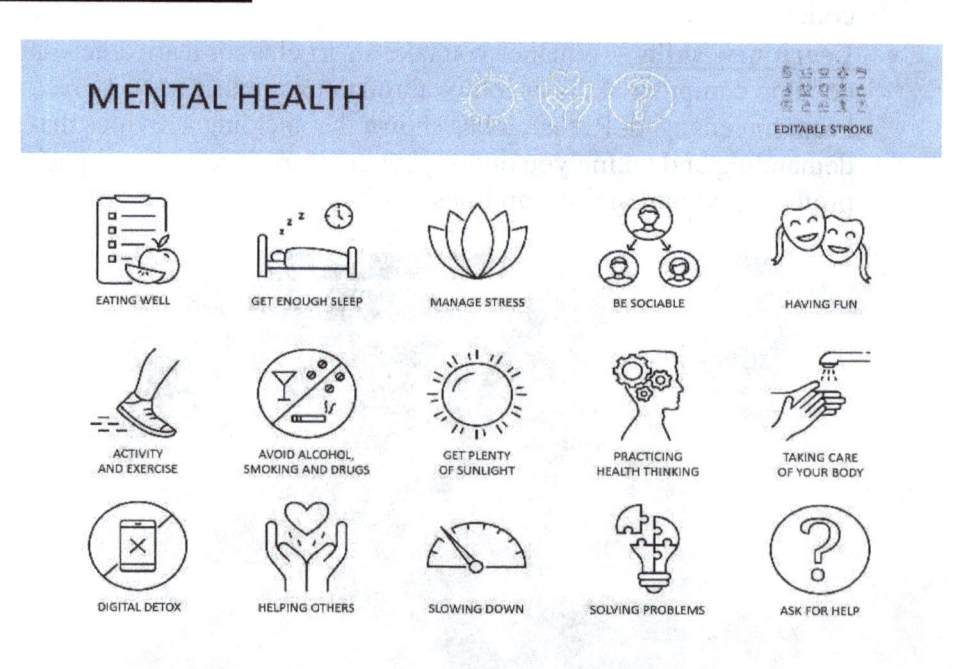

- **Have an organized environment** – Reducing clutter in your home helps decrease the amount of visual distraction. It can help you focus and assist in keeping things organized so you can find what you need quickly without wasting emotional energy.

- **Have one or more "drop spots"** – Do this for essential items like keys, wallet, mail to be posted, your glasses, and your medications. Place these items only in the appropriate spot. You will save time and aggravation and clear up mental space for more important cognitive tasks.

- **Avoid multi-tasking** – Do not buy into the myth of multi-tasking. It is not a real thing – you can only truly focus on one task at a time. Avoiding the temptation to multi-task allows you to fully engage in what you are doing, leading to more efficiency and greater enjoyment in the task.

- **Embrace lists and the use of a planner or calendar** – Avoid making the mistake of having more than one planner, which can lead to confusion and missed appointments. Instead, record all of your appointments and activities in one central place.

Conclusion

While some cognitive changes are a normal part of aging, they do not necessarily indicate the onset of dementia. Many older adults enjoy a rich intellectual life throughout their "golden years." In addition, people can take many steps to optimize their cognitive skills and reduce the impact of normal changes due to aging on their quality of life.

It is important for you to manage your physical and mental health through a healthy diet, regular exercise, adequate sleep. Additionally, you need to manage any specific physical health concerns such as heart disease, diabetes, and specific mental health concerns such as depression. Equally important to maintaining good cognitive health is to be engaged in mentally stimulating activities, foster a sense of purpose through community interactions, and avoid social isolation by regularly connecting with family and friends. Finally, maintaining a calm and organized environment is a practical change that can help.

Cognitive health is essential to the enjoyment of a good quality of life. Good cognitive health allows you to enjoy meaningful relationships, engage in pleasurable activities and participate fully in the life you have spent years building.

6.2. The Six Components of Wellness

Introduction

Wellness is a lifelong growth process that involves the integration of the mind, body, and spirit. Therefore, what a person thinks, feels, and believes impact their health and well-being. In other words, "We are what we think we are."

Independence is a critical factor for the wellness of older adults. By understanding the different components of wellness, the older adult is in a better position to maintain their independence.

Six Components of Wellness

There are six components to wellness, each of which has specific characteristics that defines it. The more you can identify with the characteristics of each component, the closer you are to achieving wellness in that particular area of your lives.

The Six Components:
1. Emotional Wellness/Intelligence
2. Intellectual Wellness/Intelligence
3. Physical Wellness
4. Social Wellness
5. Spiritual Wellness
6. Vocational Wellness.

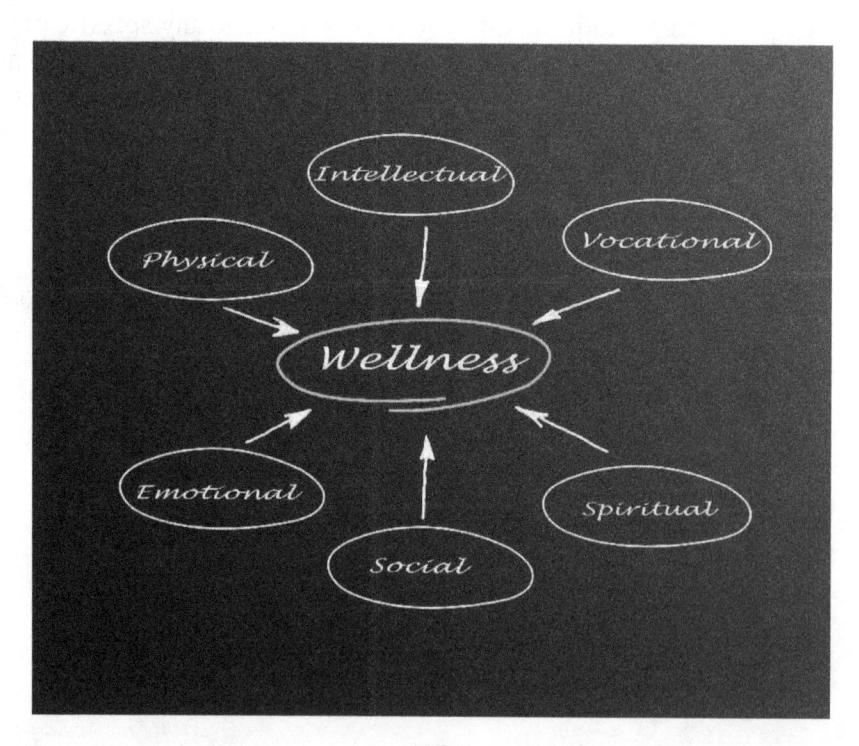

1. Emotional Wellness (Intelligence)

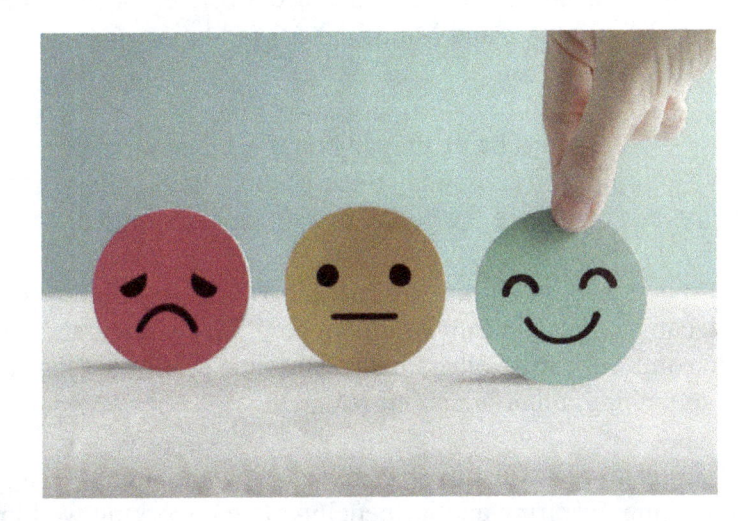

Emotional wellness involves being aware and accepting of one's feelings/emotions. It is often termed Emotional Intelligence and defined as the ability to understand, use, and manage your own emotions in positive ways to relieve stress, communicate effectively, empathize with others, overcome challenges and defuse conflict. Emotional intelligence is invaluable in helping you to build strong interpersonal relationships, which are essential in avoiding self-isolation. Social interaction significantly enhances your quality of life and longevity.

The degree to which an individual feels positive and enthusiastic about one's self and their life influences the way they;

- Recognize & express feelings
- Control stress
- Problem solves
- Manage success & failure
- Set personal expectations

Building Emotional Wellness/Intelligence involves four elements;

1. Self-management – This involves controlling emotions, impulsive feelings, and behaviors, managing stress, taking the initiative, following through on commitments, and adapting to changing circumstances.

2. Self-awareness – This means you recognize or connect to your emotions and how they affect your thoughts and behavior. To connect to your emotions and have a moment-to-moment connection with your changing emotional experience is the key to understanding how emotions influence your thoughts and actions.

Self-test:
Are emotions such as anger, sadness, fear and joy, accompanied by physical sensations in your stomach, throat, or chest?

If they do not, you may have "turned down" or "turned off" your emotions. For you to build emotional wellness, you must be able to connect and accept core emotions. The practice of mindfulness (Chapter 6.9: Mindfulness and Mindfulness Meditation), can help you reconnect to your core emotions.

3. Social awareness – This means being empathetic. By being empathetic, you can understand other people's emotions, needs, and concerns, pick up on non-verbal emotional cues, feel comfortable socially, and recognize the power dynamics in a group or organization.

Paying attention to others will not diminish your self-awareness. On the contrary, by giving attention to others, you can gain insight into your own emotions, values, and beliefs. For example, if you feel discomfort hearing others express particular views, focus on the fact that you will have learned something important about yourself.

4. Relationship management – This involves developing and maintaining good relationships, communicating, inspiring and influencing others, working well in a team, and managing conflict effectively. Working well with others is a process and involves recognizing and understanding what other people are experiencing.

To learn more about Emotional Wellness/Intelligence there are two outstanding book to reference;

1. "The EQ Edge" by Stein, Steven J. and Book, Howard E. Stoddard Publishing Co., 2000.
2. "Emotional Intelligence" by Coleman, Daniel, Bantam Books, 2012.

2. Intellectual Wellness/Intelligence

Intellectual wellness/Intelligence involves having the mental capacity to reason, plan, solve problems, think abstractly and creatively, comprehend complex ideas, desire to explore new ideas, learn quickly, and learn from experience (remember, Emotional Wellness/Intelligence is the ability to identify, assess, and control the emotions of oneself, of others, and groups). Gaining and maintaining intellectual wellness with age is essential because it expands your knowledge and skills to continue to live a stimulating life. Valuing creativity, curiosity, and lifelong learning is necessary to improve intellectual wellness.

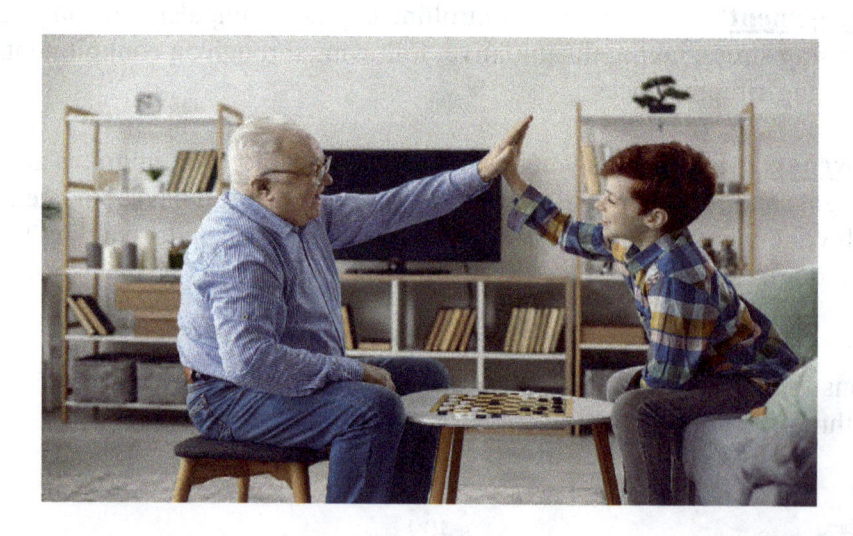

Seven Simple Steps to Increase Your Intellectual Wellness

Key Point – Intellectual wellness improvements occur as long as the mind is active.

1. Read – Reading, especially something you enjoy but are unfamiliar with, can improve your intellect by stretching your mind to think about things you usually don't think about!

2. Debate an issue with a friend, but choose the viewpoint opposite the one you hold – Supporting the opposite perspective is challenging, but the goal is to stretch oneself intellectually. When you expose your mind to opposing ideas, it expands your mind to grasp new information.

3. Learn a foreign language – When learning different ways to communicate, your mind expands.

4. Play a game – Playing board games and cards alone or with others are great.

5. Play a musical instrument – Music has a powerful impact on the mind. Learning to play a musical instrument increases intellectual wellness by learning how to create sounds and make patterns.

6. Write down your thoughts or journal frequently – Writing down or journaling thoughts and feelings often can help those who struggle with expressing their emotions. Identifying your feelings and understanding yourself better increases your intellectual wellness by exposing your mind to deeper thinking.

7. Do crossword or sudoku puzzles – Crosswords and Sudoku are leisure activities that have been proven to increase intellectual wellness. Working through puzzles or finding words in patterns uses a significant amount of brainpower.

3. Physical Wellness

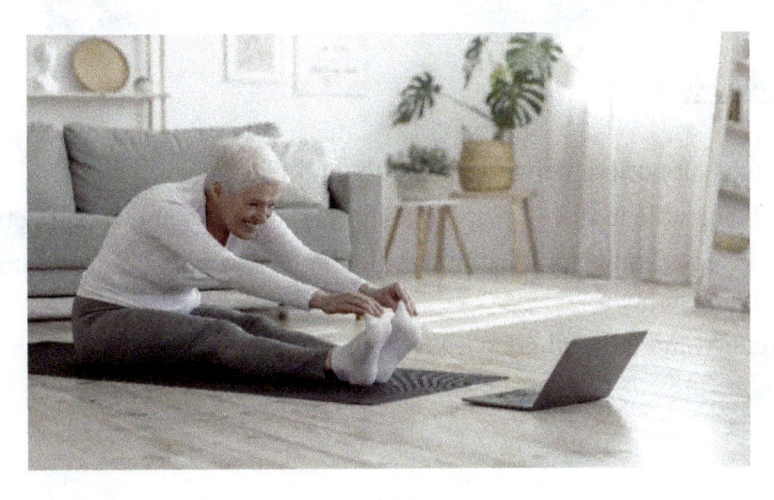

Physical wellness has many benefits and is a crucial component of your health. Even if you have existing compromising health conditions (Section 2: Studying the Opposition to the Older Adults Health), physical activity and exercise, if done with proper planning and supervision, can be practically risk-free. Research has suggested that it is the closest thing to the Fountain of Youth. Sections 4: The Offense: Getting Active the Right Way and Section 5: The Defense: Protecting Your Health and Fitness covers how to safely plan and execute a sustainable fitness plan involving cardiovascular endurance, muscular strength, agility, balance, coordination, and flexibility exercises.

Research indicates that participation in these activities will decrease chronic emotional stress and enhance your emotional and mental wellness. For physical wellness, a little bit goes a long in contributing to stronger mental health as you age.

4. Social Wellness

Social wellness is all about the creation and maintenance of healthy relationships. Social connectivity is something you need for good mental health, and a longer and higher quality of life. Research shows that people with healthy interpersonal relationships and good social support systems have better overall mood, deal better with stress, and have increased self-esteem. Conversely, people who are socially isolated, as so many older adults are, have a higher rate of illness, a higher rate of chronic disease, and 2-3 times the death rate.

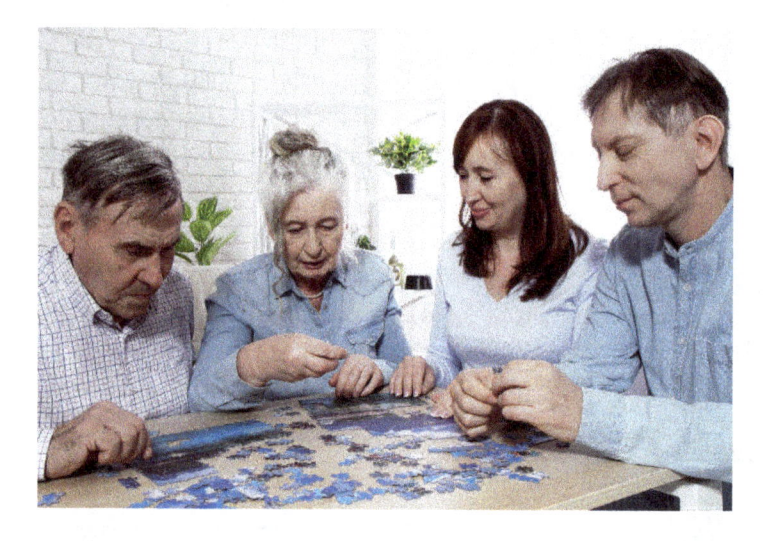

Signs of Social Wellness

- Having a strong supportive network of family and friends.
- Continually being able to develop and maintain friendships and social networks.
- The ability to create boundaries within relationships that encourage communication, trust and conflict management.
- Valuing diversity and treat others with respect.

5. Spiritual Wellness

Spiritual wellness provides us with faith, beliefs, values, ethics, principles, and morals. You do not have to belong to a formal religious group to possess spiritual wellness. A healthy spiritual practice may include examples of volunteerism, social contributions, belonging to a group, forgiveness, and expressions of compassion.

When you are spiritually healthy, you feel more socially and emotionally connected to those around you. As well, with strong spiritual wellness, you have more clarity when it comes to making everyday choices, and your actions become more consistent with your beliefs and values.

If your spiritual wellness is weak, you can slip into feelings of apathy, hopelessness, and depression, which are a common occurrence for older adults.

Ways to Improve your Spiritual Wellness

The spiritual element of wellness is the most personal component. It is healthy for people to live a life with meaning and purpose. Spiritual wellness involves owning one's values, beliefs, and purposes. These can be developed and nurtured in several ways, but the primary goal should be to identify the things in your life that bring you inner peace and tranquility so you have an understanding of what's essential in your life.

1. Explore your spiritual core and look for a deeper life meaning – For you to explore your spiritual core, you are simply asking yourself questions about the person you are and your life's meaning. Excellent questions to ask one's self are: Who am I? What is my purpose? What do I value most? What brings me the most happiness? These questions force you to think more in-depth about yourself and help you understand how you can achieve a more fulfilling life.

2. Think positively – Once you start viewing things in your life in a positive manner (glass is half full, not half empty), you will find yourself thinking differently and feeling happier all over. Eliminating negativity and re-framing how to think of certain things and situations helps give you more control over your lives.

3. Be in the Moment (Mindfulness) and Take Time to Meditate

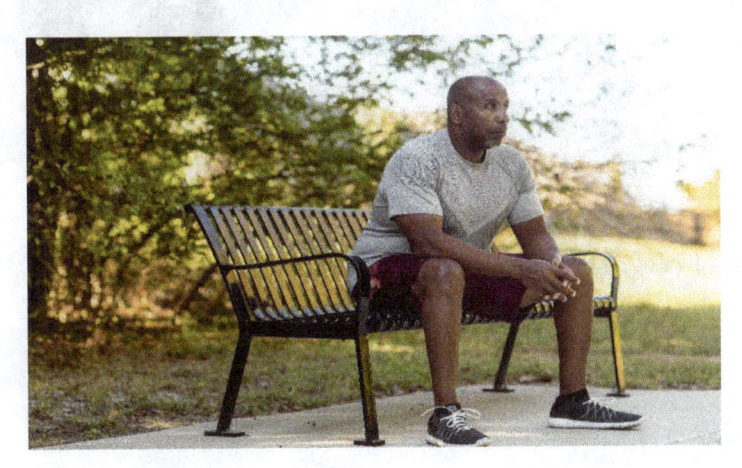

Life can be challenging and confusing, especially for older adults whose lives may change quickly due to retirement, loss of a partner or sickness. They may find their mental and physical well-being diminishing with advancing years. Consequently, it is crucial to live in the moment and devote time to connecting with oneself. Living in the moment is referred to as being mindful (refer to chapter 6.9 for a detailed discussion on mindfulness and mindful meditation).

Meditation is a precious tool to connect with your inner self. Taking five to 10 minutes to meditate each day, whether in the morning upon waking, during lunch break, or before bed, helps you relax. It takes the "hurry" out of your life and helps you focus on that particular moment. Mediation helps free your mind and foster a stronger relationship with spiritual wellness.

6. Vocational Wellness

Vocational wellness means recognizing the personal satisfaction that comes from your occupation. It's about your perception, attitude, and reaction to the type of work you do and how well you do it. Vocational wellness can be challenging for older adults since most are preparing for or are already retired. The secret is in the meaning of the word "vocation," which comes from the Latin *vocare* and means "to call." For the older adult, fulfilling "their calling" can take many forms and be pursued regardless of their employment status.

One way to understand vocational wellness for the older adults is to think of it as:

- Contributing their unique skills and talents toward activities that they find rewarding and meaningful.
- Learning new skills that they can share with others.
- Developing new interests and hobbies.

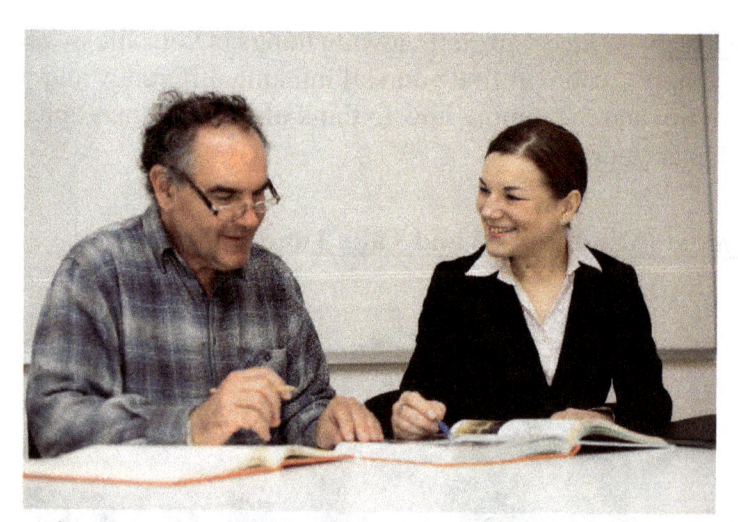

Volunteering or becoming a mentor are two ways older adults can create meaningful "work" for themselves.

Vocational Wellness Self-Assessment

The higher the score, the higher your vocational wellness. Low scores to certain questions will identify areas that need improvement:

Rate each item using this scale:
- 4 – Always True
- 3 – Sometimes True
- 2 – Rarely True
- 1 – Never True

Questionnaire:

1. ___ I am happy with how I spend my time.
2. ___ I have plans for things that I want to do.
3. ___ I do things with other people often enough so that I don't feel isolated.
4. ___ I use my time in a way that gives me meaning and purpose.
5. ___ I make good use of my strengths and experiences in the things I am doing daily.
6. ___ My daily activities are consistent with my values and interests.
7. ___ I control how I spend my time.
8. ___ I volunteer in the community or have considered volunteering.
9. ___ I look forward to my daily and weekly activities.
10. ___ The people I spend time with enjoy spending time with me.

_____ Total Score (out of a possible 40).

Improving Vocational Wellness

It is vital as you grow older that you stay relevant and have a meaningful purpose in life. Here are ways to accomplish that:

- Write out goals (Chapter 3.3: The Importance and Art of Goal Setting), and create an action plan to execute them, and then start working on implementing the plan.
- Keep motivated, don't let others deter you from what you want to accomplish.
- Increase knowledge and skills to achieve goals.
- Find the benefits and positives from what you want to do.
- Enjoy what you do, do what you enjoy.
- Create connections with your family, friends, acquaintances, and fellow retirees.

Conclusion

Understanding what wellness means and how to achieve it is vitally important for your mental health, which significantly influences your ability to maintain your independence. Each of the six components of wellness contributes to your overall sense of well-being. Therefore, if you are weak in one of these areas, attention should be given to strengthening this area.

References

http://forever-active.com/six-dimensions-of-wellness/
https://nowandme.com/blog/emotional-intelligence-and-resilience
https://www.covenanthealth.org/healthcalling/2017/july/what-is-social-wellness-/
https://brescia.uwo.ca/student_life/health_and_wellness/dimensions_of_wellness/social_cultural.php
https://spokane.wsu.edu/wellness/occupational-wellness/

6.3. Understanding Depression

Introduction

Depression is not the result of a person being mentally weak or a character flaw, and is more than just feeling sad or blue. A depressed person can't just "snap out of it." Depression is a real biological illness, a severe mood disorder with potentially many causes, some of which include a chemical imbalance in the brain, neuroplastic changes in the brain related to trauma and age, chronic or unresolved stress or conflict, abuse and medications.

The diagnosis of "Clinical depression" is made when you have trouble handling daily activities, such as sleeping, eating, and socializing, for a prolonged period. Depression affects how you think, feel, behave, and also affects your physical health because you have difficulty initiating activities and exercise.

For older adults, depression is a significant health concern. Social isolation and physical and mental/cognitive disability contribute to the onset of depression. Each of these is more prevalent in the older adult population than the general population. It is estimated that depression affects 1-5% of the older adult population and 13.5% of the elderly who require home healthcare.

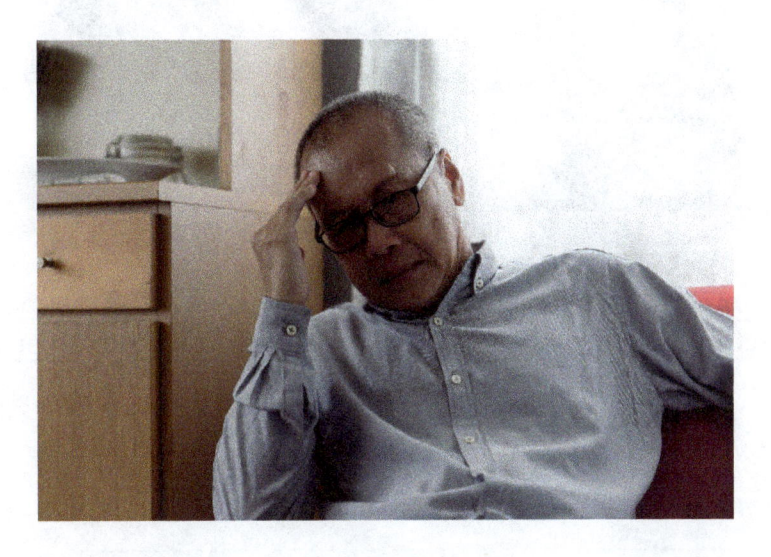

Depression can affect anyone at any age. Older adults may have had episodes of depression throughout their lives, or they may have their first episode late in life. Unfortunately, depression is often not recognized in older adults because many signs of depression can be mistaken for signs of normal aging. Older adults who are depressed may not complain about feeling low because they attribute their unhappy feelings as "just getting old." Depression may continue for months or years if left untreated. Depression, untreated, is the main cause of suicide in older adults.

Differentiating Early-Onset and Late-Onset Depression

Early-onset depression – These patients experience clinical depression before age 65 and have a strong familial (genetic) history of depression. These patients may also have a higher prevalence of personality disorders or elevated scores on personality traits such as neuroticism (the personality trait disposition to experience negative affects, including anger, anxiety, self-consciousness, irritability, emotional instability, and depression).

Late-onset depression – This is depression arising for the first time after the age of 65. Most research focuses on structural changes in the brain as the leading cause of this form of depression. Older adults with late-onset depression are more likely to have vascular risk factors, including a history of cerebrovascular disease. In addition, older adults with late-onset depression are more likely to have accompanying cognitive deficits such as memory loss, speech difficulties, attention deficits, reasoning, and decision impairment (Chapter 6.1: Understanding and Managing Cognitive Health). As well, research indicates that older adults who are depressed are more likely to develop dementia and Alzheimer's disease (Chapter 2.6: Dementia).

Early-onset v. Late-onset

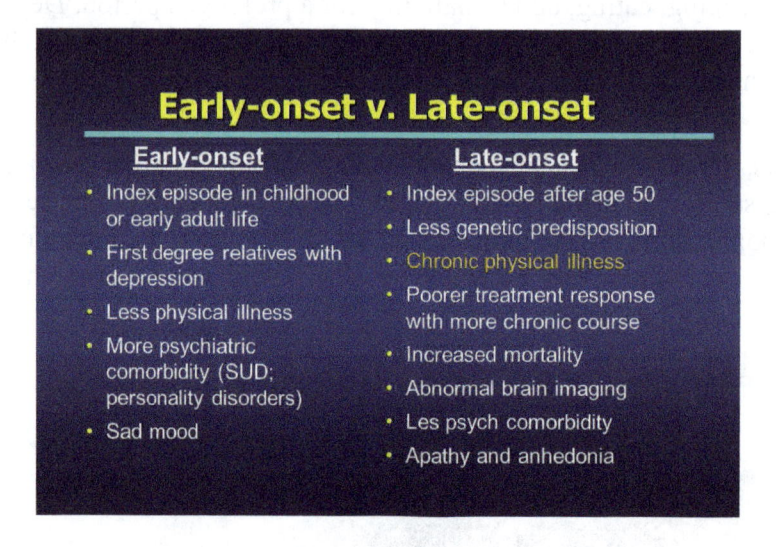

Early-onset	Late-onset
Index episode in childhood or early adult life	Index episode after age 50
First degree relatives with depression	Less genetic predisposition
Less physical illness	Chronic physical illness
More psychiatric comorbidity (SUD; personality disorders)	Poorer treatment response with more chronic course
Sad mood	Increased mortality
	Abnormal brain imaging
	Les psych comorbidity
	Apathy and anhedonia

Image source: slideplayer.com

Risk and Protective Factors and When Depression Occurs Over a Life Span

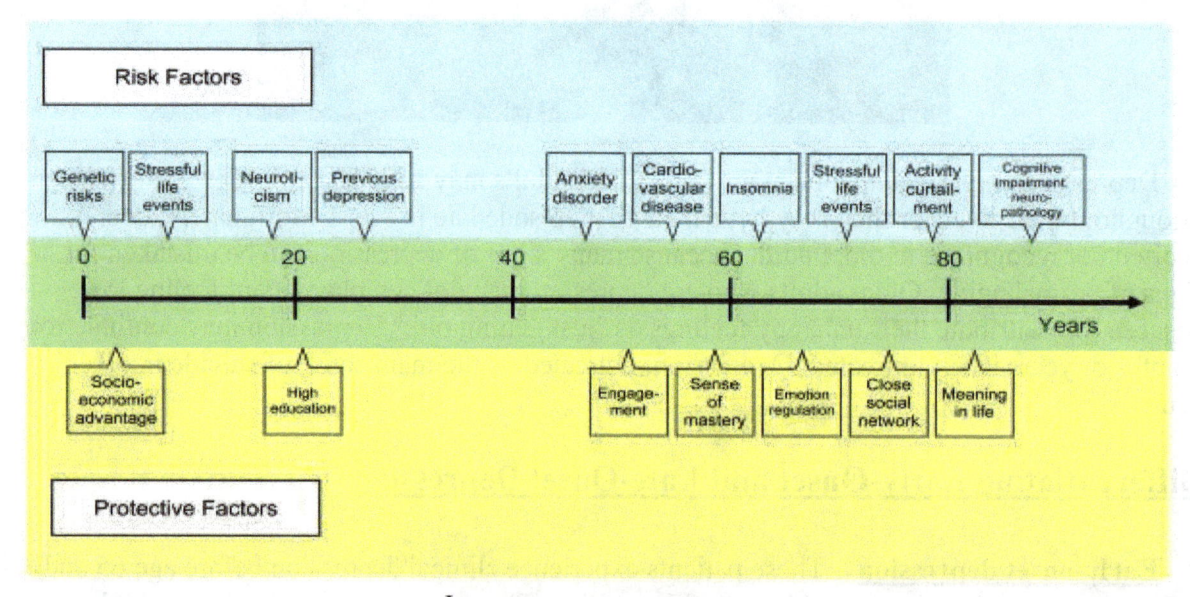

Risk Factors: Genetic risks, Stressful life events, Neuroticism, Previous depression, Anxiety disorder, Cardiovascular disease, Insomnia, Stressful life events, Activity curtailment, Cognitive impairment neuropathology

Protective Factors: Socio-economic advantage, High education, Engagement, Sense of mastery, Emotion regulation, Close social network, Meaning in life

Image source: europepmc.org

Signs and Symptoms of Depression in the Older Adult

Depression impacts older people differently than younger people. In older adults, depression lasts longer and often occurs with other medical illnesses and disabilities (heart disease, arthritis, cancer). Because depression reduces an older adult's ability to fully engage in the rehabilitation of these health conditions, there is an increased risk of death from these illnesses.

Symptoms of depression are chronic, present nearly every day and may include one or more of following:

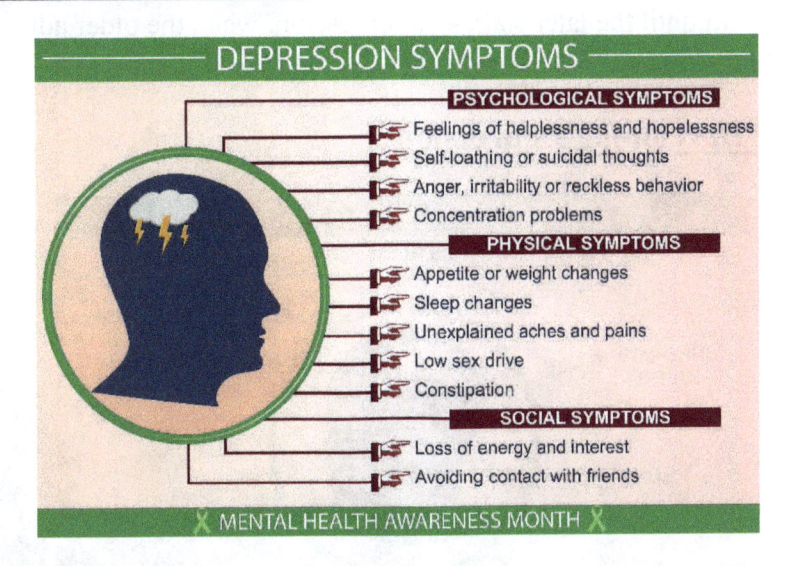

DEPRESSION SYMPTOMS

PSYCHOLOGICAL SYMPTOMS
- Feelings of helplessness and hopelessness
- Self-loathing or suicidal thoughts
- Anger, irritability or reckless behavior
- Concentration problems

PHYSICAL SYMPTOMS
- Appetite or weight changes
- Sleep changes
- Unexplained aches and pains
- Low sex drive
- Constipation

SOCIAL SYMPTOMS
- Loss of energy and interest
- Avoiding contact with friends

MENTAL HEALTH AWARENESS MONTH

- **Extreme emotions** of anxiety, agitation, restlessness, sadness, tearfulness, emptiness, or hopelessness.
- **Mood changes** including angry outbursts, irritability, and frustration, even over small matters.
- **Behavioral changes** such as loss of interest or pleasure in most everyday activities, hobbies, or sports, including sex. You often become socially isolated.
- **Sleep disturbances,** including insomnia or sleeping too much.
- **Energy depletion** like excessive tiredness. Even small tasks take extra effort.
- **Nutrition and diet changes,** such as reduced appetite and weight loss or increased cravings for food and weight gain.
- **Cognitive and motor disturbances,** this includes memory loss, slowed thinking, poor reasoning or decision making, difficulty speaking, or problems with body movements.
- **Distorted self-worth or self-esteem,** such as feeling worthlessness or guilt, fixating on past failures or self-blame.
- **Suicidal fixation,** this includes frequent or recurrent thoughts of death, suicide attempts, or suicide.
- **Unexplained chronic physical problems,** such as back pain or headaches.
- **Difficulties initiating activities,** such as feeling that you are unable to get off the couch to make dinner, clean, exercise.

For the older adult, these symptoms often go unnoticed by others because of social isolation (living by themselves) or because they think the way they feel is part of normal aging or depression has affected their reasoning and initiating skills.

Depression symptoms in older adults often occur after sorrowful events such as loss of a spouse, unexpected retirement, sudden onset of illness, or chronic disability. Because of the physical changes in the brain that occur and with advancing age, and the resulting chemical disturbances and neuro-connectivity issues (neuroplastic changes) the older adult may not emotionally and cognitively be able to overcome these life-altering events. At other times, depressive symptoms can come on slowly and insidiously and as a result, family and friends may not identify the problem until the later stages of depression, when the older adult's health is severely compromised.

Risk Factors for Developing Depression

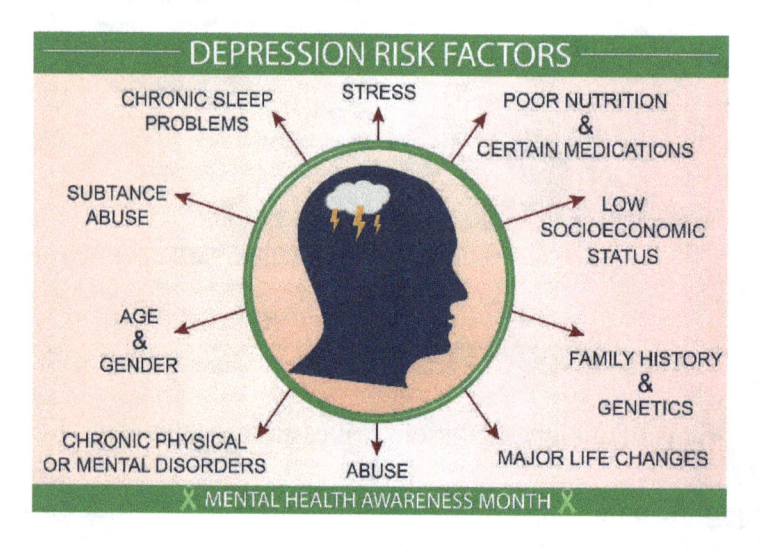

The following seem to increase the risk of developing or triggering depression:

- **Certain personality traits**, such as low self-esteem and being too dependent, self-critical, or pessimistic.
- **Traumatic or stressful events**, such as physical abuse, especially early in life, the death or loss of a loved one, a difficult relationship, or financial problems.
- **Hereditary (Genetics)** entails relatives with a history of depression, bipolar disorder, alcoholism, or suicide.
- **History of other mental health disorders**, such as anxiety disorder, eating disorders, or post-traumatic stress disorder.
- **Substance abuse**, like alcohol or recreational drugs.
- **Serious or chronic illness**, like cancer, stroke, heart disease, or chronic pain.
- **Prescription medications**, such as some high blood pressure medications or sleeping pills.

Complications that Can Result from Being Depressed

Depression is a serious disorder that can have serious consequences. Depression can worsen if it isn't treated, resulting in emotional, behavioral, and health problems that can affect every area of your life. Complications associated with depression include:

- Pain or physical illness
- Excess weight gain and obesity, which contributes to the development of heart disease and diabetes
- Alcohol or drug misuse
- Anxiety, panic disorder, or social phobia
- Family conflicts, relationship difficulties, and work problems
- Social isolation
- Suicidal feelings, suicide attempts, or suicide
- Self-mutilation, such as cutting
- Premature death from medical conditions

Treatment for Depression

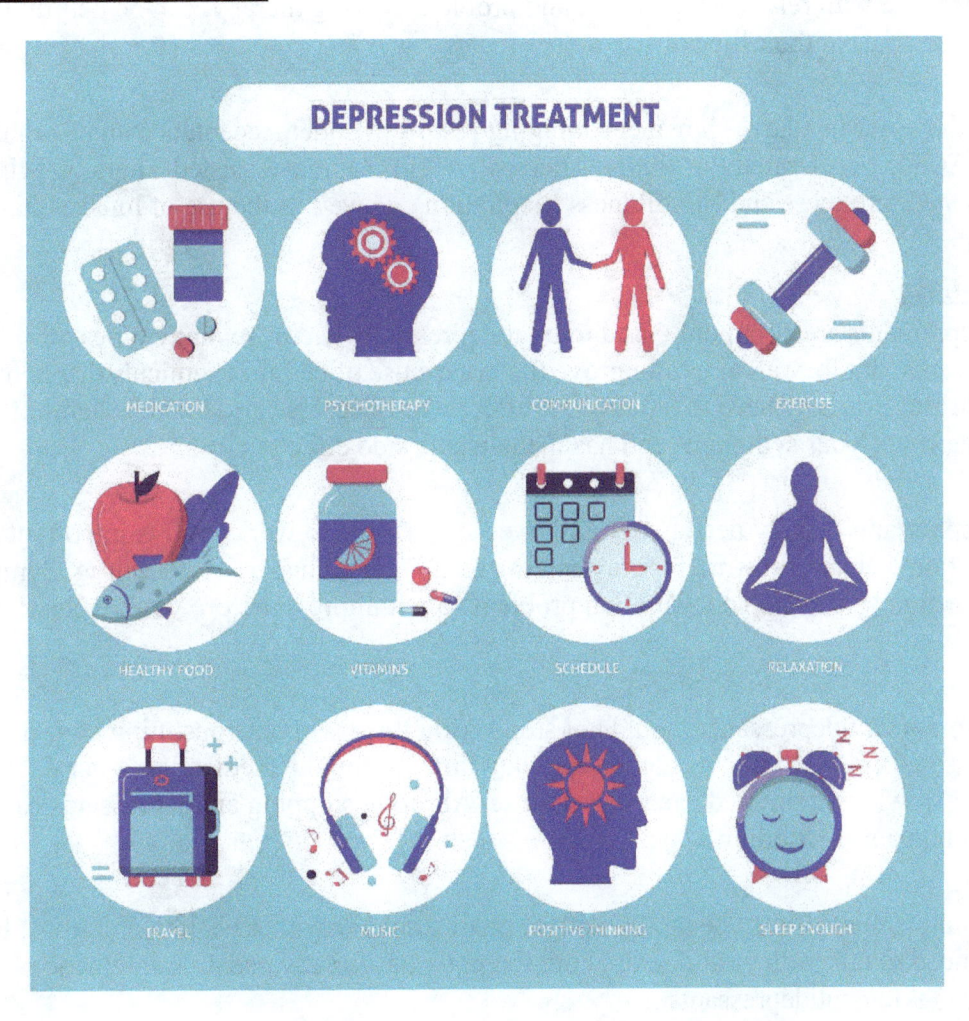

Depression can be treated; early intervention has the best results. If you suspect that you may be suffering from depression it is important that you see your medical doctor or someone specializing in diagnosis and treatment of mental health conditions, such as a psychologist or psychiatrist. Some medical conditions and medications can cause the same symptoms as depression, and these need to be ruled out. If no overt medical condition is causing the depression, you should undergo a psychological evaluation.

Treatment choices differ for each person, and often you must try multiple treatments to find one that works best for you.

Psychotherapy and medication are the most common forms of treatment for depression.

1. Psychotherapy

Psychotherapy, "talk therapy," is a proven form of depression therapy. Depending on an individual's needs, the treatment period can be short-term, 10 to 20 weeks, or much longer, possibly years.

Cognitive-behavioral therapy is a type of talk therapy used to treat depression. It focuses on changing negative thinking and behaviors that may be making depression worse. Interpersonal therapy for those with relationship issues, and problem-solving therapy, can be helpful in dealing with a loss or crisis in their life.

Other therapies that have shown encouraging results include; Acceptance and Commitment Therapy (ACT), Accelerated Resolution Therapy (ART), Animal Assisted Therapy, Mindfulness (chapter 6.9 Mindfulness and Mindfulness Meditation), as well as the use of music and art.

2. Medications

Antidepressants are commonly used to treat depression. There are many types of antidepressants, but they all aim to improve the brain's use of certain chemicals that control mood or stress. You may need to try several different antidepressant medicines before finding one that improves your symptoms and has manageable side effects.

Antidepressants usually need two to four weeks or longer to work, so it is important to give the medication a chance to work before deciding to stop or change to another drug. Symptoms such as appetite, sleep, and concentration problems often improve before your depressive mood lifts.

A person on antidepressants should not stop taking them without consulting their doctor. When it has been decided that it is an appropriate time to stop the medication, your doctor will help you to slowly and safely decrease your dose. Abruptly stopping antidepressants can cause significant unwanted withdrawal symptoms.

Older adults may already be taking several medications for other health conditions. In this case, you need to talk with your doctor about the potential for adverse drug interactions that may occur while taking antidepressants.

Preventing Depression

Prevention of depression for older adults can be challenging because of pre-existing health issues and normal biological/anatomical changes in the brain with advancing age. However, there are a few preventative steps you can take.

1. Try to prepare for significant changes in life, such as retirement or downsizing from the home lived in for many years to a condo or older adult residence.
2. Stay in touch with family and friends. Develop a solid social network. Let them know when you feel sad.
3. Plan and get regular exercise
4. Keep cognitively/intellectually active. Pick some activities you like to do and do them.
5. Eat a healthy balanced diet to avoid chronic illnesses such as heart disease, diabetes, obesity, and arthritis that can bring on disability and depression.
6. Learn new things (especially things like language, music, art or anything that involves creating something from nothing).

Conclusion

Depression can result in significant mental health issues for older adults. Suffering from chronic disabilities and social isolation leave the older adult vulnerable to developing depression. Older adults and their support team (family, friends, health team) must be aware of the risk factors and symptoms of depression. Early detection is important for successful and long-lasting management.

References

https://www.nia.nih.gov/health/depression-and-older-adults
https://www.camh.ca/en/health-info/guides-and-publications/depression-in-older-adults
https://www.medicinenet.com/depression_in_the_elderly/article.htm
https://www.mayoclinic.org/diseases-conditions/depression/symptoms-causes/syc-20356007
https://medicareworld.com/feature/insight-into-depression-in-seniors-how-medicare-can-help/

6.4. Developing Mental Fitness

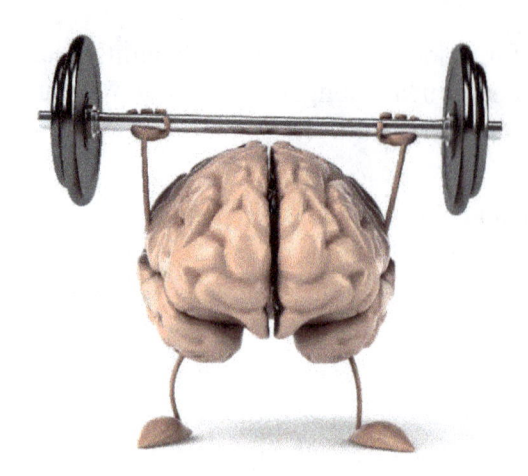

Introduction

Mental fitness means a person being in a state of well-being with a positive sense of how they feel, think and act. It also means one can overcome disappointments, stay focused and disciplined to accomplish goals, persevere under less-than-ideal physical and emotional conditions, and continue when all they want to do is quit. These are all challenges that the older adult faces regularly.

Achieving and maintaining mental fitness requires the same amount of consistent and sustained effort that physical fitness does. It takes hard work, repetition, and a conscious desire to be mentally strong. It does not just happen, and it does not happen overnight. People are not born mentally fit. It is an acquired skill that involves a continuous process of self-improvement. For older adults, being mentally fit is vital to enjoying a high quality of life.

Two Key Element to Mental Fitness

1. Confidence

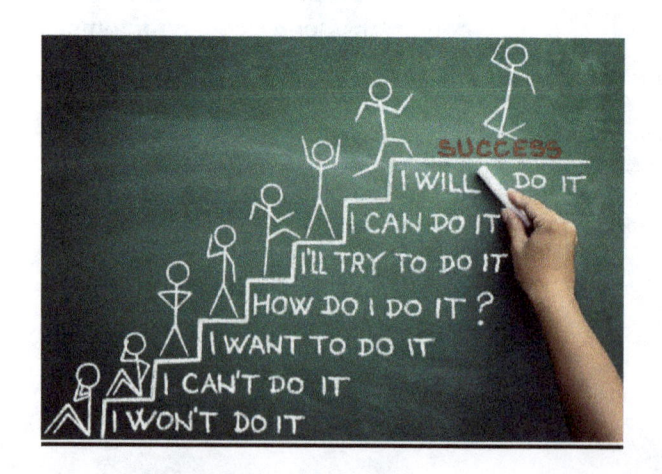

> "All I am, I am because of my mind."
> – **Paavo Nurmi** (holder of 9 golds and 3 silver Olympic medals in long distance running)

No truer words were ever spoken than the ones above. You are who you think you are. If we think of ourselves as a success, then we are a success. Conversely, if we think of ourselves as a failure, we are a failure. There is no sugar coating this fact.

As a result, you MUST have confidence in yourself, and if you don't, you must fake it until you have it. In other words, you must always act confident even if you don't feel that way at present. Therefore, it is essential to assume the posture and disposition of a confident person.

How is this done?

1. Mentorship – You need to look around and find people you admire and exude confidence. You need to study how they act and talk and then emulate these characteristics in your daily lives. The "confident" people you want to emulate got that way by studying and emulating people they admired and who had displayed confidence.

2. Posture – You need to stand tall. An individual's posture speaks a thousand words, conveying how they feel about themselves. For example, a confident person doesn't slump over looking at the ground. Instead, they stand tall and proud, and they look people in the eyes when talking to them. Your posture should shout out, "I am a confident person."

3. Communication – Listen to others and don't fall into the trap of criticizing others to elevate your personal self-esteem. Be guided by how others respond to you; communication is the response you get. Good communication starts with excellent listening skills. If you don't listen to what others say, you cannot communicate effectively with them. People want to be listened to, not lectured. Listening more and speaking less shows confidence. It shows that you are interested in what others have to say and are not just concerned about showing off what you "think" you know. Confident people know what to say, say it effectively, and most importantly, when to say it.

2. Team

Surrounding yourself with optimistic, like-minded people is vitally important for good mental fitness. There is strength in having a team to rely on for support and advice. The road ahead is much more difficult if you must go it alone. Every successful, strong, and mentally fit person has a solid supportive entourage surrounding them that will help deflect negativity and promote and reinforce self-confidence. An individual support team is there to help pick them up when they get knocked down and celebrate their victories. It is no fun celebrating alone.

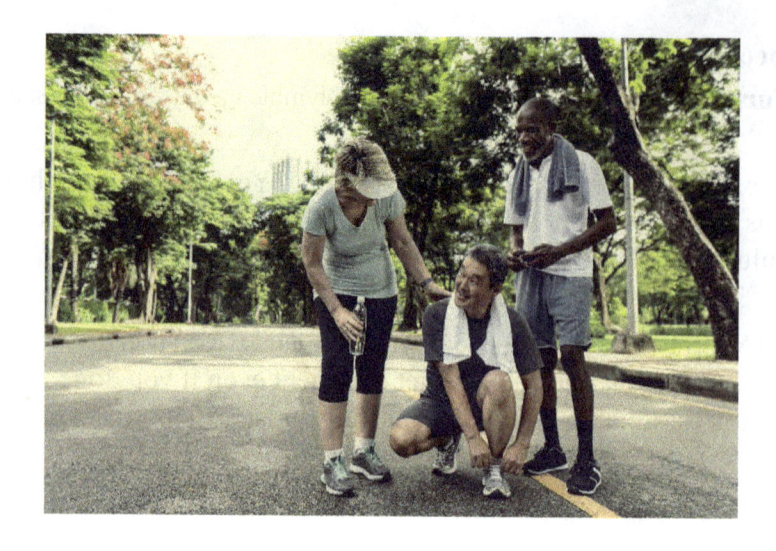

Sustained social interaction is necessary for mental fitness. Everyone needs friends; everyone needs confidants. You need to reach out to others who have expertise in areas you do not have. You become mentally stronger when you learn new things.

Equally important is that you must also be aware of and eliminate those people in your life who are not helping you achieve success and happiness. You should not share time and energy with someone if they do not contribute positively to your success and happiness?

Maintaining confidence in the face of chronic illness and deteriorating mental strength is a significant challenge for the older adult. However, the three points above (mentorship, posture, and communication) still apply and should be practiced as best as possible. Losing self-confidence and not having a support team contributes to social isolation and a significant loss of quality of life for the older adult.

Mental Skills for Mental Fitness

Developing mental fitness is a process that requires discipline and practice. However, perseverance pays big dividends if you are working on the right things. Therefore, you must work diligently on the following mental skills to achieve and maintain mental fitness, resulting in a more productive, successful, and happy life.

Some of the mental skills listed below are repeated elsewhere in this book. This reflects their importance in contributing to the older adult achieving a higher quality of life.

1. Goal Setting

You need to know what your goals are and keep them in focus. It is important to have short- and long-term goals. Goals help maintain motivation and avoid the "scatterbrain effect" or a sense of drifting through the day that often plagues the older adult's daily life. A good rule of thumb is to "Think it, then ink it." Writing down S.M.A.R.T. goals, (Chapter 3.3: The Art and Importance of Goal Setting), is the best way to do this.

S.M.A.R.T. Goals

Specific – Be as specific as possible. The more detailed the goals are, the better you can visualize the result.

Measurable – If you can't measure it, you can't do it. Therefore, you must identify specific metrics to measure their progress and achievements.

Action – What are the specific steps you are going to take to achieve your goals? These steps need to be as detailed as possible.

Realistic – Accomplishing the goal must be realistic based on the resources, time, and effort you can commit. If a goal is not realistically achievable, what will result is frustration and disillusionment. Therefore, determine how the goal can be realistically achieved.

Time lined – Set a specific time (a week, a month, a year) to accomplish your goal. Set long-term and short-term time lines for monitoring the progress towards the goal.

2. Mental Imagery

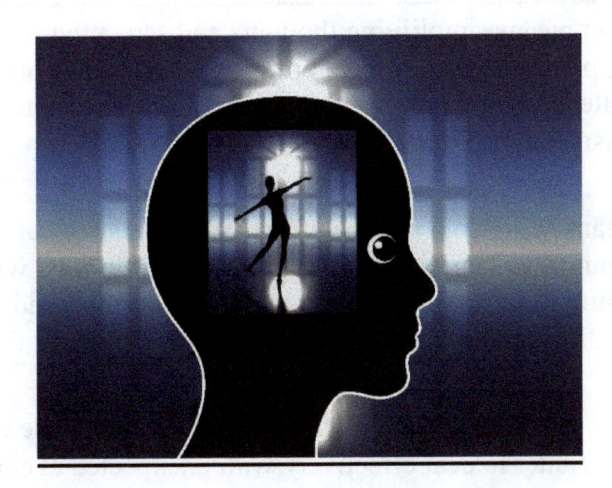

Visualize to actualize. You must see and feel yourself being successful/happy, and then enjoy being successful/happy. Athletes and performers do this all the time. The basketball player visualizes the basketball going through the hoop before he shoots. A race car driver envisions the turn before he makes it. An actor imagines their performance before the camera rolls or curtain goes up. If you want to make it happen, they have got to see yourself doing it first. That is called visualization.

3. Positive Self-Talk

You need to learn to think more positively about yourself. Gain control of your thinking process and give yourself self-compassion (Chapter 6.6: Self-Compassion: The Proven Power of Being Kind to Yourself) when things don't go as planned. Mentally beating yourself up is not productive. Behavior research has shown that positive motivational self-talk is the most effective way to get positive results.

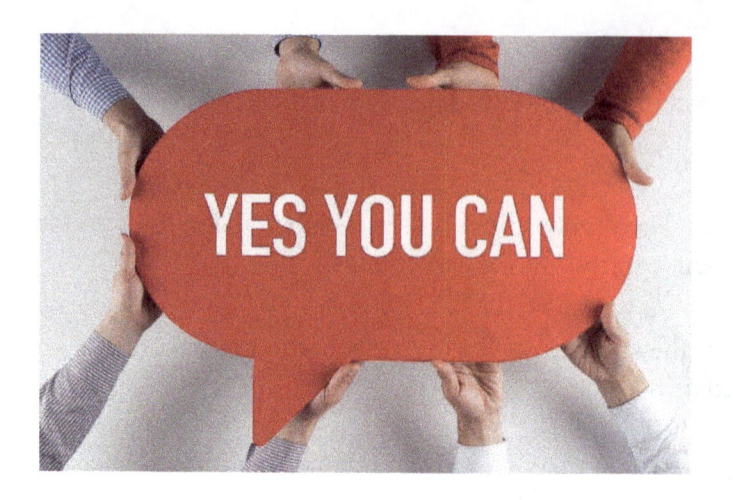

The more often you repeat positive affirmations and powerful phrases with conviction, the more concrete they will become in your mind and the more they will affect performance. Because you live and perform in the present time and not in the future, speak in the present tense rather than future tense when giving self-affirmations. In other words, use "I am, I have, I bring" vs. "I will."

4. Focus on the Present (Section 6.9.: Mindfulness and Mindfulness Meditation)

Focusing on the present means simplifying thoughts and screening out information that is not relevant at present. Being present in the moment empowers you to respond to your changing environment and any challenges confronted at the present moment. Remember, the past is history, and the future exists only in the imagination.

Being mentally fit means being able to cope effectively with stressful situations in real time. It is a helpful mental technique to "shrink your world" when confronted with stressful "out of control" situations. This simplifying skill unclutters unhelpful stimuli and allows you to focus on what needs to be done to alleviate the stressful situation at the "present" time.

Life continually throws curveballs, and you need to be mentally agile to manipulate your environment to reduce the clutter to deal effectively with unexpected events.

5. Breath Control

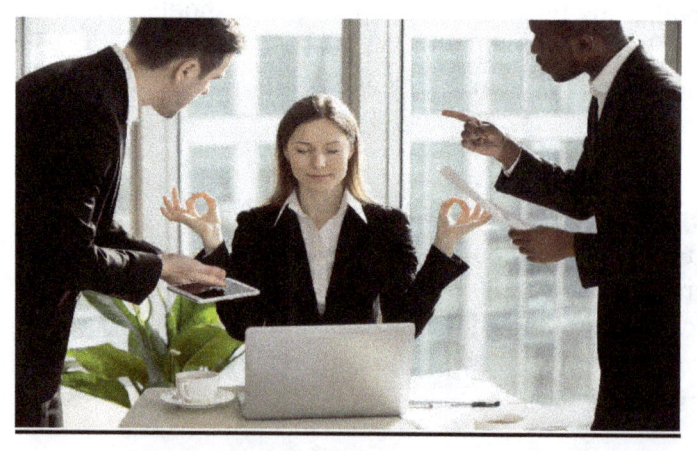

Anxiety shows its ugly face through shallow rapid breathing. Regardless of the inhalation length, you need to prolong exhalation to promote relaxation. Control your breathing to control your mind.

6. Humor and Enjoyment of the Moment is the Best Medicine

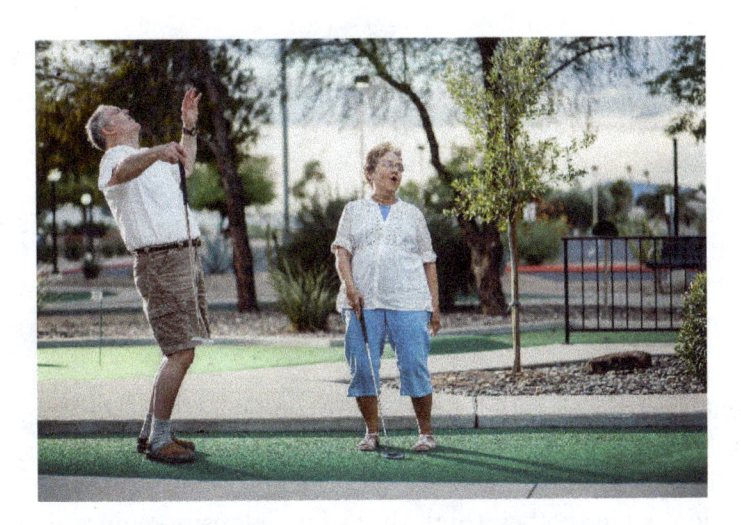

Humor – Research has overwhelmingly shown the mental health benefits of laughter. You need to find humor and enjoyment in everything you do and in every situation that presents itself. As dreadful as a situation may appear, there is usually a silver lining to be found. Finding this silver lining allows you to mentally deal with difficult situations more effectively.

Embrace the Moment – Embracing a challenge rather than avoiding or dreading it is often the best way to reduce unnecessary stress. A valuable technique to use when confronting a challenging situation is to slow things down. For example, you can tell yourself that, although you are confronting a stressful situation, you don't want this moment in time to end; you don't want the situation to end suddenly. This technique helps you gain control of the situation rather than the situation gaining control over you.

7. Good Positive Body Language speaks a thousand words

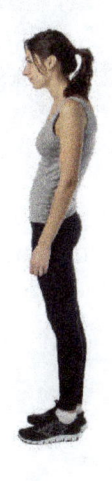

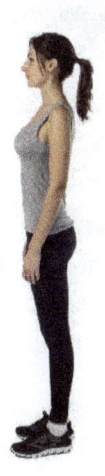

Your posture, gestures, facial expressions, and eye movements reveal thoughts and feelings. For example, positive and upbeat body language includes smiling, chin up, shoulders back and chest out, standing tall, and walking strong. These strong body gestures will reduce stress and reveal confidence.

8. Find Your Intensity Zone

Everyone has their own optimal intensity level for peak performance in any given situation. Sometimes you need to increase your intensity level, whereas at other times, it is necessary to throttle down your intensity level.

Taking forceful breaths, using powerful hand movements, repeating energizing thoughts like "Yes I can," and recalling up-tempo songs are all ways to increase intensity. Conversely, breathing slowly with long exhalations, doing passive stretches, thinking calming thoughts, and replaying calming songs help tone down the intensity level.

Stay in the present, stay emotionally under control and manage your emotional and physical intensity level (up or down) to meet the demands of the situation. Usually, the more complex the situation or more skill required to complete the task, the lower your intensity level should be. Think of kicking a field goal in football (high skill - low intensity required) vs. running back a kick-off (relatively simple skill but very dynamic situation -high intensity required).

9. Exercise, Enjoy Hobbies and Volunteer

Exercise – Research shows regular physical activity improves your mental well-being and can reduce anxiety and depression. Being a part of an exercise group or a gym reduces loneliness and connects people who share a common goal.

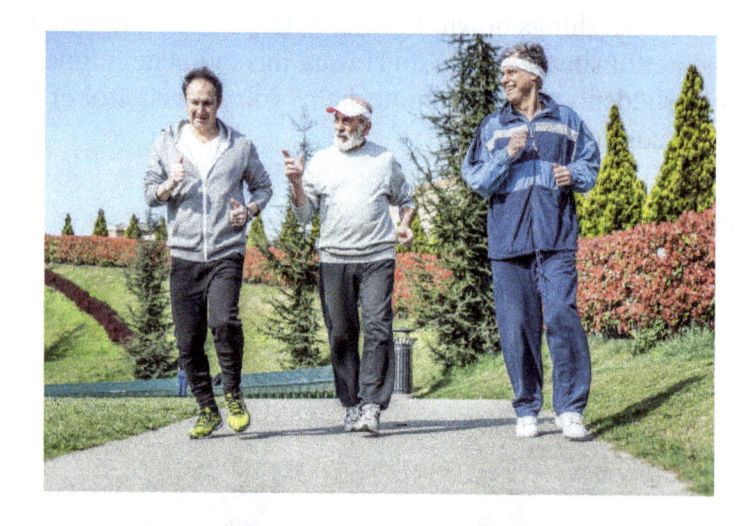

Enjoy hobbies – Taking up a hobby allows you to do something you enjoy, something you do because you want to do it, and can help free you of the pressure of everyday tasks. In addition, hobbies help keep the brain active.

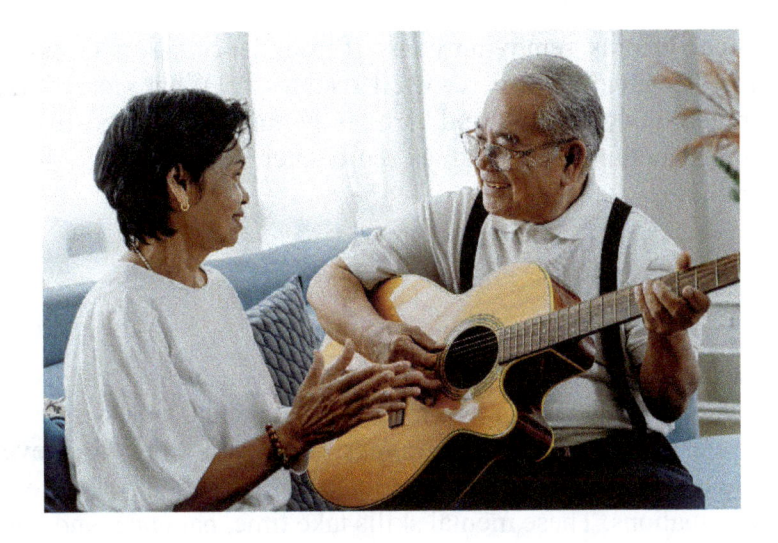

Volunteer – Volunteering is a "win-win" activity because helping others makes people feel good about themselves. It also widens your social network, provides you with new learning experiences, and can balance your lives because you are focusing on doing something for others rather than for yourself.

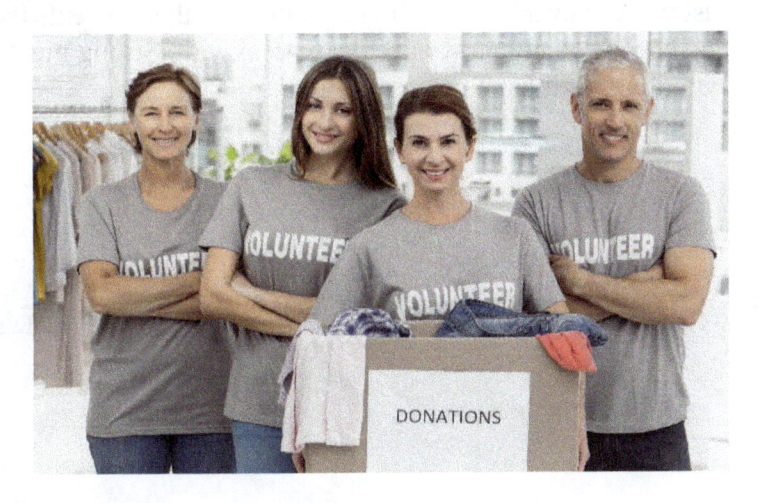

10. Control your Emotions

Learn to control emotions and not overreact to situations. You may not have control over what has happened, but you can control how they react to the situation. Controlling emotions requires good mental discipline (mental fitness).

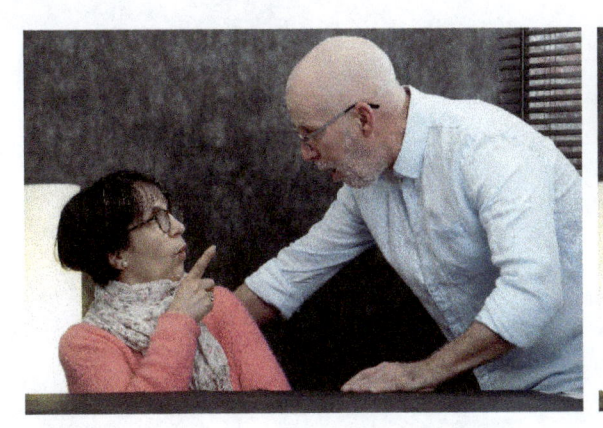

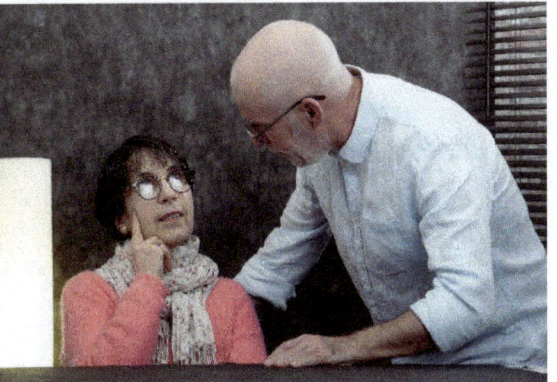

Often, by taking deep breaths, removing yourself from the situation temporarily, and letting things unfold naturally, the situation resolves itself seamlessly. What seemed like a mountain is often found to be a molehill that is easily and harmlessly managed in a positive way. Don't overreact and do or say something that you may regret later. Be in control emotionally, don't be controlled by your emotions.

Conclusion

Patience is necessary when it comes to developing mental fitness. Patience, in itself, is a cognitive skill required to be mentally fit. For most, strong mental fitness does not come easily. The mental skills/abilities discussed take time to master. For most, they are never entirely mastered. Most people have to work at being confident, mindful, and finding enjoyment and humor in challenging situations. These mental skills take time, patience, and hard work to develop. However, the more you work at developing these mental fitness skills, the easier they become to use. After a while, they will become habituated. It is important to remember that all habits need to be reinforced from time to time. This is especially true when we are under stress.

Achieving and maintaining mental fitness is a marathon event, not a sprint so be patient. It is something that you must work at every day with every situation that presents itself in your life. You should not pick and choose what you would like to deal with. Strong mental fitness means dealing productively with it all, as it happens in real-time.

References

https://joefrielsblog.com/confidence/
http://forever-active.com/wp-content/uploads/2014/01/Forever-Active-New-Years-Resolutions.pdf

6.5. Finding Meaning/Purpose in Life

Introduction

Finding meaning/purpose in life can be one of the biggest challenges for older adults as they experience retirement, an empty nest, loss of their life-long partner, declining mental and physical health. It is not surprising that, at one point or another, people of all ages wrestle with finding meaning in their lives. Life is challenging with many struggles, and at a person's most vulnerable times, they often catch themselves asking, "What is life all about?". People tell themselves that life should not be this hard, that they are entitled to a good job, good relationships, and good health. Unfortunately, for most of us, experience teaches us that life does not follow that script because adversities like layoffs, divorce, and illness happen.

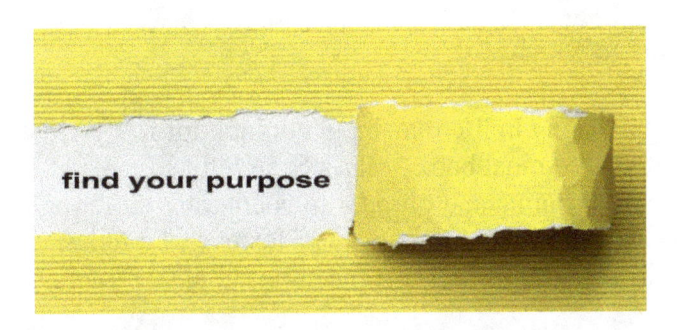

Because life is not easy but a series of never-ending challenges and obstacles, to have a fulfilling life, you must search out what life means to you. If life does not have significant meaning, why would anyone continue the struggle? Maybe that is why there is an increasing rate of suicide in both young and older adults; they have lost what life means to them. That is why finding meaning in life is an important component of mental health and deserves special attention.

Defining what "Meaning of Life" Means

Trying to define the "meaning of life" can be complicated. It can have philosophical, religious, and scientific interpretations. However, keeping with the theme of this book, let's keep it simple. Finding meaning in life is all about finding a purpose to overcome, to survive, to thrive.

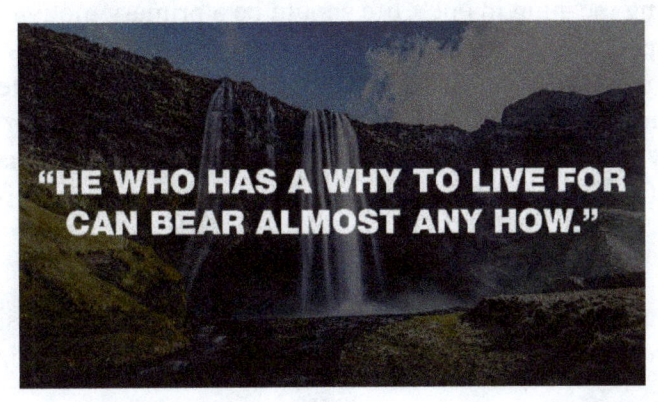

The German philosopher Friedrich Nietzsche famously said that "He who has a why to live can bear almost any how." Research and experience prove this to be true. Having a sense of meaning or purpose makes people more resilient and persistent and less affected by setbacks. Meaning and purpose in life help you to be innovative and find creative solutions to hardships. It gives you the power and courage to overcome suffering, hurt, and pain.

People who know their purpose manage stress better, and have reduced levels of anxiety and worry. They are also more decisive and have a higher level of self-esteem. People with a strong sense of "their why" are shown to likely live longer and have greater satisfaction with who they are and where they are going. Their path in life is more defined and enriched; they have embraced their meaning and purpose in life.

Finding "Your" Meaning in Life

The secret to finding meaning in life may be to not look for it. Psychiatrist Victor Frankl, a holocaust survivor, wrote the seminal book "Man's Search for Meaning." In his book, he described how he held onto meaning and purpose to counter his suffering in the concentration camps where he lived/survived for over three years. However, Frankl advised against actively searching for meaning, instead suggesting that meaning should be found as a side effect of pursuing other goals.

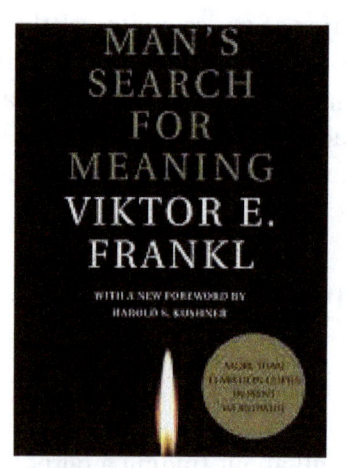

Image source: livemint.com

He stated that finding meaning in one's life should be a primary motivational force but something you should not actively search for. He stresses that finding one's meaning is a lifelong journey. To clarify his message, Frankl makes the analogy of life to a full-length movie. Each moment in life is similar to a movie frame. Each moment or frame needs to be observed and considered individually, but together; they tell a story that has meaning. Frankl stresses that the full meaning of your life may not be totally revealed until the end of your life, similar to what occurs in a movie.

This means that your purpose in life evolves throughout your lifetime, similar to a plot in a movie. As the plot matures, as your life develops, the storyline, your meaning in life, is revealed more clearly. However, your meaning is a metamorphosis, constantly changing and not fully understood until the final line is delivered, your last breath taken.

Frankl states that you can discover the meaning of life in three different ways:

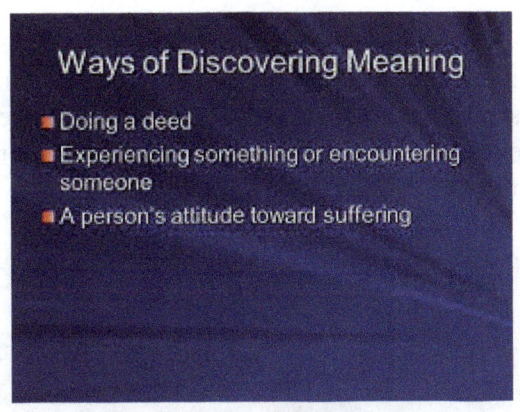

> **Ways of Discovering Meaning**
> - Doing a deed
> - Experiencing something or encountering someone
> - A person's attitude toward suffering

Image source: slideplayer.com

1. By achievement or accomplishment – This could be through your work/occupation, raising a family, volunteering.

2. Social Connections – Developing interpersonal relationships is valuable in experiencing goodness, truth, beauty, love, and togetherness.

3. The attitude you take toward unavoidable suffering – When a person suffers, there is a tendency to say, "What is the purpose of this suffering?" Frankl could have easily said this while in the concentration camps, but he suggests that there is meaning to be found in suffering. To find suffering true meaning, he states two things must happen:

First, the suffering has to be unavoidable, such as a death in the family, being held against your will, losing your job through no fault of your own. Frankl states to suffer unnecessarily is masochistic rather than heroic.

Second, you must accept the challenge to suffer bravely and believe that life has meaning throughout the suffering ordeal. So often, when you are faced with challenging situations, you cave into suffering and, as a consequence, lose hope and meaning.

Frankl states that besides the three ways stated above, finding meaning in one's life also involves making changes during your life. It means you must be adaptable. When you can no longer change a situation, you must challenge yourself to change so you can continue the pursuit of meaning. Frankl emphasizes that the choice to continue pursuing your purpose in life is always yours and to live a more fulfilling, purposeful life, you must embrace the pursuit.

Practical Suggestions to Find Your Meaning

Let your life experiences be the answer to the question, "What is my meaning/purpose in life?"

1. Choose to be Happy

Happiness is a choice that can be practiced by anyone. The challenge is to find happiness in the face of adversity. It is easier to discover one's meaning through the lens of happiness rather than despair. You must make the decision that you will be a happy person through the difficult times as well as the good times.

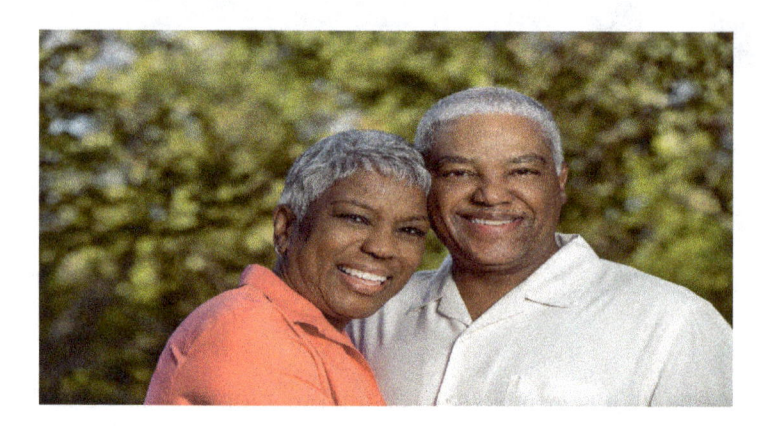

2. Identify and Utilize Your Gifts and Talents

Discovering and utilizing your gifts and talents will create experiences to help you find your meaning and purpose. You must ask yourself:

- What comes naturally to you?
- What are you doing or experiencing when you feel your best?
- How can these "good feelings" best be replicated?

3. Make Quality Social Connections

You need to spend time with the people who add value to your life. Minimize time spent with people that drain your energy or constantly give off negative vibes. Notice how you feel around others that you socialize with the most. (Hint: you should feel good). You should think of yourself as the average of the five people with whom you spend most of your time.

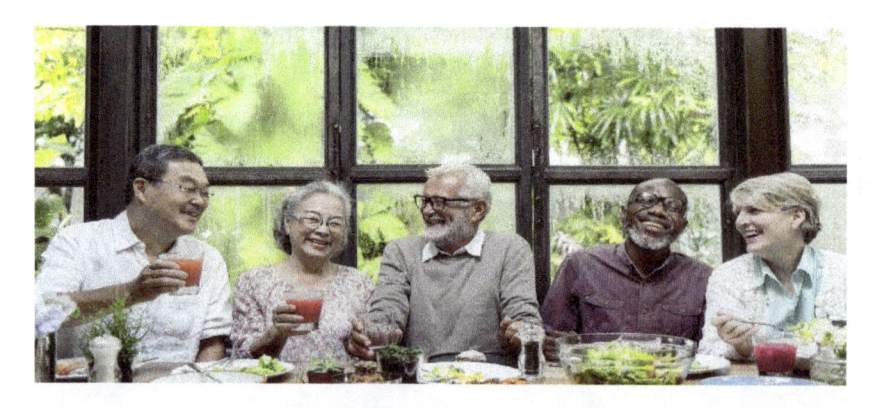

4. Goal Setting

To have meaning in life necessitates having a plan. This does not mean a plan to find meaning, but rather your meaning in life should be found as a side effect of pursuing other goals. As stated previously, finding meaning in your life should be a primary motivational force, but should not be pursued as a primary objective. Take the things you want to accomplish in life and make a plan for working towards them by writing them down and making them S.M.A.R.T. Then, most importantly, take action. Refer to chapter 3.3.: The Importance and Art of Goal Setting to learn how to establish achievable goals.

5. Help Others

Helping other people adds value to one's life. It helps you feel good and gives you a sense of meaning/purpose.

6. Do Something Different

Doing something different helps you break the cycle of just "doing" life and presents an opportunity to "experience" life. It separates you from the norm and helps bring to the forefront the realization that you may be missing out on some of life's experiences that matter.

7. Quit Watching TV

Watching too much TV can become addictive in a negative way. If you want a more interesting life, spend more time doing something stimulating, meaningful, and creative than watching the "boob tube."

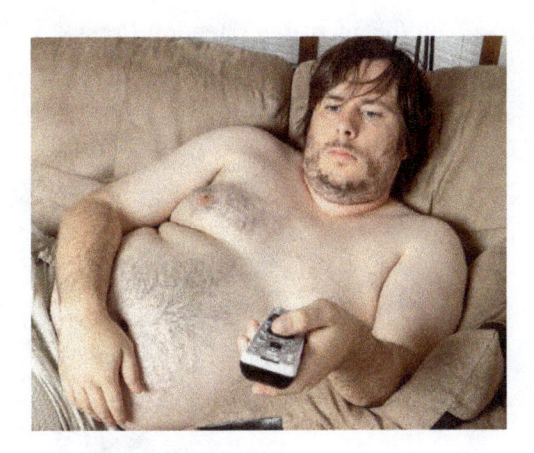

8. Do Something You Have Always Wanted to Do

Step 1. Identify your "thing."

Step 2. Do it.

It does not have to be made more complicated than that. Start today towards saving, learning, or doing whatever it will takes to make what you want to happen, happen.

Conclusion

Finding one's meaning or purpose in life is a lifelong journey of exploration. In his book "Man's Search for Meaning," Viktor Frankl presents a powerful and unique perspective on living your life purposefully and with meaning, often in the face of great suffering and adversity. His life as a Nazi concentration camp survivor is an excellent example of that.

People should not consciously search for meaning, but must let their life experiences through work, volunteering, social connections, and their attitude toward suffering reveal their life meaning. If a person does not like what they see, they need to change the dynamics of their life, and their meaning and purpose will change too. Therefore, it is essential to remember one's meaning in life will change throughout their lifetime.

Viktor Frankl found meaning and purpose for his life through the horrific suffering he endured during the holocaust. The challenge is for us to do the same throughout our lives. Finding life's meaning and purpose is especially challenging for older adults who are often retired, have raised their families are now socially isolated and are suffering from chronic aliments. However, continuing to find meaning and purpose in their lives is essential for their mental health and quality of life.

References

Frankl, Viktor. (2006), *Man's Search for Meaning,* Beacon Press
https://www.psychologytoday.com/us/blog/luminous-things/201803/finding-meaning

6.6. Self-Compassion: The Proven Power of Being Kind to Yourself

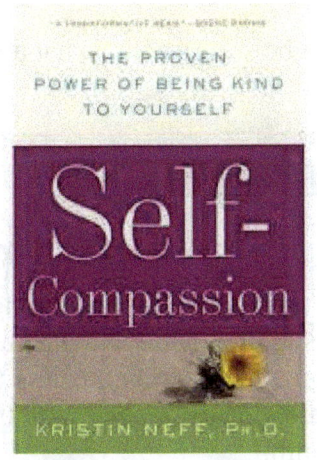

Image source: amazon.com

"Treat yourself like you would treat your best friend"

Introduction

For older adults to have good mental health, they must learn to emotionally treat themselves with kindness despite, in many cases, social isolation and deteriorating physical and cognitive health.

The quote, "Treat yourself like you would treat your best friend," sounds so easy to do, but the reality is that it is hard to execute. For example, when your best friend is suffering or distraught, you would never say, "You are so stupid. Why did you ever do that? Don't you know any better? Stop being a baby and feeling sorry for yourself." Conversely, you would most likely come up to your friend, put your arms around them and console them by saying, "It's ok, everyone makes mistakes. The world goes on, and tomorrow will be another day, another opportunity to do better."

Why is it, when we make mistakes, we often treat ourselves and engage in self-talk like the former example and not the latter? Why do we treat ourselves cruelly, expect so much more, and hold ourselves to a higher standard than we do for others? For most of us, it comes naturally to show compassion to those suffering, but it does not come so naturally to show self-compassion when we are struggling the same way.

Dr. Kristin Neff's book, "Self-Compassion: The Proven Power of Being Kind to Yourself," attempts to answer why you do not show more self-compassion to yourself and why practicing self-compassion is more important and healthier than having high self-esteem. Dr. Neff's book also explains how to implement self-compassion into your daily life effectively.

For older adults, learning and implementing self-compassion/self-love will positively change their perspective on how they should treat themselves to deal constructively with stressful and unpleasant situations.

Young and older adults alike may be surprised by what a little self-compassion can do to help them live happier and healthier lives.

Why Self-Compassion vs. Self-Esteem?

The sad truth is that there's almost no one whom you treat as badly as yourself. Self-criticism is socially accepted in society and is commonplace when things don't go as well as we expect. However, rather than improving the situation and feeling better, self-criticism results in insecurity, frustration, anxiety, and often depression. Feeling these effects of self-criticism is especially true for older adults who are already dealing with the emotional effects of deteriorating physical and mental health.

Dr. Neff, in her book, clearly illustrates that one doesn't become a better person by beating themselves up all the time when things go wrong. She states that self-criticism usually results from misperceived self-judgment due to trying to maintain a high level of self-esteem.

It is generally recognized that feeling good about yourself and protecting yourself against harsh external criticism is related to having high self-esteem, so you work hard at keeping it high. Consequently, when you fail or fall short of expectations, you belittle yourself because your positive self-esteem is threatened by failure.

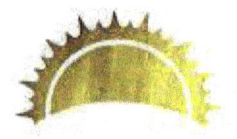

Self-esteem needs success to prove your self-worth, whereas self-compassion says you are worthy no matter what.
Shauna Shapiro, PhD

Image source: facebook.com

Dr. Neff states that you should not focus on self-esteem to achieve happiness because it is outward-looking. Self-esteem is based on comparing yourself to an external standard, often at the expense of others. In other words, for you to feel good about yourself, you must feel superior to those around you, which leads to narcissism, self-absorption, self-righteous anger, prejudice, and discrimination. These are destructive behaviors that lead to fear, negativity, and isolation.

On the other hand, self-compassion is inward-looking. It is about giving oneself kindness because people do not need to see themselves as perfect or as better than others. Self-compassion is a powerful way for you to achieve happiness, optimism, wellbeing, and contentment, which are vital elements for enhanced quality of life.

The Core Components of Self-Compassion

Practicing self-compassion entails three core components that must be implemented simultaneously:

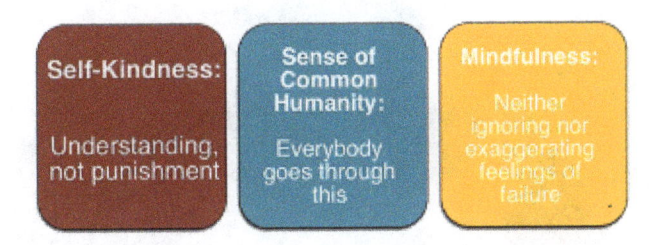

Image source: vidapsychology.com.au

1. Self-Kindness

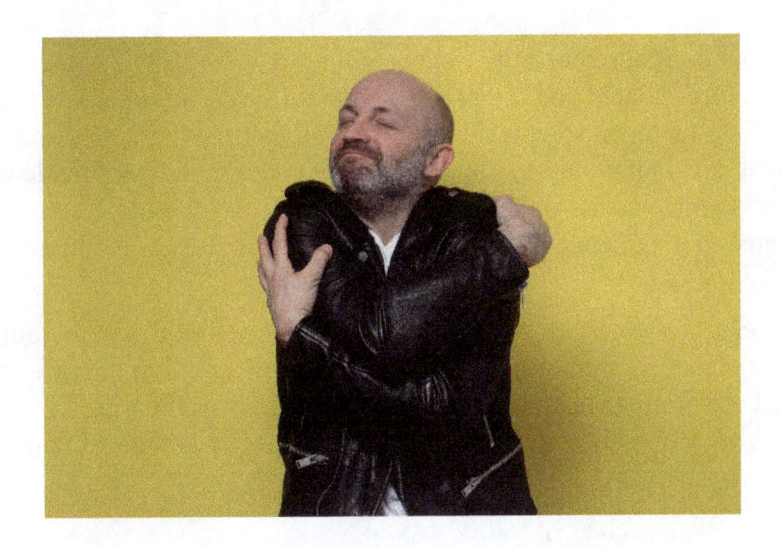

Be gentle and understanding with yourself rather than harshly critical and judgmental. Implementing self-kindness involves stopping critical self-judgment and actively comforting yourself just as you would a wounded friend. It means giving warmth, gentleness, and sympathy from yourself to yourself. Self-kindness could involve self-talk such as, "This is really difficult right now, how can I comfort myself at this moment?" or "I love and accept myself exactly as I am, the good and the not so good." It can also involve physically touching oneself compassionately with a hug or massaging one's arms, face, or gently rocking your body.

Self-kindness allows you to soothe and calm your distressed mind. When you are kind to yourself and begin to relieve your pain, you trigger the hormone oxytocin. Research has shown oxytocin strongly increases the feelings of trust, calm, safety, generosity, connectedness, and reduces fear and anxiety, helping you reduce the levels of the stress/anxiety hormone, cortisol.

People need to be aware that they don't need to look outside themselves for acceptance and security in times of trouble; it is only a self-kind word or self-hug away.

2. Recognition of our Common Humanity

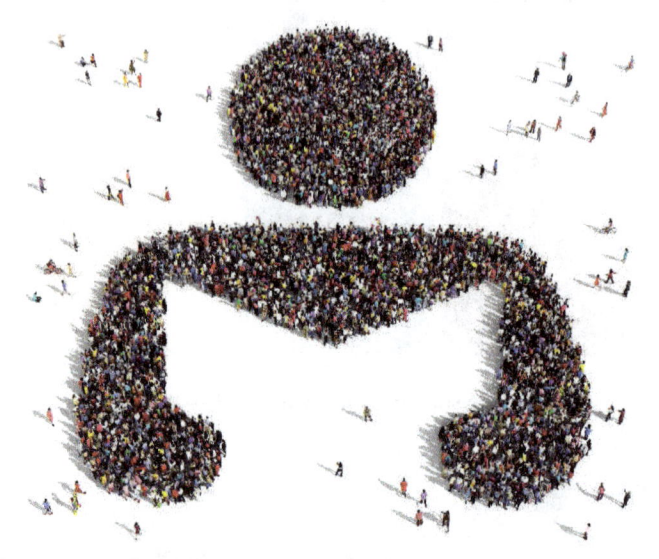

Recognition of our common humanity means feeling connected with others in the experience of life rather than feeling isolated and alienated by our suffering. In other words, everyone has similar experiences and feelings, so you should not think that the hardships and suffering you are experiencing are just happening only to you. All people share feelings of inadequacy, disappointment, and frustration, as well as happiness and joy. You need to remember that you are not alone and isolated in experiencing these emotions. You are just being human.

Loneliness comes from feeling disconnected from others, even if you are only inches away. Those who feel connected to others, who recognize that they are all in this life journey together, are not as intimated and frightened by difficult life circumstances. Feeling interconnected with others allows you to more readily roll with what life has to offer and let life unfold as it should, the good, the bad, and the ugly.

It is essential to compassionately remind ourselves in moments of difficulty that these moments are part of our shared human experience. When we do so, difficult moments become one of togetherness rather than isolation. When you recognize that you are part of the shared human experience, you begin to deal with difficult situations more calmly, effectively, and healthily.

In her book, Self-Compassion, Dr. Neff makes another compelling statement regarding interconnectedness. She states that people are all expressions of millions of prior circumstances that have all come together to shape them in any particular moment. These prior circumstances include their economic and social background, their past associations with family and friends, their culture, their genetics. This means that people do not have complete control over their thoughts and actions because prior circumstances and experiences influence their thoughts and actions. Dr. Neff states that "the illusion of being in control is just that, an illusion."

If you can embrace this understanding of yourself, that you are interconnected to previous life events before this particular moment, then you can be less critical and negatively self-judging and self-blaming in times of distress. Dr. Neff makes an analogy of our existence to that of a hurricane. A hurricane is an ever-changing phenomenon arising from a particular set of interacting conditions such as air pressure, ground temperature, humidity, etc. Like a hurricane, your life is also an ever-changing phenomenon arising out of a particular set of interacting conditions such as your genes, family, friends, education, economic and social history, etc.

Dr. Neff concludes by stating that when you recognize that you and your daily existence and circumstances are the product of countless interconnected factors, many of which are out of your control, you don't need to take your "personal failings" so personally. This allows you to have self-compassion because you are doing the best you can, given the hand life has dealt you.

3. Mindfulness

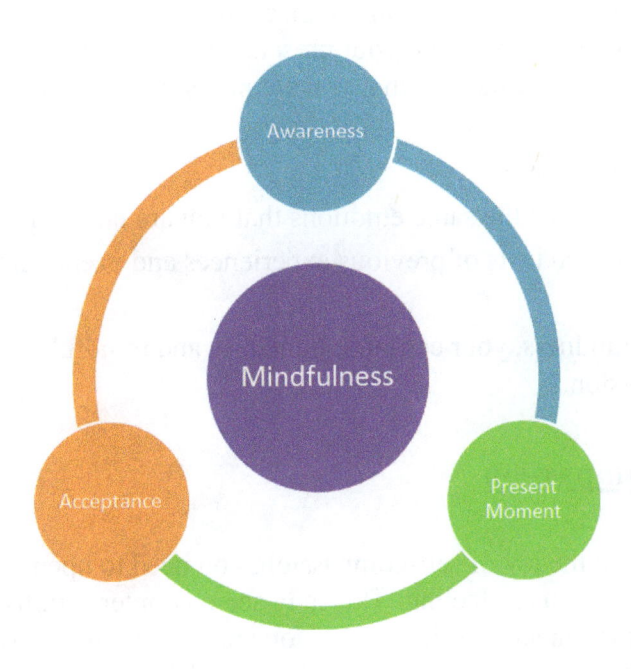

Image source: riverholistic.ie

Mindfulness (Chapter 6.9: Mindfulness and the Power of Mediation) is what you are thinking, feeling, and experiencing right now. It allows you to hold your experience in balanced awareness rather than ignore or exaggerate it. Mindfulness is necessary to successfully implement self-compassion because, if implemented correctly, it allows you to accept what is occurring in the present moment nonjudgmentally. You cannot be compassionate to yourself if you don't recognize the feelings of guilt, sadness, loneliness, and distress at the moment that they are occurring. Recognizing these feelings is difficult because we humans have an innate tendency to move away from pain, so it is difficult for us to turn toward our pain, sadness, guilt, distress, and embrace it. That is why so many people shut themselves off from their emotions. It is the natural thing to do. However, you can't begin to heal what you can't feel.

As well, humans tend to overreact to stressful situations emotionally. It is commonplace for people to make mountains out of molehills, especially when they are emotionally engaged. Mindfulness can enhance an accurate awareness of the present moment, which provides the type of emotional balance necessary to implement self-compassion.

When you see your present situation with clarity and objectivity and not get lost in the negative thoughts and emotions that narrow your ability to act wisely, you can be more compassionate to yourself and take corrective action. Mindfulness allows you to respond compassionately rather than simply react emotionally.

Implementing Self-Compassion

You need to be mindful of what you are thinking, feeling, and experiencing at the present moment. Even for just a few minutes, you need to focus on the pain associated with your failure, stress, or hardship, so you can respond with kindness, such as giving yourself a caring word or a gentle hug. As well, you need to reframe your present situation in light of your common and shared humanity. You need to embrace the fact that you are not isolated but are;

1. Interconnected with others.
2. Others have experienced the same emotions that you are now experiencing.
3. Everyone is the by-products of previous experiences and events in their lives.

By embracing self kindness, your common humanity and mindfulness, you can successfully implement self-compassion.

The Joy of Self-Compassion

For you to experience the joy of self-compassion, you need to open your heart and mind to the pain, sorrow, and distress you are feeling. This may seem counter-intuitive to feeling joy, but Dr. Neff explains that by implementing self-compassion and being kind to yourself, you can control your negative emotions in the warm embrace of good feelings. This allows you to respond, not react, in a positive and effective manner to stressful situations. For you to have control over your emotions is joyful.

Self-Compassion and Self-Appreciation

Loving Myself

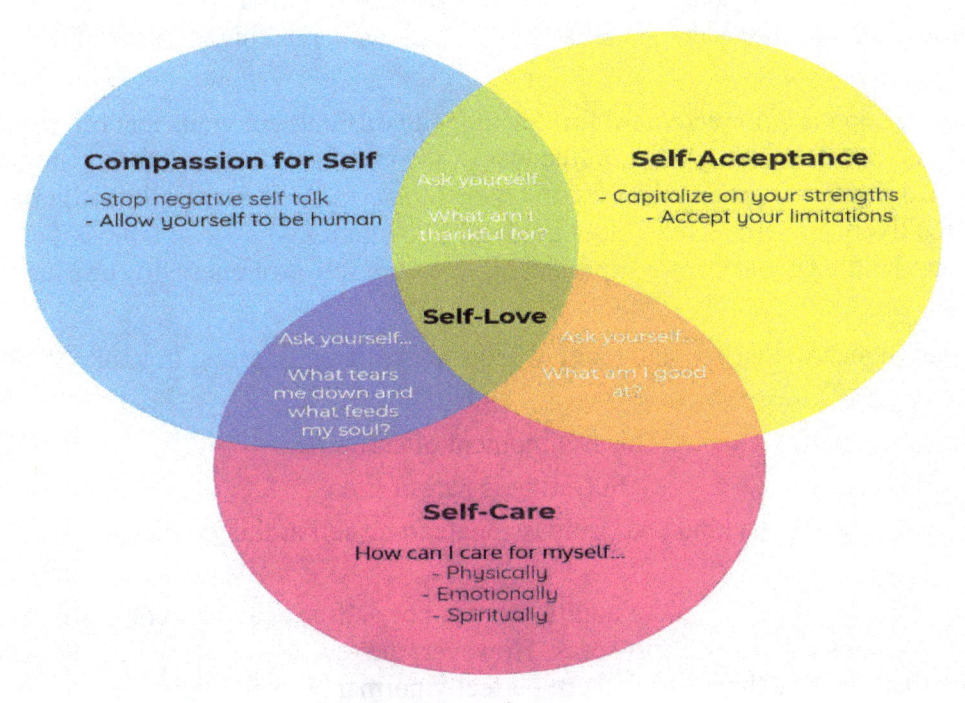

Compassion for Self
- Stop negative self talk
- Allow yourself to be human

Ask yourself... What am I thankful for?

Self-Acceptance
- Capitalize on your strengths
- Accept your limitations

Self-Love

Ask yourself... What tears me down and what feeds my soul?

Ask yourself... What am I good at?

Self-Care
How can I care for myself...
- Physically
- Emotionally
- Spiritually

Image source: noshameonu.org

    Self-compassion allows you to be self-appreciative more fully because the three basic components of self-compassion – self kindness, a sense of common humanity and mindfulness – are not just relevant to what you don't like about your life, such as suffering, sadness and feeling distress, but are equally relevant to what you do like. Dr. Neff explains that people get so caught up in problem-solving and coping with the pain in their lives that they give insufficient attention to and don't celebrate sufficiently the things that provide them with pleasure. As a consequence, people suffer more than they need to.

    Dr. Neff states that self-compassion and self-appreciation are two sides of the same coin. The first, self-compassion, focuses on you dealing with suffering, and the second, self-appreciation, focuses on dealing with what pleases you. Implementing self-compassion means accepting personal weaknesses and loving yourself despite them. Self-appreciation, on the other hand, celebrates your strengths, what you do well.

    Everyone has the capacity for resilience, growth, and happiness, simply by relating to their daily experiences, both good and bad, with appreciation and compassion. This means you can embrace both the joy and the sorrow of being human in a mentally healthy way. For the older adult, this is so important and can transform their quality of life as they enter the golden years.

Conclusion

What has been presented here is just the tip of the iceberg of the knowledge, power, and understanding that self-compassion can bring to your life. The benefits of self-compassion for older adults include emotional resilience, personal growth, and improved interpersonal relationships. Each of these is essential to improve and maintain a high quality of life.

Self-compassion is a powerful tool for dealing with difficult emotions that often occur in older adults as they deal with grief from the loss of their partner or other family members and the pain and disability from chronic illnesses and mental deterioration. By dealing with these emotions positively and effectively, older adults can rid themselves of the bonds of critical self-judgment that hold them back from experiencing accurate self-awareness, joy and happiness.

An effective mantra that you can recite when something goes wrong in your life is:

"This is a moment of suffering.
Suffering is part of life.
Let me be kind and compassionate to myself at this moment."

For most people, especially older adults, who can be self-critical, self-compassion does not come easy. Old habits are difficult to break. However, the rewards of being kind to ourselves, recognizing that what we think and feel are perfectly normal human thoughts and emotions, and being more mindful of our emotions can be immense.

Try it, and enjoy being kind to yourself.

Reference

Neff. Kristin, Morrow, William. (2011). *Self-Compassion: The Proven Power of Being Kind to Yourself,* HarperCollins

6.7. Self-Leadership

Introduction

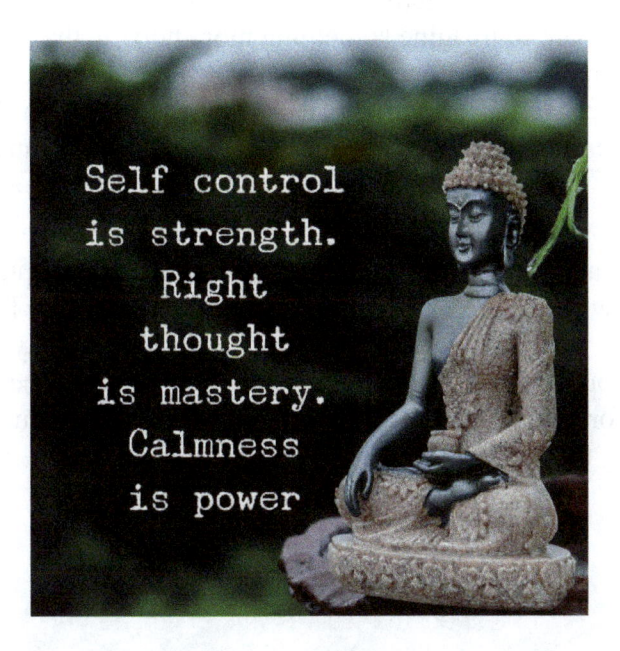

> Self control is strength.
> Right thought is mastery.
> Calmness is power

What role does leadership play in the mental health of an older adult? Leadership means being in control. A person who has strong mental health means they are mentally in control of their life. Because of the numerous and significant physical health challenges/obstacles that older adults are confronted with, (Chapter 2: The Off-Season: Studying the Opposition to Your Health), they need to be emotionally and cognitively in control of their lives. During their golden years, older adults may not be leading a corporate division, heading a volunteer committee, or being responsible for raising their children through their adolescent years. Still, they continue to be leaders by controlling of their own life. Their happiness and mental wellbeing depend on them leading well.

If the older adult, or anyone for that matter, follows the ten fundamental principles of leadership listed below, they will lead a better, more complete, balanced, accountable lifestyle. Embracing these ten principles will help eliminate "excuses" from your vocabulary. Looking for and using excuses to explain the reason why something has happened shows mental weakness and vulnerability. Making excuses can become a crutch that becomes hard to throw away. Sometimes, there are legitimate reasons why something has happened to you, but usually you own most of the responsibility.

The following ten principles will help you become accountable for what you think, say, and do. This will help you become a better person, which will help you live a higher quality of life.

The Value of Leadership in Your Life

Crap happens in our lives all the time, but what is most important is how we deal with the crap. For example, a drunk driver runs a red light, and his car slams into the side of your wife's car, and she is killed. It is hard to imagine something more horrific than that. What will be your reaction, how will you handle and respond to this horrific tragedy? You will most likely be angry at the driver. You may even want to seek revenge, "He deserves to die or live in prison for the rest of his life for what he has done." You may even experience denial and depression for what has happened.

These are expected reactions. The ten principles detailed in this chapter will suggest productive ways to deal with tragedies, hardships, and obstacles in your life. The focus of the principles listed is to help you take ownership of your emotional and physical reactions. You are never too old to learn, though learning, embracing, and implementing these ten principles will not necessarily be easy for you. However, the rewards of doing so are huge for living a happy and rewarding life during the golden years.

> "True leaders always practice the three R's: Respect for self, Respect for others, Responsibility for all their actions."
> - Anonymous

Image source: habitsforwellbeing.com

Leadership impacts all aspects of one's life. Taking leadership in life means casting no blame. Instead of complaining about illnesses, challenges, or setbacks, being your own leader means developing solutions and solving problems. Effective self-leadership means leveraging physical and cognitive assets, social relationships, and material resources available to you so you can deal productively and healthily with the issues you are dealing with. Leaders will not allow their pride or ego to control them.

Being your own leader means you control your own thoughts, words, and actions. Embracing this control means becoming accountable for everything that happens in your life. Having this type of control and accountability is very powerful to possess for older adults. If you do not have this control and are stuck with self-doubt, self-pity, and disillusionment, you become highly vulnerable to life-altering mental health issues such as depression and a diminished quality of life.

The Ten Principles of Personal Leadership

1. Extreme Ownership/Accountability

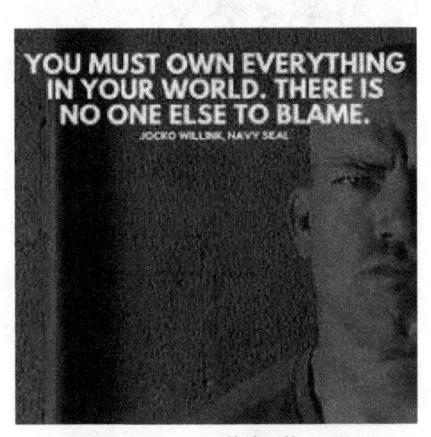

Image source: linkedin.com

Extreme ownership and accountability mean all responsibility for your happiness, success, failure, and sadness rest with only one person, yourself. To be a leader of your own life, you must own everything in your world. Therefore, ownership and accountability are the fundamental core concepts of leadership. Self-leadership requires that you do not blame others but first look in the mirror at yourself.

Taking ownership when things do not go as planned requires great humility and courage but is necessary. You must look at yourself and the challenging situations you face through the objective lens of reality, without emotional attachment or ego. You must accept responsibility for failure, admit weaknesses, and consistently build a better and effective self. Learning to take ownership and being accountable for everything that happens in your world is a lifelong project. There will be many times when you fall short of taking full responsibility. Failure to take responsibility at times should not be unexpected, especially for the older adult whose behavioral habits are ingrained and hard to change. When people fall short of taking "extreme ownership," they must remember to show self-compassion to themselves (Section 6.6. Self-Compassion: The Proven Power of Being Kind to Yourself). Change in behavior takes time.

2. No Bad Teams, Only Bad Leaders

Faults or failures rest at the top, with oneself and no one else. You are your own CEO, but you do not live in isolation. In fact, for the older adults, social isolation is one thing you need to avoid. Instead, you must get each member of your social support group to buy into the concept of supporting each member of the group in the process of enhancing one another's lives. Once this culture of support is established into your social group dynamics, the social group and each member will perform better.

> "When it comes to standards, as a leader, it's not what you preach, it's what you tolerate."

Image source: twitter.com

From a standards perspective, it is not what a leader preaches but what they tolerate that is important. If disharmony and negativism are accepted within an individual's social circle and there is no accountability for their behavior, poor social dynamics become the new standard. To be a true leader of yourself, you must tolerate only behaviors or norms from family, friends, and acquaintances that enhance your quality of life. If you tolerate anything less, it leaves you vulnerable to less-than-optimal quality of life.

3. Believe in What You Want (Understanding the "Why")

"If you understand the why, you can overcome any how." This quote was presented in a previous chapter, Chapter 6.5. Finding Meaning/Purpose in Life, but it is also applicable here. To lead oneself, you must be a true believer in what type of life you want to lead. If you don't believe it (understanding the why), you cannot live it (overcoming the how).

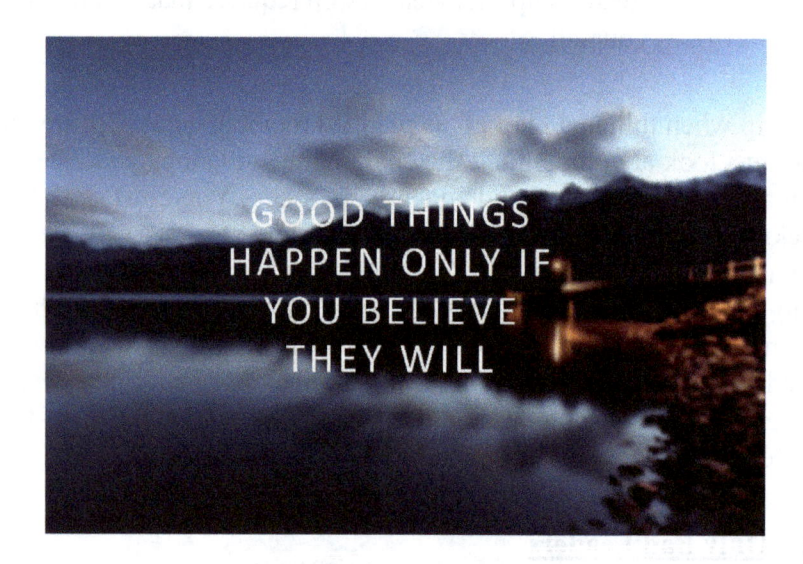

> GOOD THINGS HAPPEN ONLY IF YOU BELIEVE THEY WILL

The challenge comes when your belief is not explicitly clear. If there is ambiguity in how you want to live your golden years, your decision-making becomes more difficult. For example, "Do I want to volunteer or don't I?" or "Do I really want to travel or don't I?"

For you to be your own leader, you need a clear vision of what is important to you (short-term and long-term goals) and how you want to accomplish these goals (Section 3.3. The Importance and Art of Goal Setting). These goals can and will change over time, but believing in the goals set at present is what is necessary for them to come true.

4. Check the Ego

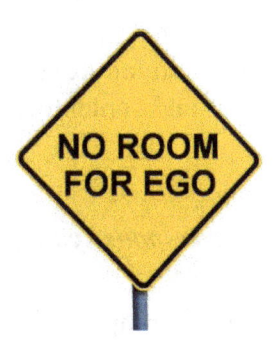

Ego disrupts everything, from planning to taking good advice to accepting constructive criticism. Everyone has an ego, and that is good. It is what allows you to set lofty goals. However, if ego is left unchecked, it can become destructive by clouding judgment and preventing you from seeing things as they are.

For older adults, this can become a real problem. Too often, the older adult becomes "set in their ways." Sometimes they perceive change as emotionally overwhelming. Other times they don't want to change because it brings about a sense of vulnerability. Unfortunately, there may be times when an older adult does not want to change just because they are too stubborn to change. "I like things just the way they are" is a phrase often heard from older adults.

Change is going to come in your life, whether you like it or not. You must embrace change, and this takes courage and leadership on your part. By dropping the ego and seeing the situation as it is, it allows change to occur more readily and productively.

Being your own leader requires humility. It requires admitting that, at times, change is necessary. You can be confident in "your way" of thinking and doing but not to your own detriment. Being a good leader of yourself means being receptive to others' opinions and making a change when it is necessary. Change is going to happen, so embrace it and enjoy the ride.

5. Developing a Strong Social Network

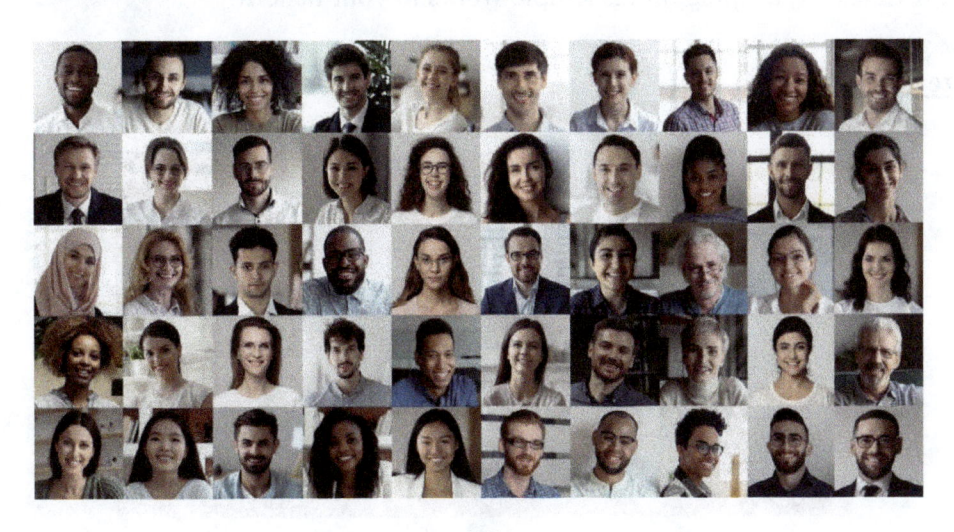

Older adults must avoid social isolation, and defensive silos must be broken down. You must recognize that operating independently of others is not always the best way. There are many times when two or more heads are better when a decision needs to be made or a goal is to be accomplished. Isolation leads to vulnerability and often failure. Being your own leader requires you to forge social relationships. Greater happiness and contentment will follow.

6. Keep It Simple

"Communication is the response you get."

Life has inherent layers of complexities and these compound issues. As your own leader, clear, concise, and simple communication of your goals is necessary. You must communicate your goals in a way that your social support team understands and embraces them. The social circle must be allowed to ask questions to clarify when they do not understand, and this must be encouraged as well as to explain to them your rationale.

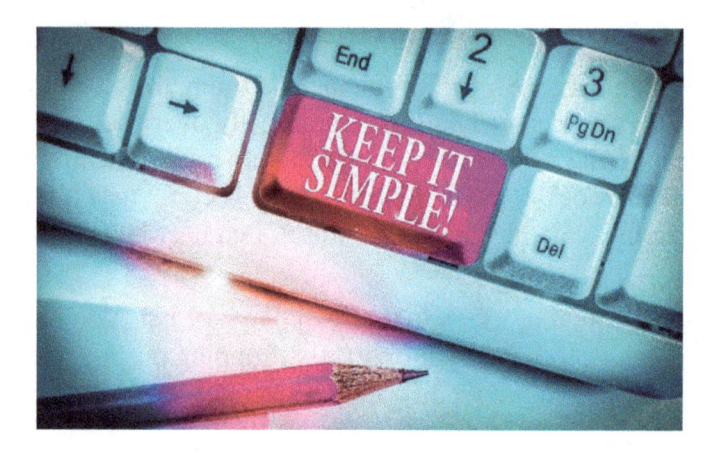

If you cannot communicate with others concisely and simply, you cannot succeed. A 30-second "elevator speech" to explain things is an excellent rule to follow. As an effective communicator, if people cannot accurately and concisely repeat what is being explained, effective communication has not occurred.

As your own leader, keeping things simple works to your benefit.

7. Prioritize and Execute

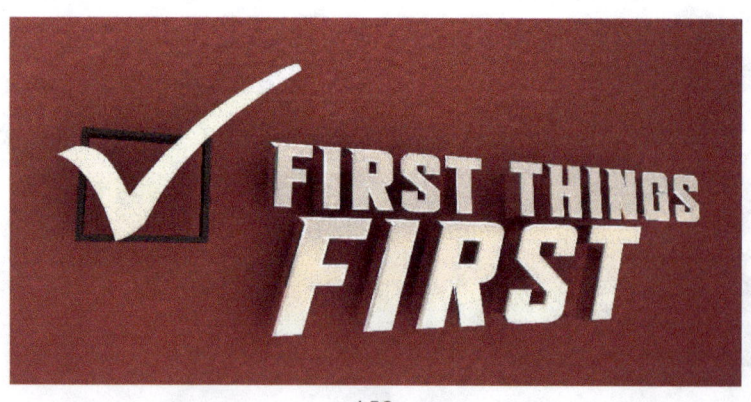

"Relax, look around, make a call"

Many challenges that present themselves feel complex and confusing for older adults because they often have little control over what is happening. Feeling confused and out of control is especially true when acute illness occurs. As an effective self-leader, you must remain calm and make the best decisions possible. It is important not to become overwhelmed and try to tackle multiple problems simultaneously, especially those out of your control. You must determine the highest priority tasks that are under your management and execute effectively.

Preventative planning is an effective way to manage challenging situations. You need to use your experience to make contingency plans in anticipation of likely challenges that could arise. Making contingency plans is especially important for older adults due to the increased likelihood of sudden sickness and injury. Having the will updated, a signed DNR (Do Not Resuscitate) form if that is your wish, and emergency instructions and contacts files are all helpful preventative measures that people should have in place.

Preventative planning shows good leadership and will communicate your wishes and reduce stress on family members who are often put into making difficult and sometimes life-determining decisions.

"Don't sweat the small stuff." It is easy to get sidetracked and lose focus on the details of a situation. A good leader will step back and look at the bigger picture to help correctly prioritize what needs to be done to achieve their short-term and long-term goals.

8. Delegate

Sometimes being a good leader means stepping back and letting others in the social circle and support team handle a problematic situation. Delegation of responsibilities is at times good and necessary but often very difficult for older adults since having a sense of being in control of their lives is extremely important to them.

Clear and open communication is vitally important. Delegation does not mean you are surrendering total control of your life. When delegating, micromanagement should not be necessary, but clear, concise communication of your wishes should be.

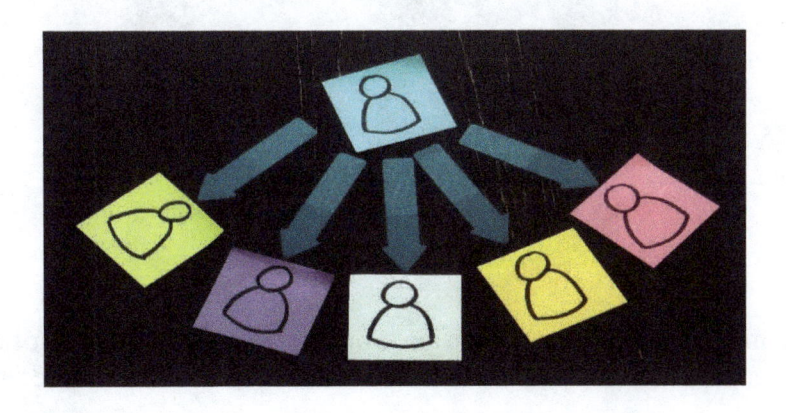

It is impossible to be a master of everything. Sometimes, deferring to specialists or consultants who are experts in the field is an effective way of managing the situation. Once again, you need to put your ego aside, show good leadership and step away when the situation warrants it.

9. Plan

Having a plan is always a good idea. Planning begins with analysis, but it is essential not to get bogged down in an overload of detail. Careful prioritization of incoming information is important. Encourage interaction with those who understand the situation best, but avoid paralysis by analysis.

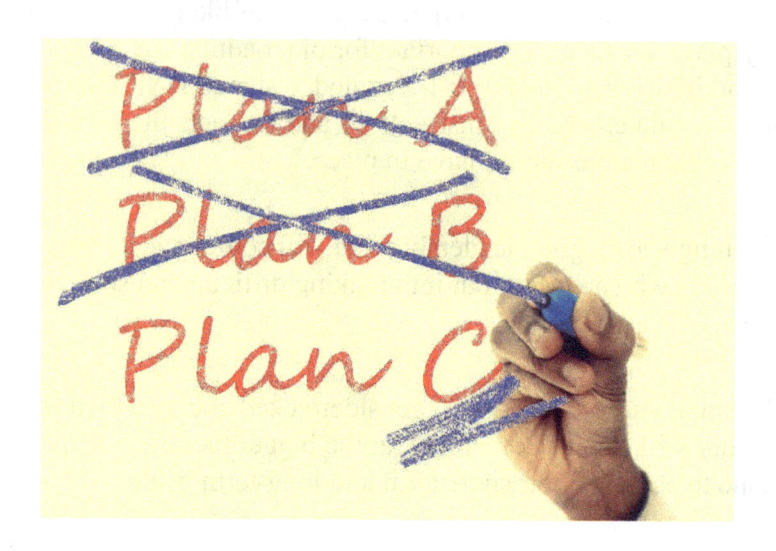

Good self-leadership requires planning for situations that you can control and developing contingency plans to help manage risk. Best practices require constant review of plans for effectiveness. You need to determine how you can adapt your plan to make it even more effective, especially as you grow older and your fitness and health change.

10. Decisiveness Amid Uncertainty

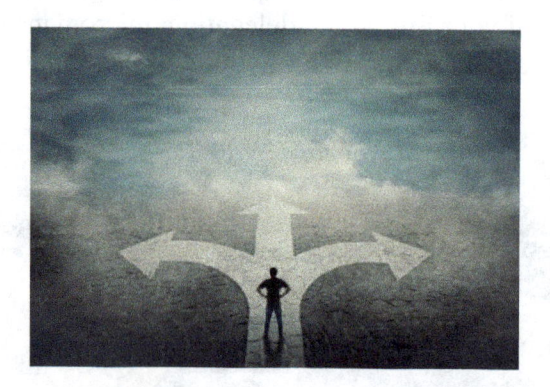

Usually, when making an important decision, you likely don't have 100% of the information needed. However, good leadership means making decisive decisions amid uncertainty. Waiting for

100% of the data often leads to delay, indecision, and an inability to execute. It is a sign of emotional insecurity. You must be prepared to make an educated guess based on previous experience, present knowledge, and likely outcomes.

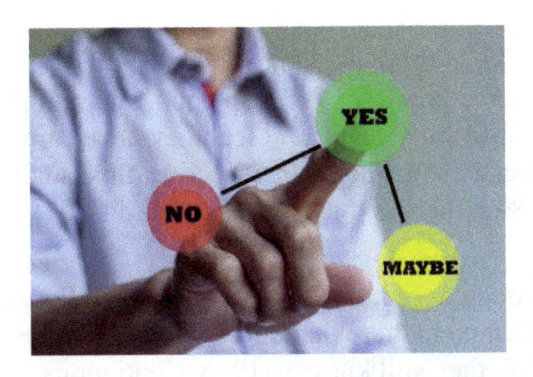

This principle applies to almost every aspect of an individual's life. Outcomes are never certain, and success is never guaranteed. You must develop the ability to be comfortable acting decisively amid uncertainty. Rarely is there a 100% correct solution, and it is essential to be ready to adjust decisions quickly based on evolving situations and new information. Effective decision-making requires good self-leadership and mental health.

Conclusion

It is not necessary to embrace all of the principles listed above. However, the more principles you can apply to your life, the better you will control the challenges that life will present. Having a sense of control for the older adult is important because it gives then a feeling of independence which will allow them to live a more joyful and productive life.

Being a leader of others is good, but being a leader to yourself is necessary.

References

Willink, Jocko, Babin, Leif. (2017) *Extreme Ownership: How U.S. Navy Seals Lead and Win.* St. Martin's Press 2nd Edition
Howell, Jon P. (2012) *Snapshots of Great Leadership*. Routledge
https://en.wikipedia.org/wiki/Leadership#Self-efficacy_for_leadership

6.8. Learn From Others Through Good Communication Techniques

Introduction

As a rule, older adults like to think they know a lot. They have lived many years and have experienced many things, some good, some not so good, and unfortunately, some ugly. They have shared many laughs, shed some tears, and feel they have earned the right to say, "I have been there, done that." From a mental health perspective, this is not the best attitude to have. Even when living in your 80's, there is much to learn and do.

A person of any age, young or old, if they take the time to listen, watch and interact with others, will quickly learn that no matter what university degree they may have or experiences they have lived and endured, they still know so little. Continuous learning is available because everyone you interact with comes from a different background and has had experiences unlike your own. You can learn so much from others. Simply through social interactions, you cannot help but learn more each day.

For older adults, continuous learning is necessary for their mental health and enhancing their quality of life. If you are not learning, you are cognitively stagnating, and stagnation leads to deterioration. Continuous learning from others is a great way to avoid mental health deterioration. Effective communication is the key that opens the door to continuous learning and good cognitive health.

The Keys to Effective Communication

1. Be Curious

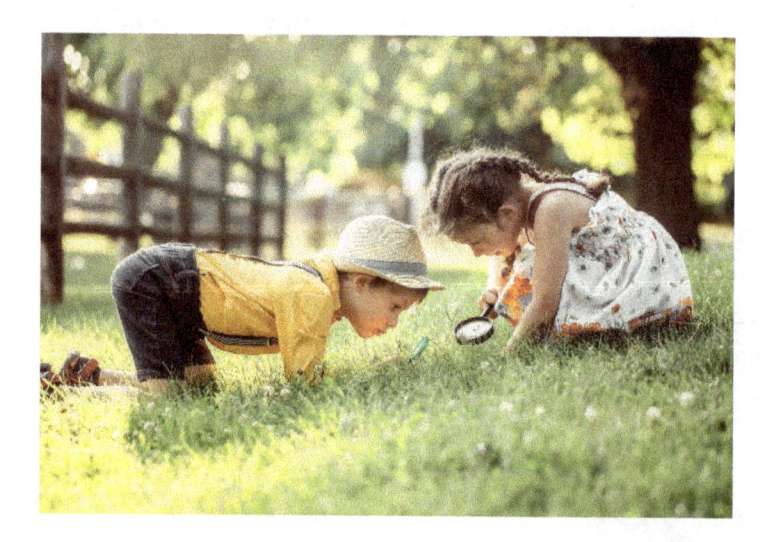

For the older adult, but really for anyone at any age, it is important to be curious about other people and what can be learned from them. There is a great book that helps illustrate this. "If I Could Tell You Just One Thing" is a compilation of 68 interviews with famous people such as entertainers Simon Cowell, Judy Dench and Jude Law; the politically powerful like President

Bill Clinton and Prime Minister Tony Blair; the spiritually influential such as The Dalai Lama and Reverend Libby Lane; the super rich such as Bill Gates and Sir Richard Branson; adventurers like Bear Grylls who summited Mt. Everest, and survivors like Lily Ebert (Auschwitz concentration camp) and Katie Piper (domestic abuse).

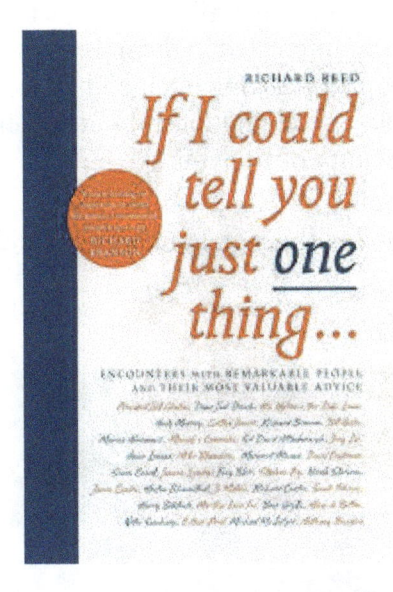

Image source: books.apple.com

Not all of those interviewed are household names, but each has his or her own unique story and nugget of gold to offer that can enrich everyone's life. "If I Could Tell You Just One Thing" covers the full spectrum of human experiences and emotions. The book allows learning from people who have made it financially to others who have endured incredible hardships and those who have witnessed the worst of what humans can do to one another.

The one question the author asks each person interviewed is the same, "Given all that you have experienced, given all that you now know and given all that you have learnt, if you could pass on only one piece of advice, what would it be?" Such a powerful question leads to powerful responses, some of which are surprisingly simple.

The author's curiosity leads to a great informative read. You personally may not get the opportunity to interview the famously rich or the politically powerful. However, there is still much to be learned from those with whom you socially interact with. Continuous learning and intellectual stimulation are two reasons it is so important for older adults to avoid social isolation. Everyone you interact with has a back story and experiences that you may not have had the opportunity to experience or, in some circumstances, have been fortunate not to have had to experience. Even in the most modest social circles, there is much to learn if you are curious enough to ask the right questions.

2. Ask Open-Ended Questions

Being curious is not an innate skill but one that you can learn. All you need to do is ask "open-ended" questions when interacting with others. Open-ended questions cannot be answered with a simple 'yes' or 'no'. Instead, they require the respondent to elaborate on their points. Open-ended questions help a person see things from another person's perspective as they get informative feedback from that person instead of stock 'yes' or 'no' answers. People learn so much more about others by asking open-ended questions.

By asking open-ended questions, not only will you learn a lot, but it will also reinforce to the recipient of the questions that you are interested in them. Everyone loves to be thought of as interesting. Showing interest in people by asking open-ended questions will strengthen the relationship between the two of you. Social relationships are essential for everyone. The stronger these relationships are, the better quality of life you will have.

Open-ended questions start with the words what, where, when, who, why and how (five W's and an H). These are powerful words and will generate interesting and informative responses.

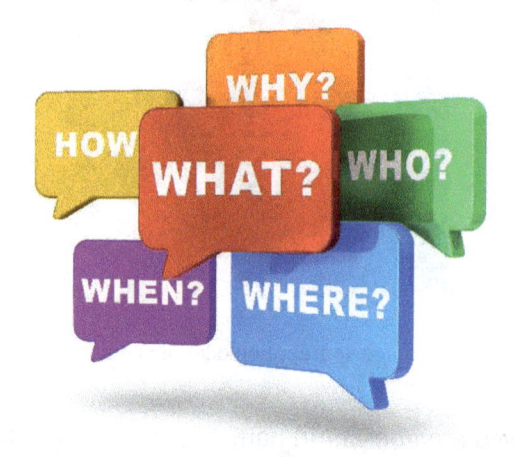

3. Active Listening

Asking the right questions is only half the battle. You must "listen" to the response to be fully engaged and learn from what the person is saying. Being fully engaged means listening "actively." By listening actively, you send a signal that you are interested in what the other has to say, and this encourages that person to "open up" more and elaborate on their response. The more information you get from another person you are communicating with, the greater the opportunity for learning on your part.

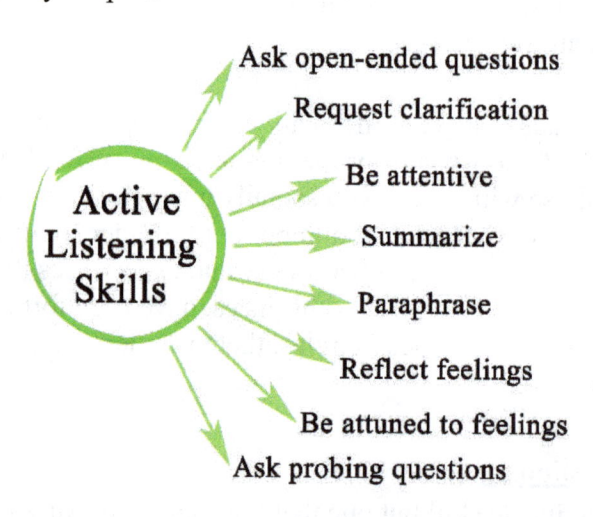

Active Listening Skills:
- Ask open-ended questions
- Request clarification
- Be attentive
- Summarize
- Paraphrase
- Reflect feelings
- Be attuned to feelings
- Ask probing questions

Active listening means doing the following:

a. Remove or avoid possible distractions – During a conversation, there should be no answering text, emails, or calls on a smartphone.

b. Pay attention – You should focus only on the person you are talking with. This focus makes the other person feel that they are the only one in the room.

c. Avoid thinking ahead – You cannot be focusing on what is communicated if you are thinking ahead to what you are going to ask next.

d. Give nonverbal cues – This is important and reinforces to the other person that you are engaged in what they are saying. Non-verbal cues include nodding your head in agreement, smiling, and making good eye contact.

e. Probe for more information – By asking follow-up open-ended questions.

f. Acknowledge feelings – Often the conversation can get quite personal with much emotion being communicated. Acknowledge these emotions by saying things such as, "It sounds like a fantastic/horrific experience," or "I can't imagine how that made you feel."

g. Pay attention to pauses and hesitancy – These may be the opportunity to ask further probing questions.

4. Clarify Understanding

It is easy for you to interpret what you hear through your personal filters/experiences. Unfortunately, this can lead to miscommunication. Good communication requires that you clarify what has been said. Getting clarity reinforces to the other person that you are interested in what they are telling you, leading to a better communication and learning experience.

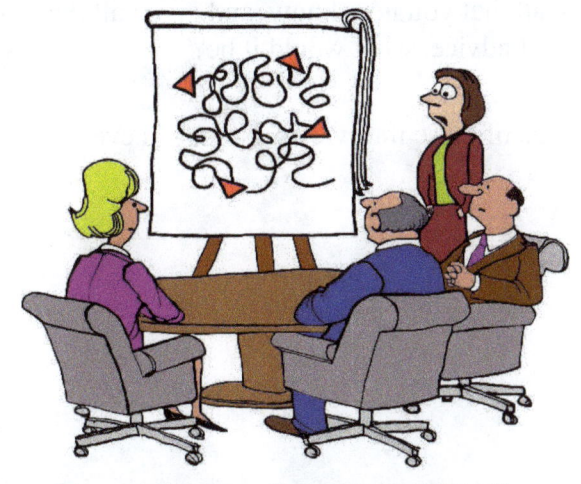

"The way forward is clear."

Clarify understanding by doing the following:
a. Ask questions to confirm that you understood what was meant to be said.
<u>Examples</u> – "Are you saying…?"

"Did you mean…?"

"Sounds like you feel…"

b. Paraphrase – Rephrase (shorter and clearly) what was heard.
– Make sure the other person confirms your interpretation of the conversation.

c. Ask for definitions or meanings of words that may have different or ambiguous meanings.
<u>Examples</u> – "What do you mean when you say…?"

"How do you define…?"

"When you say........, do you mean...?"

Conclusion

Good mental health is necessary to enhance the quality of life for older adults. Continuous learning is a crucial component for maintaining good mental health. What better way to learn than from those that surround you: family, friends, neighbours? In other words, learn from your social circle.

Learning from others requires good communication skills. Be curious and ask open-ended questions, listen actively and clarify understanding. There is much to be learned from those around you. Don't be naive, be curious.

Bonus Section

As mentioned previously, "If I Could Tell You Just One Thing" is a powerful book based on interviews with the rich, famous, politically powerful and individuals who have accomplished extraordinary things in their lives. The author asked all of them just one question, "Given all that you have experienced, given all that you now know, and given all that you have learned, if you could pass on only one piece of advice, what would it be?"

Below are excerpts of some of these interviews. No one is ever too old to learn from the advice they give.

Bill Clinton, President of the United States, 1992-2000

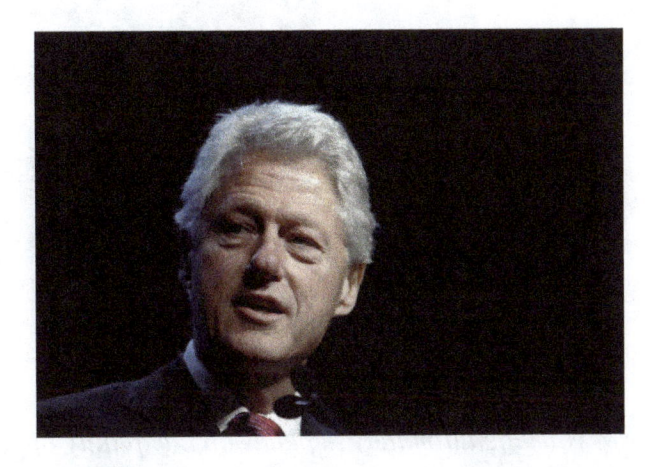

"One of the most important things is to see people. The person who opens the door for you, the person who pours your coffee. Acknowledge them. Show them respect."

Terry Waite, hostage for five years in Lebanon, four of which were in solitary confinement

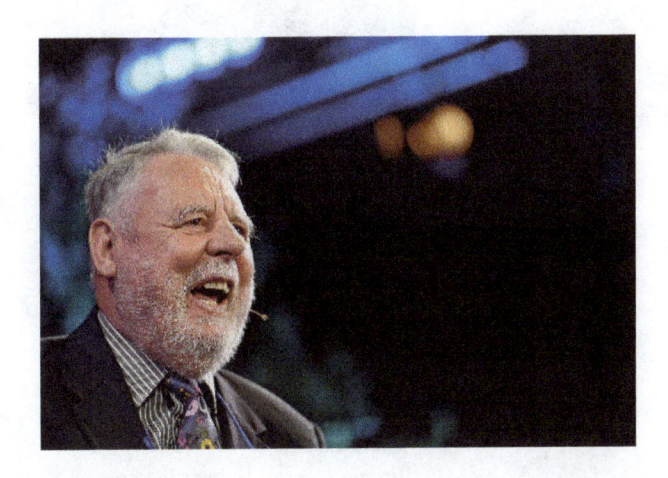

"It is the same lesson I learnt in that cell. What you have to do is live for the day, you have to say, now is life, this very moment. It is not tomorrow, it's not yesterday, it's now, so you have to live it as fully as you can. Invest in every day."

Esther Perel, the world's most renowned relationship therapist

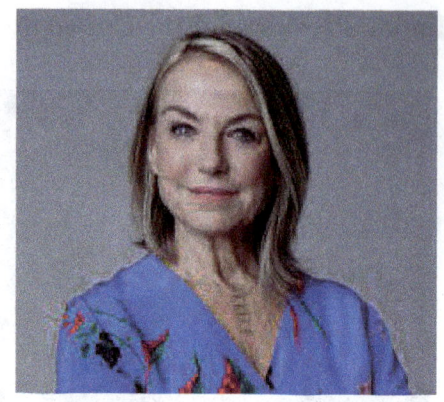

Image source: unitedtalent.com

"The quality of your life ultimately depends on the quality of your relationships. Not on your achievements, not on how smart you are, not on how rich you are…"

Simon Cowell, entertainer and entrepreneur

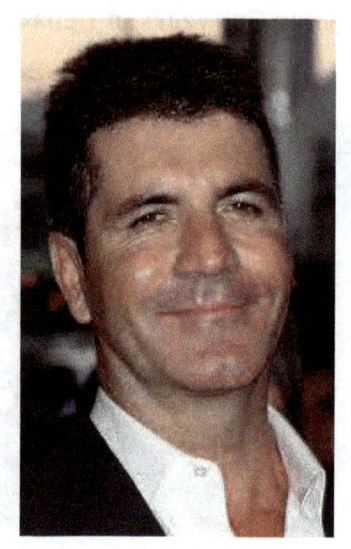

Image source: Britannica.com

"My best advice is to listen, listen rather than talk."

Shami Chakrabarti, former director of Liberty, a human right lobbying organization in Britain and who after 9/11 was given the name "most dangerous person in Britain" because of her work with terrorists and criminals

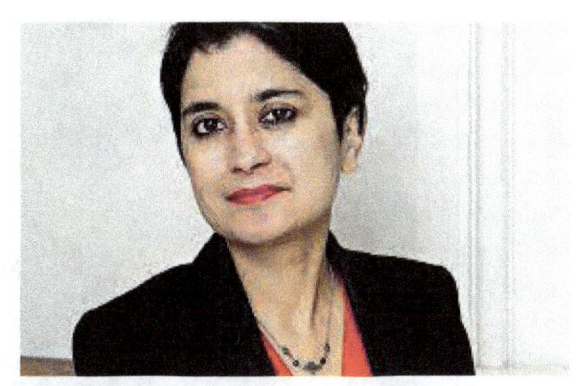

Image source: jewishnews.timesofisrael.com

"Powerful elites in the world always succeed by divide and rule, using tools like fear and racism. But solidarity, the basic human connection we can all have with one another, is stronger. It is the magic weapon to achieve change. If we remember human rights are the same as my human rights, even if we don't look the same, and if we support one another, we all benefit, we all become stronger. Ultimately, we are each other's security."

Lieutenant Colonel Lucy Giles, the first female college commander to run the Sandhurst Military Academy, the most revered military institution in Britain

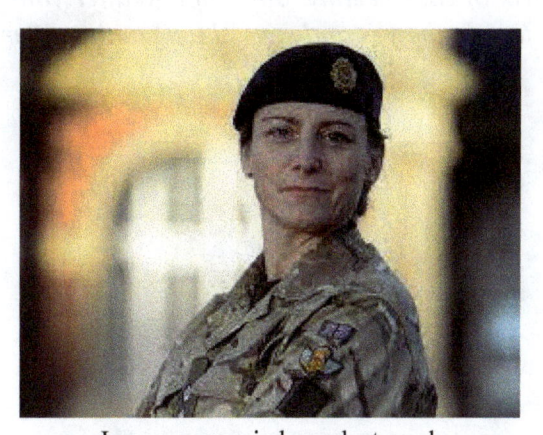

Image source: independent.co.uk

"Life is about doing the right thing, on a difficult day, when no one is looking."

Laila Ali, the most successful female boxer in history, four-time world champion, CEO of her own beauty business, best-selling author, TV host, actor, mom and daughter of Mohammad Ali, arguably the world's most famous athlete

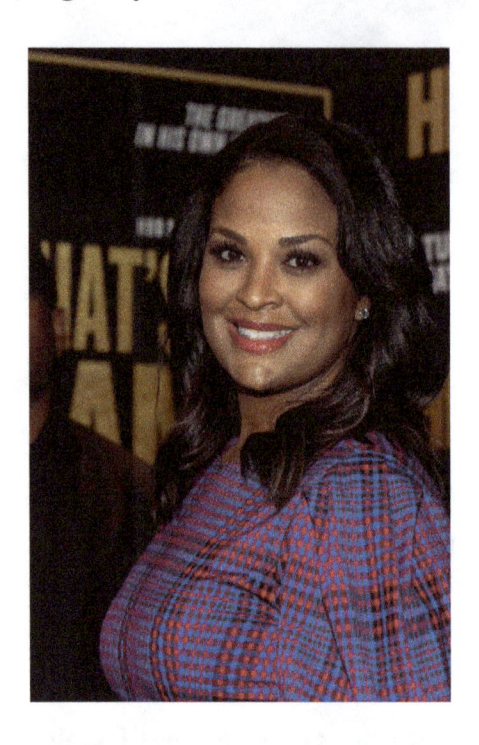

"We all have what it takes, inside us. Trust yourself, trust your intuition. Don't let someone else be in control of your destiny, don't not go after your passion because of fear. Look fear in the yes and say, "I am coming after you."

Bill Gates, one of the richest men in the world

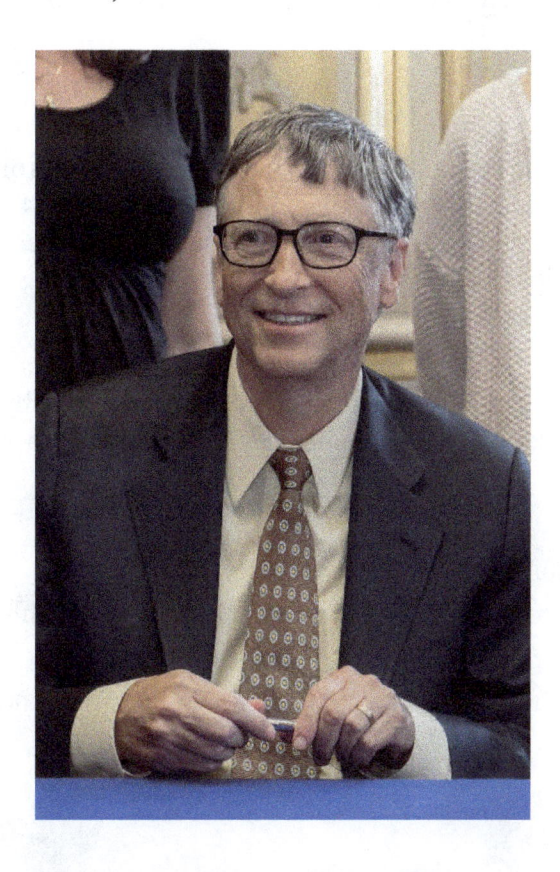

"Foster your love of reading. It's our core skill as human beings. It's the gateway to everything else. It gets you involved."

References

Richard, Reed. (2016). *If I Could Tell You Just One Thing*, Canongate Books
Zackery, Lois., Fischler, Lory. (2014). *Starting Strong: Strategies for Success in the first 90 Days.*, Jossey–Bass

6.9. Mindfulness and Mindfulness Meditation

Introduction

Older adults need good mental health so they can stay in control of their lives. As previously discussed, this means developing good mental fitness (Chapter 6.4), finding meaning/purpose in your lives (Chapter 6.5), being compassionate to yourself (Chapter 6.6), developing and practicing self-leadership (Chapter 6.7), and continuously learning from others through good communication techniques (Chapter 6.8).

Practicing mindfulness also helps nurture good mental health by encouraging you to live in the moment. Mindfulness means paying attention in a particular way:

1. On purpose
2. To the present moment experience
3. Without a judgmental attitude; you do not need to change things.

Mindfulness meditation is a technique that allows a person to practice living in the present moment.

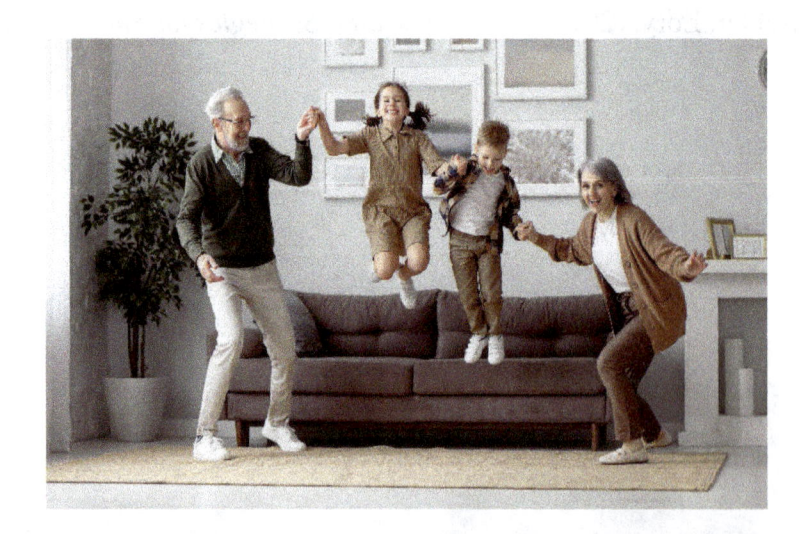

Older adults do not need to complicate their lives. With advancing age, physical and mental deterioration is already doing that for them. Older adults are often heard saying, "Life is moving too fast. Where has the day gone? Everything seems more complicated than it used to be." Practicing mindfulness regularly helps you be aware of the present moment and has the potential outcome of slowing your lives down. As a result, you are only living one moment, the present moment, at a time.

Mindfulness

Mindfulness is moment-to-moment awareness. This means being aware of the present moment experience on purpose and not judging the moment but seeing it as it is. If judgement does occur, these are noted and then dismissed as new moments of awareness arise. Think of mindfulness as the "light of awareness." It is not a tool like a light switch which you use to turn on the lights but the light itself that illuminates a room. With mindfulness, you purposely turn on the light which allows your senses to see, feel, smell, hear and touch more clearly what is in the room at the present moment. You do not judge what your senses convey to you moment-to-moment but just move on from one observation/perception to the next.

Practicing mindfulness involves stopping all the "doing" in your life and relaxing and being aware of the present without trying to fill it up with anything. Practicing mindfulness allows you to purposefully allow your body and mind to come to rest in the moment, no matter what is "on" your mind or how your body feels. Mindfulness means allowing you to be in the moment with things exactly as they are without needing to judge or change anything.

Possible Benefits of Mindfulness for the Older Adult

1. **Simplify your life** – Mindfulness means eliminating past and future clutter from your thought process. A mindful person only focuses on the present moment. It is important to note that being aware at a particular moment can include thoughts and judgments of the past or future, but by being mindful, you will not get lost or distracted in those thoughts but acknowledge them and then move on from them.

2. **Learn to be aware of oneself** – Mindfulness means you pay attention on how "you" are feeling, what "your" thoughts are at the present moment without having to judge them. Eliminating judgment often helps you reduce stress.

3. **Learn self-acceptance** – Mindfulness allows you to accept your thoughts and feelings without feeling that you have to change or manipulate anything.

4. **Self-awareness** – Mindfulness often tends to slow and clear the mind so the person can observe what their mind is up to from moment to moment.

5. **Self-control** – Mindfulness can support better decision-making because the person becomes more aware of their thoughts and feelings moment to moment.

Mindfulness Meditation (Paying Attention Right Now)

Mindfulness needs to be practiced. The more systematically and regularly a person practices mindfulness, the more likely a person will benefit. The benefits received will be unique to each person.

One of the ways you can practice mindfulness is through Mindfulness Meditation, which is about paying attention in the present moment. The challenge is that often your present awareness becomes preoccupied with the thoughts of the past or the future than in your awareness of being here in the present now. Your past or future thoughts can be so overpowering, particularly in times of crisis or emotional upheaval, that they can easily cloud your awareness of the present.

Mindfulness Meditation helps give direction of your attention to the present moment. Mindfulness Mediation is the process of observing the body and mind on purpose, of letting your experiences unfold from moment to moment, and allowing them as they are in a non-judgmental way.

How to Practice Simple Breath Focused Formal Mindfulness Meditation

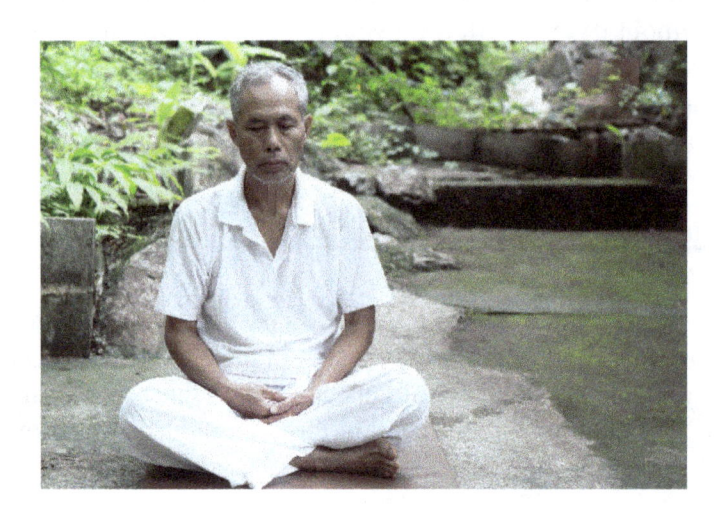

1. Position yourself in a posture so you are sitting upright in a comfortable way. If you are unable to sit upright, try to lie down with your shoulders and head elevated above the chest/torso.

2. Control your eyes. The eyes can be opened or closed. If they remain open, your gaze should be directed to a blank/neutral spot so your attention does not get distracted. The gaze should be straight ahead or slightly looking downward and blink as you normally would.

3. Bring your attention to the feeling of being there sitting. Reposition the body as you need to, but typically, you want to sit in stillness.

4. Settle your attention to the feeling of breathing. This could be the experience of your chest or lower abdomen breathing or feeling the breath at your nose.

5. Your attention should be focused on sensations that change from moment to moment. These sensations could be the feeling of your in-breath, your out-breath, and the moment between these.

6. You will notice that you will be distracted many times by your thoughts and feelings. When this happens, notice the distraction but choose to bring your attention to the feeling of breathing again. It is not necessary to stop the activity of the mind, but always choose to bring your attention back to your breathing. Distracting thoughts and feelings may continue in the background of your awareness, but your attention needs to be on your breathing.

Micro Mindfulness Meditation

Mindfulness Meditation is usually associated with the formal practice as described above. However, finding the time and an isolated place to practice formal mindful meditation is often difficult, if not impossible. As a consequence, a helpful alternative to this traditional approach is Micro Mindfulness Meditation. This involves short bursts of mindfulness meditation incorporated throughout the day. Micro Mindfulness Meditation is a shortcut attempt to try to achieve the same beneficial effects of full mindfulness meditation.

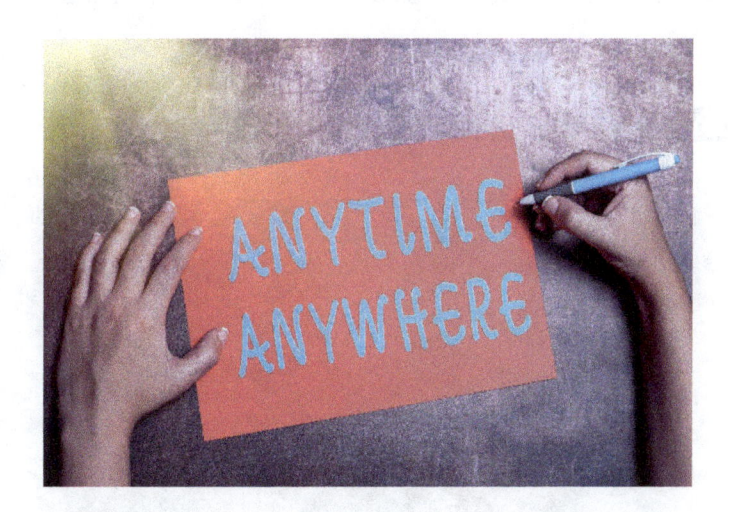

Micro Mindfulness Meditation can be done anywhere for as briefly as a few seconds. It helps to use triggers such as a physical landmark, a red traffic light, or a phone ringing in the office. When the trigger occurs, you need to take a couple of deep breaths and refocus your mind to the present, just like a person would in a formal meditation practice. During these brief few seconds, you need to bring their awareness to your surroundings and how you feel "right here, right now."

Similar to formal mindfulness meditation, the benefit you may find is to help slow your fast-paced life, which will help provide measured responses to stressful situations instead of knee-jerk reactions. These brief moments of meditation may be especially valuable for the older adult who feels that their life is always racing out of control. Micro Mindfulness Mediation has the potential to allow you to take a moment to restore calm and emotional control.

The Effectiveness In Micro Mindful Meditation

Though Micro Mindfulness Meditation is convenient and quick, the question is, does it have the same effects/benefits as traditional mindfulness meditation? Authorities in the area of mindfulness suggest that small bits of meditation are better than none at all and that the more experienced a person is at formal meditation, the more effective micro meditation will be. Most long-term mindfulness practitioners use Micro Mindfulness Mediation far more frequently than formal mindfulness mediation.

Practicing micro mindfulness mediation frequently throughout the day is often more practical than finding time to do a formal Mindfulness Meditative Practice, just as doing small bits of activity throughout the day such as walking and stair climbing is more practical for many people than finding the time for a formal cardiovascular workout session. In terms of receiving the full benefits of mindfulness meditation, micro meditation has value as an adjunct to full meditative practice, just as living an active life is to doing regularly strenuous exercise.

Just like exercise, frequent small doses of micro meditation are better than none. A person should identify triggers that they can use, such as waiting in line at a grocery store, or when the phone rings and focus on their breathing when these triggers appear. The person can then judge for themselves whether micro meditation helps them have better control over their hectic and demanding life.

Practicing Micro Mindfulness Meditation:

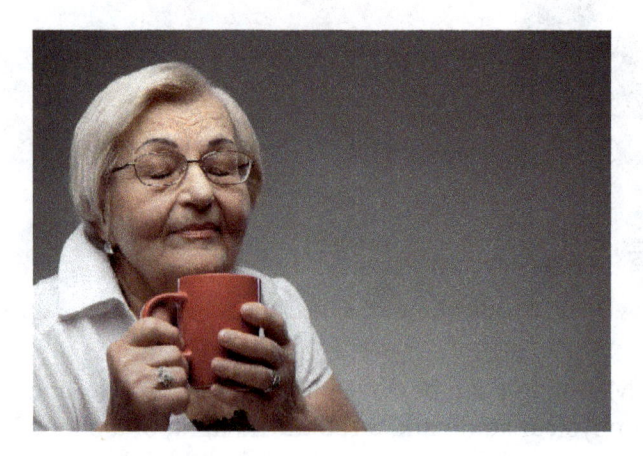

During any daily activity, such as drinking a cup of coffee, you just need to pay attention to the experience. Be attentive to your thoughts and emotional feelings and sensations such as the warmth of the cup, the aroma, and the taste of the coffee. The goal is for you to bring awareness to your surroundings at that particular moment and how you feel at that micro mindful moment. By doing this it is possible that things will slow down and you may will feel more in control of that moment.

Seven Key Elements to Successfully Implementing Mindfulness Meditation into the Older Adult's Life

1. Non-Judging – Non-judging means being impartial to one's thoughts and experiences. People naturally judge and react to everything they experience. Most of the time, these judgments have no objective reasoning and tend to dominate their thoughts.

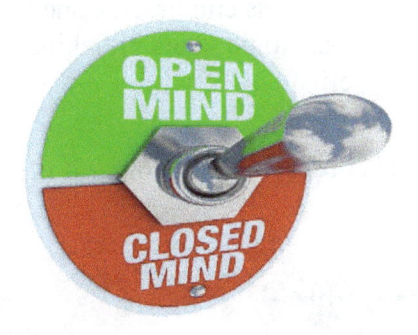

When practicing mindfulness mediation, you must be aware of these automatic judgments, prejudices, and fears that intrude your thoughts, and be impartial. To practice mindfulness, observe your thoughts without needing to judge or act on them; accept that they are present for that moment and then revert to focusing on your breath.

2. Patience – Things need to unfold in their own way and time. Patience can be a beneficial quality when the mind is agitated.

To practice mindfulness effectively, you need to be completely open to each moment and understand that things can only unfold in their own time.

Letting events unfold naturally and being non-judgmental means having more control, not less, because people are not trying to manipulate things, they possibly have no control over. People need to feel their breath, relax and let things unfold as they do. You may find that letting things unfold naturally is excellent for stress reduction.

3. Beginner's Mind – Too often, older adults fall into the trap of letting their thinking and beliefs about what they "know" prevent them from seeing things as they are.

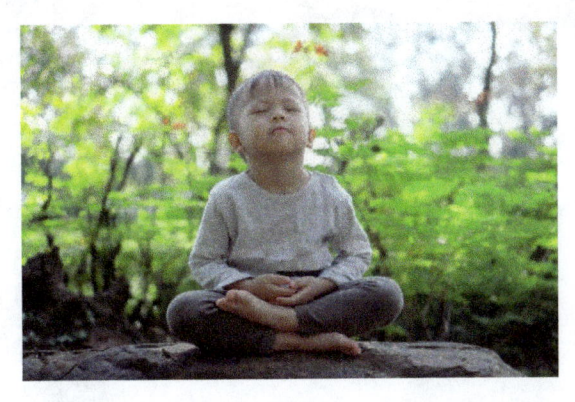

To appreciate awareness of the present moment, you must be free of expectations based on past experiences. Older adult, often find this hard to do since it is through the filter of past experiences that they see everything. The attitude of the beginner's mind invites you to open your mind and be receptive to new possibilities.

4. Trust Yourself/Practice Self Leadership – Trusting yourself is very important in all aspects of mindfulness practice. Mindfulness emphasizes one's own awareness of being your own leader, understanding what it means to be yourself, taking responsibility for being yourself, and learning to listen and trust yourself.

5. Do Nothing – Mindfulness is observing, not doing. It is simply paying attention to whatever is happening at present.

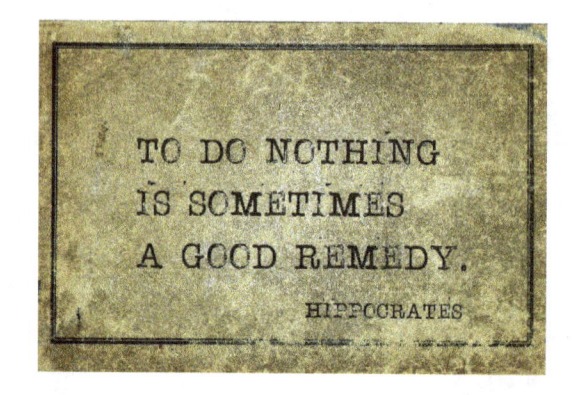

> TO DO NOTHING IS SOMETIMES A GOOD REMEDY.
> HIPPOCRATES

If you are tense, just pay attention to the tension. What is the sensation of being tense? Are you breathing more rapidly and more shallow than normal? Are you sweating in you palm or forehead? What are your thoughts and feelings while being tense? If you are criticizing yourself, then you need to observe this activity of the judging mind. Practicing mindfulness allows anything and everything that you experience from moment to moment to be there because it already is.

6. Self-accepting – This means seeing and coming to terms with and accepting things as they are in the present.

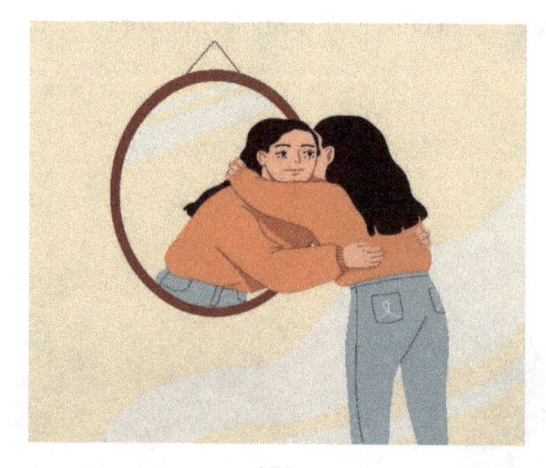

Because insecurities developed over time, you will often waste a lot of energy denying and resisting what is fact. You are trying to force situations to be the way you would like them to be. The practice of mindfulness allows you to be open to whatever you are feeling, thinking or seeing, and accepting it because it is there right now.

7. Letting Things Go (Non-Attachment) – This is the attitude of letting go which allow you to let things be and accept things as they are.

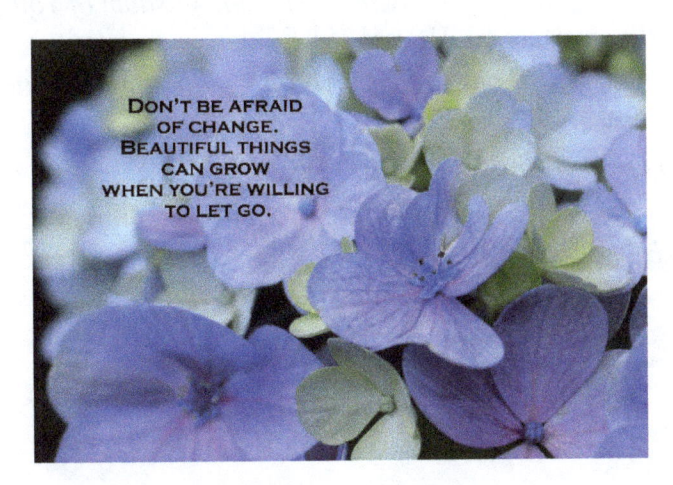

Sometimes, you will find it difficult to let something go because it has such a stronghold over your mind. Not letting things go is the origin of chronic stress.

In these instances, you need to direct your attention (mindfulness) to what "holding on" feels like, the stress it is causing, and the physical and mental consequences it has on your life. When you finally do let the stress go, you become aware of what it feels like without this stress and its positive consequences.

Turning to mindfulness frequently will allow you to benefit more from its practice. The seven key elements presented will assist you in developing a successful mindfulness practice, and this will allow mindfulness to become a "way of being," and in turn will allow the power of mental control to be put to practical use.

Conclusion

Practicing mindfulness and being mindful more frequently throughout the day can be highly beneficial to older adults' mental and physical health. A person being aware of what they are doing while doing it is the essence of mindfulness practice. A potential benefit of present awareness is being in emotional control more frequently.

Daily mindfulness mediation will encourage you to bring mindfulness into your daily life. You will likely find yourself spontaneously paying more attention to each moment of your life and not just when you are formally meditating.

Mindfulness will not directly solve any of the problems that you may encounter. However, it will allow you to see your challenges more clearly through the lens of a clear, non-judgmental mind. This will allow you to make better choices and find better solutions to your problems.

References

Kabat-Zin, Jon. (2004). *Full Catastrophe Living: Using the Wisdom of Your Body and Mind to Face Stress, Pain, and Illness.* Random House, 15th Edition.

Kabat-Zin, Jon. (2005). *Wherever You Go There You Are: Mindful Mediation in Everyday Life,* Harper-Collins, 10th Edition,

Sykes, Lucinda. (2011) *Meditation for Health: Program Workbook*

6.10. Make Life a Joyful Journey

Introduction

The presence of joyfulness in a person's life is essential for strong mental health and that is why a whole chapter is devoted to it.

Being joyful is a choice and an important choice because it affects your mental health and your quality of life. At different times in the older adult's life, as it is for everybody life, it is hard to be joyful after losing your lifelong partner, losing your job, suffering from chronic illness, or being recently diagnosed with a life-threatening event. However, being joyful or sad still boils down to making a choice. The choice is between being sad and seeing the dark side of an event or being happy and seeing hope and joy in the same event.

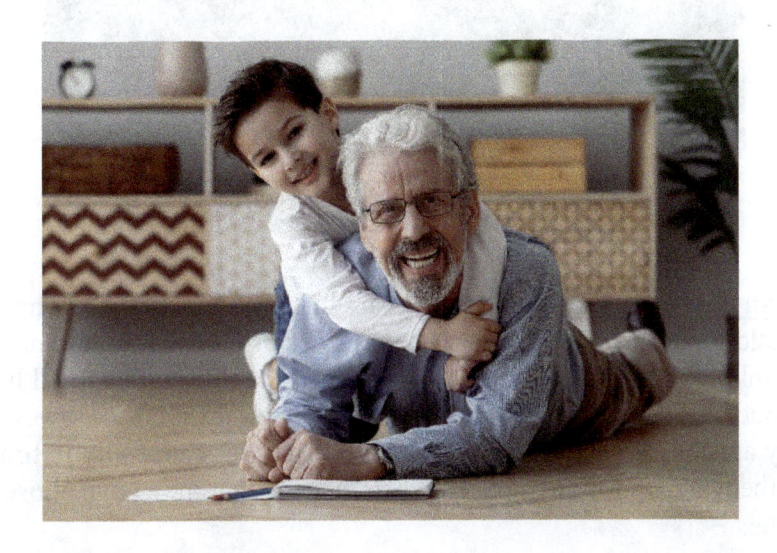

You are not alone when you feel envious of those who appear to be living a joyful life or feel frustrated when you cannot do the same. Joyfulness can be elusive, and this is especially true for older adults who are often thought of as "cranky" compared to when they were younger.

Maybe, for some, the search for joyfulness is happening in the wrong place. Perhaps it is occurring outwardly rather than inwardly. Maybe there is too much dependency on other people or material things to bring you happiness rather than searching within your own heart and soul for that elusive happiness.

Lasting joyfulness is not found in the gym, health spa, or golf course; nor does it come with new cars, new clothes, self-improvement seminars, or financial papers, but rather it is found within you. In this increasingly materialist world, it may be an innovative thought, to look inward rather than outward.

Two Key Points in the Search for Joyfulness

1. Life is like driving through the mountains – There are many highs, lows throughout life, and these are amplified in the life of the older adult. The secret to living a joyful life is closing the gap between the highs and lows. That does not mean lowering the bar on the highs but instead raising the bar on the lows. Living a joyful life means putting a different perspective on the lows, so they don't drag a person down and seem so overbearing that they dominate the person emotionally and mentally.

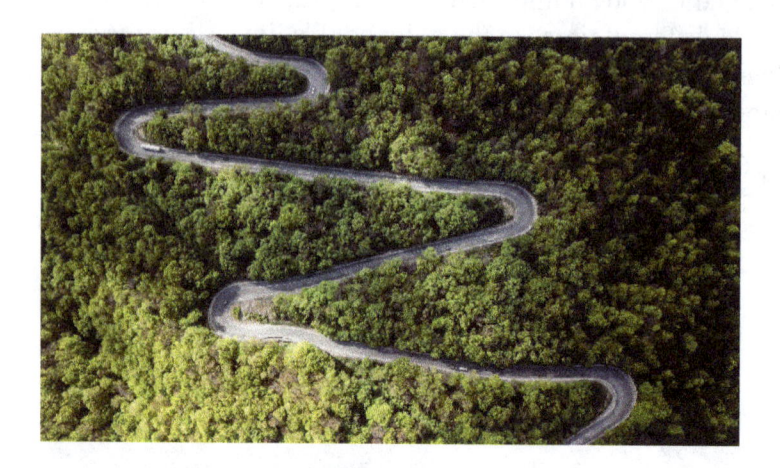

2. This is not an easy journey – It often appears that for some people, who continuously display a joyful outlook on life, it all seems to come so effortlessly. It would not be uncommon to catch oneself thinking, "Well they haven't experienced the difficulties that I have had to face," or "It has been a much harder journey for me than it has been for them." However, the reality is that, though it may appear easy for "joyful people" to be joyful, especially in times of distress, it is just as hard for them as it is for anyone. The difference is that they have chosen to be joyful rather than not to be.

Living a joyful life is not an easy choice to make. It requires thought and effort, but for those who make that choice, the rewards are just too great to pass up.

Finding Joyfulness: Five Points and the 21-day Challenge

1. Self-Reflection

Being self-reflective involves doing three things:

a. Goal Setting – Identifying what is important (what will bring joy) in your life and setting goals to achieve these things.

b. Identifying Personal Strengths – It is your strengths, not the weaknesses, that will bring you joy.

c. Identifying Negatively-Influencing People In Your Life – Identify people, events, and beliefs in your life that you perceive are holding you back from reaching joyfulness in your life.

a. Goal Setting

YES, goal setting again. If you have been reading this book sequentially, you will know that goal setting is significant in enhancing a person's mental health and quality of life.

Goal setting is all about being self-reflective. It is a process that forces you to look within yourself (that is where joyfulness comes from) to determine what is important in your life and how to enhance or optimize it.

Research has shown that the practice of writing down short- and long-term goals results in a greater opportunity to achieve these goals. Effective goal setting can be an intimidating process and often overwhelms people, especially the older adult unfamiliar with the process. However, if done precisely and strategically, it is a very effective way to redirect your thoughts and actions into achieving something special.

The secret to goal setting is to be **S.M.A.R.T.**

S – Specific
M – Measurable
A – Action orientated
R – Realistic
T – Time lined

Establishing Your Goals

(Review Chapter 3.3: The Importance and Art of Goal Setting)

Use the following table to help direct thoughts to various categories that goals could fall under but don't be limited by the categories listed here. Everyone must identify what is important in their life and what they want to achieve.

Health and Fitness	
Financial	
Business / Career	
Intellectual/ Knowledge/Creative	
Contribution and Spiritual	
Social and Family	
Travel and adventure	

Step 1 – Identify three (a person can have more if they want) short and long-term goals. The time line for short-term goals can be from a day to three months. Long-term goals typically are three months to many years in the future.

Step 2 – Once the short-term and long-term goals are established, you can utilize the table on the next page to make them S.M.A.R.T.

Take your time to think carefully about what you hope to achieve and how you will accomplish your (SMART) goals. Your first short-term goal is to set a time line of a week to complete this process.

Please Note – **It is not unusual to have difficulty organizing thoughts for SMART Goals. Effective goal setting takes practice. A person will need to revisit their goals many times and reset them as they proceed through the journey of life.**

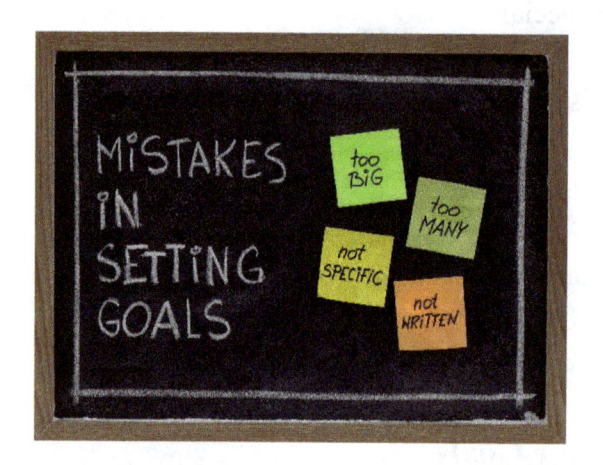

S.M.A.R.T. Goals

Specific – Be as specific as possible. The more detailed the goal, the better you can visualize the result.

Measurable – If the goal cannot be measured, it is hard to determine success. Specific metrics are needed to measure progress and achievements.

Action – What are specific actions or steps required to achieve the stated goals? Be specific.

Realistic – The goals need to be established so you can realistically accomplish them. If not, frustration, disillusionment, and failure will result. List how your goal is realistic based on the resources, time, and effort a person can commit.

Time lined – Set a specific time (a week, a month, a year) to accomplish each goal. Set a short-term and long-term timeline so you can measure your progress toward achieving the goal.

(Goal Work Sheets – refer to Chapter 9.2.6)
First Goal:

Specific	
Measurable	
Action	
Realistic	
Time lined	

Second Goal:

Specific	
Measurable	
Action	
Realistic	
Time lined	

Third Goal:

Specific	
Measurable	
Action	
Realistic	
Time lined	

b. Identify Three Strengths that You Possess.

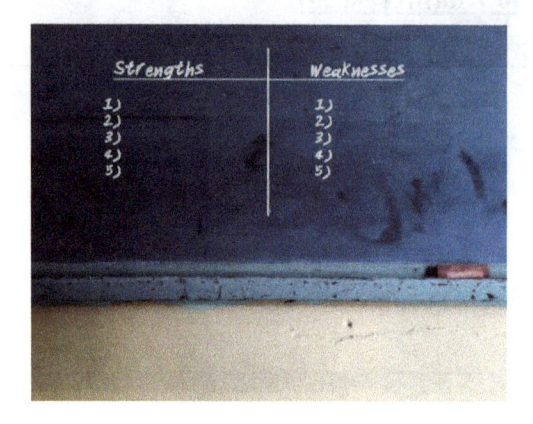

These personal strengths can be physical, emotional, and mental. Everyone has strengths that they rely on to help them achieve things in life. Unfortunately, many people focus more on their weaknesses and the things that are holding them back. Focusing on personal weaknesses is counterintuitive because if you want to live a joyful, productive life, it is your strengths that will allow you to do this. Therefore, it is essential to identify one's strengths. Doing so will enable you to focus on activities that play to your strengths, and consequently, they will be more successful in accomplishing them.

Examples of strengths that you may possess:

1. **Skills, education, social connections** – These are advantages you have
2. **Personal resources you can access** – Personal finances, property, social connections
3. **Personal achievements** – Past accomplishments you can draw confidence from

Identifying one's strengths helps you recognize your weaknesses. Identifying strengths will allow you to begin focusing on your shortcomings, so these become part of your growing list of strengths.

c. Identify People, Events, Beliefs in Your Life That Are Holding You Back

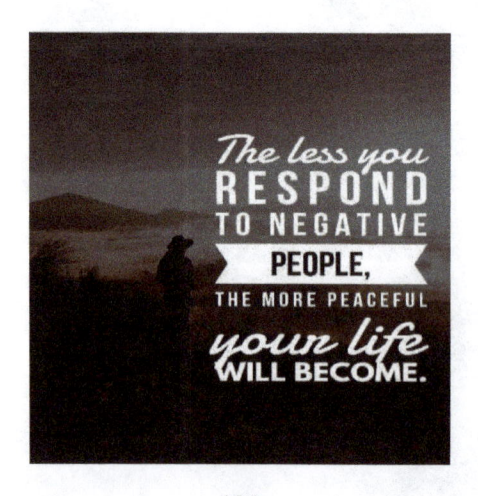

To live a joyful and productive life, it is essential that you surround yourselves with like-minded individuals and be in an environment that is conducive to joyfulness and success. Unfortunately, life often throws curve balls that can derail you from living the life you would like. Fortunately, these situations do not have to hold you back forever. Often, they are short-term events, and though dramatic, they can be overcome by recognizing what they are and formulating strategies to overcome them.

2. Perspective Is Everything

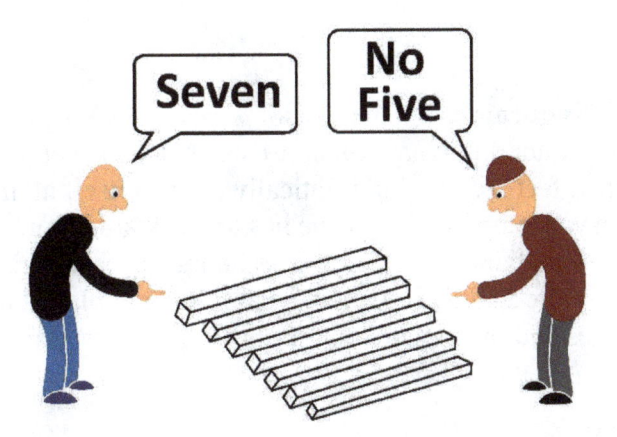

If you perceive that it is true, then it is true. There is no denying this fact. Therefore, if a person wants to live a joyful and productive life, they have to "perceive" things in a positive way. That does not mean distorting reality. Sometimes things in your life are pretty ugly, but that does not mean that they will always stay that way. Sometimes the most important thing you can do is be patient and let things unfold. Other times, it is best to be active in making a change to make things better. Regardless of the tactic used, it is the perspective that things will improve that is most important. If an ugly situation improves but you don't perceive it as improved, it has not improved. Having a positive perspective of the situation or unfolding events is the key to finding oneself living a joyful life.

3. Life is Not a Game of Perfect

One's efforts and outcomes do not have to be perfect to make a difference. Too often, we are too hard on ourselves. We expect perfection, and when perfection does not come, we persecute ourselves (Chapter 6.6. Self-Compassion: The Proven Power of Being Kind to Yourself). Too often, we compare ourselves to others unrealistically. It is unfair and unwise to compare your "hidden in the closet garbage" to everyone else's "highlight reel."

The Duck Syndrome

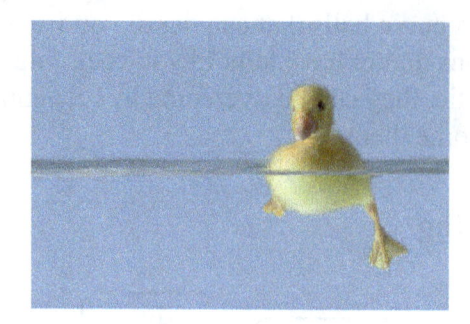

Be aware of the **Duck Syndrome**. When a person sees a duck swimming, it looks so graceful gliding along on top of the water, but what you don't see is what is happening beneath the water. The duck's legs and webbed feet are moving frantically to push itself along. Success and joyfulness rarely come easy for anyone. Everyone has to work at it. Don't be confused by what appears to be effortless; it usually has taken countless hours or years to make it look that way. Those who live a joyful and productive life realize that life is not played to perfection; instead, they recognize that mistakes and failures are opportunities for growth and personal development.

4. You Have a Choice

The path toward a joyful and productive life is full of choices. **YOU HAVE THE POWER TO CHOOSE**. Even with a choice-less event, such as a death of a family member, you have a choice in terms of how you react to it. Do you choose to wallow in the sorrow of your loss, or do you choose to remember the joy of experiencing the deceased person's life?

Dealing with fear is another excellent example of how you must choose to live a joyful and productive life. Fear sabotages the bravest of hearts. Fear is a destructive emotion that serves no joyful or productive purpose. You need to make a choice between which of the following approaches you will embrace?

F – Forget or **F** – Face
E – Everything you do or don't
A – And
R – Run or **R** – Rise

5. Mindset

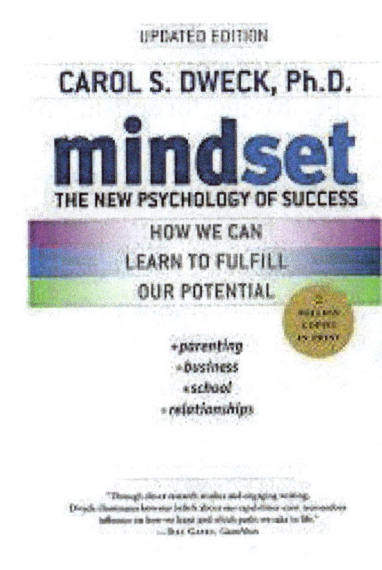

Image source: amazon.ca

There is a wonderful book called "Mind Set: The New Psychology of Success" by Carol Dweck, Ph. D. Five critical rules are listed that everyone is encouraged to follow if they want a joyful and productive life.

1. Embrace challenge – These could be physical (illness), social (need to meet new people), or psychological (overcoming a phobia).

2. Persist in the face of setback – This could involve a broken relationship/divorce, loss of a job.

3. See effort as the path to mastery – This means embracing the journey/hardships that are necessary to accomplish what a person wants to accomplish. Keep your eye on the prize as you endure the effort.

4. Learn from criticism – Don't get defensive in the face of criticism; that displays mental weakness. Usually, there is always something to be learned from being critiqued. Even if the criticism is presented harshly or is unfair or unwarranted, don't lash back at the person giving the criticism. Stay above the fray and move on (Section 6.9. Mindfulness and the Power of Meditation).

5. Find lessons and inspiration in the success of others – Learn from others (Chapter 6.8. Learning from Others Through Good Communication Techniques). You rarely have to re-invent the wheel. It is necessary to stay open-minded, use good active listening skills and embrace the wisdom that others share. There is much to be learned from others.

The 21/90 Day Challenge

For everyone, but especially for older adults, because of the physical and mental challenges they face, living a joyful and productive life is a work in progress. Therefore, regardless of a person's age, everyone should always be striving for self-improvement.

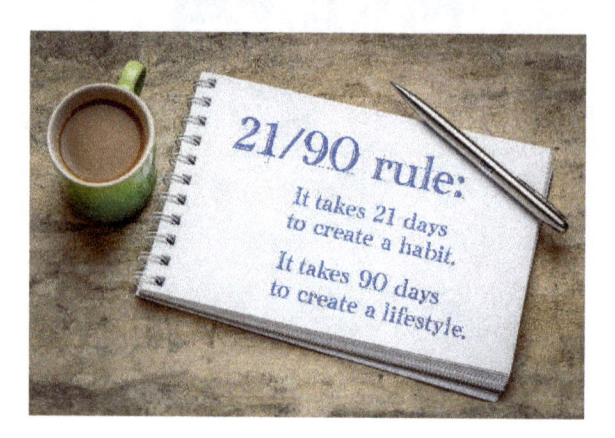

This is a challenge for anyone who wants to pursue a joyful life. For the next 21 and 90 days do the following:

Write down three different things you are genuinely grateful for each day and share these three things with family and friends.

1. Each day, remember a positive experience and write about it in detail and share the experience with others.

2. Do a minimum of 30 minutes of low to medium intensity (depending on your level of fitness and health) exercise every day. Try to vary the exercise routine each day between cardiovascular, muscular resistance, and flexibility type exercises. Refer to Section 4: The Offense: Getting Active the Right Way and Section 5: The Defense: Protecting Your Health and Fitness to help establish an excellent exercise routine.

3. Complete five minutes of formal meditation once a day and micro meditations throughout the day (Chapter 6.9: Mindfulness and the Power of Meditation). If unfamiliar with meditation, close your eyes and focus on your breathing. Accept what comes into your mind during this time, let go of these thoughts as they occur, and refocus on breathing.

4. Do a conscious act of kindness each day.

5. Deepen your social encounters with family, friends, and business associates. Avoid social isolation. Strive to surround yourself with those who make you feel joyful.

Research suggests that it takes 21 days for something to become a habit. This 21-day Challenge will help everyone make joy a habit in their life. This challenge involves a little effort for a great and joyful reward. Continue this challenge for 90 days to ensure it becomes part of who you are.

Conclusion

Change can be difficult and complex, and it takes a conscious effort and perseverance to make lasting change. Do the following to be on the path to a joyful life:

- Set goals
- Have a positive perspective on life events
- Embrace compassion (because life is not a game of perfect), recognizing that you do have a choice to be joyful or not
- Follow the five mindset rules
- Take the 21/90-Day Challenge

People need to remember that they don't need to be perfect in their execution for these steps to make a positive and joyful difference in their life.

At first, continuous joyfulness will feel awkward because most people default to pessimism and despair when things get complicated and difficult. However, over time and with conscious effort, you will become accustomed to new joyfulness and productive habits in your lives. The quality of your life depends on it.

References

Dweck, Carol. (2016). *Mind Set: The New Psychology of Success,* Ballantine Books

6.11. Dealing with Grief

Introduction

Dealing effectively with grief is a huge issue for older adults and can significantly affect their mental health and quality of life. The downside of living a long healthy life is that the older adult has a greater chance of experiencing a significant loss. This loss could involve the death of a lifelong partner, child, extended family member, friend, or casual acquaintance. It could also be associated with job dismissal, physical disability, a broken family heirloom, or the ending of a valued relationship.

If one values something and then loses it, they grieve it. Sometimes the grief felt is mild and transitory, but other times it can be substantial, prolonged, and life-altering. Your mental health is highly vulnerable to the emotional scars that sorrow and the grieving process can leave. You need to learn how to grieve in a healthy way to protect your mental health and maintain a high quality of life despite the loss you have experienced.

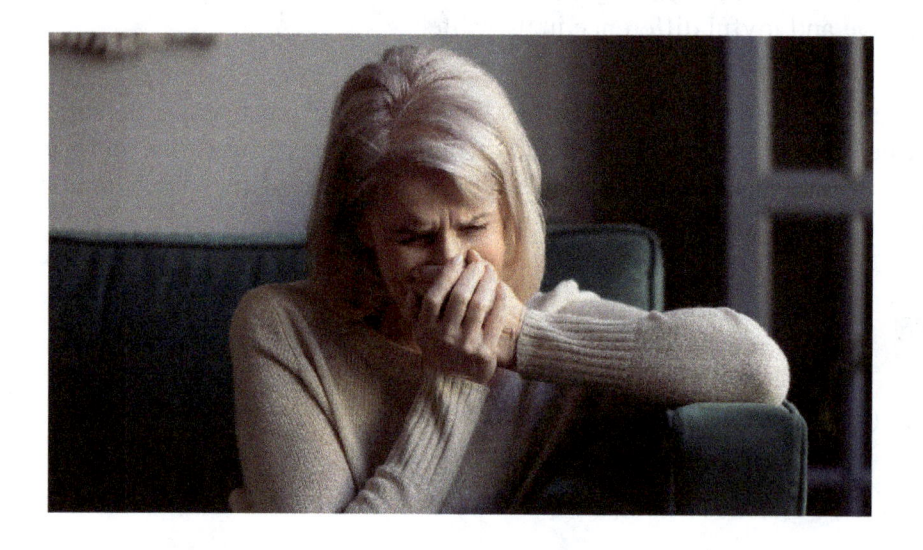

There has been much written on the topic of grief. There is no shortage of theories on why and how someone should grieve. What will be presented here is referenced from a very informative book titled, "How to Go on Living When Someone You Love Dies," written by Theresa A. Rando, Ph.D. Whether you have suffered a loss recently or several years ago, the chances are that you are still grieving that loss to a certain degree. As Dr. Rando explains, the sense of loss never really goes away. However, from a mental health perspective, the real issue is whether someone is or has been dealing with their loss in a healthy way so they can continue living their life in a joyful and productive manner.

This chapter on grief should be considered an introduction to this serious and complex topic. There is no definitive answer on how to grieve. As will be explained, grieving is very individualistic. What is a comforting and effective way for one person to manage their loss, to grieve, may not be as effective for another person, even if they are from the same family and suffer the same loss.

Consider the information presented in this chapter as one piece of the puzzle on managing grief effectively. Grief is an important topic to understand, especially for older adults, if they are to maintain good mental health.

Outline

This chapter on grief is invaluable but also intense. To better navigate your way through the information presented, here is an overview of the topics covered:

1. Grief Defined
2. Mourning
3. Types of Losses
4. The Grieving Process Is Work
5. Therapeutic Purpose of Grief/Mourning
6. The Three Stages of the Grief Response
7. How Grief Affects Us
8. Factors That Influence Grief
9. Social Recognition of the Loss
10. Timeline for Grieving
11. Unresolved Grief
12. Three Steps That You Must Go Through to Resolve Your Grief
13. Specific Actions That You Must Take for Resolving Grief
14. What "Recovery" Will and Will Not Mean

1. Grief Defined

By definition, grief is the process of experiencing the psychological, social, and physical reactions to one's perception of loss. Psychological reactions include feelings such as sadness, anger, despair, thoughts like, "I can't go on," and attitudes such as, "Why me?" Social reactions include how we behave/interact with others. Social isolation is a common and significant social reaction during grieving. Physical reactions include symptoms such as nausea, headaches and cold sweats. It is important to know that grieving is a process and changes over time. The psychological, social, and physical reactions to grief will come and go and appear different at different times throughout the grief process.

Grief is a normal, expected reaction to loss, and the absence of grief is abnormal in most cases. It is important to note that grief is the reaction to all kinds of losses, not just death, and is based upon a person's unique, individual perception of their loss.

2. Mourning

Mourning is the process of grieving that results in the gradual undoing of the psychological ties that bound someone to their loss. Mourning helps people adapt to their loss by assisting them in learning how to live healthily in the new world following their loss.

3. Types of Losses

Primary and Secondary Losses

- Primary Loss: significant loss event such as death

- Secondary Loss: come about as a result of a primary loss

Secondary Losses

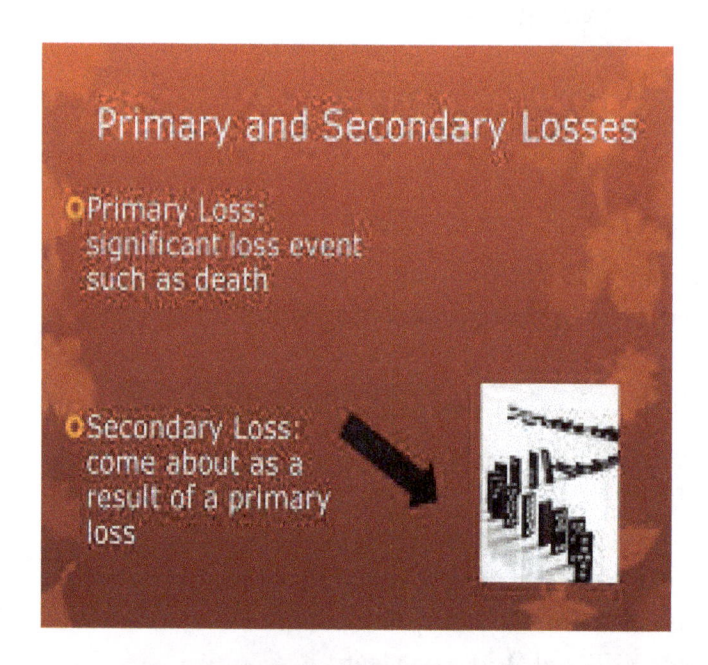

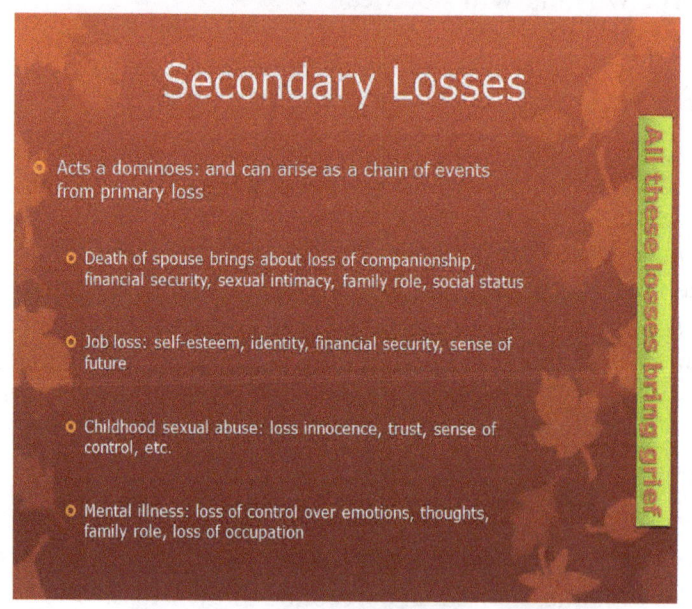

- Acts a dominoes: and can arise as a chain of events from primary loss

  - Death of spouse brings about loss of companionship, financial security, sexual intimacy, family role, social status

  - Job loss: self-esteem, identity, financial security, sense of future

  - Childhood sexual abuse: loss innocence, trust, sense of control, etc.

  - Mental illness: loss of control over emotions, thoughts, family role, loss of occupation

All these losses bring grief

Image source: slideplayer.com

1. Primary Loss
   a. Physical – A primary loss that is <u>tangible</u>, something that can be touched.
   b. Symbolic – Also a primary loss. It is <u>psychosocial</u> such as a divorce, loss of status from demotion, or a loss of a friendship.

2. Secondary Loss – These are physical and symbolic losses that <u>develop as a consequence of the primary loss.</u> This type of loss has its own grief reaction. A good example of this is if a husband or wife dies. Not only is there the primary physical loss of a partner dying and the surviving spouse can no longer hug or kiss them, and a symbolic loss of not being married any longer, but there is the secondary loss of having increased responsibility to raise and nurture children or take care of the house or business. Another example of secondary loss for the older adult is when they suffer chronic sickness or significant physical disability. These can result in the loss of bodily function and independence and force a move into a retirement or nursing home which often results in the loss of old social contacts.

It is important to note that whenever there is a change in someone's life, whether the change is perceived as positive or negative, there is some form of loss associated with it. At the very least, there is a loss of the way things were. An excellent example of this is someone getting a promotion at work. The promotion is a positive and welcomed change, something most people are looking forward to and expecting. But a promotion also involves a potential loss of the status quo with established relationships with co-workers. This is a secondary loss that could be totally unexpected and have significant emotional consequences if you are not prepared. One needs to be prepared for grief, even after a positive change, because a loss of the status quo has occurred.

Another critical point concerning loss is that a significant loss will usually resurrect old issues and unresolved conflicts. This is especially true with the loss of a parent or partner. Again, you need to be prepared, knowing that these issues/conflicts could resurface and need to be dealt with and that this will increase the intensity of the grieving process.

4. The Grieving Process is Work

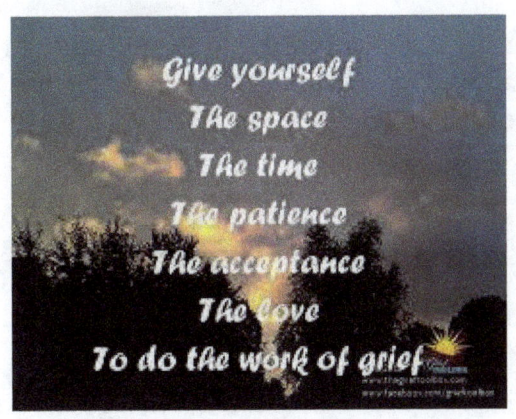

Give yourself
The space
The time
The patience
The acceptance
The love
To do the work of grief

Image source: thelifeididntchoose.com

The grieving process, mourning, requires the expenditure of physical and emotional energy. It is an active and dynamic process with specific thoughts and actions occurring if grief is to be resolved in a healthy fashion. Grieving entails not only mourning the actual loss (primary loss) but also the hopes, dreams, wishes, fantasies, unfulfilled expectations, feelings and needs (secondary losses) associated with that loss.

5. Therapeutic Purpose of Grief/Mourning

The goal of grieving/mourning is to get to the point where you can live with the loss healthily. For this to happen, four things must occur:

1. Change the relationship with what was lost – This means recognizing that the loss has occurred and developing new ways of relating to the loss.

2. Developing a new identity/how someone feels about themselves – This new identity will reflect the many changes/adaptations that a person will make after experiencing their loss.

3. Take on healthy new ways of living and socializing despite your loss – For example, you lose your job and the social contacts associated with it, but despite this, you go out and form new social circles through volunteering or finding a new job.

4. Find new people, objects or pursuits in which to put the emotional investment that you once had placed in what you lost – For example, you may have been very physically active and ran marathons or curled regularly, but because of injury, you can no longer do these activities (a significant loss). The time and energy you put into these activities must now be re-channeled into something that gives you the same positive stimulation.

6. The Three Stages of the Grief Response

1. Avoidance Stage – This early stage involves denial and disbelief, feelings of disorganization, displays of extremely uncharacteristic emotions and social isolation.

Denial – At the acute stage of grieving, this is therapeutic and functions as a buffer by allowing a grieving person to absorb the reality of the loss a little at a time rather than being completely overwhelmed. However, if denial goes on too long, it can be quite detrimental to one's mental health.

Disbelief – It is not unusual during this acute stage of grieving to have an overwhelming sense of disbelief and an urgent need to know why the loss occurred. Getting the answer as to why a loss has occurred can be very comforting.

Disorganization – This is typical during the early stages of grieving. Life feels like it is going at warp speed, and it is hard to stay focused and get things done like you are used to.

Explosion of emotions – These include anger, sadness, hysteria, tears, rage. It is important to recognize that this display of extreme emotion at this acute stage is expected and normal. What is important is how and to whom you direct these emotions.

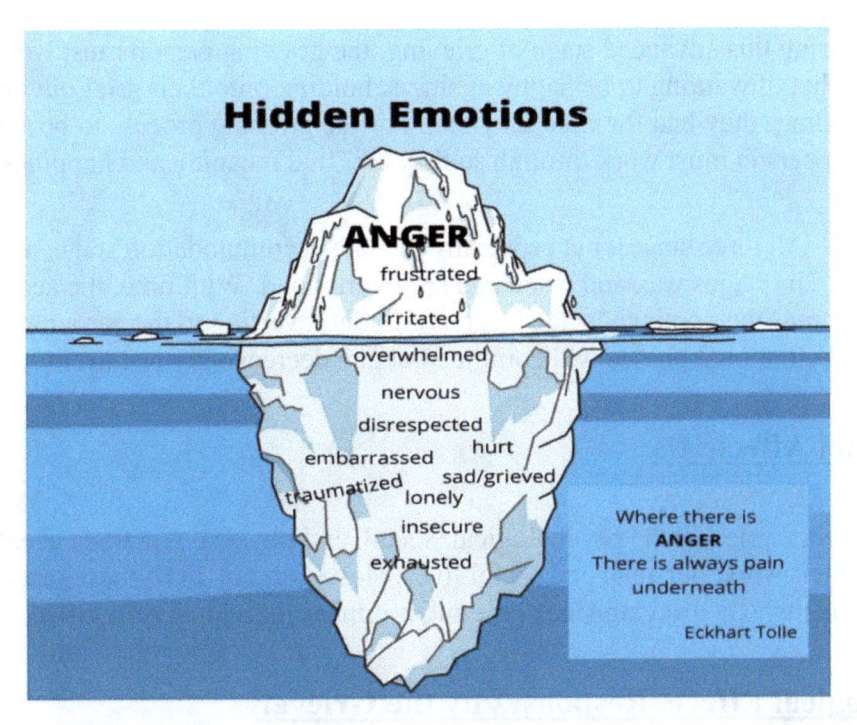

Image source: ncyi.org

Social Isolation – During the early stage of grief, a person often and quietly, socially withdraws and acts mechanically without feeling. They often feel disconnected from what is happening to them and from everyone around them, which facilitates the feeling of social isolation.

2. Confrontation/Emotional Stage – During this second stage, the grieving person repeatedly learns and accepts their loss. It is a highly emotional stage. Some people will overtly display extreme emotions of anger and sadness. In contrast, others may not readily express their emotions because they are traumatized from the loss and don't know how to express their feelings.

The emotional reactions expressed result from accepting the loss as permanent and from attempting to readjust to a new world without what they have lost.

3. Accommodation Stage – This third stage involves the gradual decline in the intense symptoms of acute grief. The grieving person tries to modify the emotional investment that bound them to their loss.

The loss is put in a special place (compartmentalized), but the loss is still allowed to be remembered. Compartmentalizing their loss frees the grieving person to go on and develop new relationships and attachments without being tied in an unhealthy way to old ones. The grieving person does not forget the old; they are just developing the new.

During this late stage, you know that you will survive the loss, although you also know that things will never be quite the same. The loss changes you, but you are coping with it and dealing with the new life that now exists.

As well, during this advanced stage of grieving, the grieving person must work through their emotional conflict of wanting to be happy again vs. holding onto their grief out of fear of "losing" the feelings they had for what they lost. For the grieving process to be successful, this is a conflict that a person must work through so they can find meaning and happiness in their life.

Key Point – All three stages, but especially the late accommodation stage, are not all or nothing stages. The stages wax and wane and are intertwined. With time, the accommodation third stage becomes the dominant stage of grieving, but reverting to the earlier avoidance and confrontational/emotional phases will continue but at a decreasingly occurrent rate.

7. How Grief Affects Us

When someone grieves, the psychological, social, and physical reactions usually show up in all aspects of their work, personal and social lives. However, not all of these reactions will show up with everyone who is grieving since grieving produces individual responses.

a. Psychological Effects/Responses by the Griever

Emotion (sadness, anger, despair) is usually a big part of grief. What makes emotions unique during the grieving process is their intensity.

Too often, people underestimate how much they are affected by their loss, and they struggle or fight themselves about the feelings they are experiencing. However, it is therapeutic just to let these emotions happen (Section 6.9: Mindfulness and Mindfulness Meditation). You need to identify your feelings, recognize you have a right to them, no matter how intense they are, and find appropriate ways to channel them.

1. Emotions of Grief

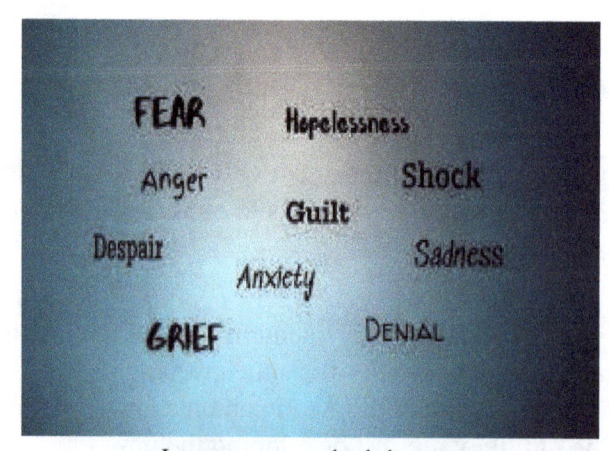

Image source: marlatabaka.com

Fear and Anxiety

These emotions can occur intermittently or can be present all the time following a loss. Any significant loss brings some fear/insecurity because of its uncertainty. Religious and ethnic social norms/guidelines on mourning and grieving can increase anxiety. Anxiety also increases with the recognition that usual coping strategies can only help you cope with your grief and not eliminate it. During the grieving process, it is normal to fear that you are losing control and going crazy.

Anger and Guilt

Anger is always present to some degree following a significant loss. It may be displaced onto other people or directed at oneself through self-hatred, guilt, feelings of worthlessness, self-punishment, and self-destructive behaviors.

Guilt may be felt by the grieving person about things that they did or failed to do. This guilt is usually related to unresolved conflict associated with the person who was lost. In the initial stages of grief (avoidance stage), the grieving person will focus on all the negative things they did and all the positive things that their loss did or how much they meant to them. As the grieving process progresses, these perceptions of positive and negative even out

Illegitimate Guilt – This is guilt that comes from one's unrealistic expectations and standards. The grieving person needs to exhibit self-compassion (Chapter 6.6. Self-Compassion – The Proven Power of Being Kind to Yourself) if they are responsible for the loss and change any unrealistic standards or irrational beliefs that contribute to their guilt.

Legitimate Guilt – This occurs if the grieving person is responsible for the loss (broke a family heirloom or caused a death). They must acknowledge this fact and make plans for restitution and atonement. If atonement is not possible, then the guilt felt must be accommodated as the grieving person learns to live with their role in the loss and not continue to punish themselves.

2. Separation of Pain, Sorrow, and Longing are normal responses to your loss.

Only with continued grief work will a grieving person overcome these dominant feelings in the early stage of grief.

3. Disorganization, Depression, and Despair

Disorganization – This occurs when the loss interrupts the grieving person's usual behavior pattern and ability to meet their needs ("paralyzed with grief").

Depression and despair – These are emotions that most people think of when they think of grief.

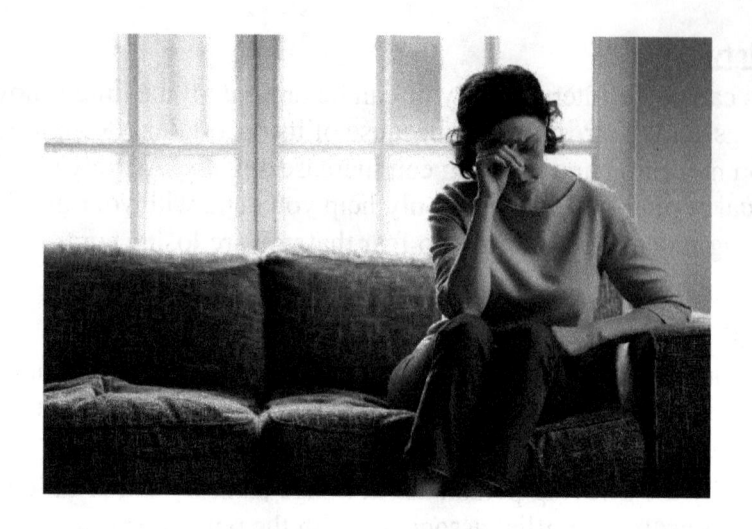

4. Confusion, Lack of Concentration, Drop in Productivity – Problems with memory and organization are common, especially in the early stage (avoidance stage) of grief. The grieving person may lose their usual assertiveness and lack clarity and certainty. It is advisable not to make major decisions too soon after a significant loss. The grieving person often finds it difficult to function at the same efficiency level as before their loss.

5. Irritability, Anxiety, Tension, Frustration, Impatience, Nervousness, Aggression – These emotions are usually due to the grieving person's anger and depression, and heightened physiological arousal.

6. Obsession with the loss – Preoccupation with a loss is a natural response. Often retrospective reconstruction of events makes the loss more manageable, especially if the loss is sudden. However, you must be careful not to hold yourself responsible for the loss incorrectly. Preoccupation with the loss becomes a problem when it dominates and interferes unhealthily with your daily activities. You need to continue to live other aspects of life.

7. Searching for Meaning – Questions about the philosophical reason why a loss happened and how it fits into the scheme of life are often difficult to answer. But accepting the fact that there is a reason, although unknown, can be therapeutic. Chapter 6.5. Finding Meaning/Purpose in Life deals with this issue.

8. Grief Spasms – This is an acute upsurge of grief that occurs suddenly and often when least expected. Small innocuous things can trigger these events. These surges can often leave the one feeling out of control. You need to be aware that this sudden burst of grief will happen and have coping strategies in place to be as best prepared as possible to handle them effectively when they do occur.

b. Social Effects/Responses Experienced by the Griever

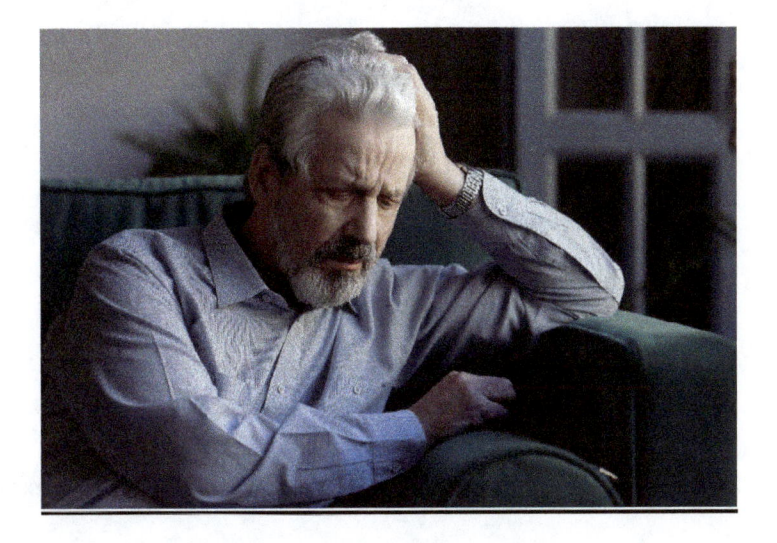

A grieving person's usual way of socially behaving can be dramatically affected since they are preoccupied with their grief, and nothing else is as important to them. Social isolation, especially for older adults, needs to be avoided.

Examples of altered social behavior due to grief:

1. Uninterested in their usual activities such as work, hobbies, and family
2. Lack of initiative, motivation, and energy to socialize resulting in social isolation

c. Physical Effects/Responses Experienced by the Griever

Often, physical manifestations of grief are the only way grief is expressed. It is important to carefully watch a grieving person's health and well-being after a significant loss.

Examples:

- Anorexia
- Gastrointestinal disturbances
- Lethargy
- Sleep difficulties
- Tearfulness and crying
- Weight gain or loss
- Trembling
- Heart palpitations
- Shortness of breath
- Dizziness
- Chest pain and tightness

8. Factors that Influence Grief

Grief and loss
- Grief and loss can be said to be part of every human life although the meaning of this experience and responses to it are unique.
- Each of us will grieve in our own unique way for the unique loss that we have suffered. There is no right or wrong way to grieve.
- Each person's unique feelings of grief and loss will be influenced by the culture and society in which they live.

Many different factors can affect the intensity of grief, and they will be experienced in very individual ways.

a. Psychological Factors that Influence the Grieving Process

I. The Meaning of the Loss

1. The severity/intensity of grief depends upon a person's perceived value of what they have lost. How meaningful was it to them?

The more roles one had in life, the functions they were responsible for, and the importance of the loss (father vs. an uncle), the more intense the mourning and larger the adaption to the loss.

2. Was there unfinished business between the grieving person and their loss?

The less unfinished business that existed, the better since there will be less emotional baggage for the grieving person to handle.

3. The more it is perceived that the deceased had a fulfilling life

This perception helps the grieving person accept the loss and complete their grief. The perception that a child's life was unfulfilled is why coping with a child's death is extremely painful.

II. The Grieving Person's Personal Characteristics

1. Coping behaviors, personality, and mental health

Adaptability – How well a person adapts to change and the strategies they use to cope with change plays a big role in their ability to cope with significant loss.

Emotional Intelligence – Typically, an empathetic or highly emotionally sensitive person experiences grief differently than someone who is more emotionally even-keeled or devoid of empathy.

Existing Mental Health – Before the loss, what was the grieving person's mental health status? For older adults, this is highly relevant. Emotional and mental health stability helps the grieving process progress appropriately.

2. Level of maturity and intelligence

The more mature/intelligent the grieving person is, the better the chance that they will understand the meaning and implications of the loss and use healthy coping resources.

3. Past experiences with significant loss

Experience with loss allows the grieving person to better expect and anticipate what they will experience throughout the grieving process and know how to utilize effective coping strategies to manage their grief.

4. Social, cultural, ethnic, and religious/philosophical backgrounds

These all influence how someone understands, expresses, and deals with their loss.

5. Sex-role conditioning

Stereotypically, women are better prepared to deal with grief

Males: In western society, males are traditionally conditioned to be in control and avoid expressions of emotions which often makes it difficult for them to cope with sadness, loss, and depression. Males tend to be more analytical and want to "problem-solve" their grief. They also want to control their pain and don't want undue reliance on others. Men tend not to have close and intimate interpersonal relationships with other men. More often, they have superficial "buddy" relationships; therefore, they have fewer support persons to share their feelings.

Females: Females tend to have a larger social circle and friends to share their feelings. Typically, they are more empathetic than males and need to explore their feelings and have their feelings recognized as legitimate by others. Females want to be listened to. They want emotional comfort and someone who can understand their pain.

6. Age
Children struggle with grief because of their lack of maturity and understanding. Adolescents have difficulty with grief because being an adolescent is already a tumultuous and stressful time.

7. Presence of concurrent stresses or crises
Additional burdens such as work/business responsibilities can sap a grieving person's energy and put extra demands on their time.

III. Specific Circumstances of the Loss
The extent to which a grieving person can accept the circumstances associated with the loss will make it easier for them to manage and resolve their grief. If the loss was untimely, sudden, or preventable, it would make the resolution of grief more difficult.

b. Social Factors that Influence the Grieving Process

1. Social support system
Dealing with grief is more difficult if others place inappropriate expectations upon the griever or withhold nurturance and support from the grieving person.

2. Education, economic and occupational status
The lack of these may magnify the stresses on a person as they grieve.

3. Rituals
Rituals (religious services) can be therapeutic if they promote realization and confirmation of a person's loss and assist them in expressing their feelings and memories and offer them social support.

c. Physical Factors that Influence the Grieving Process

1. Drugs and sedatives
Drugs will be nontherapeutic for grief if they keep you from experiencing your pain and realizing your loss. A grieving person needs to feel their pain and express their emotions when social support is most available, which is usually in the early (avoidance) stage of the grieving process.

There are times when drugs are helpful and mild sedation is warranted to prevent exhaustion, severe insomnia, and illness.

2. Nutrition
It is essential to maintain adequate nutritional balance and eating habits. Good nutrition is vital during times of emotional stress when their basal metabolism is running unusually high.

3. Rest and sleep
Some degree of sleep disturbance is typical during the grieving process.

4. Physical health
A certain amount of physical disturbance is typical, but a person must address serious physical symptoms such as high blood pressure and gastric distress with their medical doctor. Poor physical health adversely affects psychosocial function.

5. Exercise
Exercise provides an outlet for stressful emotions (aggression, tension) of grief and increases one's sense of control.

9. Social Recognition of the Loss

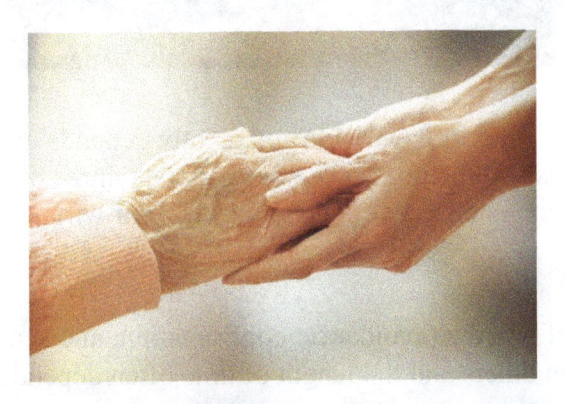

People value things differently. Death is universally accepted as a valid reason to mourn, and most people will respect a person's need to grieve the loss of a loved one. Other losses that may occur in a person's life may not be so readily accepted as a reason to mourn or to grieve to the extent that the grieving person feels it necessary to do so. This is especially true when it comes to religious and ethnic cultural differences.

When a person's loss, death or otherwise, is not socially validated or it is minimized, the grief process becomes more difficult. It is harder for the grieving person to deal with the pain of the loss and accommodate it.

For proper grieving to occur, it is vitally important that the grieving person find the necessary social support to facilitate the amount of mourning required. Rituals such as religious services as social supports are very effective in this regard.

10. Timeline for Grieving

Time helps the grieving person put things into perspective and adapt to change, but time is only helpful in the grieving process if the grieving person is actively dealing with their loss. Grieving intensity does not follow a decreasing linear pattern but will fluctuate over time. Expect a resurgence of grief any time after the initial/acute period of the loss. This resurgence of grief often occurs between the fourth and ninth months following a significant loss, but can occur years later. A resurgence of grief will become less frequent and intense over time.

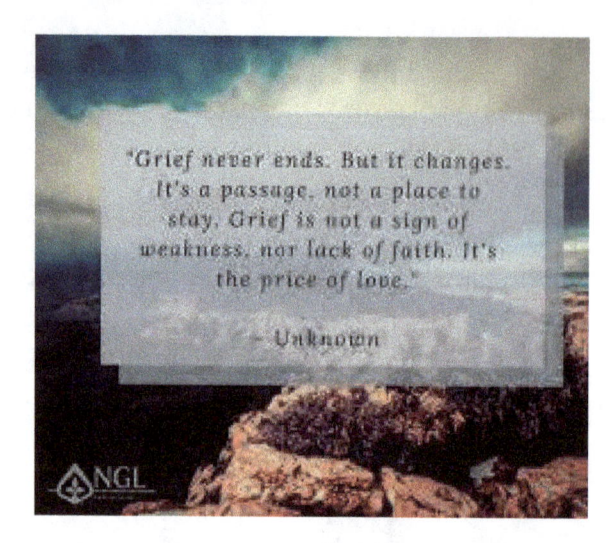

> "Grief never ends. But it changes. It's a passage, not a place to stay. Grief is not a sign of weakness, nor lack of faith. It's the price of love."
>
> – Unknown

The duration of the grief process is variable and greatly depends on the factors that are influencing the grief response. Some grief processes may take three or more years to accommodate, but most of the intense symptoms of acute grief will usually subside within 6-12 months.

Some stages of the grief process (avoidance, confrontation, and accommodation) may take longer to work through than others and the length of time often depends on:

- meaning of the loss to the person
- circumstances of the loss
- their social support
- their physical state

11. Unresolved Grief

Unresolved Grief

- Is cumulative and cumulatively negative
- Can present as anxiety, depression, stress etc..
- Based on things you wish could have been better, different or more
- Can be caused by unrealized hopes, dreams and expectations for the future
- Can be caused by undelivered emotional communications

Image source: hurondart.ca

Unresolved grief occurs when there has been some disturbance of the normal progress toward grief resolution.

Indications of unresolved Grief:

1. Absence of Grief – Emotions of grief (sadness, anger, fear, anxiety, guilt, confusion, depression, etc.) are absent because the person has denied the loss or remains in shock

2. Inhibited Grief – An ability to deal with only certain aspects of the loss and not others. For example, the grieving person accepts the loss but not the permanency of the loss.

3. Delayed Grief – This often occurs when a grieving person feels they have pressing responsibilities that don't allow them to deal with the process of grief immediately after the loss. An excellent example of this is when a person becomes a single parent due to the death of their spouse or divorce, and they now have the full responsibility of raising their children. Their complete focus is on their children and not on themselves.

4. Distorted Grief – This is an exaggeration/distortion of one or more manifestations of normal grief, such as extreme anger or extreme guilt. For example, guilt is often noted when people say that they should have been able to do more when realistically, they could have done nothing to change the suffering or outcome.

5. Chronic Grief – This involves continuously exhibiting intense grief reactions that would be normal and appropriate only in the early stages of acute grief. This form of unresolved grief often occurs when the loss is unexpected or in the death of a child.

12. Three Steps That You Must Go Through to Resolve Your Grief

Purpose of Grief and Mourning
1. To solidify the recognition that there has been a significant loss.
2. To establish the reality of the permanency of the loss and facilitate the transition to a healthy life in the new world without what or who has been lost.

Three Steps a Person Must Go Through to "Resolve" Their Grief
1. Acknowledge and understand the loss.
2. Experience the pain and reaction to the loss.
3. Adapt to the new life without forgetting the old.

1. Acknowledge and Understand the Loss
a. Acknowledge the Loss
For the grief process to begin, there must first be recognition and acceptance of the reality of the loss.

b. Understanding the Loss

Most people need to understand how the loss occurred and the reasons for the events that led to the loss. They need to have their account of the events, which explains how and why the loss happened. It may or may not be the same explanation or understanding as anyone else's, but that is unimportant as long as it satisfies the griever.

2. Experiencing the Pain and Reacting to the Loss
a. Experiencing the Pain

There is no way around the pain that you will naturally feel when you lose something of significance in life.

YOU MUST GO THROUGH THIS PAIN TO RESOLVE YOUR GRIEF!

Backing off from pain is normal and healthy. There will be times you will need to take "breaks" in your grief; times when you will need to get some distance from the pain to replenish your energies so you can cope with your grief more effectively in the future. Taking a break should include doing something that will give the grieving person a sense of control and accomplishment. This break will accelerate the re-charging of their energy to cope with the pain again.

b. Reacting to the loss

Reacting/readjusting to the new world without what a person has lost will take patience and practice. They will need to learn how to cope and adapt without the various interactions they had previously enjoyed. This coping/adaptation is very necessary when you lose your job, and the social interaction that was part of that job. You will need to change your emotional attachment. You will need to change your hopes, dreams, expectations, feelings, thoughts, and needs related to the loss and find ways to make up for these losses OR change emotionally what they meant to you and is now unfulfilled.

Coping and adaptation take time and great effort. All of your ties and emotions to what you have lost must be brought up and revived. Each one must be reviewed and felt. Only by doing this will the emotional ties be loosened or defused. Over time you as the griever will still have thoughts and memories of what you lost, but the emotional feelings accompanying that loss will loosen in intensity.

3. Adapting into the New Life without Forgetting the Old

a. Developing a New Relationship with What a Person has Lost

For the grieving person, it is essential to have a healthy relationship with what they have lost. The key is to have the appropriate acknowledgment of what is lost; and your interactions with it reflect this acknowledgment.

Having a healthy relationship with what you lost involves remembering/feeling accurately, the good and bad, the happy and the sad, the fulfilling and unfulfilling experiences of what you have lost. By doing this, you can develop an accurate image/feeling of what was, and you can use this image/feeling in interacting with your new relationship with the loss.

b. Keeping Your Loss "Alive" Appropriately
1. You must decide which parts of your old life/relationship with your loss you can and should retain.

Techniques:

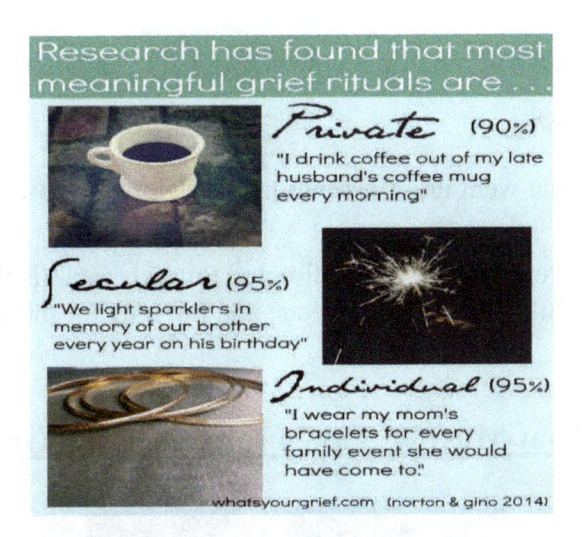

Research has found that most meaningful grief rituals are...

Private (90%)
"I drink coffee out of my late husband's coffee mug every morning"

Secular (95%)
"We light sparklers in memory of our brother every year on his birthday"

Individual (95%)
"I wear my mom's bracelets for every family event she would have come to."

whatsyourgrief.com (norton & gino 2014)

1. Rituals – Specific behaviors or activities (such as a religious service on the anniversary of a loved one's death) that give symbolic expression to the griever's feelings and thoughts. Rituals allow the griever to interact with the memory of their loved one for a limited time in a healthy way.

Rituals can be formal (such as an anniversary) or informal (going to a place you shared with your loved one). They can be frequent (daily) or infrequent (twice a year), or only once (funeral service).

2. Tangible objects – Photos, mementos.

3. Thoughts and living actions – Enjoying memories, talking about the loss, journaling.

4. Forming a New Identity – The grieving person will naturally want the world back the way it was before the loss. Still, they must develop different expectations, beliefs, assumptions, and knowledge about the world that reflects what they have lost. They need to create new hopes, expectations, experiences, and relationships. This means that they will change in different ways, and they will gain new aspects of themselves. This change is good because their world, after their loss, is different, so they must transform themselves and learn to be different.

It is necessary to acknowledge three important things;

1. <u>That which has changed</u> – recognize and grieve both the positive and negative.
2. <u>That which continues</u> – affirmation of what is.
3. <u>That which is new</u> – incorporate this into your new life

Summary of the Three Steps for Resolving Grief

1. The most crucial task in resolving grief is the emotional detachment from what a person has lost.

2. The emotional energy that went into the relationship before the loss must now be detached.

3. The detached emotional energy must be redirected towards establishing and maintaining rewarding investments in other people, objects, and pursuits for the emotional satisfaction of the grieving person.

13. Specific Actions That Must be Taken for Resolving Grief

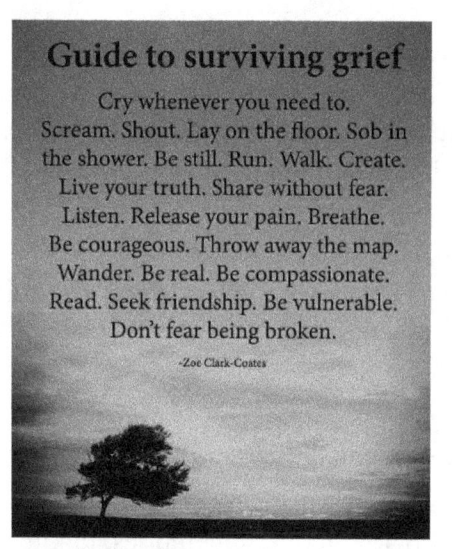

> **Guide to surviving grief**
> Cry whenever you need to.
> Scream. Shout. Lay on the floor. Sob in the shower. Be still. Run. Walk. Create. Live your truth. Share without fear. Listen. Release your pain. Breathe. Be courageous. Throw away the map. Wander. Be real. Be compassionate. Read. Seek friendship. Be vulnerable. Don't fear being broken.
> -Zoe Clark-Coates

Image source: aspirace.com

1. Give Yourself Permission to Feel the Loss and to Grieve Over It
You need to work on the grief and feel that it is acceptable to do so.

   a. Recognize and Accept the Loss – Come to an intellectual acceptance that the loss has actually occurred.

   b. Work Toward Understanding the Loss – You want and need to understand the reasons (how's and whys) for the events that led to the loss.

c. Feel and Deal with ALL of the Emotions and Thoughts About the Loss – Your focus must be on working through the negative and positive aspects of your relationship with what you have lost. So, feel your feelings, think your thoughts, and protest your pain.

d. Make a Conscious Decision to Get Through the Grief – You must commit to continuing to work through your pain and sorrow so life can be meaningful again, even if it takes a very long time and much misery before this will happen.

2. Accept Social Support and Tell Others What Is Needed

A mourner needs the support and assistance of others. They need their presence, non-judgemental listening, compassion, and concern to help them grieve.

a. Do not Socially Isolate

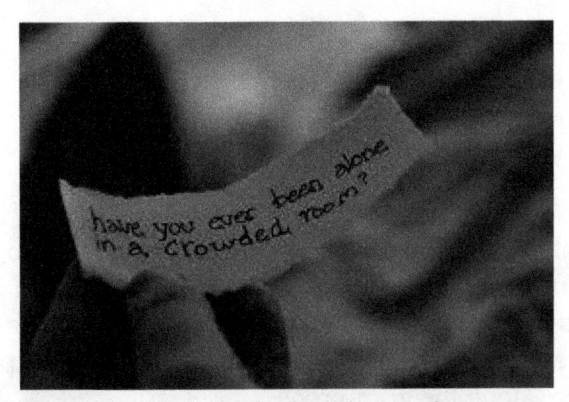

Image source: invisibleatbestblog.wordpress.com

The griever must seek social support early in the grieving process, and it is vital to maintain this support throughout. Social support helps in many ways but helping to tolerate the pain and share the burden of grief, is one of its most significant benefits. Social support is essential for the older adult who is most vulnerable to social isolation and the disabling effects this has on their mental health.

b. Accept the Help and Support of Others

The griever must be receptive when others reach out physically (hugs), socially (phone calls), emotionally (empathy), and behaviorally (bringing dinner). It is perfectly acceptable to give up some control in the early periods of grief and let others assist and nurture you.

c. Be Assertive and Tell Others What You Need and Go After What You Want

Being assertive, especially when it is not part of the griever's personality, is often difficult since the griever may have little energy to do so. Your social circle often wants to reach out and help, but often they do not know how to do so appropriately. You must educate them in what you need. For example, suppose you are grieving a death. In that case you could tell your social circle that you do not want them to avoid mentioning your loss or that your anger is a normal reaction during the grieving process and not to take your emotional outburst personally.

It is important to determine who you can reach out to early in the grieving process. Do not dismiss self-help groups; they can be very effective for social support.

It is essential to have a realistic perspective on what you can expect from others during your grieving process.

d. Be Realistic in Your Expectations as a Griever

Your expectations for yourself will influence how you experience your grief. Being well aware of the uniqueness of the grief experience and how to keep others from interfering with it is necessary. No one will grieve like anyone else, including brothers, sisters, or even an identical twin.

Have a General Understanding of Grief and a Proper Perspective on What is Realistic

1. Understanding Grief
- Its purpose
- How it proceeds
- How long it takes
- How it affects all areas of the griever's life

2. Realistic Expectations

Unrealistic expectations or negative feelings about normal psychological, social and physical reactions during the grieving process cause the majority of problems in grief. Recognize that grief will involve reactions contrary to the way a person usually is. Anger, sadness, despair, and a lack of concern for others are all normal emotions while grieving. Expect some less than positive feelings somewhere along the grief process.

Be realistic about the amount of time the grief process takes and the intensity of feelings that they will experience.

Initially, a "one day at a time" approach helps to avoid being overwhelmed by the grieving process.

3. Recognize that Grief Reactions and the Mourning Process are Unique to Everyone

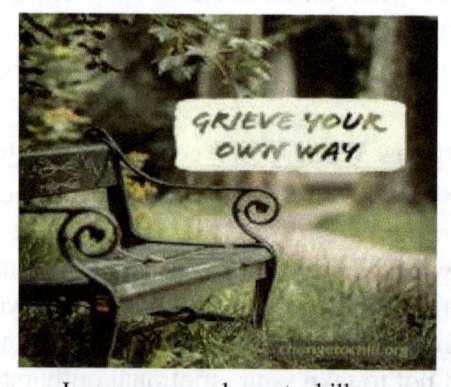

Image source: changetochill.org

You must avoid comparing your grief response to others. The uniqueness of a person's grief process is influenced by:

1. What has been lost
2. How it was lost.
3. The griever's personal characteristics
4. Social and physical factors.

The seriousness of a griever's loss and what they need to do about it can only be understood in the context of what this loss means to them. You cannot let personal judgments of others about the meaning of your loss rob you of your grief or determine how you should feel or what you should feel. You must NEVER allow anyone to minimize your loss.

There is no one correct way to grieve, so the grieving person must find the best way to go through the grieving process for themselves. The griever must be careful about following the advice of well-meaning others.

4. You Not Need to Immediately Fit Your Loss into a Religious or Philosophical Framework

It is important not to submit to the pressure of well-intentioned fellow church/synagogue/temple goers. This kind of integration takes time. If this is to occur, it must be done on your timeline.

5. Give Some Form of Expression to All Feelings

Identifying, accepting, and expressing your emotions are critical in grief.

To accept certain feelings of grief as normal, you must permit yourself to violate previously held social, cultural, ethnic, religious, or personal restrictions. A griever needs to differentiate among all of their various feelings and find ways of expressing them that are personally comfortable (e.g. talking, physical outlets such as running, hitting a punching bag, or writing/journaling).

The power of your social network comes when they will listen, non-judgmentally, as the griever expresses their feelings and emotions.

6. Repetition is Necessary

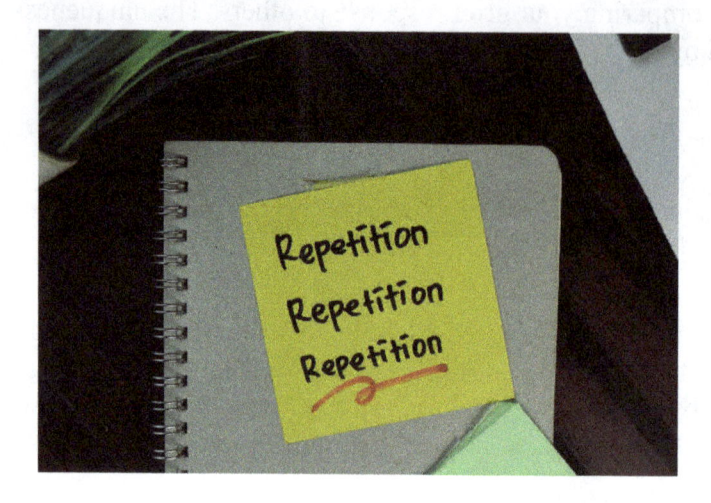

Especially in the early phase of grieving (avoidance), the griever must repeatedly allow themselves to cry and cry, talk and talk, review and review. Each story told, each memory relived, each feeling expressed represents a tie to your loved one that you must process by remembering the feelings generated by the memory and then letting the emotions go.

If you are dealing appropriately with your grief, each time you relive a memory, you feel and release associated emotions with this memory, and withdraw emotional investment in their loss, which allows more resolution of the grief.

7. Differentiate Clearly Among Various Feelings of Grief (i.e., Sorrow vs. Depression, Anger vs. Frustration, Anxiety vs. Helplessness) And the Sources of These Different Feelings

By clearly identifying your feelings, they become more manageable, giving you a better sense of control.

8. Identify Any Unfinished Emotional Issues with the Loss and Look for Appropriate Ways to Have Closure (Journaling, Ritual, Talking With Others)

Unfinished business ("emotional baggage") can prevent the griever from resolving their grief. It is essential to identify and resolve, the best you can, any unfinished issues associated with your loss.

9. Accept That You Must Go Through the Painful Process of Grief; You Cannot Avoid It

Grief cannot be delayed indefinitely; it will erupt in some way at some time, directly or indirectly. If you want to be done with your grief, you must go through the pain experienced during the grieving process.

10. Spend Quiet Time Alone

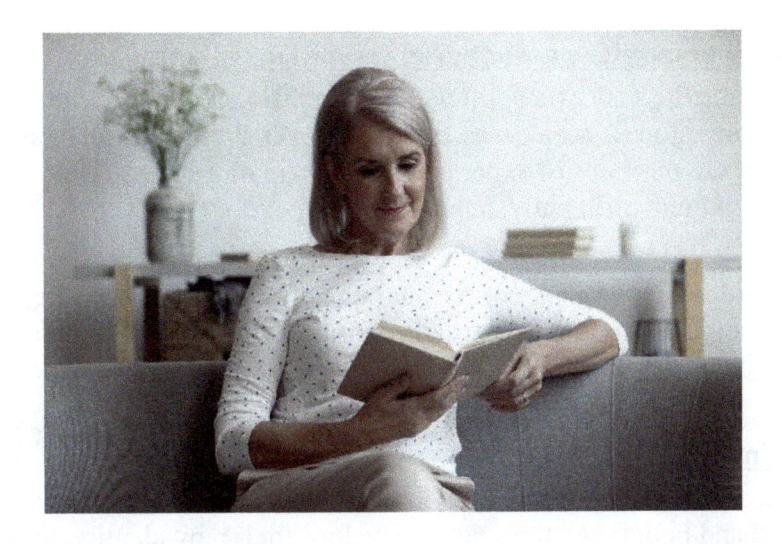

The griever must have "their time" so they have sufficient opportunity to reflect on their loss and process their feelings associated with it. You need to avoid emotional exhaustion by avoiding being constantly with others or always being on the go. A social circle is wanted and necessary for proper grieving to occur, but it should not be overwhelming. You need your space.

11. Avoid Making Snap Decisions or Significant Changes During the Initial Stages of the Grief Process

A griever's loss has already produced a significant change in their life; don't introduce more change too quickly. Remember that feeling of disorganization in the early stage of grieving (avoidance stage) is common. Introducing too much change too quickly adds to this feeling of disorganization and clutter in your life.

12. Maintain Good Physical and Mental Health

Grief is a time of high physical and mental health risk, so well-balanced nutrition, adequate sleep, and physical activity are essential. Physical activity can release stored up emotions of anxiety, despair, and depression. The intensity of the physical activity is not that important, but the emotional release of being active is priceless for the griever.

Try to avoid using medication too soon to avoid the pain of the loss; however, it is crucial not to fail to recognize when medical treatment is necessary.

13. Seek Professional Assistance if Necessary

Many people need help to navigate through the natural grieving processes or to work through conflicts impeding normal mourning.

14. Accommodate to the Loss

a. Develop a proper perspective on what grief resolution will mean
The reality is that the loss is never forgotten, but the pain associated with the loss should diminish as the grieving process progresses, and the griever should not feel guilty when this occurs. This is one of the purposes of experiencing the pain of grieving, to alleviate this pain and start living normally, though differently, again.

The grieving person will never be exactly the same after their loss, but they can recognize this fact and by grieving appropriately they can continue living without inappropriate clinging to their loss.

b. Recognize the "new person"
Following the loss, the grieving process will help the griever develop new perspectives, expectations, hopes, and beliefs. As the griever develops their new identity, they will need their social circle to validate it.

c. Recognize what aspects of the person have remained constant
Not everything changes after experiencing a loss. Recognizing what has remained constant will provide a much-needed sense of security and continuity.

d. Form a healthy new relationship with what has been lost

"If there ever comes a day when we can't be together, keep me in your heart, I'll stay there forever."
- Winnie the Pooh

Image source: indiatoday.in

It is vitally important that the griever find healthy ways to relate to their loss, such as completing rituals, recognizing anniversaries, memorial donations, photos, and journals. Maintaining this connection to the griever's past, their loss, is necessary for their healthy future.

Summary: Specific Actions to Be Taken to Resolve Grief

Resolving grief does not mean abandoning the griever's loss but instead having the griever develop a new relationship with their loss based on fond memories. The resolution of grief should allow them the freedom to move onto a healthy, productive new life. That is why it is important to endure the pain of grieving, not to forget but to renew.

14. What "Recovery" Will and Will Not Mean

Recovery from grief does not mean a once-and-for-all type of closure. What it does mean is that the griever gains abilities to function at pre-loss levels. It is essential to realize that the griever can never be totally recovered, because they will never be precisely the way they were before the loss.

Goal of Recovery

1. Learn to live with the loss – The psychological work of mourning will continue for the rest of the griever's life, but the pain and energy to do so will diminish with time.

2. Adjust to a new life in a positive, productive manner – The griever needs to learn to live with mourning in ways that do not interfere with their ongoing healthy functioning.

Adjustments to the Griever's New Life Involve:

1. Developing a new identity of themselves (Example – "I am a widow or widower", "I am a single parent").
2. Developing a new relationship with what they lost (Example - new relationship with your ex-spouse, new relationship with your deceased wife or husband).
3. Developing a new relationship with a new world means reinvesting emotional energy in new people, objects, goals, ideals, and other pursuits. (Example – joining an organization or club for those who have lost a child or spouse)

Summary to the 14 Points

Experiencing grief is inevitable. It is going to happen, maybe multiple times in multiple ways. When loss does occur, it is imperative that you are prepared and deals with your grief in the most appropriate way possible to maintain good mental health and retain a high quality of life.

To grieve appropriately means that the loss is never forgotten. Recovery will leave a psychological scar, but this scar should not interfere with your present-day functioning. However, there will be certain days/conditions when the scar will ache (Example – a birthday or an anniversary). It will remind the griever what they have lost and what they have been through.

It is necessary that the griever have coping mechanisms/strategies in place to tolerate this re-occurring pain until it passes.

Remember, the sense of loss will persist but the pain associated with this loss will subside and you should not feel guilty when this pain does subside. It is an indication that you have grieved properly and in a healthy way.

IT IS UP TO THE GRIEVING INDIVIDUAL TO DETERMINE THEIR RESPONSE TO THEIR SCAR! THEY MUST CAPITALIZE ON WHATEVER GOOD CAN COME FROM THEIR LOSS. THE GRIEVING INDIVIDUAL MUST CHOOSE NOT TO BECOME HARDENED, COLD, CLOSED, AND UNWILLING TO REACH OUT TO OTHERS. THEY MUST AVOID SOCIAL ISOLATION. THERE IS STRENGTH IN NUMBERS.

Conclusion

A griever must take the memories they have from what they lost in a healthy way, remember what should be remembered, and let go of that which must be relinquished. The griever needs to move on with their life and continue to invest emotionally in other people, goals, and pursuits.

It is appropriate to carry your loss with you but you must not allow the loss dominate your life. The grieving/mourning process will allow you developed a new sense of self and a new way of relating to the world.

By doing this, you, as the griever, have successfully grieved your loss, enriched your present, and emboldened your future life without forgetting your important past, your loss.

Reference

Rando, Theresa. (1991). *How to Go On Living: When Someone You Love Dies.* Bantam Books.

6.12. Social Intimacy

Introduction

In the preceding chapters, it has been mentioned many times that social isolation negatively affecting older adults' mental health. An older adult's ability to establish, maintain, and nurture their social circle and avoid socially isolating themselves is crucial to enhancing their quality of life through their golden years. However, social isolation at any age is not a healthy situation.

Social intimacy denotes mutual vulnerability, openness, and sharing in a relationship and is an integral part of developing strong social connections. It is a necessary ingredient in having close, loving relationships such as marriages and friendships. The term intimacy is often used to refer to sexual interactions, but intimacy in a social context means much more than just sex.

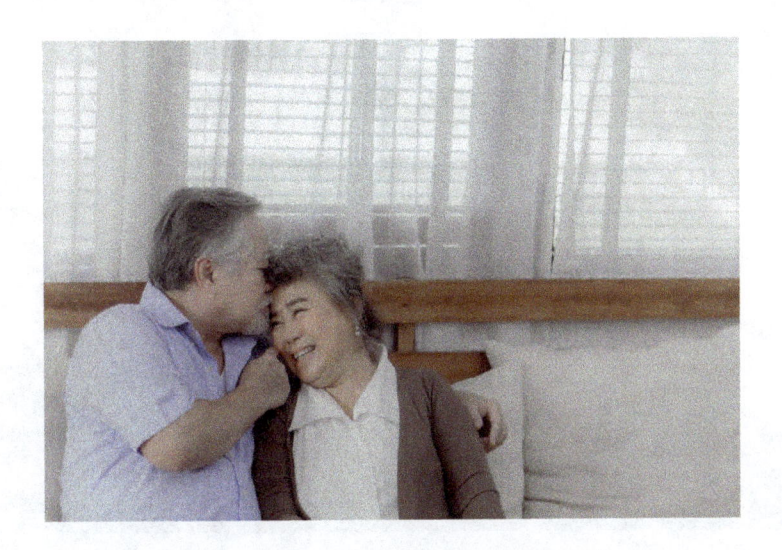

The importance and difficulty of developing socially intimate relationships for any one at any age, but specifically for older adults, should not be underestimated. Developing socially intimate relationships means nurturing and taking social relationships to a deeper understanding and mutual respect. Again, this does not necessarily imply a sexual relationship. The next chapter will deal with that topic (Chapter 6.13: Physical and Sexual Intimacy).

Developing new, socially intimate relationships, can be very difficult, intimidating, and unappealing for the older adult because they may have already lost social intimacy by the death of their partner or a good lifelong friend. Losing close, socially intimate relationships is painful and developing new personal relationships takes more time and effort than the older adult may be willing to invest.

Filling the void of intimate social relationships is healthy and essential for everyone's mental health. Your social circle is important, but finding that next level of intimacy with a friend(s) or a family member(s) can be priceless. Social intimacy means having a social relationship with a deeper layer of emotional sharing and vulnerability that facilitates cognitive stimulation, which is an important element for maintaining strong mental health.

Humans instinctively are social creatures, and getting older does not mean that the need for social interactions and social intimacy is less important. In fact, for older adults, it becomes more necessary. Retirement, and children moving away from home, means that older adults have fewer external responsibilities, contacts and social opportunities. Developing intimate relationships becomes more challenging.

For the older adult, social intimacy can be found through the development of deep interpersonal relationships with old established friends but for many, it could be found through new social interactions in their faith group (church, shul, mosque), the gym, choir, bridge or poker buddies and/or their extended family network. For many older adults, their social interaction needs are met not by a human, but by a beloved animal, and this is good and helpful. However, social intimacy means more than just social interaction. It means having a social relationship with a deeper layer of emotional sharing and vulnerability that facilitates cognitive stimulation.

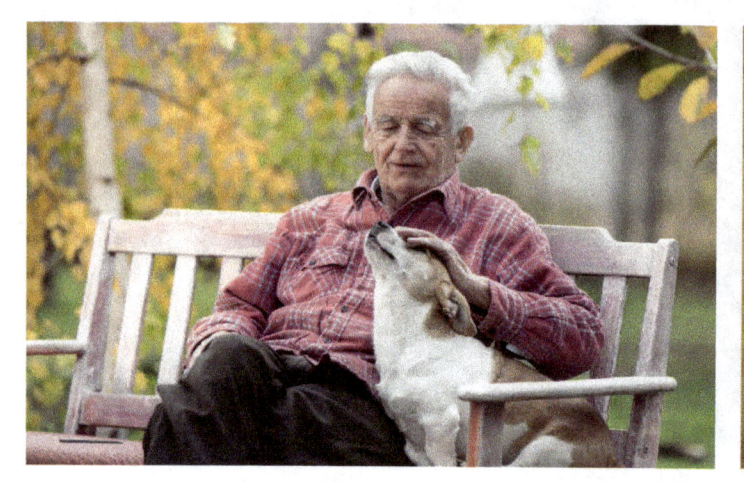

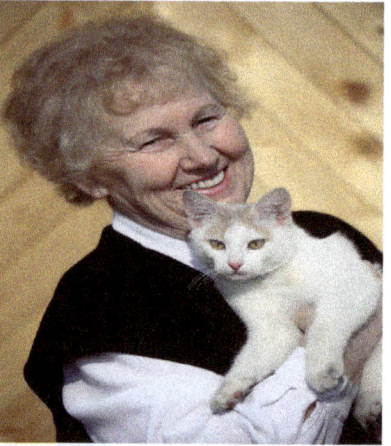

Social interaction is meaningful, but social intimacy is necessary for you to fully experience life's joys.

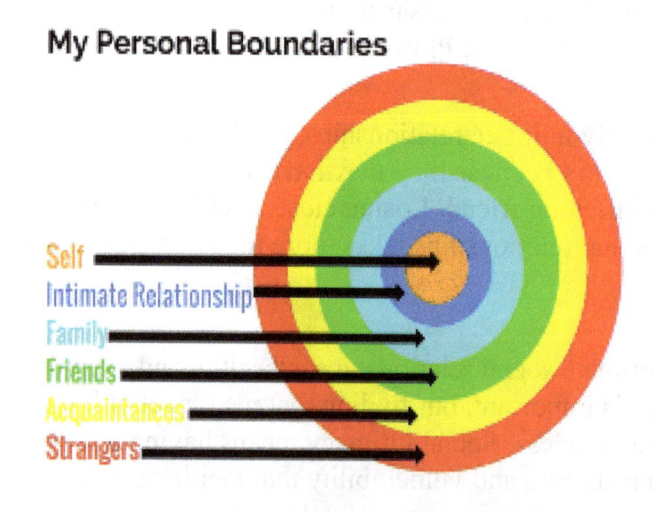

Image source: empoweredbythem.blogspot.com

Types of Intimacy

Social Intimacy develops over time. New relationships might have moments of intimacy, but building long-term intimacy is a process that requires patience and communication. Many people judge the quality of their social relationships with others based on their level of intimacy (vulnerability, openness and sharing).

There are three types of social intimacy:

1. Experience (Experiential) Intimacy – When people bond during shared leisure activities. For example, a father and son golf together every week. The more time they spend together, the stronger the bond that develops between them, and more experiences and deeper feelings are shared.

2. Emotional Intimacy – This occurs when people feel safe sharing their feelings, even uncomfortable feelings and emotions. An example is when a woman confides to her sister about her body image issues. The one sister trusts the other to offer comfort rather than using her insecurities against her.

3. Intellectual Intimacy – This occurs when people feel comfortable sharing ideas and opinions, even when there is disagreement. An example is when two friends debate an issue that is meaningful to both of them. Each friend enjoys hearing the other's opinions, and they don't feel the need to "win" the argument.

Fear of Social Intimacy

Social intimacy can help an older person feel more loved and less alone. But social intimacy also requires a great deal of trust and vulnerability, and many people, but especially older adults, often find this frightening.

Older adults can fear intimacy due to a variety of reasons. Some of the most common causes include:

- **Abandonment Issues** – Often, the older adult has already suffered the loss of intimacy through the death of a loved one. They often fear that if they become attached to someone again, eventually they will suffer the pain of lost intimacy once more.

- **Fear of Rejection** – Older adults often have feelings of insecurity concerning their appearance, cognitive abilities, and physical health. Consequently, they worry that once they reveal any flaws or imperfections, the other person will no longer want to be with them

- **Control Issues** – The feeling of independence for older adults is vitally important, and they may fear losing their independence if they become emotionally connected to others.

- **Past Abuse** – A history of abuse from family members or friends may make it difficult for the older adult to trust others.

Developing an Intimate Social Relationship

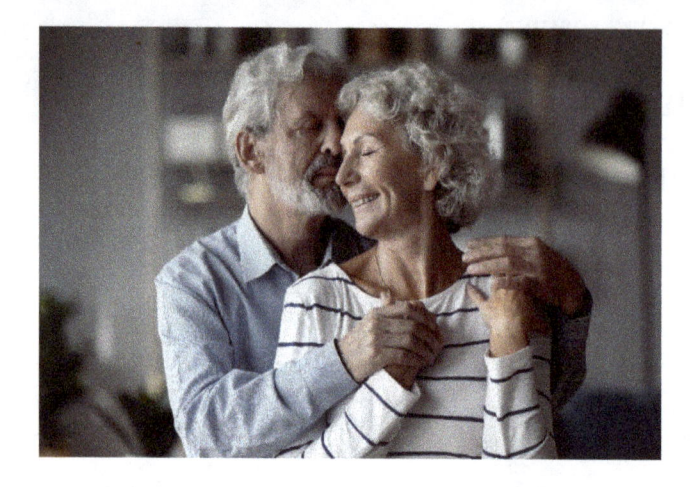

Older adults can overcome these fears of intimacy. Once they have identified the feeling that are holding them back from developing deeper social relationships, they can address them and find healthier ways to cope with them besides socially isolating themselves.

The following are suggestions to help nurture social intimacy:

1. Patience – It takes time to really get to know someone. The trust-building process is often a slow one, especially when there is hesitancy involved. Developing social intimacy is not a race. Good things take time to unfold.

2. Start with the easy stuff – A person may find it easier to talk about the past than the future since there is less uncertainty about past events in their lives. The past for many older adults is a zone of comfort and familiarity even if there is sorrow involved (Chapter 6.11: Dealing with Grief). Often, when a person shares their past, it opens the gates for them to start sharing their future dreams and goals. When you find a receptive, non-judgmental ear to talk to and share your past with, trust builds, and you may find it less frightening to speak of more complex and intimate topics.

3. Talk openly about what is needed – Misunderstandings can be prevented if you tell others plainly what you want in a social relationship instead of assuming your needs, wants, and desires are apparent.

4. Respect each other's differences – Everyone has their own identity and history to tell. Social relationships, and ultimately intimate relationships, flourish by non-judgemental communication, including listening with an open mind, asking open-ended questions, and responding respectfully (Chapter 6.8. Learning from Others Through Good Communication Techniques).

10 LEVELS OF INTIMACY IN TODAY'S COMMUNICATION

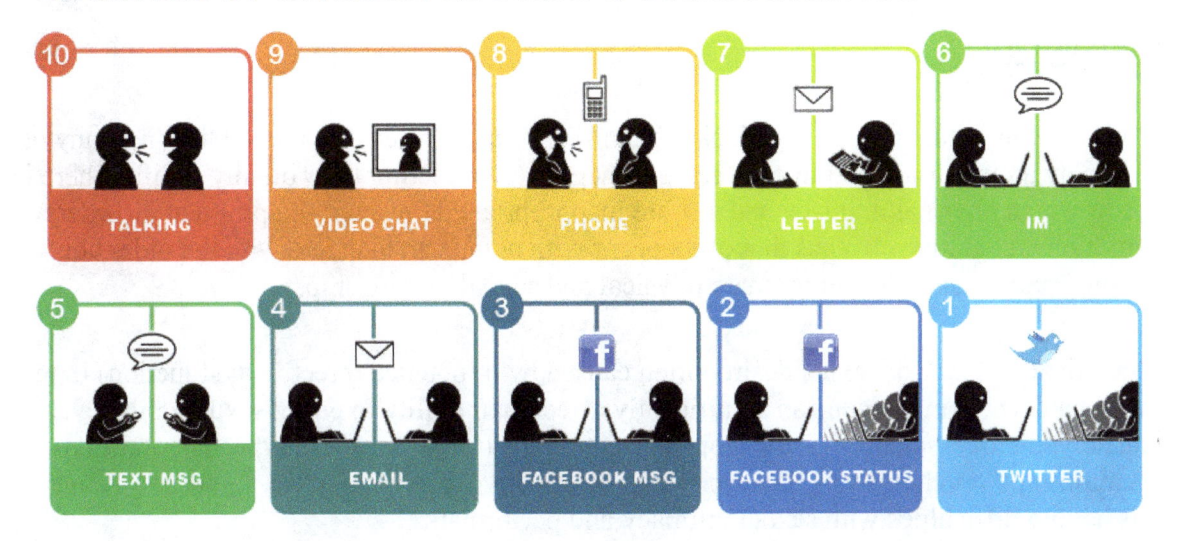

| 10 TALKING | 9 VIDEO CHAT | 8 PHONE | 7 LETTER | 6 IM |
| 5 TEXT MSG | 4 EMAIL | 3 FACEBOOK MSG | 2 FACEBOOK STATUS | 1 TWITTER |

Image source: ovrdrv.com

Conclusion

Social intimacy is taking a social relationship to a different and more intense level. It involves you being vulnerable and open in your communication by sharing your deep emotional experiences and feelings.

Developing social intimacy is often difficult for older adults to do since they may have already experienced the pain of losing intimacy through the death of a loved one. However, re-developing social intimacy is essential and contributes to an older adult having stronger mental health.

Developing and retaining strong socially intimate relationships is challenging enough in the best of times, but for the older adult, because of the social effects of declining physical and mental health, it is especially difficult. However, the emotional rewards for having strong intimate social relationships are great and should be pursued. Nothing good comes easy, and that is true when it comes to developing intimate social relationships, but the effort is well rewarded through an enhanced quality of life.

References

www.goodtherapy.org
www.merckmanulas.com
www.mayoclinic.org
www.pubmed.ncbi.nib.gov

6.13. Physical and Sexual Intimacy

Introduction

Physical and sexual intimacy, or lack of, can significantly affect the mental health of any one and can play an important part in enhancing or negatively affecting their quality of life. There is no age at which physical intimacy and sex are inappropriate. However, the physical disorders and emotional/cognitive changes that often occur with aging can interfere with the older adult developing and maintaining an intimate physical and sexual relationship.

Specifically, a lack of sexual desire, often caused by impotence (erectile dysfunction) in men, and vaginal dryness in women can significantly affect their ability to enjoy sexual intimacy. Fortunately, medical science has developed effective treatments for these types of conditions. Medications and psychotherapy have shown to be effective intervention for adults of any age who is having difficulties with sexual intimacy and performance.

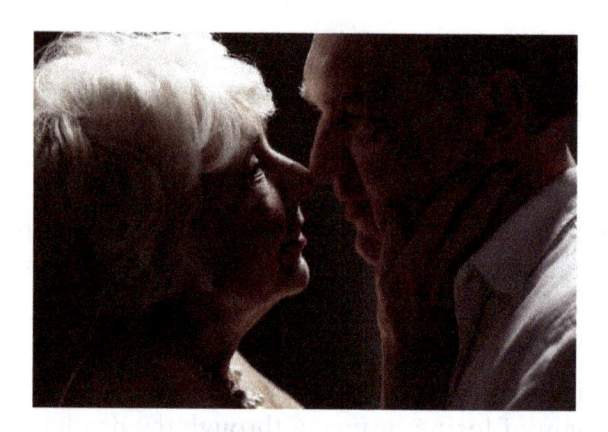

Many older people have a healthy sexual relationship well into their 80's. Social Intimacy (Chapter 6.12. Social Intimacy) and physical and sexual intimacy, can help prevent depression and improve a person's self-esteem and physical health. It is important not to underestimate the power of physical and sexual intimacy for the older adult or underestimate an older adult's ability to enjoy it.

Causes of Lost Physical and Sexual intimacy

1. Loss of a partner – Loss or absence of a partner is probably the most common age-related barrier to intimacy.

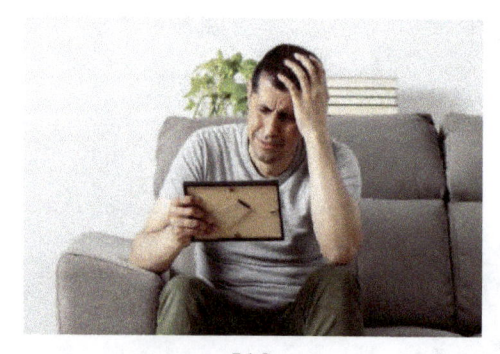

2. Physical and Cognitive Disorders – Various physical and cognitive disorders that become more common with aging can interfere with physical and sexual intimacy:

- Vascular disorders and diabetes can cause erectile dysfunction.
- Arthritis and chronic pain can limit movements and make sexual activity painful.
- Moderate to severe cognitive disorders such as dementia complicates the issues of consent to and comfort during intercourse.
- Demands of caregiving by a person's partner can create chronic stress, anxiety, depression and affect the desire for physical and sexual intimacy.

3. Use of drugs – Older adults are more likely to be prescribed medications (e.g., antihypertensives, psychoactive drugs) that may cause problems with physical intimacy such as erectile dysfunction and reduced libido (sexual desire).

4. Age-related hormonal changes – Levels of sex hormones (men – Testosterone, females – Estrogen) decrease with age, causing physical changes such as erectile dysfunction, vaginal atrophy, reduced vaginal lubrication. These changes make sexual intercourse difficult or uncomfortable. The older adult's libido may also decrease.

5. Reluctance to discuss effects of aging – Aging can result in significant self-esteem issues and social isolation issues for older adults. If the older adult develops problems that interfere with physical intimacy such as feeling embarrassed about changes in their body (e.g., wrinkles, sagging flesh/muscles, significant weight gain), it is recommended that they discuss these changes with their partner or with their health care practitioner, who may be able to suggest solutions.

6. Discrepancy in partners' expectations – One partner may want certain physical expressions of intimacy, but the other does not. This discrepancy in expectations can create stress within the relationship and social and physical withdrawal.

7. Lack of privacy – Living with family members or in a long-term care facility provides fewer opportunities for older adults to have the privacy necessary for physical intimacy.

Despite these challenges, many older people continue to have healthy physical and sexual relationships. If the obstacles to performing sexual intercourse grow too large, many older adults shift to other forms of physical and sexual intimacy such as touching, massaging, kissing, verbal expressions of affection that express familiarity, caring, or engagement with their partner.

Common Gender Specific Sexual Disorders for Older Adult

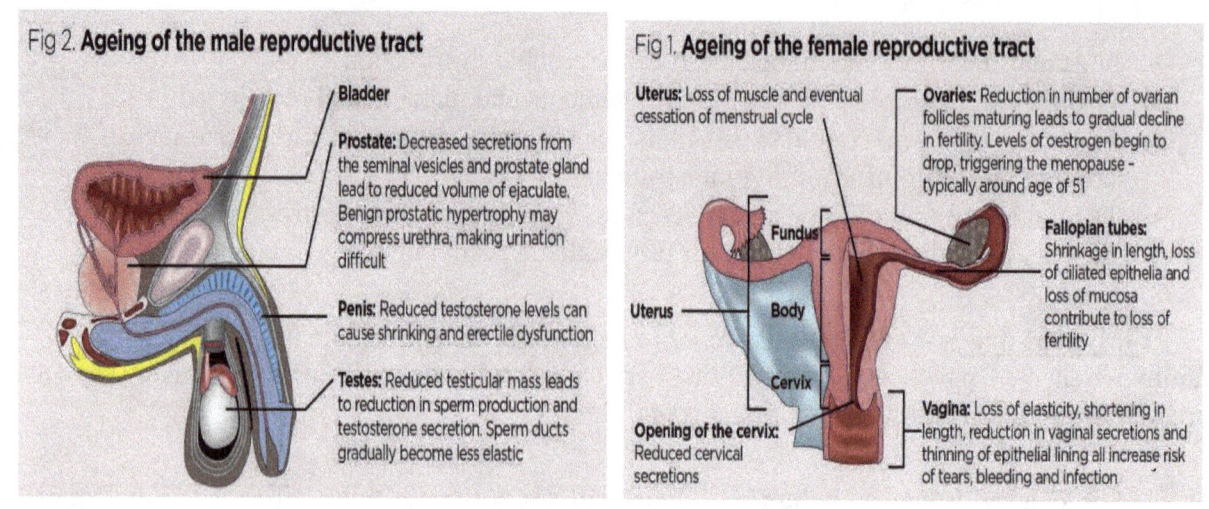

Image source: nursingtimes.net

Female sexual disorders:
- Sexual interest/arousal disorder
- Orgasmic disorder
- Genito-pelvic pain/penetration disorder

Estrogen levels decrease as women approach menopause. This decrease in estrogen levels can cause physical changes such as slower sexual arousal, vaginal dryness, thinner vaginal walls that may feel irritated during intercourse, and shorter, less intense orgasms.

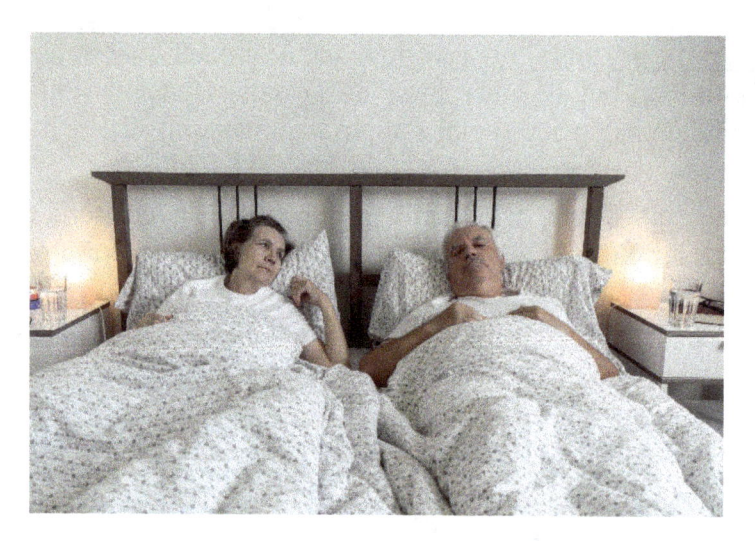

Male sexual disorders:
- Hypoactive sexual desire disorder
- Delayed ejaculation
- Premature ejaculation
- Erectile dysfunction (can't sustain an erection firm enough to have intercourse)

Testosterone levels decrease over time, starting around age 30. This lower testosterone level can lead to slower sexual response, difficulty with getting or maintaining an erection, and a longer pause between erections. It may take longer to climax.

If a woman or man suffers from any of these disorders, they should consult with their medical doctors. Most are readily treatable non-invasively by medications.

The Happiness Connection

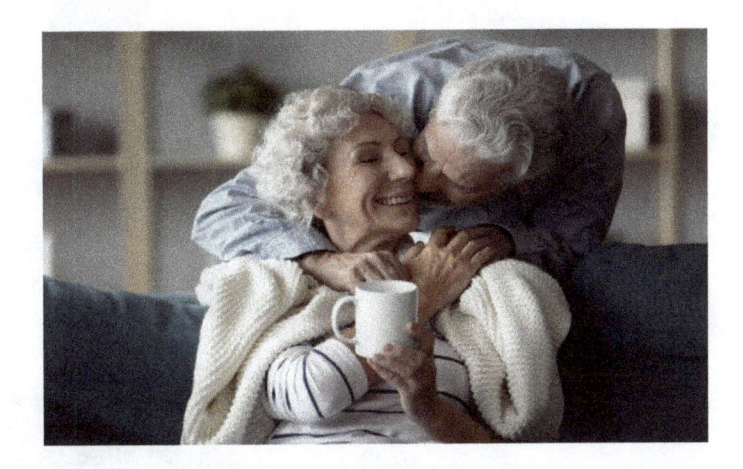

Research indicates that sexual activity by older adults is linked to their well-being and happiness. A study published in the journal Sexual Medicine in March 2019 surveyed thousands of men and women aged 50 and older and found the following:

- Sexual activity was associated with greater enjoyment of life.
- "A frequent and problem-free sex life" is linked to improved well-being.
- The less often seniors have sex, the more likely they are to experience health problems.
- Older men who are sexually active have better cognitive performance than those who do not.

The researcher's conclusion, "sexual activity helps older people live more fulfilling lives."

Conclusion

Aging does not mean the end to a person's physical and sexual intimacy. Though this form of intimacy may not be the same for an older adult as it is for a person in their 20s, but it can still be satisfying. Communication between partners is essential for maintaining an intimate physical and sexual life.

You need to talk with your partner about what you want and desire from them. It is essential to be honest about what you are experiencing physically and emotionally during physical and sexual intimacy. If an older adult feels that their medications or other health problems such as high blood pressure or chronic stress affect their sexual desire or performance, they need to talk with their doctor.

Help is not usually too far away, so let the fun begin.

References

www.mercktherapy.org
www.bayshore.ca/2020/01/10/intimacy-amoung-older-adults
www.mayoclinic.org

6.14. Finding Zen in Your Life

Introduction

This section (Section 6: Mental Health: Supporting Your Offense and Defense) has focused exclusively on defining, understanding, and developing ways to nurture and strengthen everyone's, but specifically the older adults, mental health.

By embracing the information presented in the preceding these chapters, older adults should feel empowered to improve and strengthen their mental and cognitive health continually.

Having good mental health means having cognitive control over your emotions, thoughts, problem-solving, and decision-making abilities. It means dealing with unexpected occurrences, stress, and necessary change healthily and productively.

This last chapter on mental health focuses on "Finding Zen." It is very appropriate to conclude the topic of mental health by discussing Zen teachings because when someone is in "Zen-mode," they are, by definition, mentally under control, which parallels the definition of good mental health.

Many people, and I am sure this is true for most older adults, will read the title "Finding Zen" and think this is some far-off eastern religious philosophy that has no relevance to their physical and mental well-being. Fortunately, this is the farthest thing from the truth.

What Does It Mean to Have a Zen Mind?

Zen is a school of eastern religion, Mahayana Buddhism, that originated in China. However, to have a "Zen Mind" and good mental health are the same. They both mean to be in a state of calm attentiveness in which one's actions are guided by intuition and experience rather than by uncontrolled emotionally conscious reactions. The mind is only focused on the present moment (Section 6.9. Mindfulness and Mindfulness Meditation) and not fixed on or occupied by an inner or outer thoughts or emotions, which could interfere with reasoning and judgment. In other words, when you are in "Zen Mode," you have a clear and relaxed mind. How important is that for the older adult who constantly fears the hustle and bustle that clutters their mind and makes them so confused at the very moments when they need to be sharp and focused?

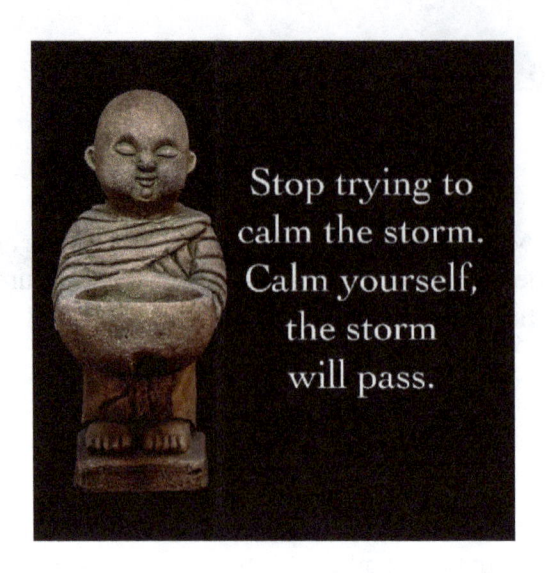

Five Ways to Unearth Inner Zen

It is challenging to feel Zen in a busy world. For many people, it has been a long time since they last felt calm and emotionally under control.

Five lessons to find Your Inner Zen:

1. Take Control of Your Thought Life – How you think directly affects how you feel. When you allow your thoughts to control their emotions and attitudes, they become unbalanced and start to move away from being in control.

2. Clear the Clutter – Clutter plays a significant role in making you feel stressed out, anxious, and scattered. Wherever there is clutter, there will be chaos. You must release everything from life that hinders you, including those in your social circle that negatively influence and prevent you from being the best you can be.

3. Replace Bad Habits with Good Habits – Bad habits impede you from feeling good about yourself. When you continue with your bad habits, you lose confidence in yourself.

4. Strive to Resolve Conflict Quickly – Nothing darkens your attitude more than letting conflict go unresolved. Conflict stems primarily from pride and anger. If you can make it a point to resolve conflict quickly, you will not have to sacrifice your peace of mind.

5. Set Sights on Reaching Goals – Here is that setting goal thing again. You need to focus, focus, focus on what makes you happy. If you are unsure of what makes you happy, you need to focus some more. Setting S.M.A.R.T. goals is the key (Chapter 3.3. The Importance and Art of Setting Goals).

Zen Teachings

Everyone who has read the previous 13 chapters in this section will find that the information just presented, "The Five Ways to Unearth Zen," was not new. That is because achieving a "Zen

Mind" and having good mental health are the same; being in control by having a clear and present mind.

An effective way of reinforcing the power of Zen teachings is through legendary fables. Some of the fabled teachings have been presented previously in preceding chapters, but a good story and their lessons are always worth repeating.

1. Empty Your Cup

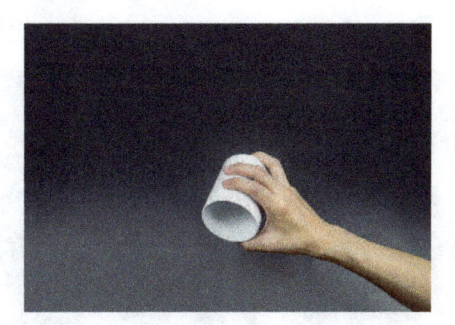

Story – A professor went to visit a famous Zen master. While the master poured tea, the professor talked about Zen. The master poured the visitor's cup to the brim and then kept pouring. The astonished professor said, "What are you doing?" and the Zen master replied, "You are like this cup; how can I show you Zen unless you first empty the cup?"

Lesson – You need to open up your mind and your heart. You need to be willing to leave what you already know, emptying your cup, so you are open to learning from others with different perspectives, more skill, and experience than yourself. You need to be a good listener, accept corrections, and act on them.

2. The Monk and the Mirror

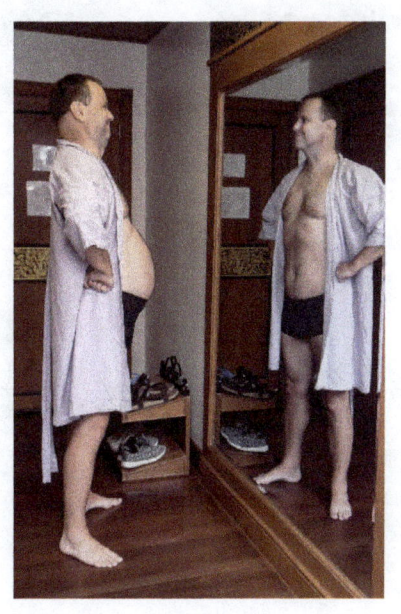

Story – There was a monk who always carried a mirror. He was asked one day why he did so. He replied, "I use it in times of trouble. I look into it and it shows me the source of my problems as well as the solution to my problems."

Lesson – You have to be accountable for who you become, never blame others, but focus instead on what you can do better.

3. The Burden – Let It Go

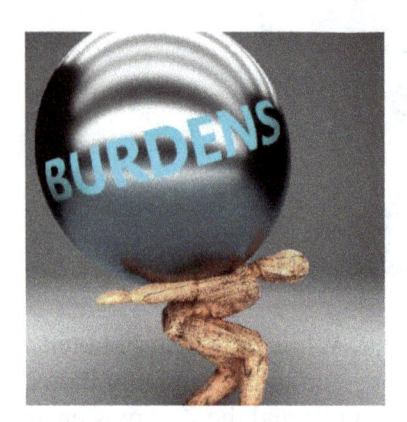

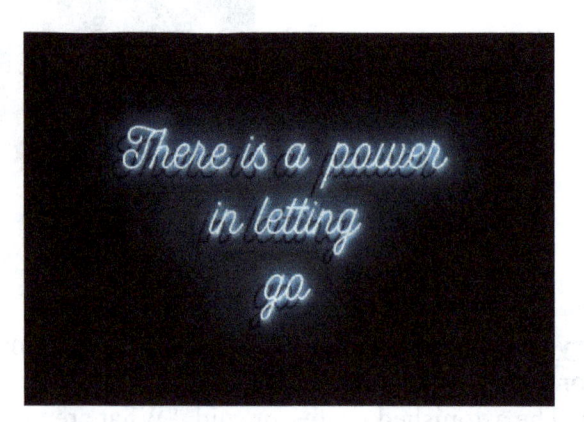

Story – Two monks were returning to their monastery in a heavy rainstorm. An elderly woman was unable to cross the road. The elder monk approached and carried the women across the road. Later in the evening, the astonished younger monk said to the elder monk, "Sir, as monks, we are not allowed to touch women, and you carried that woman across the road." The elder monk replied, "Yes, but I left her on the other side of the road, while you are still carrying her."

Lesson – Live in the present tense, focus on the process and not the result. You need to learn to quickly let go of all downfalls, defeats, and disappointments and give yourself credit and celebrate what you have done well.

4. Maybe (We Will See)

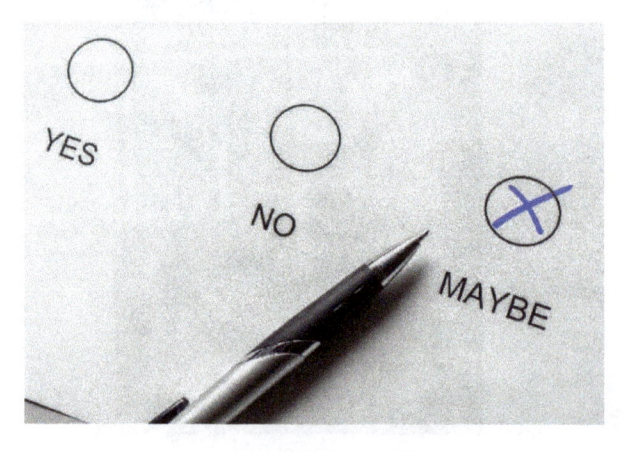

Story – A farmer was given a wild horse to train so he could plow his fields. His neighbor said to him, "What good future you have."

The farmer said, "We will see."

The next day his son tried to tame the wild horse but fell off and broke his leg. The neighbor said, "How unfortunate that your son broke his leg."

The farmer said, "We will see."

The next day military officials came to the village to draft young men into the army. Seeing the son's leg broken, they passed on him. The neighbor said, "Once again you have good fortune."

The farmer said, "We will see."

Lesson – Don't be quick to judge events as good or bad. Don't become too high or too low when events unfold, but rather stay level-headed. Always make the best of the present situation.

5. Focus on the Goal

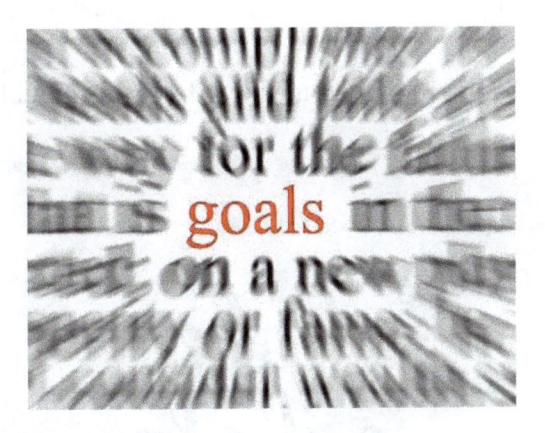

Story – An earnest Zen student approached his master and asked, "If I work really hard how long will it take for me to find Zen?"

The master replied, "Ten years."

The student then said, "What if I work very, very hard?"

The master replied. "Twenty years."

The student said, "But what if I work very, very, very hard?"

The master replied, "Thirty years."

Confused and frustrated, the student said, "Each time I say I am going to work harder, you say it is going to take me longer to find Zen. Why do you say that?"
The master replied, "When you only have one eye on the goal, you only have one eye on the path."

Lesson – Focus on the process, and the results will take care of themselves.

6. The Frog and the Centipede

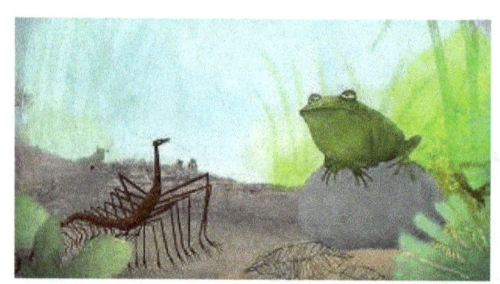

Image source: thezengateway.com

Story – A frog meets a centipede and, after watching it for a while, says, "That is unbelievable how you can walk so fast and coordinate all those legs of yours. How do you do it? I only have four and find it difficult." At this, the centipede stops, thinks about it, and finds himself unable to leave again.

Lesson – Overthinking leads to confusion and underperforming. People need to trust their skills and free their minds.

7. Breathing

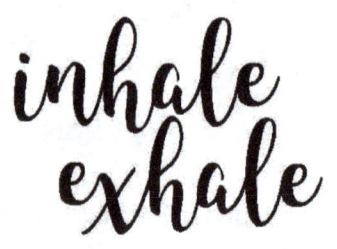

inhale exhale

Story – After a year in the monastery, a Zen monk complained, "All I have learned about is breathing." After five years in the monastery, the monk complained, "All I have learned about is breathing." When he reached enlightenment, the elderly monk smiled and said, "Finally, I have learned about breathing."

Lesson – Learn and practice the finer points of deep breathing. Breathing can become shallow when a person feels stressed. A good breathing technique to promote relaxation is to prolong exhalation, regardless of the inhalation length.

8. It Will Pass

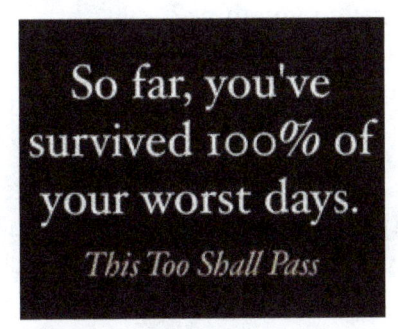

> So far, you've survived 100% of your worst days.
> *This Too Shall Pass*

Image source: pinterest.com

Story – A student went to his meditation teacher and said, "My meditation is horrible! I feel distracted, or my legs ache, or I am falling asleep. It is just horrible!"

"It will pass," said the teacher matter-of-factly.

A week later, the student came back to his teacher and said, "My meditation is wonderful! I feel so aware, so peaceful, so alive! It's just wonderful!"

"It will pass," the teacher replied matter-of-factly.

Lesson – Everything is temporary. Life is always in a state of flux. Don't panic when things are not going well; it will soon end. During those times when everything is flowing along perfectly, ride it out as long as you can. Everything passes.

9. Chasing Two Rabbits

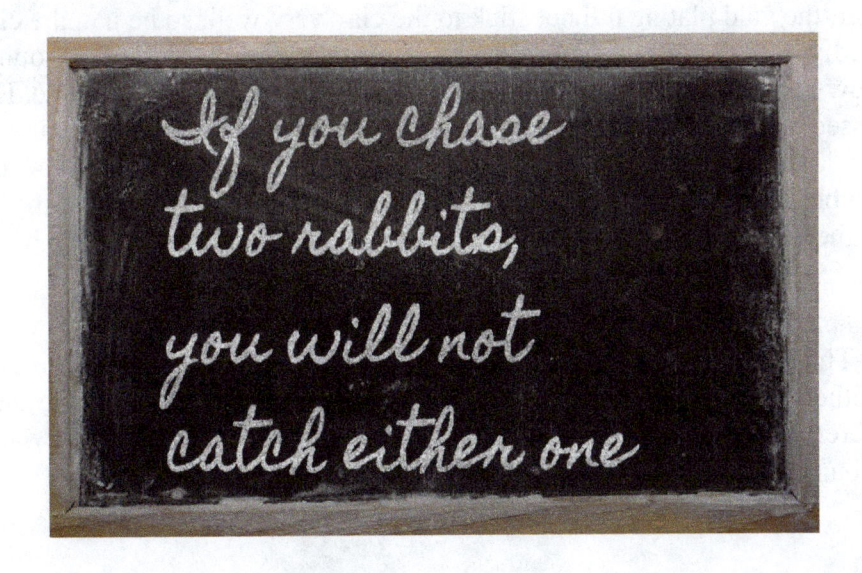

> If you chase two rabbits, you will not catch either one

Story – A martial arts student approached his teacher with a question. "I'd like to improve my knowledge of martial arts. In addition to learning from you, I'd like to study with another teacher to learn another style. What do you think?"

The master answered," The hunter who chases two rabbits catches neither one."

Lesson – The path to success and happiness is taken one step, one day at a time. You should not get ahead of yourself or try two things at once. If you try to do everything, you will end up with nothing. You need to trust your skills and training and focus all your energy and effort on doing one good thing at a time.

10. The Statue

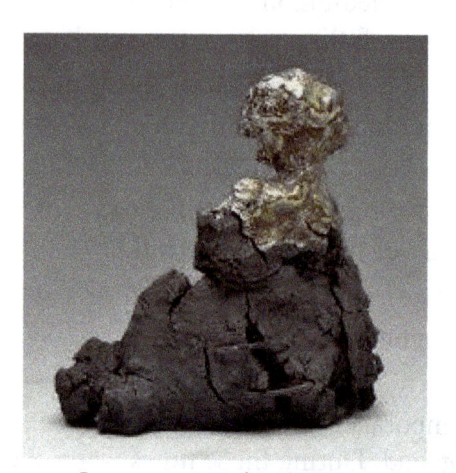

Image source: pinterest.com

Story – A young man had a clay statue, a family heirloom. However, he always wanted a bright shiny gold one instead. When he saved enough money, he had his statue covered with gold. However, the gold plating did not stick to the clay very well, so he had the clay statue gold plated repeatedly. One day his grandfather returned from a long journey. The young man was excited to show his grandfather how he had made the clay statue into a gold one. However, he was embarrassed because the clay was showing through in many spots. The grandfather smiled, held the statue lovingly and gently rubbed it, and gradually dissolved some of the clay. Underneath, a bright yellow colour shone through. The grandfather stated, "Many years ago, before your time, the statue must have fallen into the mud and was coated with it. Your statue has been gold from the very beginning."

Lesson – The key to success and happiness in a person's life lies within them. If you can spot greatness in others, you already possess some of that greatness. Remove self-doubt and other mental interference, and let your gold shine through. You have inner greatness waiting to be unleashed. You need to tap into that potential.

Conclusion

Possessing a Zen Mind means maintaining good mental health. There is much to be learned through eastern religious teachings that are valuable and practical for your mental health.

The goal is to have a clear and present mindful approach, so you can cognitively function effectively and have control over your environment and life. As the years go by, this becomes an increasingly bigger challenge for the older adult to achieve.

Older adults can do a lot to help slow the effects of aging on their cognitive and mental health. You need to embrace what has been presented in these 14 chapters. Your mental and physical health and quality of life depends on it.

Reference

Afremow, Jim. (2013). *The Champions Mind: How Great Athletes, Think, Train and Thrive.* Rodale Books,

Section 7

The Post-Season – The Playoffs and Super Bowl – Raising Your Expectations

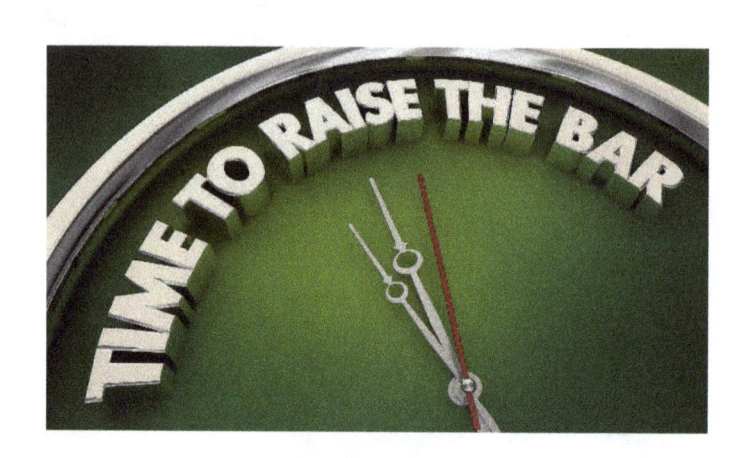

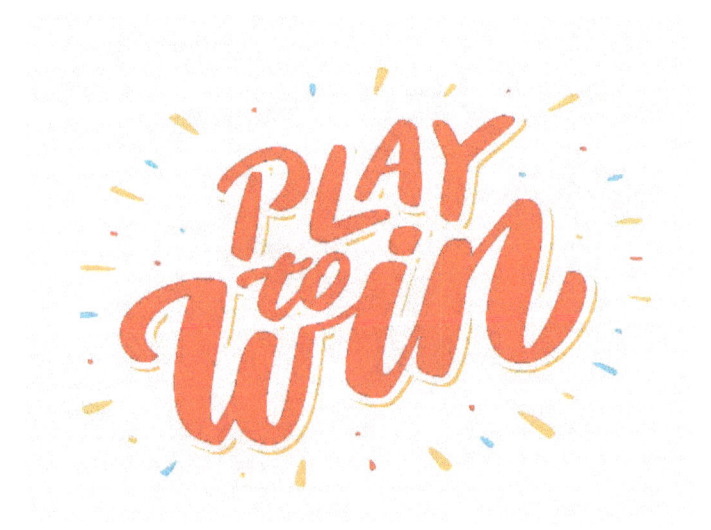

7.0. Introduction: The Post Season – Raise Your Expectations

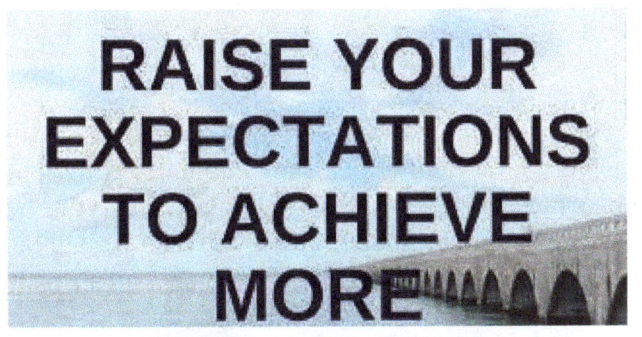

Image source: meaningfullife.com

Introduction

It is playoff time. In football, it is time to win or go home. For the Forever Active Older Adult Health and Fitness Playbook, it means raising expectations so positive changes in physical, nutritional, and mental health can occur. If not now, then when?

Your goal should not be to try. It MUST be to win. Winning is the purpose of this book. Giving the best information in a format that is easy to follow and practical to use, so you can succeed at something that so many others have failed at doing. Winning means developing a health and fitness plan that is sustainable so you can enjoy a healthier life this year than last year.

This section will suggest ways to compete and help level the playing field against all the health barriers that can get in your way of succeeding.

Review: What Has Been Presented So Far

It's playoff time, or as they say in football, *crunch time*. So, it is an excellent time to review what we have learned so far to help you achieve your fitness and health goals.

Section 2: The Off-Season – Studying the Opposition
This section focuses on the opponent, health conditions that you must be ready to compete against, to maintain a high quality of life as you grow older. These conditions include: arthritis, heart disease, cancer, diabetes, obesity, dementia, oral and dental problems, and visual and hearing impairments.

Section 3: Pre-Season – Preparation Time for Best Performance
This section focuses on preparing for game time, by learning how to execute one's personalized health and fitness plan successfully. It covers:

- The Eight Golden Rules of Training
- Learning to Overcome the Five Internally Generated Obstacles to Exercise

- The Importance and Art of Goal Setting
- Visualization for Motivation to Promote Change

Section 4: The Offense – Learning How to Stay Active

This section covers two critical components of physical health—cardio vascular fitness and muscular strength, and the very important topic of maintaining agility, balance, and coordination for fall prevention. You become more functional by strengthening your heart and body muscles, and improving agility, balance, and coordination. You will also be in a better preventative position to fight off chronic illnesses that plagues older adults and strips away their quality of life.

Section 5: The Defense – Protecting Your Health and Fitness

This section focuses on the preventative measures of flexibility, nutrition, and sleep. Improving each of these areas builds a solid defensive wall against chronic illness. The defense must support the offense if you are going to win the game.

Section 6: Special Teams – Mental Health: Supporting Your Offense and Defense

This section focuses on the mental components of your health. The role and importance mental health plays on your overall well-being cannot be overstated. No matter how strong and flexible you are physically, or how well you eat and sleep, you cannot take advantage of these positive physical attributes if you are not mentally healthy.

The review is over. It is now time to learn how to implement what has been taught – to learn how to be successful in creating a healthy lifestyle. In other words: *to win*.

7.1. How to Play to Win

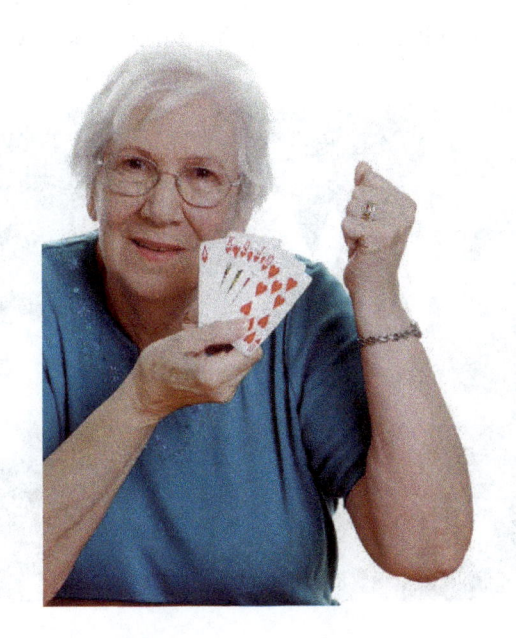

Introduction

Playing to win is based on confidence. Playing to lose is rooted in fear. Fear can sabotage the best of intentions. You need to have confidence in yourself to make positive changes in your life. It is never too late for you to make positive, life-altering changes in the way you live your daily life.

Learning how to win is important. Many great athletes have never won **"The Big One"** because they never knew how to. It takes more than great athletic ability to be a champion, and it takes more than good intentions to make positive health changes. You can have a solid game plan for your offense, defense, and special teams, but if you don't understand how to implement the plan successfully, you are more likely not to be successful, especially in the long run. In football, the goal is not just making it to the playoffs but to win the Super Bowl. If you want to make positive health changes in your life, the goal must be to achieve consistency and sustainability in executing your fitness and health plan. The points discussed in this section will help you achieve this goal.

Before tackling the nitty gritty of this chapter, one last point needs to be emphasized. You must not limit yourself to small goals, and you must not be discouraged if you don't succeed fully initially. The 80/20 rule is important to remember. A realistic goal is for you to achieve 80% compliance. If you do so, you should consider yourself successful. Moreover, don't think of setbacks as endpoints but rather transform them into new beginnings. Keep pushing towards long-term goals. Repeatedly succeeding at short-term goals leads to accomplishing long-term goals. Celebrate successes, even small ones, and NEVER undervalue them.

1. Take Ownership

The attitude with which you approach life's challenges will determine your ability in handling them in a positive productive manner. You must take ownership of this attitude.

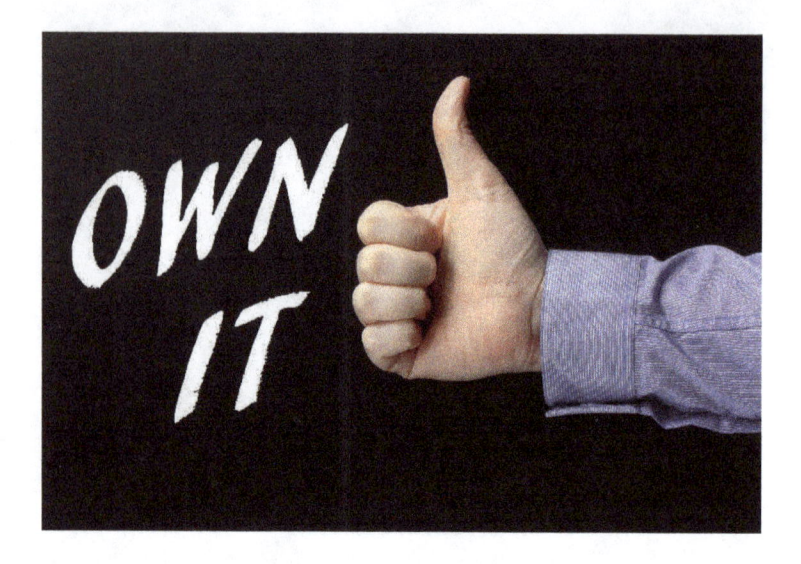

Taking ownership involves taking responsibility for all your thoughts, words and actions. Nobody but yourself is responsible for these. For example, when things do not go as planned such as not achieving a short-term weight loss goal of losing four pounds in a month, it requires great humility and courage to take the responsibility of owning the reasons for this disappointment. It takes discipline not make excuses as to why the short-term goal was not achieved. Taking ownership of your own thoughts, words, and actions is necessary for self-improvement.

Taking ownership requires you to look at yourself and a failed situation through the objective lens of reality, without emotional attachment or ego. You must accept responsibility for failure, admit weaknesses, and consistently improve yourself.

Taking ownership of failures and disappointments is why it is essential to take ownership and celebrate successes no matter how small. Celebrate every success because there will be setbacks along the way that could potentially discourage and derail your plans for positive change. Celebrating successes helps balance out the disappointments of failures.

2. Learn to Love the Grind

Rarely, from one day to another, are you on your "A" game. It is impossible and unrealistic to expect yourself to perform at your best all the time. As a result, you must figure out how to "close the deal" on each given day. On those days when you are not at your best, you must focus all your energy on execution, not self-analysis of results. The mental challenge is to focus on the process and you will surprise yourself on how well the results turn out. You need to be willing to adapt and problem-solve when the unexpected happens. Winning ugly is always better than not winning at all. People only remember who won, not how they won.

A good rule of thumb if you're struggling to start executing your fitness plan on a particular day is to tell yourself, "I will give it 10 minutes; if after 10 minutes I still don't want to do it today, I will stop and look forward to tomorrow." You will be surprised by how many times you'll finish a workout or a meditative session once you have started.

3. Pressure is a Privilege, not a Problem

Reframe any situation that is creating tension and stress in your life. Life will throw many curve balls that will get in your way of executing your health and fitness plan. Think of these situations as an opportunity to thrive, not fail. Welcome the challenge to overcome any obstacle that lies in the way of accomplishing goals. You must trust your plan, preparation, determination, and mental toughness to overcome formidable challenges that get in your way. Your mindset should be that you have nothing to lose and everything to gain. Remember, you only need to be successful 80% of the time.

4. True Happiness Comes from Within

Happiness is an inside job. Don't assign anyone else that much power over your life
—Mandy Hale

Image source: unbrokenself.com

You need to make executing your daily, weekly, and monthly health and fitness plans your primary activity and your biggest reward. You need to find happiness in your participation and accomplishments, knowing you have made an effort to do your best and to become the best that you are capable of becoming.

Finding happiness in what you do and accomplish is a conscious decision. It comes from within. Unfortunately, many people consciously decide to only see the glass as half empty even if they have accomplished something great.

A good example of this is Tiger Woods, the best or second-best golfer who has ever played the game. I was watching a golf tournament one Sunday, and one of Tiger's competitors finished a round of 65, an excellent score, especially on a Sunday when the course set up is at its hardest. This golfer, who should have been elated, was interviewed as he came off the course and said, "Yup, it was an okay round, but I left a lot of good scoring opportunities out there." He saw his cup as being "half empty." When Tiger finished, he had shot a round of 74, way below his standard and expectation for the day, and as a result, he had no shot at winning the tournament. When he was interviewed and asked about his round, he saw his cup as "half full" by saying, "Yup, tough scoring day, but I hit a lot of really good shots, which will give me confidence for the next tournament."

The difference between the two golfers' attitudes is notable. The "half-empty" comment came from an average golfer who had a great round, and the "half-full" comment came from one of the greatest golfers who had a poor round. How you perceive things within your heart and mind makes a difference in your long-term success and happiness.

People, especially older adults, need to find internal joy and happiness in what they are doing to live a healthier life. They will enjoy their journey more, and it will make a big difference in their success and quality of life.

5. Manage Your Limitations

You need to focus on your strengths and find ways to reduce the impact of any limitations you may have. You need to forget about your shortcomings quickly. Remember, 80% compliance is the goal. Even if you do not accomplish 80% of what you wanted to for the week or month, you should not worry about it. Remember and repeat the mantra, "do your best and forget the rest." There is an old Buddhist saying, "The arrow that hits the bull's eye is the result of a hundred misses." Failure breeds success. It is essential that you should not be intimidated or discouraged by not accomplishing something, but rather be motivated by the possibilities of doing it.

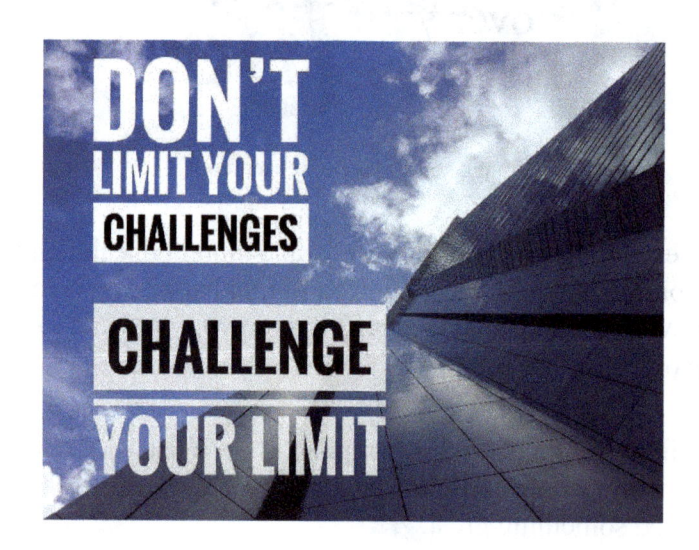

6. Accept Yourself Unconditionally (Self-Compassion)

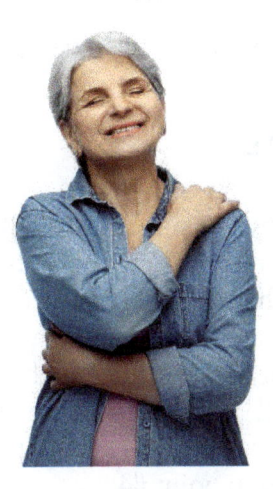

You are more than a performance outcome. You should not identify yourself singularly because you are so much more than a single entity. You are the sum of your life experiences, and you need to focus on the positive ones, for those are the experiences that will form the foundation upon which a you build your tomorrows.

Having unconditional self-compassion (Chapter 6.6: Self-Compassion: The Proven Power of Being Kind to Yourself) will help you bounce back from disappointments quickly and move toward your goals.

7. Never Stop Learning

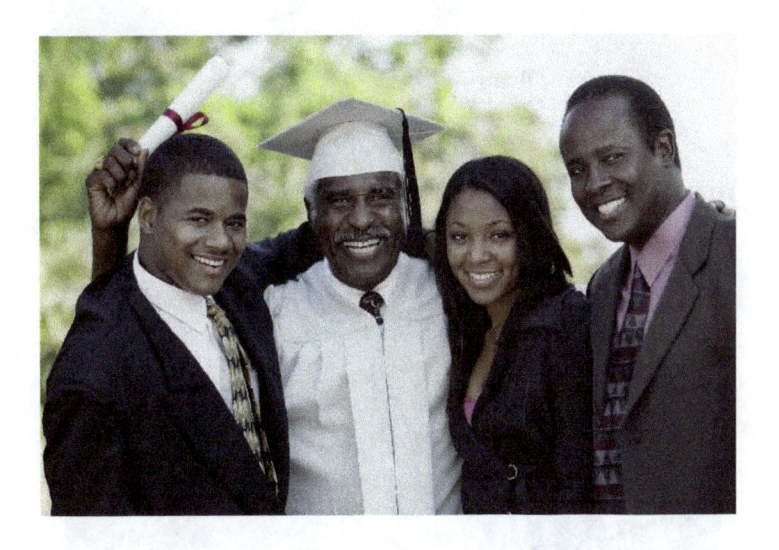

Embrace the Zen idea of "always a student." Your willingness to learn and evolve is invaluable for attaining personal excellence and fulfillment. You will achieve more success and happiness by understanding that you can progress in every area of your life, including your health and fitness. Reading Forever Active Older Adult Health and Fitness Playbook should be just a starting point for your quest to become healthier, and to attain a higher quality of life as you grow older.

"Never Stop Learning" is crucial to good robust mental health. Embrace it.

8. Maintain a Great Perspective

Always put things in perspective by considering the BIGGER picture. Looking at something, such as a particular workout session or a week of workouts in isolation, is misleading. Good or lousy compliance to your fitness and health plan usually doesn't just happen, but happens because of prior thoughts, words, and actions. Consider what these thoughts, words, and actions were, how they influenced the good or bad result, and what you can do in the future to improve the outcome. But most important of all, keep the good, the bad and the ugly in perspective. Most of the time, things are never as good or bad as they first appear. Perspective is everything. Remember the Tiger Woods story told in point #4.

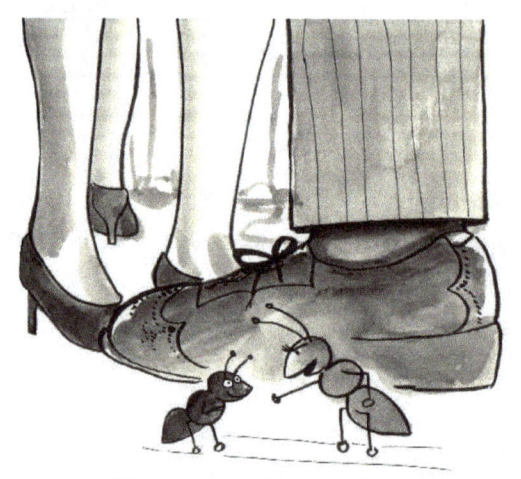

"Be proud you're an ant ... and don't let anyone step on you!"

9. Possess Self Control and Patience

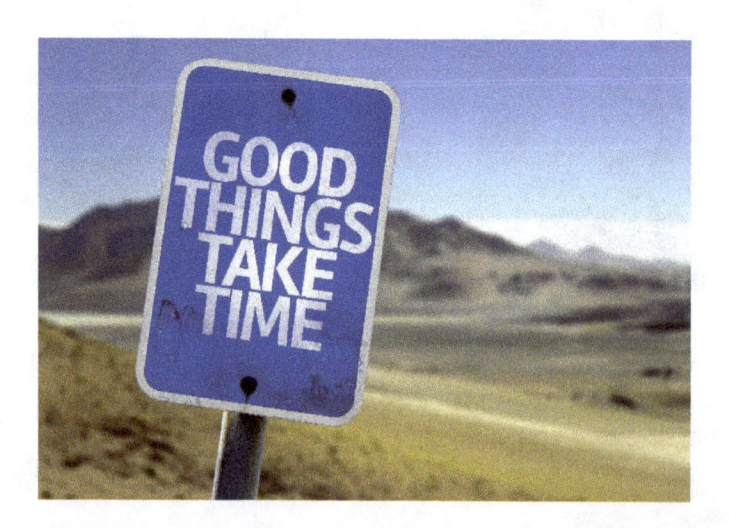

Today's society focuses on instant gratification, especially true for fitness and health. Most people want to train so they can go from 0 Km to being able to run 10 km in a month or lose 10 pounds a week every week. Physiologically, the body does not work this way. Your body, even the older adult's body, has an incredible ability to adapt to the physical stress that is placed upon it. However, this adaption takes time. If you go too hard, too fast, too much, too soon, your body and mind (emotional burnout) will break down. This is especially true for the older adult or anyone who has not been regularly exercising for the past several years. Be patient, use self-control and go low and slow. This point is discussed in detail in chapter 3.1: The Eight Golden Rules of Training.

10. Be Grateful

Expressing gratitude is not showing weakness but is showing the strength of character. The Greek philosopher Plato wrote, "A grateful mind is a great mind which eventually attracts to itself great things." Being thankful is one of the strengths most strongly correlated with well-being.

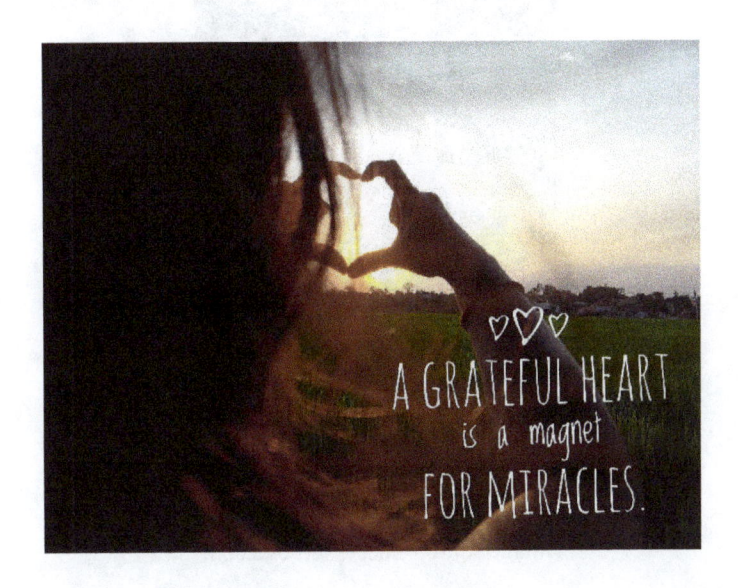

You need to reflect on things in your life daily that you can be thankful for. You should keep a "Gratitude Journal" that you can refer to when you are challenged negatively about continuing with your health and fitness plan. Gratitude is an effective mood enhancer and motivator. It is an excellent way of seeing the glass as half-full. It will help you realize all the good things in your life and that any current challenge is temporary. Remember what the Zen master said in Chapter 6.14, "It will pass."

11. Have a Daily Game Plan

It is essential to have a daily mental game plan that allows, in a productive way, the handling of any obstacle that may present itself. By creating a daily readiness plan/routine, you will always be in total control, even if you have to make some adjustments. It provides reassurance and predictability.

Developing a daily routine involves reflecting on past experiences. What were the best times to get workouts in? What works on Monday, Tuesday or Wednesday may be different than what works best later in the week or on the weekends. Over time, you will find out what works best for you. If a particular day did not go as planned, what could have been done better or differently to produce the desired results?

It is important that you feel in control so you can do your best and be more productive. Having a daily game plan will allow you to do this.

12. Personal Pep Talks

Positive pep talks can help ease obstructive situations and eliminate doubt and fear.

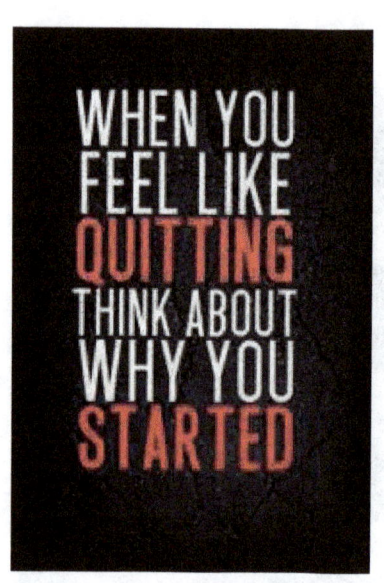

Image source: successgroove.com

Here are some tips for you to take into consideration:
1. Keep it simple but powerful – For example, "I always feel better after I exercise, even if I only did half a routine."

2. Evoke previous successes for confidence – For example, "I have done this before. I can do it again."

3. Tell yourself to focus and stay in the present – For example, "What I have to do later in the day doesn't matter. It is only right now that I have to focus on."

4. Tell yourself how much you enjoy the challenge regardless of the time and effort it is taking – For example, "I love this, bring it on."

Conclusion

"The toughest thing about success is that you have got to keep being a success."
— Irving Berlin

Developing a champion's mindset to achieve the goal of consistent, and sustained health and fitness, and maintaining mental strength through adversity is a marathon, a lifelong endeavour. It is not easy, but the 12 points listed above will help as a guide. There can be no let-up. To win, and there is no other alternative but to win when it comes to your health, you have to think long term. That has to be your mindset. New challenges will constantly present themselves, and you must keep pushing yourself to meet these challenges with a champion's mind daily.

Success and winning are not random acts. They are earned through tenaciously implementing what has been discussed here. By embracing the twelve points presented, you'll have the tools to succeed, but they must be implemented. Like any new skill, it is a learning process to master, but you will get better at using these skills/tools/techniques every time you use them.

References

Afremow, Jim (2013). *The Champions Mind: How Great Athletes Think, Train, and Thrive* Rodale Inc

Fitzgerald, Matt. (2015). *How Bad Do You Want It: Mastering the Psychology of Mind over Muscle.* Velopress.

Neff, Kristin. (2011). *Self-Compassion: The Proven Power of Being Kind to Yourself.* William Marrow.

Willink, Jocko., Babin, Leif. (2015). *Extreme Ownership: How the U.S. Navy Seals Lead and Win.* St. Martin's Press.

Section 8

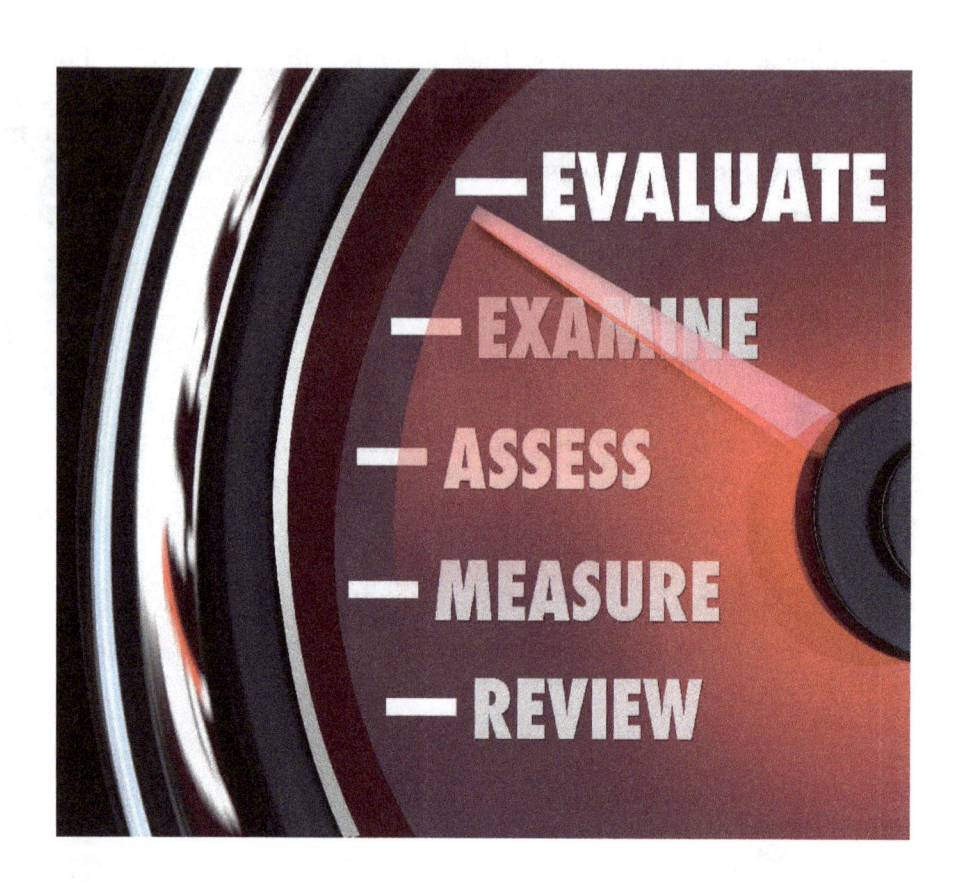

Post-Season Wrap-up – Measuring Progress and Success

8.0. Evaluation of Effort – Measuring Progress and Success

Introduction

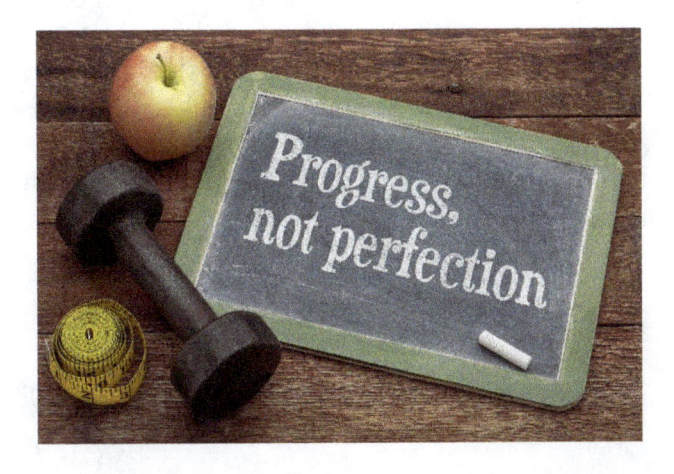

Evaluation of effort is necessary. There is nothing more motivating for you than seeing progress at something you are working at. Seeing progress is especially true when it comes to exercising and nutrition. People love to feel themselves getting stronger (walking or running farther and lifting boxes that they struggled with before), becoming more flexible (being able to touch their toes or reach a higher shelf in the cabinet), or losing a few pounds. Ironically, however, the real power of measuring progress is discovering that progress that you are expecting is not happening. Finding this out early in the process allows you to re-evaluate your health and fitness plan and determine what is not working, and make the necessary corrections before wasting too much time and effort. Remember, "Progress is not perfection."

Developing an effective health and fitness plan is as much an art as it is a science. It will usually take many repeated efforts before determining what works best. Everyone, but especially older adults, has special needs and health challenges that must be taken into account in order for their health and fitness plans to be effective. Unfortunately, there is no one size fits all plan. Because of the individuality of health and fitness plans, evaluation and continuous re-evaluation of effort and results are important.

Time Frame for Evaluation and Re-Evaluation

An individual's fitness and health plan should be evaluated and re-evaluated regularly. The time between re-valuations must be long enough to allow physiological and emotional changes to occur but not so long that regression can happen without being detected. Making progress initially and then having unexpected regressing can be very discouraging.
Re-evaluating your progress every six weeks is the appropriate time frame to allow positive adaptations to occur and catch regressions early enough.

Types of Evaluations

Physical activity and fitness, nutrition, and holistic health are the three main components of your plan and the areas that need to assessment regularly. Your level of physical activity, quality of their diet, and holistic health are accurately and most easily evaluated through a questionnaire. Your physical fitness can be measured through a comprehensive fitness test. The goals you set can be evaluated through self-reflection. To repeat, you should do these re-evaluations regularly, every six weeks. If you are not consistent about completing your re-evaluations, the results will not be accurate or reliable. Like implementing your health and fitness plan, evaluating your progress needs to be done consistently to be valuable.

Questionnaires

Each of the questionnaires presented here are included in Worksheet 9.2.6: Re-evaluation

1. Physical Activity Evaluation

(Reference: Can-Fit-Pro - *Nutrition and Wellness Specialist Certification Manual*, March 2007)

Date:_____

(Assessment of Current Physical Activity Level)

Physical activity level is described as maintaining a physically active lifestyle. Listed below are 20 statements that refer to physical activity. Use the scale, and respond to each question by circling the number that best describes your current lifestyle.

Description	Great	Good	Fair	Needs Attention
1. Amount of energy every day.	4	3	2	1
2. Cardiovascular endurance.	4	3	2	1
3. Ability to perform continuous activity for 30 minutes.	4	3	2	1
4. Accumulate at least 30 minutes of physical activity most days of the week.	4	3	2	1
5. Muscular strength and endurance.	4	3	2	1
6. Upper-body strength.	4	3	2	1
7. Ability to lift and carry heavy objects.	4	3	2	1
8. Perform resistance exercise regularly.	4	3	2	1
9. The range of motion in joints.	4	3	2	1
10. Ability to move arms and legs with minimal pain and limitations.	4	3	2	1
11. Participation in stretching and flexibility activities regularly.	4	3	2	1
12. Posture and low back strength.	4	3	2	1
13. Physical appearance.	4	3	2	1
14. Body weight.	4	3	2	1
15. Amount of body fat versus muscle.	4	3	2	1
16. Live an active lifestyle.	4	3	2	1
17. Ability to engage in activities with a moderate amount of effort or intensity.	4	3	2	1
18. Level of current physical fitness.	4	3	2	1
19. Physical condition for age.	4	3	2	1
20. Overall assessment of health and wellbeing.	4	3	2	1
Totals				

Total Physical Activity SCORE _____/80

2. Nutritional Balance Evaluation

(Reference: Can-Fit-Pro - *Nutrition and Wellness Specialist Certification Manual*, March 2007)

Date: _____

(Assessment of Current Nutritional Choices and Health)

Nutritional balance is the ability to make intelligent and beneficial dietary choices. Listed below are 25 statements that refer to nutritional balance. Use the scale, and respond to each question by circling the number that best describes your current lifestyle.

Description	Great	Good	Fair	Needs Attention
1. Amount of energy every day.	4	3	2	1
2. I enjoy eating a diet with lots of variety.	4	3	2	1
3. I eat at least 3.5 to 5 servings of vegetables daily.	4	3	2	1
4. I eat a variety of vegetables (lots of different colours).	4	3	2	1
5. I eat at least 3.5 to 5 servings of fruit each day.	4	3	2	1
6. I eat a variety of fruit.	4	3	2	1
7. I eat 6 to 8 servings of grain products each day.	4	3	2	1
8. I attempt to eat whole grain products and avoid refined (white flour) grain products.	4	3	2	1
9. I am careful to eat appropriate serving sizes of grain products.	4	3	2	1
10. I consume 2 to 3 servings of milk products daily.	4	3	2	1
11. I avoid milk products that are high in fat.	4	3	2	1
12. I eat 2 to 3 servings of meat and alternatives each day.	4	3	2	1
13. I have reduced my consumption of red meat.	4	3	2	1
14. I eat beans and legumes.	4	3	2	1
15. I eat seafood/fish at least once a week.	4	3	2	1
16. I choose healthy snacks and avoid snacks that have low nutritional value.	4	3	2	1
17. I drink at least 8 to 12 glasses of water daily.	4	3	2	1
18. I take supplements to balance my diet.	4	3	2	1

19. I read labels and am careful about the food I serve.	4	3	2	1
20. I am happy with my body weight.	4	3	2	1
21. My body's ratio of fat versus muscle is appropriate.	4	3	2	1
22. I avoid eating fast food.	4	3	2	1
23. I am pleased with my physical appearance.	4	3	2	1
24. Generally, my diet is balanced.	4	3	2	1
25. Overall assessment of my health/well being.	4	3	2	1
Totals				

Total Nutritional Balance SCORE _____/100

3. Holistic Wellness Evaluation

(Reference: *Can-Fit-Pro - Nutrition and Wellness Specialist Certification Manual,* March 2007)

Date: _____

Holistic wellness is the ability to develop balance and harmony in life. Listed below are 25 statements that refer to holistic wellness. Use the scale, and respond to each question by circling the number that best describes your current lifestyle.

Description	Most of the Time	Frequently	Sometimes	Rarely or Never
1. I have a good relationship with my family	4	3	2	1
2. I am involved in my community	4	3	2	1
3. I do something for fun and for myself every week.	4	3	2	1
4. I provide support for others.	4	3	2	1
5. My life has meaning and direction.	4	3	2	1
6. I have life goals and I strive to achieve them.	4	3	2	1
7. I look forward to the future.	4	3	2	1
8. I have a sense of peace in my life.	4	3	2	1
9. I feel positive about myself and my life.	4	3	2	1
10. I learn from my mistakes.	4	3	2	1
11. I can say no without feeling guilty.	4	3	2	1
12. I find it easy to laugh	4	3	2	1
13. I cope with life's changes in a healthy way.	4	3	2	1
14. I prepare ahead of time for events that may cause stress.	4	3	2	1
15. I schedule enough time to accomplish what I need to get done.	4	3	2	1
16. I participate in activities that relieve stress.	4	3	2	1
17. I stay calm and patient under pressure.	4	3	2	1
18. I know what my values and beliefs are.	4	3	2	1
19. I have interest outside my work.	4	3	2	1
20. I am interested in learning new things.	4	3	2	1
21. I make time to relax regularly	4	3	2	1
22. I cope well with changes in my life.	4	3	2	1
23. I feel that things often go my way.	4	3	2	1

24. I get enough sleep and have little trouble going to sleep.	4	3	2	1
25. I am happy and enjoy life.	4	3	2	1
Totals				

Total Holistic Wellness SCORE _____ **/100**

Interpretation of Questionnaire Results

When you look over the results of your physical activity, nutritional balance, and holistic wellness questionnaires, you should do the following:

1. Look at your overall score for each component (Physical activity, Nutritional Balance, Holistic Wellness). Is it above or below average? This will give a good idea whether you need to give more attention to this component of your health.

Score	Physical Activity Category
70 - 80	Excellent
60 - 69	Good
50 - 59	Average
< 49	Needs Improvement

Score	Nutrition Balance Category
85 - 100	Excellent
75 - 84	Good
65 - 74	Average
< 64	Needs Improvement

Score	Holistic Wellness Category
85-100	Excellent
70-84	Good
55-69	Average
<54	Needs Improvement

2. Identify specific areas of strength (scores 3 or 4) and areas of weakness (scores 1 or 2) in each of the components of health.

3. Try to determine why you are weak in specific areas.

4. Establish a **S.M.A.R.T.** goal (Chapter 3.3.: The Importance and Art of Goal Setting) to improve the area of weakness This means that you establish a strategy/ action plan that is **S**pecific, **M**easurable, **A**ction oriented, **R**ealistic and **T**ime lined.

Physical Fitness Evaluation

1. Resting Heart Rate

Take your radial (wrist) or carotid (neck) pulse for 10 sec and multiply by 6.

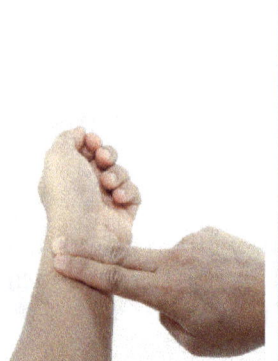

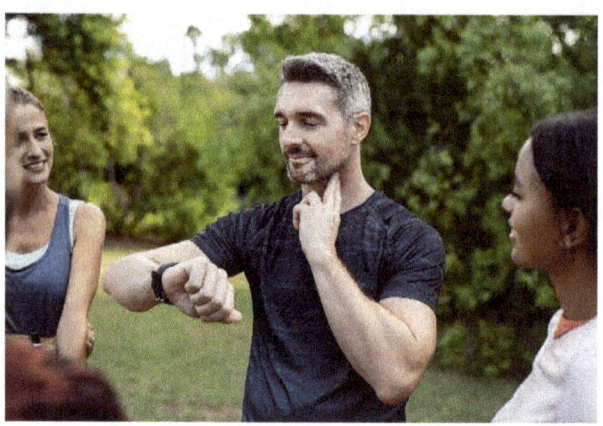

	Initial			
Date				
Resting Heart Rate				

Comment: Even though the reading of a resting heart rate can vary by about 10%, a lowering in your resting heart rate is a positive sign because it is usually an early indication of improved fitness. On the other hand, a higher resting heart rate could be an indication of infection, chronic stress or a heart condition, and would warrant further investigation.

(A person should take their heart rate just before they get out of bed in the morning three to five days in a row to get an accurate reading of your resting heart rate).

2. Resting Blood Pressure

Everyone should have a self-administered blood pressure monitor at home.

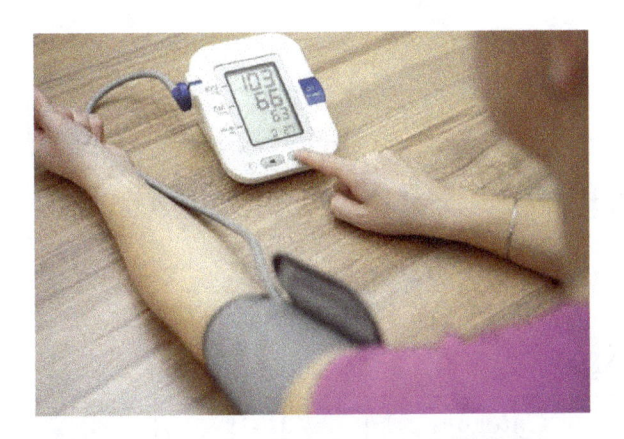

	Initial			
Date:				
Resting Blood Pressure				

Comment: 120/80 is considered a normal resting BP. The systolic pressure (the top value) can vary quite a bit, for example 180, due to excitement, anxiety and exertion. However, the diastolic pressure (the bottom value) remains relatively constant. A diastolic pressure over 90 would indicate borderline hypertension and require further investigation and possible medication.

3. Body Composition
1. Body Mass Index

Purpose: Use as a guideline to determine if you are carrying an acceptable amount of weight for your height.

(Major Limitation – It does not take into account the amount of muscle development a person may have).

Weight   **Height**

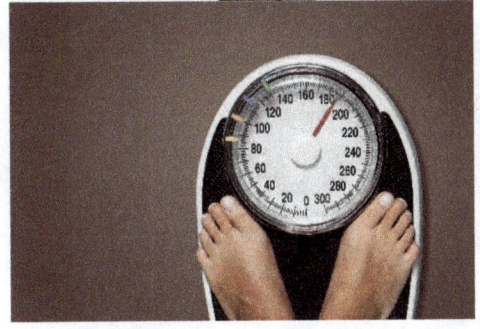

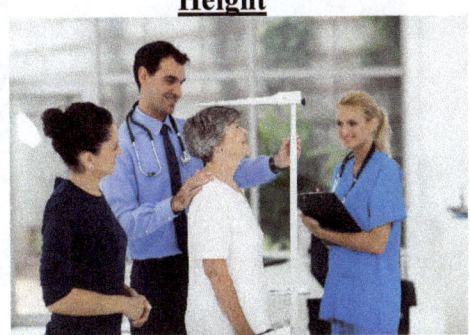

	Initial			
Date				
1. Weight (Kg.)				
2. Height (M)				
BMI (wt/ht^2)				

Example Calculation – Ht 1.55M (6'1"), wt. 91 kg (200 lbs)

Formula BMI = wt (Kg)/Ht^2(M)
$$= 91/(1.55)^2 = 91/2.4 = 37.9 \text{ (Obese 2)}$$

Evaluation of BMI

Category	BMI
Underweight	<18.5
Normal	18.5 – 24.9
Overweight	25.0 – 29.9
Obese 1	30.0 – 34.9
Obese 2	35.0 – 39.9
Extreme Obesity	>40.0

2. Waist-to-Hip Ratio

Purpose – Recent research indicates that it is the distribution/areas of fat on the body and not the amount of body fat that determines the cardio-vascular health risk of obesity. Fat carried internally in the abdominal area carries the greatest risk.

Waist Measurement　　　　　　　　**Hip Measurement**

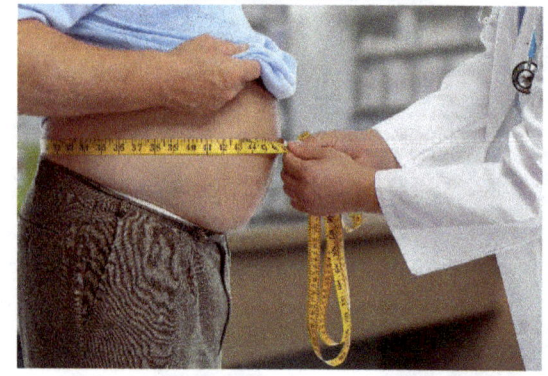

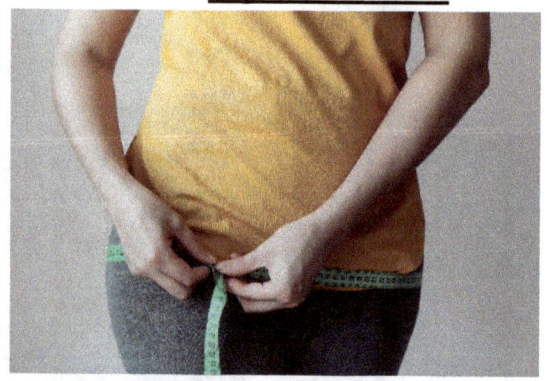

Initial

	Date				
1. Waist Girth (Measure around your belly button) (inches)					
2. Hip Girth (Measure 2" below iliac crest) (inches)					
Waist/Hip Ratio					

Example calculation – waist 40" & Hip 38" (50-year-old male)

<u>Formula</u> – waist measurement (inches)/hip measurement (inches)
= 40/38 = 1.05 (very high risk of heart disease)

	\multicolumn{8}{c}{Risk for Heart Disease}
	Low		Moderate		High		Very High	
Age	Men	Women	Men	Women	Men	Women	Men	Women
20-29	< 0.83	< 0.71	0.83 - 0.88	0.71 - 0.77	0.89 - 0.94	0.78 - 0.82	> 0.94	> 0.82
30-39	< 0.84	< 0.72	0.84 - 0.91	0.72 - 0.78	0.92 - 0.96	.79 - 0.84	> 0.96	> 0.84
40-49	< 0.88	< 0.73	0.88 - 0.95	0.73 - 0.79	0.96 - 1.00	0.80 - 0.87	> 1.00	> 0.87
50-59	< 0.90	< 0.74	0.90 - 0.96	0.74 - 0.81	0.97 - 1.02	0.82 - 0.88	> 1.02	> 0.88
60-69	< 0.91	< 0.76	0.91 - 0.98	0.76 - 0.83	0.99 - 1.03	0.84 - 0.90	> 1.03	> 0.90

4. Flexibility Evaluation

Purpose – To detect muscle imbalances (one side of body less flexible than the other side) and joint instabilities (excessive mobility).

1. Upper Body Flexibility Evaluation

Evaluation – do you feel/notice one arm is stiffer (can't scratch as far on the back as the other side)

Initial

Date:				
1. External Rotation (Upper back scratch)				
2. Internal Rotation (Lower back scratch)				
3. Abduction (Lifting arms over your head)				

556

2. Lower Body Flexibility Evaluation

Initial

Date:				
1. LB Forward Flexion (Standing and touch toes without bending your knees) Evaluation – Inches/cm from to toes/floor				
2. LB Extension (Standing and lean back at the waist) Evaluation - Do you feel restricted				

3. Quadriceps (Lie on stomach and bend heel to buttocks) <u>Evaluation</u> – Inches/cm from heel to buttocks				
4. Groin (Sit on mat with heels touching) <u>Evaluation</u> – Inches/cm from bottom of knee to floor.				
5. Ankle and Calf <u>Evaluation</u> - Does one ankle feel more restricted than the other. (Extension/Flexion) **Extension** **Flexion**				

6. Hip extensors

1. Gluteus Medius

(Lie on floor and bring knee to opposite side chest)

Evaluation – Inches/cm from knee to chest.

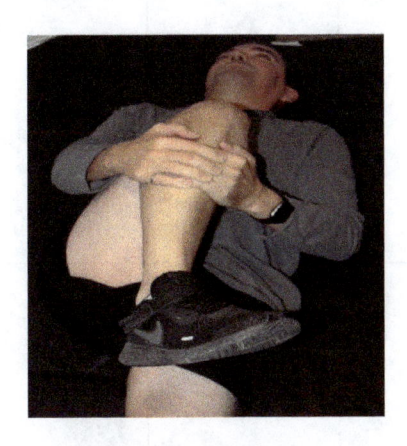

2. Gluteus Maximus)

(Lie on floor and bring knee to same sided chest)

Evaluation – Inches/cm from knee to chest.

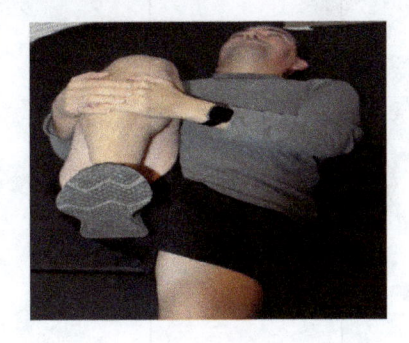

7. Hip Flexors (Lie on floor and bring one knee to chest) <u>Evaluation</u> - Observe if opposite leg raises off the floor/table				
8. Trunk Rotation (Sitting, arms crossed against the chest and rotate shoulders in both directions) <u>Evaluation</u> - Observe if there is restriction on rotation in either direction.				

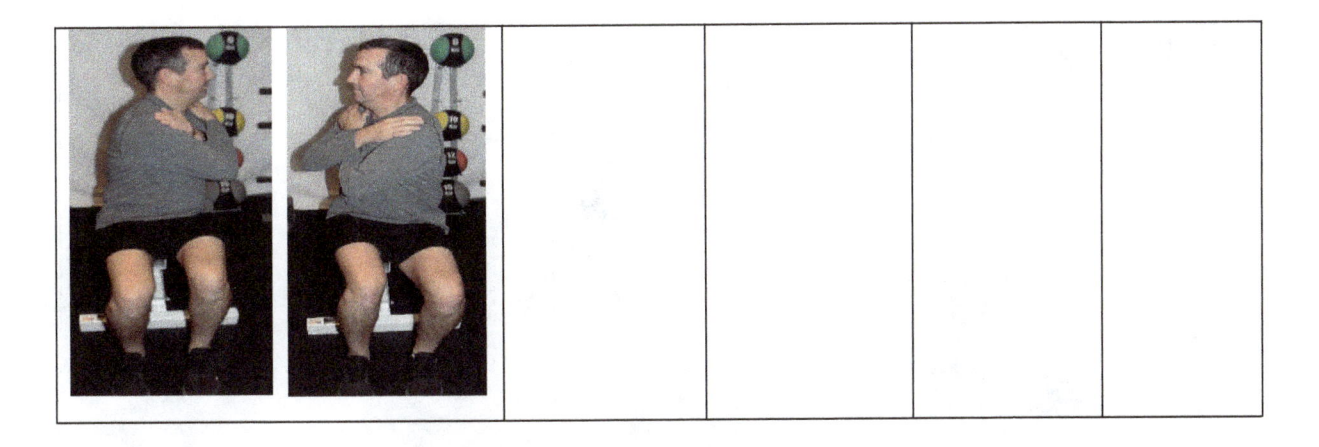

5. Agility, Balance and Coordination Evaluation

1. Agility and Coordination Evaluation

Evaluation - Put a check mark in the appropriate box)

Initial

	Date:			
	Test	**No Hesitation/ Stumbles/ Difficulties**	**Moderate Hesitation/ Stumbles/ Difficulties**	**Significant Hesitation/ Stumbles/ Difficulties**
	Walking Drills:			
	1. Walk Forward 10 steps			

2. Walk Backward 10 steps			
3. Walk Sideways 10 steps			
4. Walk sideways crossing your legs 5 steps (Alternate the crossing leg going in front and then behind the other leg.) (Do a second time with the opposite leg crossing over)			

Hop Drills:			
1. Forward Hop Drills:			
1. Double leg forward hop 5 x's			
2. Single leg forward hop 5 x's (Repeat with opposite leg 5 x's)			
3. Feet wide then narrow hop scotch			

4. Scissor hop in a stationary position			
2. Sideways Hop Drills:			
1. Double leg hop sideways			
2. Single foot hop sideways			

3. Rotational Hop Drills			
1. 90° rotation hop			

2. Static Balance Test – Eyes Open and then Closed

Evaluation - Stand on an unsupported leg for maximum of 10 seconds)

Eyes Closed

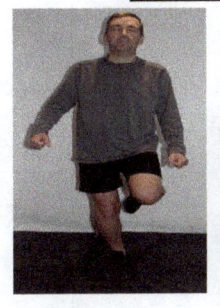

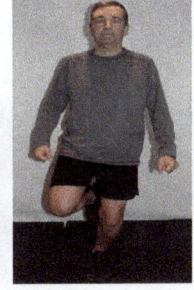

Initial

Date:				
Eyes Open (sec.)	R- - L -	R- L -	R- L-	R- L-
Eyes Closed (sec.)	R- L-	R- L-	R-. L-	R- L-

6. Muscular Strength and Endurance Evaluation

(<u>Note</u> - **All exercises listed below are described in detail and illustrated in Appendix 9.1.2.2.1**)

1. Muscle Strength Evaluation

<u>Initial</u>

Date:							
<u>Exercise</u>		<u>Weight Lifted (lbs.)</u>	<u>Reps</u>	<u>Weight Lifted (lbs.)</u>	<u>Reps</u>	<u>Weights Lifted (lbs.)</u>	<u>Reps</u>
1. Leg Extensions / Lunges (Quadriceps) **Machine** - Single leg or **Double Leg Extension** or **Bench Balance Lunge**	**Machine:** **Single Leg** **Double Leg**		R- L-		R- L-		R- L-

566

	Balance Lunge:					
2. Leg Curls (Hamstrings) **Machine** - Single leg or Double Leg Curl or **Stability Ball** Supine Single Leg or Double Leg Curl	**Machine:** **Single Leg** **Double Leg**		R- L-		R- L-	R- L-

	Stability Ball Curl:		R- L-		R- L-		R- L-
3. Chest Press (Pectoralis Major) **Machine** Chest Press or **Dumbbell** Chest Press	**Machine:** **Dumbbells**						

4. Shoulder Pull-Downs (**Latissimus Dorsi**) **Machine** **Lat. Pull Down** or **Dumbbells** **Lying Down Overhead Two-Handed Vertical Raise**	**Machine:** **Dumbbells:**						

5. Overhead Press (Trapezius) Machine Overhead Shoulder Press or Dumbbells Overhead Press	Machine Dumbbells						

6. Rows (Rhomboids) **Machine** Cable Rows or **Dumbbells** Bent Over Rows (Standing or Sitting on Stability Ball)	**Machine:** Cable Rows **Dumbbells** **Bent Over Rows:**						

7. Lateral Raises (Deltoids) Shoulder Abduction (Can use dumbbells or rubber resistance bands)	**Dumbbells**						
8. Arm Curls (Biceps) **Machine** Arm Curls or **Dumbbells** Arm Curls	**Machine:** **Dumbbells:**						

9. Arm Extensions (Triceps) **Machine** Triceps Arm Extensions or **Lying** **or** **Sitting** Double Triceps Extensions	**Machine** **Standing Double Arm Extensions**							

2. Muscle Endurance Evaluation

	Date:	**Initial**			
1. Push-ups **Regular** **Wall** **Modified (on knees)**					
Number completed					

3. Core Strength Evaluation

<u>**Initial**</u>

Date				
1. Full Sit-ups **Stabilize the feet**				
Number Completed				

7. Cardiovascular Fitness Evaluation
1. Walking Fitness Test

Initial

Date:				
Heartrate at end of a one-mile walk				
Time it took to complete the walk				

Rate of Perceived Effort
    7 – very, very light
    9 – very light
    11 – light
    13 – somewhat hard
    15 – hard
    17 – very hard				

Interpretation of Physical Fitness Evaluation (What Do the Results Mean)

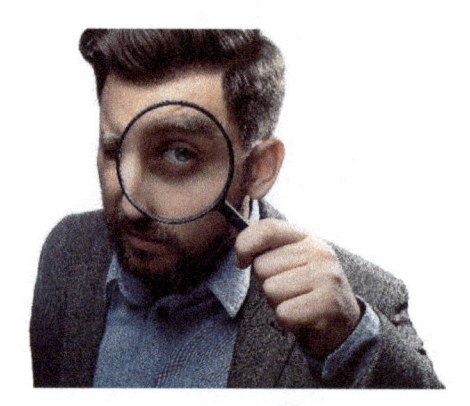

When evaluating the physical fitness results, the focus should be on looking for trends in the performance. The actual number of sit-ups, push-ups, or weights lifted is not as significant as whether you have done more or less over the past two or three re-evaluations. For example, if the number of sit-ups a person competed has dropped over the last three re-evaluations, they need to focus more on core exercises. The same holds for all muscle strengthening exercises or flexibility. If a person finds that the distance to touch their toes has increased over the last three re-evaluations, it is a signal to them to increase the amount of effort spent on hamstring and lower back stretches.

You must not get hung up on the specific numbers on a particular re-evaluation day. It is not be a big deal if you did not do as many chest presses or bicep curls on one specific re-evaluation. It might be that your chest muscles or arms were more tired on that particular day. It is impossible to give a gold medal performance on each test. One particular re-evaluation day may show terrible results across all muscle tests, and there could have been many reasons for this.

That is why you should focus on trends. If your performance has decreased over two or three re-evaluations, you need to investigate why.

When interpreting physical fitness results, it is also important to look for general tendencies such as whether one arm is weaker than the other, or the hamstrings are significantly weaker than the quadriceps. For example, there should be a 3 to 2 ratio between the strength of the quadriceps and hamstrings and a 1 t 2 ratio between the strength of the biceps and triceps (Chapter 4.2.: Muscular Resistance Training: Developing Muscular Strength and Endurance). When a person notices these imbalances, they can focus more on these imbalanced areas when developing their next six-week strength program.

Goal Setting Evaluation

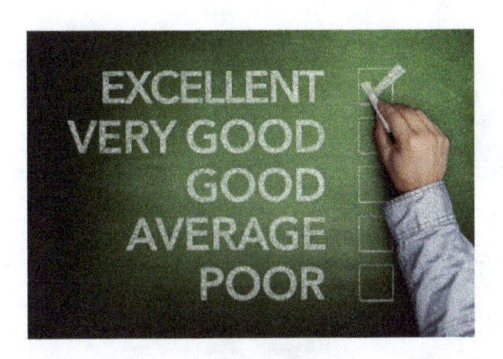

Section 3.3: The Importance and Art of Goal Setting explicitly covers the topic of goal setting. However, no matter how good or diligent you are at establishing short and long-term goals, setting goals serves no real purpose if you don't evaluate your success in achieving them.

Evaluating success at accomplishing set goals makes a person accountable, and that is the true power of goal setting; being responsible for doing something that you felt important enough to write it down as a goal. Research shows a much higher probability of achieving a goal if it is written down in a S.M.A.R.T. format and evaluated for achievement in the time line(T) established.

If you determined that a set goal was not accomplished it is necessary to determine why. What factors got in the way of achieving this particular goal? Was the goal important enough to make it a priority? Was the goal set too high, or was it set too low if accomplished with little effort? A critical element of setting goals is being realistic (R) in what can and cannot be achieved in the timeline established.

Goal setting is a powerful tool to give direction and help a person accomplish great things, but you must evaluate your success in reaching these goals to exploit its true value fully.

Goal Evaluation

First Goal:

Specific	
Measurable	
Action	
Realistic	
Time lined	
Evaluation (if not accomplished, why? What can you do better to be more successful?)	

Second Goal:

Specific	
Measurable	
Action	
Realistic	
Time lined	
Evaluation (If not accomplished why? What can you do better to be more successful?)	

Third Goal:

Specific	
Measurable	
Action	
Realistic	
Time lined	

Evaluation **(If not accomplished, why?** **What can you do better to** **be more successful?)**	

Conclusion

Evaluating progress and success, or lack of success, is vitally important and contributes significantly to making fitness and health plan sustainable. Only by re-evaluating the results of your effort will you know if you are on the right track to accomplish your goals. Why spend the time and effort exercising and managing diet if it will not allow you to become stronger, more flexible, and lose weight? Only through consistent evaluation of the results of effort can you be assured that you are doing everything right.

Evaluation and re-evaluation are vital components to successfully implementing your fitness and health plan and ensuring an improved quality of life. Do it consistently, and good things will happen.

Reference

www.forever-active.com
Can-fit-Pro, (2007), *Nutrition and Wellness Specialist Certification Manual*, Canadian Fitness Professionals Inc.
Can-Fit-Pro,(2008), *Foundations of Professional Training*, Human Kinetics.
Can-Fit-Pro, (2003), *Older Adult Fitness Specialist Certification Manual*, Human Kinetics, June 2003.
Rose, Debra J.(2010), *Fall Poof: A Comprehensive Balance and Mobility Training Program, 2nd Edition*, Human Kinetics

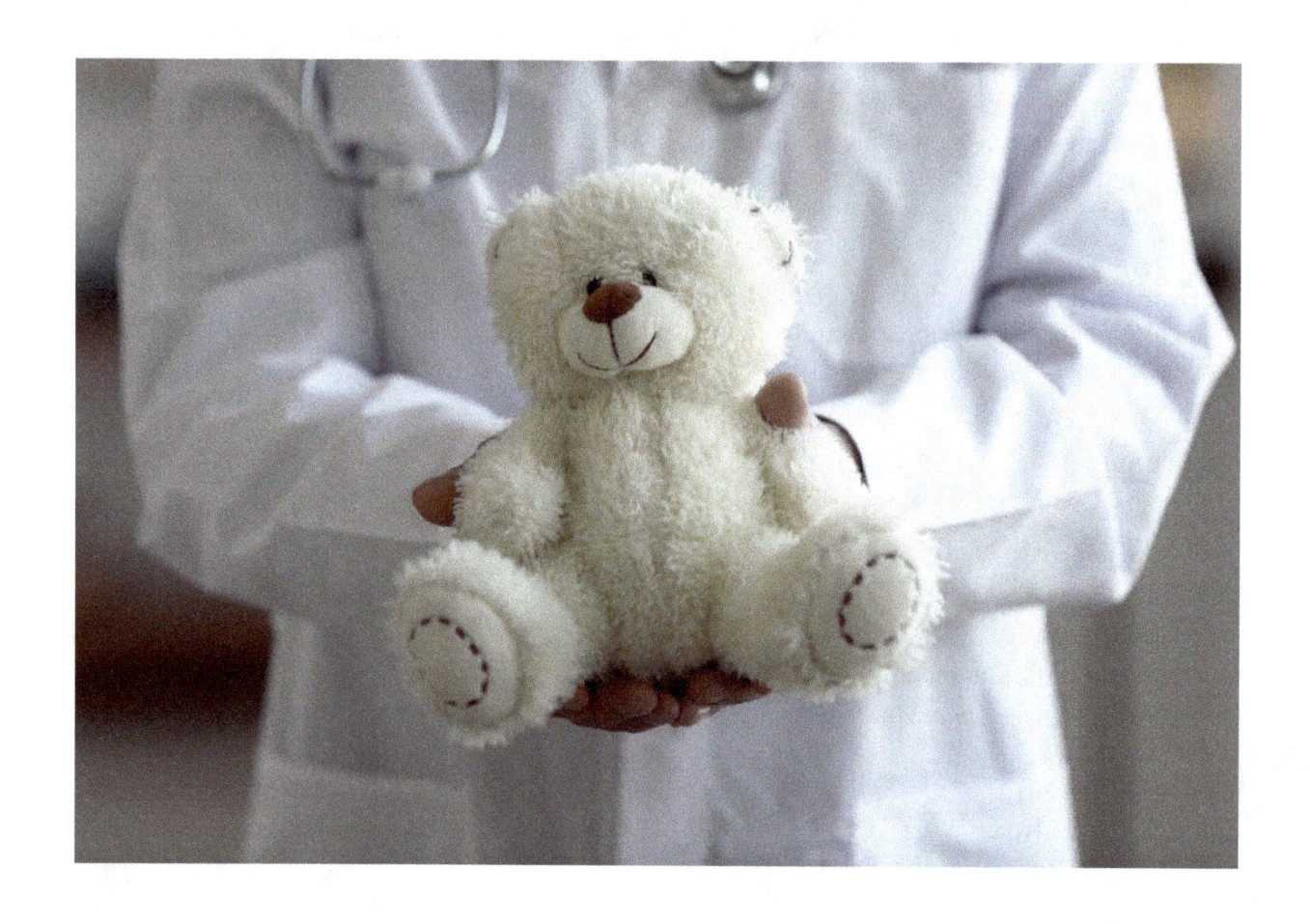

Section 9

The Support Staff

9.0. Introduction: The Support Staff

It takes more than a great offense, defense, and special teams to make a champion football team. And this is true for making The Forever Active Older Adult Health and Fitness Play Book a great health and fitness resource. The information covered in this book is accurate (edited by professionals in their particular fields), comprehensive, and relevant for today's older adults. In fact, it is perfect for anyone who wants to improve their level of health and fitness.

Section 9: The Support Staff, plays an integral role in making this book complete and practical for anyone to use. The information provided in the various chapters is only valuable if utilized properly. This section aims to allow the reader to effortlessly implement practical applications of the information provided in the text, so they can use it purposefully.

On a football team, the support staff's responsibility is to make it possible for the players and coaches to perform at their best to beat the opposition. The same is true for this book. The support staff in this section includes appendices, workout sheets, a link for online support, and a reference library to help combat an older adult's opposition to their health (Section 2: The Off-Season: Studying the Opposition to the Your Health).

Whenever relevant, supporting documentation is referenced in the appendix and workout sheets, so it can be easily found in the appropriate text chapters. It can then be readily accessed and used to design and implement your personalized fitness and health program.

The Forever Active Older Adult Health and Fitness Playbook aims to present relevant information so older adults can develop sustainable health and fitness plans. The support staff (appendices, worksheets, online support, and reference library) purpose is transformational, to help convert theory into practical applications.

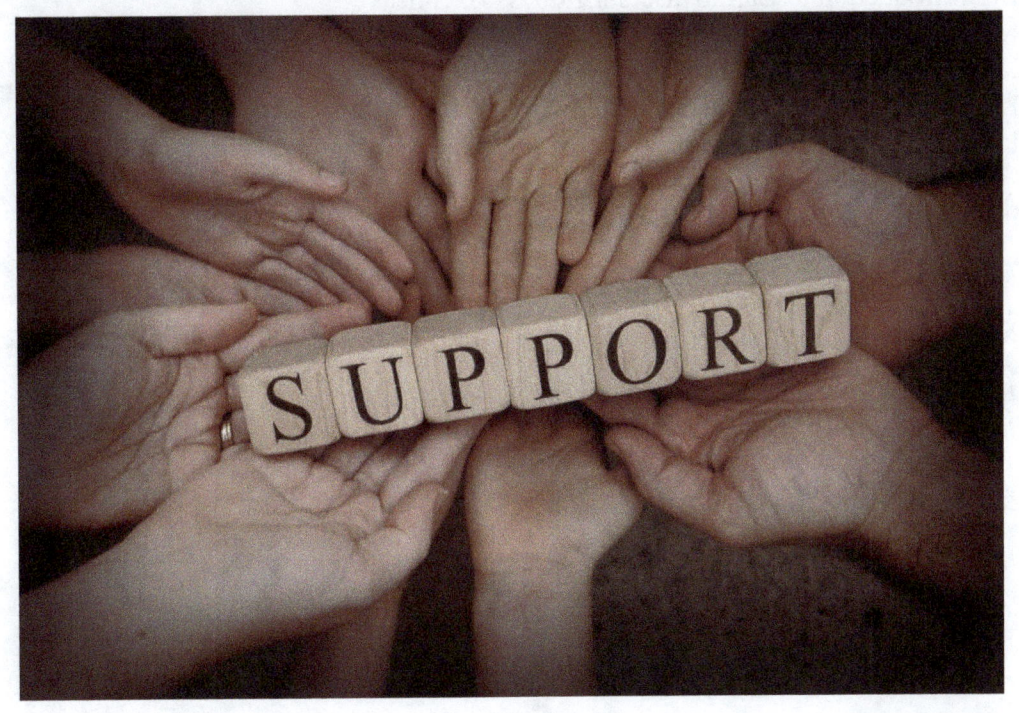

9.1. Introduction to the Appendices

The appendices, as part of the Support Staff section, are a vital resource and will make Forever Active Older Adult Health and Fitness Playbook unique and invaluable. The appendices are there to support the information presented in various chapters of the book.

Because safety is essential when exercising, the appendices illustrate and give in-depth descriptions of the various exercises that should be implemented into an older adult's fitness routine. There should be no ambiguity when doing exercises. There is a specific way of performing each particular exercise and, to minimize the risk of injury, each exercise movement needs to be performed as described.

To complement the appendices, Chapter 9.2's workout sheets organize the exercises described in the appendices into various workout routines. The workout sheets are in table form so the workout routines can be efficiently followed and recorded.

Recording workouts and evaluating progress every 5-6 weeks is essential to ensure steady progress and achievement of your S.M.A.R.T Goals.

Listed below is an outline of the appendices:

9.1.0. Appendices

9.1.0. Introduction: The Appendices

9.1.1. Cardiovascular Fitness Exercises

    9.1.1.0. Introduction to Cardiovascular Fitness Exercises
    9.1.1.1. Walking with Good Posture
    9.1.1.2. Developing Proper Running Form
    9.1.1.3. Cycling Safely: Good Sizing, Good Posture, Follow Safety Guidelines
    9.1.1.4. Swimming: Knowing How to Swim Makes it Easier and More Enjoyable

9.1.2. Muscular Strengthening/Resistance Exercises

    9.1.2.0. Introduction: Muscular Strengthening/Resistance Exercises

    9.1.2.1. Core

        9.1.2.1.0. Introduction: Core Exercises
        9.1.2.1.1. Core Exercises Described and Illustrated

    9.1.2.2. Whole Body Strengthening Exercises

        9.1.2.2.0. Introduction: Whole Body Strengthening Exercises
        9.1.2.2.1. Whole Body Strengthening Exercises Described and Illustrated

    9.1.2.3. Bodyweight Muscular Strengthening/Resistance Training

9.1.2.3.0. Introduction: Bodyweight Muscle Resistance Training
9.1.2.3.1. Bodyweight Muscle Resistance Exercises Described and Illustrated

9.1.3. Agility, Balance and Coordination Exercises

9.1.3.0. Introduction to Agility, Balance and Coordination Exercises
9.1.3.1. Agility, Balance and Coordination Exercises Described and Illustrated

9.1.4. Flexibility/Stretching Exercises

9.1.4.0. Introduction to Flexibility/Stretching Exercises
9.1.4.1. Stretching Exercises Described and Illustrated
9.1.4.2. 10 Minute Dynamic and Static Routine Described and Illustrated
9.1.4.3. Yin Yoga Described and Illustrated
9.1.4.4. Myofascial Self Massage Utilizing a Roller Described and Illustrated

9.1.5. Resistance Band Exercises Described and Illustrated

9.1.6. Stability Ball Exercises Described and Illustrated

9.1.7. BOSU Exercises Described and Illustrated

9.1.8. TRX Exercises Described and Illustrated

9.1.9. Medicine Ball Exercises Described and Illustrated

9.1.10. Floor Slider Exercises Described and Illustrated

Appendix 9.1.1.0. Introduction to Cardiovascular Fitness Exercises

Any type of movement is a good movement because being active requires the heart to work harder than just sitting or lying down. However, not all activities deliver the same cardiovascular fitness benefits. As explained in Chapter 4.1.1. Cardiovascular Fitness Training, for effective cardiovascular training, the activity must be intense enough to raise the heart rate within a specific target heart rate zone for a minimum of 20 minutes.

Walking, running, cycling, and swimming are four of the most effective activities to accomplish this goal. That is not to say that golfing, tennis, downhill skiing (cross-country skiing is excellent for cardiovascular training), and yoga are not great exercises to participate in, but they don't reach the threshold of elevating the heart for the sustained period of time required to effectively train the heart.

This appendix will explain how to walk, run, cycle, and swim properly and safely, so a person can achieve maximum training benefit and enjoyment from each activity.

Walking

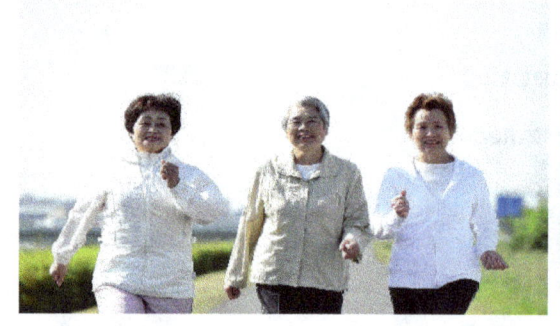

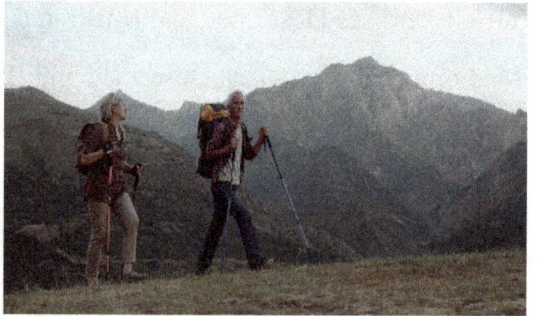

Running

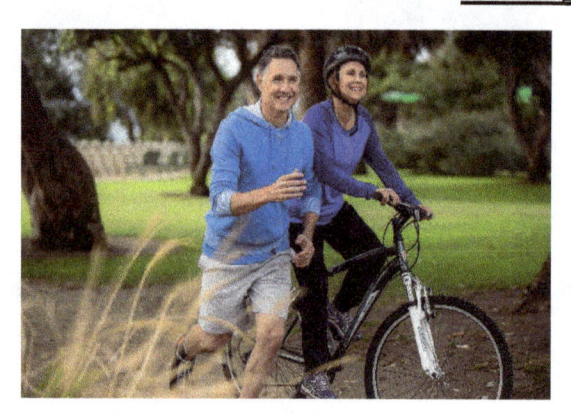

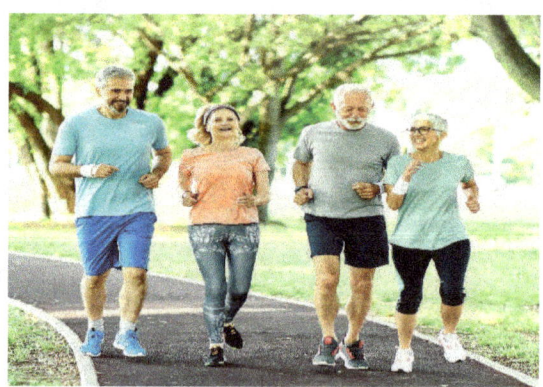

Cycling

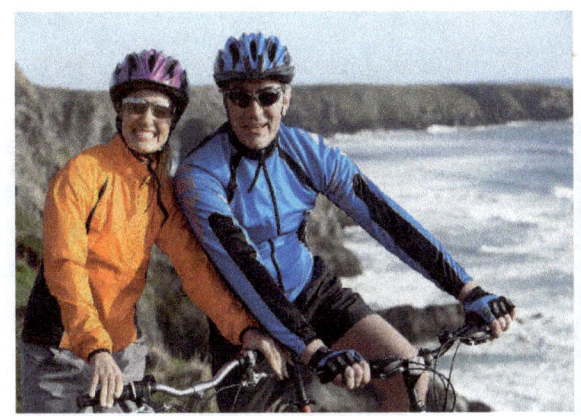

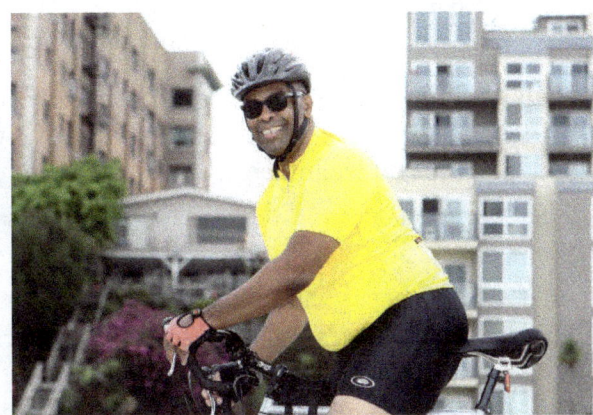

Swimming

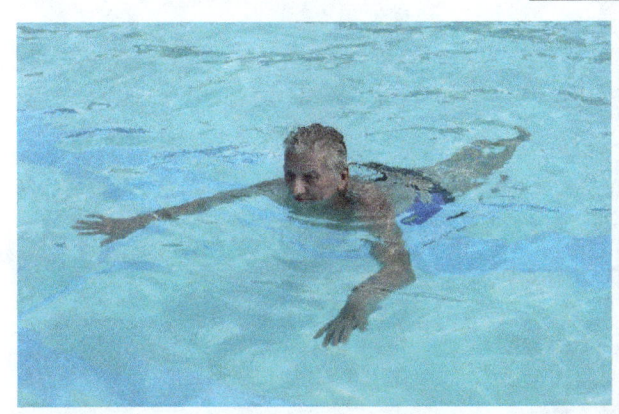

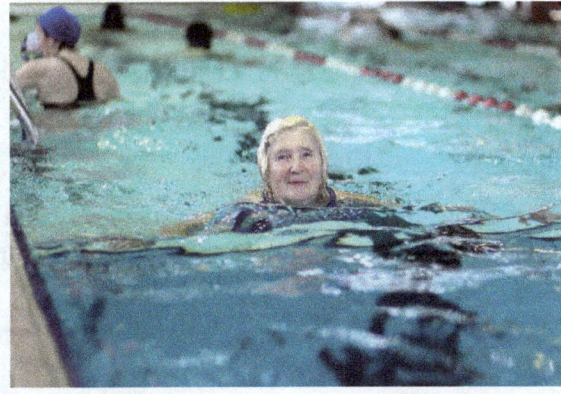

Appendix 9.1.1.1. Walking with Good Posture

Introduction

Walking is an excellent, low impact activity, for an older adult to engage in, especially if they are just beginning a regular and dedicated physical activity routine. Unfortunately, good walking posture and technique are not given much attention. Walking using a good posture nd technique can help:

- Keep bones and joints aligned properly
- Decrease wear and tear on joints, muscles, and ligaments
- Prevent back, hip, neck, and leg pain
- Reduce muscle aches and fatigue
- Reduce the risk of injuries
- Improve stability and balance

Walking with the right technique involves being mindful of how you move.

Tips for Walking Properly

Walking properly involves using the entire body so to walk correctly, it is necessary to focus on proper walking mechanics for each part of the body.

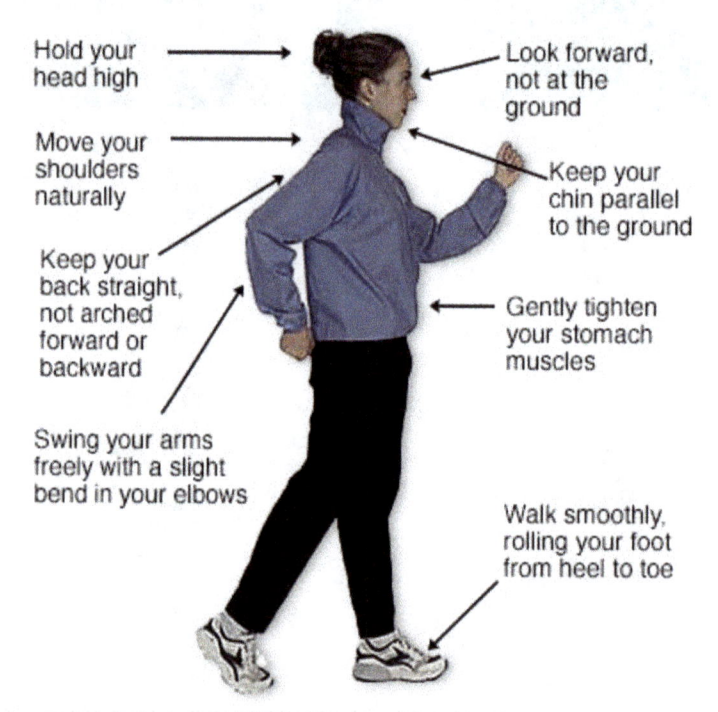

© MAYO FOUNDATION FOR MEDICAL EDUCATION AND RESEARCH. ALL RIGHTS RESERVED.

1. Head Position

Keep your head up and focus on standing tall with the chin parallel to the ground, and ears aligned above your shoulders. A good image to use is imagining your head being pulled up gently by an invisible piece of string that's attached to the ceiling. This image will help prevent your head from dropping onto your chest while you walk. Walking with your head up also improves your ability to breathe as you walk by opening up your airway. This is very important for any older adult who may have difficulty breathing from a pre-existing lung condition.

2. Eyes
The eyes and gaze should be looking forward, focusing on an area about 10–20 feet ahead, while walking. Avoid looking down at your feet or the sidewalk. As mentioned previously, a head down position compromises breathing as well as putting additional strain on your neck, and shoulders.

3. Lengthen Your Back (Tall Spine)
Stand tall and elongate the spine/posture while walking. Avoid slouching, hunching, or leaning forward, which puts unnecessary stress on your upper and lower back muscles.

4. Keep the Shoulders Down and Back (Shoulder Blades Coming Together)
The shoulders have a key role in proper walking posture and technique. If the shoulders are tense or hunched forward, it puts strain on the joints and muscles in the neck, upper back, and shoulders.

Do the following to ensure that the shoulders are correctly aligned while you're walking
- Raise the shoulders in a shrug-like motion, then let them fall and relax. Shoulder shrugs relieve tension, and help put the shoulders in a natural position, which allows the arms to move freely and easily.

It is important to have relaxed shoulders. They should not be held in a shrugged position toward the ears, or slouched forward, so the upper back is rounded. Doing occasional shoulder shrugs while walking helps keep the shoulders relaxed and in the right position.

5. Engage the core
Engage the core muscles by pulling the belly button in toward your spine. Engaging the core muscles when walking helps maintain stability and balance, and helps relieve stress and pressure on your lower back.

6. Swing the arms
Gently and freely, swing the arms back and forth at your sides as you walk. Swing the arms from the shoulders and not from the elbows.

Do not swing the arms across your body or swing them too high. Keep the height of the arm swing around the midsection and below the ribs and not as high as the chest.

7. Step from heel to toe
Walk by hitting the ground heel first, then rolling through your heel to your forefoot, and pushing off the big toe. Avoid walking flat-footed or striking the ground with the toes first.

What Not to Do While Walking

To prevent injury or physical stress on the muscles and joints, avoid the following habits:

Don't look down – Looking down at your feet or phone too frequently can put unnecessary strain on the neck and compromises breathing.

Don't take very long strides – The power in walking comes from pushing off the rear leg. Overstriding can put too much stress on the lower leg joints.

Don't roll the hips – The hips should stay as level as possible while walking. There should not be large vertical or horizontal oscillations.

Don't slouch – To avoid back and shoulder strain, keep the shoulders down and back (think of trying to squeeze your shoulder blades together) when walking or standing, and focus on keeping your spine elongated.

Don't walk in the wrong shoes – DON'T compromise on the quality of your shoes. It is important to wear shoes that fit comfortably, are well cushioned to absorb the shock of your feet hitting the ground. As well, they should have good arch and heel support.

Conclusion

Walking properly with good technique and posture helps reduce unnecessary stress and strain on the joints and muscles, prevent back pain, and reduces the risk of injuries in the feet, lower legs, knees and hips.

It is difficult to break old habits. Walking with the correct gait and posture may take some practice. This is especially true for the older adult who may have been walking improperly for years, or whose posture is already compromised, due to weak spinal and core musculature and arthritis.

To enjoy walking more, walk tall, keep the head up, shoulders relaxed and the core tight.

References

www.healthline.com

Stanton, John, (2009), *Walking: A Complete Guide to Walking for Fitness, Health and Weight Loss,* Penguin Canada.

Appendix 9.1.1.2: Developing Proper Running/Jogging Form

Introduction

Running/Jogging is a step-up on the intensity ladder vs. walking and, as a result, increases the chance of injury. Having a basic understanding of proper running/jogging form will help lessen injury.

Jogging is thought of as a slower pace running. When people say they are going for a run, they are actually going for a jog.

There is no "perfect" running/jogging form. Biomechanical studies of elite marathon runners clearly show that there is no one size fits all approach when it comes to running/jogging form. However, there are well-established dos and don'ts, concerning your running form that will make the running/jogging experience safer and more enjoyable.

For older adults, past injuries, arthritis, and engrained poor running/jogging technique will influence their ability to adapt and improve their running mechanics.

Running/Jogging Form

Below are a few suggestions for improving a person's running/jogging form to boost their running economy (less wasted energy), improve performance, and lower their risk for injury.

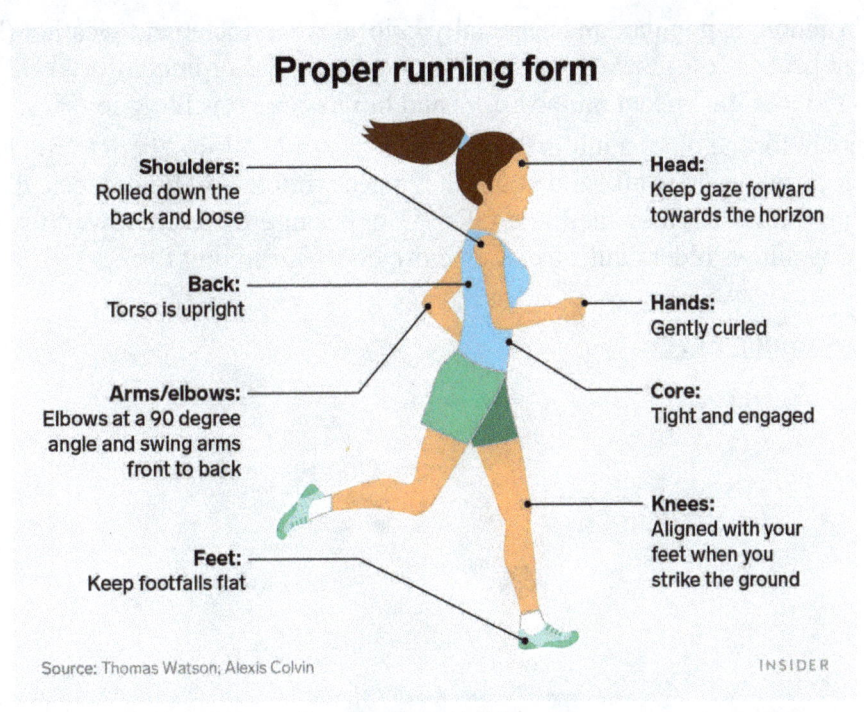

Image source: Insider.com

- Maintain a good upright posture with a slight forward tilt of the body.
- Engage the core (pull the belly button into the spine)
- Head up to a neutral position with the eyes focused forward approximately 10–15 feet.
- Avoid tilting the head up, down, or to one side
- Avoid rounding and slumping your shoulders.
- Widen the chest, and keep it lifted (run proud) as the shoulders are drawn down and back (think of squeezing the shoulder blades together).
- Keep the hands loose. Imagine holding a potato chip lightly between the thumb and middle finger.
- The arms need to be relaxed with the elbows bent approximately $90°$. The arms should be swinging effortlessly forward and backward to the height of the belly button. Avoid crossing the arms in front of the body.
- It is best to use a midfoot strike and avoid hitting the ground with your heel to prevent injuries to your lower body. The foot lands directly under the hips with a mid-foot strike as the body moves forward.
- Avoid long strides that encourage heel strike vs. mid foot strike. A heel strike causes the legs to slow during the stride and increases the stress on the knees.
- Visualize minimizing contact time on the ground. Visualize the feet just tapping the ground.
- Minimize vertical oscillation of the body to avoid wasting energy.
- Use relaxed deep breathing to avoid hyperventilating or creating stress in the shoulders.
- On toe off press up and forward from the ground.

Treadmill Running

Treadmill running is popular, and especially helpful when inclement weather (heavy snow, ice, rain, severe heat or cold) makes running outside dangerous or uncomfortable. Running on a treadmill also reduces the impact on the knees and hip joints, preventing injuries.

A great advantage for the older adult is that treadmill running allows them to run on a smooth surface vs. bumps in the sidewalk, and at a steady pace without any hindrances, distractions, or necessary sudden stops that may facilitate falls. Also, because there are fewer distractions, treadmill running allows older adults to focus more on their running form.

Treadmill Running Form:

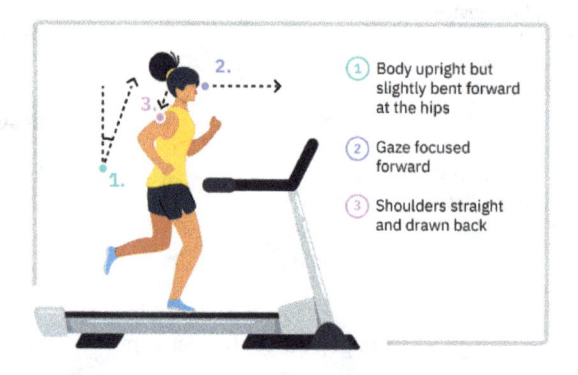

Image Source: treadmillreviews.net

- Shoulders are drawn back, and the core is engaged with a slightly forward body lean.
- The spine is straight, erect, and the shoulders are directly over the hips.
- Arms are relaxed, gaze straight ahead, and avoid looking down or at the monitor or the feet.
- Use short strides/small steps. Running on a treadmill will force a shorten stride since overstriding may cause a person to kick the front of the treadmill.
- Unless there are balance concerns, avoid hanging on to the treadmill's rails.

Your Feet

You run on your feet so you have to take care of them.

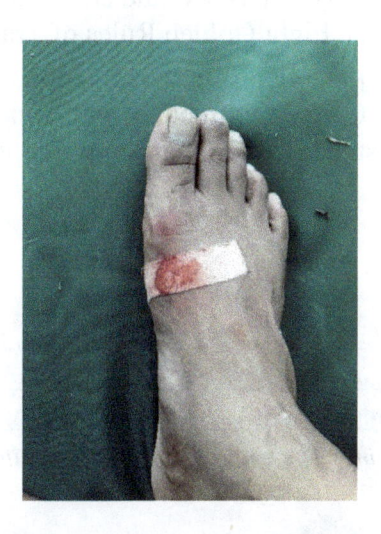

1. Shoes

Invest in good, proper-fitting running shoes. Buy shoes only from a professional running shoe retailer that can examine the feet and determine if they are fitted best with a neutral fitting shoe, or a shoe that will help with pronation, or supination of the feet.

It is a good idea for a person to bringing in their old running shoes so the sales person can see the wear pattern.

2. Socks

Invest in good, properly fitting socks. Cotton socks are recommended since they help reduce friction and help prevent blisters. Do not reuse dirty socks to avoid fungus infections (athletes' foot.)

3. Foot Care

Good management of the toenails will help prevent ingrown toenails, and the toenails irritating the other toes.

Conclusion

Running/jogging is a great and enjoyable way to improve your cardiovascular fitness. However, a person must do it safely. Improving running/jogging form and wearing good shoes and socks are the best ways to avoid injury and enjoy running. Good dynamic stretching before and static stretching afterwards helps with injury prevention too. Refer to Chapter 5.1.0: Flexibility, to learn about flexibility and Appendix 9.1.4.0 for appropriate flexibility exercises and stretching techniques.

It is very frustrating to injure yourself after starting a running/jogging program. Consistency and sustainability are important to see the best results and avoid injury. The body will adapt to the stress of running/jogging, if you start low and slow, and do it consistently over a sustained period of time (Chapter3.1: The Eight Golden Rules of Training).

Being aware of your running/jogging posture, use a good mid-foot strike, and having a strong, engaged core (Chapter 4.2.2: Core Strengthening and Appendix 9.1.2.1.1: Core Strengthening Exercises Described and Illustrated) will enhance your running/jogging activity.

References

www.healthline.com/health/exercise-fitness/proper-running-form
www.newsnetwork.mayoclinic.org/discussion/tuesday-tips-6-ways-to-check-your-running-technique
www.runnersworld.com/beginner/a20811257/proper-running-form-0

Stanton, John, (2010), *Running: The Complete Guide to Building Your Running program*. Penguin Canada

Appendix 9.1.1.3. Cycling Safely: Good Sizing, Good Posture, Follow Safety Guidelines

Introduction

Cycling is a great cardiovascular alternative to walking and running for older adults. Its most significant advantage is that it is a non-impact activity on the knee and hip joints. The disadvantages are the need to purchase a bike and the increased need for good agility, balance, and coordination to ride safely, compared to walking and running. Because of the physical demands for agility, balance, and coordination, having a bike that fits properly is paramount.

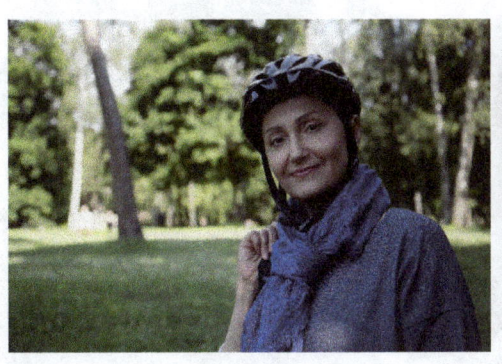

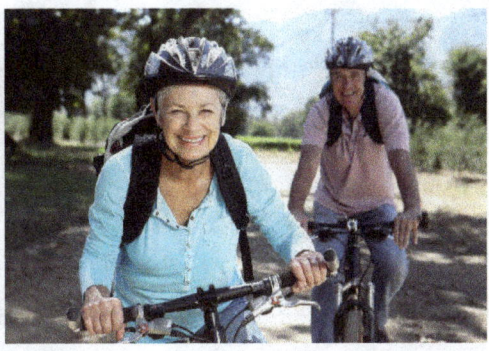

Proper Bike Sizing

Hybrid and Fitness Bike Sizing Chart

Rider Height		**Suggested Frame Size**		
Feet and Inches	**Centimeters**	**Size**	**Inches**	**Centimeters**
4' 10" – 5' 1"	147 – 155	XS	13 – 14	47 – 49
5' 1" – 5' 5"	155 – 165	S	15 – 16	50 – 52
5' 5" – 5' 9"	165 – 175	M	17 – 18	53 – 54
5' 9" – 6' 0"	175 – 183	L	19 – 20	55 – 57
6' 0" – 6' 3"	183 – 191	XL	21 – 22	58 – 61
6' 3" – 6' 6"	191 – 198	XXL	23 – 25	61 – 63

Proper Bike Posture

Whether an individual is riding a road bike (pictures below), mountain/gravel bike, or recreational bike, the riding posture is the same.

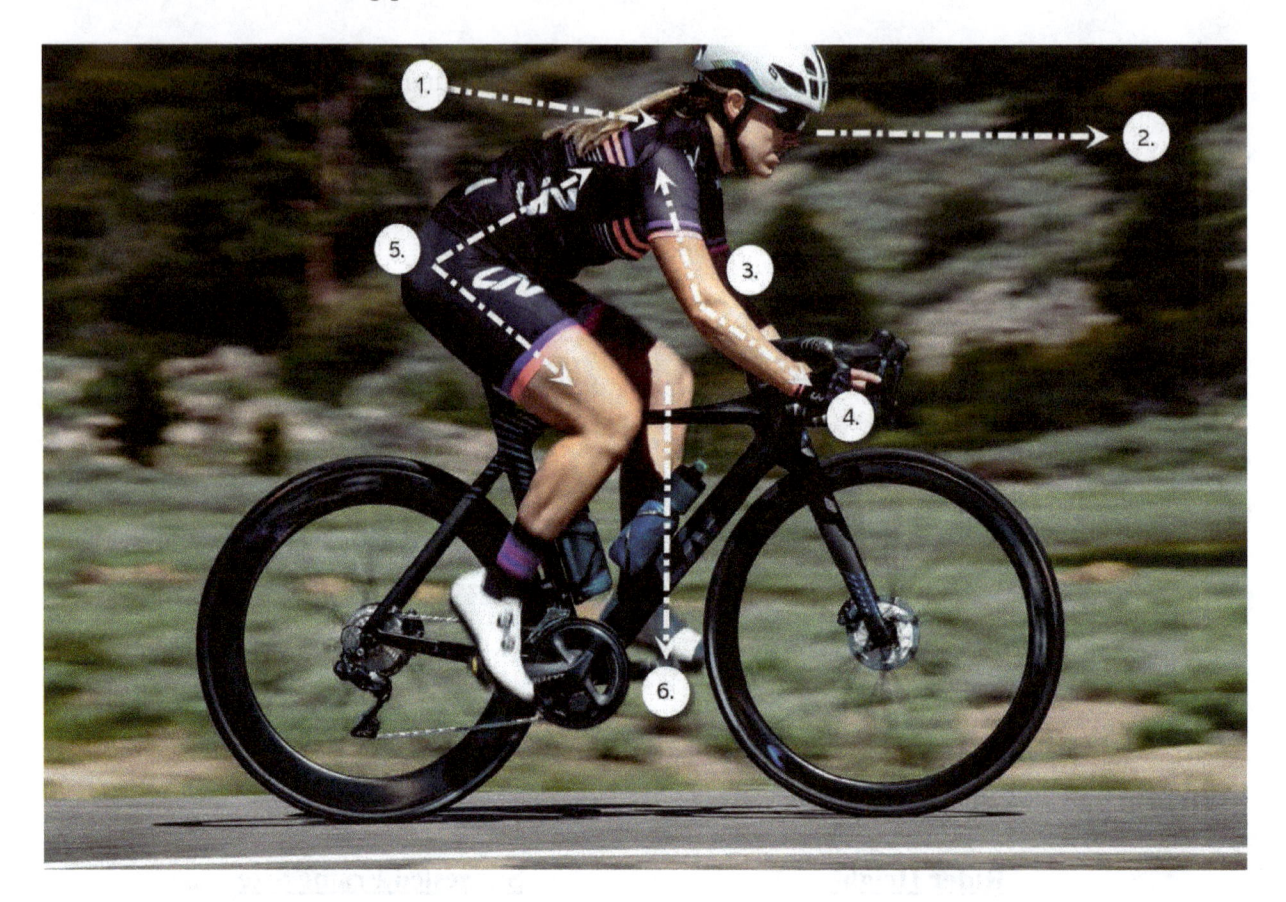

Saddle Height – the knees should be 25–30 % bent on extension (foot at the lowest position when pedaling)

Sitting – the sit bones in the buttocks are the point of contact on the seat.

1. Relax The shoulders – The shoulders should be dropped and away from the ears. If pushing hard to climb a hill, be aware that the shoulders may begin to stiffen and start to creep up again.

2. Free Up Your Head – Lowering the shoulders away from the ears will help with this. If the neck is loose, it makes it easier to turn and look for traffic.

3. Bend Your Elbows – Riding with relaxed, bent elbows allows the arms to act as shock absorbers. The arms can help absorb impact from hitting a pothole or bump in the road. The elbows should be tucked into the sides of the body near the ribs instead of spreading wide.

Having the elbows bent will also reduce strain on your shoulders and allow riding with less pressure on the hands.

4. A Straight Line Should Be Maintained from The Elbow Through to The Fingers – There should be no significant extension (hands bent upwards) in the wrists on the handlebars. If this position is difficult to achieve, a modification in the bike setup might be necessary.

5. Maintain A Neutral Spine – The back should be relaxed, keeping a reasonably straight line between the hips and shoulders.

6. Knee Tracks Over the Ball of The Foot/Pedal – If the knees points out to the sides when riding, it may look a little funny, but more significantly, it could cause inefficiency and pain in the knee.

Safety Tips

1. Helmet – Always wear a properly fitted helmet.

HELMET SIZING GUIDE

EYES — Only TWO fingers should fit in the space between your eyebrows & the bottom of your helmet

EARS — Line your TWO fingers up with the straps; the V of your fingers should be right at your earlobe

CHIN — Hook TWO fingers between your chin. There should be no extra space

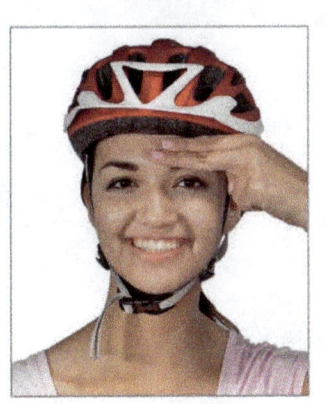

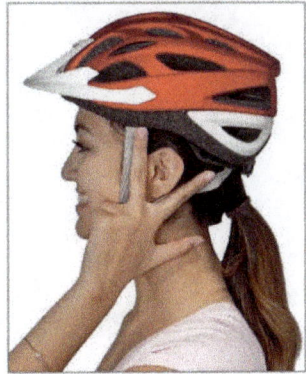

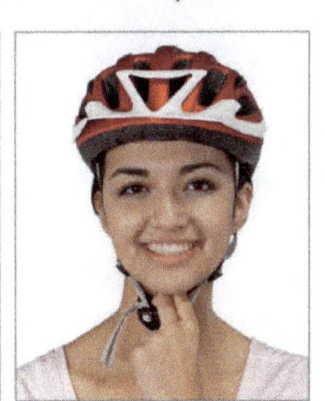

Image source: it-recruitment-house.blogspot.com

2. Front Brake Is Your Friend – Don't be afraid to use the front brakes in conjunction with back brakes.

3. Braking Hard – The more forcefully there is a need to brake, the farther a person needs to move the body back (move your buttocks backwards) and stay low (lower your center of gravity.)

4. DON'T Break in Corners – Feather the brakes if there is a need to brake in corners.

5. Road Surfaces – Know or anticipate the road surfaces. Be aware of how rough the roads are (potholes) and how much grip the tires will have (gravel vs. asphalt vs. cement.)

6. Ride at Comfort Level – Whether a person is riding in a group or alone, they should never ride faster or on routes (busy streets, steep declines) or rough terrain (trails) that makes them feel uncomfortable.

Conclusion

Cycling is a popular and great way for older adults to get good cardiovascular exercise. To cycle safely, it is essential that an individual has a properly fitting bike, utilizes good posture habits, and never exceeds their riding capabilities.

References

www.bicycling.com/training/a20027599/how-to-start-cycling
www.lifebestbrand.com/proper-riding-posture
www.liv-cycling.com/global/camapigns/peoper-body-position-on-a-road-bike/20716

Appendix 9.1.1.4. Swimming: Knowing How Makes It Easier and More Enjoyable

Introduction

Swimming is another excellent cardiovascular exercise but is not as popular as walking, running, and cycling. Three major reasons for this are; that not everyone has convenient access to a pool or open water to swim, fear of the water, and swimming is more physically demanding than walking and running. As well, most people grew up walking, running, and biking but not swimming. Swimming is a much more technical activity than walking, running, and cycling, and for someone who did not learn to swim well as a child, swimming can be challenging to learn as a person gets older.

However, swimming has excellent health benefits. Swimming is a great cardiovascular activity. When a person swims, they use almost all the muscles in the body. The more muscles used and the larger the muscles used during an activity, the more forcefully the heart has to work to deliver blood to all the working muscles. Swimming requires both upper and lower body muscles, whereas walking and running are primarily lower body activities. Also, swimming is a non-weight bearing activity, so it is less stressful on the hips, knees, and ankles than walking and running.

Swimming Technique

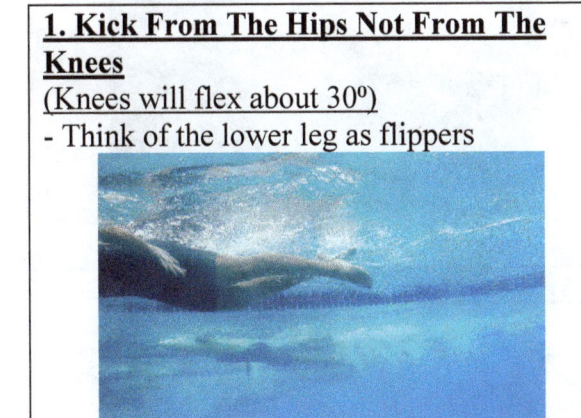

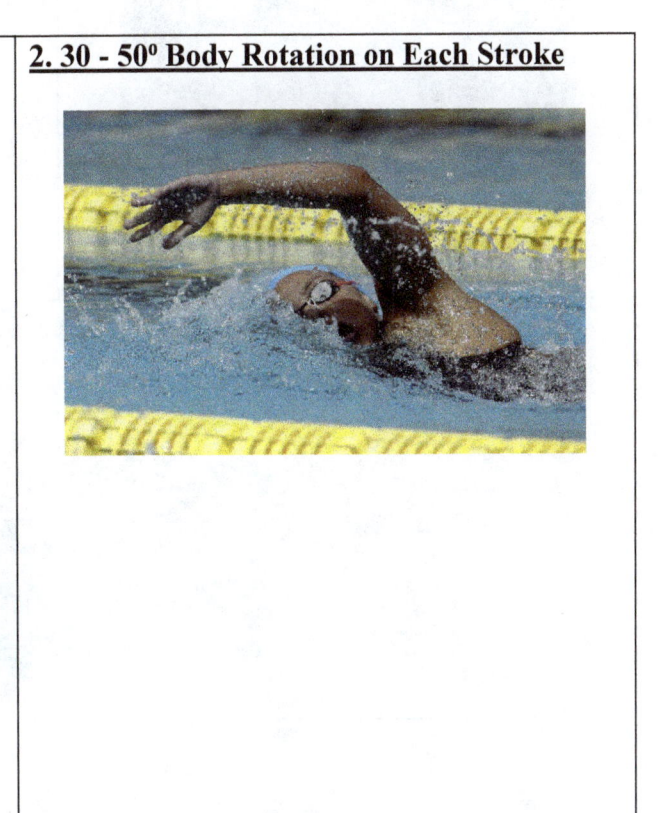

1. Kick From The Hips Not From The Knees (Knees will flex about 30º) - Think of the lower leg as flippers	**2. 30 - 50º Body Rotation on Each Stroke**

3. Fingers Spear the Water on Entry (One Hand is Always In Front Of Head- DON'T Over Extend The Entry)	**4. Underwater Hand Extension** - The hand and arm are extended forward underwater and is driven by the body rotation
5. Fingertips Below Wrist and Wrist Is Below Elbow. Arm In-Line with Shoulder	**6. Catch (arms move backwards) – Initiates the Stroke by slight Bending Of The Elbow And Starting To Press The Water Backwards** - The "Catch" - starts with dipping of the wrist - The "Pull" – Accelerates under the head and body and produces most of the stroke power

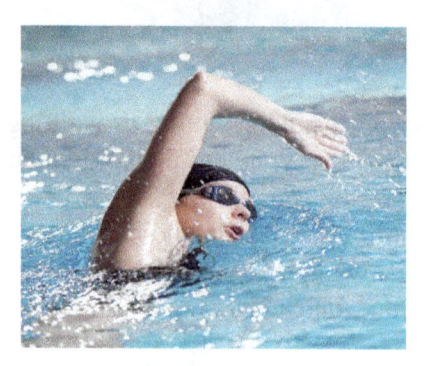

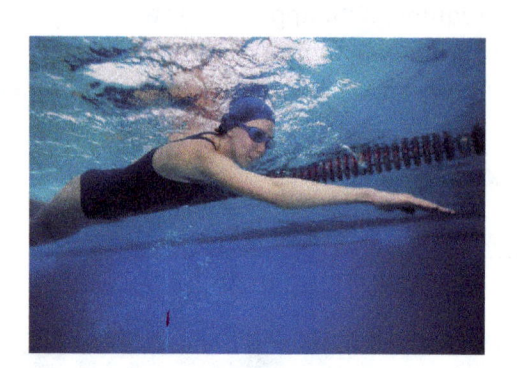

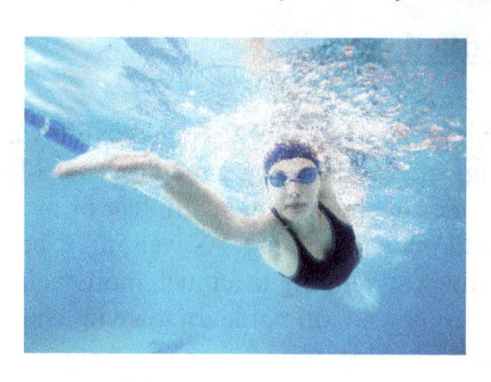

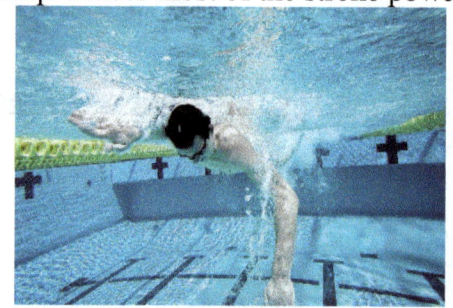

7. Classic High Elbow with Arm Out Of the Water

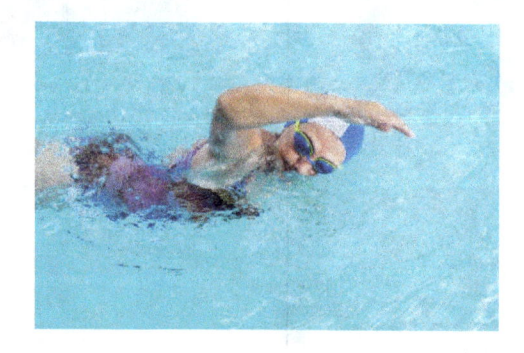

Summary of Swim Technique

Key Point – One hand is always in the front quadrant (in front of the head).

Terminology:
- **Catch (Pull) Hand** – Front arm and hand pull back from in front of the head to the hips.
- **Recovery hand** – Back arm and hand exit the water at hips and move toward the front of the head.
- **Entry Hand** – Hand enters the water in front of the head.

Key Technical Swimming Points
1. Start "catch" with bending of the wrist as "pull hand" leaves the water
2. Hands pass each other in front of the head
3. Recovery hand enters the water as the catch/pull arm is under the shoulders
4. As the "entry hand" extends out and down due to body rotation (body rotates back and forth 30 -50°);
    The "pull hand" continues pulling back to the hip with the
    Pull hand medially rotated and the thumb brushes against the hip
5. Hold this "Glide" position until recovery hand is at head level and the extended arm begins the "catch"
    - Think long and lean as you glide – stretch between the pelvis and rib cage. (Swim as if you are in a cylinder)
6. Keep legs together (Kick comes from the hips, knees stay relatively straight (Quadriceps stay contracted)
7. Don't lift head too far out of the water to breathe when you rotate
8. Don't forget to breathe out (you are either inhaling or exhaling all the time)
9. Stay relaxed

Conclusion

Swimming is great fun and a great cardiovascular and musculature endurance exercise if you can sustain your strokes for 5, 10, 15, 20 minutes, or longer. Once you understand how to swim (swim mechanics), all it takes is practice to perfect your stroke and get stronger in the water.

Stay Relaxed and Enjoy

Reference

Newsome, Paul. Young, Adam. (2012), *Swim Smooth: The Complete coaching Program for Swimmers and Triathletes*, Fernhurst Books.

Laughlin, Terry. (2004). *Total Immersion: the Revolutionary Way to Swim Better, Faster, and Easier*. Simon and Schuster

Appendix 9.1.2.0. Introduction to the Muscular Strengthening/Resistance Exercises

Muscular strength/resistance exercises are vitally important to older adults because of age-related muscle loss (Sarcopenia). After age 25, this muscle loss averages .5 to 1%/year, and the rate accelerates after the age of 65. Only by keeping the muscles active and safely applying the overload principle (applying more resistance to the muscle than it is used to) can the older adult slow muscle loss.

The following chapters will describe and illustrate how to perform core, whole-body, and bodyweight resistance strengthening exercises safely and effectively. The instructions need to be followed precisely to avoid tendon, ligament, and muscle injury.

Remember to follow the golden rule of progressing slowly. Increase resistance and repetitions only after your body and mind have adapted to the stress applied. As well, be as consistent as possible in doing your muscle resistance routine. Being consistence and sustainability provides the best results.

Muscle resistance exercises need to be an essential part of you daily and weekly routine. Your quality of life depends on it.

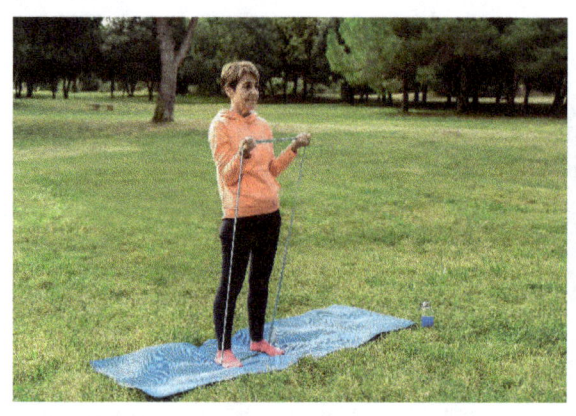

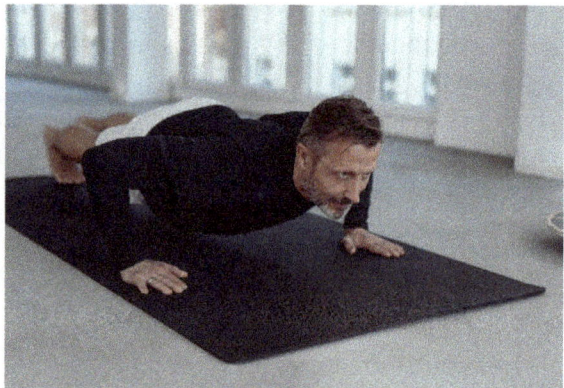

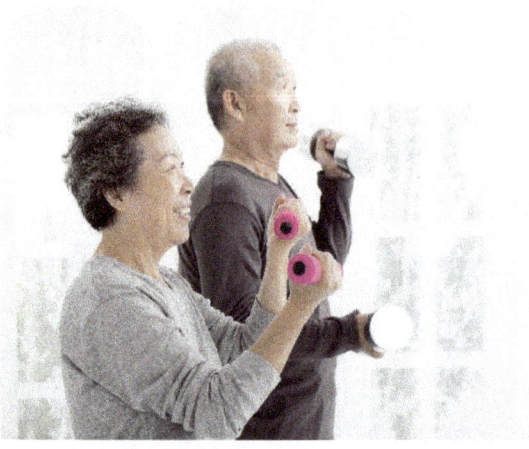

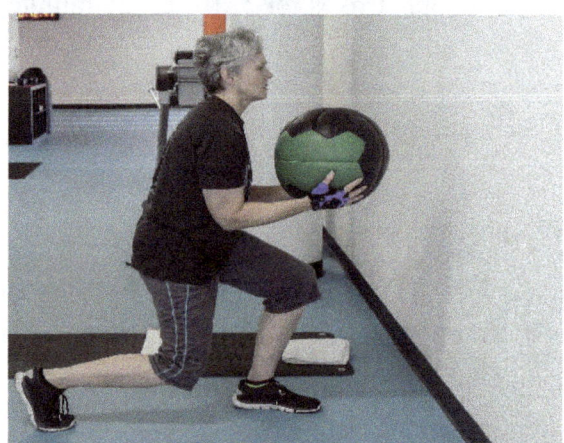

Appendix 9.1.2.1.0. Introduction to Core Strengthening Exercises

Identifying "The Core", its functional importance, and what exercises are best to help condition and strengthen the core has been confusing and often misleading. "The Core" is basically the front and back torso. Specifically, these muscles include;

Front and Sides:
- Erectus abdominis (what you think of when you think "abs")
- Transverse abdominis (the deepest internal core muscle that wraps around your sides and spine)
- The internal and external oblique (the muscles on the sides of your abdomen)

Back and Hips:
- Erector spinae (a set of muscles in your lower back)
- Gluteal muscles (hip musculature)

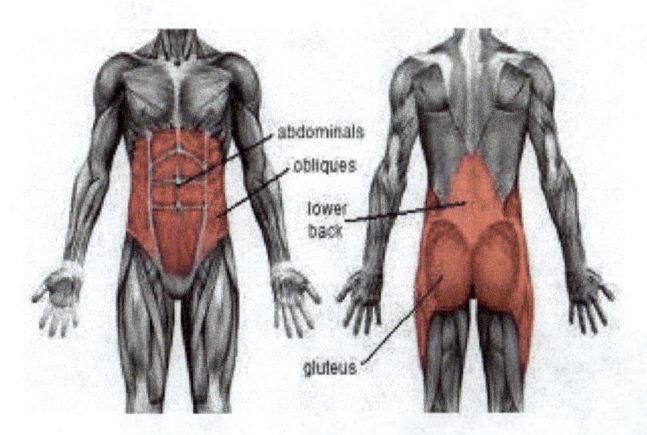

Image source: setforset.com

"The Core" is very important to the older adult in maintaining good posture and helping stabilize the spine during functional movement such as walking, bending, twisting, reaching, and lifting.

To perform core exercises safely, follow the description and illustrations in Appendix 9.1.2.1.1.

Any exercise that involves stabilizing the trunk and maintaining good posture (abdominal bracing) will engage the core muscular and helps condition these muscles, even if the primary purpose of that specific exercise is to target another specific muscle group such as the biceps when doing bicep curls.

Having a well-conditioned core is important to help prevent lower back injuries and maintaining good functional capacity and high quality of life.

Appendix 9.1.2.1.1. Core Strengthening Exercises Described and Illustrated

Key Points;

1. **Abdominal Bracing** – Basic technique used during core exercise training.
   – Pull the navel into the spine
2. **NEVER** hold your breath
3. **Go Slow** – The slower an exercise is done and the longer each repetition is held the more effective and beneficial will be the exercise.

1. Isolate Lower Abdominal Muscles (Hip flexors will be engaged as well):	
1. Flutter Kicks 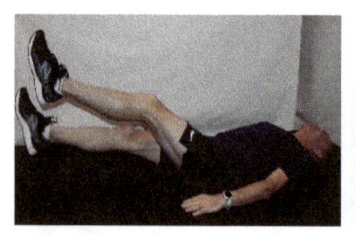 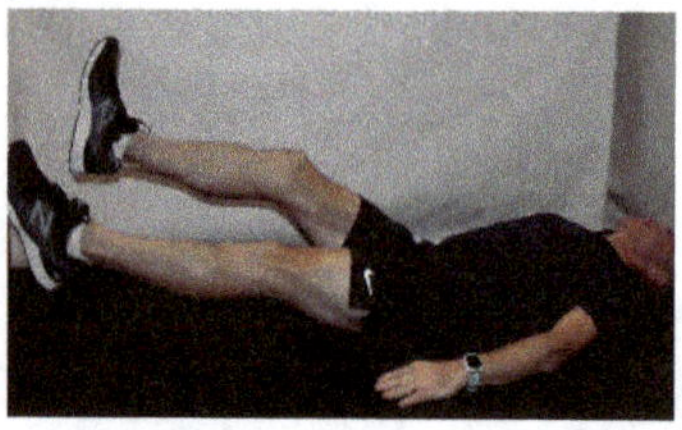	Supine - hands under bum and head and shoulders up looking. - Keep knees straight and lift feet off the mat one foot. - flutter kick - alternatively and repetitively move your legs up and down 1 to 2 feet, at a moderate pace
2. Pilates 100's **Start** 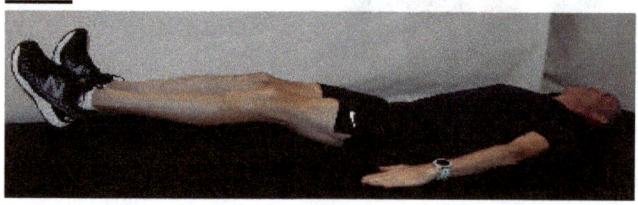 **Hands Tapping** 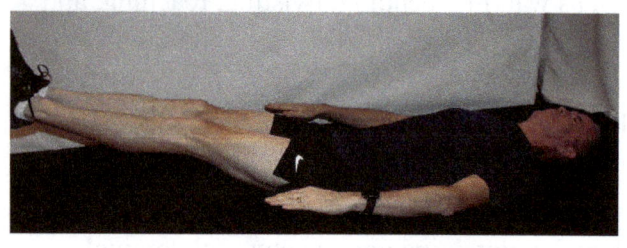	Supine - hands besides buttocks and lift both feet 30º - 60º off floor one foot and they stay still. - Tap your hands on the mat 100 times Advanced - with the feet elevated they do a small flutter kick (feet move up and down 1 to 2 feet) to 100 as your hands tap the mat.

3. Straight Leg Raise to 90º **Legs alone** **Small Ball between Ankles** 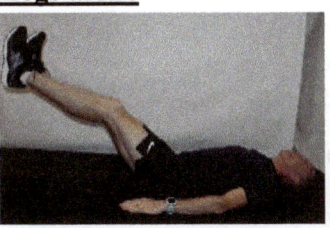 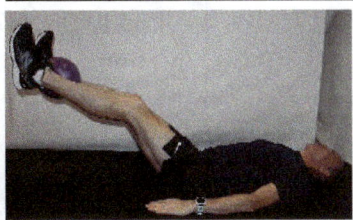 **Stability Ball between ankles** 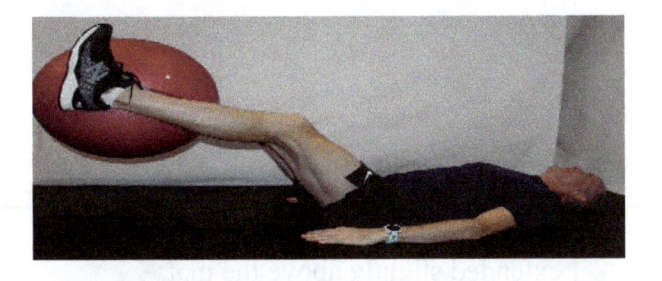	Supine - Lift legs up as high as possible but no more than to 90º and then lower to just above the mat. (Keep the knees as straight as possible) Advanced Perform with small ball or stability ball between ankles
4. Scissors 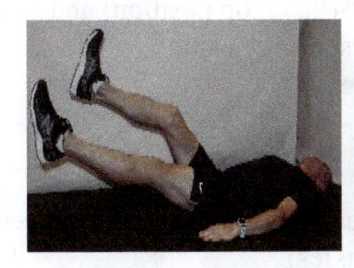 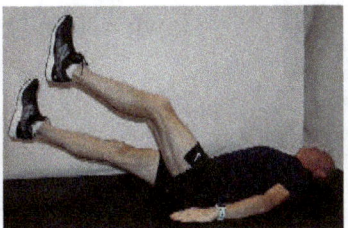	Supine - shoulders and head supported on mat - start with legs slightly off floor and <u>alternately</u> raise legs to 90º trying to keep legs as straight as possible. - to protect the lower back, you can lift shoulders and neck slightly off matt (to help keep the neck in neutral position you can support the neck with your hands.)
5. Pendulum - Vertical Straight legs rotate to each side 90º **Rotate to Left** **Rotate to Right** 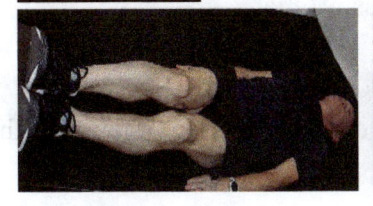 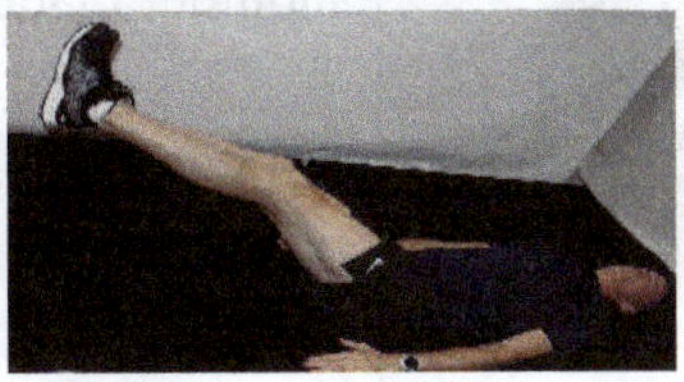	Supine – legs straight and elevated as high as possible but not greater than 90º - Keeping knees straight rotate legs to one side and then to the other in a pendulum like motion. Advanced - small ball or stability ball between ankles

6. Heel Taps 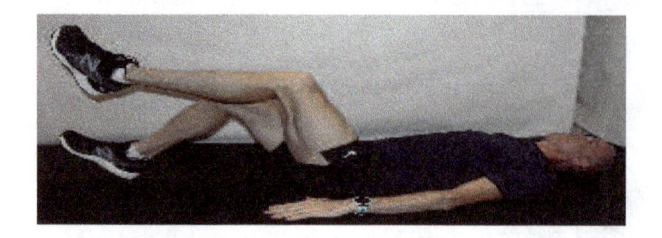 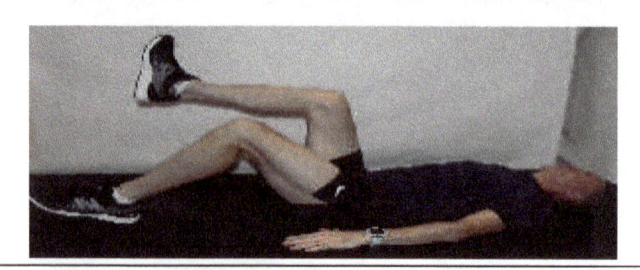	<u>Supine</u> - hips and knees bent 90º - Slowly lower one bent knee so heel touches the floor. - Then repeat with opposite leg.
7. Supine Reverse Crunch 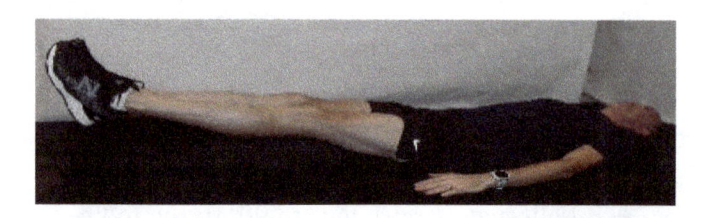 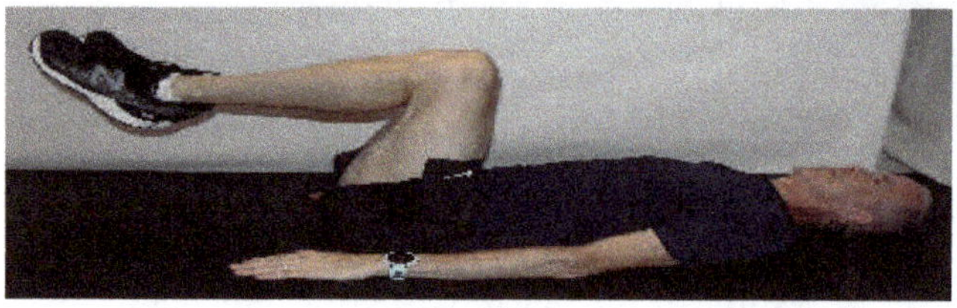	<u>Supine</u> - lying on your back with legs extended slightly above the mat. - Slowly bend hips and raise knees toward chest to 90º-100º (table top position) and slowly return to starting position. <u>Advanced</u> - put a stability ball or medicine ball between legs (knees or ankles)
8. Bicycles 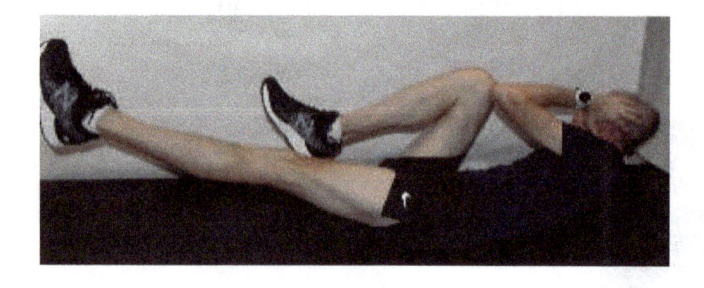	<u>Supine</u> - legs extended and off the mat a foot. - Hands behind head for support and shoulder blades off mat. - Simultaneously bend one knee to 90º and raise opposite elbow and attempt to touch the bent knee. - Return to starting position and repeat with opposite knee and elbow.

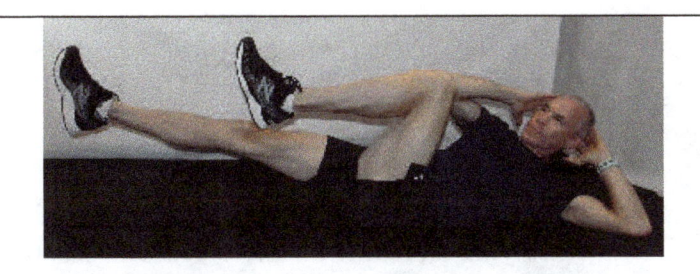

9. Prone Stability Ball (SB) Reverse Crunch

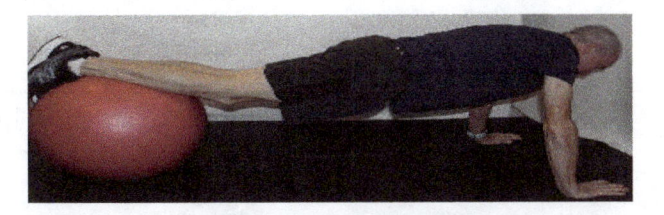

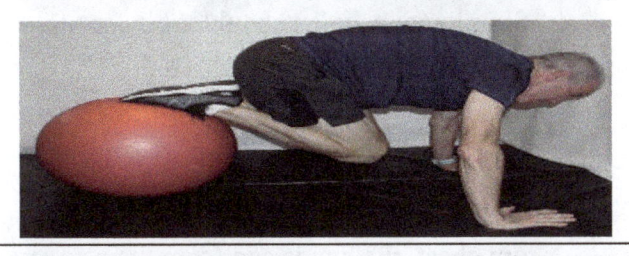

Prone on SB - top of feet on SB and body in plank position with hands or forearms on mat.

- Bend knees to bring SB toward your chest and then return to starting position

2. Crunch/Sit-Ups (Trying to Isolate Rectus Abdominis and Abdominal Oblique):

1. Crunches:

1. Abdominal Crunch

Straight Crunch

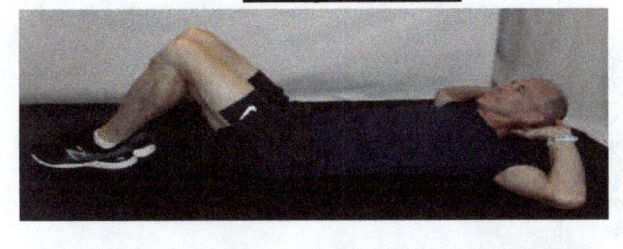

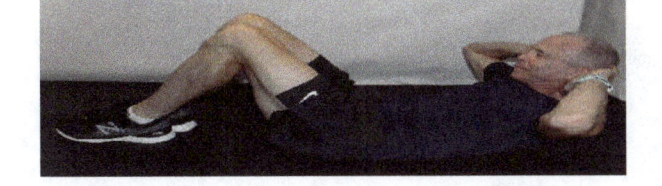

Supine - knees bent, feet on the mat and arms extended in front of chest or behind head for support

- Keep neck in neutral position and lift head and shoulder blades straight up off floor as a unit.

One Leg in Air 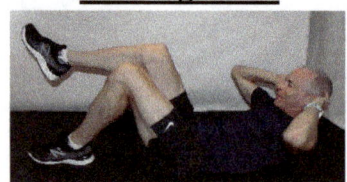 **Feet on Stability Ball** 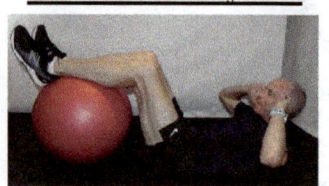	Modifications: 1. Lying on mat with knees bent and feet on mat but one leg lifted off ground 45° 2. Lying on mat with, knees bent and feet on SB, hips at 90° 3. Lift one leg into the air as you crunch, then lift alternate the opposite leg).
2. Supine Double Crunch 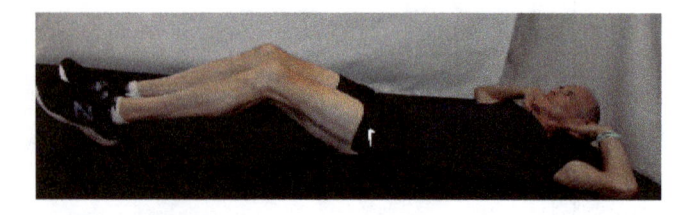 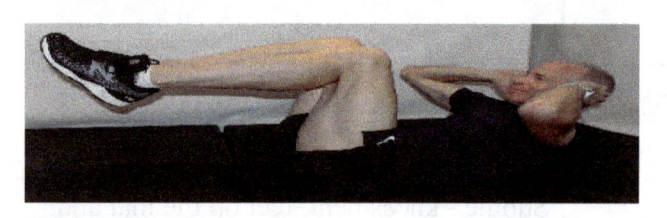	Supine - hands at ear level or extended out in front of chest. - Simultaneously lift shoulder blades off ground and bent knees into chest. (If hands start at ear level attempt to have the elbows touch knees as they approach the chest. If the hands and arms are extended out from chest, the hands can wrap themselves around the knees as they approach the chest to ensure a good crunch.)
3. Supine Oblique Crunch 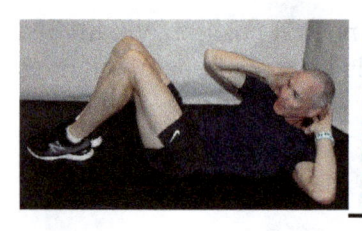 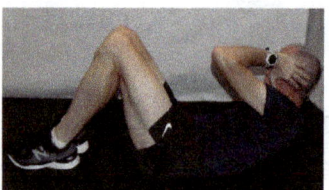 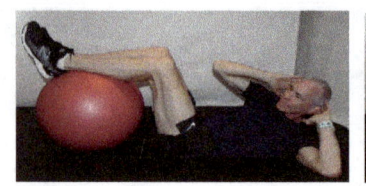	Supine – feet on the mat, knees bent, arms extended in front of chest or behind head. - Lift head and shoulder blades off floor at an angle toward one knee, return to start position and repeat to the other knee. Modifications: 1. Lower legs on SB 2. Legs cross in fig 4 position (oblique crunch all done to one side and then to the other)

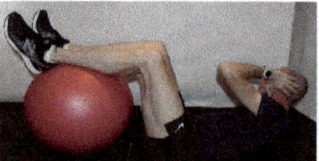

4. ½ Lateral Oblique Crunch 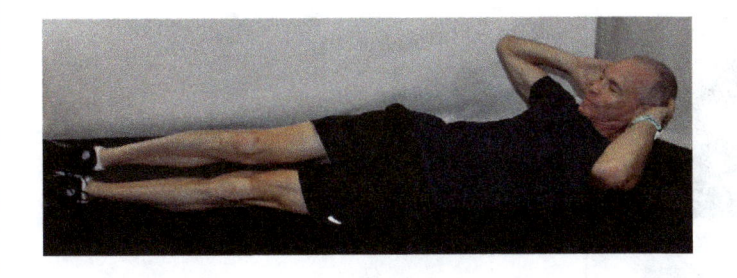	Sit obliquely (1/2 way between the bottom of your buttocks and the outside side of your hip) on your hip - Hands behind head for support and legs flat on ground. - Lift bottom shoulder blade off floor straight up toward top leg.
5. Lateral Crunch on BOSU 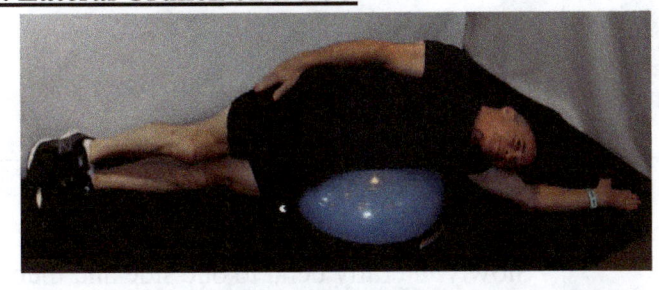 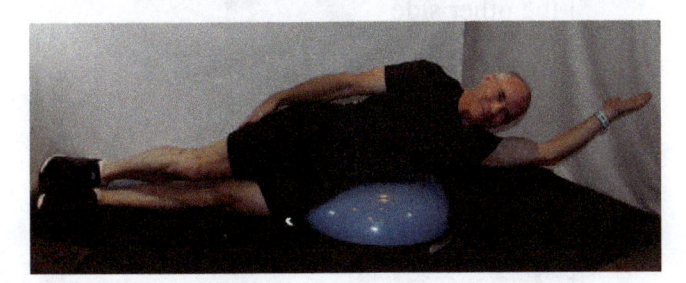	Lying on your side with the BOSU between the lower ribs and top of hips. - Bottom arm extended along the floor and top arm extended along the side of the body. - Lift trunk and bottom arm off floor as high as possible and then lower to just above mat level and repeat. Try not to touch the floor when lowering arm Notes: 1. Avoid the hips rotating backwards. The body needs to be vertical on the BOSU. 2. The higher the hips are on the BOSU the harder the exercise (more unstable) Advanced Put weight in the hand of the extended arm

6. Twisting Lateral Plank Crunch 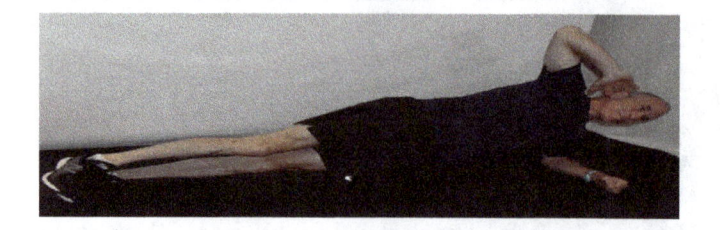 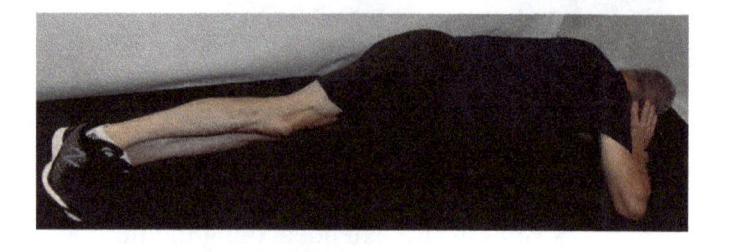	Lateral plank position (on hand or forearm) - Top hand at ear level - Bring elbow down to floor by twisting the torso toward the floor.
7. Standing Lateral Crunch 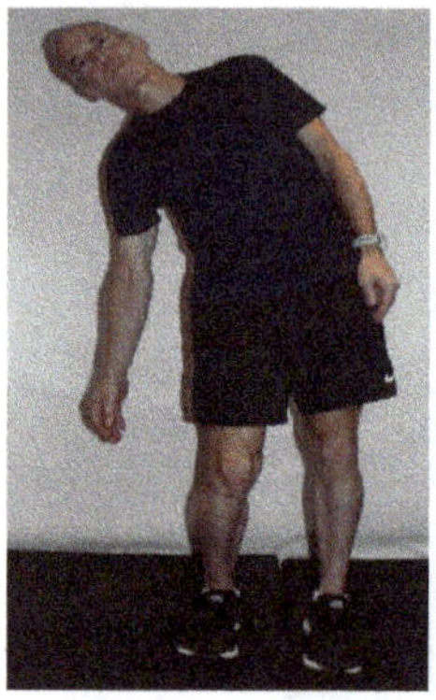 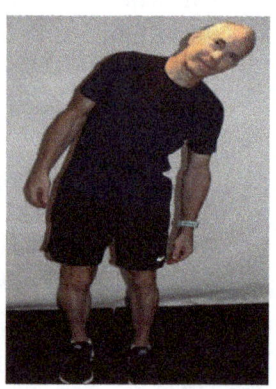 **Elbow to Knee Lateral Crunch** 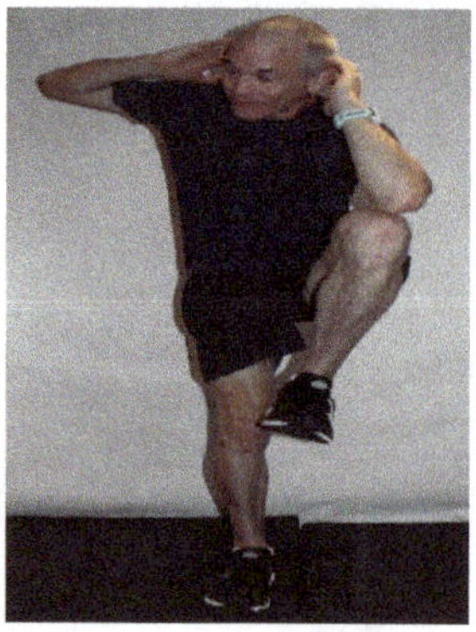	Stand erect - Slowly laterally bend to one side and then the other side Advanced; 1. Hand weights in the hands 2. Hands behind head and raise one knee as laterally bend to the side and have the elbow touch the raised knee at around hip level.

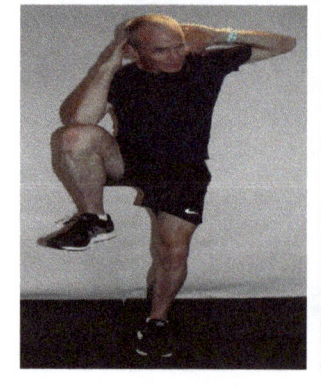

2. Sit-Ups:

1. Full Sit-Ups **Anchor Feet - Full Sit-up** 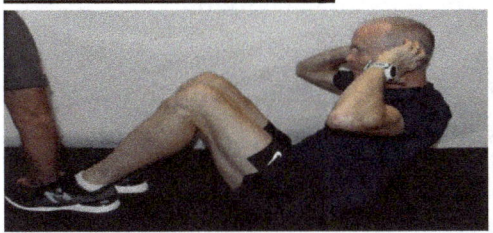 **No Anchor Full Sit-up** 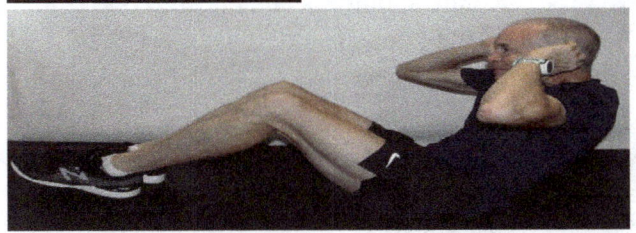	<u>Supine</u> - Hands in front of chest or behind neck, knees bent and feet anchored under something or held and come up vertically so lower back is completely off the floor <u>Modifications:</u> 1. Try with no anchor of feet or feet in butterfly position (soles of feet together and knees wide apart) 2. Raise one foot off the floor as you do the full sit-up
2. Vertical Toe Touches 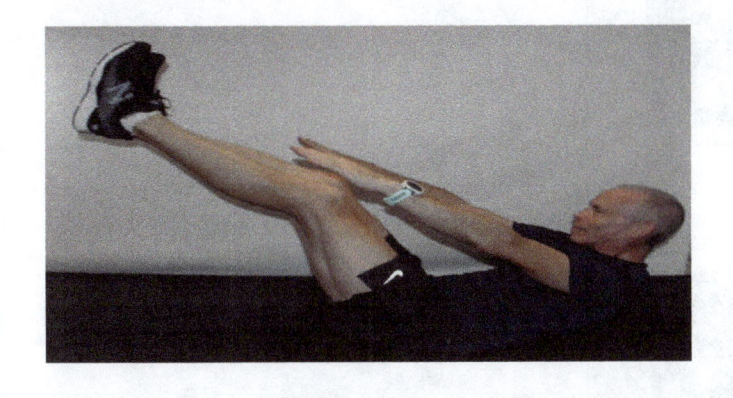	<u>Supine</u> - hips bent 60 - 90° so legs are in the air. The knees can be slightly bent. Hands are extended in front of chest. - Come up straight with hands and attempt to touch the toes.
3. V Sit-Ups 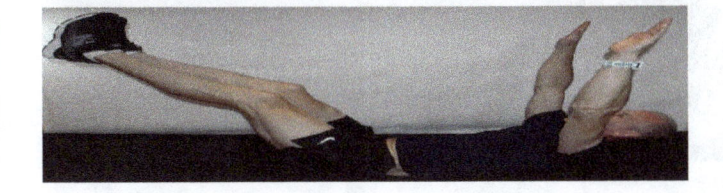	<u>Supine</u> - arms extended over your head and flat on the floor. The legs are extended. - Simultaneously, lift your arms, chest and legs into the air as high as possible as if you are forming a "V" <u>Modification</u> - only lift one leg up on each crunch

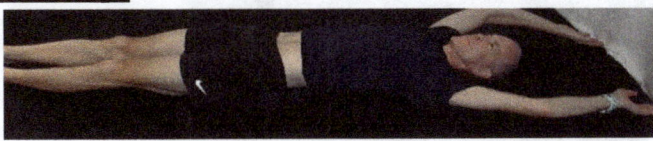

4. Jack Knife	Supine - arms extended over the head and flat on floor.
	- Lift one arm, chest and opposite leg up and attempt to touch hand to foot.
	- Lower to starting position and repeat same side or alternate sides

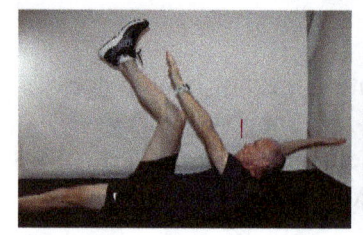

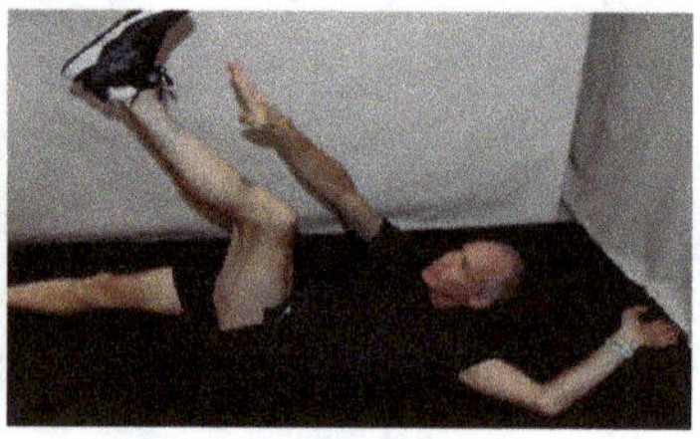

3. Twisting exercises to isolate the abdominal oblique:

1. Russian Twist	Sitting on mat or BOSU with feet on or off (advanced) the ground
	- Rotate shoulders and chest to one side and then the opposite side.
	Note - keep hands tight in front of the chest (small rotations of shoulders) or extended in front of the chest so can swing the arms to touch the floor behind you (big rotation of shoulders)
Medicine Ball (MB) Russian Twist	Advanced
	1. Hold medicine ball (MB)tight in front of chest and do small shoulder rotations.
	2. Hold MB with arms extended in front of chest and as you rotate the shoulders swing MB to touch mat behind. (Big rotation of shoulders)

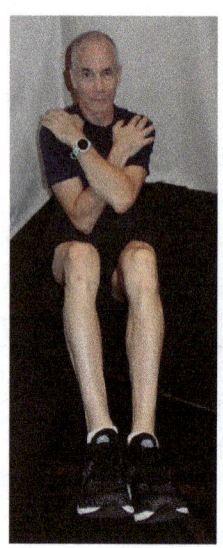

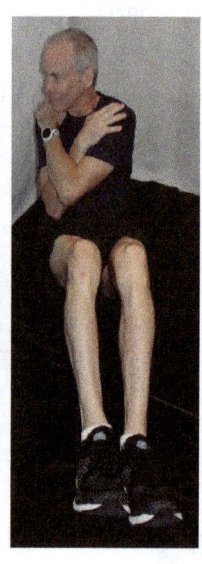

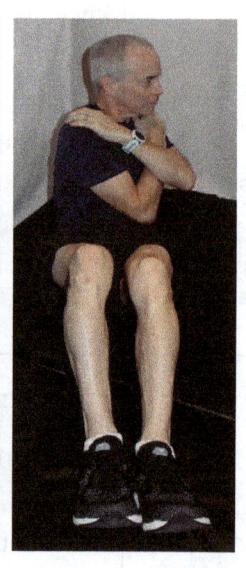

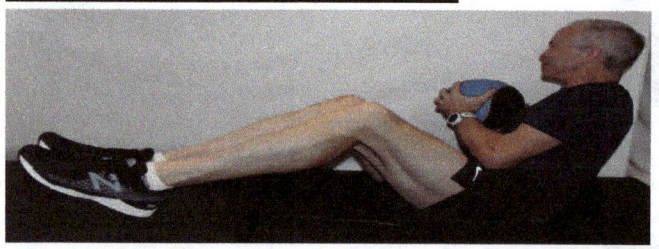

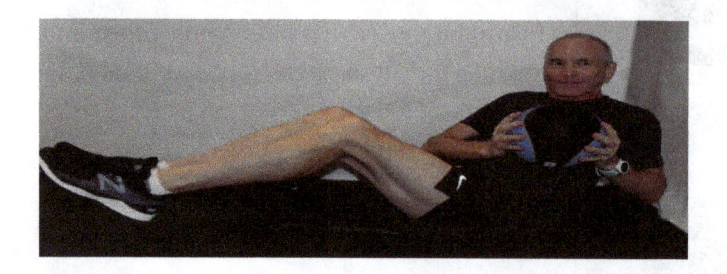

2. Woodchopper

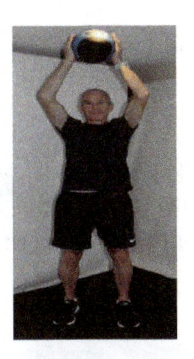

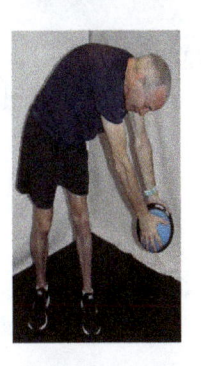

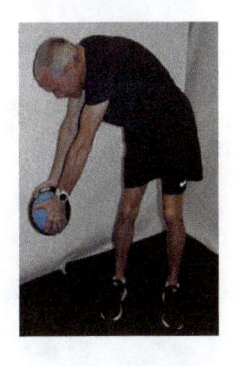

Standing or kneeling

- Start with arms extended above the head and hips and shoulders slightly twisted to one side.

- Uncoil the hips and shoulders and bring the hands down diagonally toward the floor outside the opposite foot (if standing) or knee (if kneeling.)

- Your knees may bend slightly so the hands finish about 1 foot above the mat.

- Return to starting position and repeat

Advanced:
- Hold a medicine ball for resistance.

3. Cross Body Twist (Standing Russian Twist)

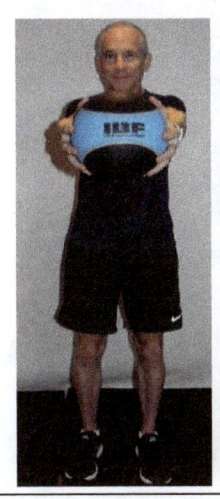

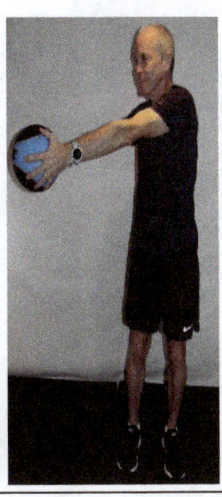

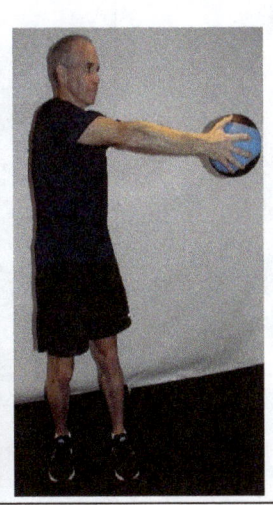

Standing or kneeling

- Start with shoulders and hips rotated to one side and arms extended in front of the chest.

- Uncoil and twist so the hips and shoulder are now facing the opposite direction.

- Repeat by twisting back to starting position.

Advanced
- hold medicine ball for resistance.

4. Pendulum

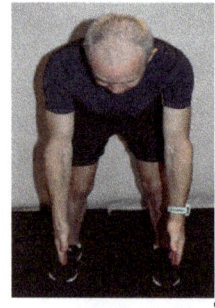

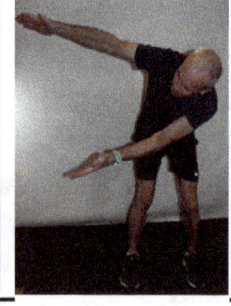

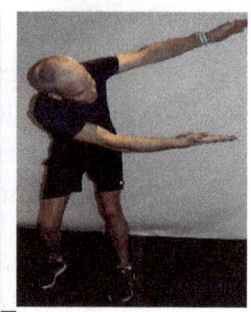

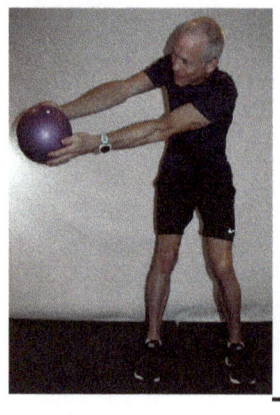

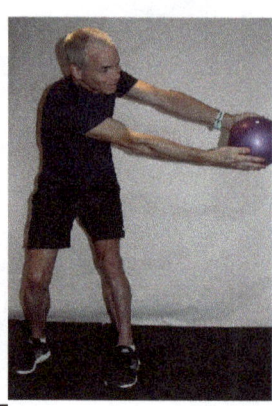

Start in standing semi squat position

- Bend forward at the hips 45° and with arms extended down between your knees.

- Diagonally twist shoulders and arms to one side up to shoulder height or higher if able. Repeat motion to opposite side.

Advanced
 - hold medicine ball for resistance

4. Planks and Variations (Isolates Arms-Biceps, Triceps, Shoulders-Deltoids, Chest - Pectorals Major, Core, Hips - Gluts And Hip Flexors, Legs - Quadriceps, Hamstrings)

1. Standard Planks **Low Plank (On Forearms)** 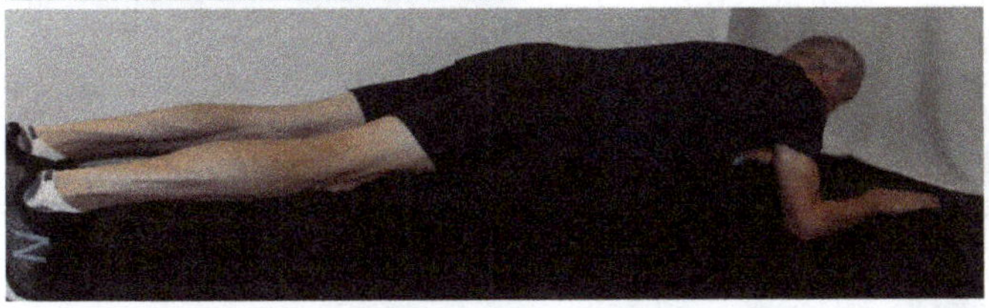 **High Plank (On Hands)** 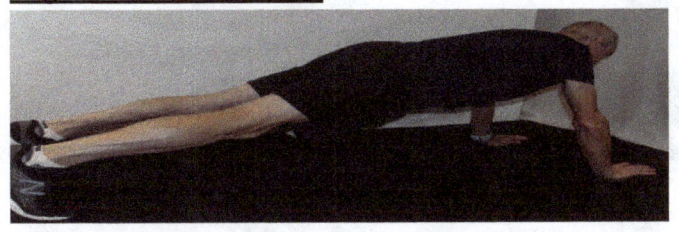 **Lateral Plank on Forearm (Low Plank)** 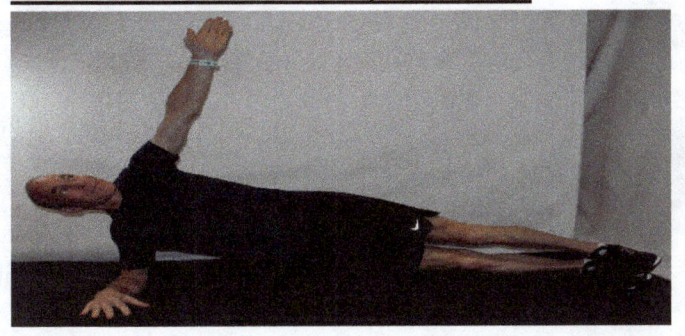	Prone (face down) and Lateral plank positions - Low planks - on forearms and toes - High planks - on hands and toes, Advanced - hands or forearms on SB or BOSU.
2. Bird 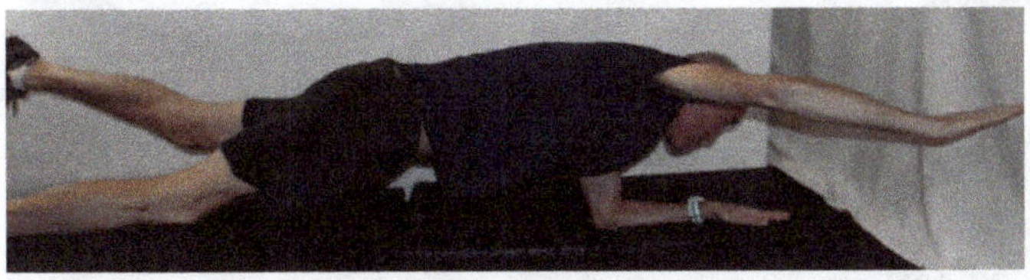 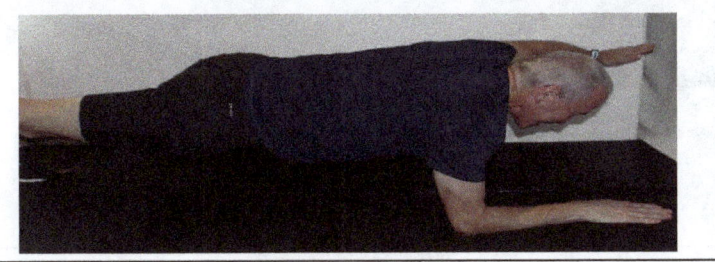	Low or high prone plank position - Elevate the opposite arm and leg to horizontal position, hold for 3-5 sec and then repeat with the other arm and leg. Easier modifications - extend only one arm or one leg at a time Advanced -Forearms or hands on SB or BOSU

3. Mountain Climber 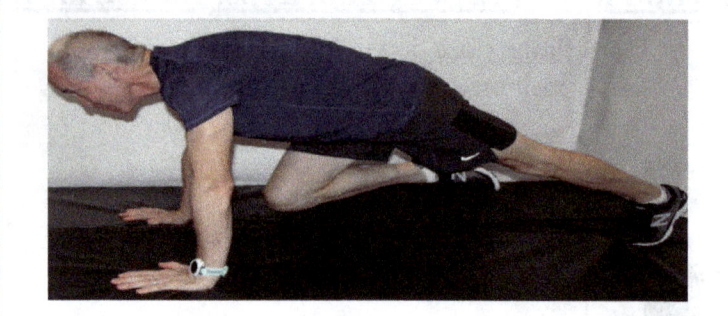 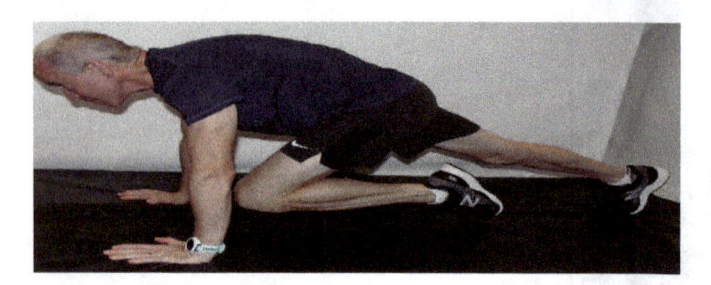	High prone plank position (on hands and toes) - Draw one knee between the hands to same side and alternate quickly with opposite knee. Advanced - draw knee to outside of same side arm vs. the inside of the same side arm.
4. Cross-Body Mountain Climber 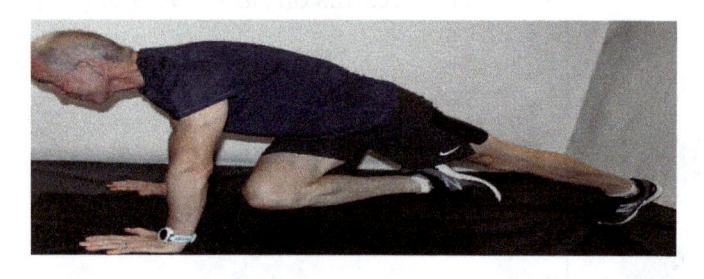 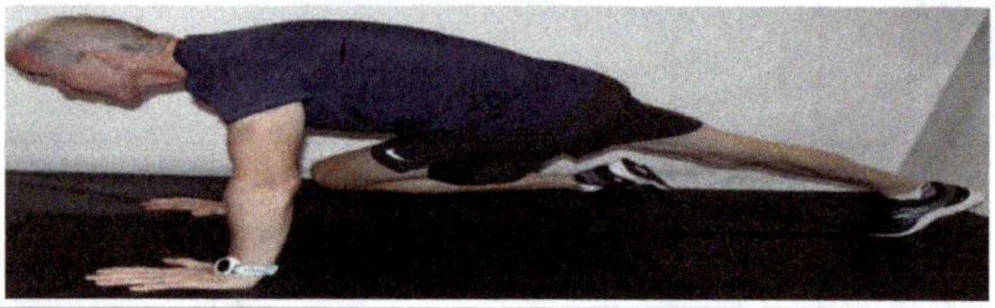	High prone plank position - Draw one knee to opposite chest and the alternate quickly with opposite knee. Advanced - draw the knee to the outside of the opposite arm
5. Thread the Needle 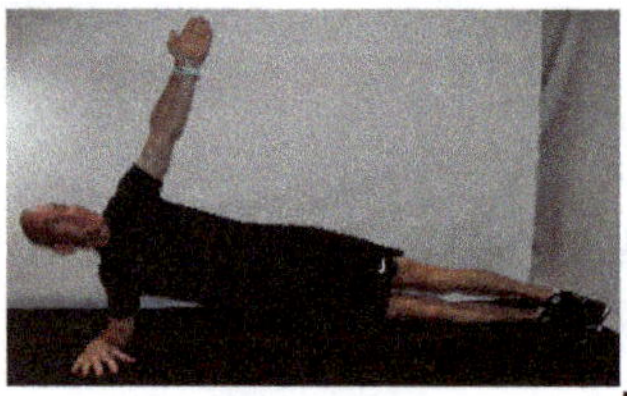 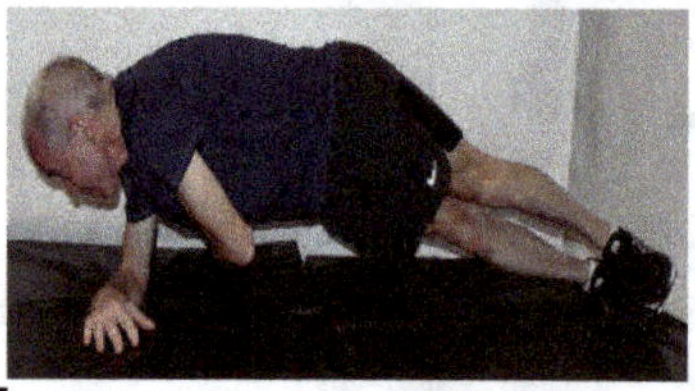	Lateral Plank position - Support yourself by lying laterally on forearm and lateral aspect of lower foot - Take top hand and twist down and under the ribs as far as possible. You are "threading" your hand through the open space underneath the opposite arm. - Then rotate arm back and twist and reach up to the ceiling with the arm extended. (Starting position)

6. Plank with Alternating Shoulder Touches	<u>High or low prone plank</u> - Alternate one hand touching opposite shoulder. <u>Easier Modification</u> - start with hands, knees and toes on mat and then do alternating shoulder taps.
7. Lateral Plank with Top Leg abduction **Low Lateral Plank Position** **High Lateral Plank Position**	<u>Low or high (Advanced) lateral plank</u> - Slowly lift the top leg as high as possible. - Hold 3 secs and then return to starting side plank position and repeat.

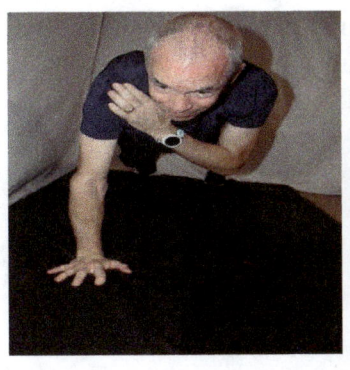

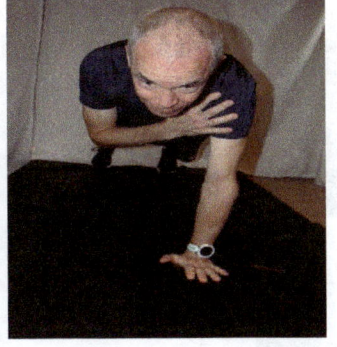

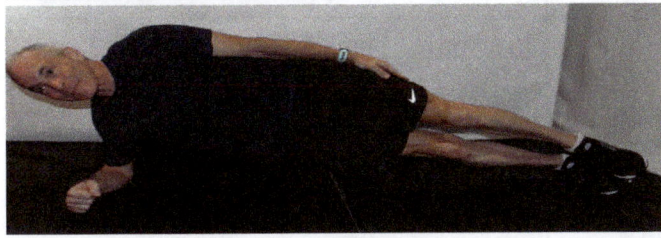

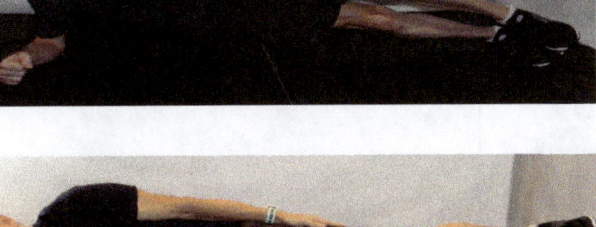

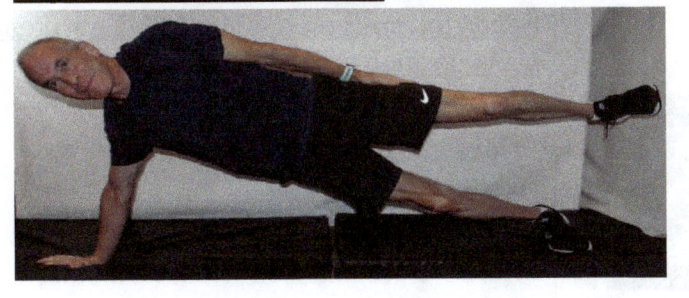

8. Lateral Hip Dip 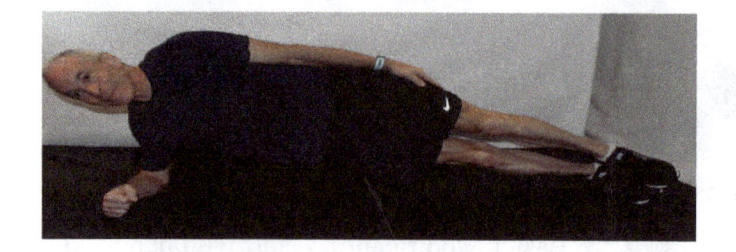 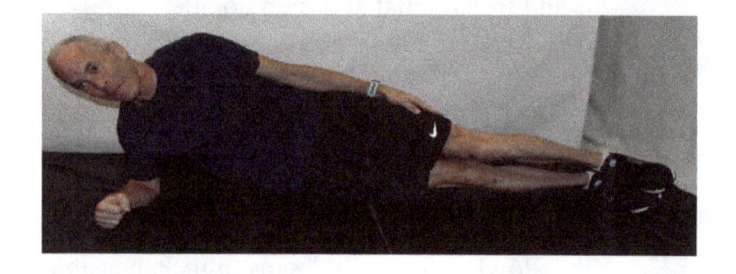	Low lateral plank or High (Advanced) - Lower your hips to just above the ground and raise hips up again.
9. Plank Jacks 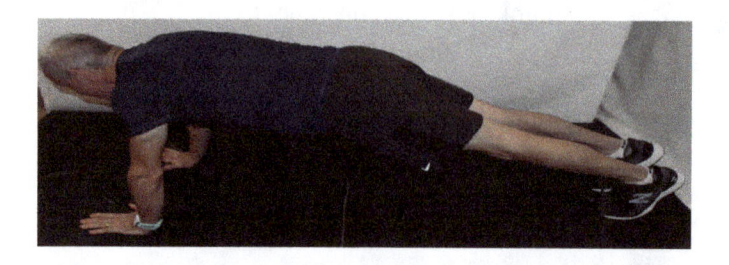 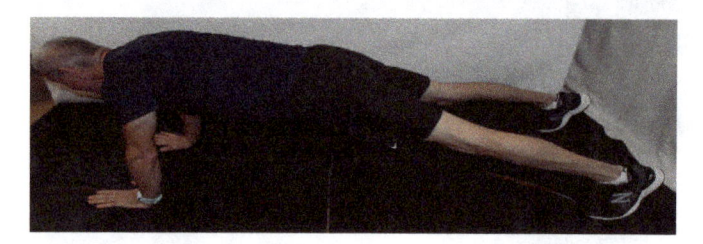	Low prone plank position High (Advanced) - Hop (abduct) legs/feet out wide and then back to original position.
10. Stability Ball Rollout 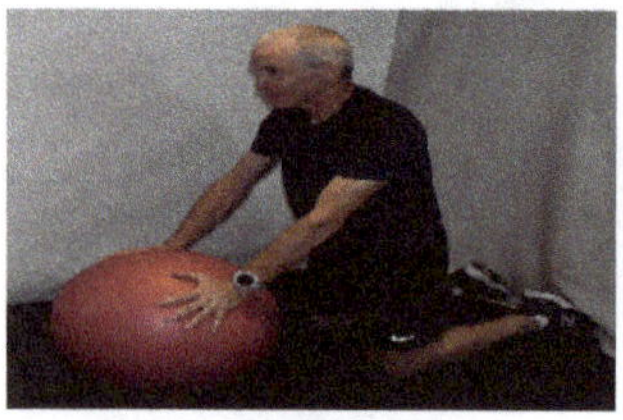 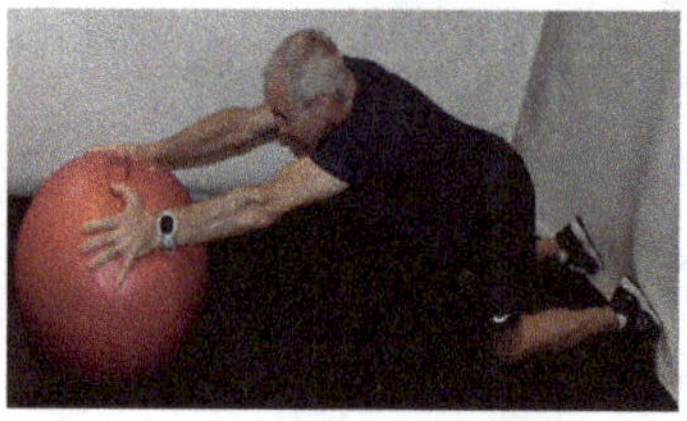	Hands/forearms on stability ball (Low prone plank position or High (Advanced)) - Slowly roll or push SB forward a few inches to comfort level. - Hold 3-5 sec and then return to starting plank position.

11. Abdominal wheel	Kneeling on your knees on edge of the mat with both hands on the abdominal roller in front of you
	- Roll slowly out to an extended position and then roll back.
	Key - only rollout and extend as far as feels comfortable.

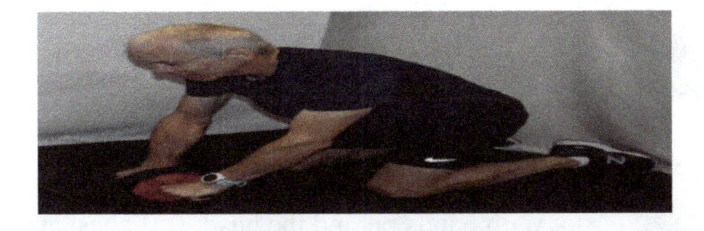

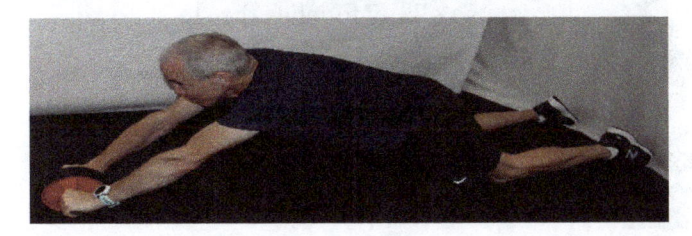

5. Back Extensions (Isolate the Back Erector Spinae Muscles)
(These can be done on mat, stability ball or BOSU)

1. Back Extensions	Prone
Lift Chest off the Ground (feet stay on the ground)	- Hands behind head or resting on lower back and lift chest off ground and return to the ground
	Advanced:
	1. Use stability ball or BOSU under your belly button
	2. Oscillate with chest off the ground
BOSU	3. Lift legs off ground (chest stays flat on the ground)

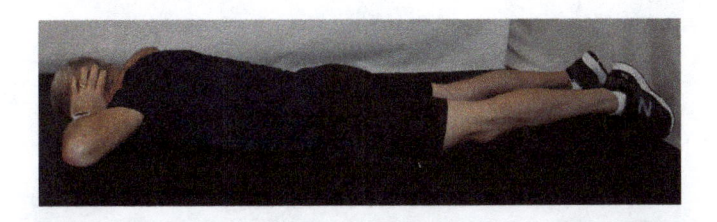

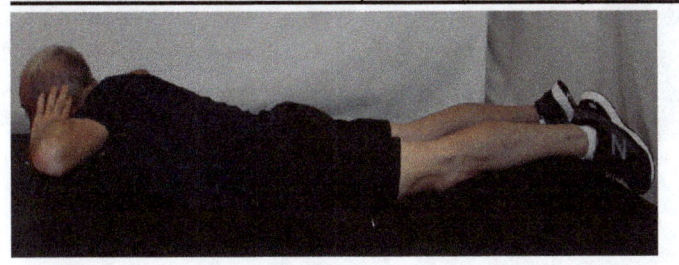

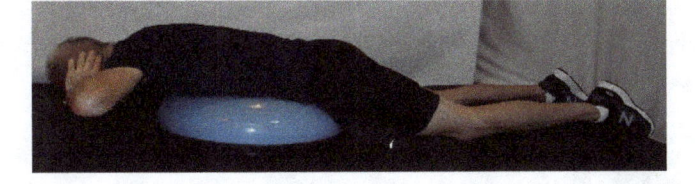

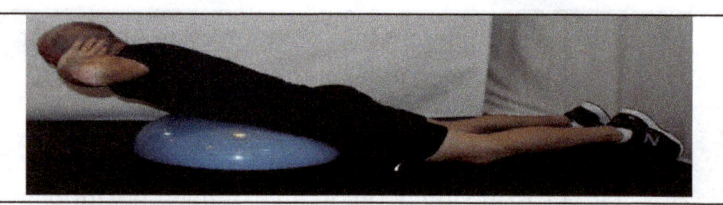 **2. Back Extensions with small Rotation BOSU** 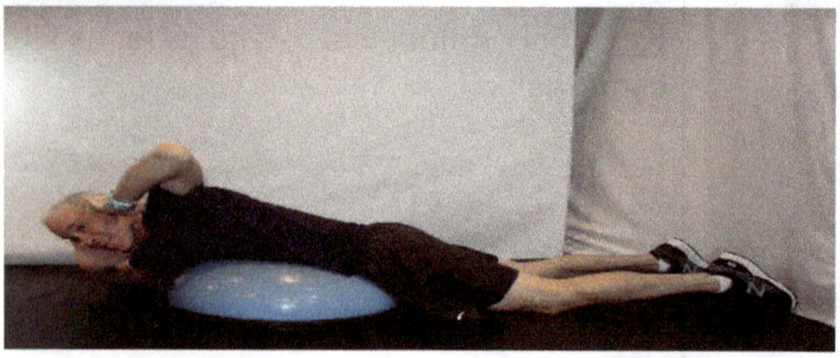 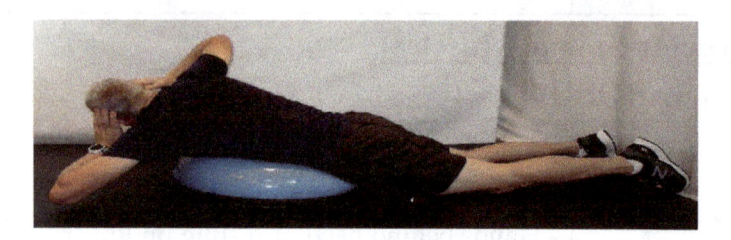	<u>Prone</u> - With hands behind the head. Lift chest and rotate so elbow touches the floor, lower chest and repeat with the other elbow.
3. Superman's **Chest and Feet off the ground** 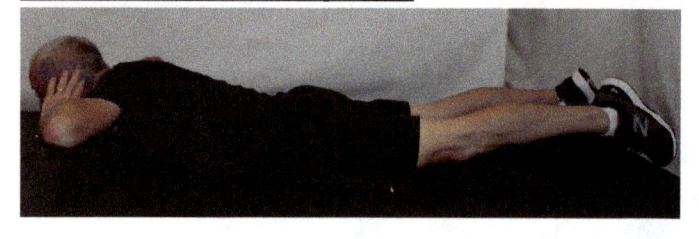	<u>Prone</u> - With hands extended out in front of head, or beside or behind the head or on small of back. Lift chest and thighs off ground and return to ground. <u>Advanced</u> - Oscillate with chest and thighs off
4. Bridges 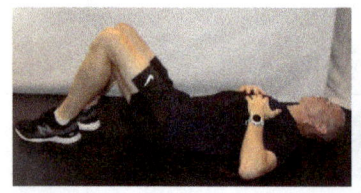 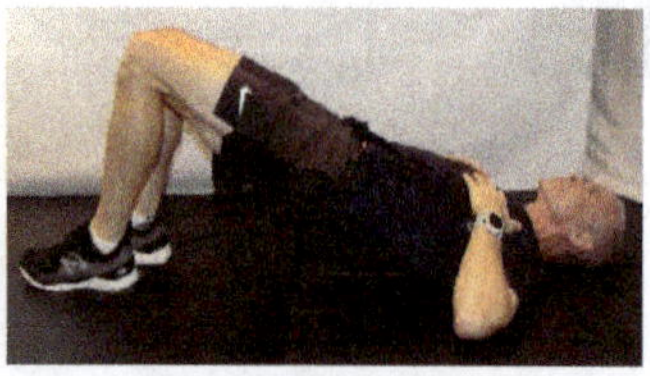	<u>Supine</u> - Both feet on ground, hands resting on lower abdominal. Lift buttocks off mat and hold 5 - 10 sec.

BOSU

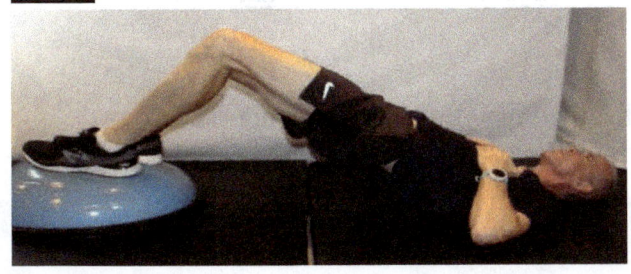

Stability Ball

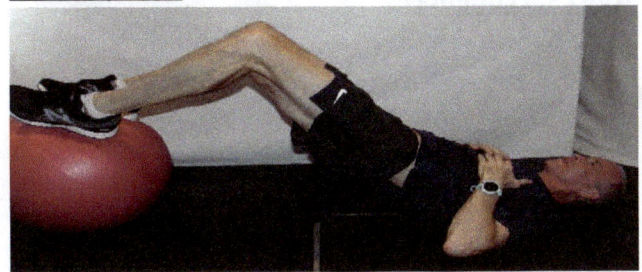

Modification
- Put feet on SB, BOSU to perform the bridge)

Advanced:

1. Oscillate hips up and down while in bridge position

2. Extend one leg while in bridge

3. One leg bridge (other leg in figure 4 position)

Appendix 9.1.2.2.0. Introduction to Whole Body Muscular Strength Training Exercises

As a person ages, they lose muscle mass. Medically, this is called Sarcopenia. The rate of loss accelerates with age. After age 30, the rate of muscle loss is approximately .5 % per year. After 50, the loss rate is 1% per year and doubles to greater than 2% per year after age 70. Muscle loss with age results from a lack of exercise and a decrease in the hormones Testosterone and Growth Hormone.

Muscle Loss with Age (Sarcopenia)

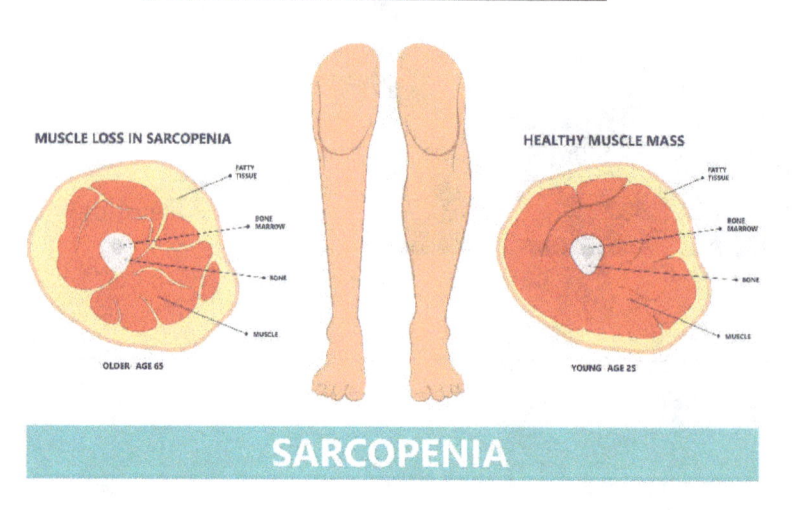

The loss of muscle mass and strength in the older adult affects their ability to be functionally active and leaves them vulnerable to falls.

Strength training is necessary to slow the rate of muscle loss in older adults. However, unlike core strength training, strength training of the chest, shoulders, arms, hips, and legs needs to be very specific. To maximize the effectiveness of a strength training exercise, the person needs to isolate the target muscle specifically. As a result, proper positioning to start the exercise and correct biomechanics while performing the exercises are of the utmost importance.

Appendix 9.1.2.2.1. describes and illustrated the various whole-body exercises that can strengthen the different muscle groups of the body.

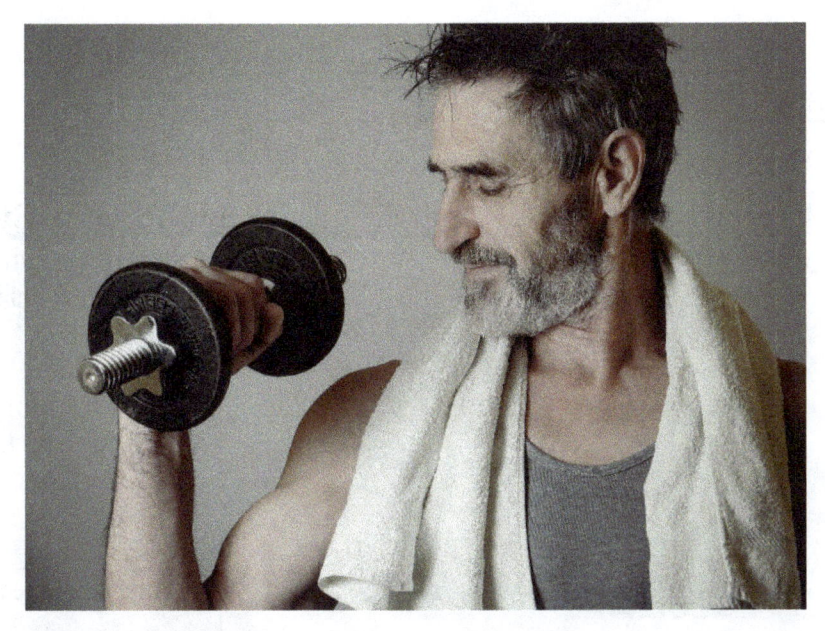

Muscles get stronger based on the overload principle. However, doing too much too soon leaves a person vulnerable to injury. It takes time to make positive strength changes. Start with light resistance and progressively increase the resistance slowly. It takes patience to re-conditioning muscles, tendons and ligaments.

The best advice is to:

1. Start with low resistance
2. Progress slowly with adding additional weight and increasing the number of repetitions and sets
3. Perform your exercise routine consistently
4. Make strength training a lifelong commitment. You will lose it if you don't do it, so do it!

"Success is in the Doing"

Appendix 9.1.2.2.1. Whole-Body Muscular Strength Training Exercises Described and Illustrated

1. Shoulder Exercises (Deltoids, Upper Trapezius and Rotator Cuff)

1. Weighted Circles with Dumbbells

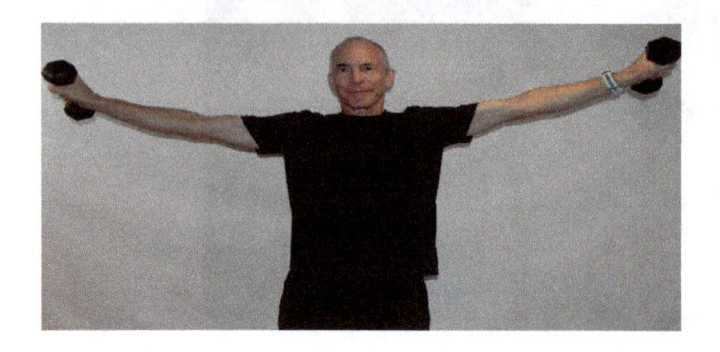

- Stand erect with weights at your side. Lift the weights laterally to shoulder height.

- Rotate the arms in a forward small circle 8-10 times and then in a backward small circle 8-10 times.

- Drop the weights to side for a 10 sec rest or continue a second set without any rest.

2. Straight Overhead Shoulder Press with Dumbbells (I's)

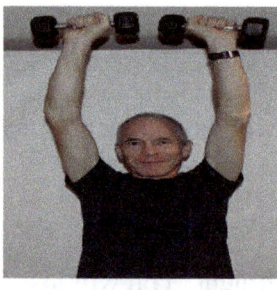

Start   **I's**

Y's

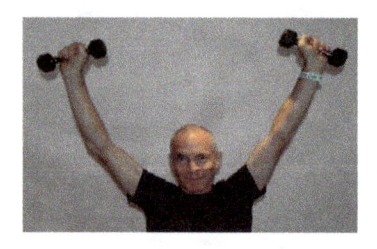

Alternating

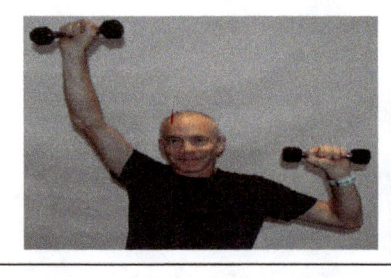

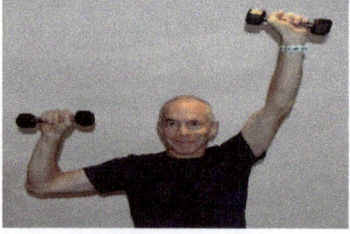

- Standing erect with weights lifted to ear level.

- The weights are turned and face toward the front.

- Lift the weights up vertical as high as you comfortably can.

- The inside of each weight can touch each other at the top and the arms should be felt against your ears.

Modifications:
1. Y's - lift weights so arms are 60-70° from horizontal at the top.

2. Alternating Overhead Press - alternate lifting arms up over your head to the straight "I" position.

Swimmers

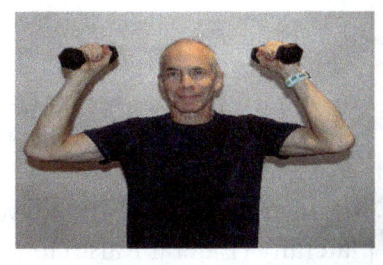

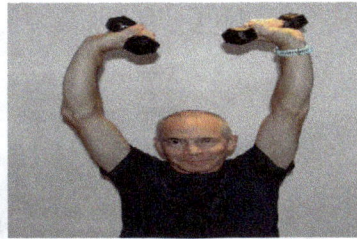

3. <u>Swimmers</u> - weights start facing your ears and as your lift them up vertically the arms twist so at the top they face outward (180º rotation).

3. Lateral Raises with Dumbbells

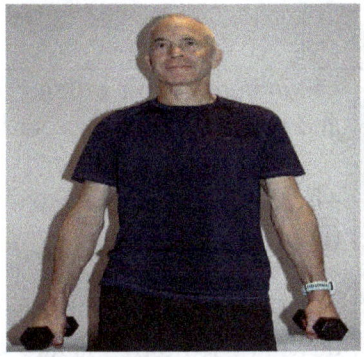

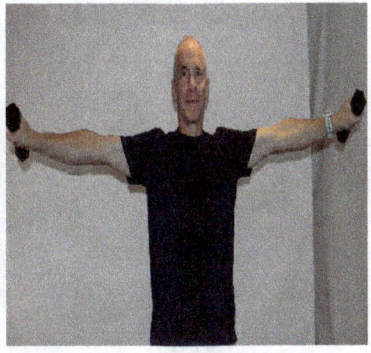

- Stand erect with weights at your side facing toward your body.

- Lift the weights up laterally with arms extended to shoulder height.

<u>Modification</u> - Start with elbows bent 90º (weights are pointing inward) and lift the arms up laterally to shoulder height with elbows still at 90º.

4. Angle Raise with Dumbbell

Start   **Anterior lift at 45º**

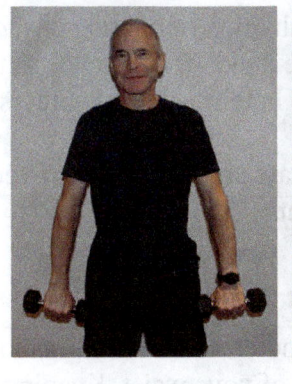

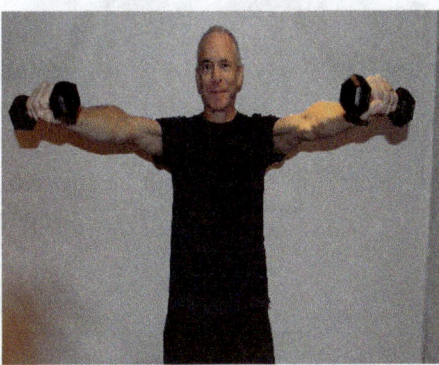

- Stand erect with arms at your side but ½ between the side and front of your bodies.

- Turn your hands so thumbs are pointing toward your legs.

- Lift one or both arms outward diagonally to shoulder level.

- Return to starting position and repeat.

5. Anterior Raise with Dumbbells

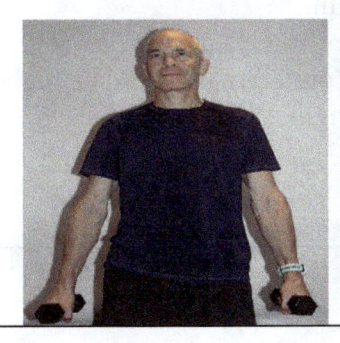

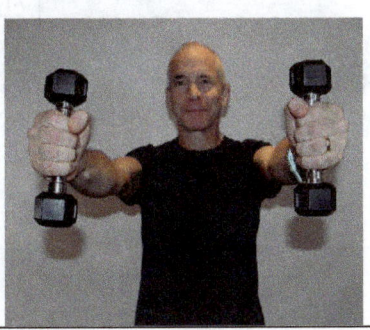

- Stand erect with arms at side of body with weights facing your body.

- Lift the arms up anteriorly in front of the body to shoulder height.

6. In's and Out's with Dumbbells In's Out's	- Stand erect with weight at your side and facing your body. - First - In's - Lift the weights to the front of you to shoulder height (Anterior Raise) and then return the weights to your side. - Second - Out's - Lift the weights laterally (Lateral Raise) to shoulder height and then return to starting position.
7. Pours with Dumbbells	- Stand erect with weights at your sides and pointing towards your body. - Laterally lift weights to shoulder height (lateral raise). - Rotate the arms so the weights point down. (The motion is like you are pouring a bottle of wine.)
8. Scarecrows with Dumbbells	- Stand erect and lift weights to shoulder height with the elbows at 90°. - With arms remaining at shoulder height rotate hands forward 90° so they are at the same height as the shoulders. - Rotate arms back 90° to vertical and repeat.
9. Upright Rows with Dumbbells	- Stand erect with weights together in front of your waist. Keeping the weights together lift the weights to just under your chin. (Your elbows should be higher than the height of the weights.)

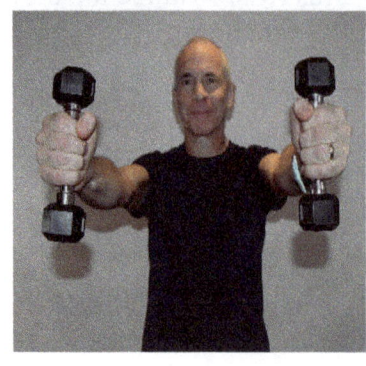

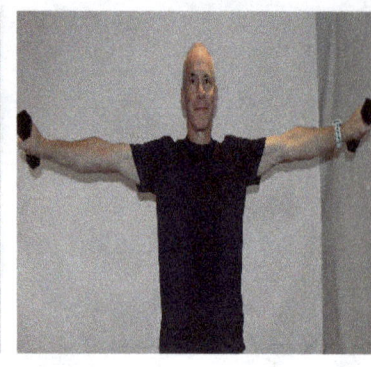

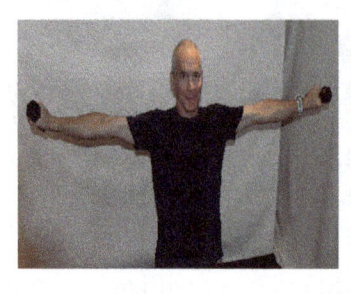

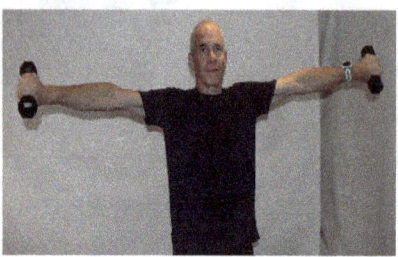

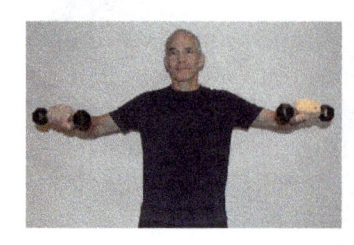

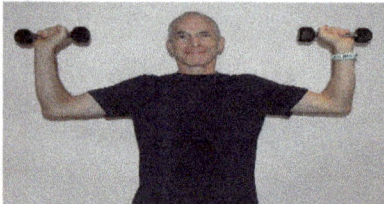

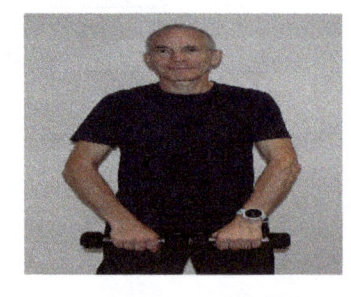

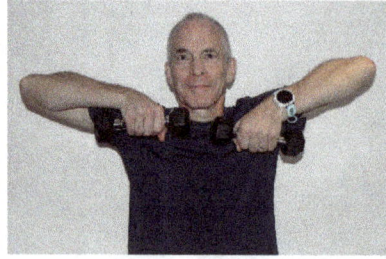

10. Fly-Row-Press with Dumbbells
 	
Fly   **Row**
 	
Press
	- Stand erect with weights at the side of your body.
	
	    1. Do a lateral raise
	    2. Do a upright row
	    3. Do an overhead "I" press from the top of the upright row position. Rotate the weights so they are pointing vertical and then do an overhead press.
	
	- Return to original starting position and Repeat the three lifts.

11. External and Internal Rotation Arm at Side of Body **Start** **External Rotation** 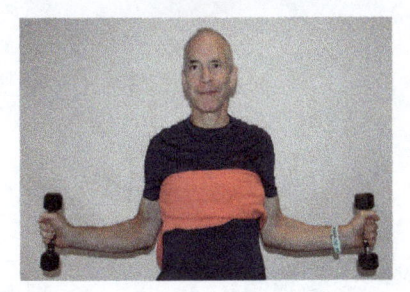 **Internal Rotation** 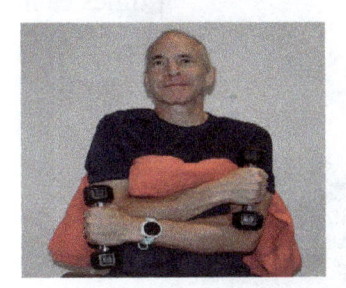	- Stand erect with elbow bent 90º and weight facing inwards. - Use a towel to keep your elbows tight against your ribs. **External Rotation** - Keep your wrist in neutral position and elbows at 90º and rotate arm laterally 60-80º. **Internal Rotation** - From external rotation position rotate arms across the body.

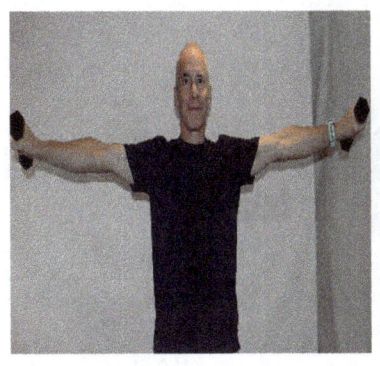

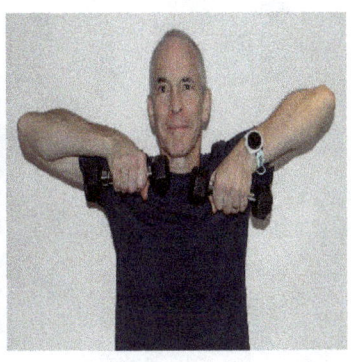

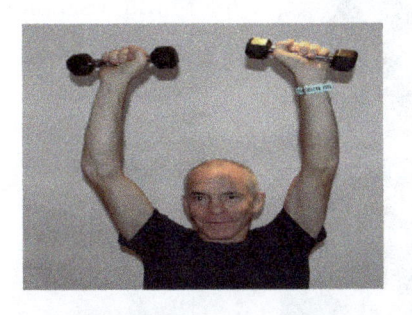

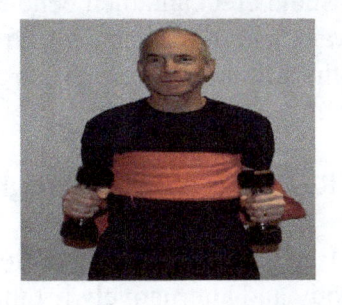

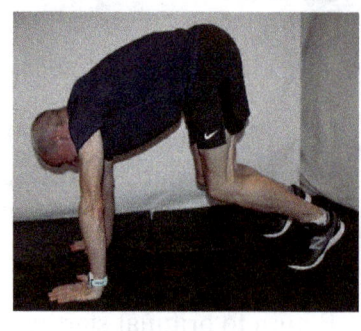

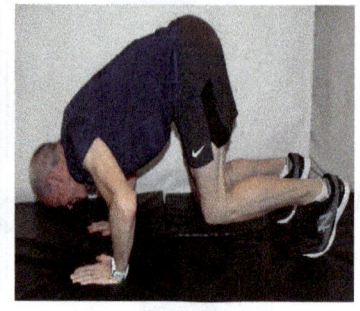

12. Pike Press	- Start in push-up position. Prone plank position)
	- Raise your buttocks as high as you can so body looks like an upside-down V and head is pointing down toward the floor.
	- Do a push-up until forehead is about to touch the floor and then return to starting position.
13. Shoulder Shrugs	- Stand erect and weight at side of body.
	- Squeeze or lift the top of your shoulder (Upper Trapezius) toward your ears and hold 3 seconds.

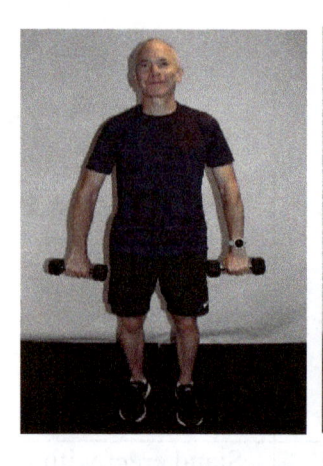

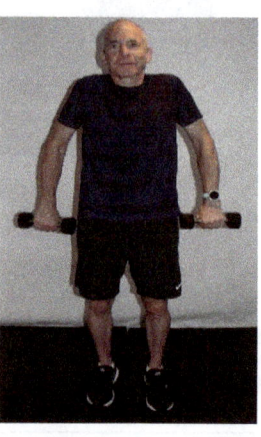

2. Upper Back (Rhomboids and Middle to Lower Trapezius and Latissimus Dorsi)

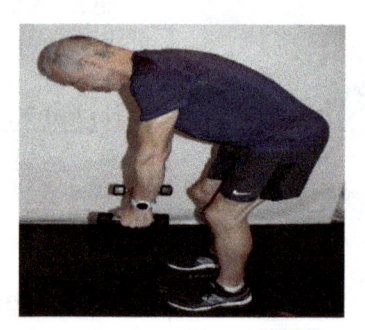

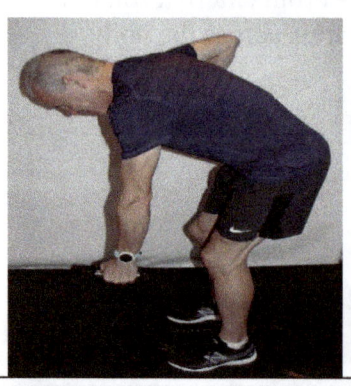

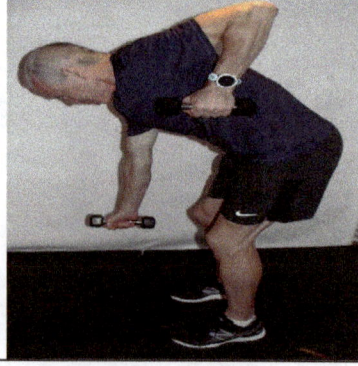

1. Locomotives	- Stand erect and then bend forward at the waist and move one leg in front of the other (Straddle position.) or shoulder width apart (picture)
	- Reach down for both weights.
	- Bend the elbow, keep it close to the body and alternatively lift the weights up to rib level in quick succession for 20 times each arm.

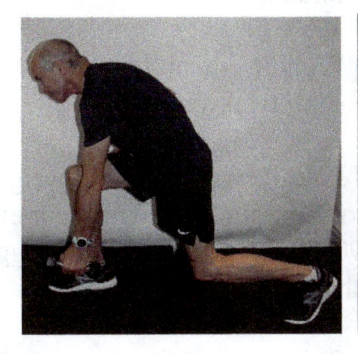

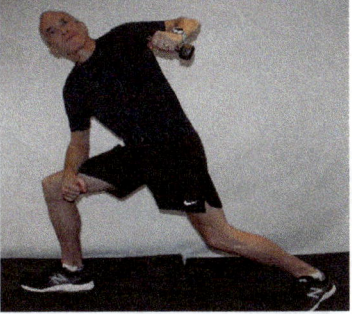

2. Lawnmowers	- Stand erect, then bend forward at the waist and move one leg in front of the other. Rest your elbow on the forward knee. - Reach down for the weight. - Bend the elbow, keep it close to the body and lift the weight up while rotating your trunk to the side that you are lifting the weigh on. - Return the weight to just above the floor and repeat.
3. Bent over Rows	-Sit on a bench, stability ball or stand with one leg in front of the other or shoulder width apart. - Bend over at the waist 90°. - With a slight bend of the knees reach for the weight on the floor. - Bend your elbows, keep the elbows close to your ribs and lift both weights to rib level. (You should feel your shoulder blades squeeze together.)
4. Bent over Shoulder Flies	- Sit on a bench or stability ball or stand with one leg in front of the other or shoulder width apart. - Bend over at the waist 90°. - With a slight bend of the knees reach for the weight on the floor. - Lift both arms laterally while in bent over position. The elbows may bend a bit. (Feel the shoulder blades squeezing together.)

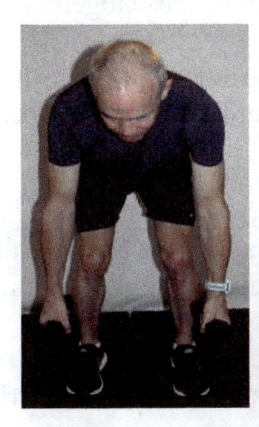

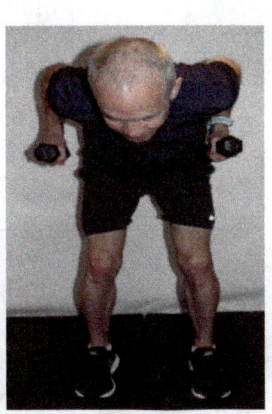

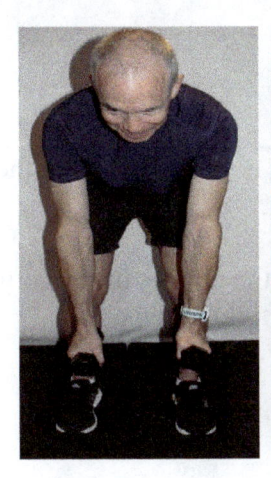

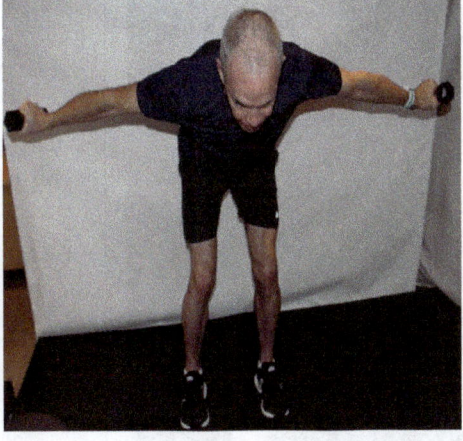

5. Two Angle Shoulder flies

1. Standing Erect

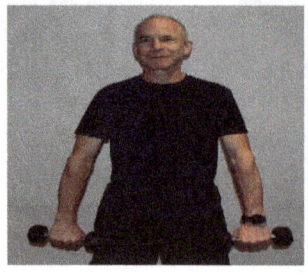

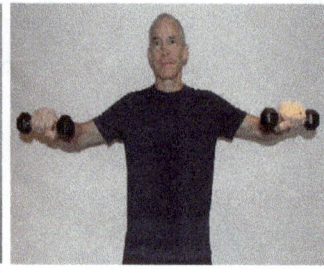

2. Bent Over

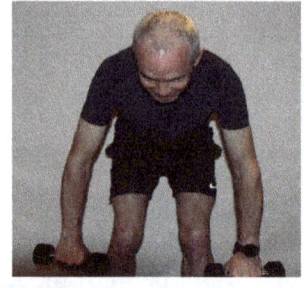

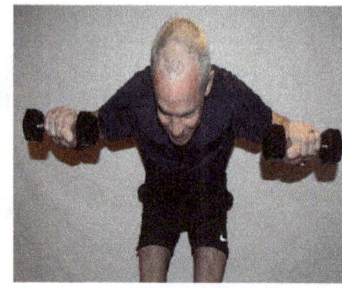

- Sit on a bench or stability ball or standing erect.

- Weights are at the side of your body facing backward.

1. While erect lift both weights laterally to shoulder level with your elbows bent 90º. (feels like you are shrugging your shoulders)

- Return to starting position.

2. Bend forward 90º at the waist and laterally lift weights to shoulder level with elbows bent 90º. (feel the shoulder blades squeeze together)

- Return to starting position and get back into erect posture to repeat the exercise.

6. Machine Low Rows

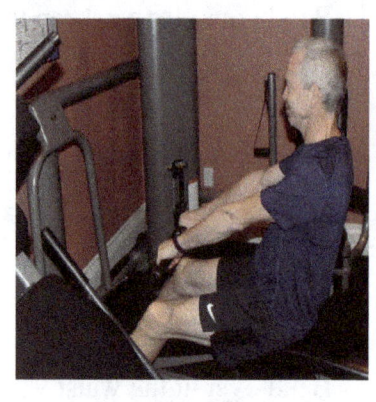

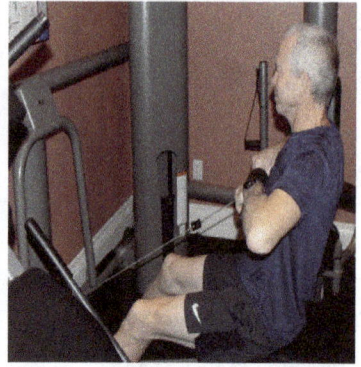

- Sitting on the bench with the back straight but slightly leaning backwards

- Keep the elbows close to ribs and pull the bar to bottom of the rib cage.

7. Machine High Rows

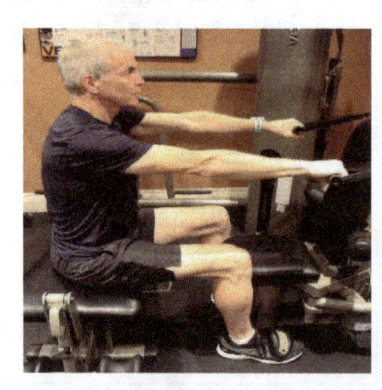

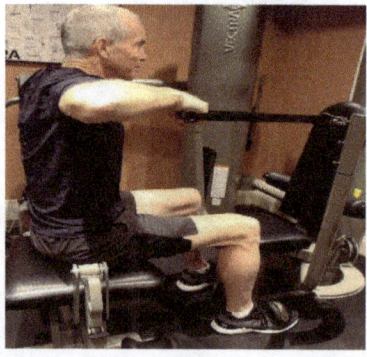

- Sitting on the bench with the back straight.

- Keep the elbows high and wide and pull the bar tight to the chest.

8. Stability Ball Reverse Flies (Prone "T's") 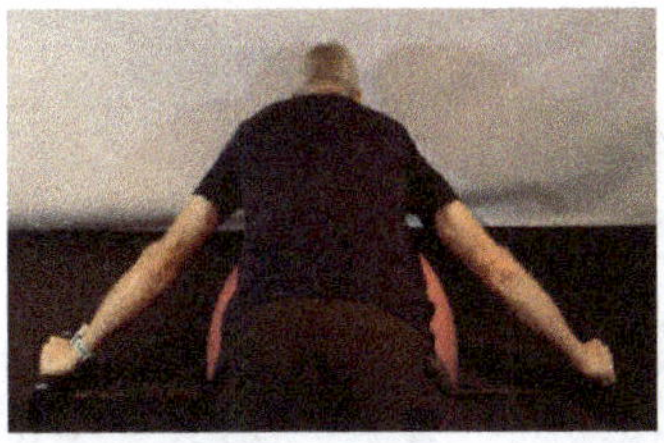	- Lying prone (face down) with stability ball at lower abdominal level. - Grab both weights and with arms extended lift the weights to shoulder level. - Try to keep the elbows as straight as possible while lifting the weights. - Avoid lifting or extending your neck. You chin should be slightly tucked into your chest. - Lower the weights but do not let the weights touch the ground before repeating the exercise.
9. Standing Resistance Band "T's" 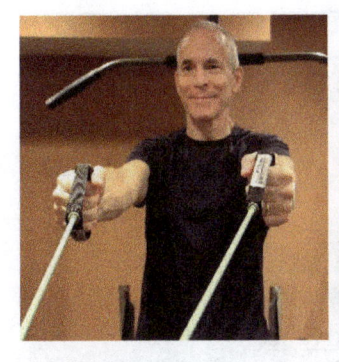	- Stand erect in front of mid anchor with arms extended in front of the chest. - Pull resistance bands wide until arms are in line with the body (feel the shoulder blades squeeze together).
10. Machine Pull Downs **Start** **Regular Grip** 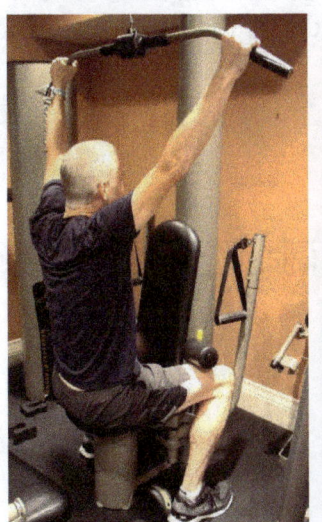	- Use the pull-down machine. - While sitting pull down to your upper chest level. Note - DO NOT pull down behind you head. Three hand positions: 1. Regular Wide Grip - hands face away and on the wide rubber grips 2. Reverse Grip - Hands face toward you and narrower than wide grip.

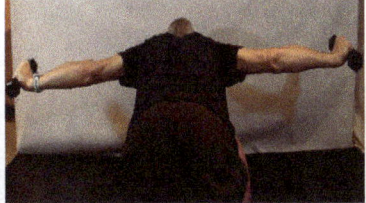

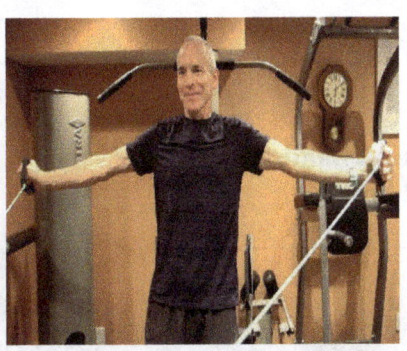

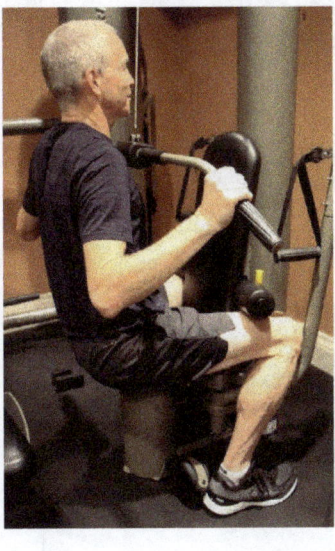

Reverse Grip **Close Grip**	3. <u>Closed Grip</u> - hands face away and very close to the center of the bar

<u>Modifications:</u>

1. <u>Straight Arm Pull Downs</u> - Standing and use the mid-width grip and with elbows extended pull down the bar to thigh level.

2. <u>Use a high anchor resistance band to do straight arm or regular pull downs</u> - This can be done with both arms together or pull down with the arms alternatively (one arm pulls downs at a time.)

The hands can be facing toward you or away from you. |
| **3. Chest** | |
| **1. Push–ups**
  – Strength exercises in a plank position
<u>Note</u> – all push–ups can be done on hands and toes or modified by being on hands and knees | |
| **1. Regular** | - Hands shoulder width.

<u>Advanced</u>
- Hands on stability ball or BOSU. |
| **2. Military** | - Hands along sides of your ribs (narrow) and slightly behind shoulders. |
| **3. Wide** | - Hands out wide as you feel comfortable |

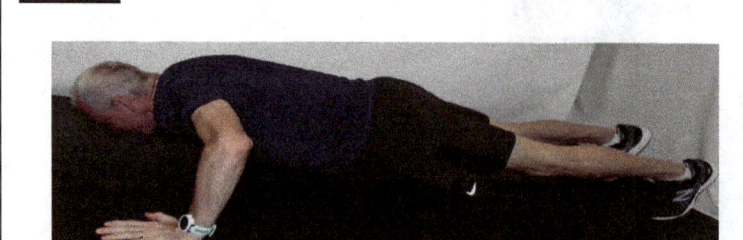

4. Diamond 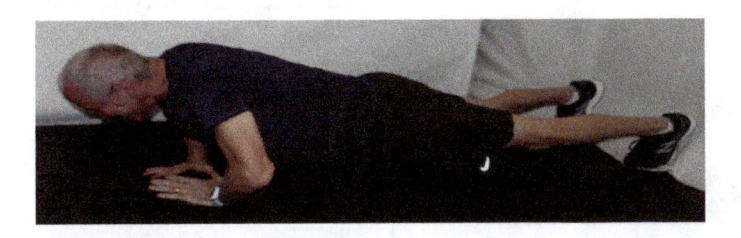	- Hands under your chest with index and thumbs of each hand touching to make shape of a diamond.
5. Under the Fence 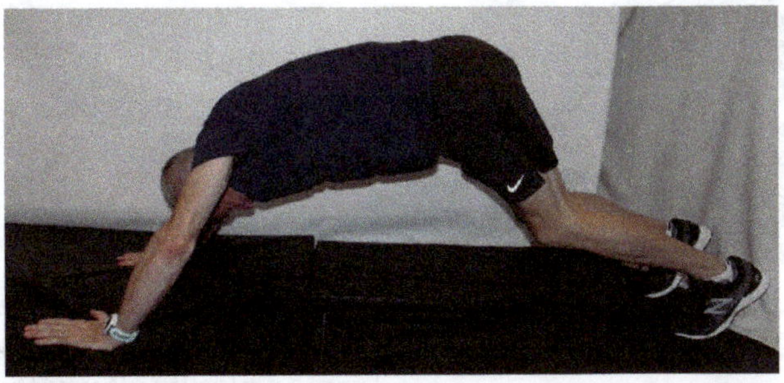	- As you do your push-up, pretend you are crawling forward under a fence and then moving backward under the fence.
6. Decline 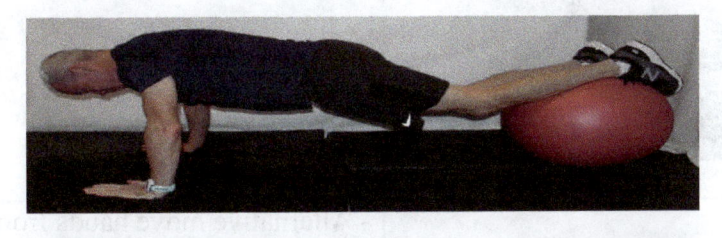 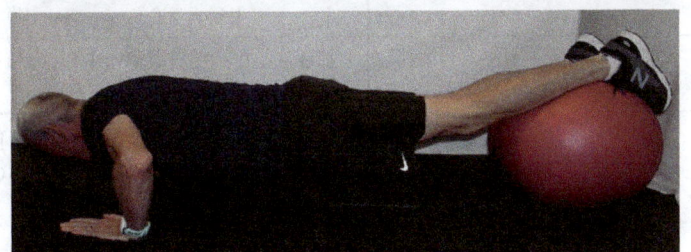	- Feet are elevated on a bench or stability ball.

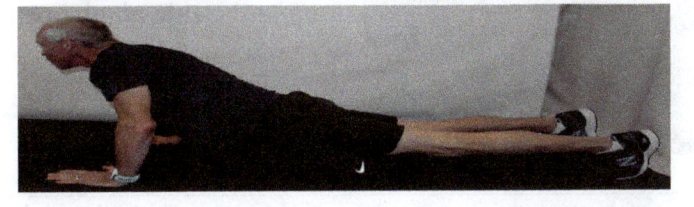

7. Incline	- Hands are positioned higher than hips on a bench, stability ball or BOSU.
8. Push-up to one arm side plank position	- Do regular push-up and then rotate into a side plank (alternate sides on each push up to the side plank position).
9. Plange Push-ups	- Hands next to ribs and face outward.
10. Floor Fly Push-ups	- Alternative move hands from narrow to wide position after every 4th push-up.
11. Two Twitch Speed Push-Ups	- Do 4 fast and then 4 slow (4 beats down and 4 beats up).
12. Side-to-Side Push-Ups	- move to one side and do a push-up and then move to the opposite side and do a push-up
13. Three-in-one push-ups	- Do 2, 3, or 4 military push-ups, followed by same number regular and wide push-ups. (Going from narrow to wide)

2. Chest Press <center>**Dumbbells**</center> <center>**Machine**</center> <center>**Resistance Band**</center>	Supine 1. <u>Dumbbells on Bench</u> (flat, decline or incline) or on stability ball. - Press upward from just above your chest. Don't lock your elbows when you extend your arms. 2. <u>Machine</u> 3. <u>Resistance Band</u> - standing with back to mid-anchor and press forward.
3. Cross Body Chest Press	Supine - on stability ball or bench - Start with weights just above your chest and with alternating arms, press up and across your chest. - Don't lock your elbows when you extend your arms.

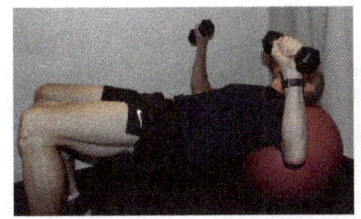

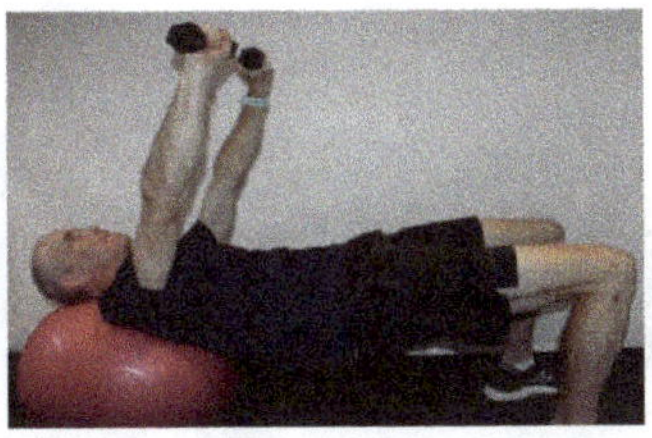

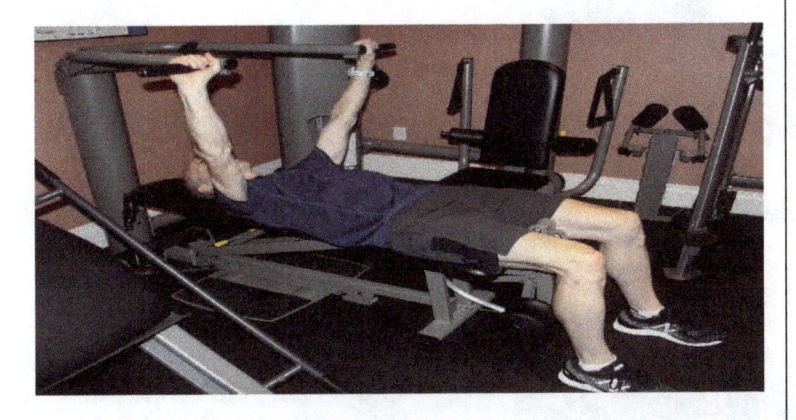

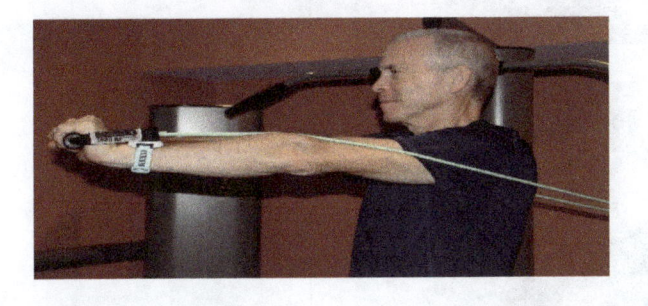

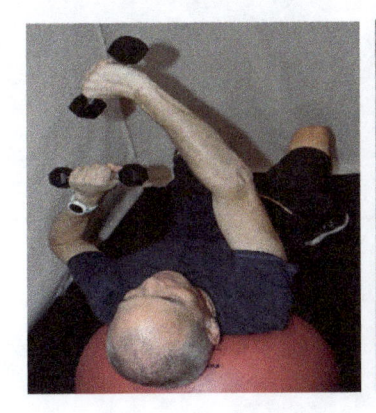

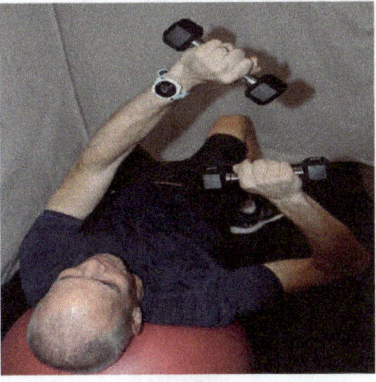

4. Chest Flies

Dumbbells

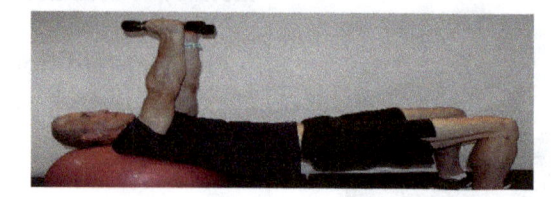

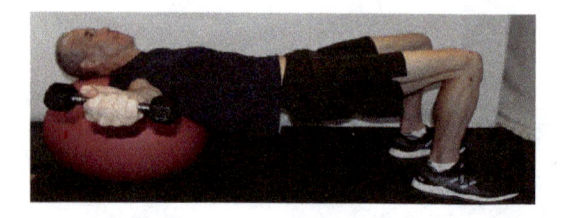

Machine

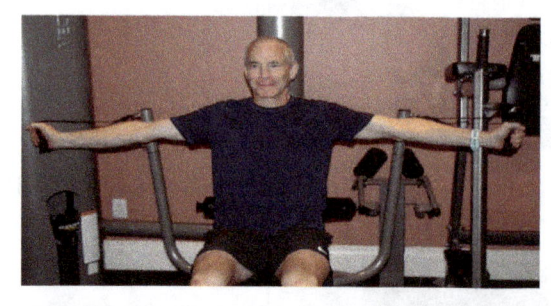

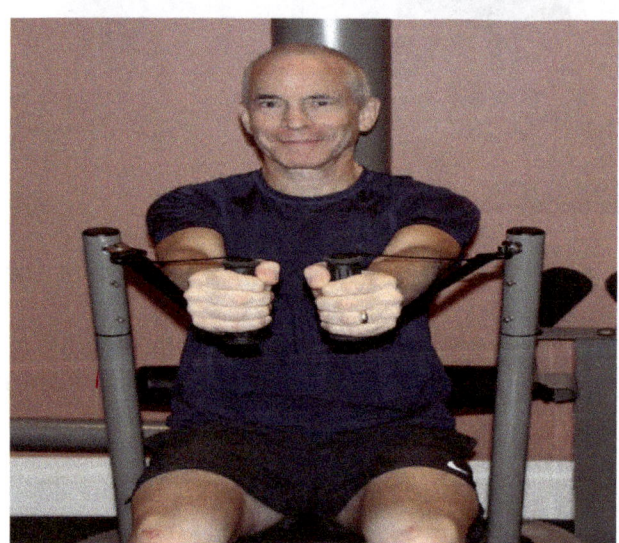

Supine

1. Using Dumbbells on Stationary Bench (flat, decline, incline) or stability ball.

- Lying supine and with arms extended above the chest lower arms to horizontal position.

(Try to keep elbows as straight as possible.)

2. Machine - Sitting or standing and with arms extended wide pull extended arms inward toward mid-line and hold for 1 second.

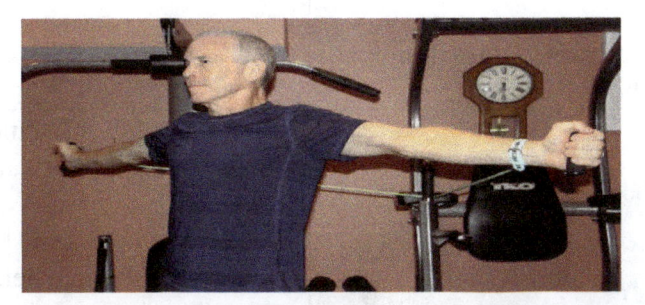

Resistance Band	3. <u>Resistance Band</u> - standing with back to mid-anchor, arms are wide and press the hands together.
5. Standing Front Extended Arm Pull Downs with Resistance Band	- With back to high Anchor and arms extended over your head pull resistance down in front of chest. - Stop at chest level or pull all the way down to thigh.

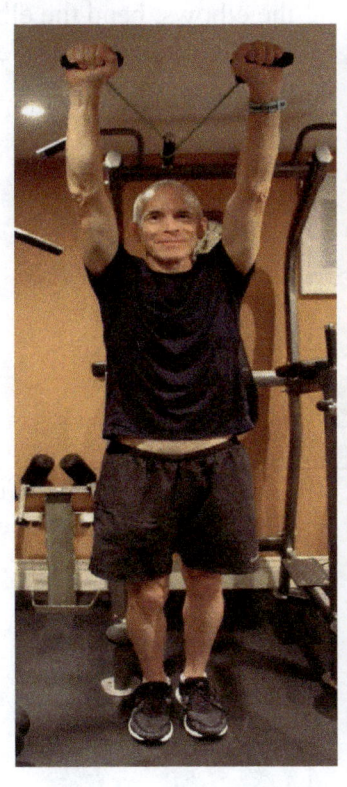

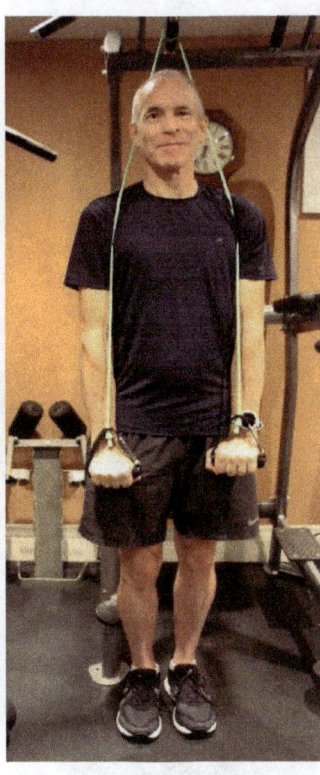

4. Arm Exercises (Biceps, Triceps)

Biceps:

Note – all bicep exercises can be performed with dumbbells resistance band or sitting on a Stability Ball.

1. Regular Curls

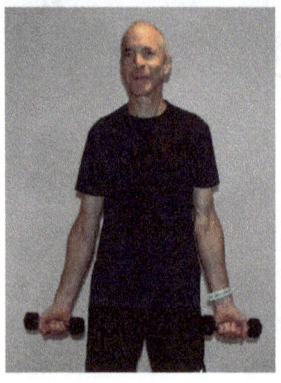

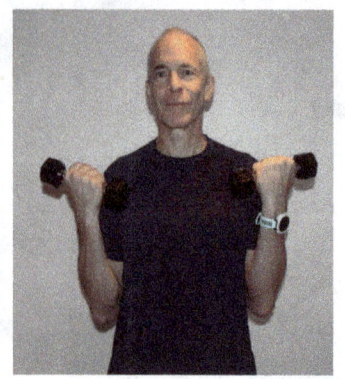

- Standing with resistance at side of body. Hands are facing forward.

- Without swaying the body or swinging the elbows forward, bend the elbows and raise the resistance to shoulder level and against the upper arm.

Modifications
 - Can be done on a machine

2. Out Curls

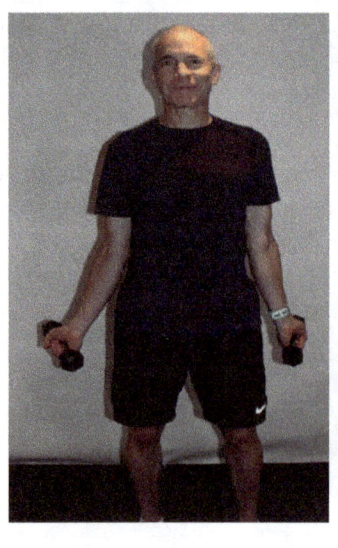

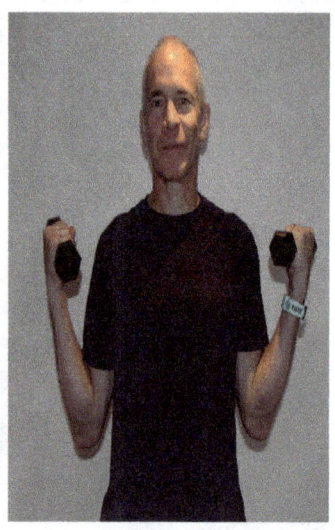

- Standing with resistance at side of body but arms are turned out 45º.

- Without swaying the body or swinging the elbows, bend the elbows and raise the resistance to shoulder level and against the upper arm.

3. In's and Out's

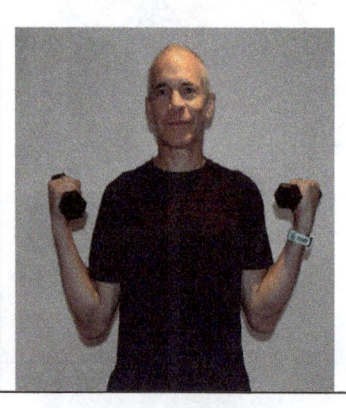

In's   Out's

- Alternate a Regular Curl (In's) and Out Curl (Out's) as one repetition.

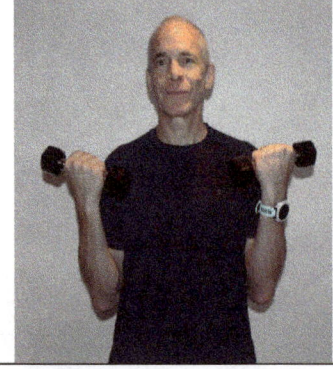

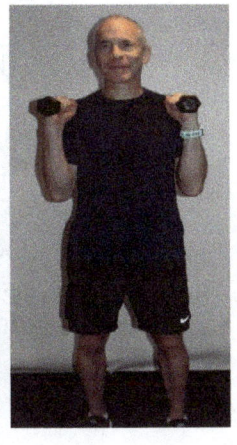

4. Hammer Curls 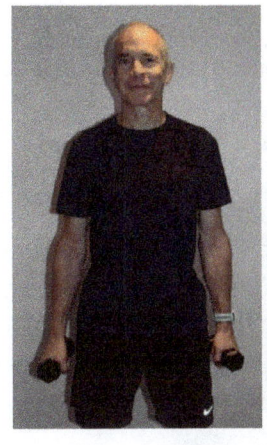	- Standing with resistance at side of body. - Turn the hands so that are facing toward the body. - Without swaying the body or swinging the elbows forward, bend the elbows and raise the resistance to shoulder level and against the upper arm.
5. Out Hammer Curls 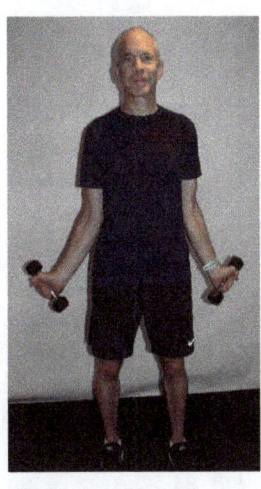	- Standing with resistance at side of body and the hands facing the body - Now turn the arms out 45º. - Without swaying the body or swinging the elbows, bend the elbows and raise the resistance to shoulder level and against the upper arm.
6. In's and Out's Hammer Curls In's Out's 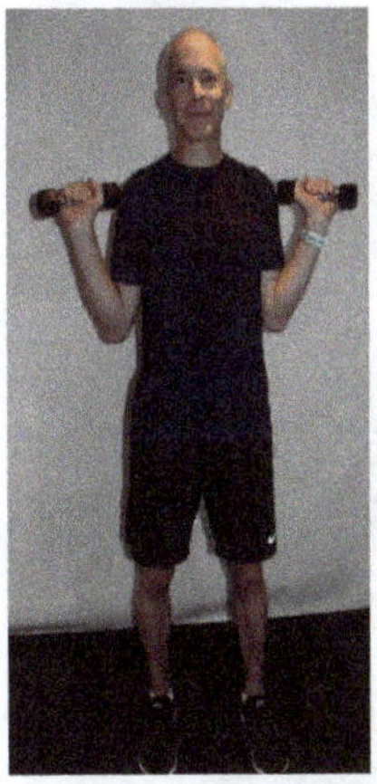	- Alternate between Regular Hammer Curls (In's) and Out Hammer Curls (Out's) for one repetition.

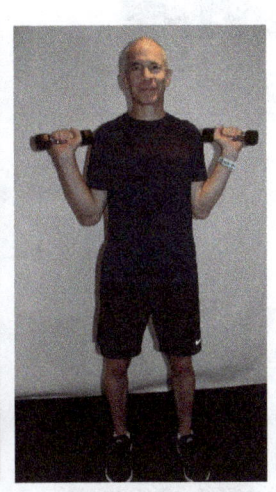

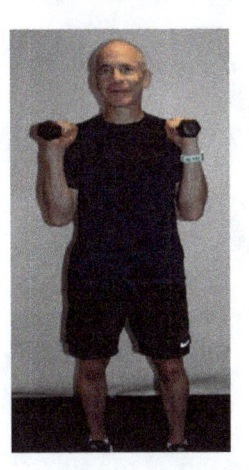

7. Curl Up and Hammer Down	- Do a regular Curl up and Hammer Curl down.
8. Cross Body Curls	- Standing with resistance at side of body. - Hands are facing forward. - Without swaying the body or swinging the elbows forward, alternate bending of elbows and raise the resistance across the chest to the opposite shoulder.
9. Alternating Arm Corkscrew Curl	- Standing with resistance at side of body. - Turn the hands so that are facing backwards. - Without swaying the body or swinging the elbows forward, simultaneously bend the elbows and raise the resistance to shoulder level while twisting the arm so resistance ends up finishing like a Regular Curl against the upper arm.
10. Twenty-ones Lower ½ Curl Upper ½ and full Curl	- Do 7 lower ½ regular curls. - 7 upper ½ regular curls. - 7 full regular curls.

11. Static Arm Curls	- Standing erect and holding weight in one hand at mid curl position do 8 regular curls with the other arm. -Then repeat with the opposite arm. - Repeat this sequence twice for a total of 32 repetitions.
12. Crouching Curls	- Spread your legs wide and do ¾ squat. - Place the elbows inside the top of the knees so weights are in the middle. - Do a regular curl from this position.
13. Concentration Curl	- Sitting on a stationary bench or SB bent at the waist, place elbow inside the thigh just above the knee. - Do a regular curl with one arm for ½ the set and then change arms to complete the set.
14. Strip Set	- Do 4 rounds of 8 Regular Curls but drop the weight on each round by 2.5 lbs.

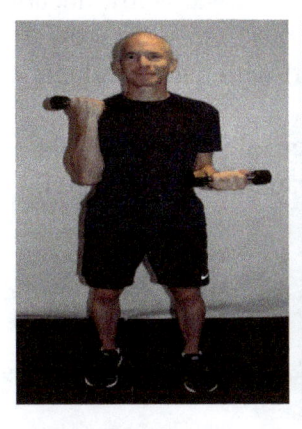

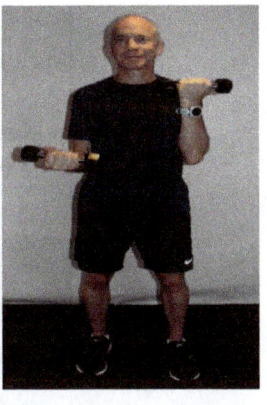

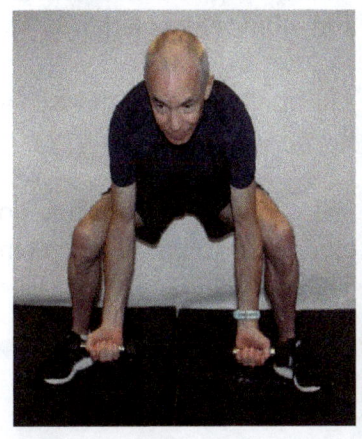

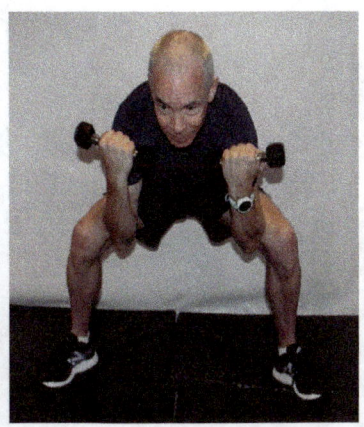

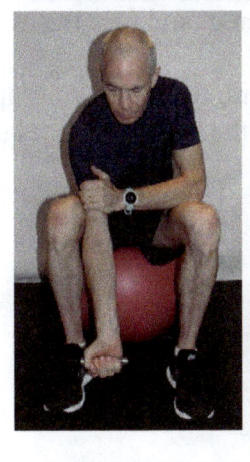

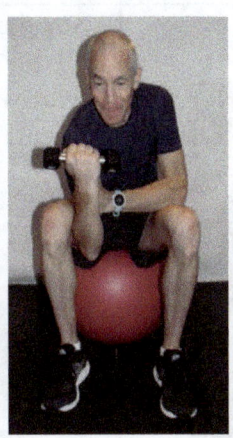

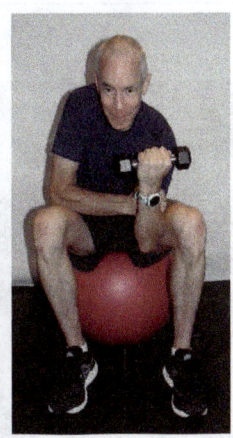

15. Resistance Band Curl	- Stand on the resistance band or face away or towards low anchor. - Start with hands at thigh level. - Keep elbows close to the ribs and curl the band up to chest level.
16. Standing Curls TRX	- Face a high anchor with arms extended and elbows elevated. - Keep the elbows elevated as you bend the elbows to do a curl. - Slowly return to starting position with elbows elevated but keep tension on the TRX bands
17. Machine Bicep Curl	- Stand erect and face the machine. - Start with the bar at your upper thighs and curl the bar like a regular curl

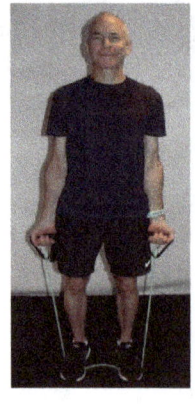

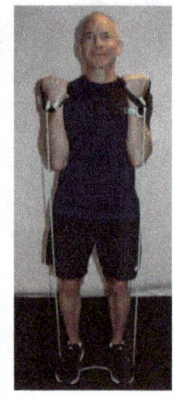

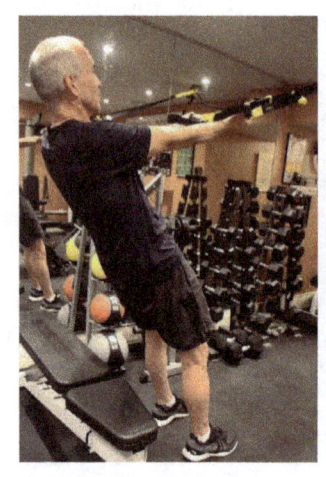

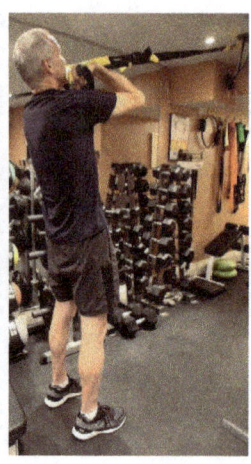

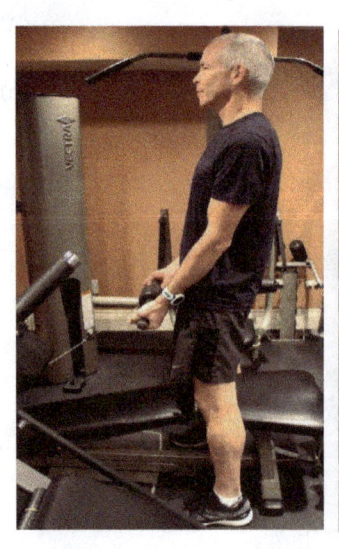

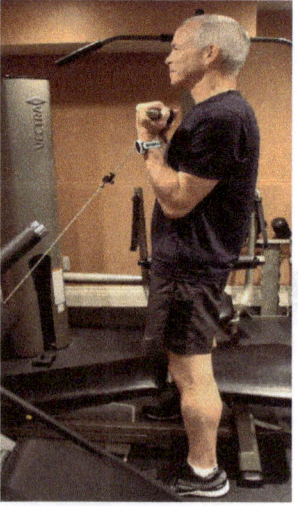

Triceps:

1. Machine Triceps Extensions

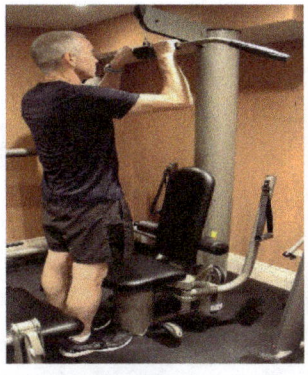

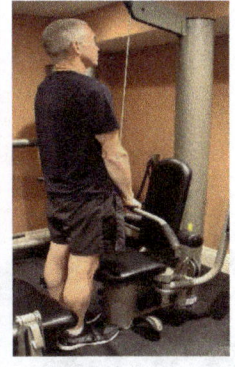

- Standing erect facing the machine.

- Starting with bar at head, shoulder or chest level pull down to thighs.

<u>Note</u> - Make sure you don't go pass your chest when returning the bar to starting position.

2. Two Arm Triceps Kick backs

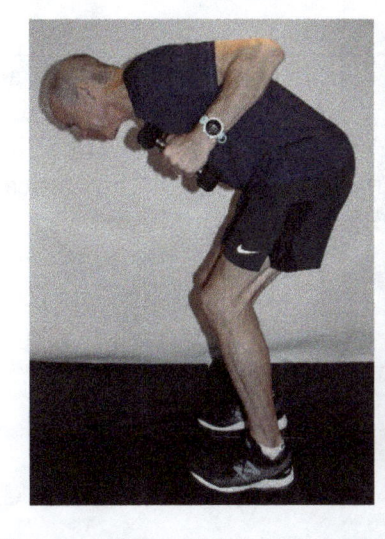

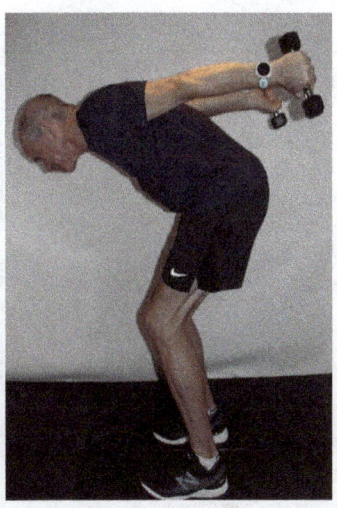

- Bend at the waist and lift elbows up so they are level with the trunk.

- Hands are pointing toward the body.

- Keep the elbows high as you extend the elbows (kick back).

3. Flip Grip Triceps Kick Backs

Palms Facing Upward

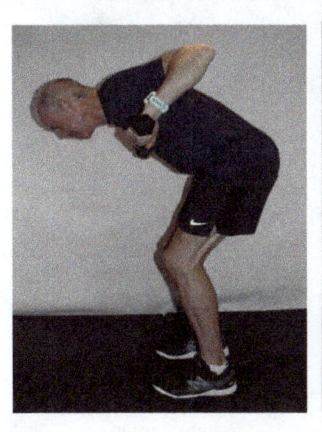

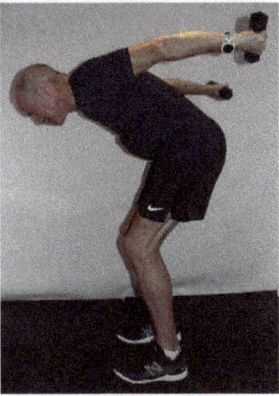

- Bend at the waist and lift elbows up so they are level with the trunk.

- Hands are pointing upward.

- Keep the elbows high as you extend the elbows (Kick back.)

- When you return to the starting position you flip the hands over so hands are facing downward

- Keeping the elbows high extend the elbows again (Flip gripped kick back.)

Palms Facing Downward

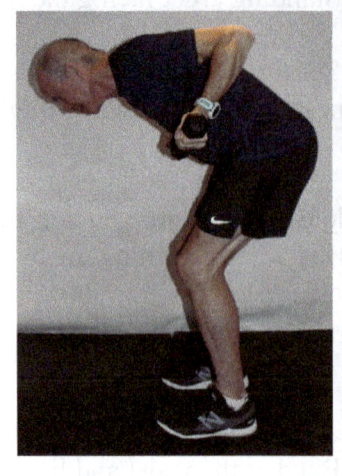

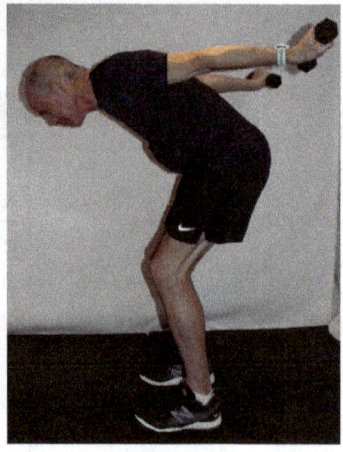

4. Sitting Two Arm Triceps Extension

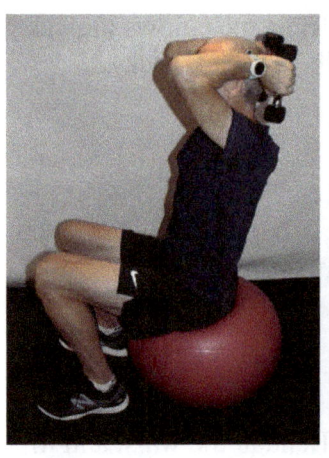

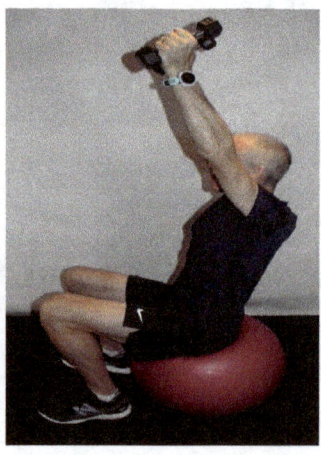

- Sitting erect on bench or stability ball place both arms over your head with elbows bent/flexed. Both Elbows are pointing as straight up/vertical as you shoulder flexibility allows.

- Extend both elbows and then return to starting position (flexed elbow.)

5. Sitting One Arm Triceps Extension

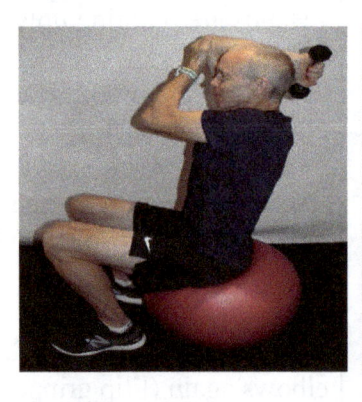

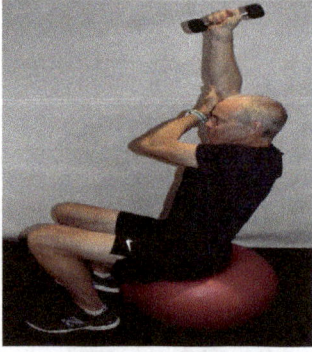

- Sitting erect on bench or stability ball place one arms over your head with elbow bent/flexed.

- The raised elbow is pointing straight up and supported by the opposite hand.

- Extend the elbow and then return to starting position (flexed elbow.)

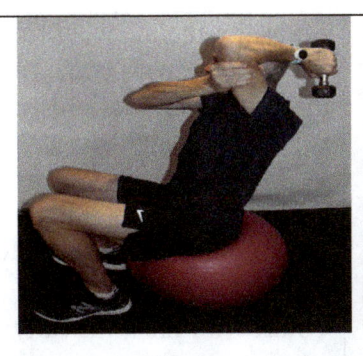

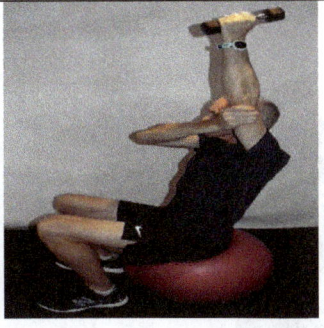

6. Throw the Bomb

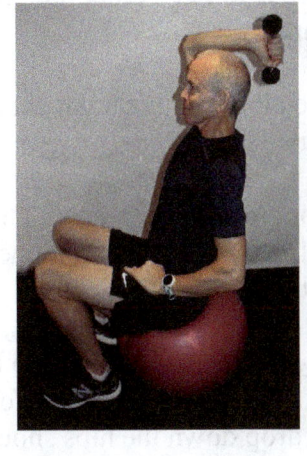

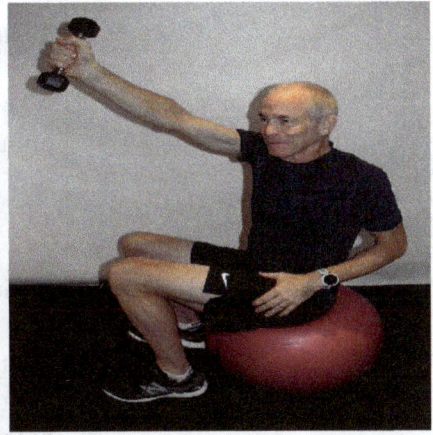

- Sitting erect on a bench or stability ball.

- Body is turned slightly to the raised arm side.

- The front arm is extended out in front of you or at your side and the opposite arm is raised with the weight to shoulder level with elbow bent.

- Initiate the motion by slightly rotating the body so your shoulders become square to the imaginary target as you extend the back elbow as if you were throwing a football or baseball.

7. Lying Two Arm Triceps Extension

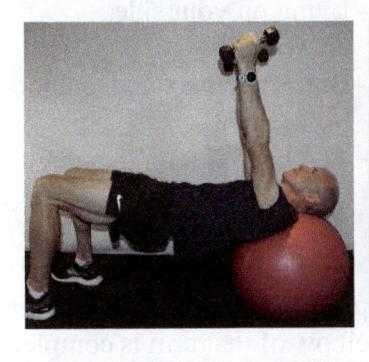

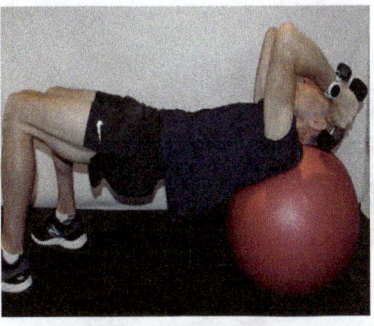

- Lying supine (flat) on bench or stability ball place both arms over your head so elbows are bent and pointing vertical at your head level.

- Extend both elbows and then return to flexed elbow position keeping the elbow pointing vertical

8. Lying One Arm Triceps Extension

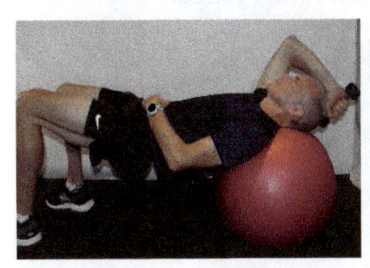

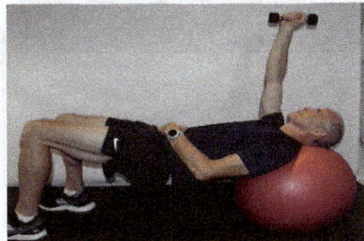

- Lying supine (flat) on bench or stability ball place one arm over your head so elbow is bend and pointing vertical.

- Extend the raised elbow and then return to flexed elbow starting position keeping the elbow pointing vertical.

- you can support the raised elbow with the opposite hand

9. Chair Dips

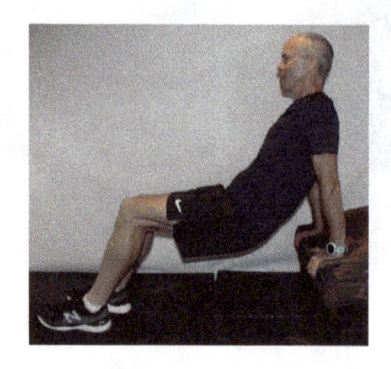

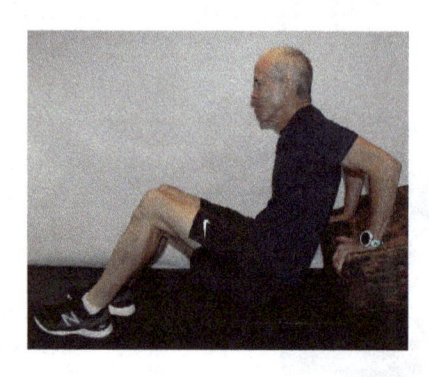

- Start by facing away from the edge of a bench/chair with both arms slightly wider than shoulder width resting on the edge of the bench/chair.

- The legs are either bent at the knees or fully extended in front of you (advanced).

- Start with the arms fully extended.

- Bend the elbows and slowly lower your buttocks to just before touching the ground.

- The elbow at this point should be bent about 90°.

- From this position extend the elbows and lift the buttocks up to the starting position.

Note - It is important not to let your hips drift too far from the bench/chair. As the hips drop down the hips should stay relatively close to the bench/chair to take stress off the shoulders.

10. Side Tri-Rise

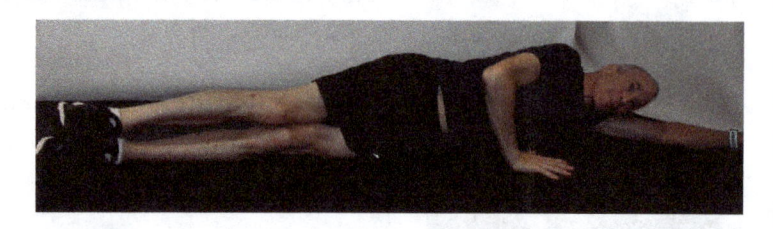

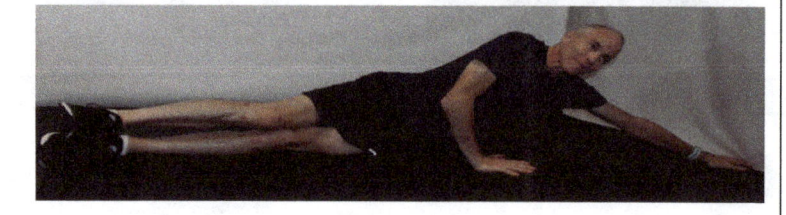

- Lying on your side.

- Bottom arm extended under your head.

- Top hand flat on the mat in front of your chest.

- Lift the upper body off the mat by pushing down on the front hand until elbow of that arm is completely straight. Bend elbow to return to starting position and then repeat.

11. Standing Resistance Band Triceps Extension 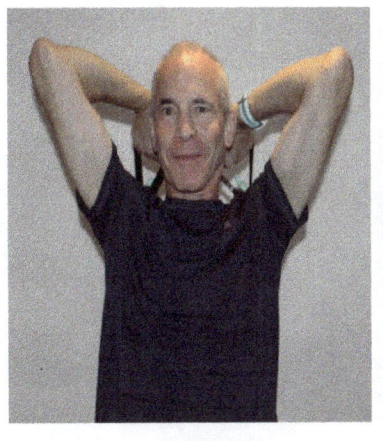	- Stand erect with back to high anchor. - Lift bent elbows high so they are at head level. - Keeping the elbows high straighten both elbows and then slowly bend them back to original starting position.
12. TRX Triceps Extension	- Standing with your back to the anchor - Lean forward and bend the elbows as far as you can - Straighten the elbows but keep the elbows as high as possible

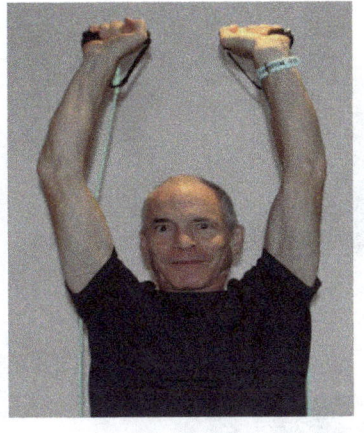

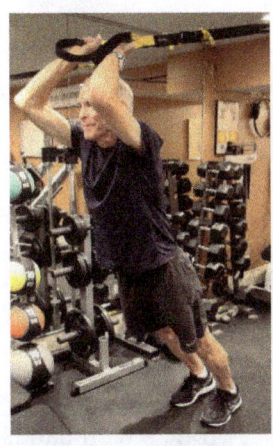

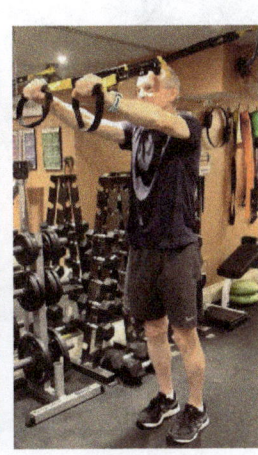

5. Lower Back Exercises (Also Covered under Core Exercises (Appendix .9.1.2.1.1)

1. Back Extensions (Isolate the back Erector Spinae muscles) (can be done on mat, Stability Ball or BOSU)

1. Back extensions Start 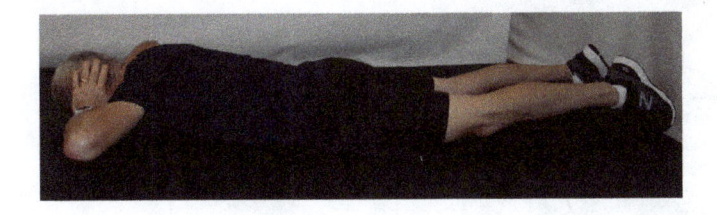	- <u>Prone</u> - hands behind head or resting on lower back - Lift chest off ground and return to the ground - can be done on BOSU or Stability Ball <u>Advanced</u>: 1. Oscillate with chest off the ground. 2. Lift legs off ground (chest stays flat on the ground)

Lift Chest off the Ground (feet stay on the ground)

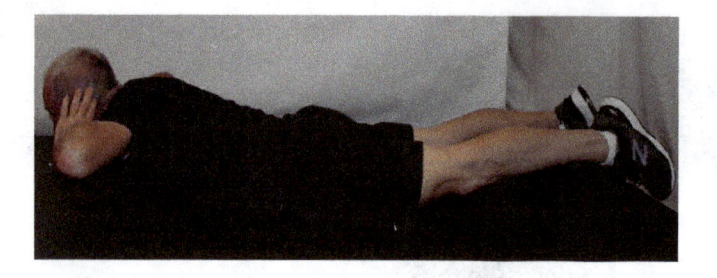

BOSU

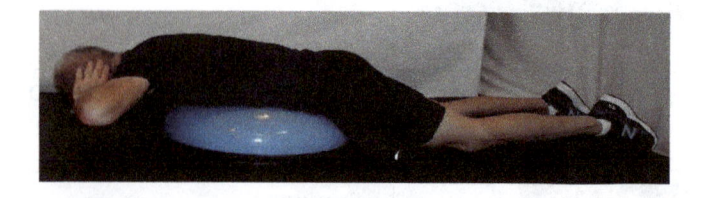

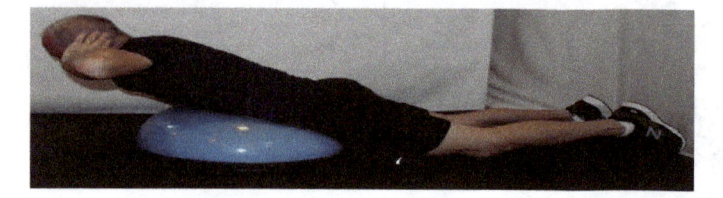

2. Back Extensions with Small Rotation

BOSU

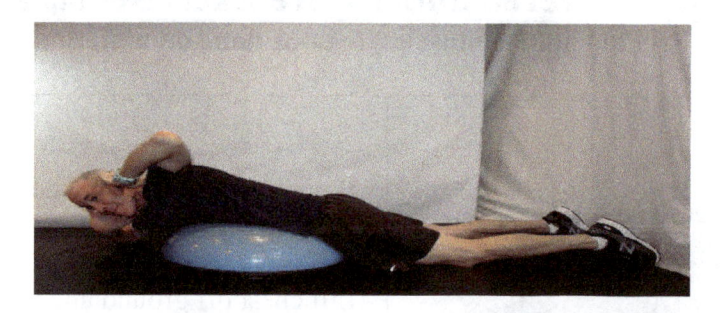

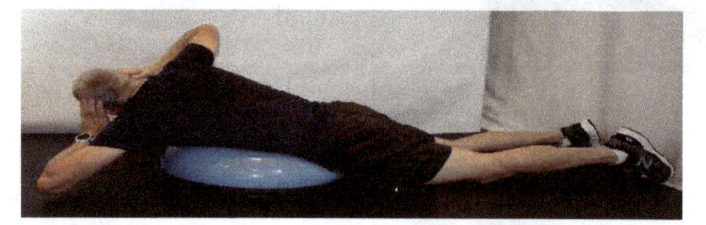

- <u>Prone</u> - with hands behind the head.

- Lift chest and rotate so elbow touches the floor, lower chest and repeat to the opposite side.

3. Superman's Chest and Feet off the ground 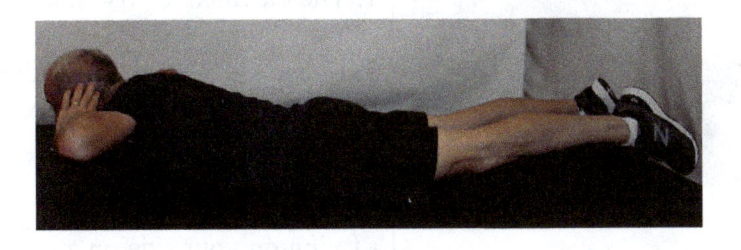	- Prone - with hands extended out in front of head, behind or beside the head or on small of back. - Lift chest and thighs off ground. (Advanced - oscillate with chest and thighs off the ground
2. Bridges 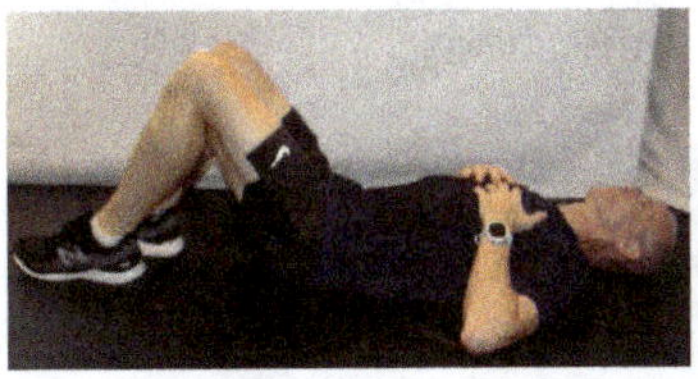 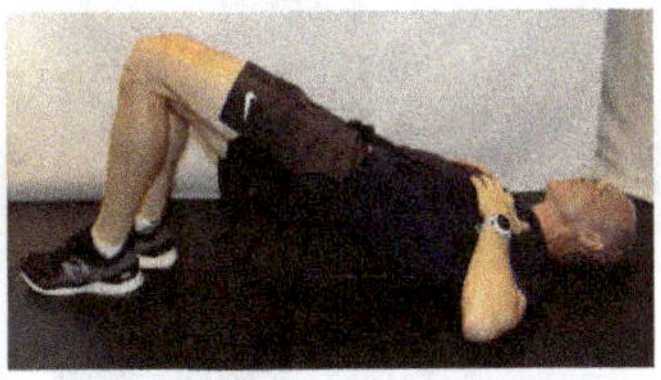 BOSU 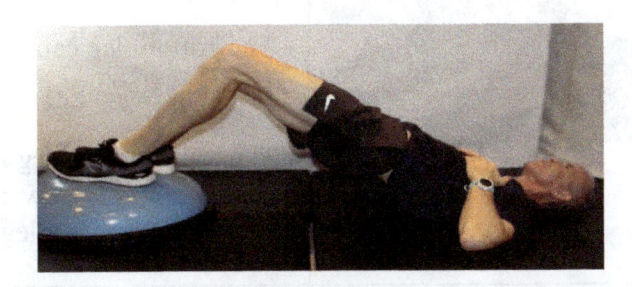 Stability Ball 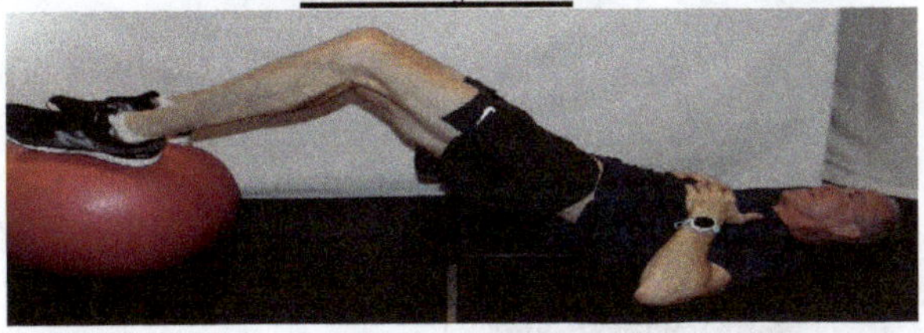	Supine - Both feet on ground, hands resting on lower abdominal. - Lift buttocks off mat and hold 5-10 sec. - Can put feet on SB, BOSU to perform the bridge Advanced: 1. Oscillate hips up and down while in bridge position. 2. Extend one leg while in bridge. 3. One leg bridge (other leg in figure 4 position).

6. Hips (Gluteus Medius, Gluteus Maximus, Tensor Facia Lata)

1. Prone Stability Ball Hip Extensions 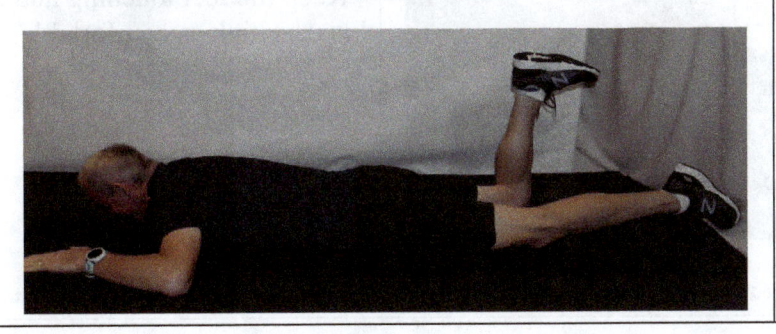	- Lying on floor or Stability Ball at lower abdominal area. - Have one leg touch the floor for stability. - Bend the opposite leg knee to 90° and lift to just past horizontal. - Lower the bent knee and repeat.

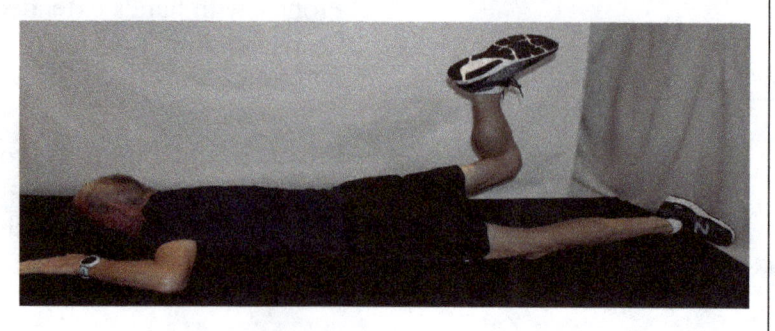

Advanced:
1. The elevated leg oscillates 4-6"

2. Use ankle weights for additional resistance when lifting the bent knee.

2. Side Lying Hip Abductions

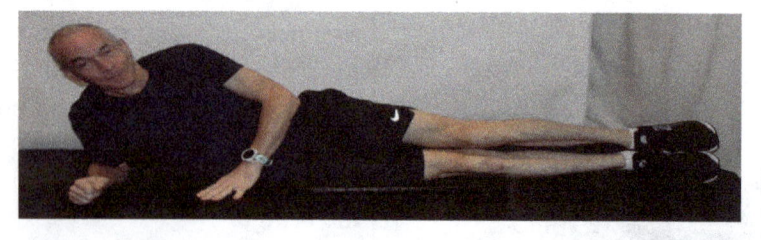

- Lying on your side on a mat.

- Bottom arm straight and supports the head or bent and forearm supports the upper body.

- The opposite arm lies along the side of the body.

- The legs are stacked one on top of the other.

- The bottom leg can be bent at 45° for additional stability.

- The top extended leg is lifted up as high as comfortable. - Lower the raised leg to just above the lower leg and repeat.

3. Clam Shell

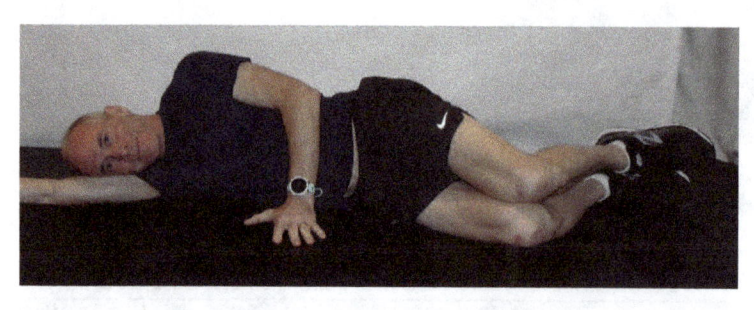

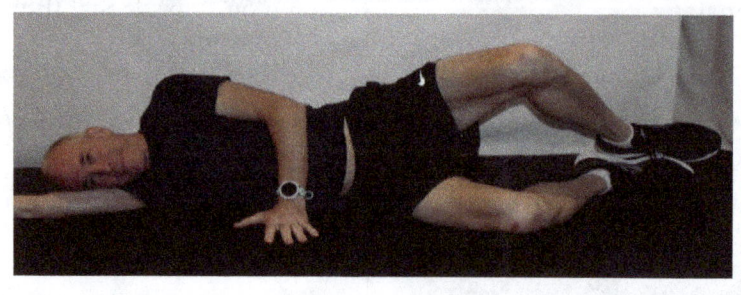

- Lying on your side on a mat.

- Bottom arm bent and supports the head

- The opposite arm lies along the side of the body or in front of the chest.

- The hips and knees are bent 45° and stacked on top of each other.

- Keep the feet touching and lift the top knee as high as comfortable.

Resistance Band 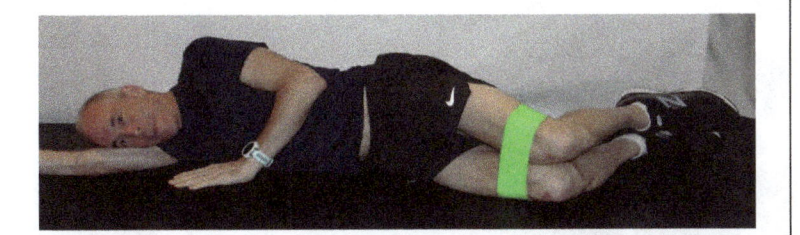 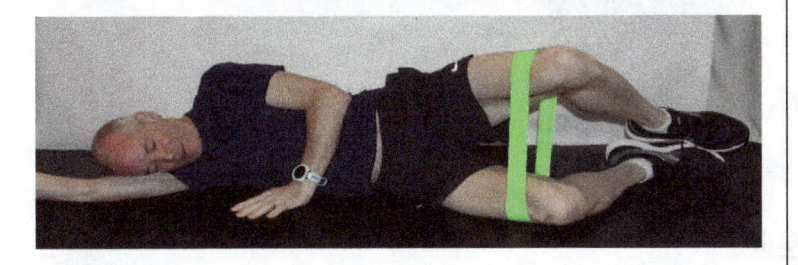	Advanced - Place resistance band around the knees
4. Fire Hydrant 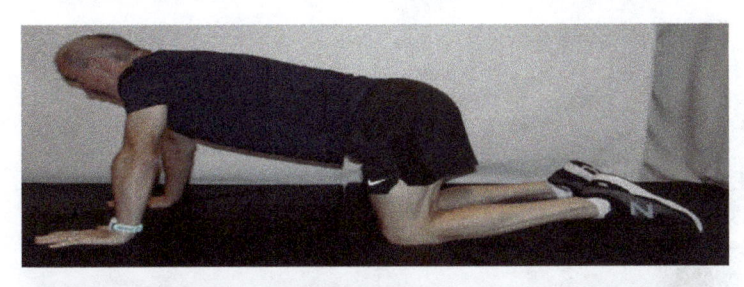 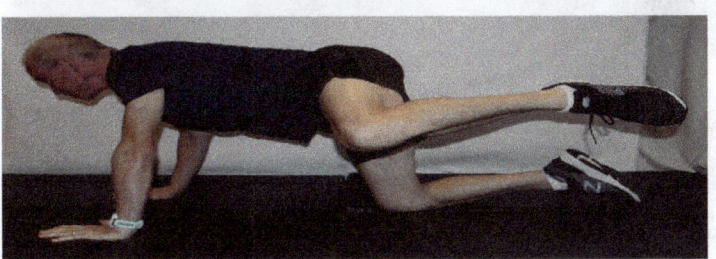 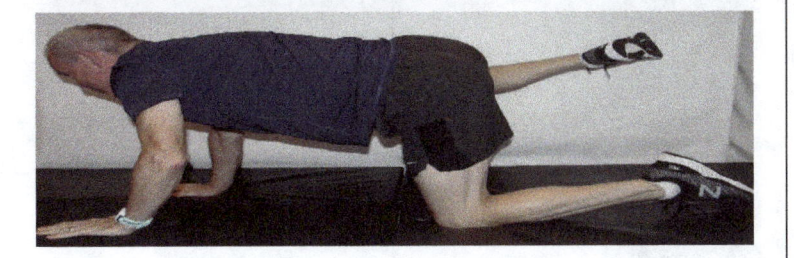	- Start on with hands and knees on the mat and abduct (lift sideways) one leg to horizontal position. Knee is bent 90°.

5. Resistance Band at Ankles Forward and Backward Walk

Forward Walk

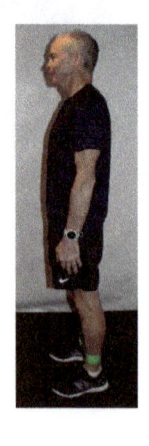

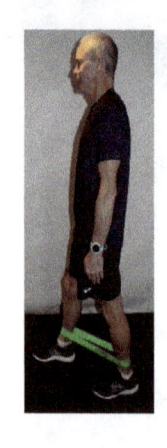

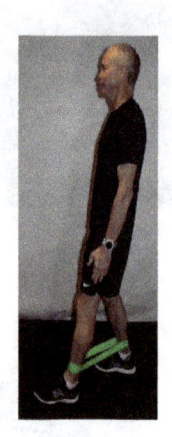

Backward Walk

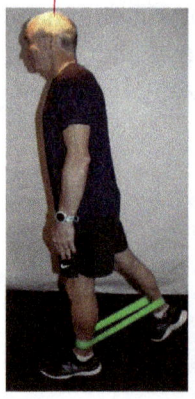

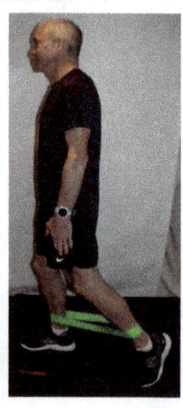

Resistance Band Above the Knees

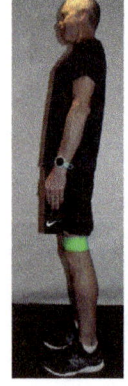

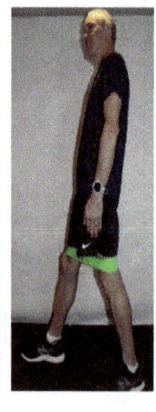

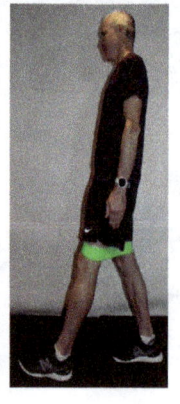

- Stand erect and place resistance band around both ankles.

- Walk forward with knees as straight as possible 10 steps and then walk backward with knees as straight as possible 10 steps.

Advanced
- Have resistance band on the thighs just above knee level

7. Resistance Band at Ankles Lateral Walk 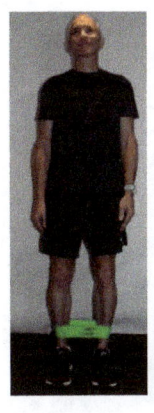 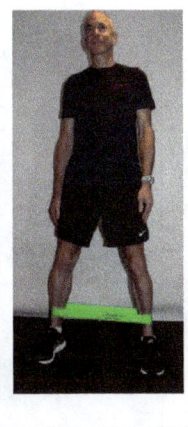 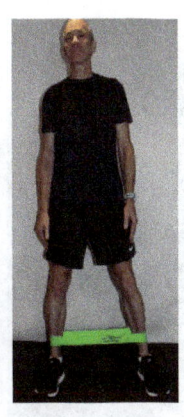	- Stand erect and place resistance band around both ankles. - Walk laterally with knees as straight as possible 10 steps, and then walk laterally in the opposite direction 10 steps with knees as straight as possible. Advanced - Have resistance band on thighs just above knee level.
8. Machine Hip abduction, 45º abduction and hip extension **45º Angle Abduction** 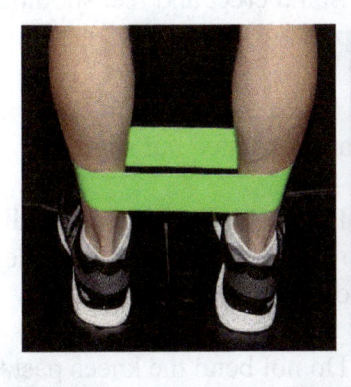 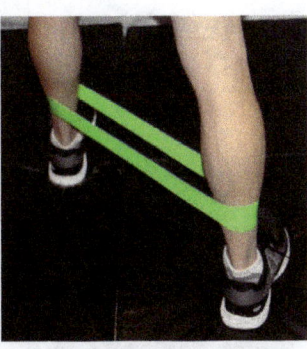	- Stand erect with foot in the loop. - step backward by abducting the hip (moving it laterally) at a 45º angle.
9. Machine Leg Press and Squat **Leg Press**	- Don't bend the knees greater than 90º.

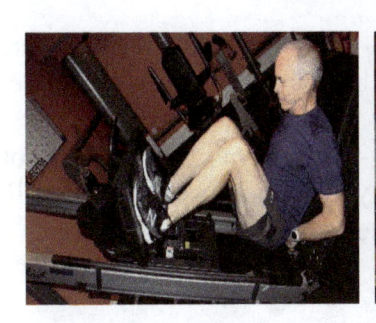

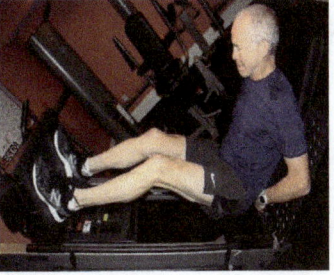

Machine Squat

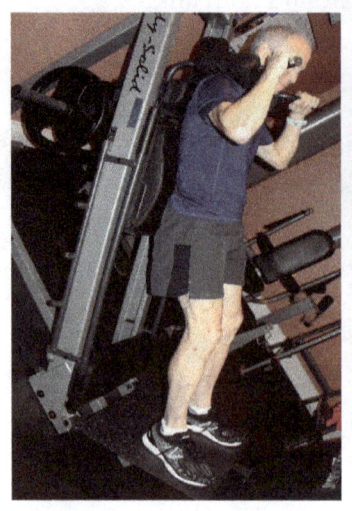

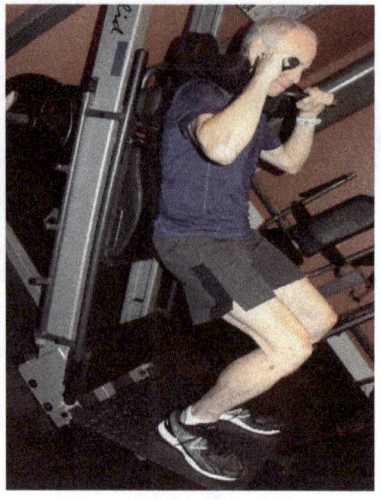

10. Squats

Standard Squat   **Squat with Weights**

- Stand erect and feet shoulder width apart.

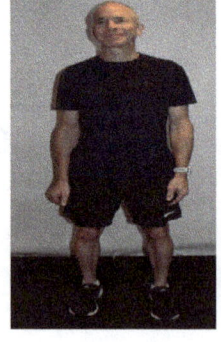

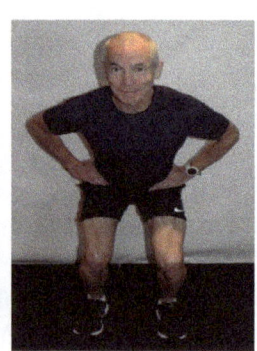

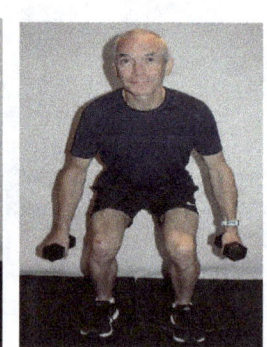

- The knees can be pointing straight or can be rotated out slightly.

- Begin the exercise by bending the knees to a depth that is comfortable. (Pretend you are sitting in a chair.)

- Do not bend the knees past 90º.

- The knees should not go forward past your toes.

- Your chest will lean forward slightly for balance as you move into the squat.

- You may extend the arms out in front of you for additional stability. Return to erect position and repeat.

Advanced:

1. Weights in your hands

2. Squat on an unstable surface like a BOSU or wobble board

Sumo Squat

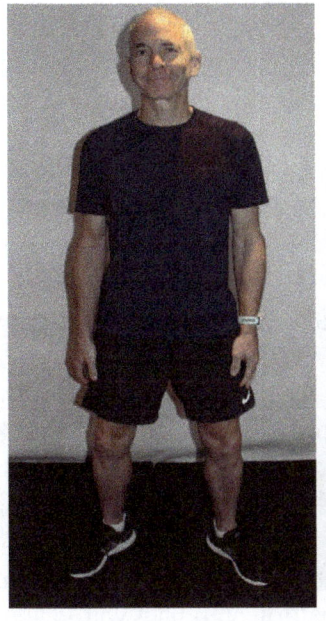

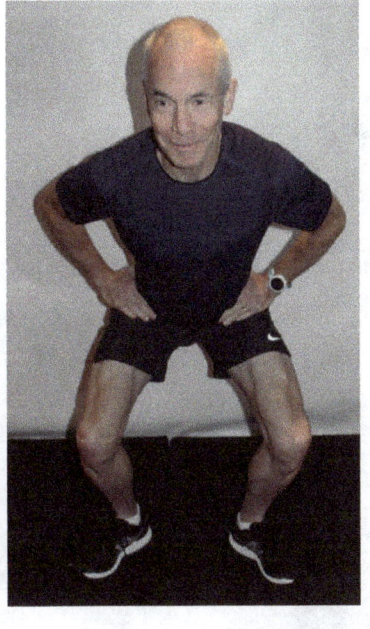

Variations of standard Squat:

1. <u>Stability ball between the lower back and wall</u> as you do the squat

2. <u>Sumo Squat</u> - Feet are wider and feet and knees point out 45º.

11. Lunges

Forward Lunge

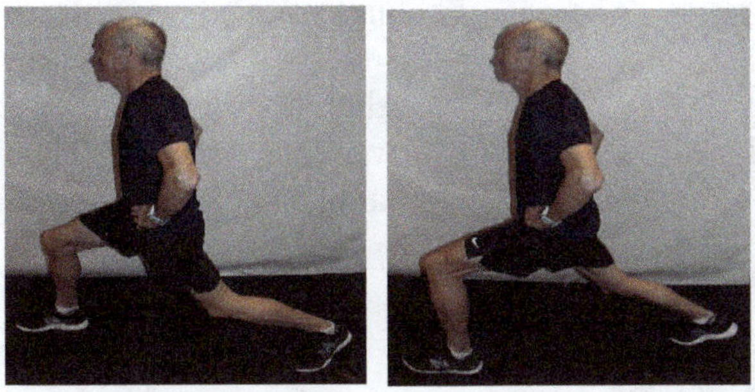

Horizontal Twist

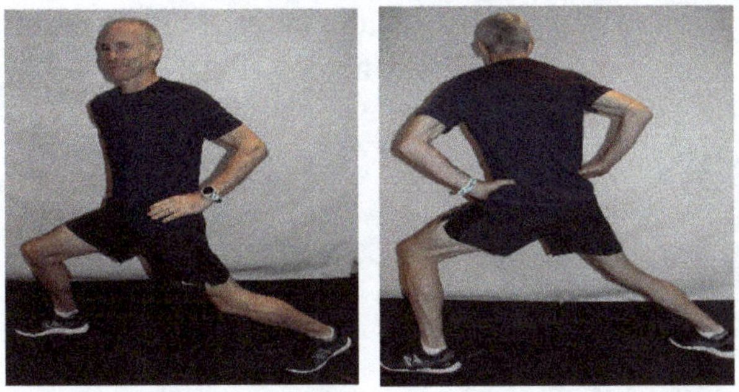

- Stand erect and feet shoulder width apart.

- Step forward with one leg and bend the knee no farther than 90º (back leg knee almost touches the ground).

- The knee should not go forward pass the toes.

- Your back should stay erect as you go deep into the lunge.

Advanced:

1. <u>Weights</u> in your hands

2. <u>Horizontal twist</u> to one side

3. <u>Vertical twist</u> so one arm reaches to the sky and the opposite touches the floor.

4. <u>Elevating both arms</u> above the head.

5. Forward lunge onto an <u>unstable surface</u> like a BOSU

Vertical Twist

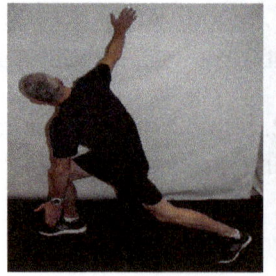

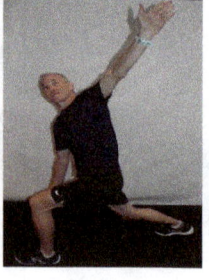

Elevated Arms

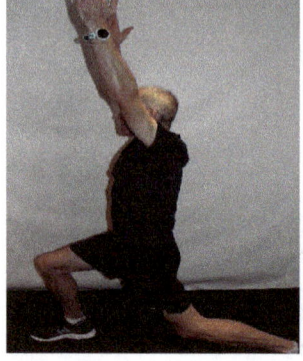

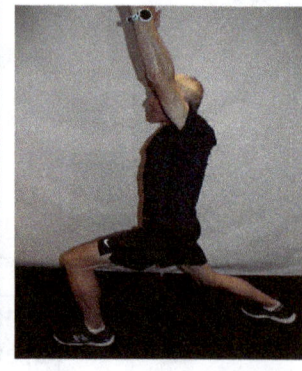

Lateral Lunge

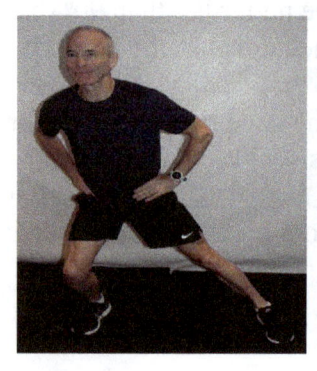

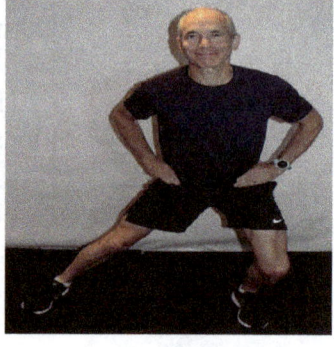

Variations of Standard Lunge:

1. <u>Alternating Leg Pulse Lunge</u> - once in lunge position go up and down about 2-4 inches rather than returning to erect position immediately. Do not do the pulses fast.

2. <u>Walking Forward Lunge</u> - continue to walk forward with each lunge.

3. <u>Alternating Leg Backward Lunge</u> - from erect position step backwards and lunge and repeat with opposite leg

4. <u>Alternating Leg Backward Cross Over Lunge (Cutesy Lunge)</u> - from erect position step backwards and cross the rear leg behind the front leg and then proceed to do a lunge.

5. <u>Rear Foot Elevated Lunge (Balanced Lunge)</u> – put one foot on a chair or bench behind you and perform a lunge.

6. <u>Alternating Leg Lateral Lunge</u> - facing forward step laterally. The foot and knee should be angled out about 45º.

12. Alternating Leg Step Ups

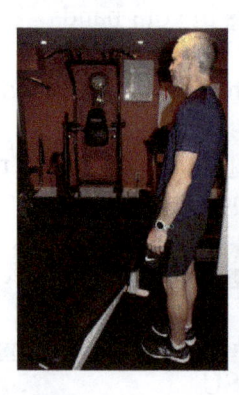

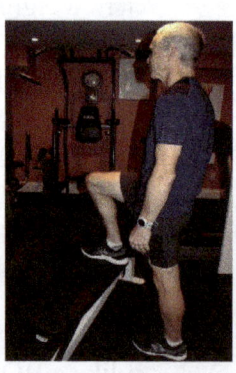

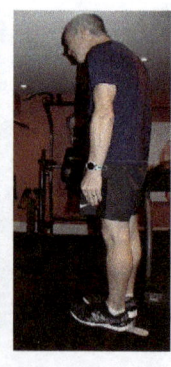

- Stand erect and step up onto an elevated surface of 12-18".

7. Legs (Quadriceps, Hamstrings, Calves, Tibialis Anterior)

Please Note – Alternating step-ups, squats and lunges, which are covered under hip exercises, are multi leg muscle exercises and therefore activate the leg muscles (quads, hamstrings, gastroc and soleus) as well as the hip musculature (gluts and hip flexors)

1. Quadriceps:

1. Machine Single or Double Leg Extensions **Start**　　　　**Double Leg** **Single Leg**	- Focus on complete extension of the leg with a slight a pause before returning to starting position.
2. Alternating Leg Step ups	- Stand erect and step up onto an elevated surface of 12-18".

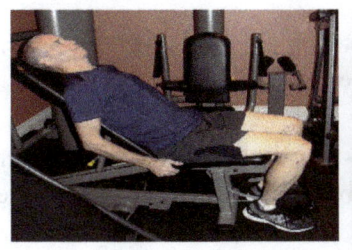

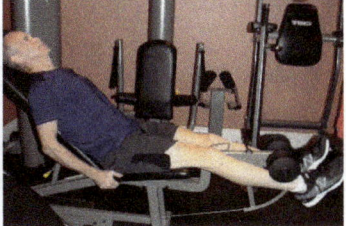

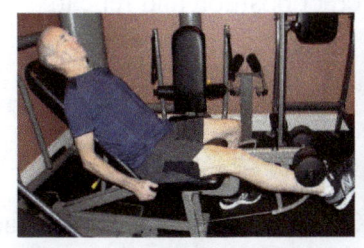

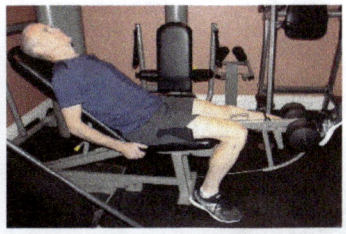

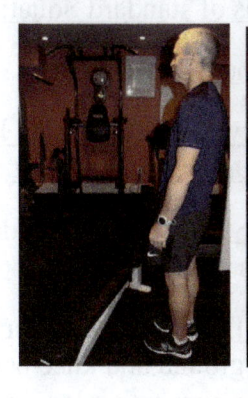

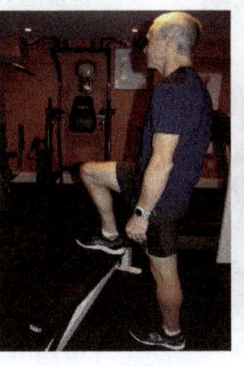

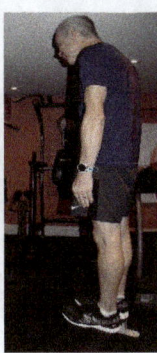

3. Squats

Standard Squat   **Squat with Weights**

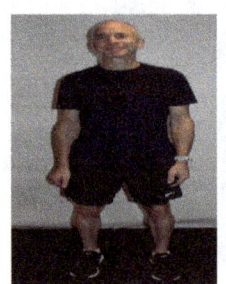

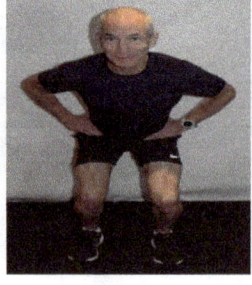

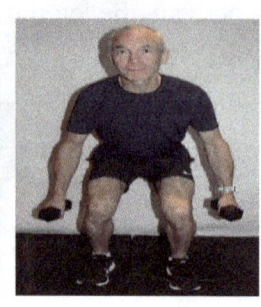

Sumo Squat

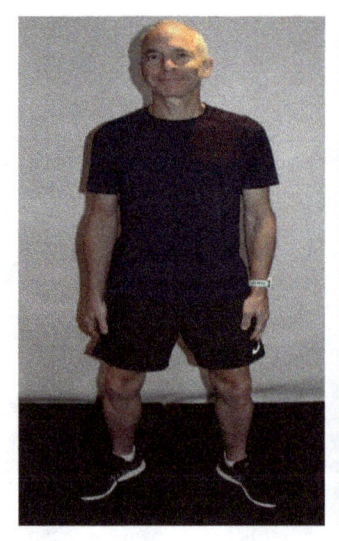

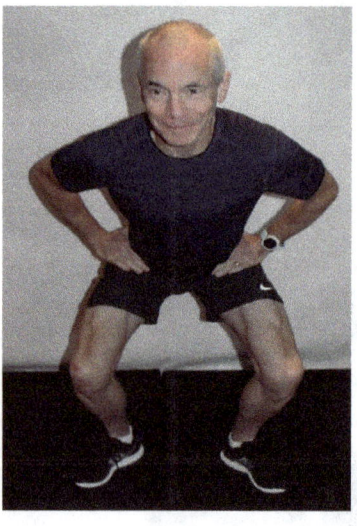

- Stand erect and feet shoulder width apart.

- The knees can be pointing straight or can be rotated out slightly.

- Begin the exercise by bending the knee to a depth that is comfortable. Do not bend the knees past $90º$.

- Pretend you are sitting in a chair.

- The knees should not go forward past your toes.

- Your chest will lean forward slightly for balance as you move into the squat.

- You may extend the arms out in front of you for additional stability. Return to erect position and repeat.

Advanced:

1. Weights in your hands.

2. Squat on an unstable surface like a BOSU or balance board.

Variations of standard Squat:

1. Machine Squat

2. Stability ball between the lower back and wall as you do the squat

3. Sumo Squat - Feet are wider and feet and knees point out $45º$.

4. Single Leg Squats - non supporting leg is off the ground and knee bent, wrapped around the supporting leg, in a figure four position across the supporting leg or extended out in front of you (Pistol squat and does not touch the ground.

5. Pulse Squat - Once deep into your squat rather than returning to erect position you go up and down about 2-4 inches. Do not do the pulses too fast.

4. Lunges

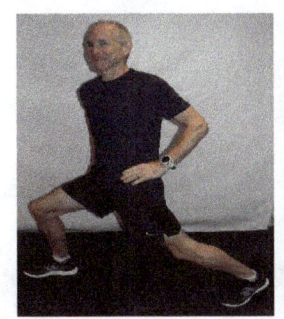

Forward Lunge

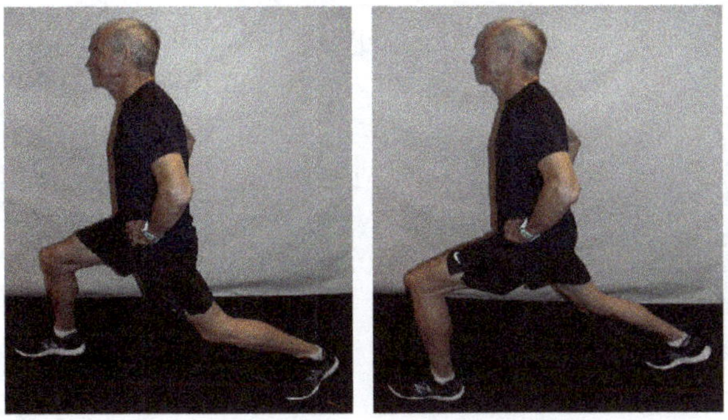

Horizontal Twist

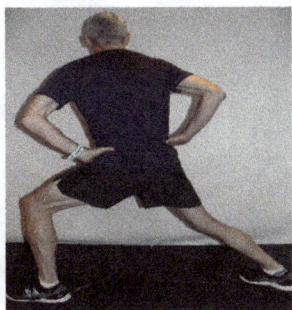

Vertical Twist

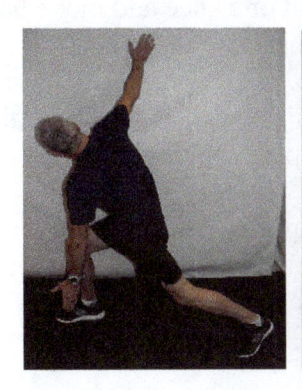

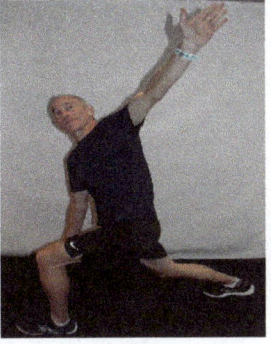

- Stand erect and feet shoulder width apart.

- Step forward with one leg and bend the knee no farther than 90º (back leg knee almost touches the ground).

- The knee should not go forward pass the toes.

- Your back should stay erect as you go deep into the lunge.

Advanced:

1. Weights in your hands.

2. Horizontal twist to one side or both sides.

3. Vertical twist so one arm reaches to the sky and the opposite touches the floor.

4. Elevating both arms above the head.

5. Forward lunge onto an unstable surface like a BOSU

Variations of Standard Lunge:

1. <u>Alternating leg Pulse Lunge</u> - once in lunge position, go up and down about 2-4 inches rather than returning to erect position immediately. (Do not do the pulses fast.)

2. <u>Walking Forward Lunge</u> - continue to walk forward with each lunge.

3. <u>Alternating Leg Backward Lunge</u> - from erect position step backwards and lunge and repeat with opposite leg.

4. <u>Alternating Leg Backward Cross Over Lunge (Cutesy Lunge)</u> - from erect position step backwards and across the

Elevated Arms

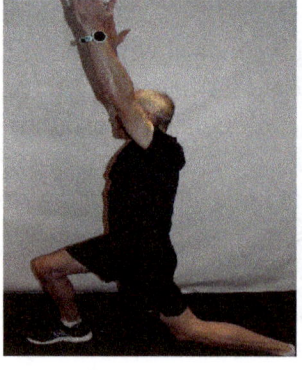

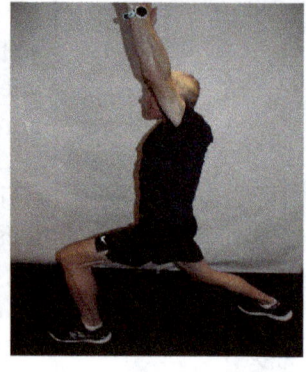

Lateral Lunge

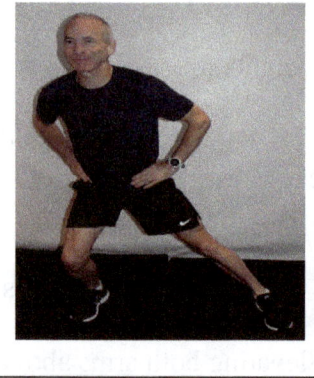

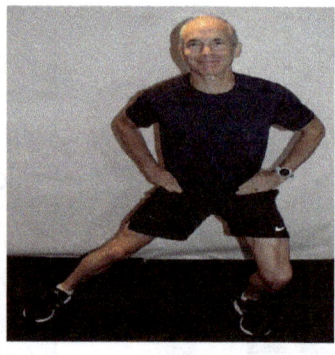

rear leg behind the front leg and then proceed to do a lunge.

5. <u>Rear Foot Elevated Lunge (Balanced Lunge)</u> - put one foot on a chair or bench behind you and perform a lunge.

6. <u>Alternating Leg Lateral Lunge</u> - facing forward step laterally. The foot and knee should be angle out about 45º.

2. Hamstrings:

1. Standing Hamstring Curl

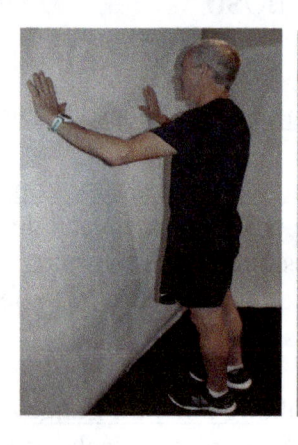

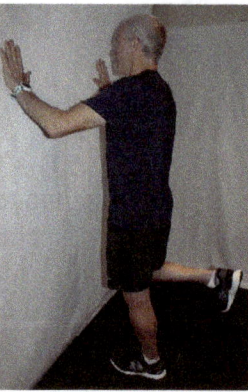

- Stand erect and face the wall and place hands at chest level against wall for balance.

- Bend one knee and move heel toward buttocks.

- Don't bend the knee more than 100º (Just past horizontal.)

<u>Advanced</u>
- Use ankle weights for increased resistance.

2. Machine Single of Double Hamstring Curl **Start** 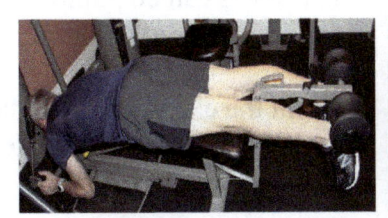 **Double Leg** 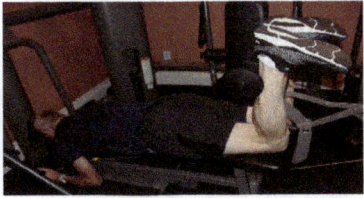 **Single Leg** 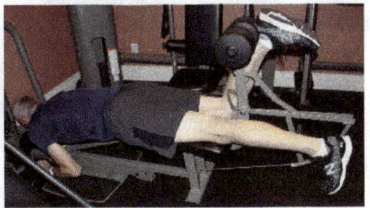	- It is important not to curl the legs pass 100º (just past vertical for the leg).
3. Stability Ball Hamstring Curl 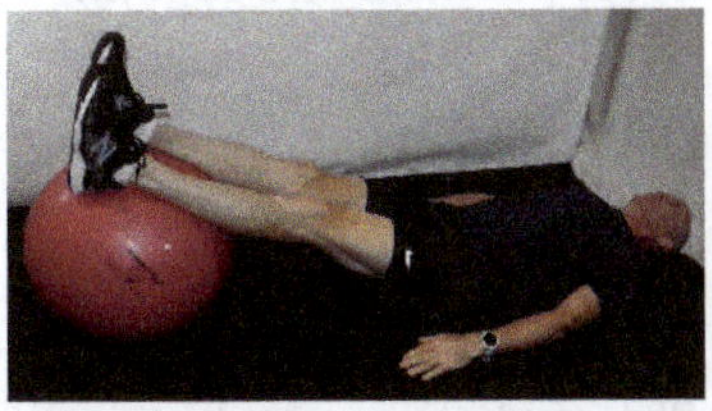 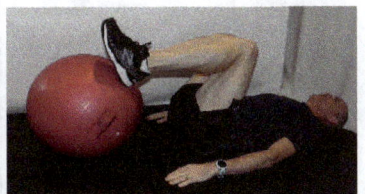	- Lying on your back place your lower calves and heels on a stability ball. - Lift your hips into a bridge position and then roll the stability ball toward you. - Hold for 1 sec and then return to bridge position and repeat.
4. Dead Lifts 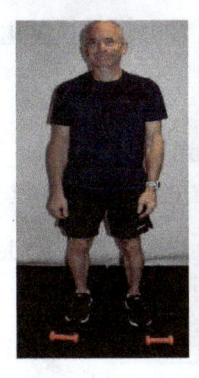 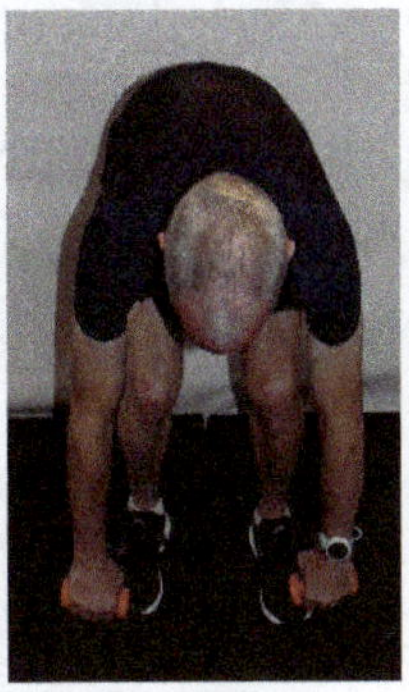 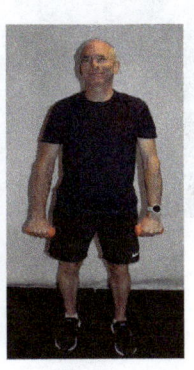	- Stand with your mid-foot under the barbell or dumbbell and bend over and grab the weight. - Lift your chest up and straighten your lower back. <u>Note</u> - Do not hold your breath as you are lifting the weight - Hold the weight for a second in the extended back position. - Return the weight to the floor by moving your hips back while bending your legs. Avoid bending at the waist. <u>Note</u> - It is important that your lower back stay in neutral position to avoid injury

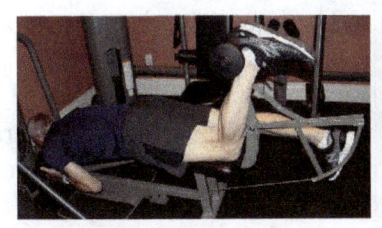

5. Squats

Standard Squat **Squat with Weights**

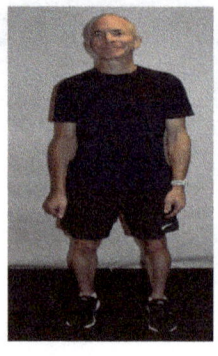

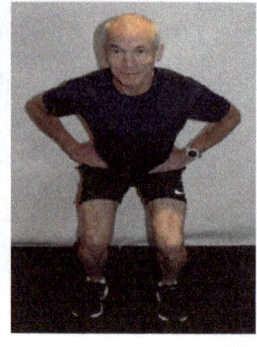

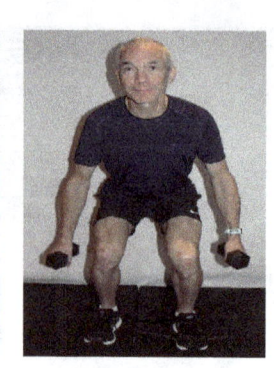

Sumo Squat

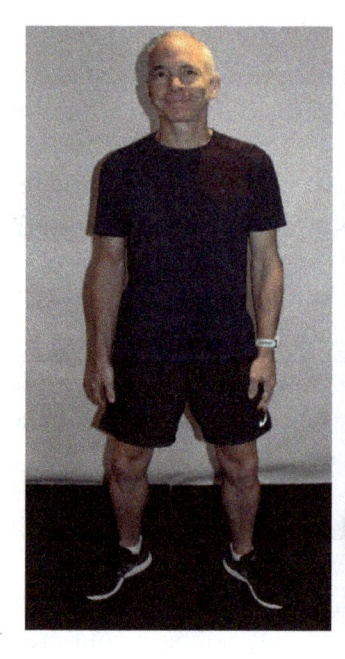

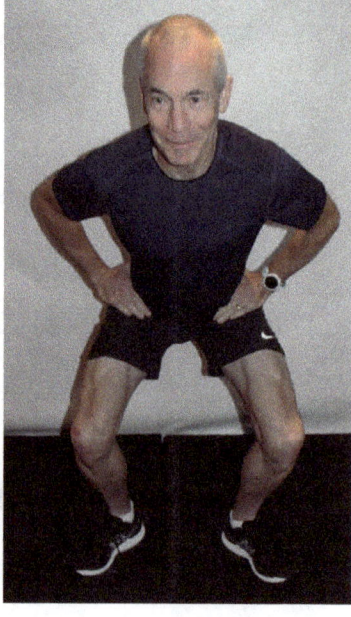

- Stand erect and feet shoulder width apart.

- The knees can be pointing straight or can be rotated out slightly.

- Begin the exercise by bending the knee to a depth that is comfortable. Do not bend the knees past 90º.

- Pretend you are sitting in a chair.

- The knees should not go forward past your toes.

- Your chest will lean forward slightly fo balance as you move into the squat.

- You may extend the arms out in front o you for additional stability. Return to erect position and repeat.

Advanced:

1. Weights in your hands.

2. Squat on a unstable surface like a BOSU or balance board.

Variations of standard Squat:

1. Machine Squat

2. Stability ball between the lower back and wall as you do the squat

3. Sumo Squat - feet are wider and feet and knees point out 45º.

4. Single Leg Squats - non supporting leg is off the ground and knee bent, wrapped around the supporting leg, in a figure fou position across the supporting leg or extended out in front of you (Pistol squat and does not touch the ground.

5. Pulse Squat - once deep into your squa rather than returning to erect position you go up and down about 2-4 inches. Do not do the pulses too fast.

6. Lunges

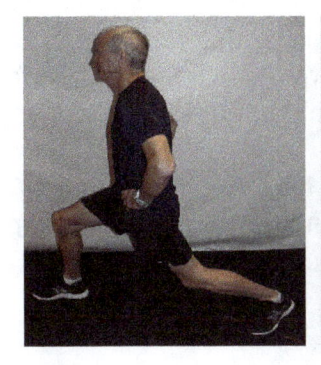

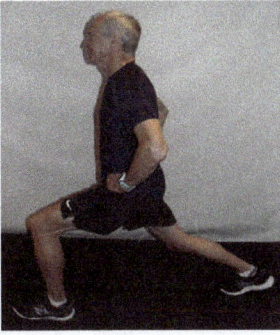

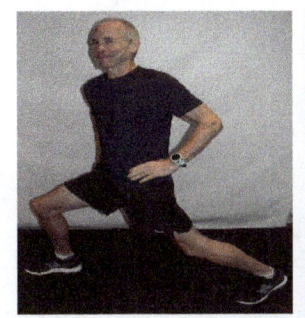

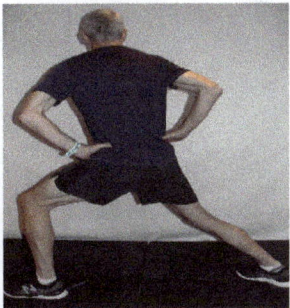

Forward Lunge

Horizontal Twist

Vertical Twist

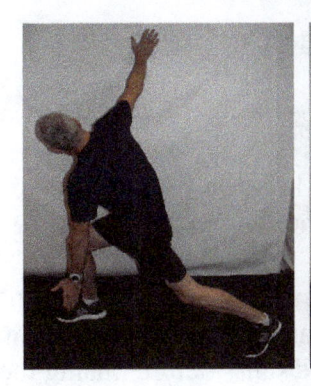

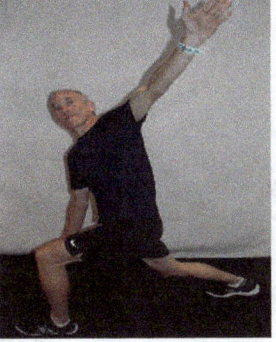

- Stand erect and feet shoulder width apart.
- Step forward with one leg and bend the knee no farther than 90º (back leg knee almost touches the ground).
- The knee should not go forward pass the toes.
- Your back should stay erect as you go deep into the lunge.

Advanced:

1. Weights in your hands.

2. Horizontal twist to one side or both sides.

3. Vertical twist so one arm reaches to the sky and the opposite touches the floor.

4. Elevating both arms above the head.

5. Forward lunge onto an unstable surface like a BOSU.

Variations of Standard Lunge:

1. Alternating Leg Pulse Lunge - once in lunge position go up and down about 2-4 inches rather than returning to erect position immediately (do not do the pulses fast).

2. Walking Forward Lunge - continue to walk forward with each lunge.

3. Alternating Leg Backward Lunge - from erect position step backwards and lunge and repeat with opposite leg

4. Alternating Leg Backward Cross Over Lunge (Cutesy Lunge) - from erect position step backwards and across the rear leg behind the front leg and then proceed to do a lunge.

Elevated Arms

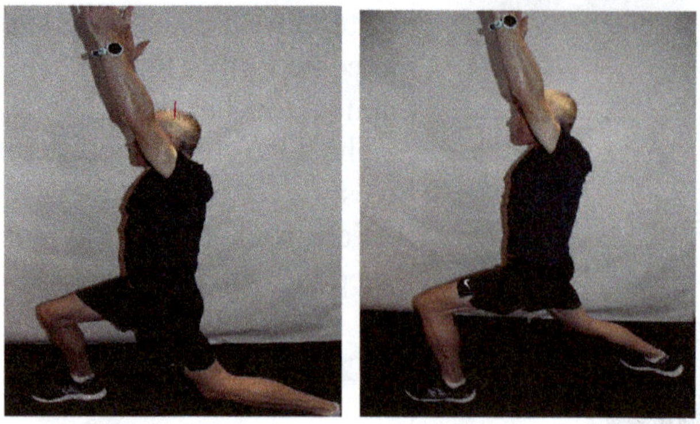

Lateral Lunge

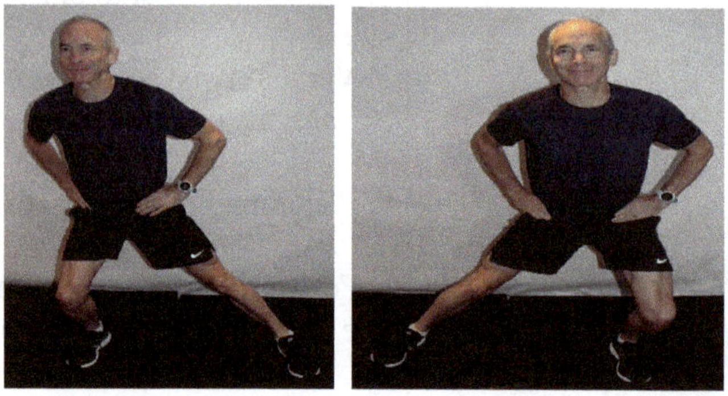

3. Calves

1. Single or Double Standing or Seated Heel Raise

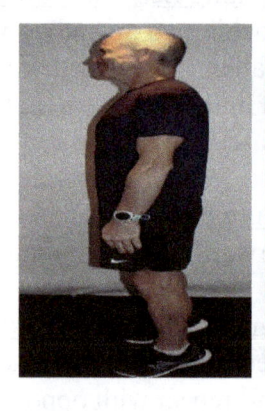

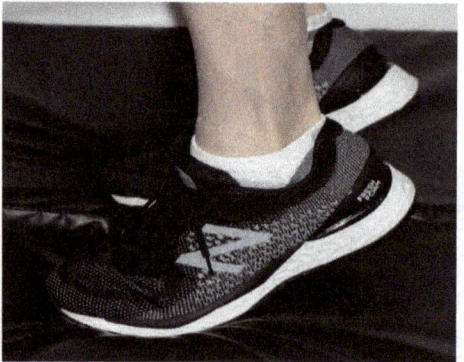

2. Toe Walking

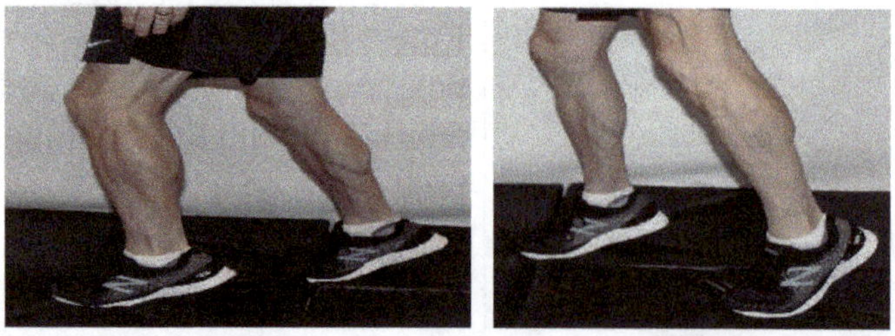

5. <u>Rear Foot Elevated Lunge (Balanced Lunge)</u> - put one foot on a chair or bench behind you and perform a lunge.

6. <u>Alternating Leg Lateral Lunge</u> - facing forward step laterally. The foot and knee should be angle out about 45º.

7. <u>Alternating Leg Rotational Lunge</u> - facing forward and rotate hips and trunk 90º and step into a lunge.

- Stand erect and stand on your toes, hold for 1-2 sec and return to starting position.

<u>Advanced</u>:

1. <u>Toes walking</u> - focus on keeping your heels high as you walk.
- Do beside a wall in case you lose your balance.

2. <u>Single or Double Heel Raise</u> - on edge of stairs. Drop your heels lower than edge of the stairs before raising the heels up.

4. Tibialis Anterior

1. Standing Toe Raises 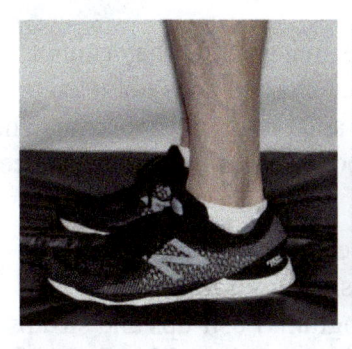 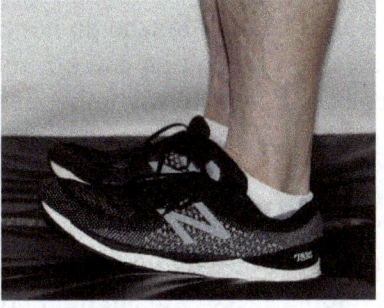	- Stand erect. Use wall or chair for stability. Raise your toes as high off the ground as possible.
2. Walking Toe Raise 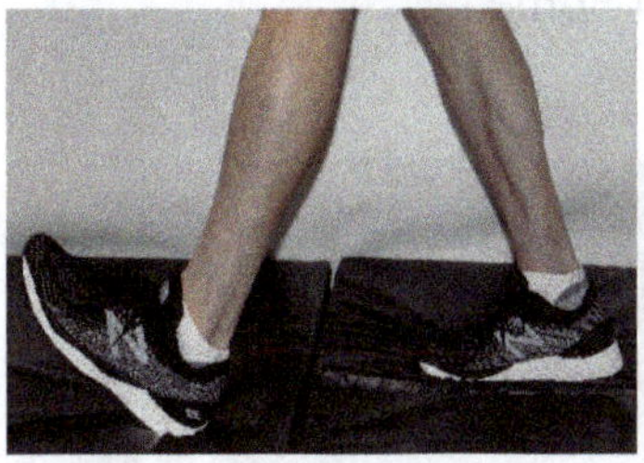 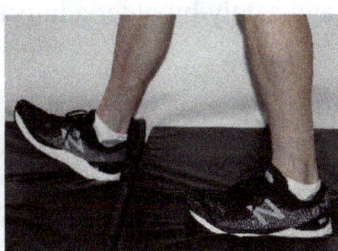	- Walk on your heels with the toes as high in the air as possible for 10 steps. - Do beside a wall in case you lose your balance.

Appendix 9.1.2.3. Introduction to Bodyweight Muscle Strength Training

One of the most common excuses used by people who do not exercise is that they cannot afford a gym membership or buy home exercise equipment. Fortunately, one does not need to spend money on either of these to get a good muscle strengthening and endurance workout. The solution is simple and not fancy. A person needs only to use their body weight as the resistance.

By utilizing one's body weight as the load and implementing the "overload" principle of strength training (a greater than normal stress or load on the body is required for training adaptation to occur), a person can develop a successful strength program. Push-ups and sit-ups are the most commonly known and used bodyweight strength training exercises. This form of resistance training is excellent at developing tone and endurance in the muscles. Most importantly, it can be done efficiently and safely by older adults at home.

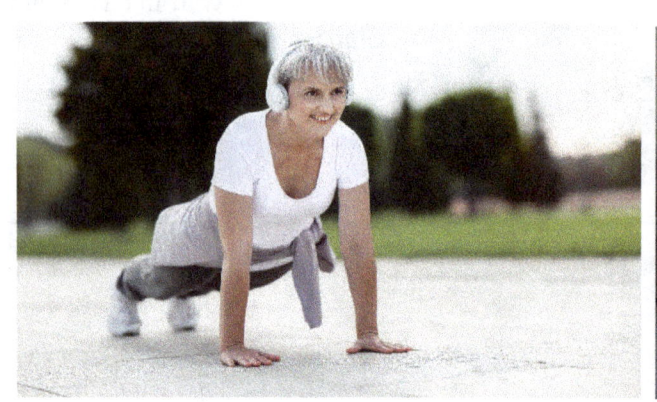

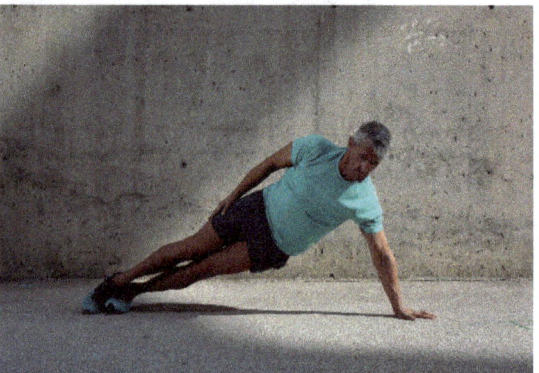

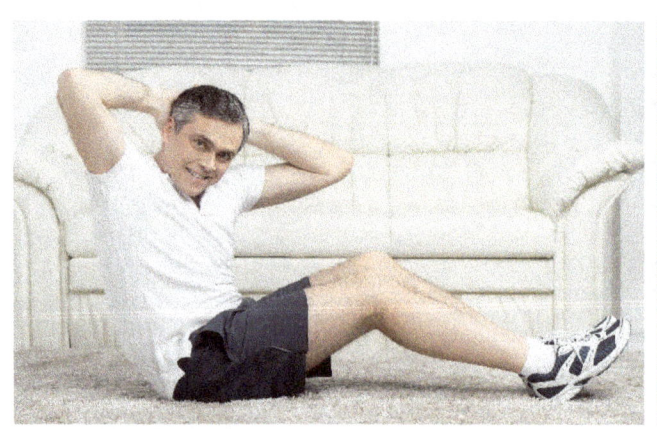

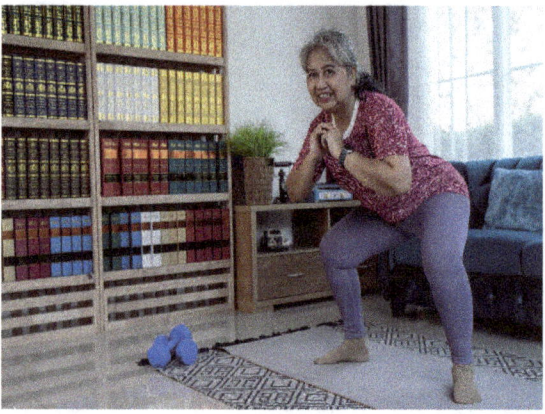

Appendix 9.1.2.3.1: Bodyweight Muscle Strengthening Exercises Described and Illustrated

Most of these exercises have several variations/modifications that can be performed to make them more or less challenging.

Name	Muscle Group	Description
1. Chest		
1. Push-Ups Regular	Chest (Pectoralis Major and Minor), Triceps and Biceps	- In a prone (face down) position, the body is raised and lowered using the arms while the back remains straight and the toes remain on the ground.
Easier Push-Up Modifications:		
1. Knee Assisted		1. Knees are resting on the ground.
2. Push Against a Wall		2. Push-up against a bench or wall. Hands are at shoulder level.

Harder Push-up Modifications:		
1. Feet on an Incline		- Feet are on an incline so the upper body must now support more weight.
2. Underneath the Fence		- Simulate going forward under a fence as you do your push-up. - Return to starting position by pretending you are going backward underneath a fence.
3. Diamonds		- The hands are shaped as a diamond (thumbs and index fingers touch) under the chest.

4. Wide-fly		- The hands are 3" wider than normal or as wide a s feels comfortable.
5. Military		- The hands underneath the shoulders & arms and elbows tight to the ribs.
6. Alternate Speed		- Perform regular push-ups 4 repetitions fast (1 count down and 1 count up) & 4 repetitions slow (4 counts down and 4 counts up).
7. Side-to-Side		- Move arms to one side and do push-up & then move arms to opposite side & do push-up.

8. One-Arm Balance		- Following a push-up rotate body so one arm is pointing skyward and balance on one arm & then repeat the rotation on the other side after a full push-up.
9. BOSU or Stability Ball (Unstable Surface) **Stability Ball** **BOSU** **Dome side up** **Dome side down**		- Push-up on unstable surface. Hands or feet can be on the unstable surface.
2. Arms		
1. Dips	Triceps and shoulders (Trapezius)	- Facing away from bench or chair & hands resting on bench/chair. - With arms extended and the shoulders positioned above the hands, lower the body until the arms are

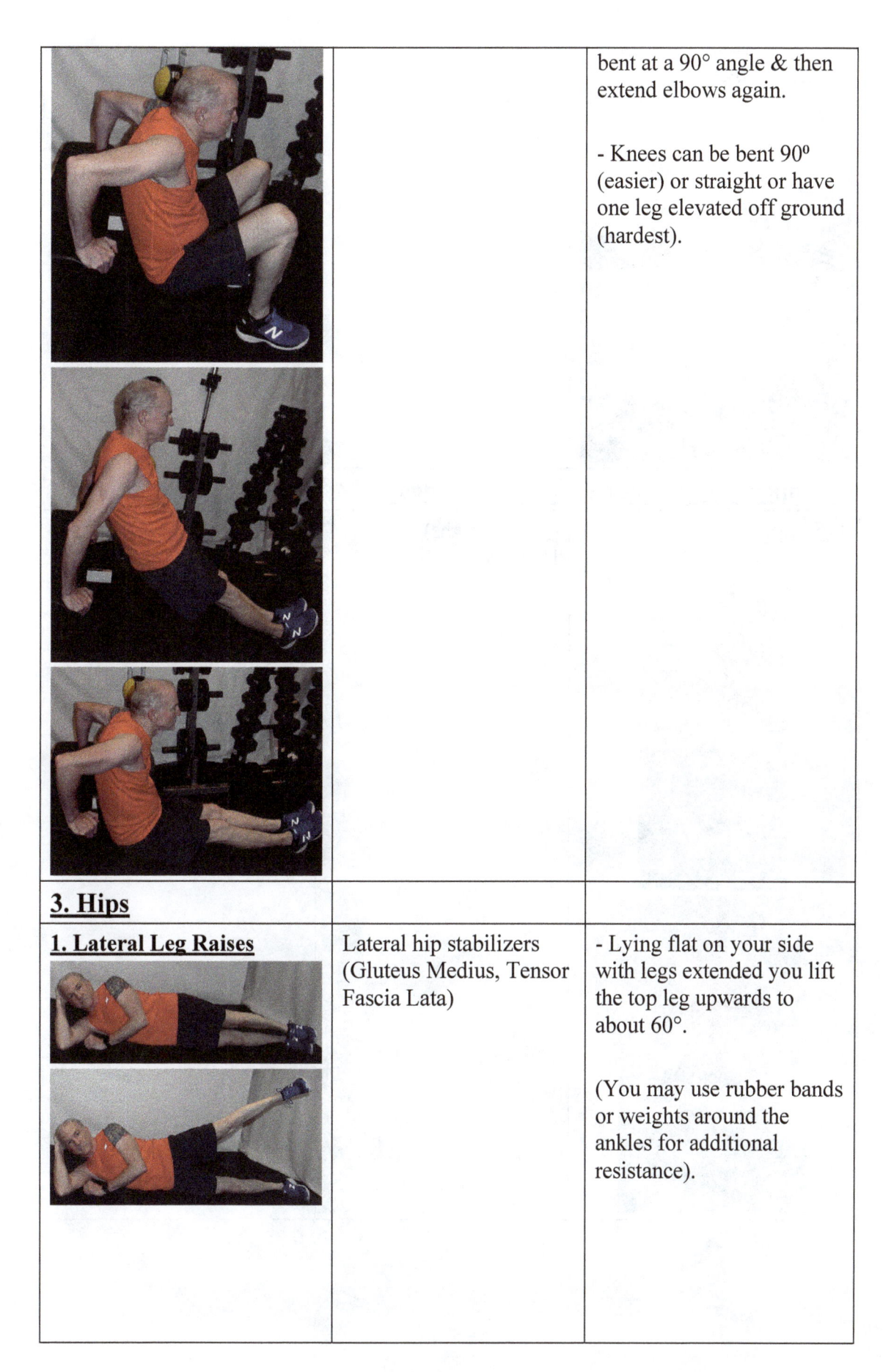

		bent at a 90° angle & then extend elbows again. - Knees can be bent 90º (easier) or straight or have one leg elevated off ground (hardest).
3. Hips		
1. Lateral Leg Raises	Lateral hip stabilizers (Gluteus Medius, Tensor Fascia Lata)	- Lying flat on your side with legs extended you lift the top leg upwards to about 60°. (You may use rubber bands or weights around the ankles for additional resistance).

| 2. Hip Extensions | Hip extensors (Gluteus Medius and Maximus) | Lying on your hands and knees.
-with the knee bent 90º lift one foot/leg toward sky keeping
- repeat with other foot/leg. |

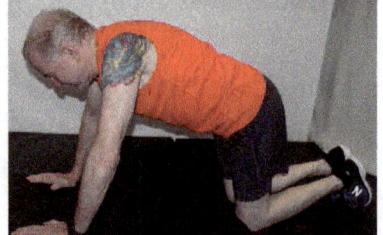

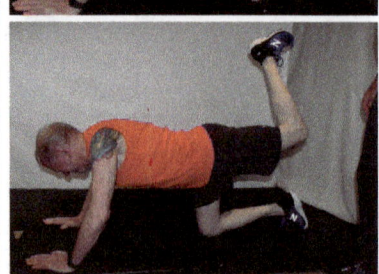

4. Upper Legs (Quadriceps, Hamstrings)

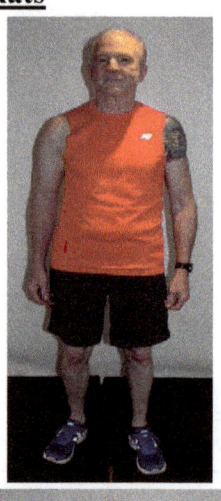

| 1. Squats | Quads (thighs), Hamstrings, Glutes | - Standing up straight, bend the legs at the knees and hips and lower the buttocks between the legs. The torso will lean forward to maintain balance.

(Pretend you are going to sit in a chair) |

Squat Modifications:		
Unstable Surfaces **BOSU**		- With a BOSU you may use the ball side (blue) or flat side (black). - You may also put an object in your hands for additional resistance.
2. Lunges **Forward Lunge**	Quads (thighs), Hamstrings, Glutes	- Stands on flat surface and steps forward with one leg and bends the forward knee down until the it is at a 90° angle and the back knee almost touches the floor while keeping the upper body straight (minimal forward bend). - You then push down with the front leg and return to a standing position - Repeats the exercise with the alternate leg.

Lunge Modification:		
1. Lunge with a Twist		- Do a forward lunge lunge with a twist to the forward lunge leg side.
2. Lateral Lunge		- Lunge (step laterally and bend the knee) to one side and then step and lunge to the other side.

3. Unstable Surface **BOSU** **Dome side up** 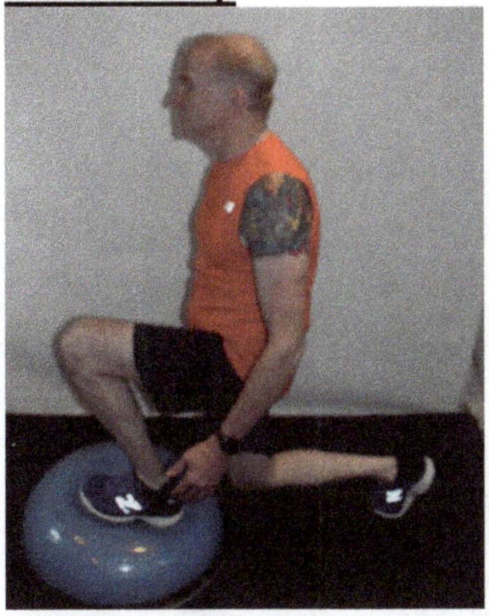 **Flat Side Up** 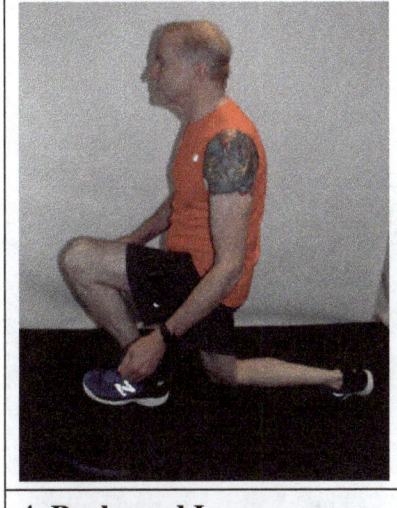		- The person can do the forward or lateral lunge by stepping onto the unstable surface. Requires more balance and coordination.
4. Backward Lunge 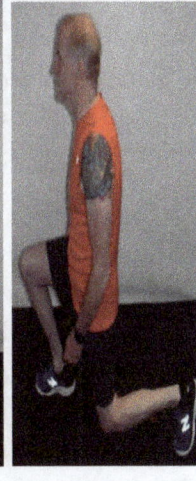		- The person steps backwards and then bend's the knee. Requires more balance.

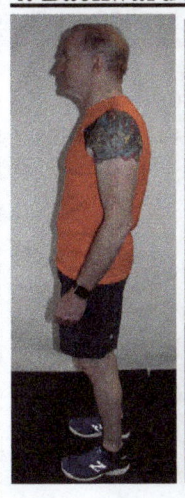

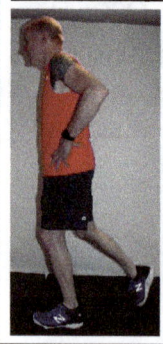

5. Walking Lunge 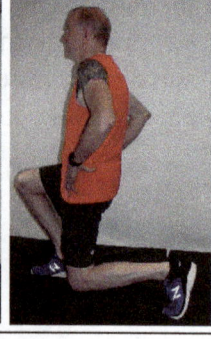		- The person does a forward lunge as you step forward but rather than push back to straighten up you straighten the front leg as you move forward in a walking motion.
6. Balance Lunge 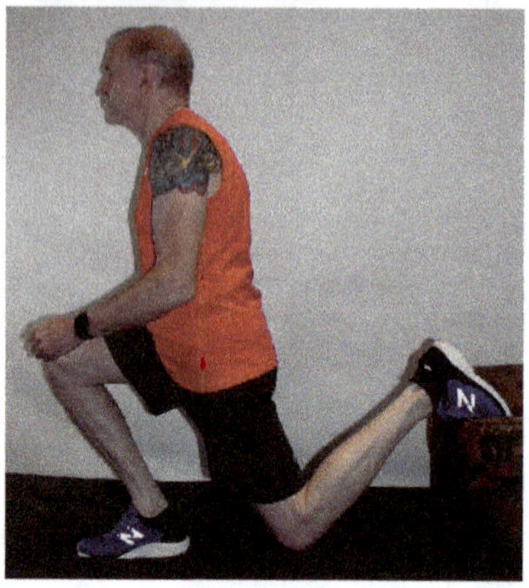		- The back leg is on a bench or chair as you perform the lunge.
5. Lower Legs (Gastrocs and Tibialis Anterior)		
1. Heel Raises 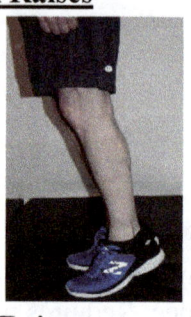 **2. Toe Raises** 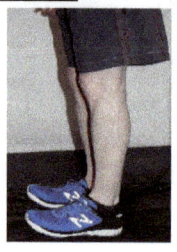	Gastrocs and Soleus	**Heel Raise** - Standing calf raises are executed with both feet on a flat surface or raised surface (heel lower than the toes). -The exercise is performed by raising the heel as high as possible. (You may need to stand beside a chair or wall for balance) **Toe Raise** - stand on flat surface and extend or lift your toes as high as possible. (You may need to stand beside a chair or wall for balance)

6. Core		
1. Planks **High Plank (on Hands)** **Low Plank (on Forearms)**	Core (abdominals, back and shoulders)	- Lying on the stomach and lifting the body and keep the toes and on the ground. -hold for 30 seconds or more. (<u>Easier modification</u> – kneel on knees rather than being on your toes)
Plank Modifications:		
1. Lateral Planks **Low Lateral Plank**		- Lie on forearm or hand. The feet may be stacked on top of each other (harder) or behind each other (increased stability).
2. Supine (face up) Planks **Low Supine Plank** **High Supine Plank**		- Facing upwards with hands shoulder width apart.

3. Planks on Unstable Surface **Stability Ball** **BOSU** **Flat Side up**		- The person does a standard plank on unstable surface such as BOSU or Stability ball. - Hands or feet can be on the unstable surface.
4. One Arm Plank		- Lift one arm off the supporting surface, hold and then alternate to the opposite arm.
5. One Leg Plank		- Lift one leg/foot off the supporting surface, hold and then alternate to the opposite leg/foot.

2. Crunches and Sit-Ups		
1. Crunch	Rectus Abdominus, Internal and external obliques	**Crunches** – - Lying face up on the floor. - Shoulders are curled upward towards the pelvis while the lower back remains flat against the floor. - Focus is on contracting the abdominal muscles as you rise yourself up.
2. Full Sit-Up **Feet Supported Full Sit-Up**		**Full Sit-ups** - Lying with the back on the floor, with the knees bent to reduce stress on the back muscles and spine. - Lift the chest towards the knees - Both the upper and lower will be off the floor (Only the buttocks is touching the ground).
Crunch/Sit-up Modifications:		
1. Oblique Crunch		- Twists (elbow to opposite knee) as you come up. - Lower back stays on the ground.

2. Oblique Full Sit-Up		- The person twist as they come up. - The lower back comes off the floor.
3. Russian Twist **Feet On Ground** **Feet Off Ground** **Holding Medicine Ball**		- Starts with knees bent and feet on or off ground and in upper sit-up position and then twist to each side repetitively. <u>Advanced</u> - hold a weight or medicine ball in your hands in front of your chest.

4. Crunch on Unstable Surface **Crunch on Stability Ball** **Oblique Crunch** **Side Lying Lateral Crunch on BOSU**		- Do a regular crunch on Stability ball or BOSU for Sit-up/Crunches. **Stability Ball** - Lying on stability ball between bottom of ribs and top of hips. **Side Lying on BOSU** - Side lying on BOSU between bottom of ribs and top of hips.

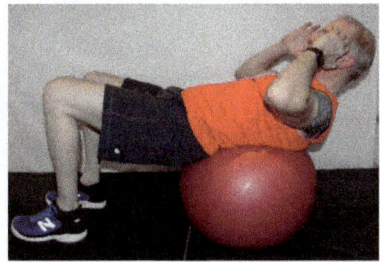

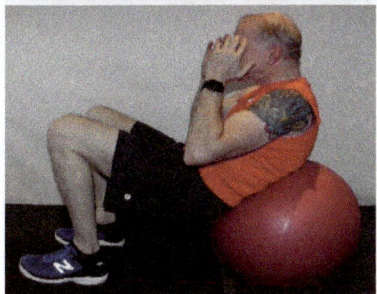

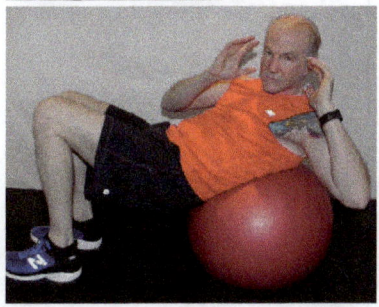

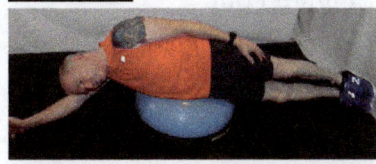

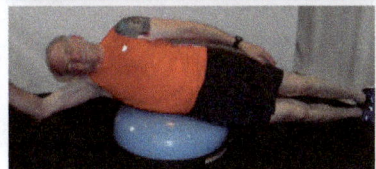

5. Table Top Crunches		- Hips and knees are bent 90°. (Table top position) Lower back stays flat on the mat during crunch.
Stability Ball Supported Table Top Crunch		Stability Ball Supported Table Top - Lower legs supported by stability ball.
Figure Four Straight Crunch		Figure Four - Cross one leg over the other in a figure four configuration.

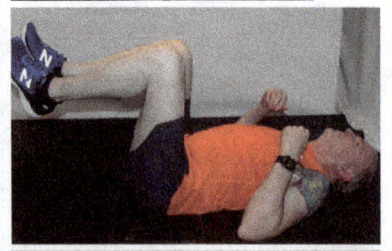

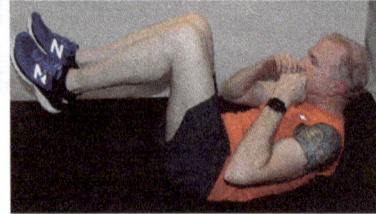

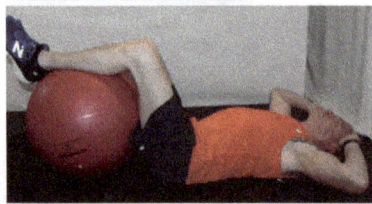

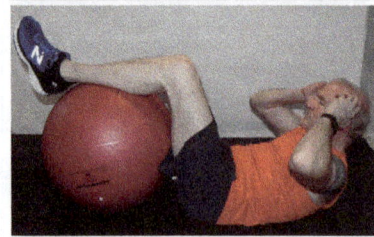

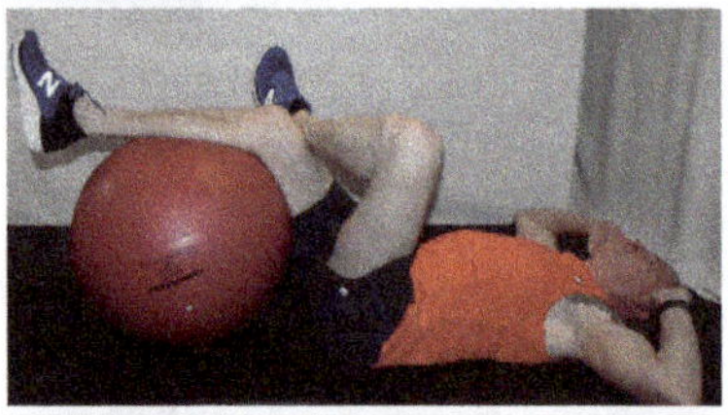

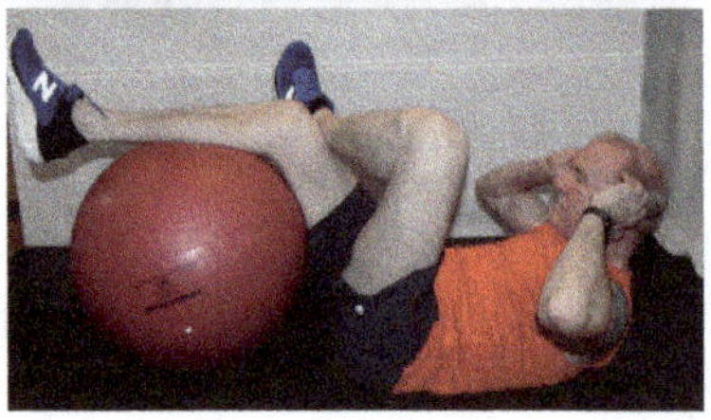

680

Figure Four Oblique Crunch		Oblique Crunch - As you crunch, move one elbow towards opposite (crossed over) knee.
6. Double Crunch		Double Crunch - Bend knees toward chest while lifting extended arms towards the knees and pretend to wrap arms around knees.
7. Bicycle 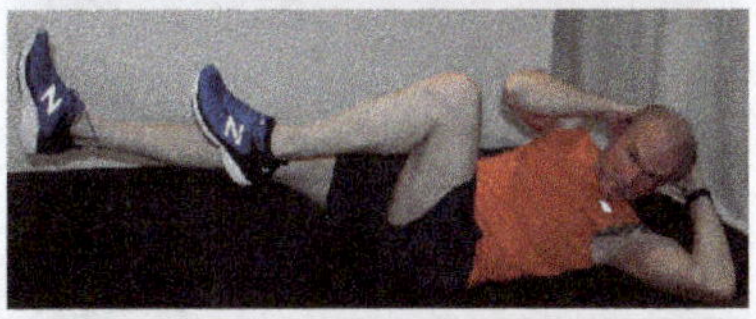 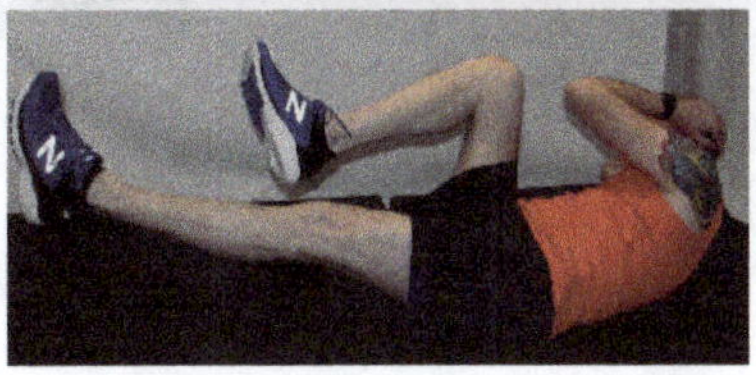		- Start with lifting legs and upper back off the ground. - Flex one knee to chest and lift opposite elbow to meet that knee and then repeat with opposite knee and elbow.

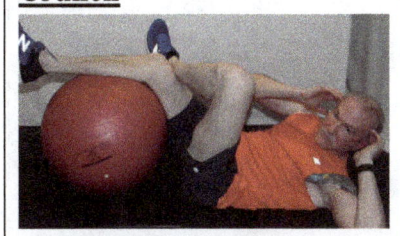

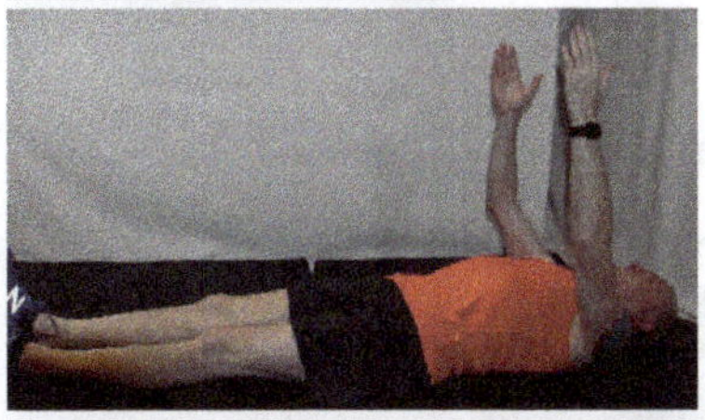

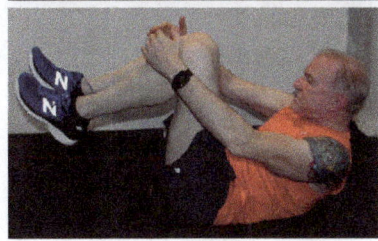

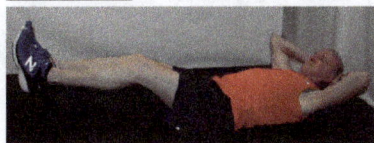

8. Mountain Climber		- Lying face down on your hands and toes you bend one knee and bring it up to your chest and then do that same with the opposite leg.
9. Pendulum **Rotate to Left** **Rotate to Right**		- Legs extended and lifted up 90° and then rotated and dropped to one side and then the other.

Ball Between Ankles

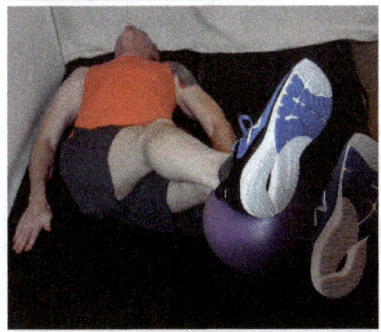

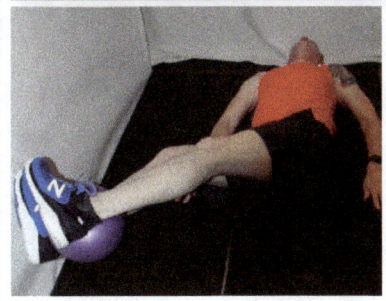

Advanced
- place a small ball or stability ball between the ankles.

10. Straight Leg Raise

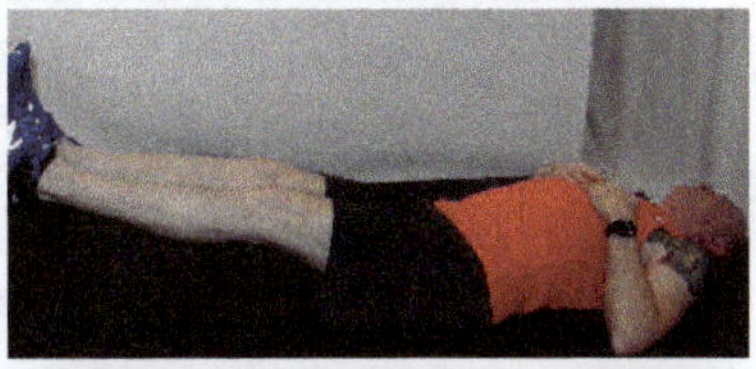

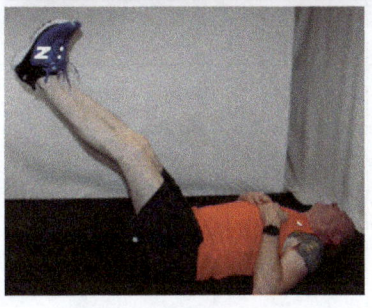

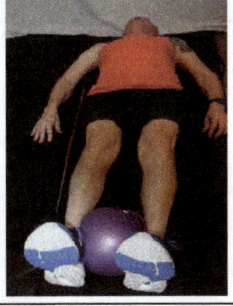

- Lie on the floor on your back. Keep the lower back in contact with the floor and place hands to sides or under lower back for support.
- Lift legs upward as far as possible. Lower down to starting position slowly and with control.
- Make sure the back stays flat on the floor and that the abdominal muscles stay tight.

Advanced
- place small ball or stability ball between ankles

Small Ball Between Ankles

Stability Ball between lower legs

- place stability ball between lower legs

3. Back Extensions Exercises	Erector Spinae	
1. Back Extensions **Chest only lifted off mat**		- Lying flat with hands behind the head lift chest off floor. Advanced - done on unstable surface such as a Stability ball or BOSU.

Stability Ball		
2. Superman **Chest and legs lifted off mat** **BOSU**		- Lying flat with arms extended forward lift chest and legs (thighs) off floor and hold. Advanced - done on unstable surface such as a Stability ball or BOSU
3. The Bird **Stability Ball**		- Face down and resting on hands and knees. Extend one arm out in front and lift and extend opposite leg back and hold. Then repeat with other arm and leg. Advanced

		- done on unstable surface such as a Stability ball or BOSU.
4. Bridge (Hip Raises) **Bridge (Hip Raise) on Unstable Surface** **Stability Ball** **Knees Bent** **Knees Straight**		- Lying flat and face up. Bend knees 90° and then lift hips up as high as possible and hold. Advanced - done on unstable surface such as a Stability ball or BOSU.

5. Combination Exercise		
1. Burpees *a b c d e*	Legs (Quads, Hamstrings), Hips (Hip Flexors and Extensors), Core, Shoulders	- (a) Start from a standing position. - (b) the person drops to a squat with hands on the floor - (c) thrusts legs back to assume push-up position. - (d) returns legs to squat position -(e) return to standing position
Burpee Modification:		
Burpee with Push-up		- Do a push-up when in the push-up position - Do jumping jack after you stand up. Note - you can alternate doing a push-up or jumping jack on each rep or do whatever combination you would like.
Burpee with Push-up and Jumping Jack		

6. Dynamic Exercises (only recommended for an older adult with advanced fitness level)		
Plyometrics **Stationary Double Knee Jump** **Double Leg Jump onto a bench**	Legs	- Plyometrics, also known as "jump training" or "plyos", are bodyweight resistance exercises based around having your leg muscles exert maximum force in as short a time as possible, with the goal of increasing both speed and power. - Plyometrics is an advanced lower body exercise routine that requires strength, balance, coordination, agility, and endurance.

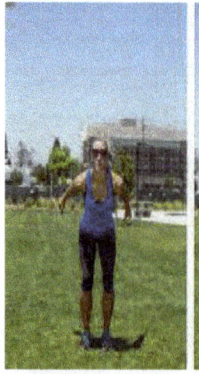

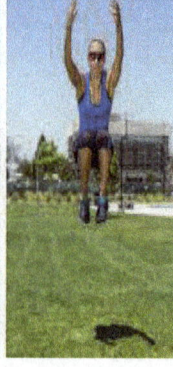

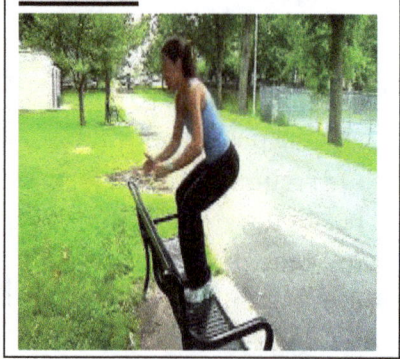

Appendix 9.1.3.0. Introduction to Agility, Balance and Coordination Exercises

This appendix complements information presented in Chapter 4.3. Fall Preventions: Agility, Balance and Coordination Training. The goal is to reinforce which exercises are necessary to develop muscular strength and improve the older adult's agility, balance and coordination to help minimize the threat of falling.

In workout sheets 9.2.4 these exercises are presented again, but in a table format to be copied and used to record and track daily, weekly and monthly accomplishments and progress. By accurately monitoring progress, you will know when it is best to add progressively more challenging exercise to your routine to enhance fall prevention.

Agility

Balance

Coordination

Appendix 9.1.3.1. Agility, Balance and Coordination Exercises Described and Illustrated

Table 1: Muscular Strengthening Exercises to Improve Agility and Balance

Note – all standing exercises can be done beside a chair or wall to help with balance.

Core Exercises:	
1. Abdominal Crunch Lie down on the floor on the back with knees bent. Place the hands behind the head or across the chest. - Pull the belly button inward towards the spine abdominal bracing), and flatten the lower back against the floor. - Slowly contract the abdominals, raising the shoulder blades about one or two inches off the floor. - Exhale as the shoulder blades come up and keep the neck straight, chin up. - Hold at the top of the movement for a 1-2 second count, breathing continuously. - Slowly lower back down, but don't let the abdominal muscles relax at the bottom, keep the abdominals contracted.	
2. Back Extensions and Superman's **Back Extensions** Lie down on the stomach and raise the chest off the floor with the arms extended in front (beginners may place their hands behind their head or in the small of their backs).	**Start**

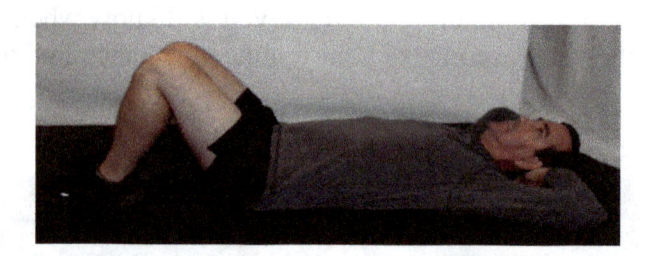

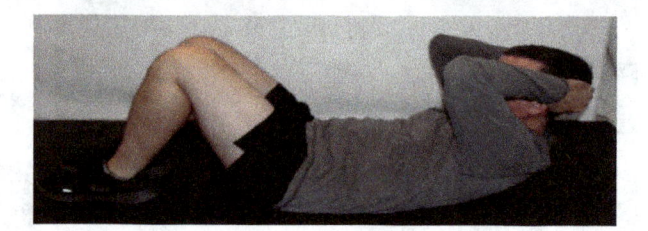

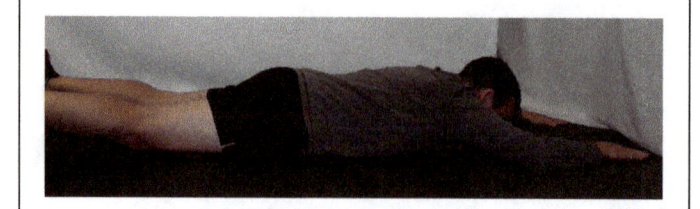

- Hold for 5-10 seconds. Lower the chest to the ground to complete one rep. Rest for 3-5 seconds and repeat.

Superman's

For an advanced exercise, lift the legs and chest off the ground.

Superman's chest and thighs are off the mat

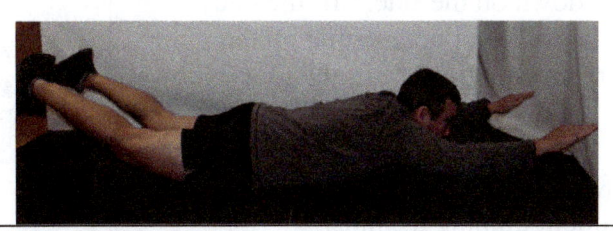

3. Lateral Hip Raises/Dips

Lie down on your side.

- <u>Hip Raise</u> - Lift the body (hips) off the floor, supported by the forearm (elbow at 90° degrees) and the side of the foot. Keep the body in a straight position.

- Hold for 2 seconds

- <u>Hip Dip</u> - Return hips to just above the floor.

<u>Advanced</u>
For added difficulty, lift one foot in the air.

Lateral Hip Raise

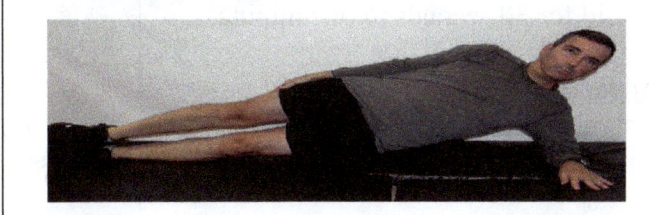

Hip Dip

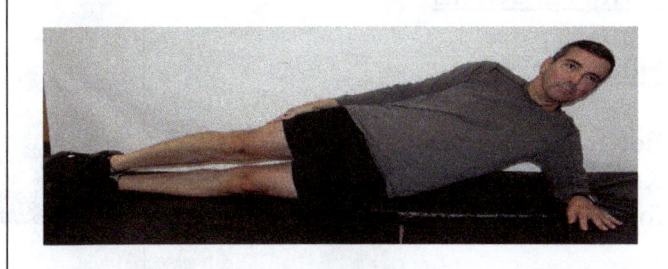

4. Planks

Lie down on the stomach. Lift the body off the floor, resting on the forearms and the toes (low plank) (elbows at 90° degrees) or on your hands (high plank).

- Keep the body in a straight position (without arching the back) and hold for 30 seconds to one minute.

<u>Advanced</u>
Lift one foot in the air for added difficulty.

Low Plank (lying on forearms)

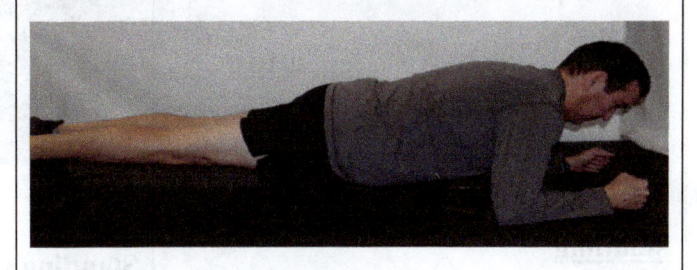

High Planks (hands on mat)

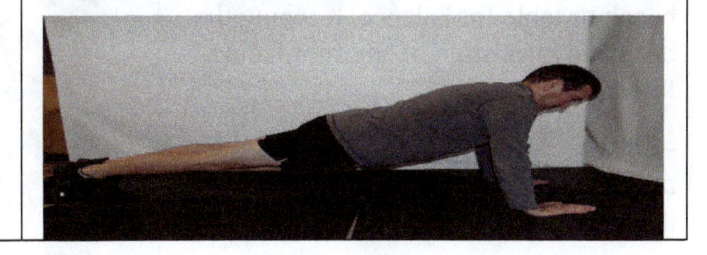

5. Side Plank

Lie down on the side. Lift the body (hips) off the floor, resting on the forearm and the side of the foot (elbows at 90° degrees).

- Keep the body in a straight position without dipping the hips.

- Hold for 30 seconds to one minute.

Advanced
Lift one foot in the air for added difficulty.

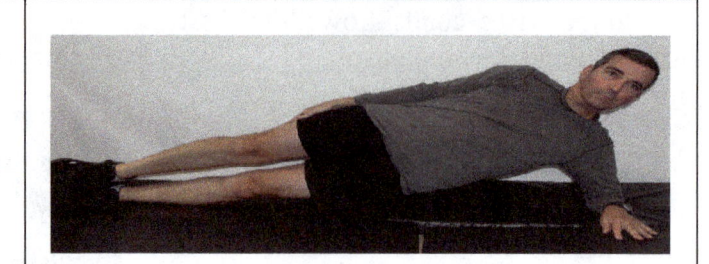

Hip Exercises:

1. Hip abductions

Side lying

Begin this exercise lying on the side. Keeping the back and knee straight and foot facing forwards

- Slowly lift the top leg as high as possible pain-free.

- Hold for 2 seconds and repeat 10 times.

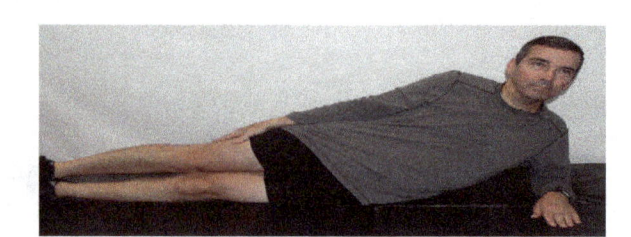

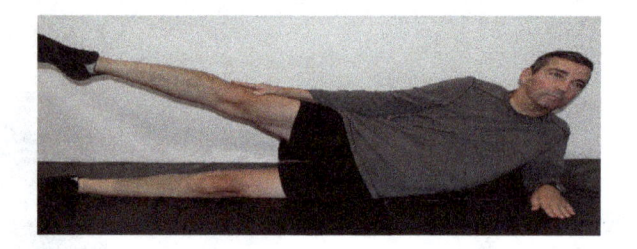

Standing

Begin this exercise standing beside a bench or table for balance. Keeping the back and knee straight and foot facing forwards.

- Slowly move the outer leg to the side, tightening the muscles at the side of the thigh/hip (abductors).

- Hold for 2 seconds and repeat.

- Move the leg to the side as far as possible pain-free.

Standing Chair assisted

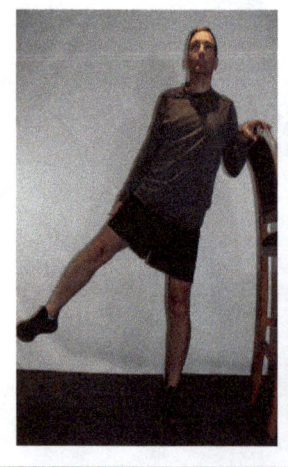

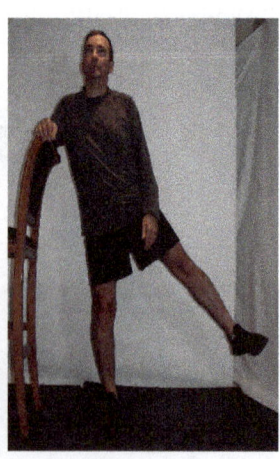

2. 45° Hip Abduction (Gluteus Medius)

Begin this exercise standing at a bench or table or facing a wall for balance. Keeping the back and knee straight and foot facing forwards.

- Slowly move one leg back and laterally at a 45° angle. Hold for 2 seconds and repeat.

- Move the leg at a 45º angle as far as possible pain-free.

3. Hip Extensions (Gluteus Maximus)

Begin this exercise lying on the stomach.

- Keeping the knee straight or bent 90º slowly lift one leg, tightening the buttocks muscles (gluteals).

- Hold for 2 seconds and repeat.

Advanced
– Balance on hands or forearms and knees and lift straight leg or bent knee to hip level and hold for 2 seconds.

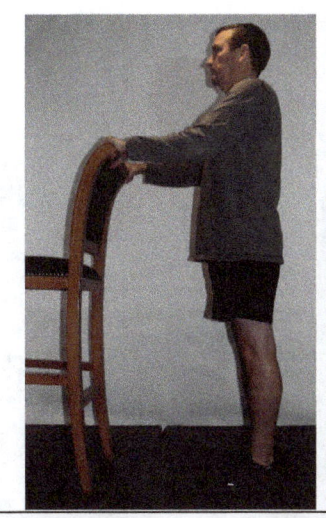

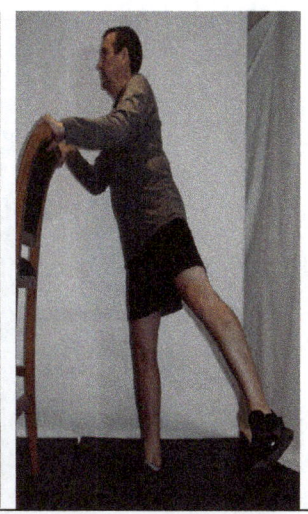

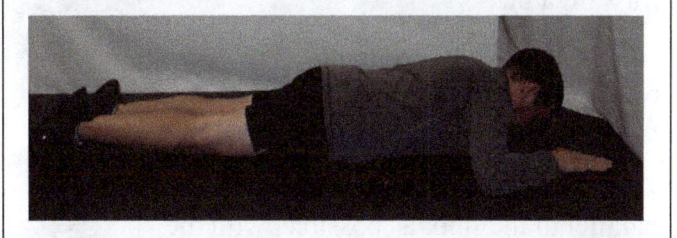

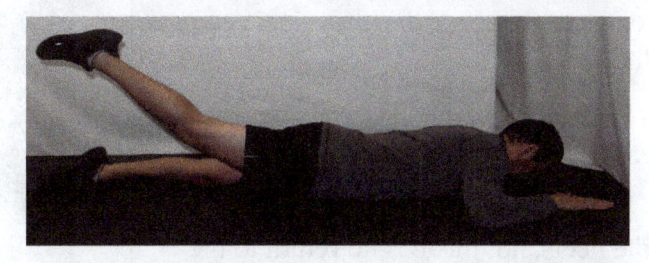

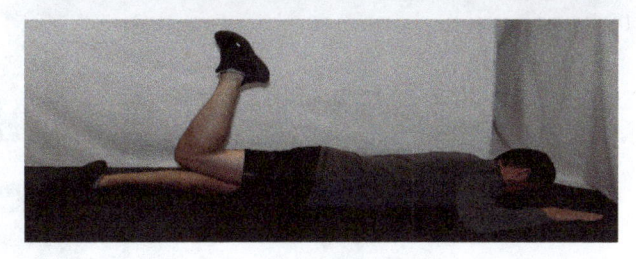

Leg Exercises
1. Squats

Stand with the head facing forward and the chest held up and out. Place the feet shoulder-width apart or slightly wider.

- Extend the hands straight out in front of the body to help keep balance.

- Sit back and down like sitting into an imaginary chair. Keep the head facing forward as the upper body bends forward a bit.

- Rather than allowing the back to round, let the lower back arch slightly while lowering into the squat.

- Squat down so the thighs are as parallel to the floor as possible, with the knees over the ankles (they don't go past the toes).

- Press bodyweight back into the heels rather than forward onto the toes.

- Keep the body tight and push through the heels, not the toes, to return to the starting position.

Note – use a chair to balance if necessary.

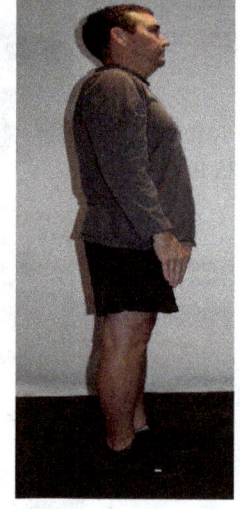

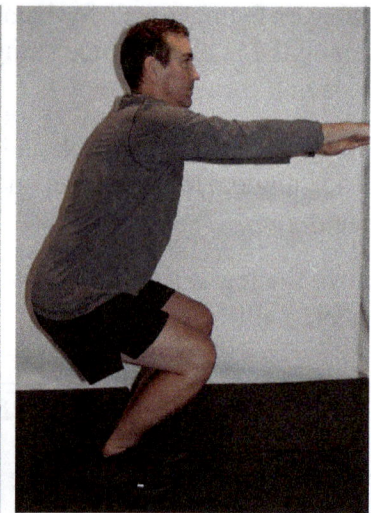

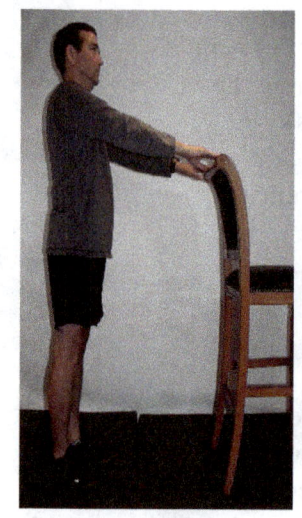

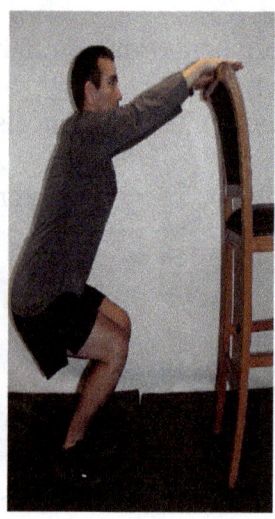

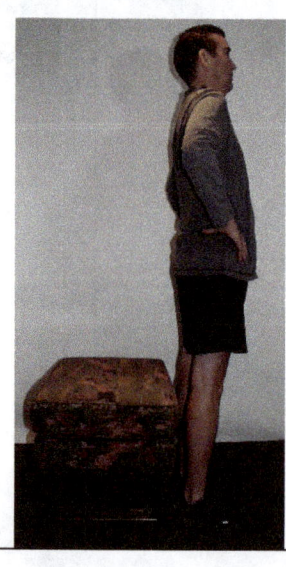

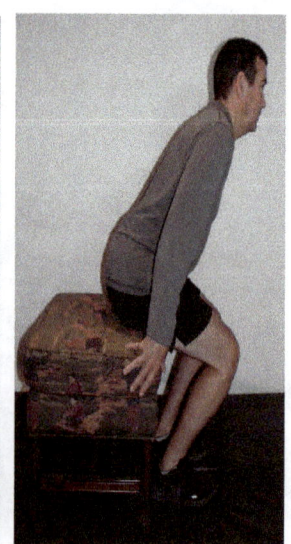

Lunges

Keep the upper body straight, with the shoulders back and relaxed and chin up (finding a focal point straight ahead to look at can help keep the gaze forward and up). Always engage the core (tighten up the belly).

- Step forward with one leg, lowering the hips until forward knee is bent at about a 90° angle.

- Make sure the front knee is directly above the ankle, not pushed out too far, and make sure the back knee doesn't touch the floor.

- Keep the weight on the front heel and return to the starting position.

Additional lunge exercises that require more strength and balance;

Backward Lunge – step backwards and lower the hips and back knee.

Side Lunge – Stand with the feet and knees together, hands on the hips.

- Take a large step with one foot to the side and lunge toward the floor.

- Make sure the lunged knee does not extend past the toes and keep the opposite leg relatively straight.

- Push off through the lunged foot to return to the start to complete one repetition.

Forward Lunge

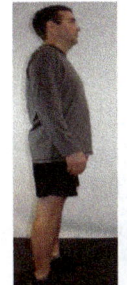

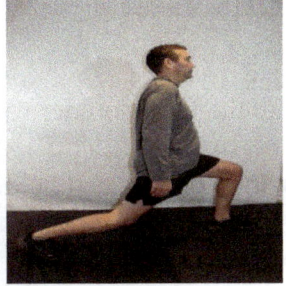

Chair Assisted forward Lunge

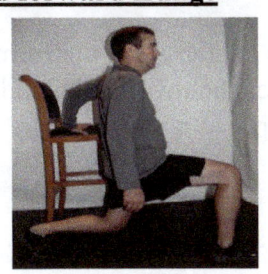

Backward Lunge

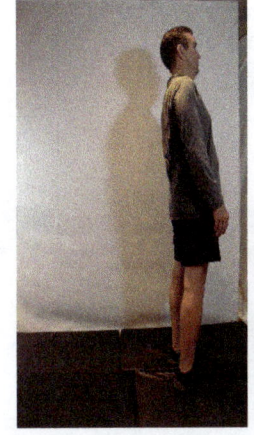

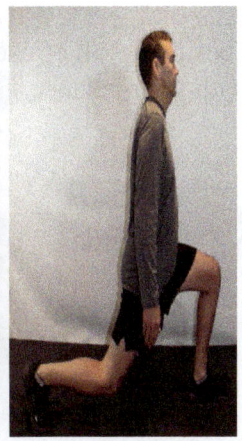

Side Lunge

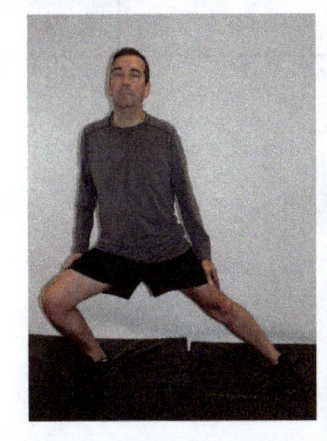

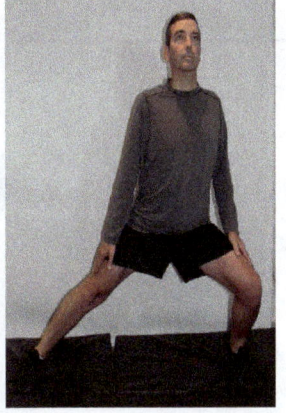

Heel and Toe Raises **Heel Raise** Stand with the feet shoulder width apart. - Lift up onto the toes and hold for 2 seconds and then return so the feet are flat onto the ground. Advanced – stand on edge of stairs or a platform and drop the heels below parallel and then lift heels up. **Toe Raise** Stand with feet shoulder width apart. -Lift your toes as high as possible while balancing on your heels. (Stand beside a wall or use a chair to assist with your balance.)	**Neutral Position** **Heel Raise** **Toe Raise** **Chair Assisted** **Heel Raise** **Toe Raise**

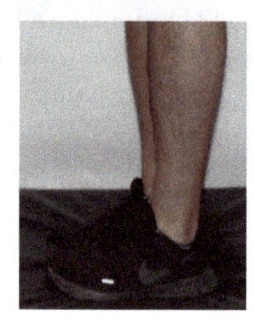

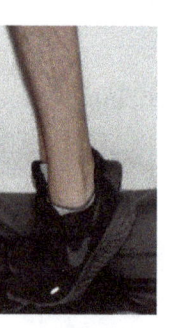

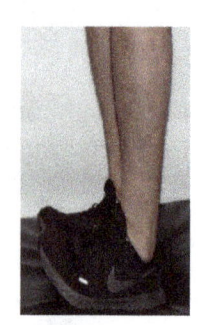

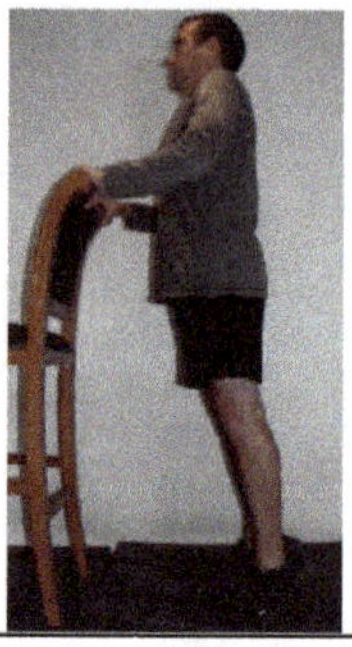

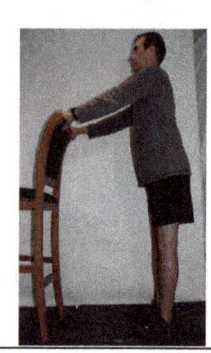

Table 2: Balance Exercises to Improve Stability

Notes:

1. Balance exercises should not be attempted until you have completed 4 to 6 weeks of muscular resistance exercises (Table 1) to ensure adequate core and leg strength.
2. The following balance exercises are in order of increasing difficulty. They can be made more challenging (progression) by changing feet position or the stability of the surface you are standing on (inflatable disc, wobble board or BOSU). Progression to the next level of instability should only occur when you can safely complete the series of balance exercises without significant swaying or fatigue.

Levels of Progression

1. .Feet shoulder or hip width apart.
2. Staggered Step Position – one foot takes a step forward. The feet are shoulder width apart
3. Split position 1 – one foot is one step ahead but directly in front of the back foot.
4. Split position 2 – same as split position 1 but heel of forward foot is touching the toe of the back foot, therefore a narrower base of support.
5. Stand on single leg.
6. Stand on unstable surface (inflatable Disc, wobble board or BOSU).

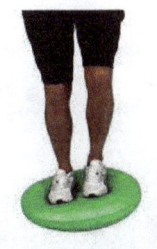

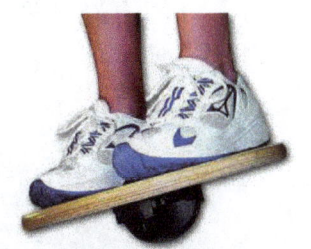

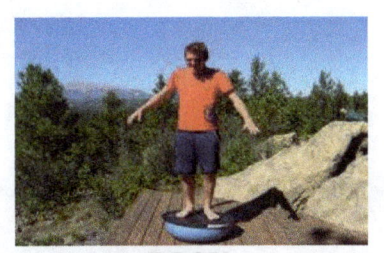

Inflatable Disc   **Wobble Board**   **BOSU**

3. When doing each balance exercise, it is important to keep the core tight (Abdominal bracing - abdominals/belly button tucked in) and feel the hips and buttocks muscles working to keep stability. The goal is to minimize swaying as you perform each exercise.

Progression when doing balance exercises

1. The goal is to progress so you can hold each position for 10-20 seconds or can do 10 reps of each exercise.
2. To add an additional level of difficulty, do each exercise with your eyes closed or moving your head back and forth sideways or up and down. This confuses the ocular (eyes) and/or vestibular (ears) proprioceptive reflexes

Precaution – Make sure you are standing next to a chair or wall that you can use to regain your balance if attempting a balance exercise with your eyes closed.

Balance Exercises

<u>Note -</u> Progress SLOWLY and have a chair or wall close by to help if there is a loss of balance

1. Standing on Both Legs;

1. Move both arms overhead & hold.

Progressions

1. Drop one arm to the side so it is at shoulder height & hold.

2. Bend torso to the dropped arm side & hold.

3. Straighten up and move the arm to the front of the body and bend forward & hold.

4. Do each of the previous exercises with the eyes closed and/or a more challenging foot position.

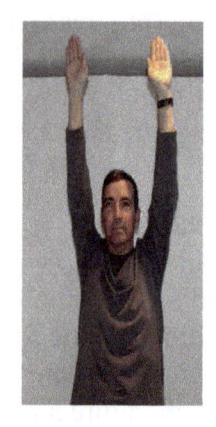

Progressions

1. Drop one arm

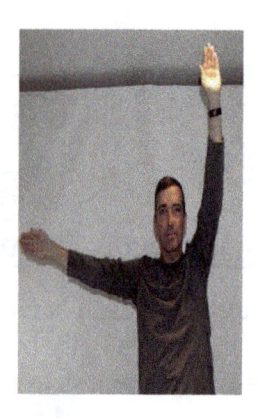

2. Bend to the dropped arm side

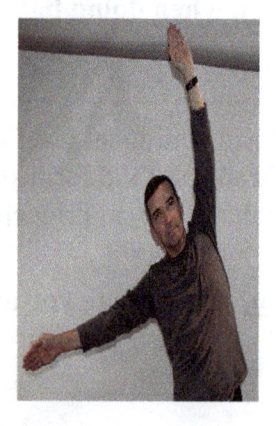

3. Move arm to front of body and bend forward

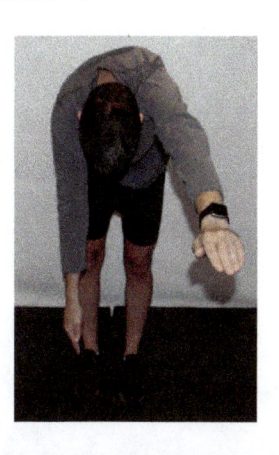

2. Raise a finger to eye level and follow it with the eyes while moving it up and down and to the sides.

Progressions:

1. Follow the moving finger with the eyes while allowing the head to move.

2. Keep the eyes closed while the head turns simultaneously with the finger movement.

3. Change to a more unstable foot position.

Follow the Moving Fingers

(Eyes open and then closed)

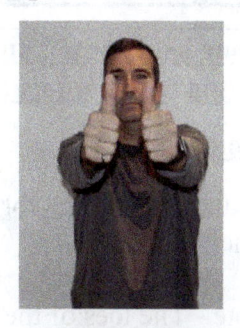

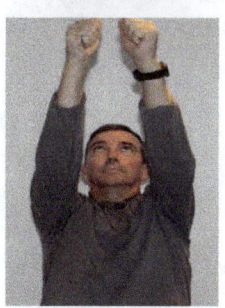

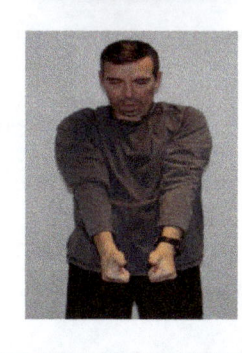

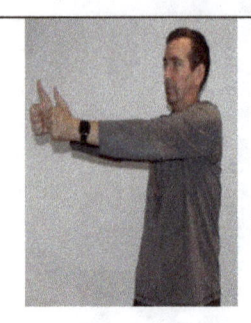

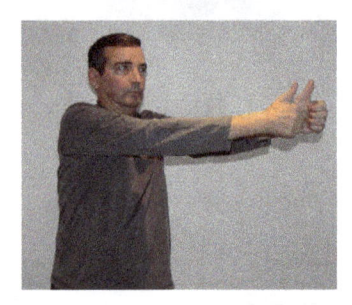

2. Standing on One Leg;

1. Swing one leg forward and back with the opposite arm swinging in the opposite direction of the leg.

Progression;

- As the arm swings forward, reach down and touch the floor.

    Note - The toes of the swinging leg do not touch the floor.

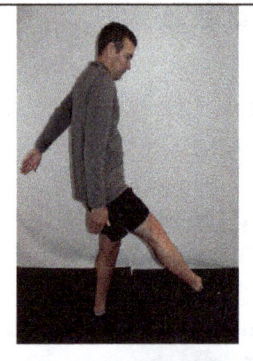

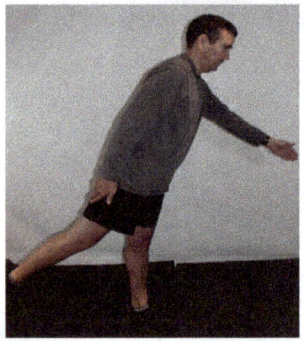

2. Swing one leg out to the side and then across the body.

Progression

The opposite arm swings in the opposite direction of the leg.

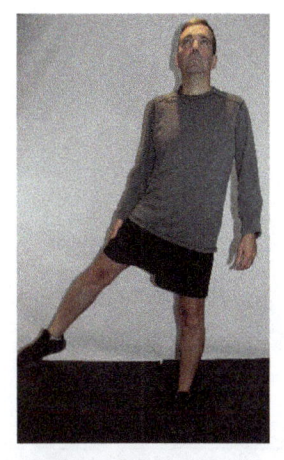

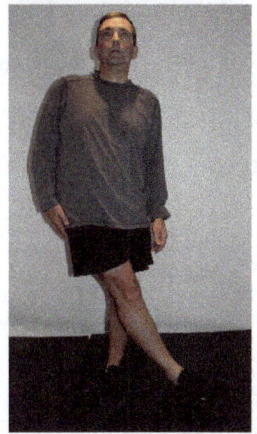

3. Swing the leg out to the side and across in front of the body, and then around and across the back of the body.

Progression

– The opposite arm swings in the opposite direction of the leg.

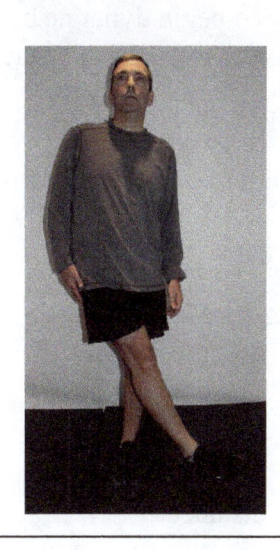

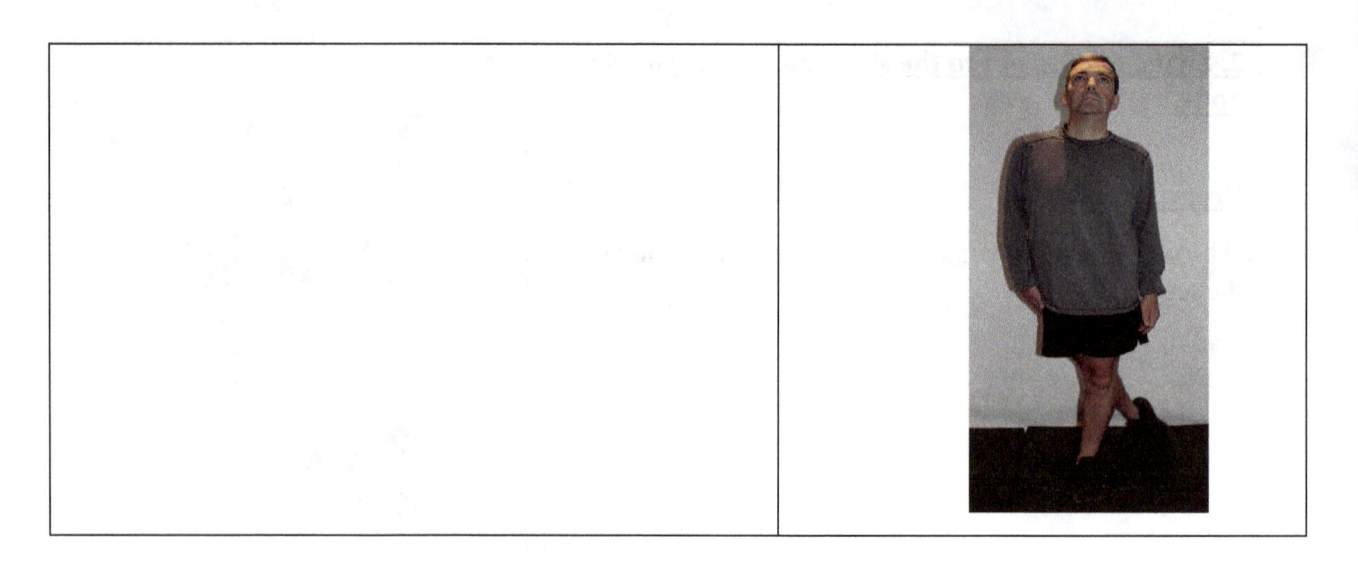

Table 3: Agility Exercises (Dynamic Balance Exercises)

Agility exercises are basically dynamic balance exercises. In other words, instead of standing still the person is moving forward, sideways or backwards. They are an advanced form of balance exercises and require a greater amount of leg strength and neurologic coordination (proprioceptive reflexes) than static balance exercises in Table 2.

As with static balance training, remember to start simple and slowly increase the complexity of movement. All movements should be slow in the beginning and increase in speed when progression is appropriate. A person should **never** overestimate their skill level when increasing the level of difficulty. Progress slowly.

To begin dynamic balance activities, find a flat, soft surface. Perform each agility exercise by moving a specific distance forward and then the same distance in the opposite direction.

Recovery time between agility exercises should be between 45 to 60 seconds. As the person progresses, they can reduce recovery time to 30 or 15 seconds.

Key Points:
1. Progress slowly.
2. The most important point in agility training (dynamic balance training) is to master proper form, *not* speed.
3. To make the agility exercises more difficult as you progress, increase the speed and/or distance.
4. For the older adult, focus is on maintaining good balance when performing the agility exercises.
5. For the athlete, focus on mimicking movements that are essential to your sport of choice. For example, if you are a soccer player, incorporate more side-to-side movements. If you are a golfer, focus on how to maintain balance while moving and twisting.
6. The agility exercises illustrated below can be used with or without an agility ladder.

Agility Ladder

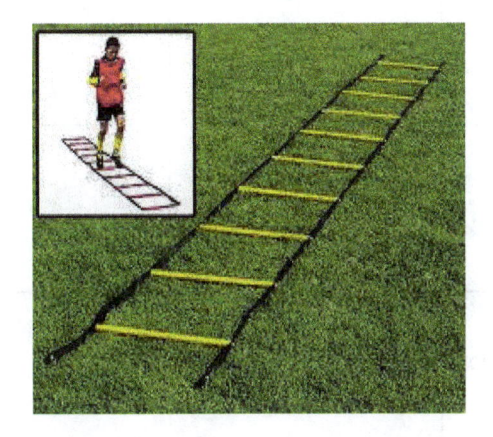

Agility Exercise Evaluation Chart

Agility exercises are listed below in chart form. You can use the chart to grade yourself on how proficient you are at performing the various drills.

It is not necessary to perform each of the exercise. You may pick and choose as you progress down the list. Under each category the exercises progress from easy to hardest.

Refer to workout sheet 9.2.4 for agility, balance and coordination exercise routines.

Test	No Hesitation/ Stumbles/ Difficulties	Moderate Hesitation/ Stumbles/ Difficulties	Significant Hesitation/ Stumbles/ Difficulties
Walking Drills (Forward, sideways and cross-over):			
1. Forward Walking: (Start facing forward)			
1. Regular Walking Forward			
2. Take one step forward and then the opposite leg catches up Before you take the next step			

2. Sideway Walking: (Start facing sideways)			
1. One foot walking sideways and then the other foot catches up. **(Return to start position with other leg leading the sideways walk).**			
2. Front cross-over moving sideways (Which ever foot is the leading cross-over foot it always crosses in front) **(Return to start position with other leg leading the cross-over walk).**			
3. Carioca (Start facing sideways) (The leading crossing foot alternates between going in front and then behind the other leg) **(Return to start position with other leg leading the cross-over)**			
Hop Drills:			
1. Forward Hop Drills: (Each Starts facing forward)			
1. Both feet hop forward.			
2. One leg every square hop forward.			
3. Two Feet narrow hop and then wide hop (hop scotch). (Hop scotch – Hop forward with feet together and then hop forward separating the legs)			

2. Sideways Hop Drills:

(Each starts facing sideways)

(Return to start position with the opposite leg leading the hop)

1. Both feet hop sideways.			
2. One foot hop sideways.			

3. Scissors Hop

(Facing forward)

1. Start with feet together and on hopping forward the legs split and land with one leg in front of the other. On the next hop the opposite leg lands in front.			

4. Diagonal Hop

1. Two feet Hop diagonally			
2. Hop diagonally alternating feet			

(Hop to the right diagonally with the right foot and then to the left with the left foot)

5. Rotational Hop Drills:

1. 90° Two-legged Hop Rotation

- Hop and rotate with feet together 90°
- do a hop and 90° rotation in opposite direction

2. 180° Two-legged Hop Rotation

- Hop and rotate 180° with each hop
- do a hop and 180° rotation in opposite direction

Example of an Agility Workout

Note – Start with 3 reps of each exercise and progress depending on your proficiency.

Workout #1	Workout #2
1. Front cross-over sideway walking 2. Carioca 3. Two feet hop forward 4. Scissors hop 5. 90° rotation hop	1. Side-way walking – one foot catches up with the lead foot 2. Two feet side-way hop 3. One foot side-way hop 4. Hop diagonally alternating feet 5. 180° rotational hop

Appendix 9.1.4.0. Introduction to Flexibility/Stretching Exercises

Maintaining flexibility in older adults cannot be minimized. Part of the physiological process of aging is the muscles and connective tissues (ligaments, tendons, and fascia) become less elastic. The tightening of the soft tissues leaves the older adult vulnerable to injury. A lack of flexibility also leaves the body's joints susceptible to injury and increases the chance of falling.

Flexibility is the third and equally important fitness component, together with cardiovascular fitness, and muscle strength and endurance. Consistently stretching is the best way to maintain and improve a person's flexibility. It is important to remember that it is better to stretch for shorter periods frequently during the day than to do it for a prolonged period once a day. Everyone, but especially an older adult, should make stretching part of their daily routine.

Appendix 9.1.4.1. illustrates and describe a complete range of stretches for every joint in the body. A 10-minute stretching routine is presented in Appendix 9.1.4.2. Yin Yoga (holding a particular position/pose for two to four minutes) is an excellent and meditative way of introducing stretching into your daily routine. Appendix 9.1.4.3. illustrates these positions/poses. Myofascial self-massage with a roller is an effective way to soften and improve the pliability of the muscles and fascia. Appendix 9.1.4.4. describes and illustrates this technique.

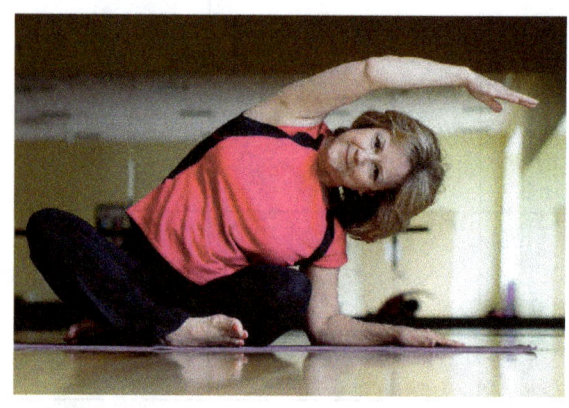

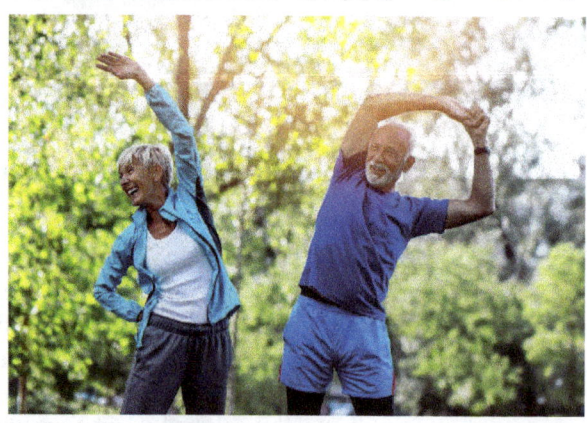

Appendix 9.1.4.1. Stretching Exercises Described and Illustrated

Flexibility is the most overlooked and ignored of the three components of fitness. Cardiovascular/aerobic fitness and strength training get far more attention. However, as a person ages, having a good level of flexibility in their muscles, tendons, and ligaments is necessary to achieve and enjoy a good quality of life. Life is much more difficult if a person cannot bend over to tie their shoes, reach behind to put on their coat, or reach high for a plate on the top shelf in the kitchen.

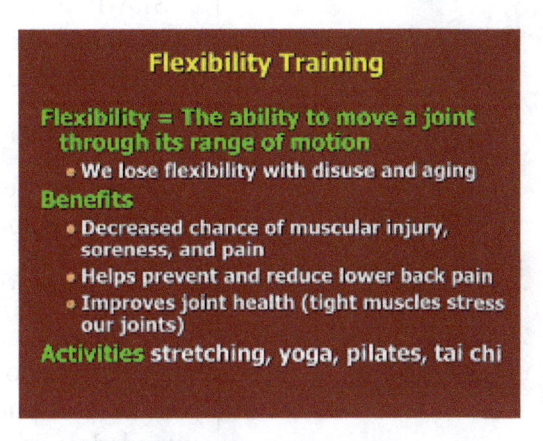

Image source: slideplayer.com

To maintain flexibility, a person must stretch. Stretching involves dynamically moving and statically holding our muscles and joints in specific directions and positions. Breathing is an essential element for effective stretching because it allows the person to relax and "move into" a deeper stretch.

Stretching is not as glamorous as going to a spin class or running with friends to improve aerobic fitness or pumping weights for strength gain. However, regular stretching helps maintain flexibility to help prevent injury as we participate in those other components of fitness. It also helps reduce soreness and stiffness that often result from these other forms of exercise.

The secret to effective stretching and improved flexibility is doing stretching exercises as described and illustrated and doing them frequently and consistently. It is better to spend 5 minutes three times a day stretching than to stretch for 15 minutes only once a day. Doing flexibility exercises correctly and frequently is the key.

Make stretching a part of your daily routine, and you will reap the benefits every time you move.

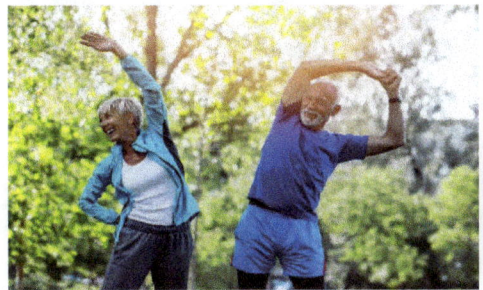

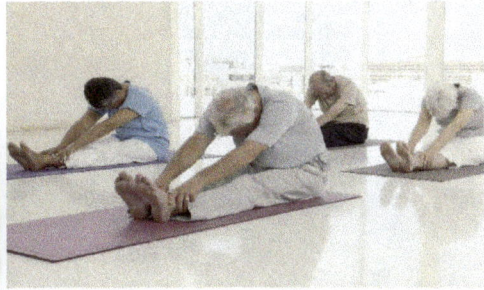

Dynamic & Static Stretches for Neck, Shoulders, Lower Back, Hips, Legs

1. Neck

1. Semi-circle Head Rotations (Dynamic) 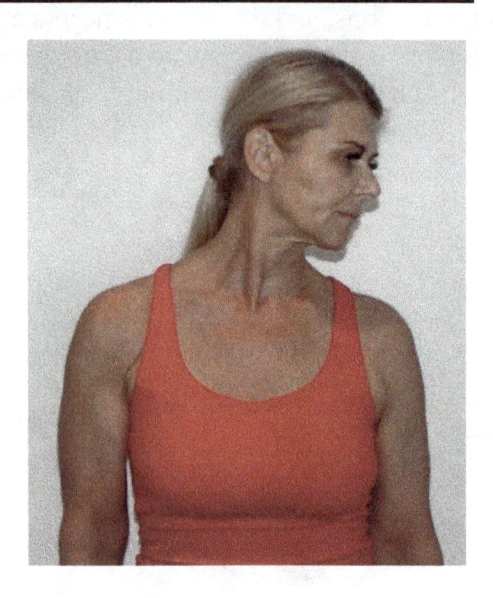	Target: Lateral and Extensor Neck and Trapezius
	1. Drop your chin to your chest. 2. Slowly rotate your chin along your chest to one shoulder or until you feel stress in the neck muscles. Hold for 1-2 seconds. 3. Slowly rotate your chin along your chest to the opposite side and hold. 4. Repeat 3-5x's. Note – never do a full 360º rotation of your neck or put your neck in an extended position.
2. Side/lateral Head Pull to the shoulder with the Hand (Static) 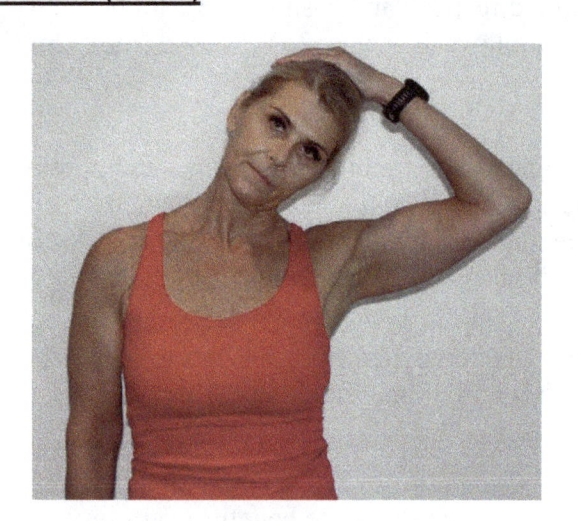	**Target: Lateral Neck and Trapezius** 1. Laterally tilt your head to one side and hold 3-5 seconds. Advanced – Increase the stretch by: 1. Having the arm reach over the top of the head, and gently pull the head farther toward the shoulder. 2. Sit and anchor the arm that is opposite to the tilt side under the buttocks and then pull neck laterally to opposite side.

2. Shoulders

1. Shoulder Rolls (Dynamic)

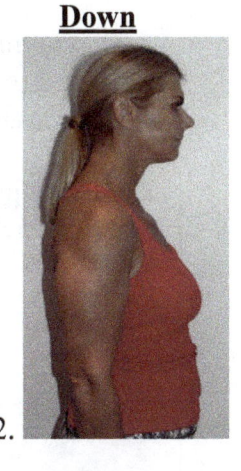

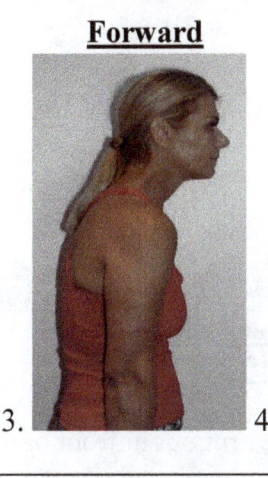

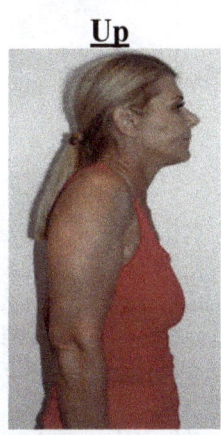

Back **Down**

Forward **Up**

Target: Rotator cuff, Traps, Chest (Pectoralis Major)

1. Stand with feet shoulder width apart and arms are along the side of the body.

2. Move shoulders back, down, to the front and then up for one complete rotation.

3. Repeat 5 rotations in one direction and then 5 in the opposite direction.

2. Standing Huggers (Dynamic)

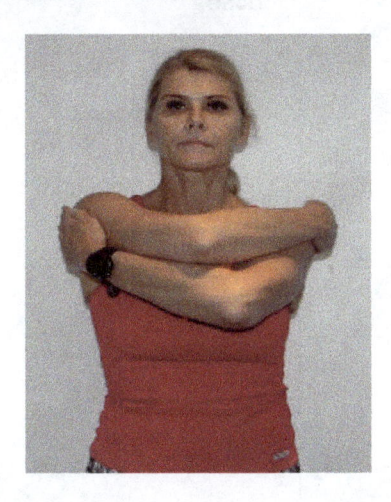

Target: Rotator Cuff and Chest (Pectoralis Major)

1. Stand upright and lift your arms to shoulder height.

2. Move the arms across your body and hug yourself. Hold the hug for 1-2 seconds.

3. On each hug alternate which arm goes on top of the other.

3. Standing Arm Circles (Dynamic)

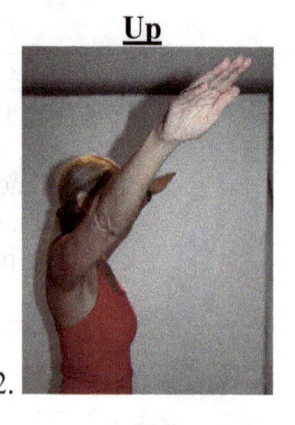

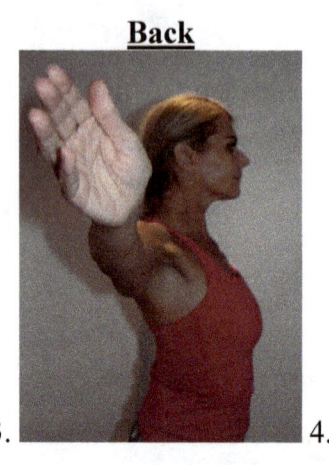

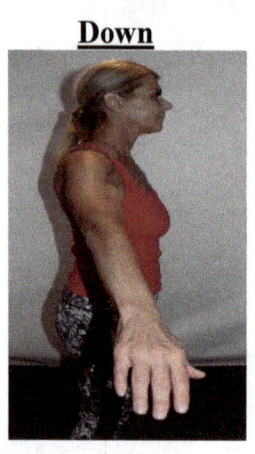

Forward | Up

1. | 2.

Back | Down

3. | 4.

Target: Rotator Cuff and Chest (Pectoralis Major)

1. Standing upright and lift your arms to shoulder height.

2. Slowly rotate your arms in a forward direction 10x's and then in a backward direction 10x's

3. Slightly increase the size of the circle on each rotation.

4. Single Arm Reach Across Your chest (Static)

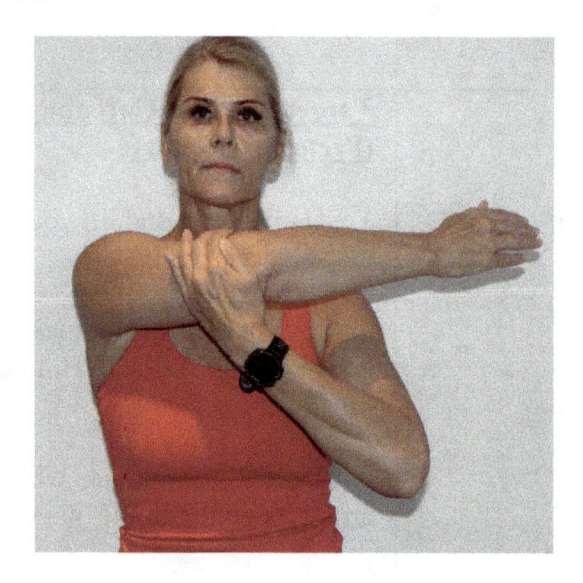

Target: Posterior Shoulder (Rotator Cuff)

1. Extend one arm out in front of you and then move it across your chest.

2. With the opposite hand push the extended arm closer to the chest.

Hold for 5 seconds.

5. Hands Behind Your Head and Squeeze Your Shoulder Blades Together (Dynamic)	**Target: Chest (Pectoralis Major)**
	1. Put both hands behind the base of your head.

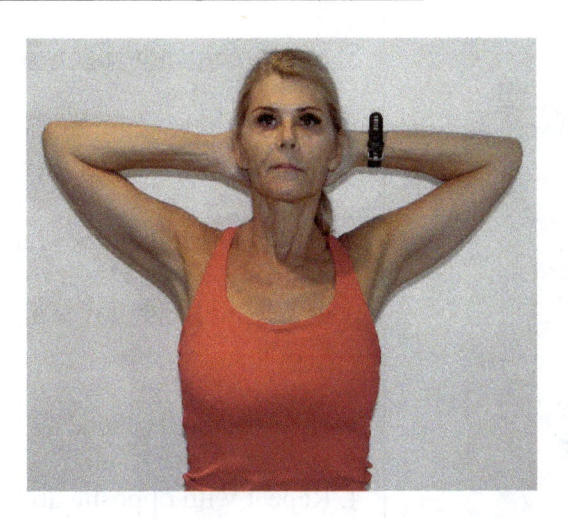

2. Actively pull both elbows back and feel the shoulder blades coming together.

3. Hold for 1-2 seconds.

4. Release and repeat trying to move your arms farther back and squeezing the shoulder blades closer together with each repetition. |
| **6. Single Arm Chest Stretch Utilizing the Wall (Dynamic and Static)** | **Target: Chest (Pectoralis Major)** |
| | 1. Stand perpendicular to a wall.

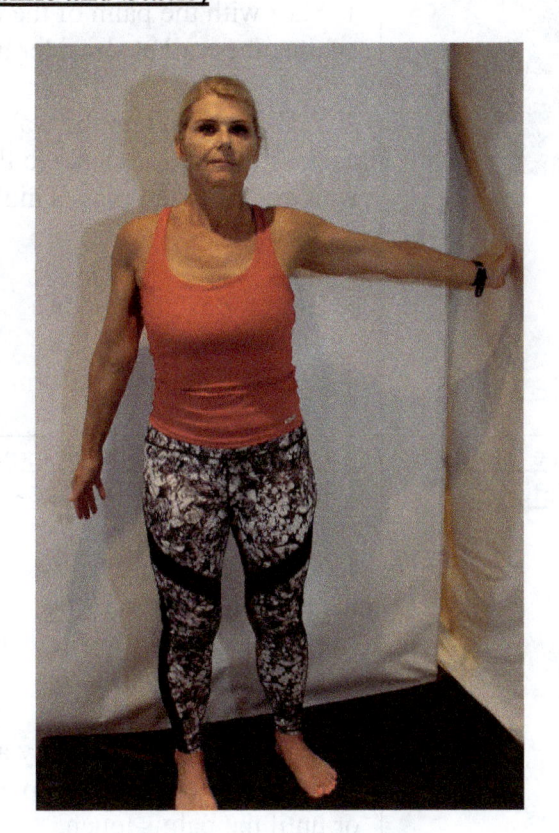

2. Raise arm closest to the wall to shoulder level.

3. Move the arm backward along the wall as you move your body closer to the wall.

4. Keep the chest perpendicular to the wall.

5. Continue to move closer to the wall with the arm extended back along the wall until you feel a stretch in your chest.

6. Hold for 5-20 seconds and then lower the arm and repeat with the opposite arm. |

7. Single Arm Abduction – Perpendicular and Facing the Wall (Dynamic and Static) **Perpendicular to Wall** **Facing Wall**	**Target: Lower Rotators and Latissimus Dorsi** Standing perpendicular to a wall; 1. Start with the palm of the hand against the wall at shoulder height. 2. Walk the hand up the wall as far as possible. Move closer to the wall as your hand moves higher on the wall. 3. Hold for 5-20 seconds. 4. Repeat with opposite arm Standing facing the wall; 1. Start with the palm of the hand against the wall at shoulder height. 2. Walk the hand up the wall as far as possible. Move closer to the wall as your hand moves higher on the wall. 3. Hold for 5-20 seconds. 4. Repeat with opposite arm.
8. Arms Lifted Laterally and Reach Above Your Head and Palms Touch (Dynamic and Static)	**Target: Lower Rotators and Latissimus Dorsi** 1. Stand up straight with head over the shoulders. (You can stand with your back and head against a wall) 2. Raise your arms laterally and above your head as far as possible or until the palms touch. 3. Try to keep the elbows straight and arms in line with your head and shoulders and not out in front of your head.

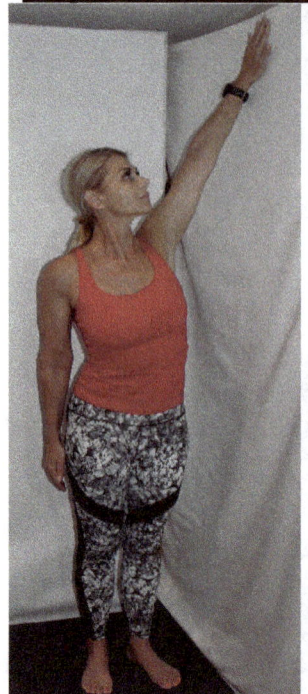

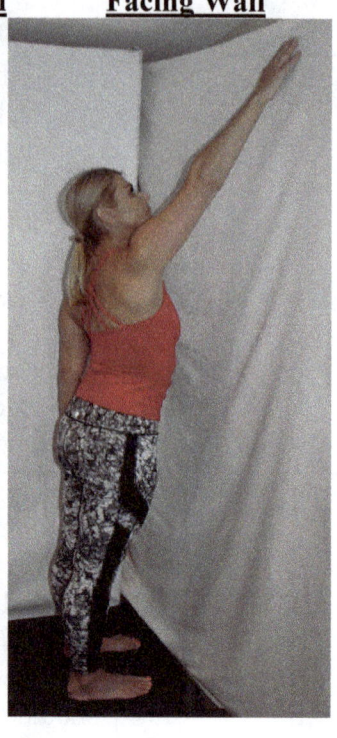

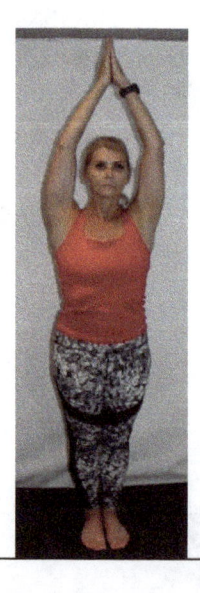

	4. Hold for 5-20 seconds. Advanced – At the top cross your hands and interlock your fingers increase the stretch.
9. Single Arm Over the Same Shoulder and Scratch Upper Back (Dynamic and Static) 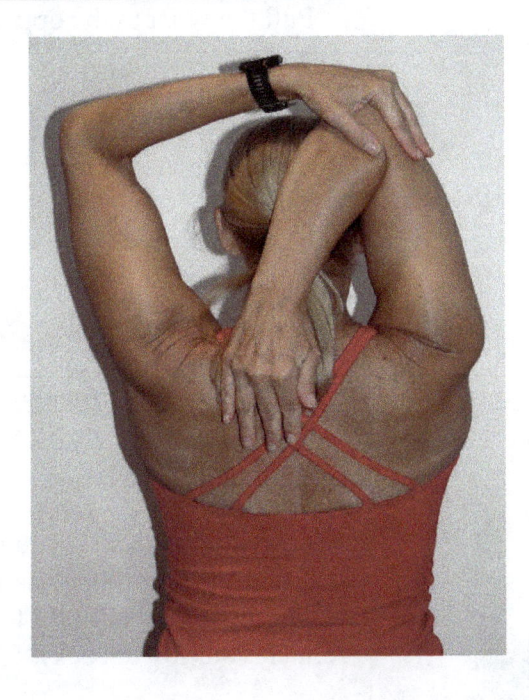	**Target: Lower Rotators and Latissimus Dorsi** 1. Stand up straight and raise one arm over the same side shoulder. 2. Reach as far down the spine as possible as if you are trying to scratch your upper back between your shoulder blades. Advanced – Use the opposite hand to push back on the elbow to increase the stretch.
10. Palms Together and Fingers intertwined behind the Lower Back and Pull Arms Down (Dynamic and Static) 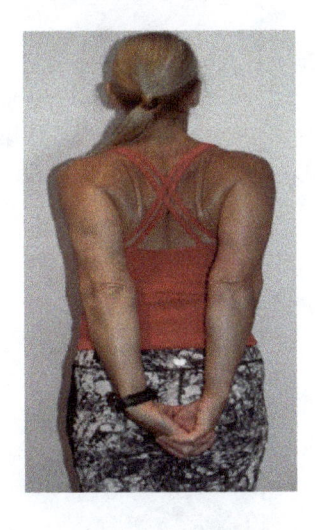	**Target: Chest (Pectoralis Major) and Shoulder (Anterior Deltoids)** 1. Stand straight and look forward. 2. With elbows slightly bent reach behind and interlock your fingers and push the heels of hands together. 3. Pull down on the hands until you feel a stretch in the front of your shoulder and chest. 4. Hold for 5-20 seconds.

11. Arm/Wrist Grab and Pull to Side (Dynamic and Static)	**Target: Lateral Deltoids, Trapezius and Lateral Neck** 1. Stand straight and look forward. 2. Grab the wrist of the opposite arm that is extended and behind your back. 3. Pull the wrist to the opposite side. 4. Laterally tilt your head to the side that you are pulling the arm toward. 5. Hold for 5-20 seconds
12. Underneath Lower Back Scratch (Dynamic and Static)	**Target: Chest (Pectoralis Major) and Anterior Shoulder (Anterior Deltoid)** 1. Take one arm and rotate it underneath toward the small of your back (as if you want to scratch your lower back). 2. Move the hand up the spine as high as possible. 3. Hold 5-20 seconds Advanced – To increase the stretch, you can take the opposite hand and grab the hand that is scratching the lower back and pull it further up the spine.

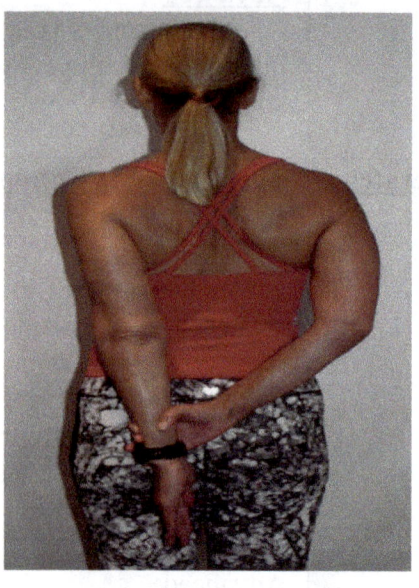

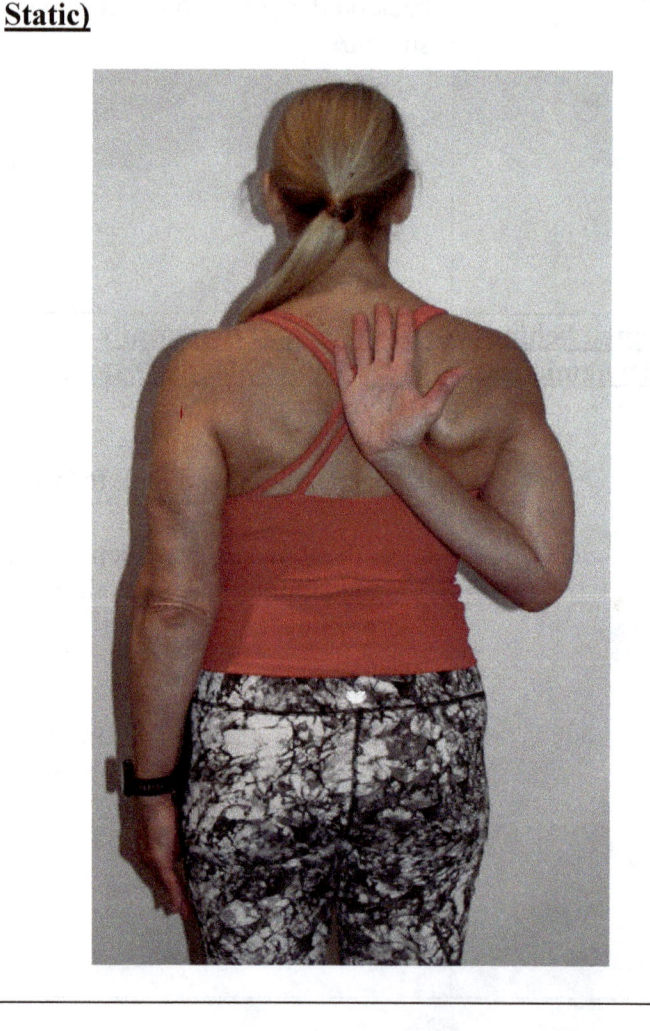

13. Touch Both Hands/Fingers Behind the Back (Dynamic and Static)

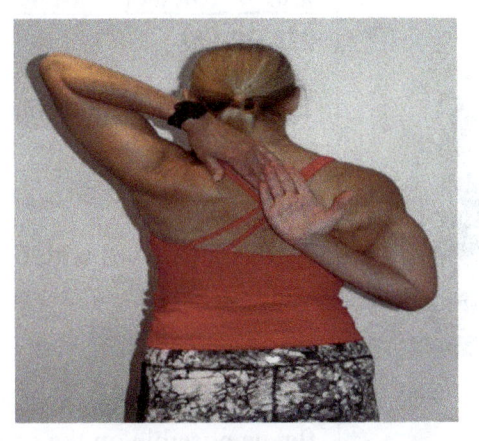

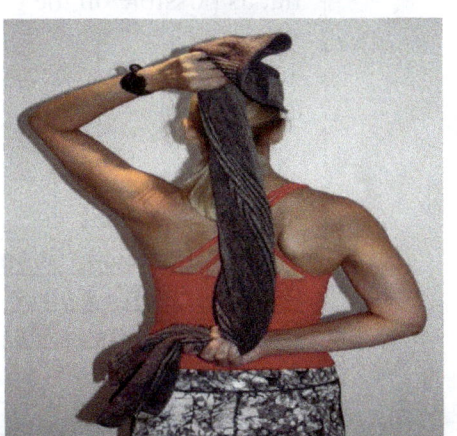

Target: Lower Rotators and Latissimus Dorsi

This is a combination of the two scratch stretches that were done previously.

1. One hand scratch the upper spine and the opposite hand scratch the lower spine.

2. Move both hands as close to each other as possible along the spinal column so the fingers can touch.

3. Hold 5-20 seconds.

Note – if you have significant restriction of shoulder movement you can grab both ends of a towel and pretend to dry your back.

14. Child Pose with a Cushion (Static)

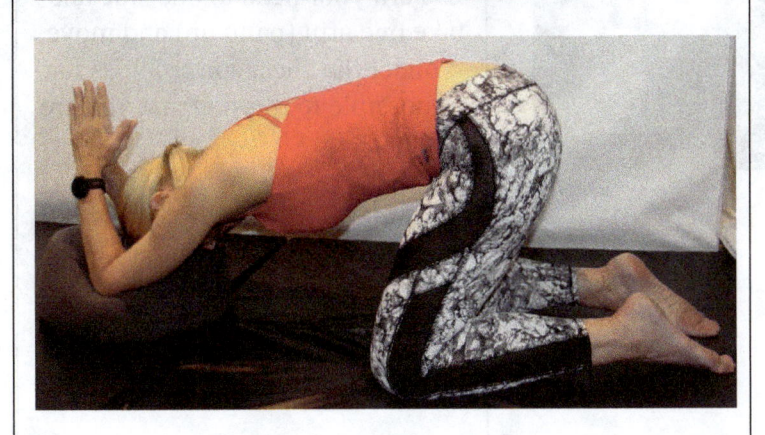

Target: Lower Rotators and Latissimus Dorsi

1. Start in a kneeling position with your elbows on a cushion.

2. Point your forearms vertical with palms touching.

3. Drop your head between your arms and move your buttocks towards your heals.

(Avoid your head being in an extended position)

4. Hold 5-20 seconds.

15. Child's Pose (Static)	**Target: Lower Rotators and Latissimus Dorsi, Lower Back and Buttocks (Gluteus Maximus)**
	1. From a kneeling position move your buttocks back to sit on your heels. 2. Reach forward with both arms (shoulder width apart) as far forward as possible. 3. Keep the palms forwards and as flat as possible on the ground. 4. Drop your head between your arms. 5. Hold 2-20 seconds.
16. Thread the Needle (Static)	**Target: Posterior Shoulder (Rotator Cuff), Lower Back and Buttocks (Gluteus Maximus)**
	1. From a kneeling position drop your chest and head to the floor. 2. Turn your head to one side and take one arm (palm up) and move it under the chest and reach as far as possible to the side that you are facing. 3. Buttocks can stay hi or dropped toward your heels. 4. Hold 5-20 seconds.

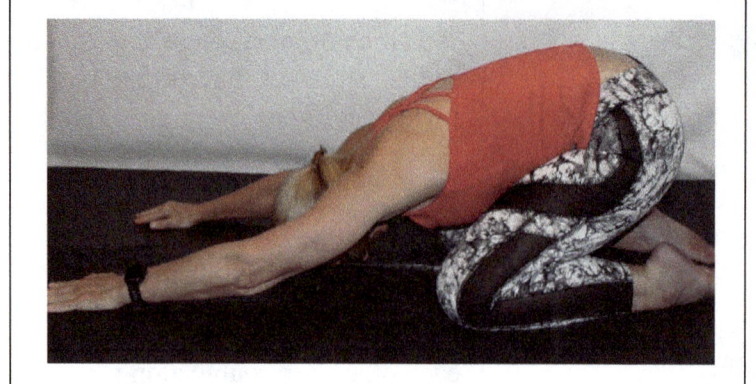

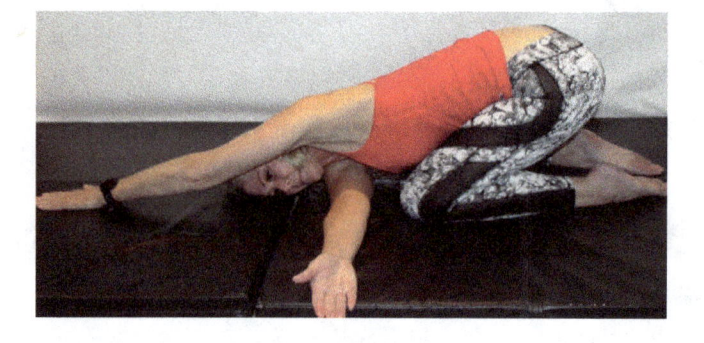

17. Eagle Arm (Static)	Target: Posterior Shoulder (Rotator Cuff)
	1. This pose can be done either standing in or seated on the mat. Either way, keep your upper back straight and look forward. 2. Hook the right elbow under the left, and wrap the hands so that your palms meet. Note – This is an advanced stretch. You may not be able to get your hands touching. Do the best you can. Advanced – Raising your elbows to deepen the stretch.

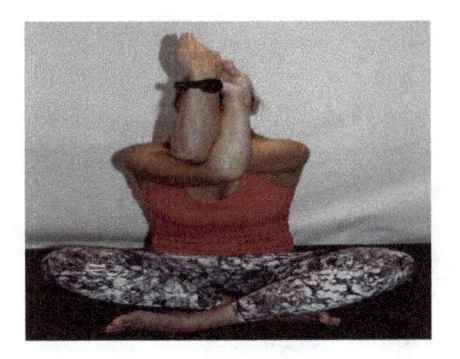

3. Trunk

1. Wide Stance Truck Rotations (Dynamic and Static)	Target: Trunk rotators
	1. Stand with feet shoulder width apart. 2. Hands can be on your hips, or arms can be extended out lateral or in front of the body as shown. 3. Rotate shoulder to one side as far as comfortable. 4. Hold for 5-20 seconds. 5. Rotate to the opposite side.

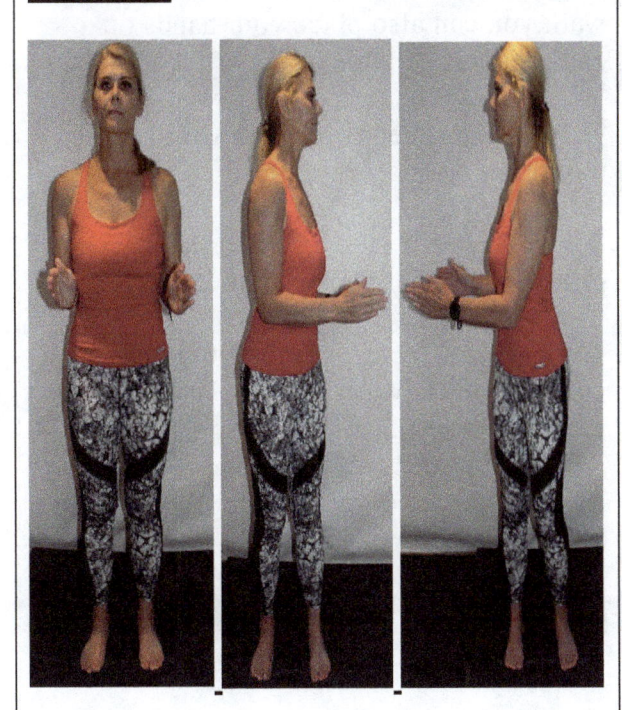

2. Wide Stance Side Lateral Bending (Dynamic and Static)

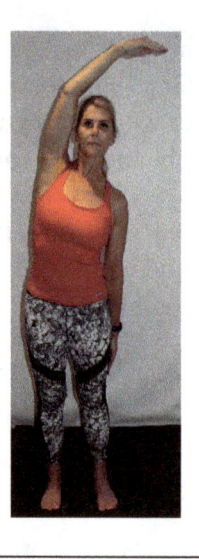

Target: Lateral benders of the trunk

1. Stand with feet shoulder width apart.

2. Bend laterally by running your hand down the side of your leg as far as comfortable.

3. Opposite arm can reach over your head or stay at your side.

4. Hold for 5-20 seconds.

5. Laterally bend to the opposite side.

4. Lower Back

1. Forward Bend at the Wall (Static)

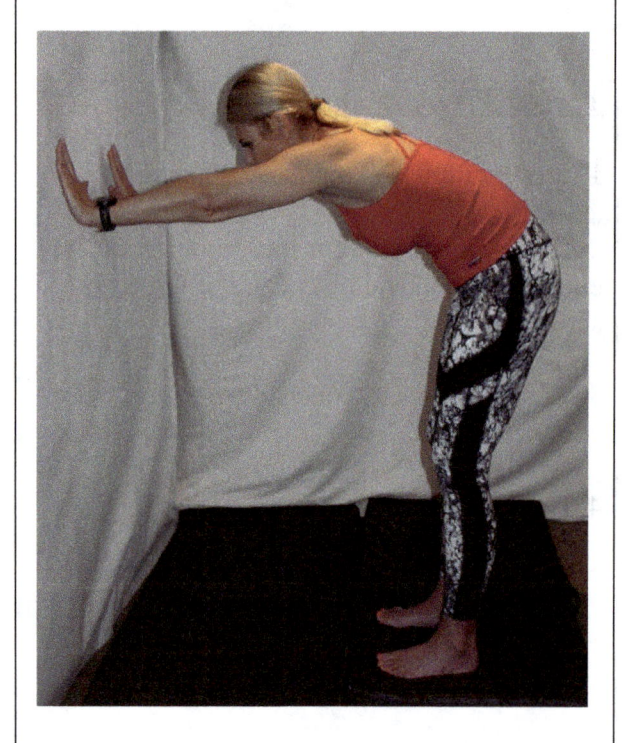

Target: Shoulders (Latissimus Dorsi), Lower Back and Hamstrings

1. Place your hands to the wall at chest height, shoulder-distance apart.
(Note - If you don't have access to a clear wall, you can also place your hands on a chair, bench, or table).

2. Walk your feet away from your support until your arms are straight.

3. Position your feet hip-distance apart and place a slight bend in your knees.

4. Press your hands into the support, and pull your hips away to lengthen your torso.

5. Put your head and neck in a position that follows the line of your spine.
(Do not extend your neck)

6. Hold for 5-20 seconds.

2. Rag Doll (Static)	**Target: Lower Back and Hamstrings**
	1. From standing position, feet shoulder width apart, bend forward at the waist.
	2. Have a slight bend in your knees initially. They may straighten once you have completed your forward bending.
	3. Have your arms hang down toward floor and cross the forearms in front of you and relax.
	4. Hold for 5-20 seconds.
	Caution – With your head hanging down toward the floor you may feel a rush of blood to the head. If you feel uncomfortable or lightheaded straighten yourself up and relax and Do Not repeat this exercise.
3. Child Pose with or without Blocks (Static)	**Target: Shoulders (Latissimus Dorsi), Lower Back and Buttocks (Gluteus Maximus)**
	1. If necessary, place two flat blocks shoulder-distance apart at the front of your mat.
	2. Bring your palms onto the blocks, and press your hips back and down toward your heels.
	3. Press your palms into the blocks, straighten your arms, and lengthen through the sides of your torso.
	4. Hold 5-20 seconds.

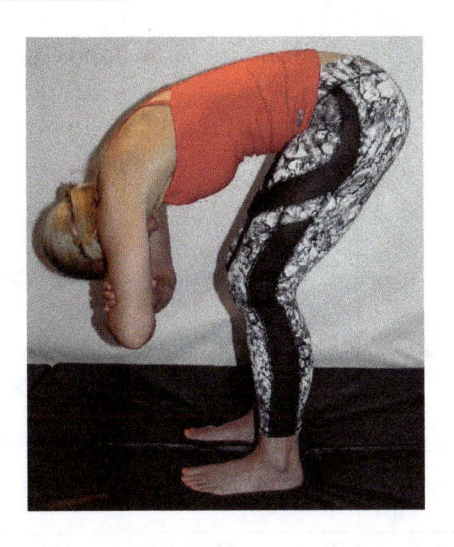

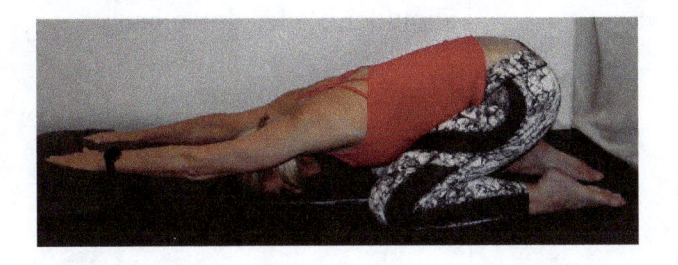

4. Cat Cow Pose **(Dynamic and Static)**	**Target: Lower Back** 1. Start on your hands and knees. 2. Arch your back downward. 3. Hold 5-20 seconds. 4. Round your back upward. 5. Hold 5-20 seconds.
5. Cobra **(Dynamic and Static)**	**Target: Hip Flexors (Quads) and Lower Back** 1. Lie face-down, forehead resting on the floor. 2. Place hands on either side, at middle of ribcage. Draw legs together, pressing tops of feet into floor. 3. Press evenly through hands as you draw elbows close to ribcage and using strength of back (not arms), lift head and chest, sliding shoulder blades down back. (Avoid hyperextending of the neck) 4. Hold for 5-20 seconds.

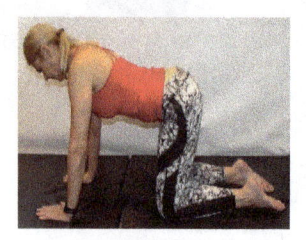

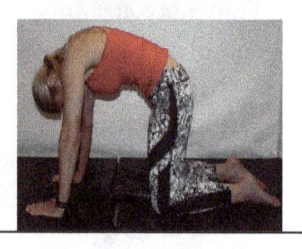

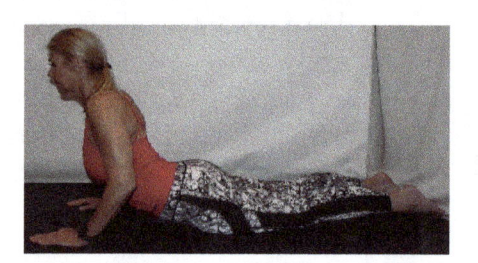

6. Sitting Butterfly with or without Blocks (Static) 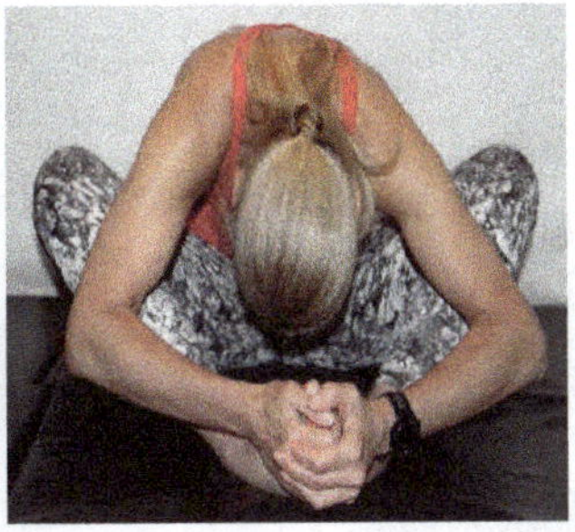 **Blocks to support head** 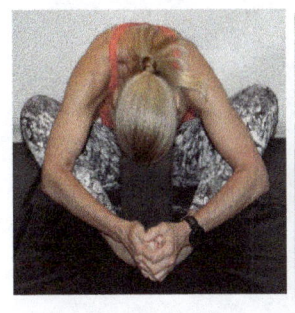 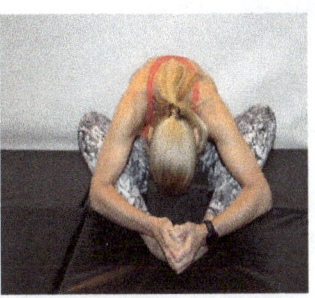	**Target: Inner Thighs (Groins) and Lower Back** 1. Sitting on buttocks or a block with feet facing each other and knees spread apart. 2. Lean forward at the hip. Use the block to support your head if you can bend that far forward. 3. Hold 5-20 seconds.
7. Supine Twist (Dynamic and Static) 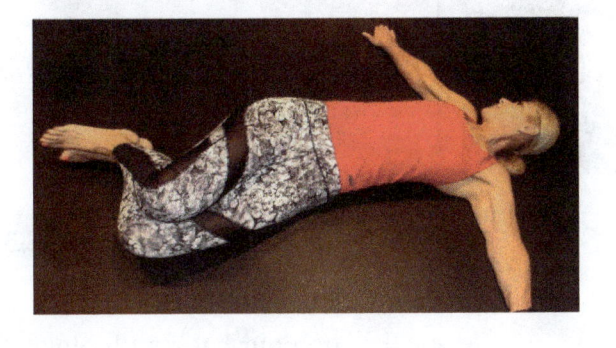	**Target: Lower Back Rotators** 1. Lie on your back. 2. Bend your knees 90° and rotate both of your legs to one side. Your knees should be stacked on top of each other with the bottom knee resting on the ground. 3. Do not force your knees down to the ground if you feel discomfort or too much stretch. If this is the case, tuck a pillow or block under your bottom knee for support. 4. Stay in this position for 5-20 seconds and then repeat on the other side.

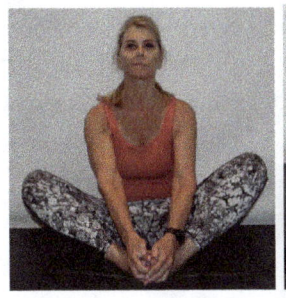

8. Bridge with or without Block at Lower Back	Target: Hip Flexors
With Block (Dynamic and Static) 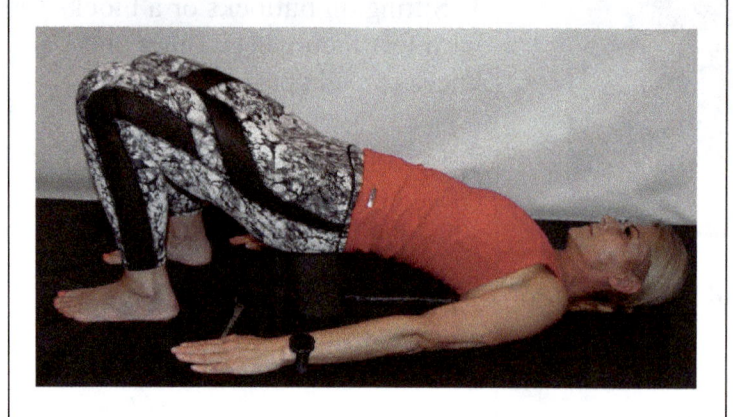 **Without Block** 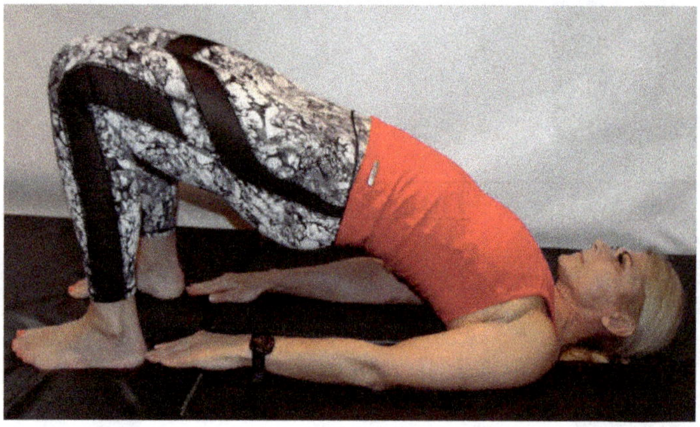	1. Lie down on your back with your knees bent 90º, feet are hip distance apart. Heels are under the bent knees. 2. Press your feet down and lift your hips. 3. Place one or two blocks under your hips. 4. Hold for 5-20 seconds.
9. Upper Back Block Stretch (Static) 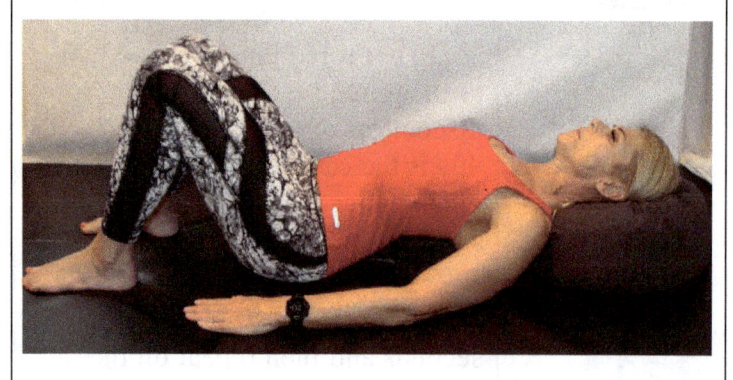	**Target: Upper Spine, abdominals and Chest (Pectoralis Major)** 1. Lie on your back with block positioned at shoulder blade level. The block can be positioned length or crossways. 2. Lean backwards and rest your head on another bock or a pillow for support. 3. Hold for 5-20 seconds. Advanced – Rest head on the ground.

10. Seated Spinal Twist (Static)	**Target: Lower Back Rotators and Buttocks (Gluteus Medius)**
	1. Sit on buttocks with straight & heels resting on the ground in front of you. 2. Cross one bent leg over the other extended leg. 3. Rotate trunk to side of bent leg and place opposite side elbow on the outside of bent knee. 4. Reach back as far as possible with bent knee side arm and placed on the ground. 5. Keep the back as straight as possible. 6. Hold for 5-20 seconds.
11. Lunge with a twist (Dynamic and Static)	**Target: Lower Back Rotators**
	1. From your hands and knees position, step one foot forward and place a tall block under the opposite hand. 2. Press into the ball of your back foot to straighten that back knee. 3. Place the hand on the side which the leg is forward on our hip or extend it up toward the ceiling and twist to the forward leg side (Imagine a line from your tailbone to the crown of your head, and rotate along that axis). 4. Hold for 5-20 seconds. 5. Bring the front foot backwards to return to the knee and hand (all fours) position. 6. Repeat with the opposite leg.

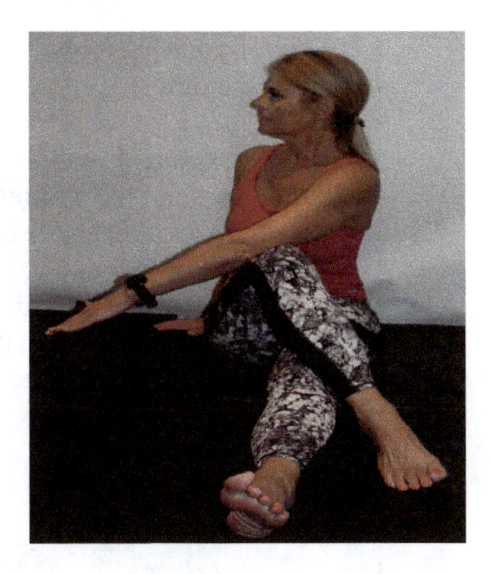

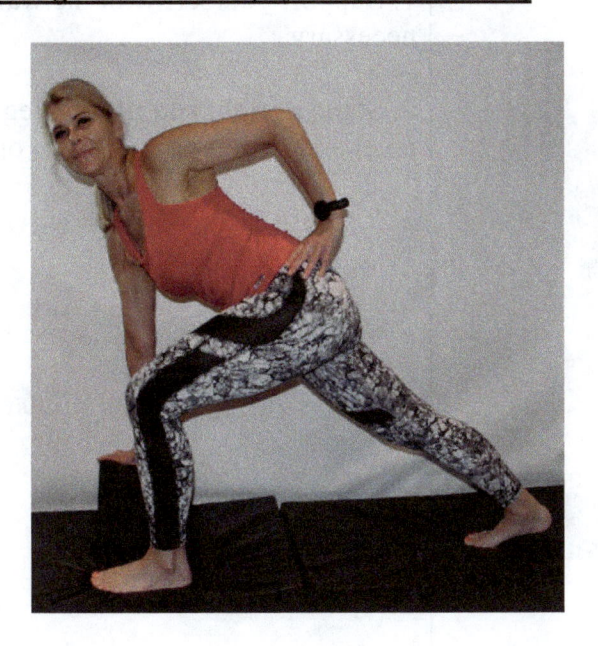

12. Triangle Pose (Dynamic and Static)	**Target: Lower Back Rotators**
	1. Scissor your legs (one leg in front of the other). 2. Reach down and with the arm opposite the lead leg and reach down to the level of the lead foot. 3. Twist your trunk toward the lead leg side and extend that side arm toward the ceiling. 4. Hold for 5-20 seconds.

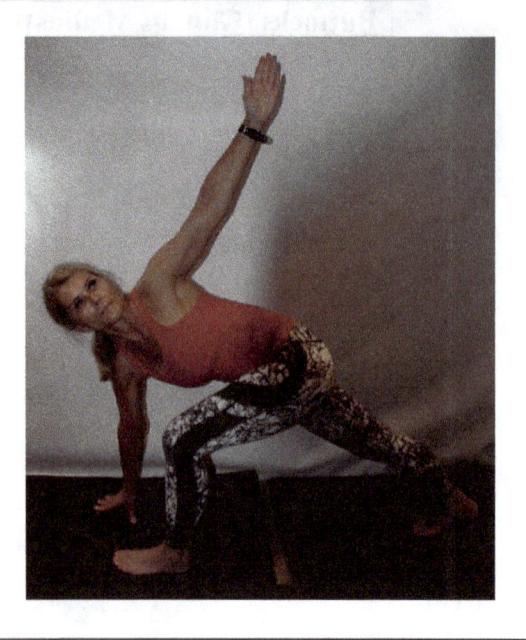

5. Hips

1. Marching (Dynamic)	**Target: Hip Flexors and Extensors**
	1. Support yourself with the wall or chair if necessary. 2. Stand upright and lift one leg to waist level and then repeat with the opposite leg. 3. Repeat 10x's with each leg

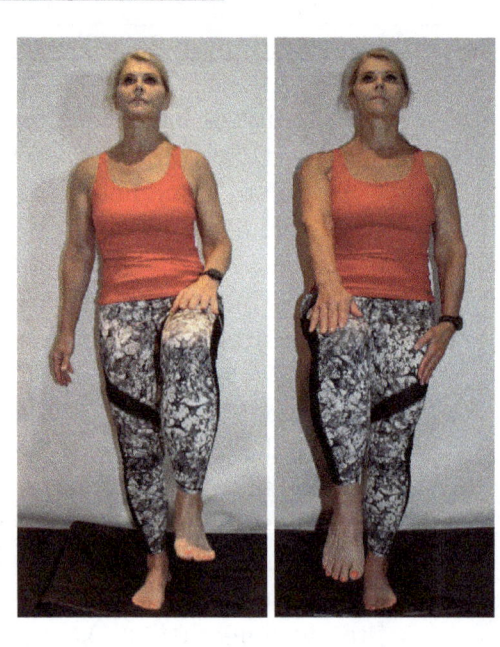

2. Leg Swings (Dynamic)

Forward and backward

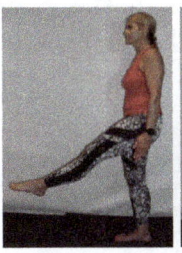

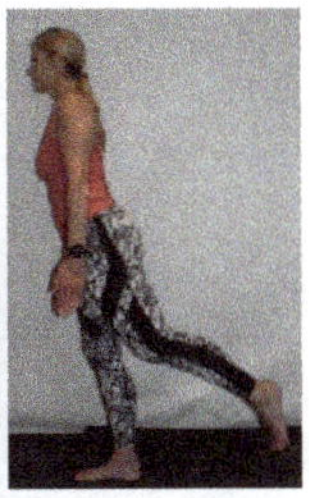

Side to Side

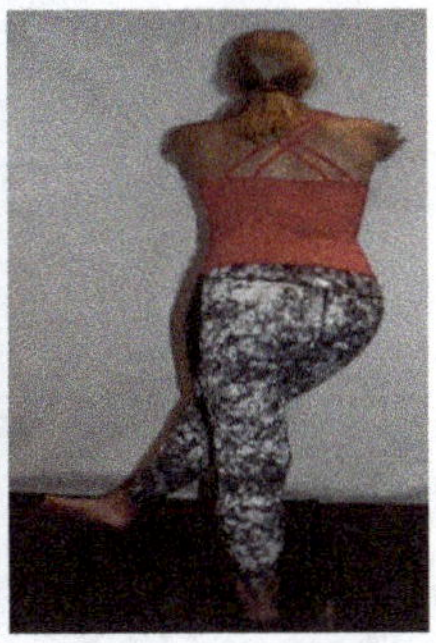

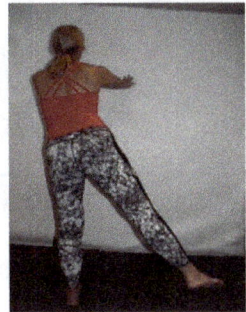

Target: Hip Lateral Stabilizers

Support yourself with the wall or chair if necessary.

Forward and Backward Swing

1. Swing one leg forward and backward.

2. Start the swinging of the leg small but try to progress to a larger swing with each repetition.

3. Do 10 reps in each direction with one leg and then repeat with the opposite leg.

Side to Side Swing

1. Swing one leg across your body and then out to the side laterally.

2. Start each swing small but try to increase the size of the swing with each repetition.

3. Do 10 reps with one leg and then repeat with the other leg.

3. Knee to Chest (Static)

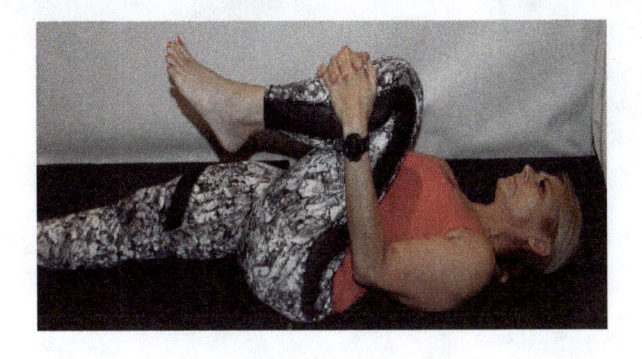

Target: Buttocks (Gluteus Maximus)

1. Lie on back and bring knee to same side chest.
(Try to keep the opposite leg flat on the floor)

2. Hold for 5-20 seconds.

4. Knee to Opposite Chest (Static)	**Target: Buttocks (Gluteus Medius)**
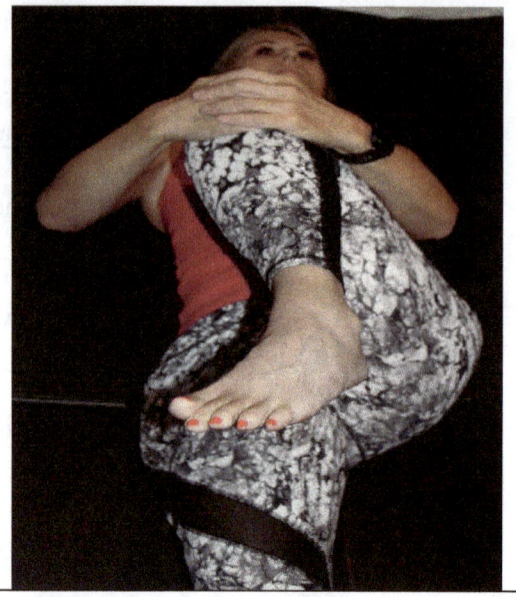	1. Lie on the floor and bring knee to opposite chest. (Try to keep opposite leg flat on the floor) 2. Hold for 5-20 seconds.
5. Lying Leg Crossover (Static)	**Target: Buttocks (Gluteus Medius)**
	1. Lie on the floor and cross one extended leg across body. 2. Extend arms out and look away from the crossed leg. 3. Try to get the cross over foot as close to the floor as possible. 4. Hold for 5-20 seconds.
6. Sitting Leg Crossover (Static)	**Target: Buttocks (Gluteus Medius)**
	1. Sit tall on buttocks. 2. Cross one leg over the opposite leg and pull the knee in towards the opposite shoulder. 3. Twist the upper body towards the crossed knee. 4. Hold for 5-20 seconds.

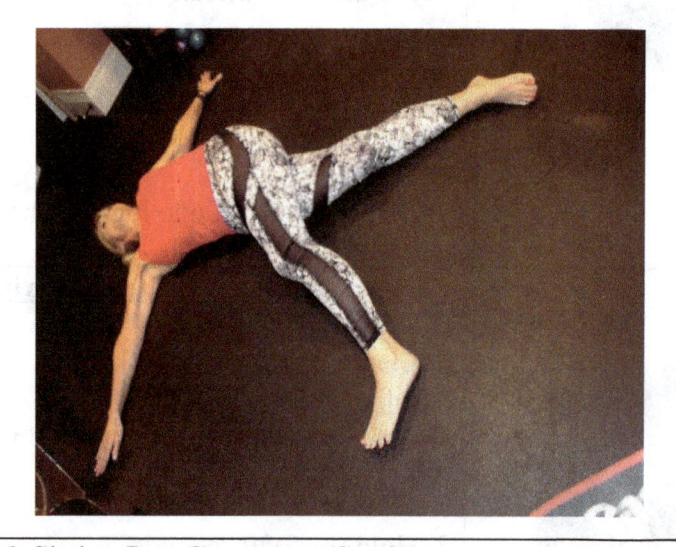

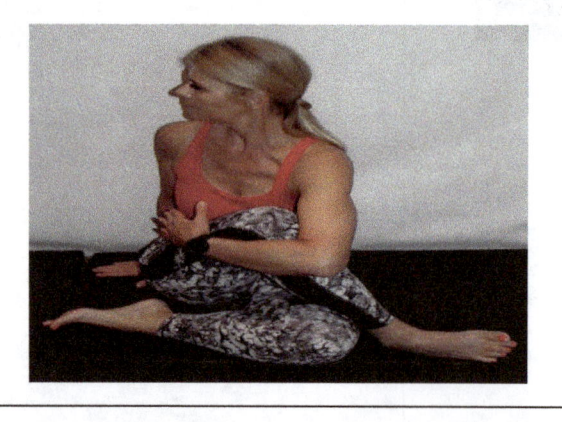

7. Thread the Needle (Static)	**Target: Buttocks (Gluteus Maximus and Medius)**
	1. Lie on your back with your knees and hips bent 90º.
	2. Place one ankle right above the opposite knee, creating a "four" shape with one leg.
	3. Thread arm through the opening you created with the crossed over leg and clasp hands behind opposite knee.
	4. Pull that knee toward chest.
	5. Hold for 5-20 seconds.
8. Happy Baby Pose (Static)	**Target: Inner Thighs (Groins) and Buttocks (Gluteus Maximus)**
	1. Lie on the mat and pull your knees to your chest.
	2. Place hands on outsides of feet, opening your knees wider than your torso.
	3. Press your feet into hands while pulling down on feet, creating resistance.
	4. Hold for 5-20 seconds.
9. Recline Butterfly (Static)	**Target: Inner Thighs (Groins)**
	1. Lie on your mat with your knees bent 90º.
	2. Bring soles of feet together and let knees fall out to sides as far as possible.
	3. Place hands on your chest
	4. Hold for 5-20 seconds.

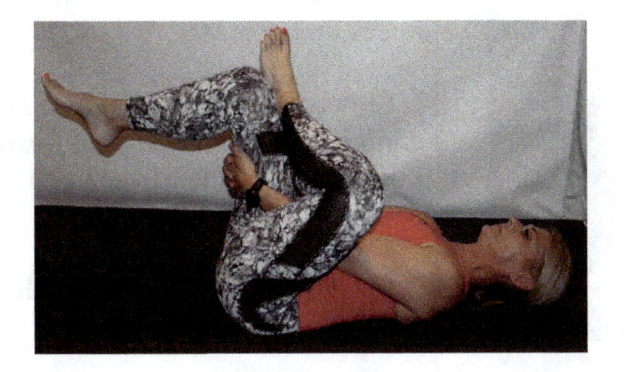

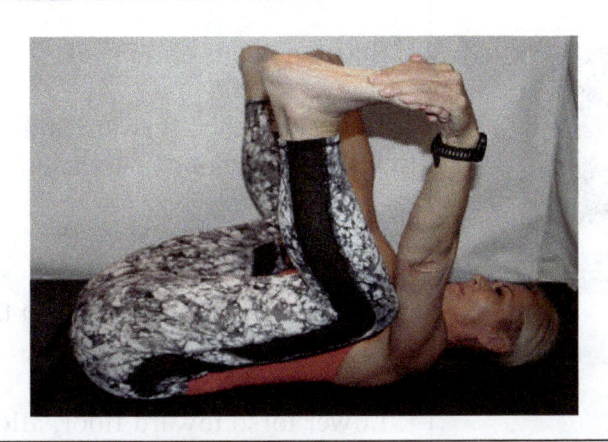

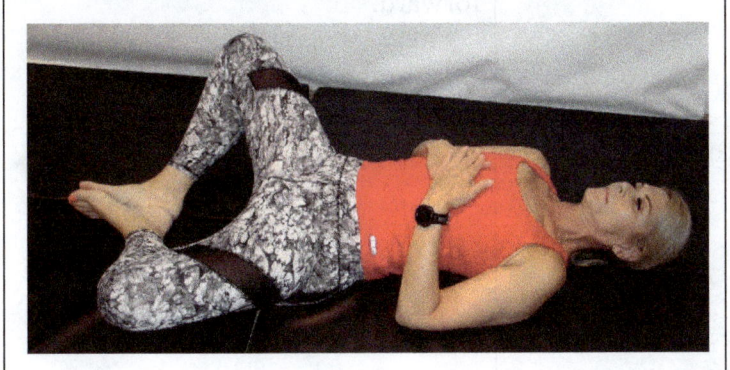

10. Frog Pose (Static)	**Target: Inner Thighs (Groins)** 1. Get down on all fours, with hands and knees on the mat. 2. Slowly widen your knees until you feel a comfortable stretch in your inner thighs, keeping the inside of each calf and foot in contact with the floor. 3. Make sure to keep your ankles as wide as your knees. 4. Lower your chest towards the mat. 5. Hold for 5-20 seconds.
11. Half Pigeon (Static)	**Target: Buttocks (Gluteus Medius)** 1. Start on hands and knees. 2. Move one knee forward and cross the lower leg in front of pelvis. 3. The crossed leg rest on the floor. (Your hips should be square to the front of the room) 4. Lower torso toward floor, allowing head to rest on floor with arms extended forward. 5. Hold for 5-20 seconds.

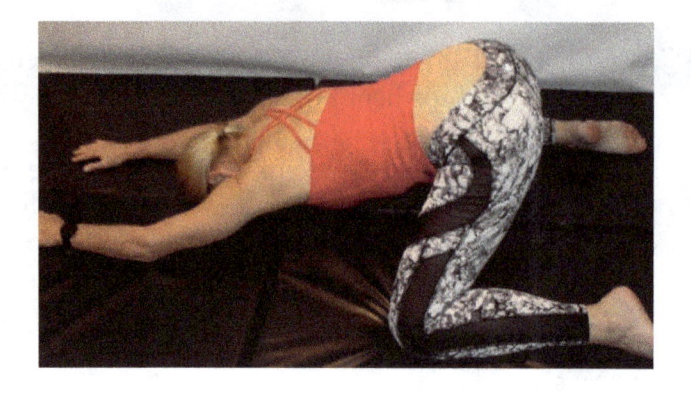

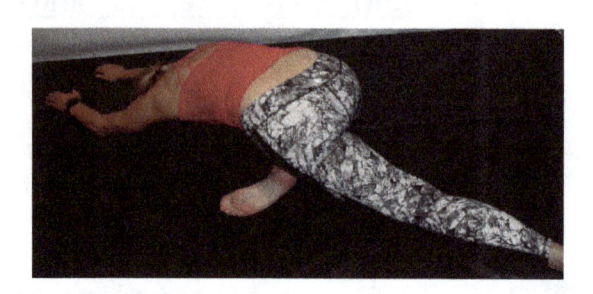

12. Double Pigeon (Static)	**Target: Buttocks (Gluteus Medius)**
	1. Sit on the floor with knees bent and shins stacked with one leg on top of the other. 2. Use your hand to position the top ankle onto bottom knee. (Ideally, the top knee will rest close to the floo, but if your hips are tight, your top knee may point up toward the ceiling (overtime, as your hips become more open, your knee will lower). Advanced – Keeping your hips squared to the front of the room, hinge at the hips and slowly walk hands slightly forward to feel a good stretch in the lower back.
13. Camel Pose (Dynamic and Static)	**Target: Hip Flexors (Quads)**
	1. Kneel on a mat with knees hip-width apart. (Toes should be lying flat to the ground) 2. Put hands on lower back with fingers pointing down and palms resting above glutes. 3. Lift your chest and slowly start to lean backwards. 4. Attempt to have hands reach and touch your heels. Press thighs forward so they stay perpendicular to the floor. 5. Keep head in neural position. DON'T let it extend backwards. 6. Hold 5-20 seconds. (Come out of the pose by bringing your hands to your hips and slowly lift your torso to starting position).

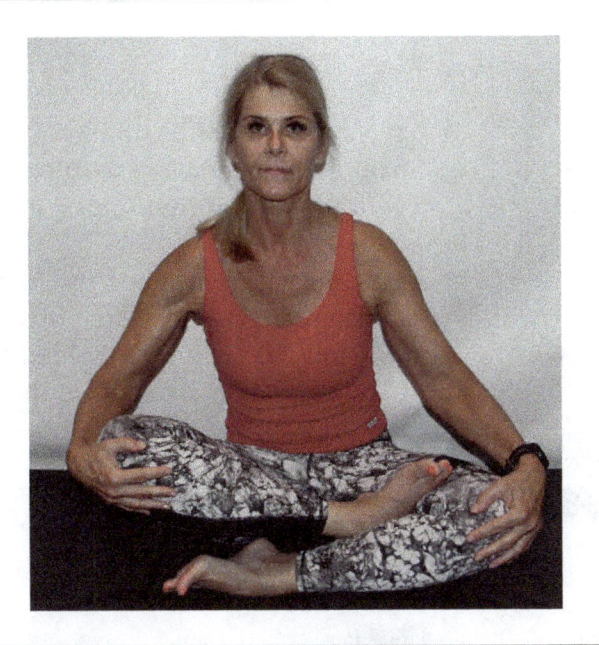

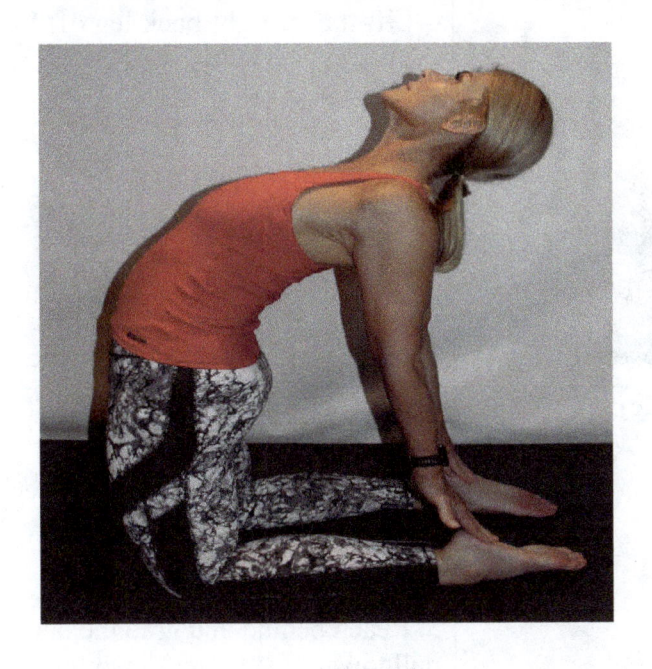

14. Low & High Lunge (Static)
Low Lunge

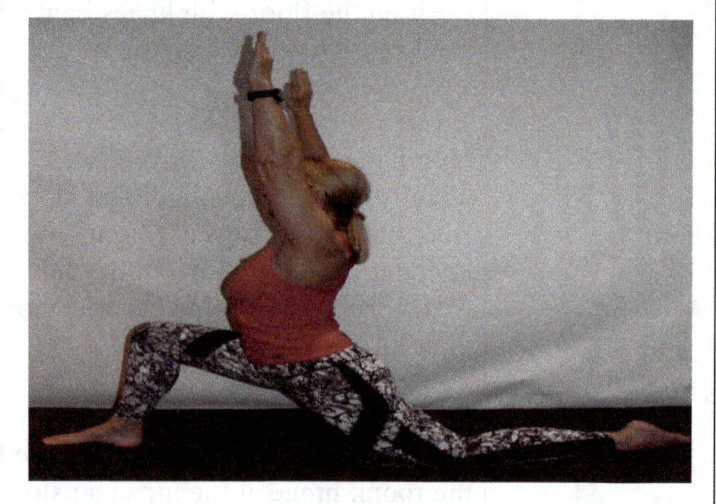

Target: Hip Flexors (Quads)

Low Lunge:

1. Start with one leg forward with knee over ankle and the opposite knee on ground with top of that foot flat on the mat.

2. Slowly lift chest and rest hands lightly on front thigh. Lean hips forward slightly, keeping the front knee behind the front toes, and feel the stretch in the rear leg hip flexor.

Advanced:
1. Raise arms overhead.

High Lunge

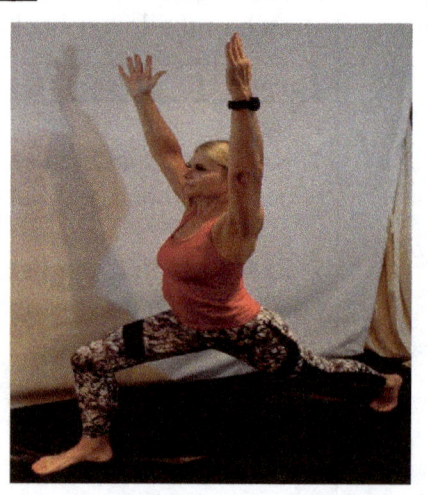

High Lunge (Advanced)

– Lift the straight back leg off the mat.

15. Low Lunge with Ankle Grab (Static)

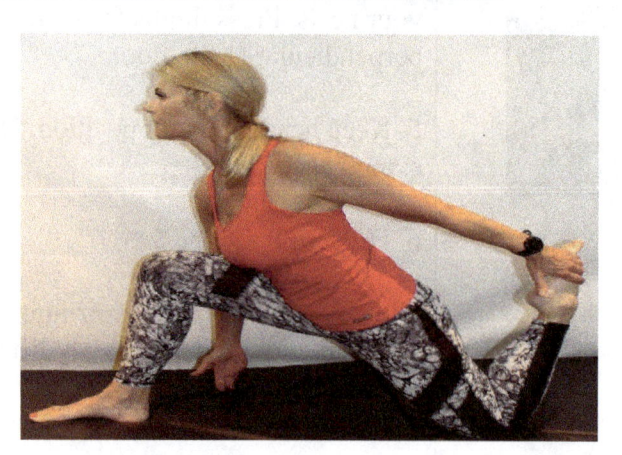

Target: Hip Flexors (Quads)

1. Get into a low lunge position (#14 above)

2. Bend the back knee

3. Reach behind and grab the back ankle and pull toward the buttocks while you lean forward onto the opposite front leg.

3. Hold for 5-20 seconds.

16. Sitting Pose With or Without Block (Static)	**Target: Quads, Anterior Shins (Tibialis Anterior) and Anterior Ankles (Ankle Dorsi Flexor Tendons)** 1. Kneel on your mat with thighs perpendicular to the floor and the tops of your feet facing down. 2. Place a yoga block between your feet and under the buttocks. 3. Bring your inner knees together and slide your feet apart so they are slightly wider than your hips. 4. Slowly lower your buttocks sit down on the yoga block. 5. Rest your hands on your thighs. Advanced – Remove the block so your buttocks rest on the mat between your feet.
17. Reclining Hero Pose (Static)	**Targets: Quads, Anterior Shins (Tibialis Anterior) and Anterior Ankles (Ankle Dorsi Flexor Tendons)** 1. Kneel on your mat with your thighs perpendicular to the floor and tops of your feet facing down. 2. Bring your inner knees together & slide your feet apart so they are slightly wider than your hips. 3. Slowly lower buttocks between your feet and slowly lower upper back to the booster. 5. Use a booster to support your head as well. 6. Hold for 5-20 seconds Advanced - Lower the upper back and head to the floor.

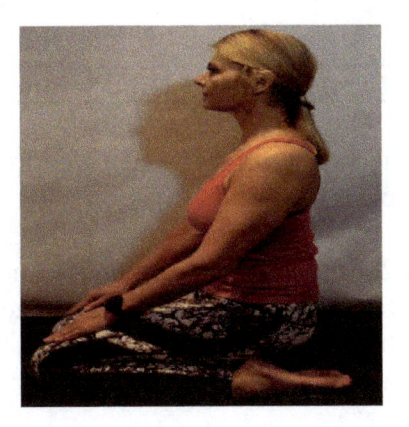

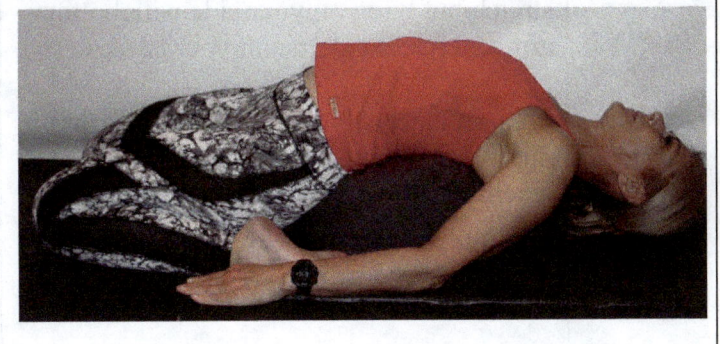

6. Legs

1. Quadriceps

1. Supported Standing Heel to Buttocks (Static)	**Targets: Quads, Hip Flexors**
	1. Stand upright beside or in front of a chair or wall for balance. 2. Simultaneously bend one knee and raise heel toward buttocks while reaching behind and gripping the raised foot or ankle. 3. Squeeze the foot/heel toward buttocks while maintaining an erect posture. 4. Hold for 5-20 seconds. (The thigh should be pointing vertical toward the ground and in line with the supporting/opposite leg).
2. Side Lying Heel to Buttocks (Static)	**Targets: Quads and Hip Flexors**
	1. Very similar to standing heel to buttocks stretch but lying on your side with bottom arm extended underneath your head. 2. Simultaneously bend the top knee and move your heel toward buttocks while reaching behind with the top hand and gripping the foot or ankle. 3. Squeeze the foot/heel toward buttocks. 4. Hold for 5-20 seconds. (The thigh should be horizontal and in line with the opposite leg which is lying extended on the mat).

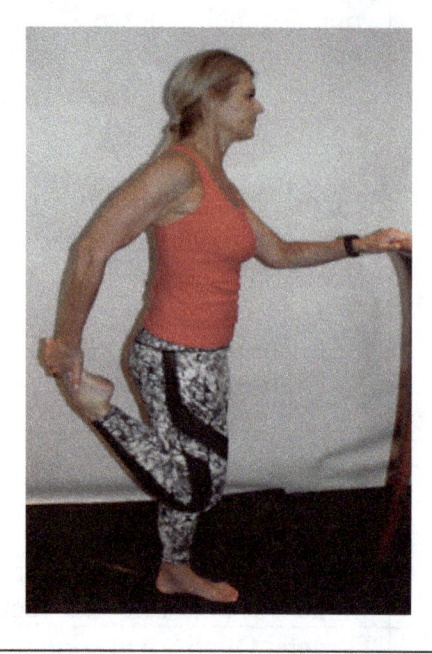

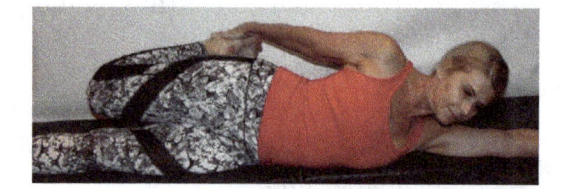

3. The following are Quad Stretches which are listed and Explained under Hip Stretches:

1. Camel Pose (Static)	**2. Low Lunge (Static)**
	High Lunge (Static)

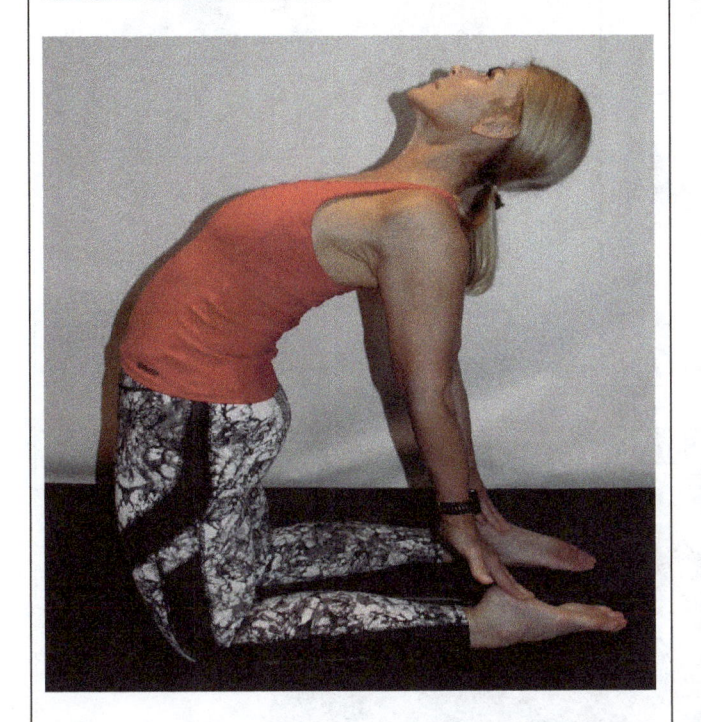

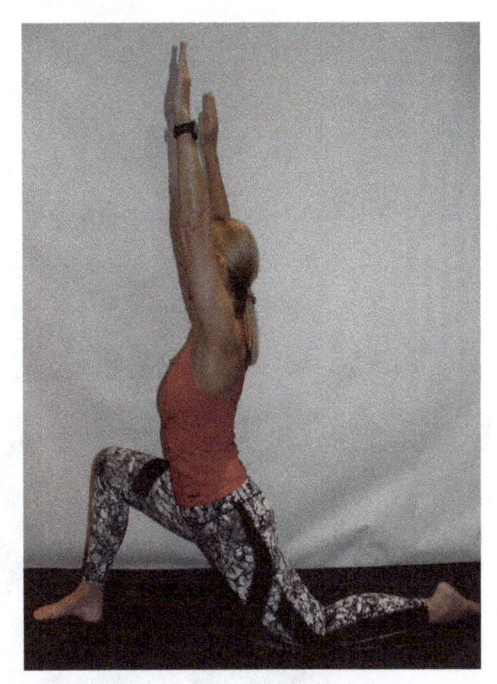

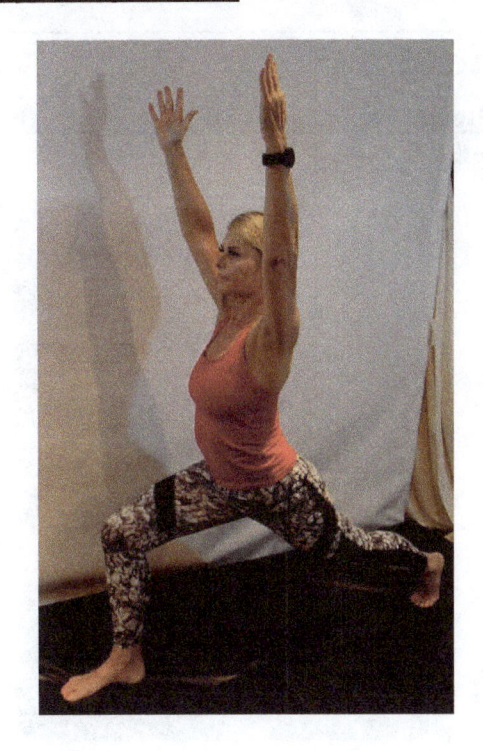

3. Low Lunge with Ankle Grab (Static)

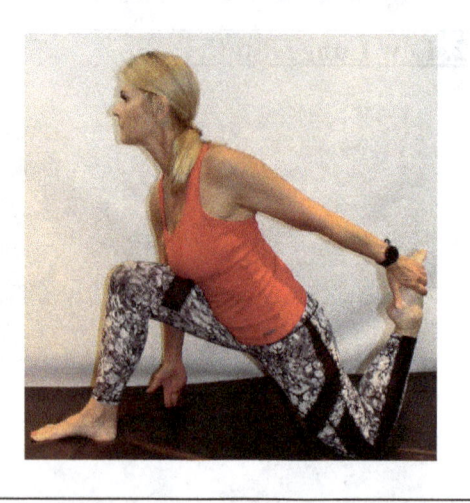

4. Sitting Pose with Block (Static)

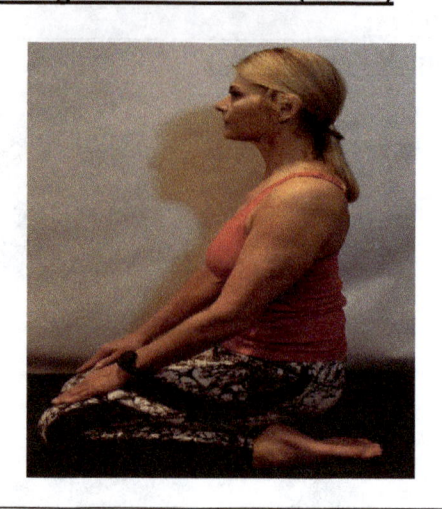

5. Reclining Hero Pose with or Without Support (Static)

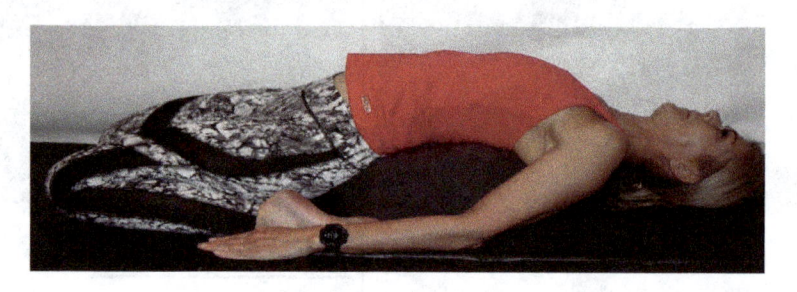

2. Hamstrings

1. Bend Over at Hips 90° and Touch the Wall (Static)

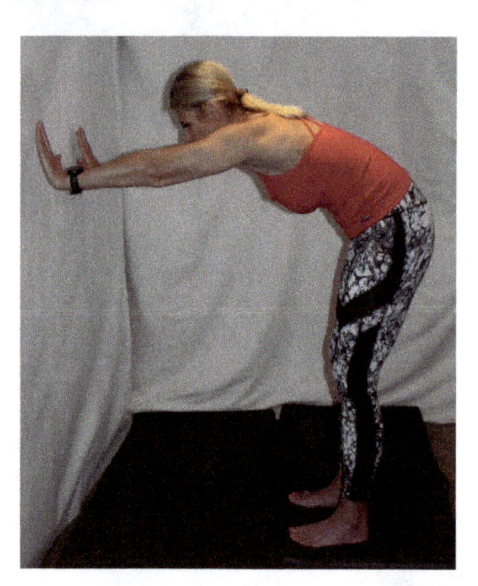

Target: Shoulders (Latissimus Dorsi), Lower Back and Hamstrings

1. Bring your hands to the wall at chest height, shoulder-distance apart.

2. Walk your feet away from the wall until your arms are straight. Bring your feet hip-distance apart and place a slight bend in your knees.

3. Press your hands into the wall, and pull your hips away to lengthen your torso.

4. Place your head and neck in a position that follows the line of your spine.

5. Hold for 5-20 seconds.

(Note - If you don't have access to a clear wall, you can also place your hands on a chair, bench, or table).

2. Standing Toe Touch (Static)	**Targets: Hamstrings and Lower Back**
	1. Stand erect with feet shoulder width apart. 2. Slowly bend forward at the hips and run your hands down the front of your legs and attempt to touch your toes (only go down as far as you are comfort). 3. Hold for 5-20 seconds and then slowly return to an upright position. 4. Repeat. Try to go a bit further down towards the toes on each repetition.
3. Modified Standing Toe Touch (Static)	**Targets: Hamstrings and Lower Back**
	1. Stand erect and place one foot in front of the other. 2. Bend forward at the waist, running your hands down the front leg to the knee that is extended in front and keep the knee of the other leg slightly bent and its foot flat on the mat. 3. Hold 5-20 seconds.
4. Standing Foot on Bench (Static)	**Targets: Hamstrings and Lower Back**
	1. Stand facing the side of a bench (18" high) or stairs. 2. Place one foot on the bench or on the second step so the foot is about 18-24" off the floor. 3. Bend slowly forward at the hip and try to touch the foot that is on the bench/stairs while maintaining good balance. 4. Hold for 5-20 seconds.

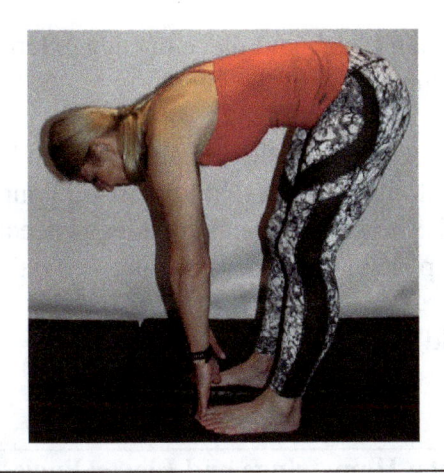

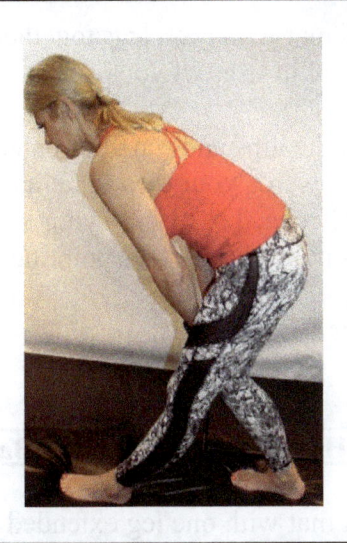

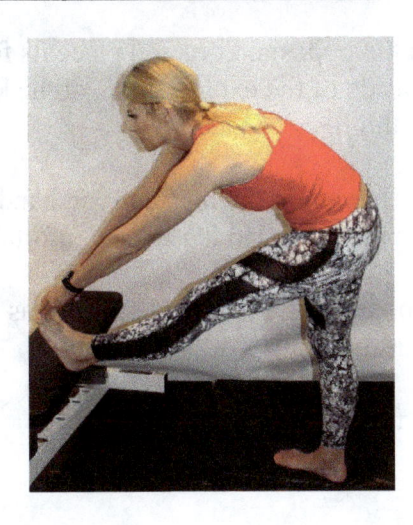

5. Sitting One leg Bench Hamstring Stretch (Static) 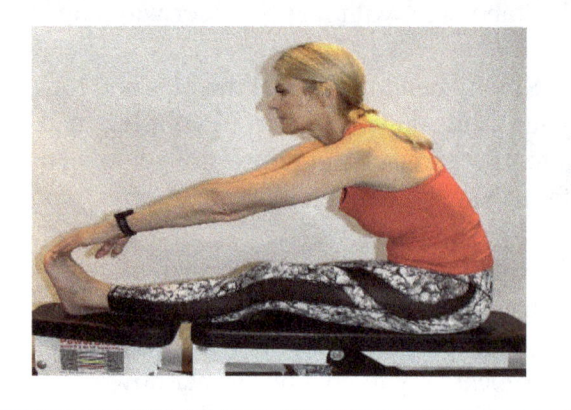	**Targets: Hamstrings and Lower Back** 1. Sit on a bench and place one leg extended along the length of the bench. 2. Bend forward at the hip and run both hands down along the extended leg toward your toes. Try to keep the extended legs knee as flat as possible and toes pointing vertical. 3. Hold for 5-20 seconds.
6. Sitting Double Leg Hamstring Stretch (Static) 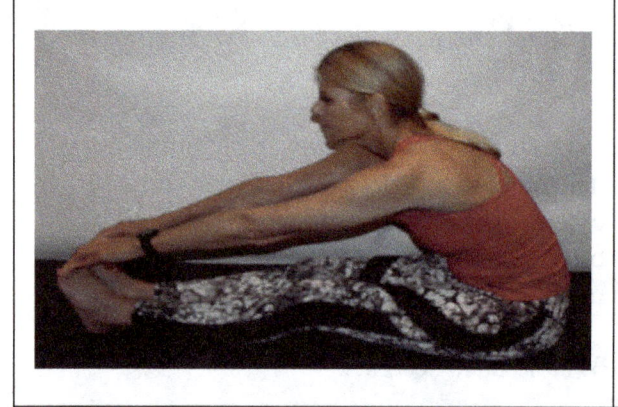	**Targets: Hamstrings and Lower Back** 1. Sit on a mat with both legs together and extended out in front of you. 2. Bend at the hips and run your hands down your legs towards your toes as far as you comfortably can. Try to keep your knees as straight as possible and toes pointing vertical. 3. Hold for 5-20 seconds.
7. Sitting Floor Hurdler Stretch (Static)	**Targets: Hamstrings and Lower Back** 1. Sit on a mat with one leg extended out in front of you. 2. Bend the opposite knee and place its foot on the inside of the extended leg, at the knee or inner thigh. 3. Bend forward at the hips and run hands as far down the extended leg as is comfortable. 4. Try to keep the extended legs knee as straight as possible. 5. Hold for 5-20 seconds.

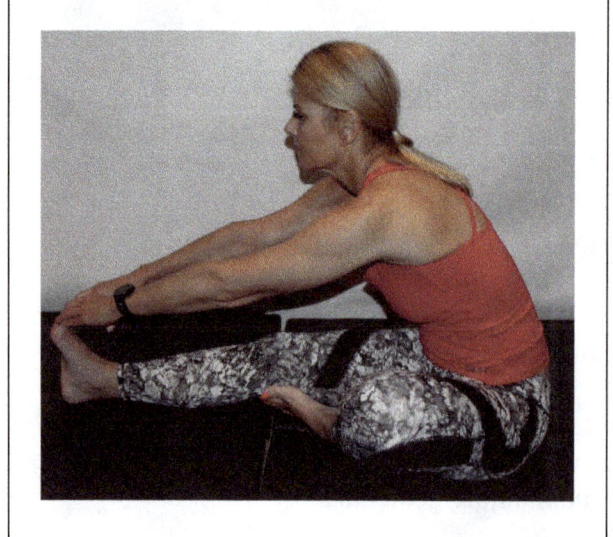

8. Lying Floor Rubber Band/Towel Stretch (Dynamic and Static) 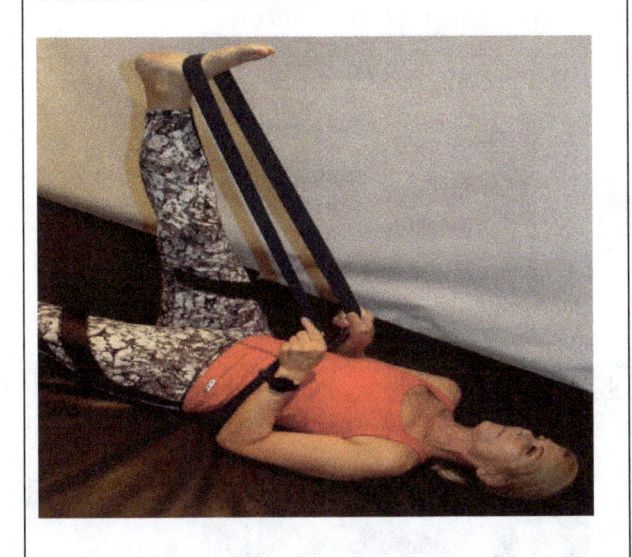	Targets: Hamstrings and Calves
	1. Lying on your back flat on a mat. 2. Place an elastic resistant rubber band or towel around the arch of one foot. 3. Lift that foot up as high as possible while trying to keep the knee as straight as possible. 4. Once you reach your extended limit pull down on the rubber band/towel to try to get a little extra stretch in the hamstring. 5. Hold for 5-20 seconds. **Advanced Stretch** – Once in the maximum stretched position push the extended leg against the rubber band/towel for 10 seconds and then pull on the rubber band/towel to get a little extra stretch.
9. Wall Hamstring Stretch (Static) 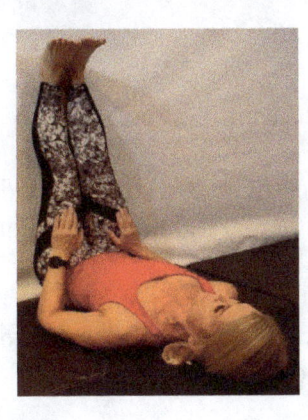	Targets: Hamstrings
	1. Lying on your back move your hips as close to the wall as possible and extend your legs up onto the wall. 2. Keep inching your hips closer to the wall and moving your legs farther up the wall. 3. Try to keep your knees as straight as possible. 4. Hold for 5-20 seconds.

3. Abductors (Groins)

Abductor Stretches illustrated and Explained under Hip Stretches	
1. Frog Pose (Dynamic and Static) 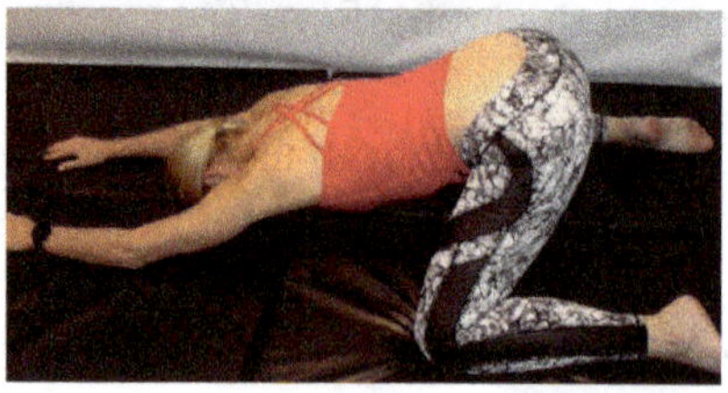	**2. Recline Butterfly (Dynamic and Static)** 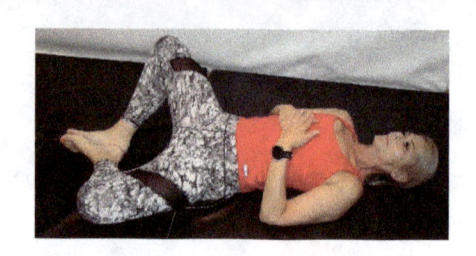
3. Baby Pose (Dynamic and Static) 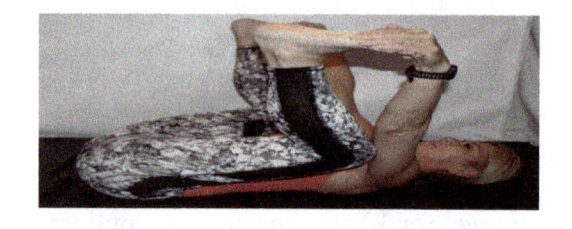	**4. Half Happy Baby Pose (Dynamic and Static)** 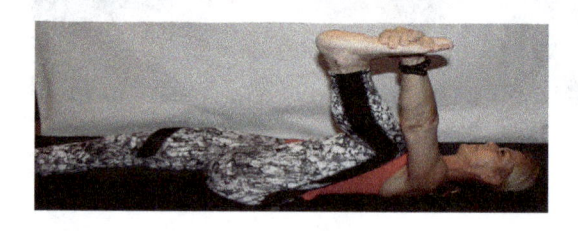

4. Gastrocs and Soleus (Calves and Achilles Tendon)

1. Wall Lean with one Knee Bent (Static)	**Targets: Gastrocs, Soleus and Achilles Tendon**
	Gastrocs:
	1. Facing the wall.
	2. Take a step back with one leg and keep the knee of that leg straight and heel flat on the ground.
	3. Lean forward against the wall and bend the knee of the other leg which is closest to the wall.
	4. Hold for 5-20 seconds.
	Soleus (Achilles Tendon):
	1. Similar to Gastroc stretch but the back knee is bent to stretch the deeper Soleus muscle and Achilles Tendon.

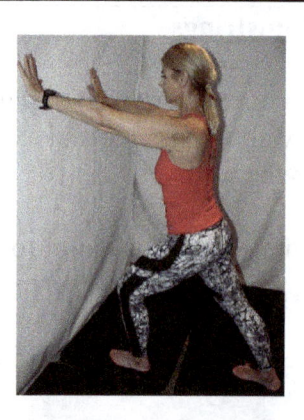

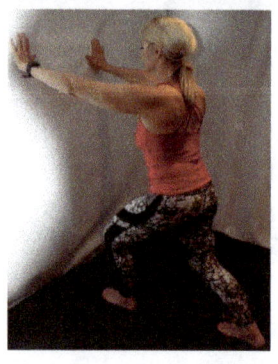

5. Tibialis Anterior (Anterior Shin)

1. Toe Drag (Dynamic and Static)	Targets: Tibialis Anterior and top of the foot
	1. Stand next to a chair or wall for balance. 2. Point toes of one foot down to floor and lean forward slightly as if you are going to drag the toes along the floor. 3. Hold for 5 -20 seconds
2. Sitting Pose with or without Block (Static)	Target: Quads, Anterior Shins (Tibialis Anterior) and Anterior Ankles (Ankle Dorsi Flexor Tendons)
	1. Kneel on your mat with thighs perpendicular to the floor and tops of your feet facing down. 2. Place a yoga block between your feet. Bring your inner knees together and slide your feet apart so they are slightly wider than your hips. 3. Slowly sit down on the yoga block. Allow the backs of your hands to rest on your thighs. 4. Hold for 5 -20 seconds Advanced - remove the block and move buttocks down so it is sitting on the mat.

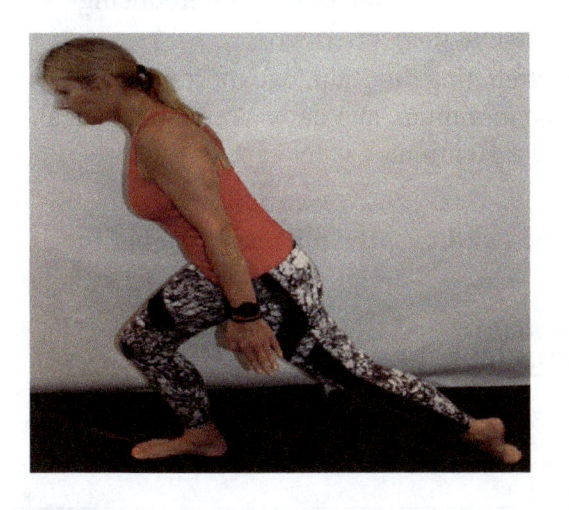

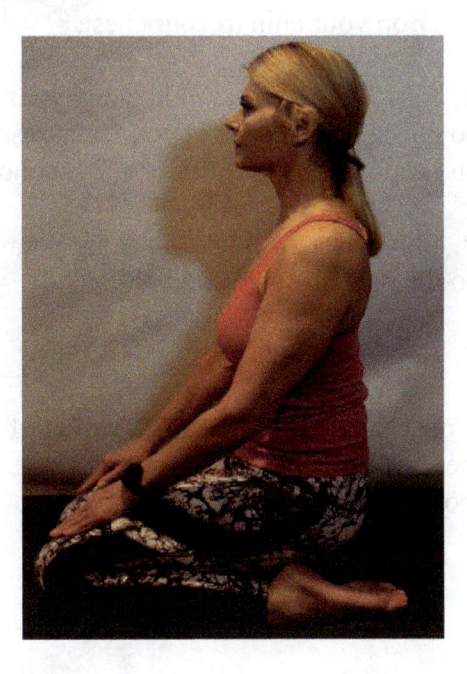

Appendix 9.1.4.2. 10 Minute Dynamic and Static Stretching Routine

The 10-minute stretching program illustrated below is an effective way of introducing stretching and improving flexibility in a very time-efficient manner.

Key Point – to gain maximum benefit from any stretching program, one must perform it frequently and consistently. Three times a week is the minimum, and daily stretching is ideal. Spending 10 minutes a day stretching could be the best 10 minutes spent each day.

Remember to hold each static stretch for 20 seconds and breathe normally during the stretch.

Dynamic & Static Stretches for Neck, Shoulders, Lower Back, Hips, Legs

Dynamic Stretches

1. Neck:	
1. Semi-circle Head Rotations	**Target: Lateral and Extensor Neck and Trapezius**
	1. Drop your chin to your chest.
	2. Slowly rotate your chin along your chest to one shoulder or until you feel stress in the neck muscles. Hold for 1-2 seconds.
	3. Slowly rotate your chin along your chest to the opposite side and hold
	4. Repeat 3-5 x's
	Note- Never do a full 360° rotation of your neck or put your neck in an extended position

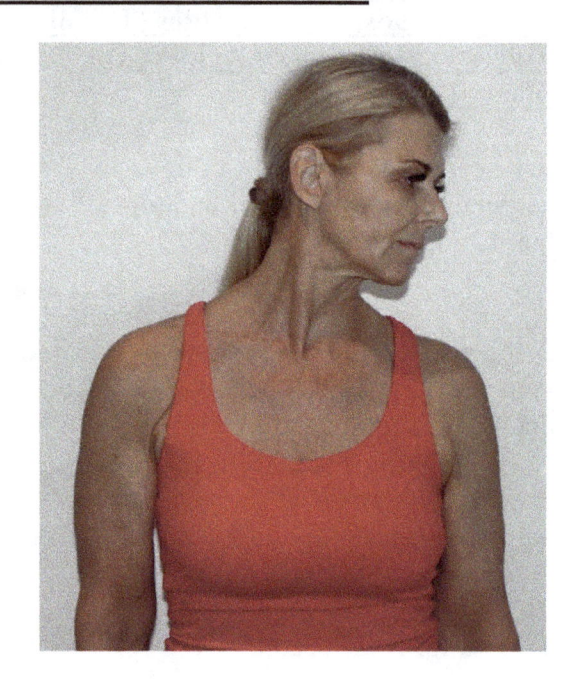

2. Shoulders:

1. Shoulder Rolls

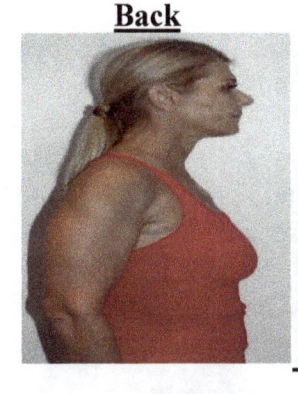

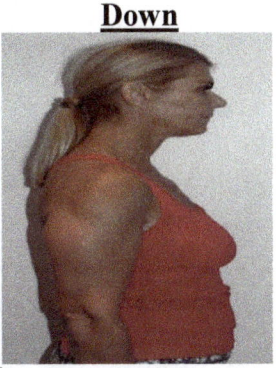

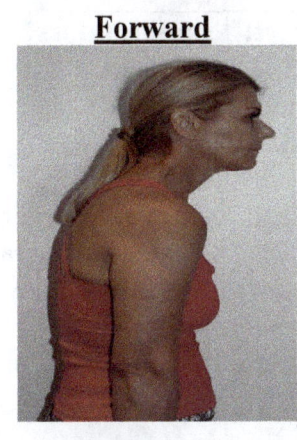

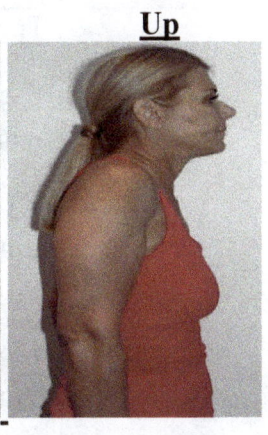

Back — Down — Forward — Up

Target: Rotator cuff, Traps. Chest (Pectoralis Major)

1. Stand with feet shoulder width apart and arms are along the side of the body.

2. Move shoulders back, down to the front and then up for one complete rotation.

3. Repeat 5 rotations in one direction and then 5 in the opposite direction.

2. Standing Arm Circles

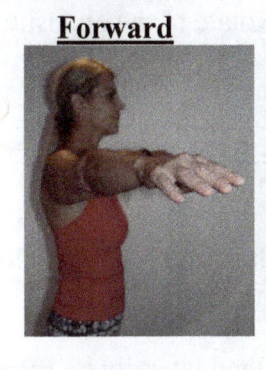

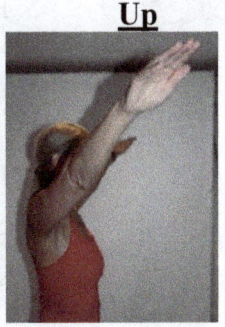

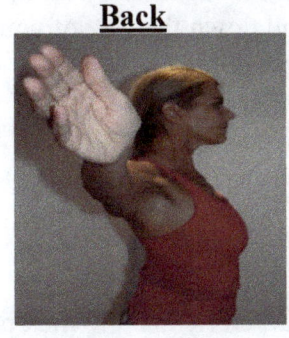

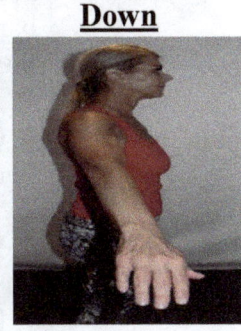

Forward — Up — Back — Down

Target: Rotator Cuff and Chest (Pectoralis Major)

1. Standing upright and lift your arms to shoulder height.

2. <u>Slowly</u> rotate your arms in a forward direction 10x's and then in a backward direction 10x's

3. Slightly increase the size of the circle on each rotation.

3. Standing Huggers	**Target: Rotator Cuff and Chest (Pectoralis Major)**
	1. Stand upright and lift your arms to shoulder height. 2. Move the arms across your body and hug yourself. Hold the hug for 1-2 seconds. 3. On each hug alternate which arm goes on top of the other.

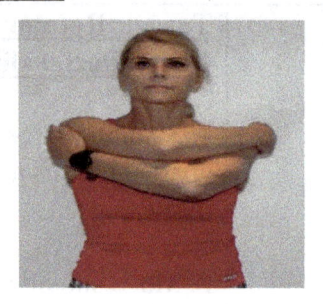

3. Trunk:

1. Wide Stance Truck Rotations	**Target: Trunk rotators**
	1. Stand with feet shoulder width apart. 2. Hands can be on your hips, or arms can be extended out lateral or in front of the body as shown. 3. Rotate shoulder to one side as far as comfortable. 4. Hold for 5-20 seconds. 5. Rotate to the opposite side
2. Wide Stance Side Lateral Bending	**Target: Lateral benders of the trunk**
	1. Stand with feet shoulder width apart. 2. Bend laterally by running your hand down the side of your leg as far as comfortable. 3. Opposite arm can reach over your head or stay at your side. 4. Hold for 5-20 seconds. 5. Laterally bend to the opposite side.

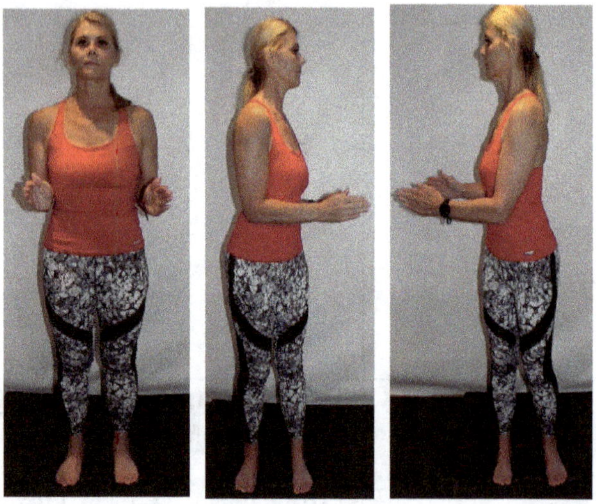

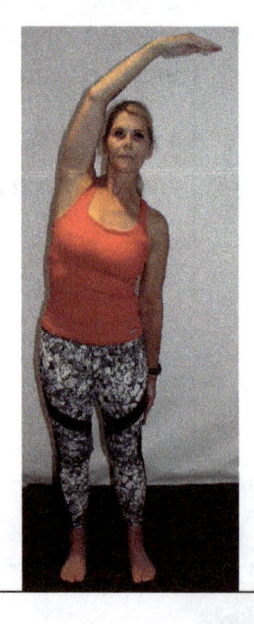

4. Legs and Hips:

1. Marching

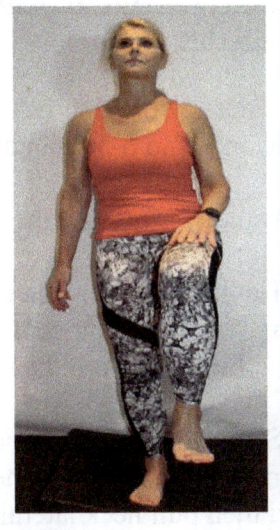

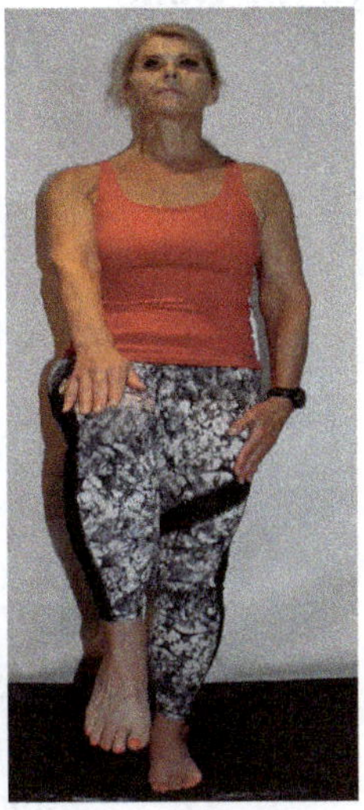

Target: Hip Flexors and Extensors

1. Support yourself with the wall or chair if necessary.

2. Stand upright and lift one leg to waist level and then repeat with the opposite leg

3. Repeat 10 x's with each leg

2. Leg Swings

Forward and backward Swing

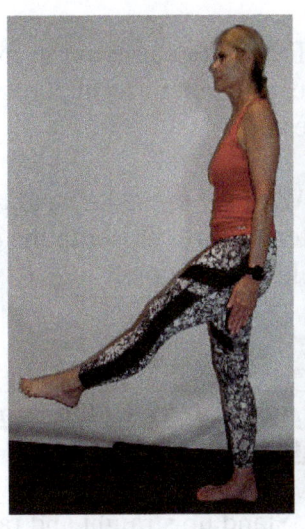

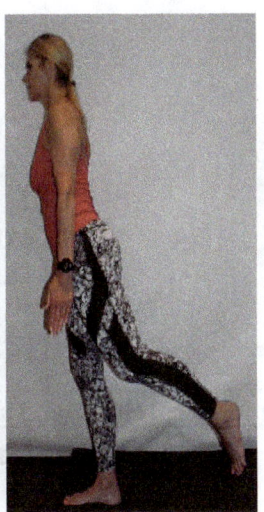

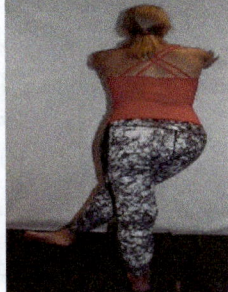

Target: Hip Lateral Stabilizers Forward and Backward

1. Support yourself with the wall or chair if necessary.

2. Swing one leg forward and backward.

3. Start the swinging of the leg small but try to progress to a larger swing with each repetition.

4. Do 10 reps in each direction with one leg and then repeat with the opposite leg.

Side to Side Swing

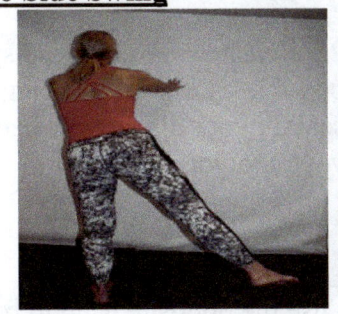

Side to Side

1. Swing one leg across your body and then out to the side laterally.

2. Start each swing small but try to increase the size of the swing with each repetition.

3. Do 10 reps with one leg and then repeat with the other leg.

Static Stretches

1. Neck:

1. Side/lateral Head Pull to the shoulder with the Hand

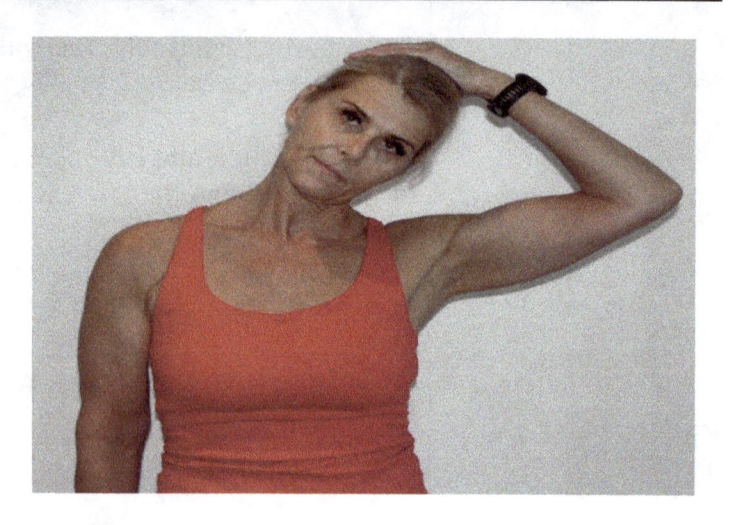

Target: Lateral Neck and Trapezius

1. Laterally tilt your head to one side and hold 3-5 seconds.

Advanced - increase the stretch by:

1. Having an arm reach over the top of the head and gently pull the head farther toward the shoulder.

2. Sit on the hand and anchor the arm that is opposite to the tilt side and then pull neck laterally to opposite side.

2. Shoulders:

1. Single Arm Reach Across Your chest

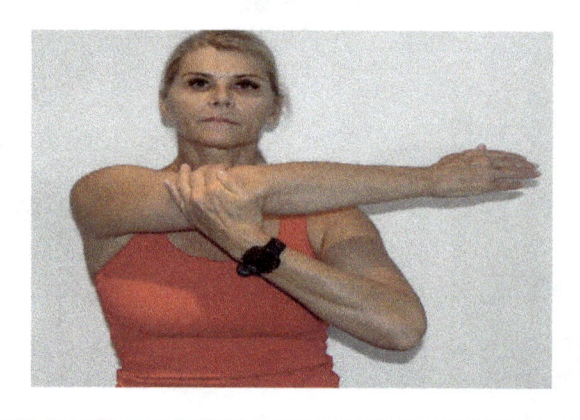

Target: Posterior Shoulder (Rotator Cuff)

1. Extend one arm out in front of you and then move it across your chest.

2. With the opposite hand push the extended arm closer to the chest. Hold for 5 seconds.

2. Single Arm Over the Same Shoulder and Scratch Upper Back

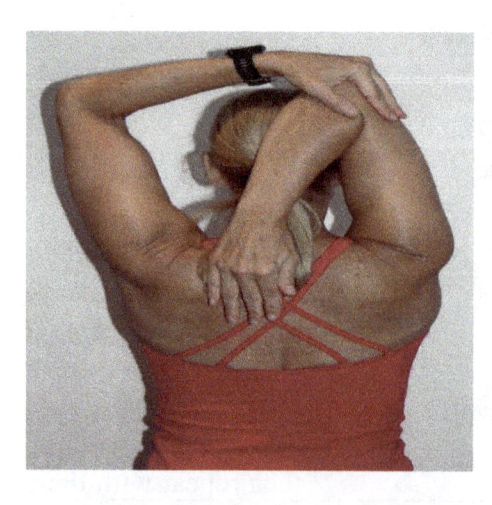

Target: Lower Rotators and Latissimus Dorsi

1. Stand up straight and raise one arm over the same side shoulder.

2. Reach as far down the spine as possible as if you are trying to scratch your upper back between your shoulder blades.

Advanced
- use the opposite hand to push back on the elbow to increase the stretch

3. Underneath Lower Back Scratch

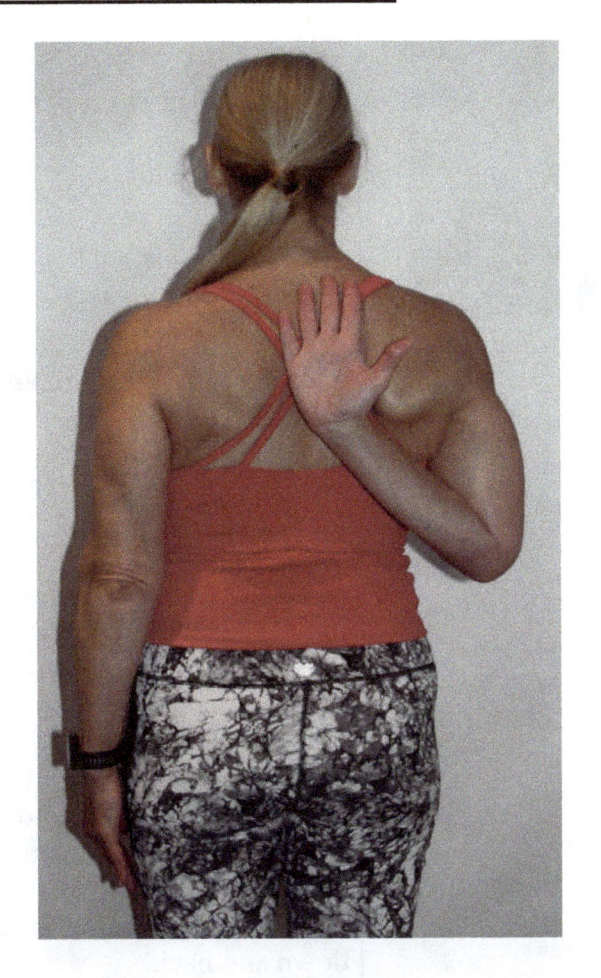

Target: Chest (Pectoralis Major) and Anterior Shoulder (Anterior Deltoid)

1. Take one arm and rotate it underneath toward the small of your back (as if you want to scratch your lower back).

2. Move the hand up the spine as high as possible.

3. Hold 5-20 seconds

Advanced
- To increase the stretch, you can take the opposite hand and grab the hand that is scratching the lower back and pull it further up the spine.

3. Lower Back:
1. Child Pose with or without Blocks

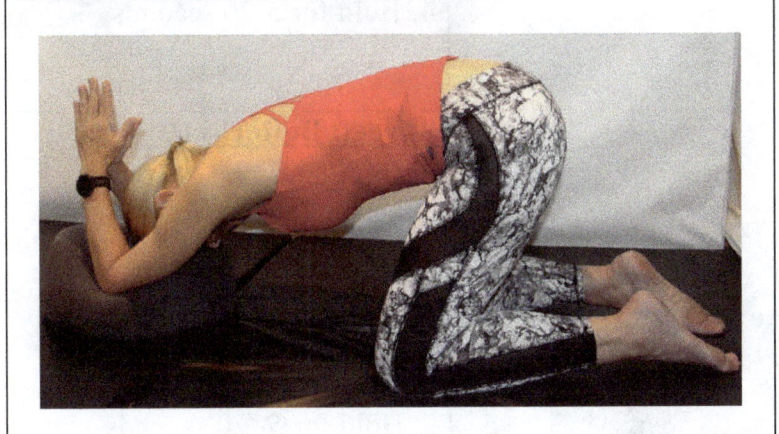

Target: Shoulders (Latissimus Dorsi), Lower Back and Buttocks (Gluteus Maximus)

1. If necessary, place two flat blocks shoulder-distance apart at the front of your mat.

2. Bring your palms onto the bolster, and press your hips back and down toward your heels.

3. Press your palms into the bolster, straighten your arms, and lengthen through the sides of your torso.

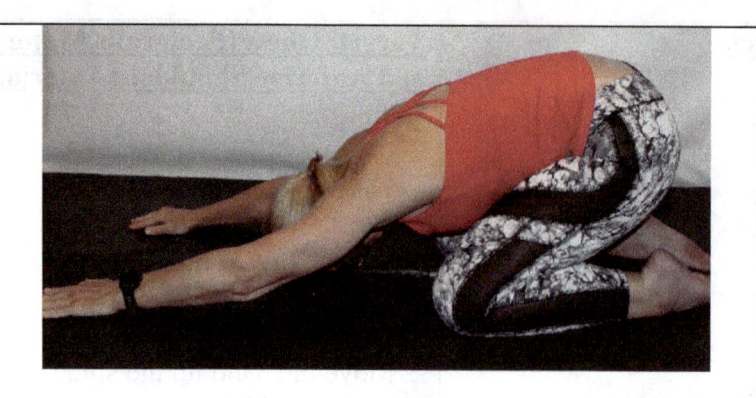

4. Hold 5-20 seconds.

Advanced
- use no bolster to support the arms

2. Cobra/Upward Dog

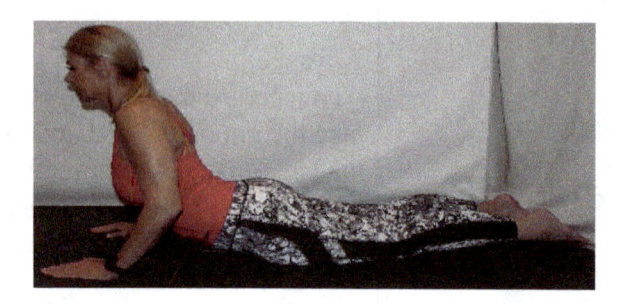

Target: Hip Flexors (Quads) and Lower Back

1. Lie face-down, forehead resting on the floor.

2. Place hands on either side, at middle of ribcage. Draw legs together, pressing tops of feet into floor.

3. Press evenly through hands as you draw elbows close to ribcage and using strength of back (not arms), lift head and chest, sliding shoulder blades down and back.

(Avoid hyperextending of the neck)

4. Hold for 5-20 seconds

4. Hips:

1. Knee to Chest

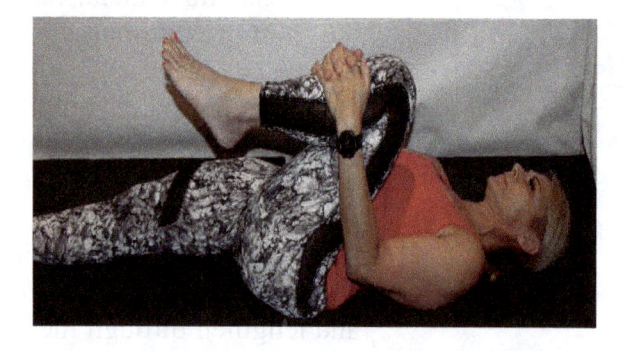

Target: Buttocks (Gluteus Maximus)

1. Lie on back and bring knee to same side chest.
(Keep the opposite leg flat on the floor)

2. Hold for 5- 20 seconds

2. Knee to Opposite Chest 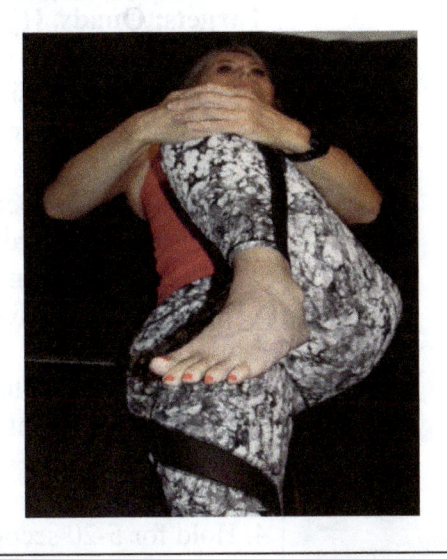	**Target: Buttocks (Gluteus Medius)** 1. Lie on the floor and bring knee to opposite chest. (Keep opposite leg flat on the floor) 2. Hold for 5-20 seconds
3. Sitting Butterfly with or without Blocks 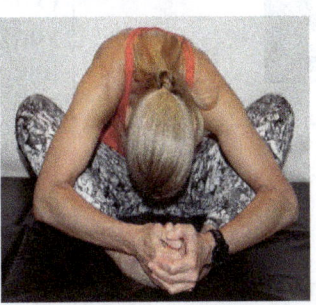 **Blocks to Support Head** 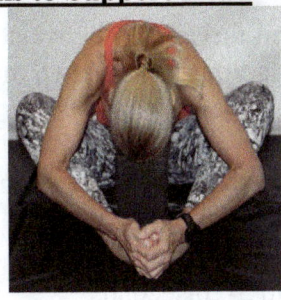 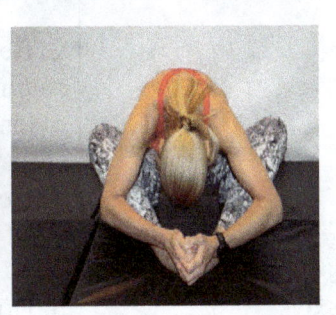	**Target: Inner Thighs (Groins) and Lower Back** 1. Sitting on buttocks or a block with feet facing each other and knees spread apart. 2. Lean forward at the hip. Use the block to support your head at your comfort level if necessary. 3. Hold 5-20 seconds

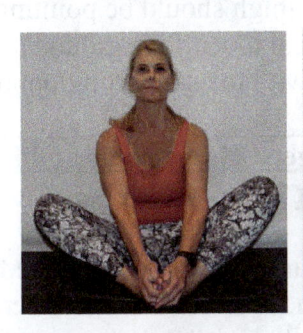

5. Legs:

1. Supported Standing Heel to Buttocks

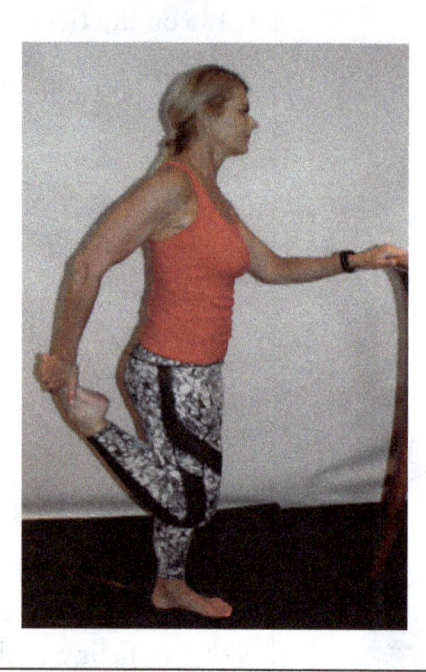

Targets: Quads, Hip Flexors

1. Stand upright beside or in front of a chair or wall for balance.

2. Simultaneously bend one knee and raise heel toward buttocks while reaching behind and gripping the raised foot or ankle.

3. Squeeze the foot/heel toward buttocks while maintaining an erect posture.

4. Hold for 5-20 seconds.

(The thigh should be pointing vertical toward the ground and in line with the supporting/opposite leg)

2. Modified Standing Toe Touch

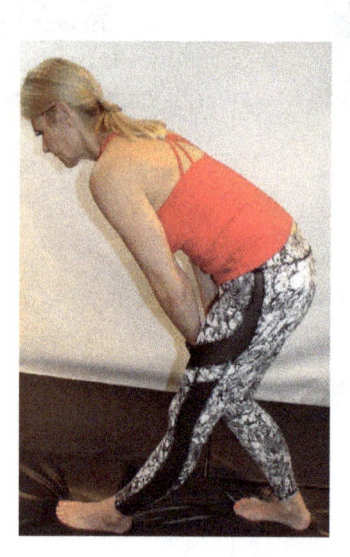

Targets: Hamstrings and Lower Back

1. Stand erect and place one foot extended in front of the other. The other leg is slightly bent.

2. Bend forward at the waist running your hands down the front extended leg.

3. Keep the foot of the extended front leg flat on the mat.

3. Hold 5-20 seconds

3. Single Leg Bench Hamstring Stretch	**Targets: Hamstrings and Lower Back**
	1. Sit on a bench and place one extended leg along the length of the bench. 2. Bend forward at the hip and run both hands down along the extended leg toward your toes. Try to keep the extend legs knee as flat as possible. 3. Hold for 5-20 seconds
4. Wall Lean with Front Knee Bent	**Targets: Gastrocs, Soleus and Achilles Tendon** **Gastrocs:** 1. Facing the wall. 2. Take a step back with one leg and keep the knee of that leg straight and heel flat on the ground. 3. Lean forward against the wall and bend the knee of the front leg 4. Hold for 5-20 seconds. **Soleus and Achilles Tendon:** 1. Similar to Gastroc Stretch but the back knee is also bent to stretch the deeper Soleus muscle and Achilles Tendon.

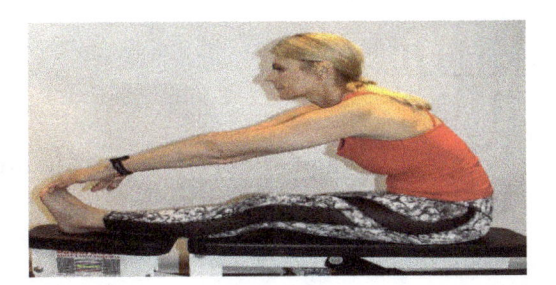

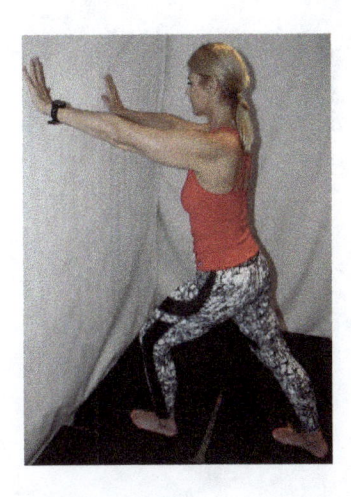

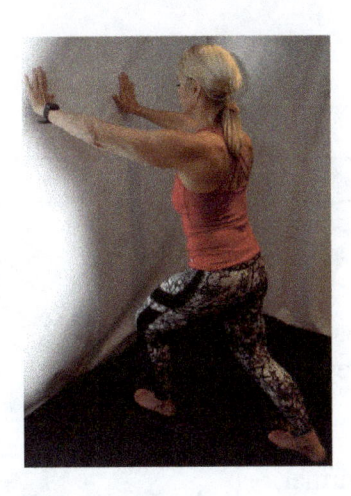

Appendix 9.1.4.3. Yin Yoga Poses Illustrated and Described

Summary of Yin Poses for Lower Back and Hips

Lower Back:	**Number of Poses**	**Minutes/Pose**
1. Bent over Butterfly (Groin and Back)	1	4
2. One Legged Butterfly (Hamstring and back)	2	4 each = 8
3. Child Pose (Shoulders and Back)	1	4
4. Seal (Back Extensions)	1	4
5. Sitting or lying spinal twist	2	4 each = 8

Hips:		
1. Dragon (Hip flexors)	2	4 each = 8
2. Swan (Hip flexors, Gluteus Medius and TFL)	2	4 each = 8
3. Single/ Half Saddle (Quads, Tibalis Anterior, dorsal ankle)	2	4 each = 8
4. Double Saddle (Quads, Tibalis Anterior, dorsal ankle)	1	4
	Total Time	**56 minutes**

Yin Yoga Poses: Lower Back and Hips

Note

1. Hold poses from 2-4 minutes

2. Breath slowly and rhythmically.

3. Gradually move deeper into the pose

Pose	Technique	Illustration
1. Lower Back:		
1. Butterfly - Both Legs - Stretches the lower spine and groin	- Sit with the soles of the feet touching and lean forward. - If you start with the feet closer to your groin, your groin muscles will be stretched more. - If you start with your feet further from your groin, the lower spine will be stretched more.	

	- you can use a bolster to support your head	
2. One Legged Butterfly - Stretches the hamstrings and lower back	- Sit with one leg stretched forward and the other leg folded, with the foot near the opposite groin - Drop your chin to your chest, lean forward and try to grasp your ankle or foot. - The knee of the extended leg may be bent as long as you can feel the stretch in the back of your leg.	
3. Dragonfly - Stretches the hamstrings, groins and lower spine	- Sitting with your legs spread out 45-60° or more apart. - To increase the stretch, begin to lean forward, first touching your hands, your elbows, and eventually your forehead to the floor. - may use a bolster to support your head	**Bolster Support**
4. Caterpillar - Stretches the legs and entire spinal column	- Sit with both legs out in front of you, with your feet either together or hip width apart. - Drop your chin to chest and lean forward to grasp your ankles or feet. - Try to keep your legs straight but don't overdo it. A slight bend in the knees is okay as long as you feel the stretch.	

5. Child - Stretches the spine	- Kneel with your buttocks on your heels and lean forward to rest your head on the floor. - Arms should rest comfortably beside you or in front of you.	
6. Seal - Re-establish the lumbar curve and stretch the hip flexors	- Lie on your stomach with your hands on the floor in front of and to the sides of the shoulders. The hands should be turned slightly outwards. - Straighten your elbows and lift your chest and belly off the floor. <u>Note -</u> if you keep your legs apart, the stress will be more localized to the lower back. If you keep your legs together the stress is more evenly distributed along the entire spine.	
7. Lying Spinal Twist - Stretches the lower back and lateral hip extensors	- Lie on your back and bend both knees to 90º. - Twist both legs to the opposite side. - Extend the opposite arm away from the twist, and turn your head away from the side your legs have twisted to increase the stretch of the twist. The goal is to try to get that opposite shoulder as close to the floor as possible. (You can do this pose by just twisting/moving top leg)	

| 8. Sitting Spinal Twist | - Bend one knee so foot is close to your buttocks.
 - Cross your other leg (top leg) over and place its foot next to the thigh that is flat on the ground.
- The cross-over foot should stay planted on the floor and square your hips so they remain even.

- The arm of your cross over leg (top leg) is placed behind you and with your fingertips on the floor.

- Gently twisting your body to that side.

- Hook the opposite arm around your bent top knee.

- With each exhale, twist your body further.

- repeat in the opposite direction | |

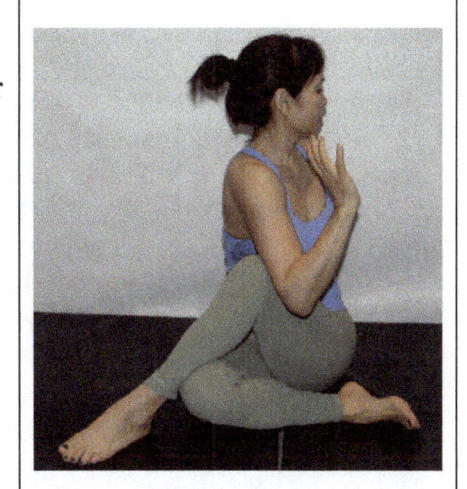

2. Hips

1. Hip Flexors:

1. Dragon - One Leg - Stretches the groin, ankles and hip flexors.	- Place one foot forward in front of you and rest the opposite knee on the floor behind you. - Slowly lower the thigh of your rear leg to the floor so you feel a stretch on the top and front of the thigh. Advanced – Twist to the forward leg side and elevate your arm.	**Block Support** **Twist and Arm Elevated**

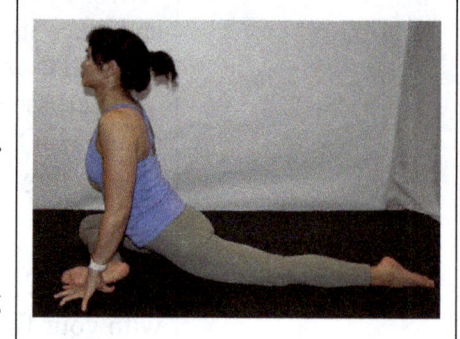

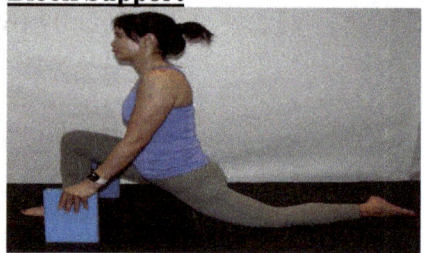

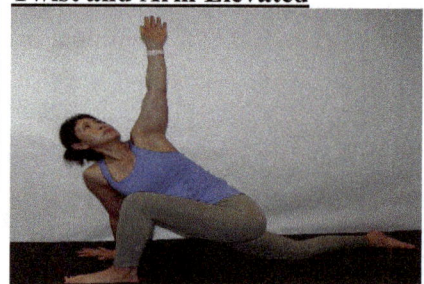

2. Groin:

1. Frog	- Start in tabletop position on the mat. - Allow the knees to move out to the sides of the mat, keeping the ankles and feet in line with the knees. - The elbows and forearms drop to the floor with the palms flat – the hips push slowly backward.	

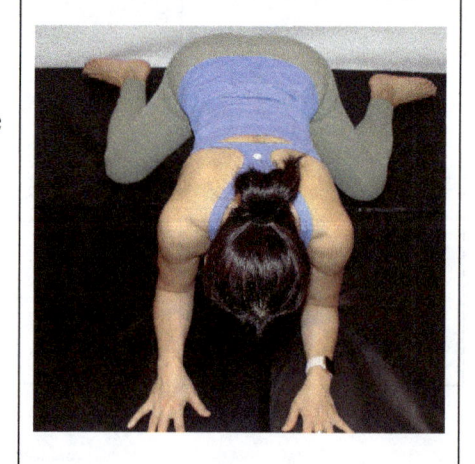

3. Glutes Medius and Tensor Fascia Lata:

1. Sleeping Swan - Externally rotates and opens up the hip and stretches piriformis, tensor facia lata and ilio tibia band.	- Get on your hands and knees and then move one knee back roughly a foot. - Place the opposite foot in front of the first knee and then slide the first knee backwards as far as possible so your pelvis lowers towards the floor. - Lean forward - you can use a bolster to support the arms and head	
2. Swan - Externally rotates and opens up the hip, and stretches the hip flexors of the straight leg and piriformis of the bent knee leg	- Get into the sleeping swan position - Use your arms to push the chest up and extend as far back as you can.	

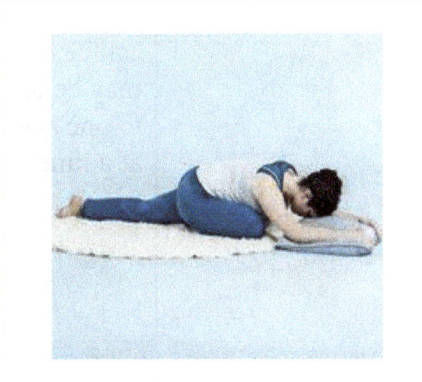

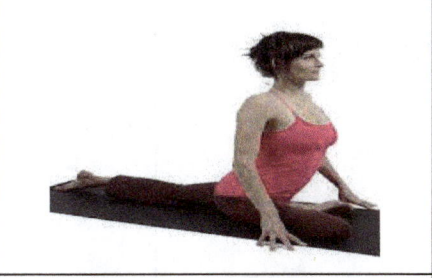

3. Quads, Ankle & Tibialis Anterior:

1. Saddle - both legs or one leg at a time - Stretches the feet, knees, thighs and hip flexors	**Double Leg** - Sitting on your feet and shins (lower legs) with your knees spread apart. Advanced - As your flexibility improves, try to lower yourself backwards and support your weight first on your hands, then your forearms and finally on your upper back. - you can use a bolster to support your buttocks, lower and upper back and neck and head **Single Leg** - one leg is extended and opposite leg is flexed back. - sit up straight Advanced - try to lean back as far as possible. - use a bolster for support	**Double Leg** **Bolster Under Buttocks** **Bolster under shoulders and neck**

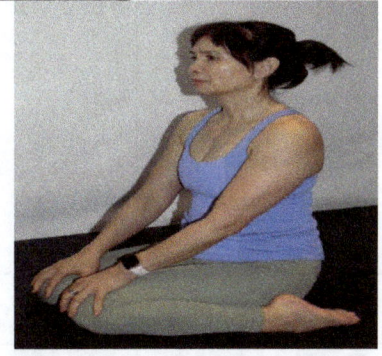

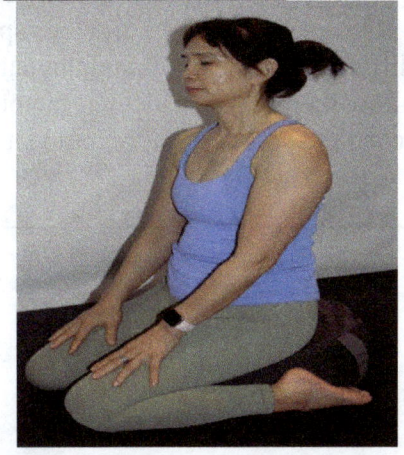

755

	Note - coming out of these poses can be challenging, and for many it may be less stressful to roll or lean to one side and unfold your legs one at a time.	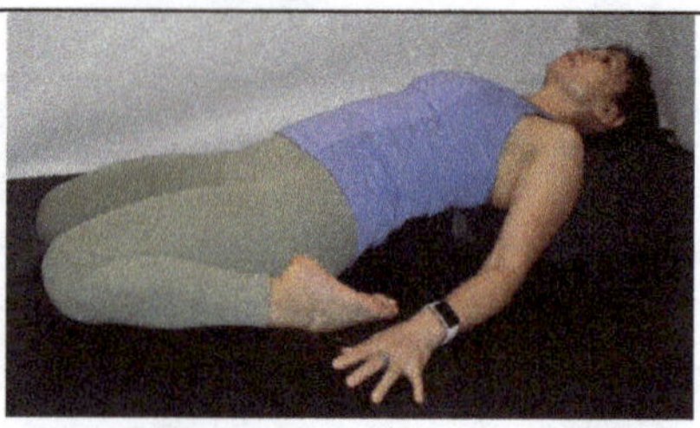 **Bolster under Lower and Upper Back and neck** 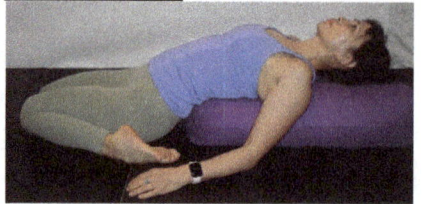 **Half (Single Leg) Saddle** 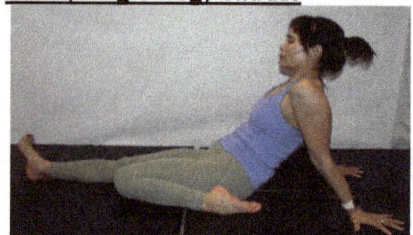 **Single Leg Bolster Support** 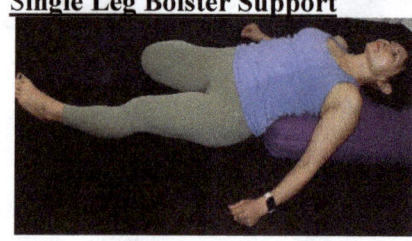

4. Ending Pose:		
1. Pentacle - Used between difficult poses to allow the body to relax and recover.	- Lie on your back with your arms and legs spread out in a comfortable and unguarded position - Close your eyes and let your recumbent body sink into the floor	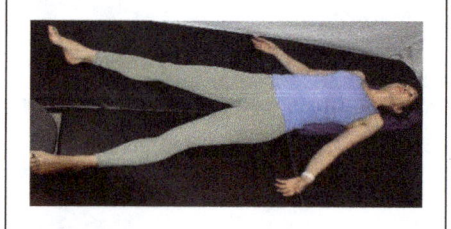

756

Yin Yoga Poses: Upper Back, Chest and Shoulders

Summary of Yoga Poses for Upper Back, Chest and Shoulders

	Number of Poses	Minutes / Pose
Upper Back		
1. Bow Tie	1	4
Chest Openers		
1. Sphinx	1	4
2. Supportive Fish	1	4
Shoulders		
1. Child Pose	1	4
2. Side lying Chest Opener	2	8
3. Thread the Needle	2	8
4. Cow Face Arms	2	8
	Total Time	**40 minutes**

Yin Yoga Upper Back, Chest and Shoulders Illustrated

Pose	Technique	Illustration
1. Upper Back		
1. Bow Tie (Straight Jacket)	- Lie prone. - Cross one arm in front of the other at shoulder level & reach to the sides as far as possible. - Elbows are stacked in front of each other. - Palms of hands facing downward. - Place forehead on mat or block or bolster - Repeat with opposite arm in front.	

2. Chest

1. Sphinx	- Lie prone on the floor legs shoulder width apart. - Rest forearms on the floor with elbows under the shoulders. - Lift chest off the ground into a back bend.	
2. Supportive Fish	- Lie supine with bolster or block between shoulder blades. - Lie back and rest head on bolster or block. - Arms and legs are extended and lying comfortably on the floor.	

3. Shoulders

1. Child Pose	- Kneel with your buttocks on your heels and lean forward to rest your head on the floor. - Arms should rest comfortably beside you or in front of you. Advanced - interlock hands in front of the head	
2. Side Lying Chest Opener	- Start in prone position. - Extend one arm to support head. Or - Have it extended behind you along the floor. - Rotate onto the hip on the same side as the extended arm. - Hips and knees are bent 90° or straight.	

3. Thread the needle	- Start on hands and knees. - Slide one arm underneath your chest with your palm facing up. - Let your shoulder come all the way down to the mat. Rest your ear and cheek on the mat. - Keep your hips back or raised. - Do not press your weight onto your head; instead, adjust your position so you do not strain your neck or shoulder.	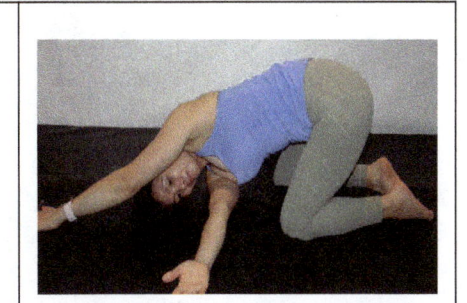
4. Cow Face Arms	- Scratch as far down the upper back with one hand (external rotation). - Scratch as far up on the lower back with opposite hand (internal rotation). - If hands cannot touch, use a towel and grab both ends	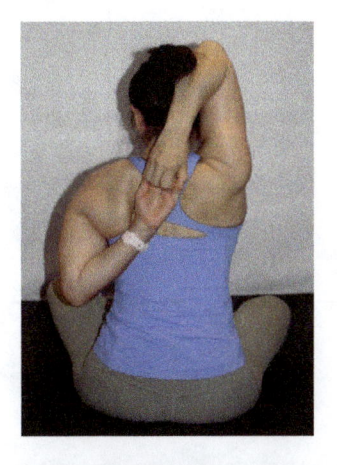 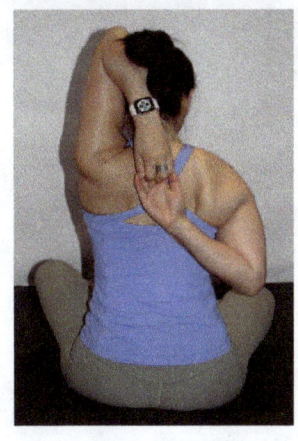

		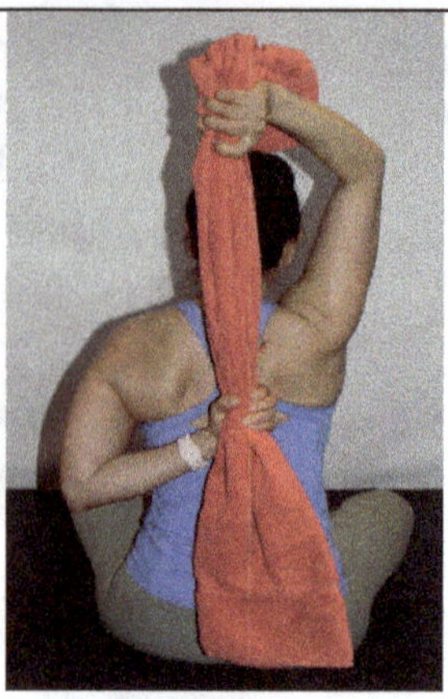 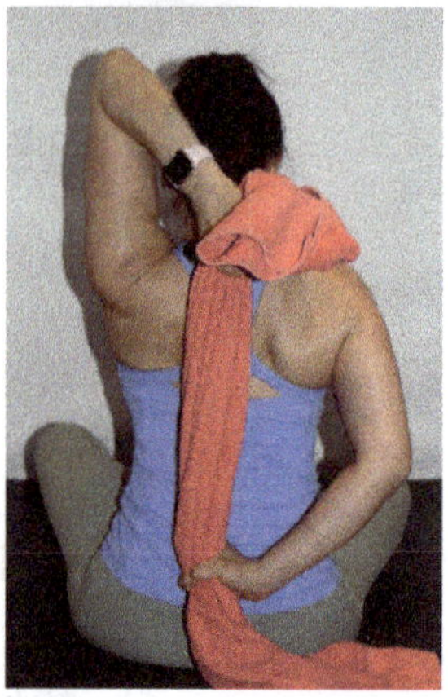

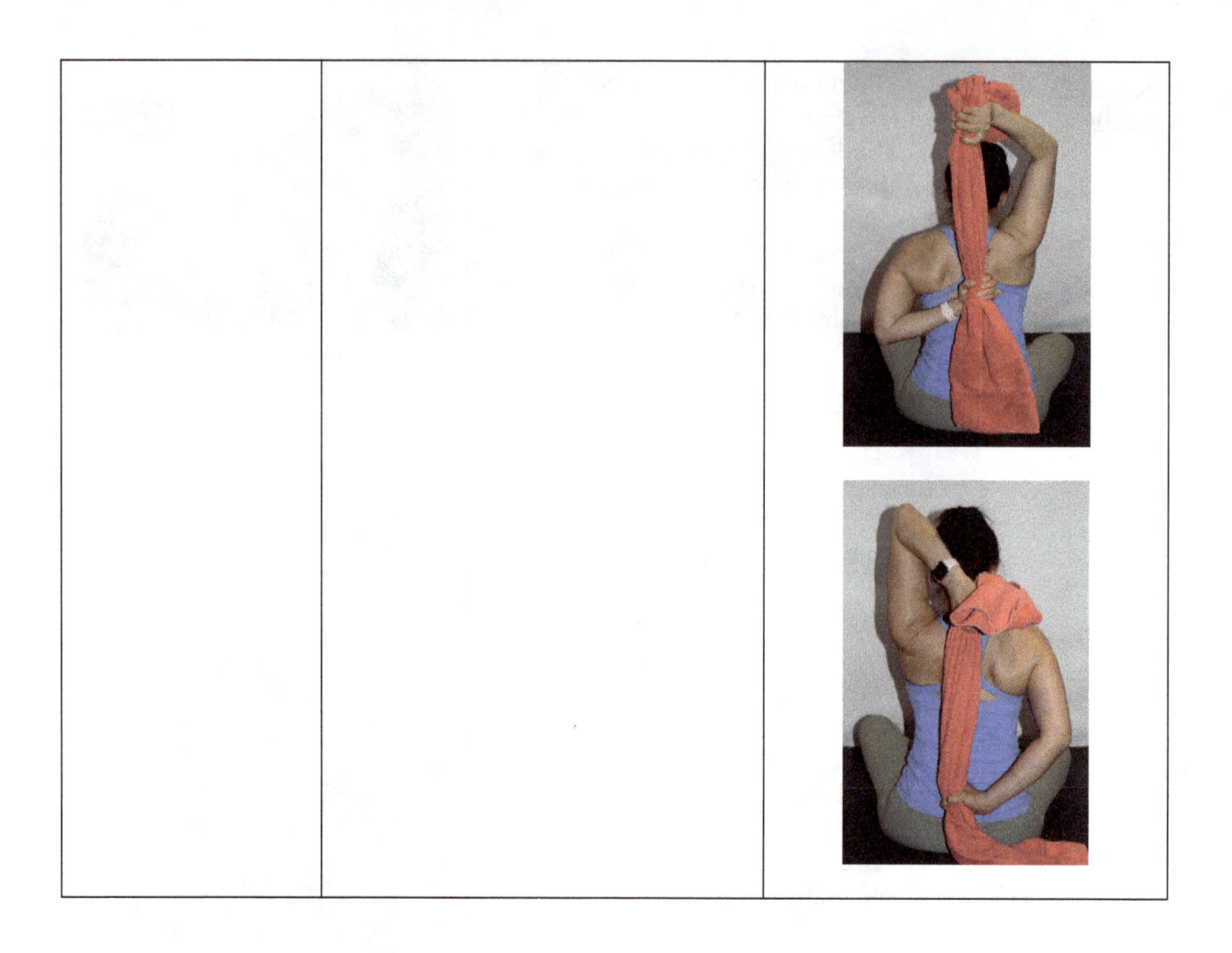

Appendix 9.1.4.4. Myofascial Self Massage Utilizing a Roller

Key points:

1. Never use a roller over joints or bony prominences or inside the upper arms.
2. All movements (rolling) are done slowly with gentle to deep pressure for a count of 10.
3. Focus on deep, controlled breathing in rhythm with the rolling.
3. If there is a sensitive area, apply pressure over this area with the grid for 10 to 30 seconds.
4. Correct posture and positioning of the roller are necessary for effective results.
5. It will take practice to learn how to perform each movement correctly.

1. Supine (Face Up) Position

Position	Illustration
1. Calf (Posterior lower leg) **Body position:** - Seated or hips off the floor with one or both legs straight on the grid in front of you - Hands on the floor beside or slightly behind the hips - Body leans slightly back **Grid Position:** - At upper end of calf near knee **Action:** - Flex and extend the knee of the leg on the grid so roller moves along the lower leg Or Move whole body back and forth so grid moves along the lower leg (calf from knee to ankle). (Can do with both legs on roller)	**Hips are sitting on mat** **Hips off mat**

761

2. Hamstring
(Posterior upper leg)

Body Position:
- Seated with one or both legs on grid.

Grid Position:
- Half way between lower buttocks and knee

Action:
- Lift hips off the floor and move hips back and forth so grid moves over hamstrings from knee to buttocks.

(Can do with both legs on roller)

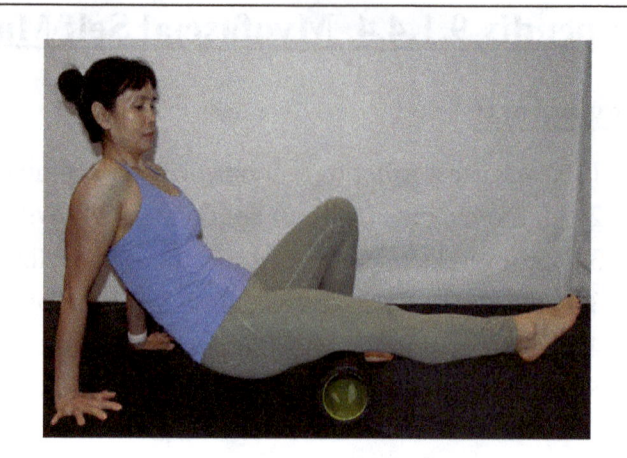

3. High Hamstring
(Posterior leg near buttocks)

Body position:
- Seated with one or both legs straight and on the roller.

Grid Position:
- Beneath lengthened leg at base of glute.

Action:
- Small rolling of grid through high hamstring.

(Can do with both legs on roller)

Single Leg on Roller

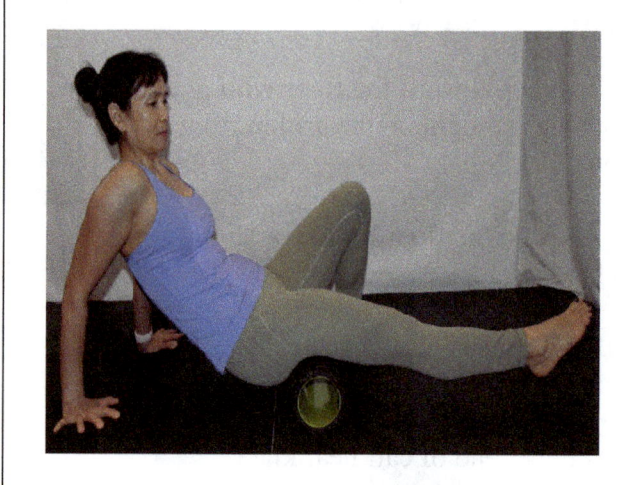

4. Glutes
(Buttocks)

Body Position:
- Seated with one buttock on grid with knee bent and other legs knee bent in figure 4 position over other knee

- Lean slightly back with hands supporting you on the floor

Grid Position:
- In middle of one or both buttocks.

Action:
- Roll back and forth between iliac crest (top bony rim of the pelvis) and "sit bone" in lower buttocks.

(Can do with both buttocks on roller)

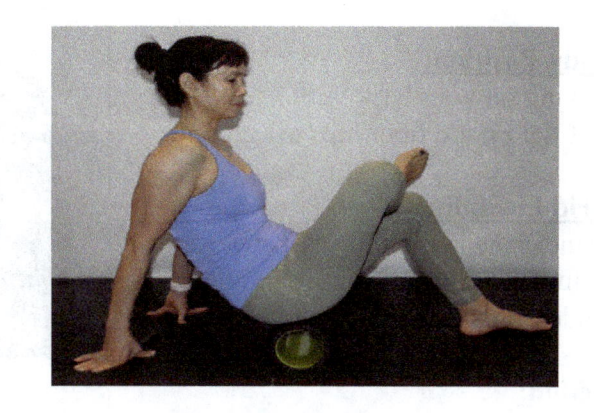

5. Piriformis
(Posterior lateral aspect of the buttocks)

Body Position:

- One hip is seated on grid with lower leg on or off floor & top leg knee bent and foot on the floor.

- Body leans back slightly with hands behind and supporting you.

Grid position:
- Mid - Lateral over the area of the buttocks that your back pocket would be.

Action:
- Push hips back and forth through the lateral region of the glutes.

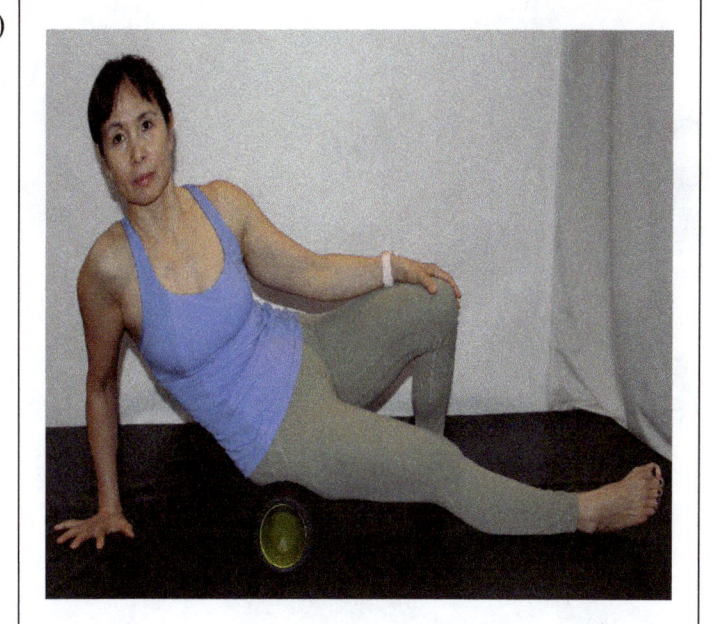

6. Mid to Upper Back
(Shoulder blade area)

Body Position:
- Lying on your back with knees bent, feet flat on the floor hips off ground.

Grid Position:
- Under the body midway between top of lumbar spine and lower shoulder blades.

Action:
- Using your feet move back and forth with grid moving from top of lumbar spine to upper mid shoulder blade area. **DON'T ROLL ONTO LUMBAR SPINE OR NECK**

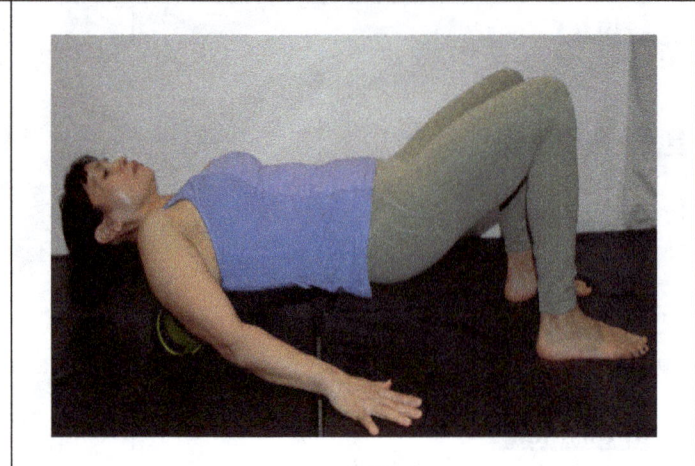

2. Side Lying

1. Peroneal
(Lateral aspect of lower leg)

Body Position:
- Side plank position with elbow directly underneath the shoulder.

- Top leg foot in front of body on the ground.
or
- Top leg on top of bottom leg.

Grid Position:
- Between ankle and knee on lateral portion of lower leg.

Action:
- Push body forward and back 2-3 inches so grid rolls along the peroneal muscles.
Note - hip can stay on ground if side plank position is too difficult.

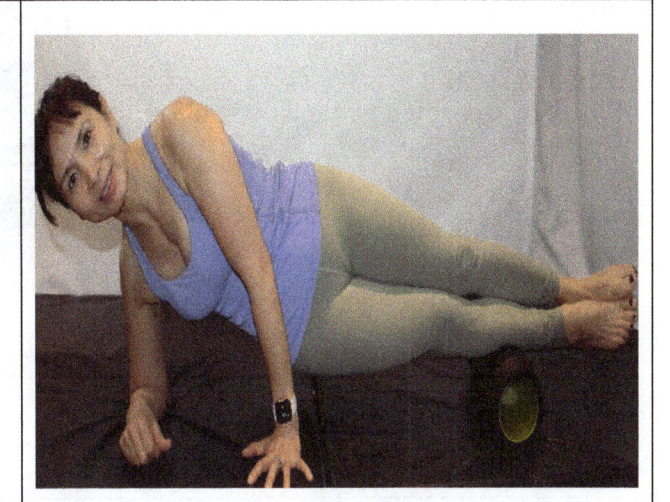

2. Side Plank- IT band and Vastus Lateralis
(Upper Lateral leg)

Body Position:
IT Band:
- Side plank position and elbow underneath shoulder.

Vastus Lateralis:
- Side plank position with body rotated 10-20° towards floor and elbow underneath shoulder.

Grid Position:
- Between hip and knee on lateral portion of thigh.

Action:
- Push body forward and back 2-3 inches and grid moves along the IT band or Vastus Lateralis.

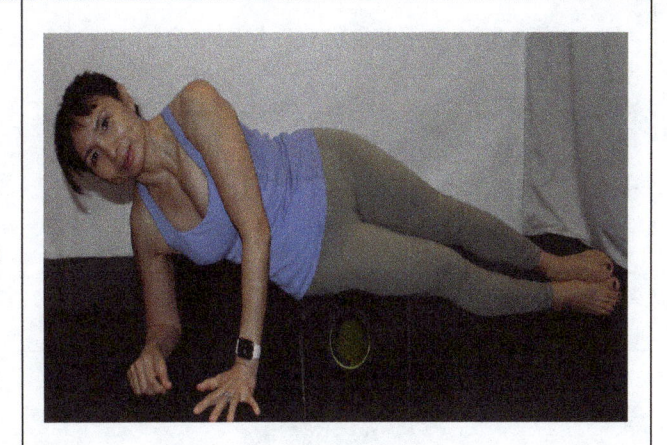

3. Tensor Fascia Lata (TFL)
(Lateral buttocks)

Body Position:
- Side plank position with elbow underneath the shoulder.

Grid Position:
- On lateral side of hip between upper rim of iliac crest and hip bone.

Action:
- Push body forward and back 1-2 inches (very small movement) so grid moves along TFL.

4. Latissimus Dorsi
(Upper lateral back under the arm pit)

Body Position:
- Lying laterally on hip and outstretched on the floor, top foot planted in front of body.
Or
On top of the lower leg.

- Bottom arm extended beyond the top of the head.

Grid Position:
- Just below arm pit.

Action:
- Move grid from arm pit to upper ribs (small movement)

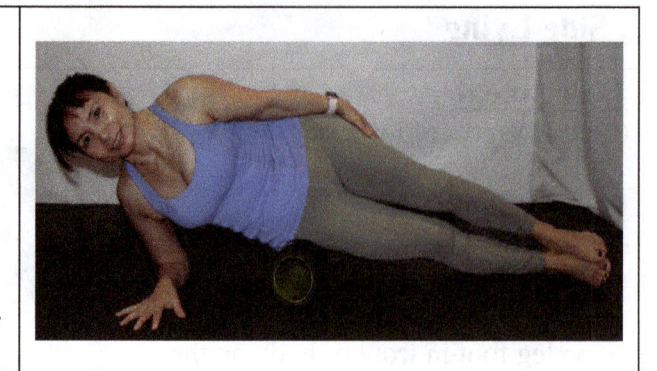

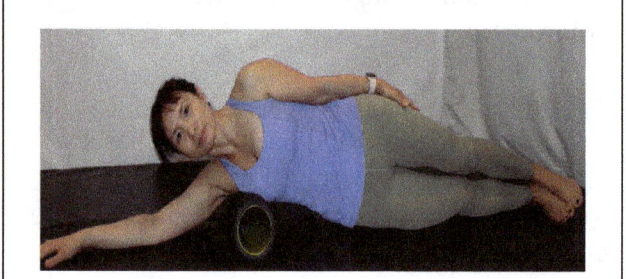

3. Prone

1. Tibialis Anterior
(Lateral/Front of shins)

Body Position:
- Front plank with elbows or elbows underneath the shoulder.

- Toes are rotated in.

Grid Position:
- Grid on one leg or both legs.

- Just below the knees and just lateral to the shins.

Action:
- Bend the knee toward chest (reverse crunch movement) or whole body can move forward and backward so grid moves along the lateral shins

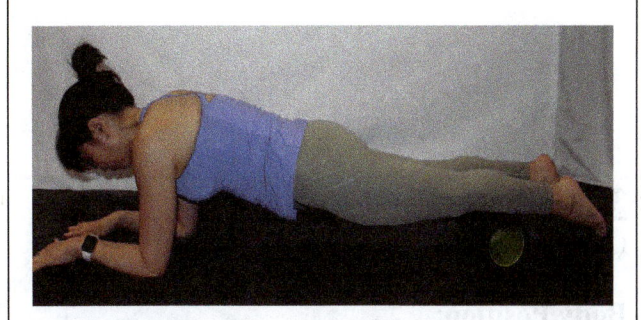

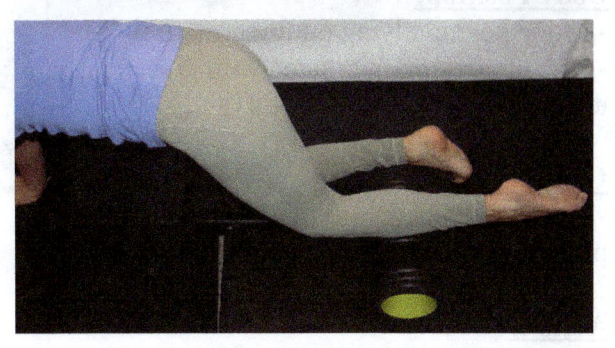

2. Quadriceps
(Front of upper leg (Thighs))

Body Position:
- Prone plank position, elbows planted directly beneath shoulders.

Grid Position:
Basic:
- On quads 2-3 inches above the knees
- knees can be extended or bent 90º

Action:
- Push body forward and backwards from elbows, 2-3 inches which allows grid to roll through quads region with knees extended.

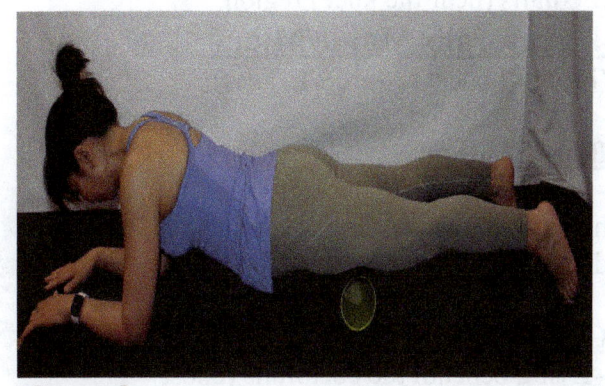

Advanced

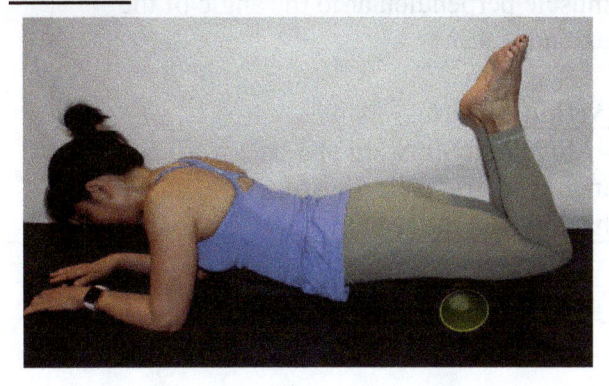

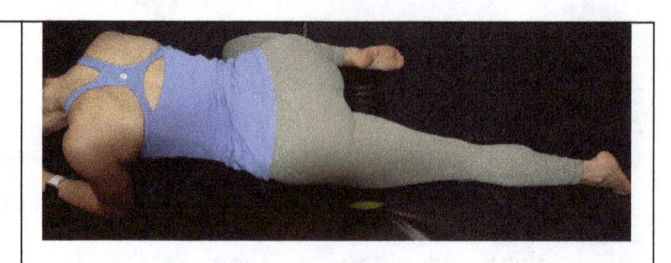

3. Adductors and Vastus Medialis
(Inside of upper leg)

Body Position:
- Prone position lying on forearms.
- One hip externally rotated with knee bent towards hip.

Grid Position:
- Grid perpendicular to thigh beneath inner portion of bent leg between hip and knee.

Action:
- Move bent leg away and toward the body so grid moves through adductor and Vastus Medialis (near the knee) region.

4. Pectoralis Major/Minor
(Front of chest toward shoulder)

Body Position:
- Lying prone with one arm extended out halfway between straight laterally and directly over your head.

Grid Position:
- Lying beneath the pectoralis (chest) muscle perpendicular to the angle of the extended arm

Action:
- Move body forward and backward 1-2 inches so grid rolls toward shoulder and back (small movement)

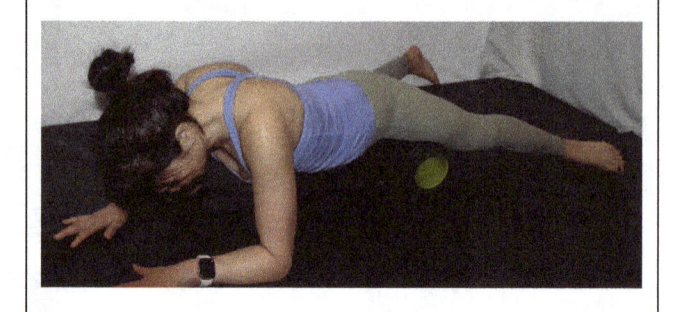

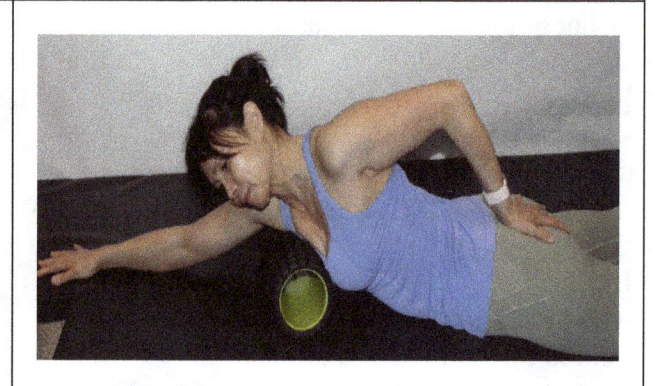

Appendix 9.1.5. Resistance Band Exercises Described and Illustrated

Introduction

Using resistance bands is convenient, especially if a person is traveling or has limited space to store their exercise equipment. They are an economical way of doing resistance training. Resistance bands target upper and lower body muscles. They come in different resistances or strengths based on the thickness of the tubing, so regardless of a your fitness or strength, you can get a challenging workout.

Muscle confusion, targeting specific muscle groups in different ways, is a critical component of effective training programs. Resistance bands can be an alternative to using traditional forms of resistance like machines, barbells, and dumbbells. Resistance bands are a great way of introducing variety into a person's exercise routine.

As with every type of exercise, proper technique is fundamental when using resistance bands to ensure safety and effectiveness. Adhering to the guidelines listed beside each exercise in the table below is essential to ensure proper use and safety. Performing each exercise in a biomechanically correct way makes sure that a person will get the most of each repetition and set.

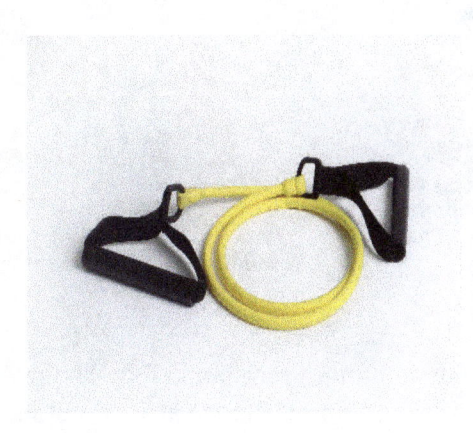

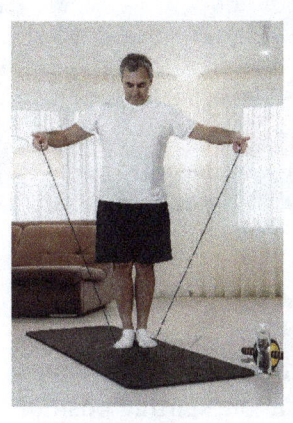

Color Coding the Resistance of Resistance Bands

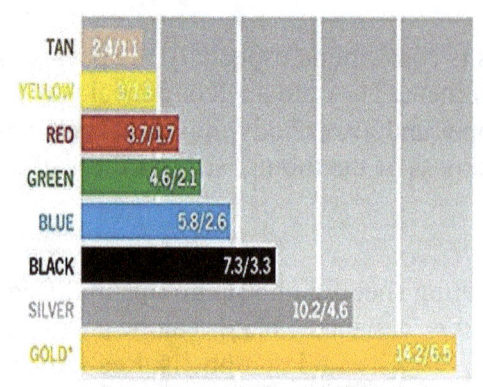

Image source: walmart.ca

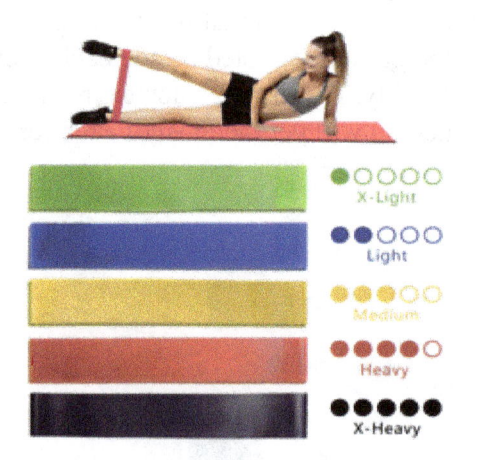

Image source: ebay.ca

Image source: amazon.com

Key Points:

1. Stretching the resistance band changes the amount of resistance felt. The resistance increases from very light at the starting position to maximum resistance at 100% elongation.

2. As a person stretches the resistance bands to 100%, they will feel the increase in resistance and feel a bit of instability or variability as they control the stretching of the resistance band. Feeling this instability is a good thing. It forces the muscle and joint proprioceptive system to control the motion to make it smooth during the movement to a much greater degree than when using free weights. Weight machines eliminate all this instability during the lift.

3. With resistance bands, it is VERY important to control the stretch/movement at all times. Because there is very little resistance at the beginning of the movement, it is easy to generate momentum and stretch the resistance band too quickly. Stretch the band SLOWLY to its full length (concentric contraction – muscle is shortening) and then slowly control the motion as it returns to the starting position (eccentric contraction - muscle is lengthening). Because of the tension built up in the resistance band when stretched 100%, the resistance band will

want to "spring" back to its original position. DO NOT let this happen. One of the outstanding advantages of using resistance bands is that they force the person to resist and control this "spring" tendency after full lengthening of the rubber band has occurred (full concentric contraction of the muscle).

4. Never hold your breath during the exercise's contraction phase (resistance band elongation phase). Exhale as you elongate the resistance band (increase resistance) and inhale as the band is shortened and returned to its starting position (decreased resistance).

Resistance Tubing Exercises

Please Note:

1. The exercises listed below target each major muscle group; however, the exercises illustrated are only a sampling of the various types of movement a person can perform with the resistance bands to target these muscles.

2. With many resistance band exercises, an anchor will be used. The anchor is what the resistance band wraps around to perform the exercise. There are three positions for the anchors, high (above your head), mid height at chest level, and low, which is just above the ground.

Resistance Band Exercises Described and Illustrated

Chest

Mid-line Chest Press (Mid anchor) 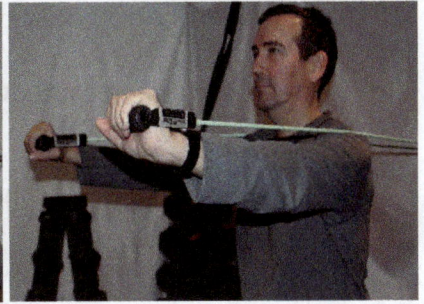	- Stand erect facing away from the anchor. - Hands chess level and shoulder width apart. - Press both hands forward to complete extension. - Slowly control the recoil of the arms back to starting position.
Incline Chest Press (Low anchor) 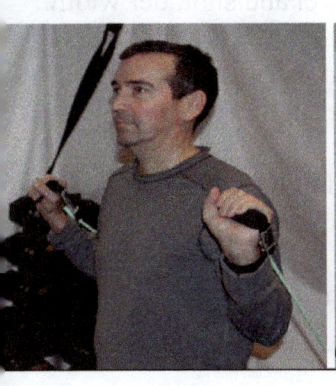	- Stand erect facing away from the anchor. - Hands lower than chest and beside your ribs. - Press upward over your head a slight diagonal motion. - Slowly control the recoil of the arms back to starting position.

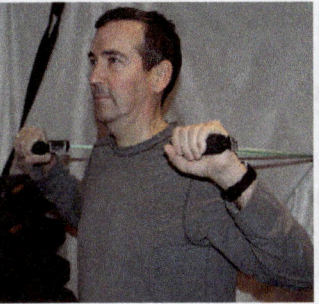

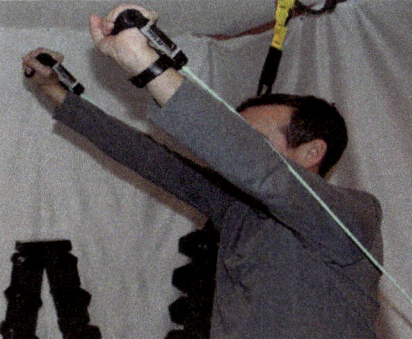

3. Decline Chest Press **(High anchor)** 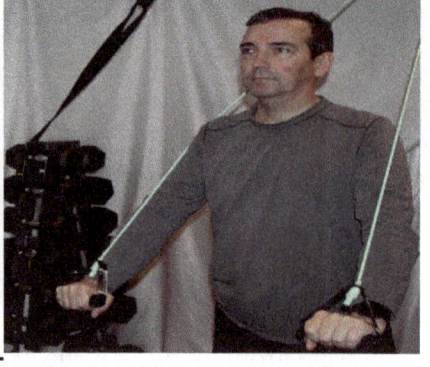	- Stand erect facing away from the anchor. - Hands are at shoulder level and shoulder width. - Press downward in a slight diagonal direction to complete extension. - Slowly control the recoil of the arms back to starting position.
4. Chest Fly **(Mid anchor)** 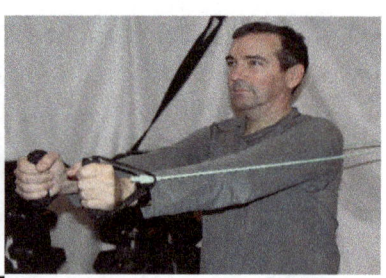	- Stand erect facing away from the anchor. - Hands are at chest level and extended out to the sides of the body. - With the elbows staying extended, slowly move the arms medially toward the mid-line until the hands touch. - Slowly control the recoil of the arms back to starting position.
5. Alternating Arm Diagonal Incline Chest Crossover Fly **(Low anchor)**	- Stand erect facing away from the anchor. - Hands lower than chest and beside your ribs. - Press one arm upward over your head a slight diagonal motion. - Slowly control the recoil of the arms back to starting position. - Repeat with the opposite arm.
6. Alternating Arm Diagonal Decline Chest Crossover Fly **(High anchor)** 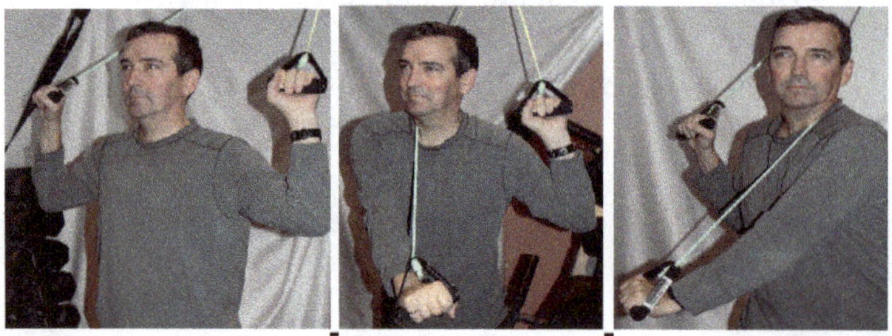	- Stand erect facing away from the anchor. - Hands are at shoulder level and shoulder width. - Press one arm downward in a slight diagonal direction to complete extension. - Slowly control the recoil of the arms back to starting position. - Repeat with opposite arm.

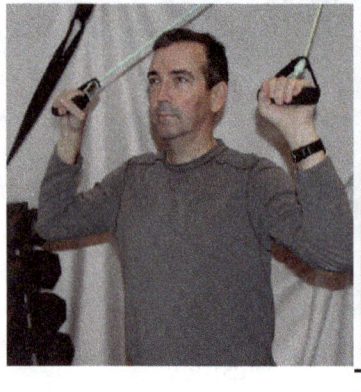

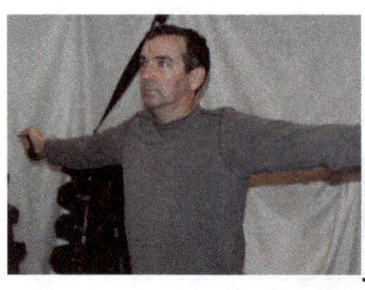

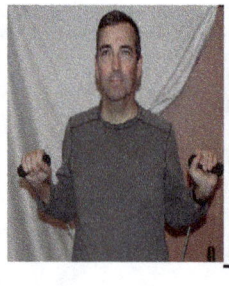

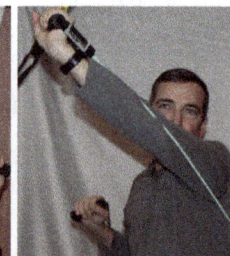

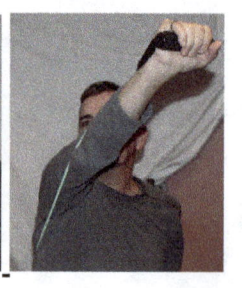

houlders

Standing Double Arm Lateral Raise (ow anchor or under feet) 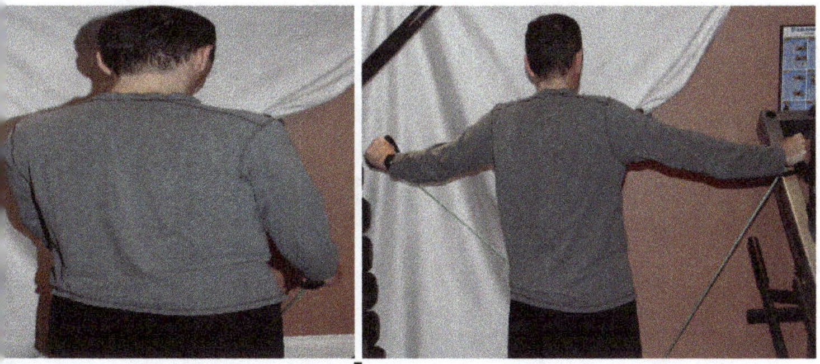	- Stand erect facing the anchor. - Hands are positions at the side of your hips and are facing the body. - Laterally raise both hands to shoulder level. Hands will now be pointing donward. - Keep the elbows as straight as possible. - Slowly control the recoil of the arms back to starting position.
Standing One Arm Lateral Raise (ow anchor or under feet) 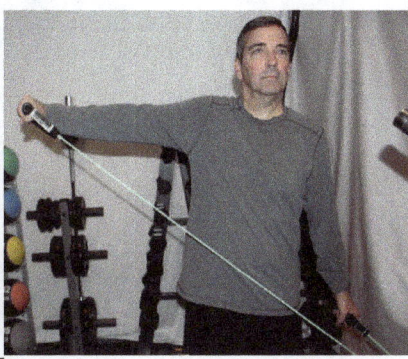	- Stand erect facing the anchor. - Hands are positioned at the side of your hips. - Laterally raise one hand to shoulder level. - Keep the elbows as straight as possible. - Slowly control the recoil of the arm back to starting position.

Standing Anterior Raise (ow anchor or under feet) wo hand positions:
Hands facing inwards   **Hands facing downwards** 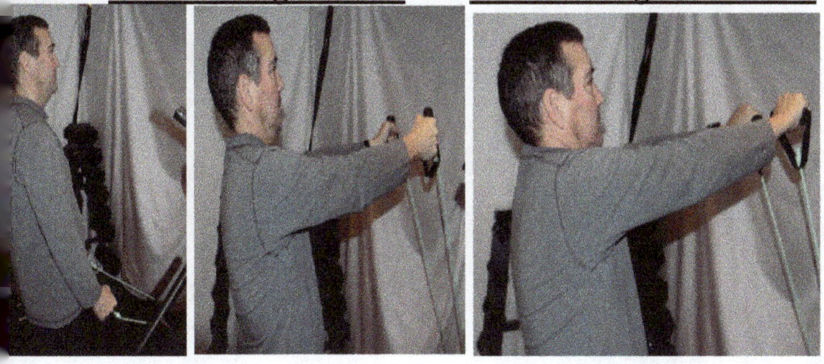
	- Stand erect facing the anchor.
	
	- Hands are beside your hips in one of two positions:
	
	  1. Hands facing medially toward the body
	
	  2. Hands facing downward toward the floor.
	
	- Raise the arms forward and up to shoulder level.
	
	- Keep your elbows straight.
	
	- Slowly control the recoil of the arm back to starting position.

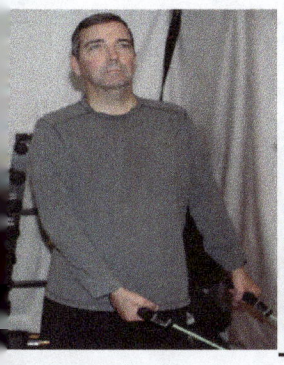

4. Standing Shoulder Raise
(Low anchor or under feet)

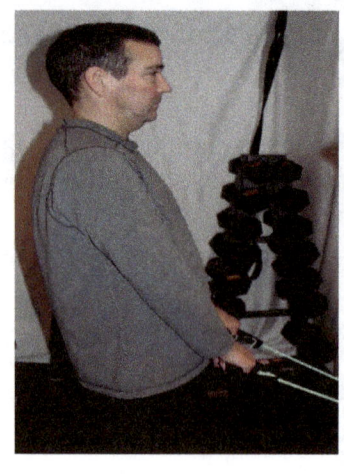

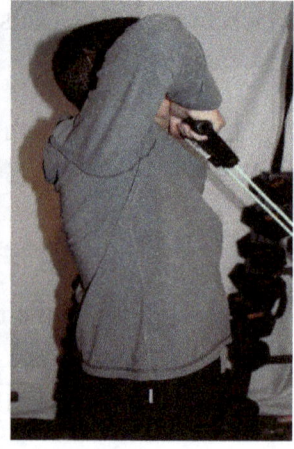

- Stand erect facing the anchor.

- Hands are together in front of the hips.

- Bending your elbows and raise both hands up to just under your chin. (Try to keep elbows above ha[nd] level when hands are under the chin).

- Slowly control the recoil of the arm back to starti[ng] position

5. Standing Horizontal Internal Shoulder Rotation
(Mid anchor)

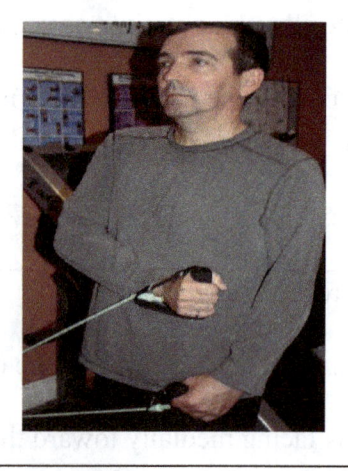

- Stand erect sideways to anchor.

- The hand to be exercised is closest to the anchor.

- Hand is facing forward and elbow is bent 90º.

- Move the hand medially across the chest (away from the anchor).

- Slowly control the recoil of the arm back to starti[ng] position.

6. Standing Horizontal External Shoulder Rotation
(Mid anchor)

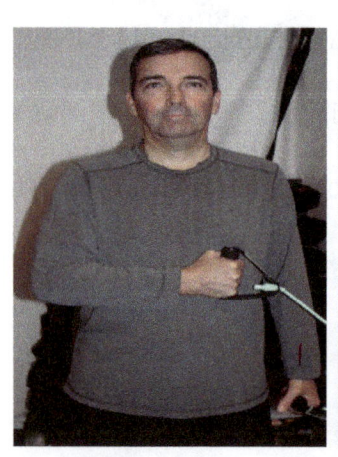

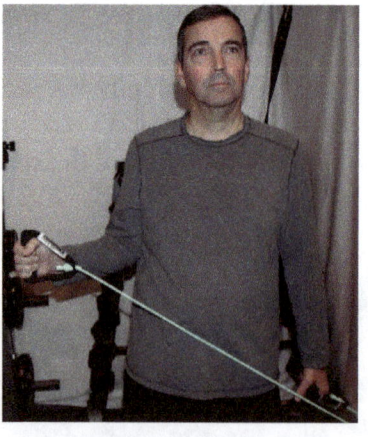

- Stand erect sideways to anchor.

- The arm to be exercised is farthest away from the anchor.

- Elbow is bent 90º and hand is positioned across th[e] chest.

- Move the hand outward away from the anchor.

- Slowly control the recoil of the arm back to startin[g] position.

Upper Back

Standing Reverse Fly (Mid anchor)

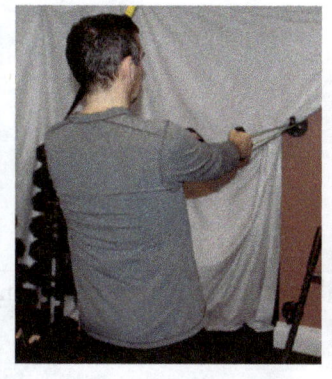

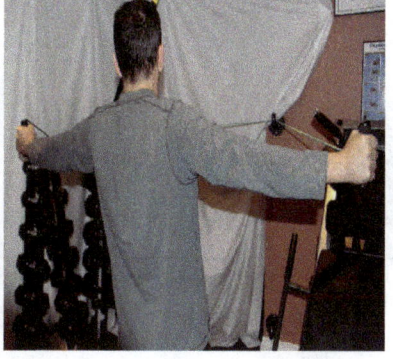

- Standing erect facing the anchor
- Hands extended (elbows straight) in front of the body.
- Move the arms laterally until they are in line with the body.
- Slowly control the recoil of the arms back to starting position.

Bent over Reverse Fly (Low anchor or under your feet)

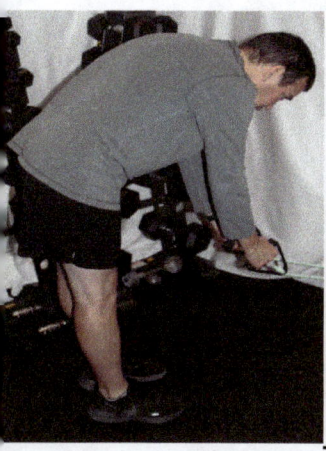

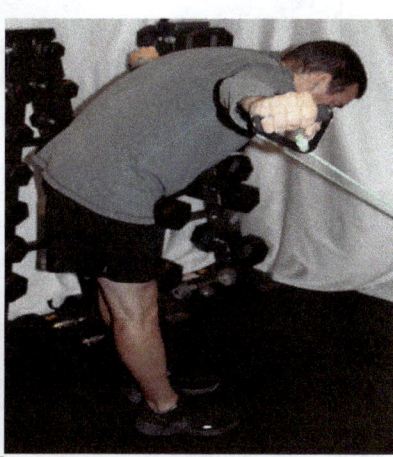

- Stand erect, facing the anchor and bent at the waist 90º
- Arms are extended down to the floor.
- Move the arms laterally upward with elbows straight.

(Feel the shoulder blades squeeze together).

- Slowly control the recoil of the arms back to starting position.

Standing Rows (Mid and High Anchor)

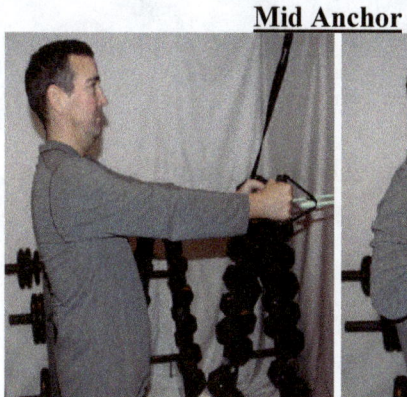

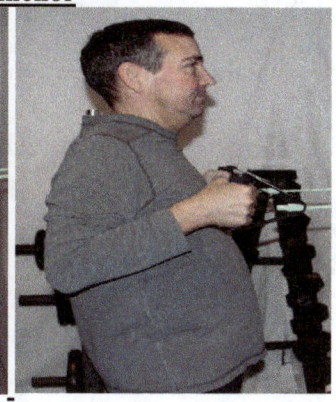

Mid Anchor

- Stand erect facing the anchor.
- Arms are extended out in front of the body.
- Bend the elbows and move the hands towards and beside the ribs.
- Slowly control the recoil of the arms back to starting position.

High Anchor

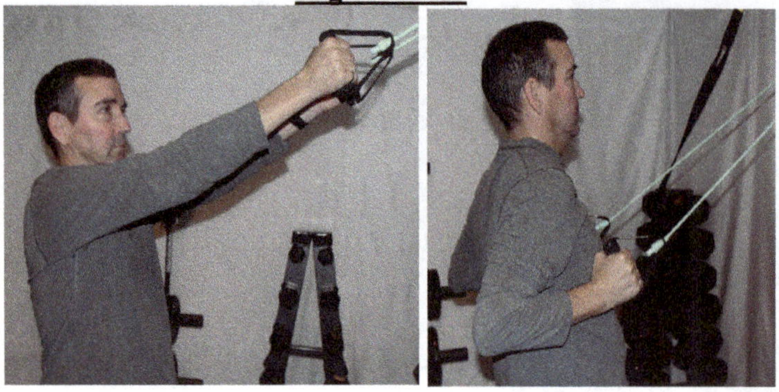

4. Over Head Pull Downs (High anchor)
(Hands face Down and Up)

Hands facing down *Hands facing up*

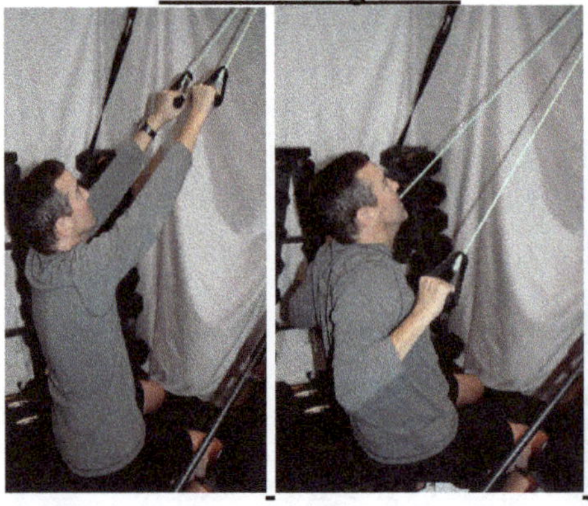

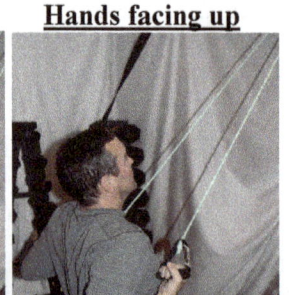

- Sitting on a bench, stability ball, kneeling or sitting on buttocks.

- Arms extended over your head.

- Pull down with both hands to shoulder level.

- Slowly control the recoil of the arms back to starting position.

Biceps

1. Standard Curl
(High, mid, low or standing on Band anchor)

High Anchor

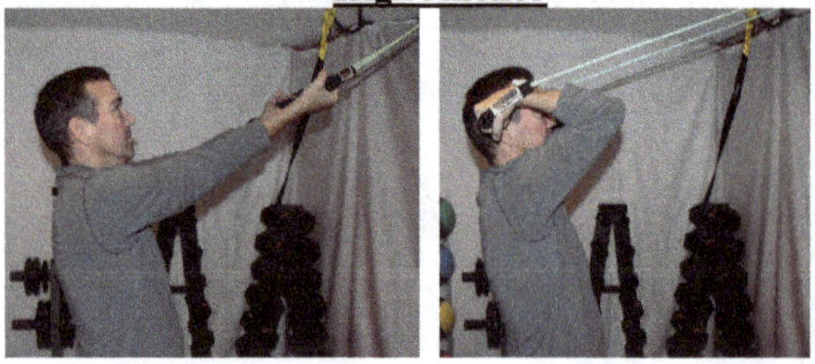

Mid Anchor *Low Anchor*

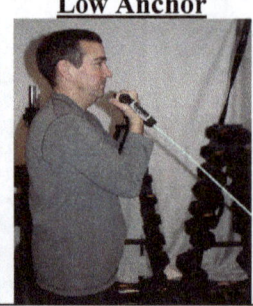

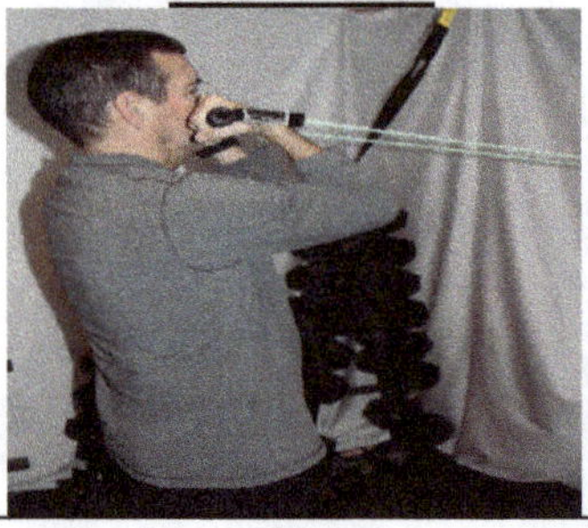

- Stand erect facing the anchor.

- Hands beside the hips facing forward.

- Bend the elbows and raise the hands to shoulder level.

- Avoid swinging of elbows.

- Slowly control the recoil of the arms back to starting position.

Standing on the Band

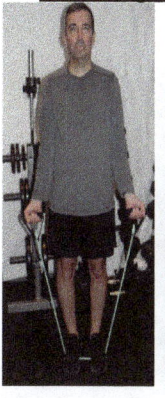

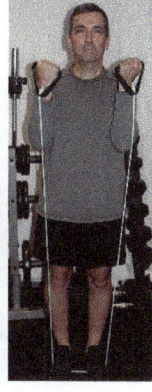

Hammer Curl
(High, mid, low or standing on band anchor)

High Anchor

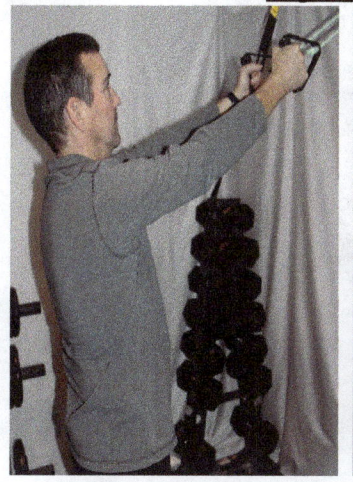

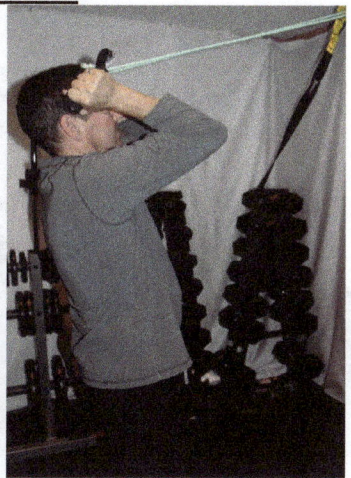

Mid Anchor   Low Anchor

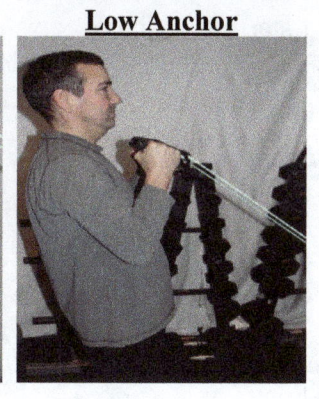

- Stand erect facing the anchor.

- Hands beside the hips facing medially toward the body.

- Bend the elbows and raise the hands to shoulder level.

- Avoid swinging of elbows.

- Slowly control the recoil of the arms back to starting position.

Standing on Band

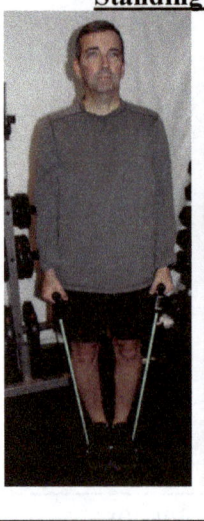

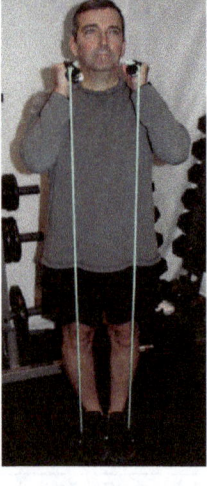

3. In and Out Standard or Hammerer Curl
(Low, Mid, High Anchor or standing on the band)

Standard Curls (Standing on the band)
In's   Out's

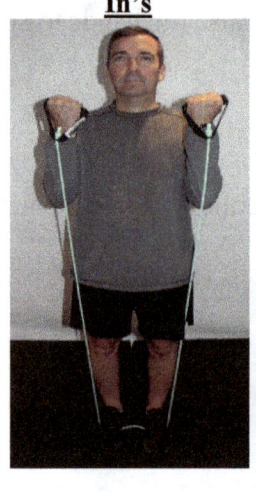

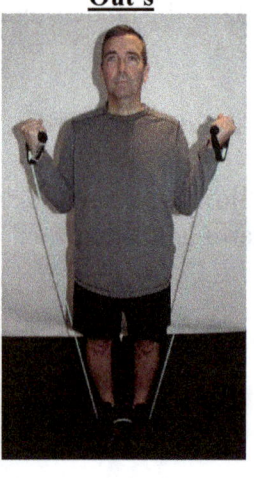

Hammer Curls (Standing on the band)
In's   Out's

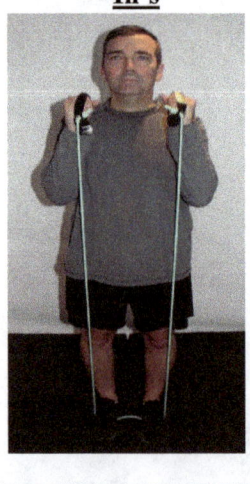

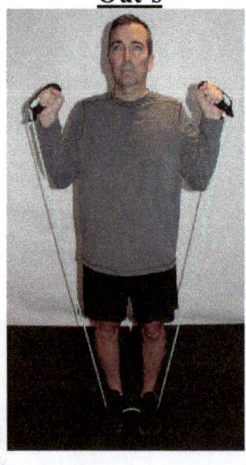

- Stand erect facing the anchor.

1. (In's) Hands beside the hips facing forward (Standard curl) or medially toward the body (hammer curl).

- Bend elbows and raise the hands to shoulder level.

- Slowly control the recoil of the arms back to starting position.

2. (Out's) Rotate hands laterally 45º or as far as possible.

- Bend elbows and raise the hands to shoulder level.

- Slowly control the recoil of the arms back to starting position.

- Rotate hands back to original starting position beside the hips.

Triceps
Over Head Triceps Extensions
(Mid, High Anchor)

High Anchor

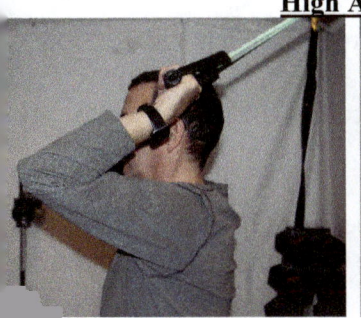

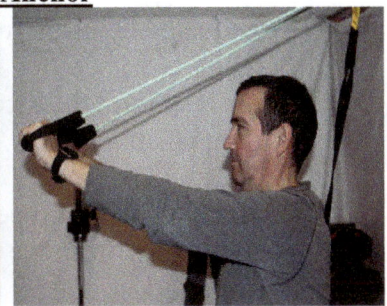

Mid Anchor

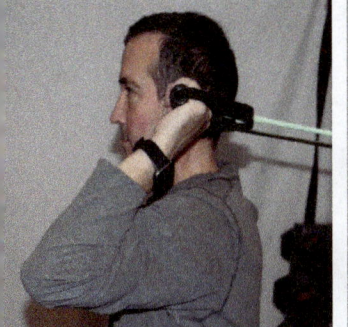

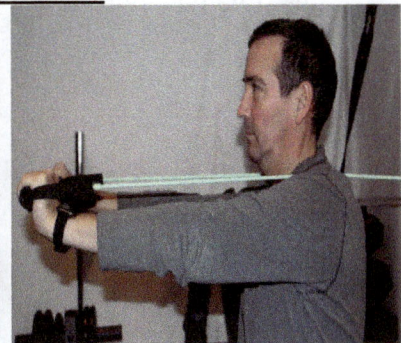

Standing on Band

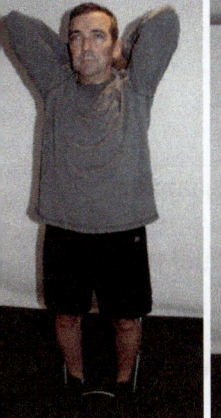

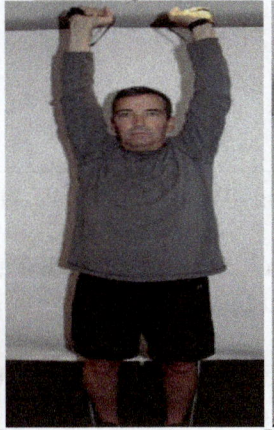

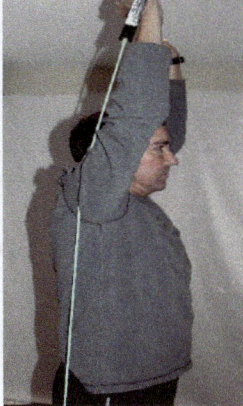

- Stand erect or sitting facing away from the anchor.

- Raise the elbows to shoulder height.

- Extend the elbows while keeping them at shoulder height.

- Slowly control the recoil of the arms back to starting position.

Core

1. Standing Over Head Arm Extended Lateral Bend (High Anchor)

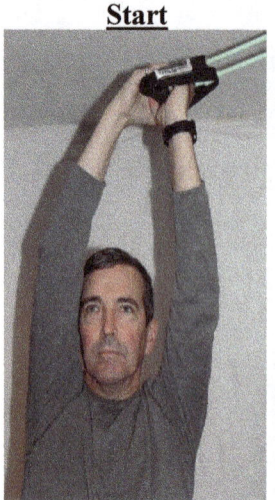

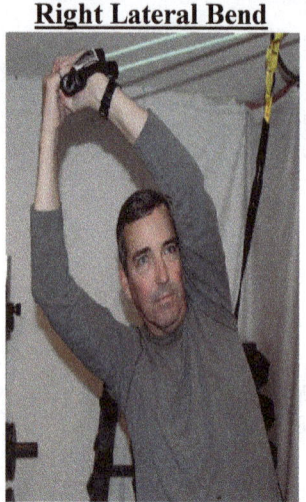

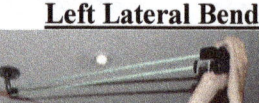

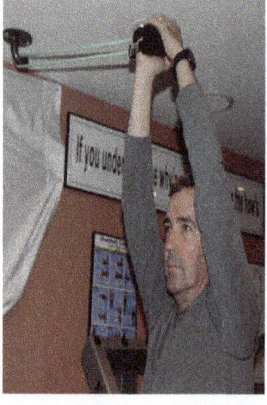

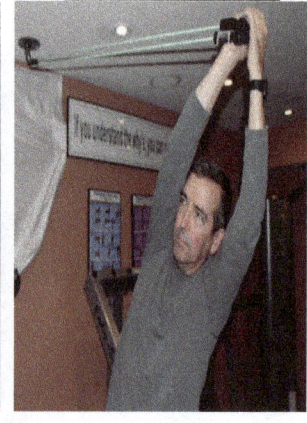

Start   Right Lateral Bend

Start   Left Lateral Bend

- Stand erect facing sideways to the anchor.

- Arms are extended over your head.

- Bend laterally away from the anchor.

- Slowly control the recoil of the arms back to starting position.

- After a number of repetitions turn 180º and bend laterally away from the anchor to exercise the other side.

- Slowly control the recoil of the arms back to starting position.

2. Standing (Arms Straight) Trunk Twist (Mid Anchor)

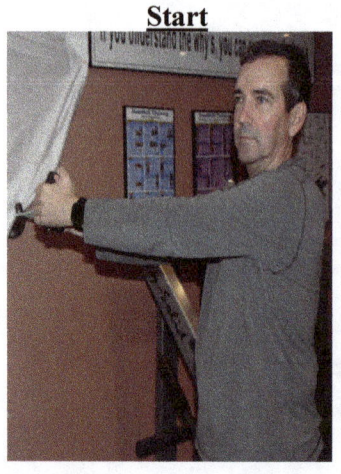

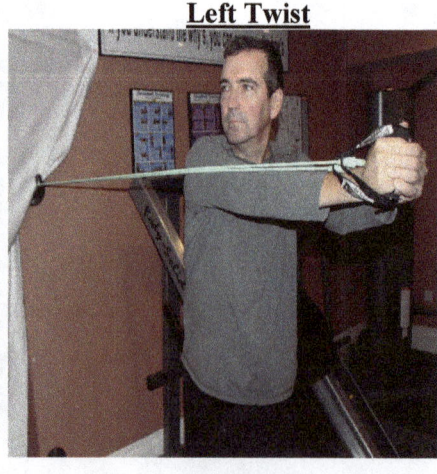

Start   Left Twist

- Stand erect facing sideways to the anchor.

- Arms are at chest level extended and trunk is rotated toward the anchor.

- With arms extended and at chest level, rotate away from the anchor as far as possible.

- Slowly control the recoil of the arms back to starting position.

- After a number of repetitions, turn 180º and repeat to exercise the other side.

- Slowly control the recoil of the arms back to starting position.

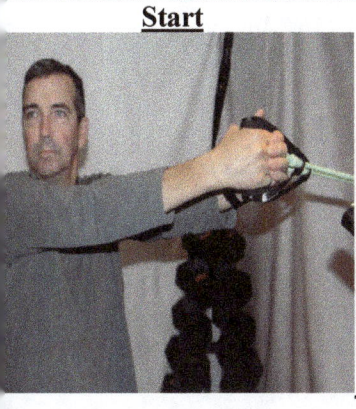

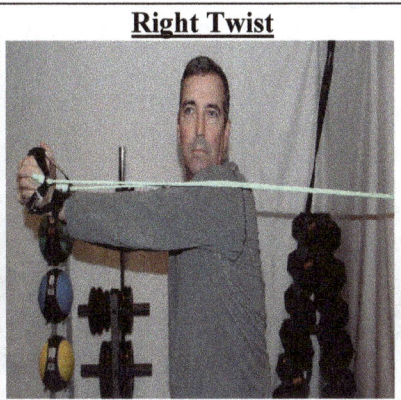

Standing (Arms Bent) Trunk Twist (Mid Anchor)

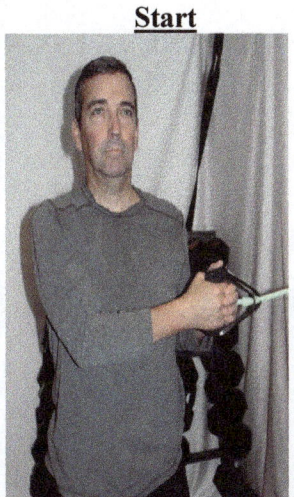

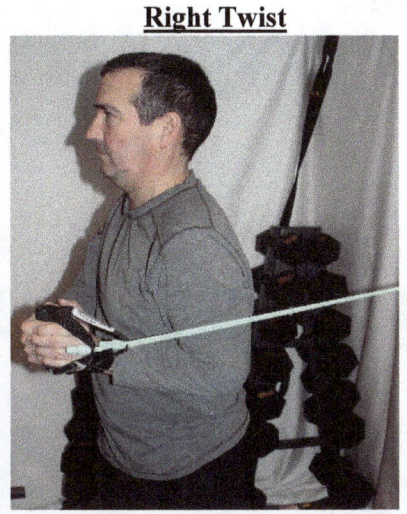

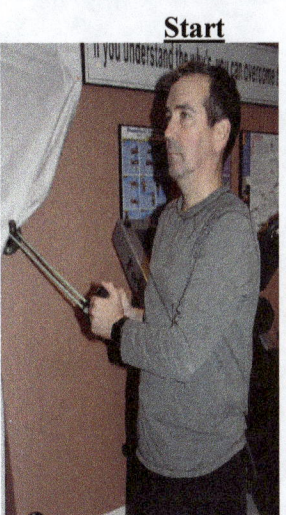

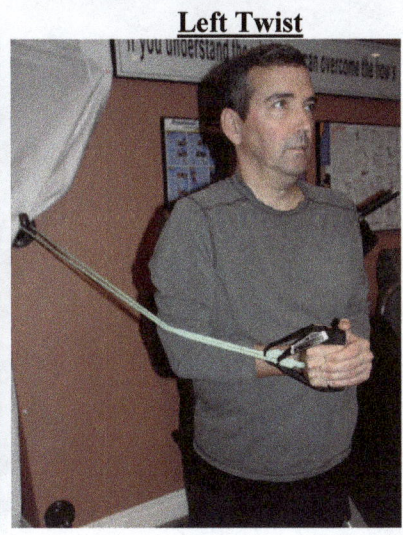

- Stand erect facing sideways to the anchor.

- Arms are at chest level bent and tight against the chest and trunk is rotated toward the anchor.

- Rotate away from the anchor as far as possible.

- Slowly control the recoil of the arms back to starting position.

- After a number of repetitions, turn 180° and repeat to exercise the other side.

- Slowly control the recoil of the arms back to starting position.

4. Standing Low to High Wood Chop (Low Anchor)

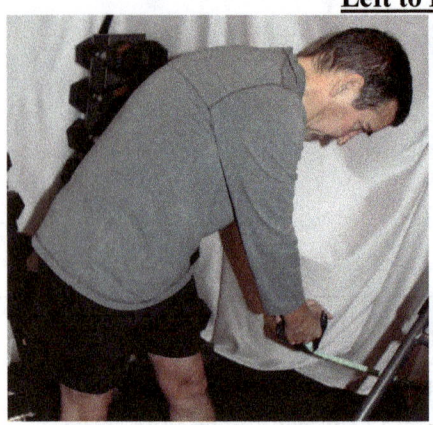

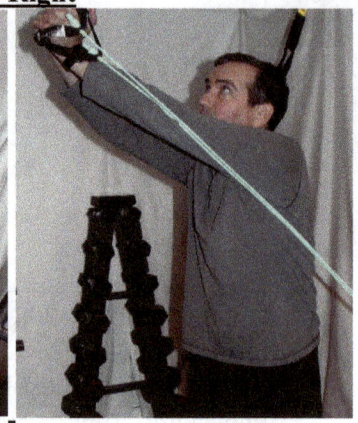

Left to Right

Right to Left

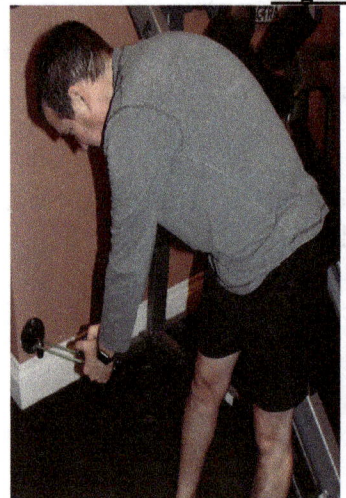

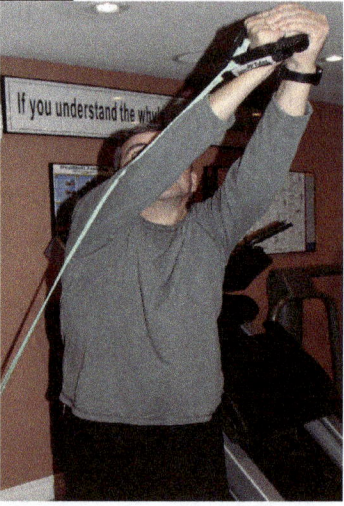

- Stand erect sideways to the anchor.

- With arms extended bend at the waist 90º and rotate toward the anchor.

- Knees are slightly bent.

- With elbows as straight as possible, diagonally raise the hands, stand up and rotate the trunk so hands end up extended over your head and you are facing away from the anchor.

- Slowly control the recoil of the arms back to starting position.

- After a number of repetitions, turn 180º and repeat to exercise the opposite side.

Standing High to Low Wood Chop (High Anchor)

Left to Right

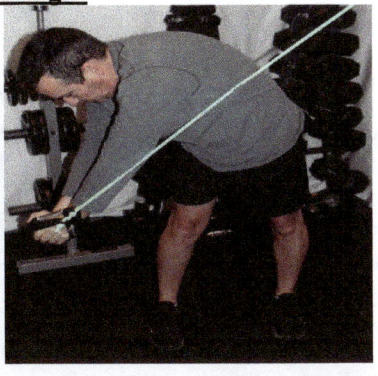

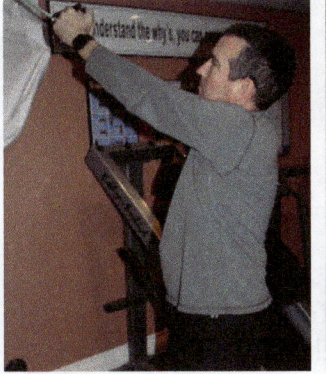

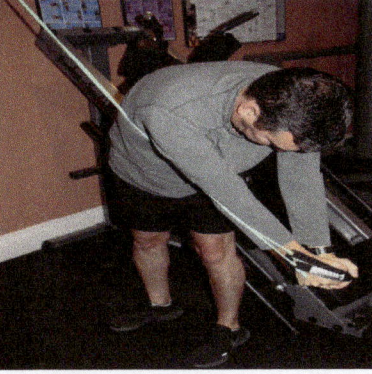

Right to Left

- Stand erect sideways to anchor.

- Arms are extended over your head and trunk is slightly rotated toward the anchor.

- Keeping your arms relatively straight pull down diagonally with the hands, rotating your trunk and bending at the waist so hands end up outside the foot farthest from the anchor and you are facing away from the anchor.

- Slowly control the recoil of the arms back to starting position.

- After a number of repetitions, turn 180^0 and repeat to exercise the opposite side.

Kneeling Abdominal Crunch (High Anchor)

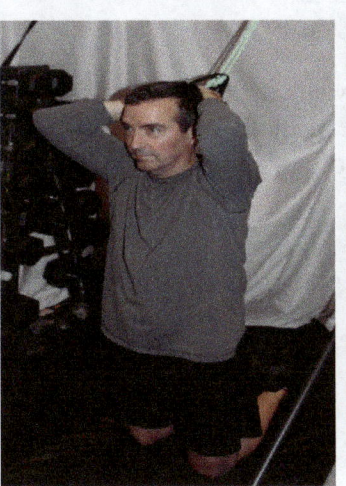

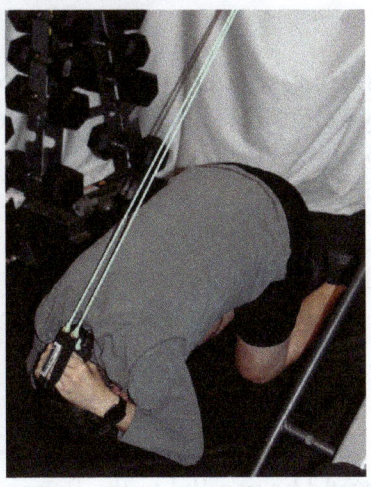

- Kneeling upright and away from the anchor.

- Arms are raised over your head with elbows bent. - hands are resting on top of your head.

- Bend forward so head moves toward floor.

- Slowly control the recoil of the arms back to starting position.

References

McNeely, Ed., Sandler, David, (2006). *The Resistance Band Workout Book*. Burford Books

Potvin, Andre Noel., Jespersen, Michael, (1999). *The Great Stretch Tubing Handbook*. Productive Fitness Products Inc.

Appendix 9.1.6. Stability Ball Exercises Described and Illustrated

Introduction

The Stability Ball was first developed to rehabilitate neurological disorders such as spinal cord and stroke injuries. However, since the nineties, it has become standard exercise equipment in exercise facilities.

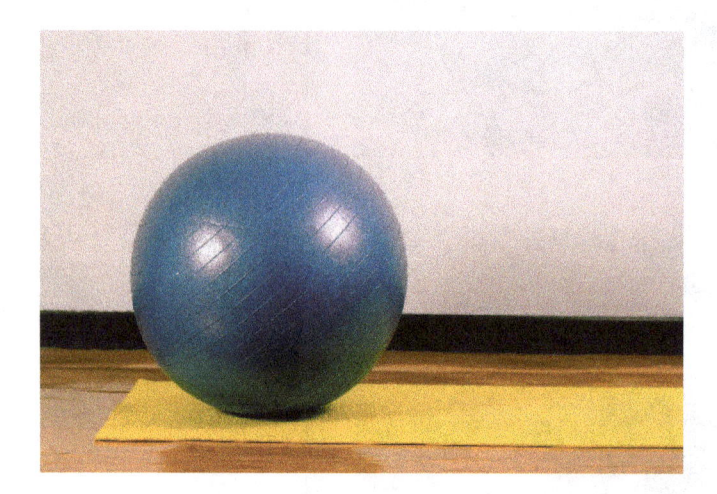

When used correctly, the Stability Ball, originally known as the Swiss Ball from the country it originated, introduces instability into a person's exercise routine. As a result, the muscles, especially their core musculature, must work harder to keep the ball stable while doing a particular exercise movement. Providing this instability challenges a person's balance, flexibility, coordination and strength.

The Stability Ball is a very practical piece of exercise equipment. It is inexpensive, takes up very little space, can be used on its own for bodyweight resistance exercises, especially core exercises, or used to enhance results from the combined use with other forms of resistance such as free weights, resistance bands, and the medicine ball.

As with all types of exercise, using the stability ball properly is necessary for safety and to maximize its effectiveness. Use the illustrations and descriptions listed beside each exercise to ensure proper use.

Selecting the Correct Ball Size

When you sit on top of the ball, the thighs should be parallel to the floor and the knees should be at a 90º angle.

Size Chart

Person's Height	Ball Size
5' - 5'7"	55 cm
5'-8" – 6'2"	65 cm
6'3" – 6'9"	75 cm
Over 6'10"	85 cm

Inflation

Inflate the ball to its correct height (55 cm, 65 cm, 75 cm, 85 cm).

Depending on a person's fitness and skill level:

1. Inflate the ball less, and it becomes more stable for the beginner.
2. Inflate the ball more, and it becomes livelier and more unstable for advanced training.

Stability Ball Exercises Described and Illustrated

Core:	
1. Pelvic Tilt/Shift:	
a. Front and Back Tilts *Forward Tilt* *Backward Tilt*	- While sitting erect on the ball move your hips forward and backwards slowly.
b. Side to Side Lateral Tilts *Right Tilt* *Left Tilt*	- While sitting erect on the ball move your hips slowly side to side.

2. Abdominal Crunch	- Start by sitting erect on the ball. - Slowly slide your hips forward on the ball until the ball is positioned in the small of your back. - Place your hands across your chest or beside your ears. - Slowly squeeze your abdominal muscles and lift your chest half way to vertical. Keep your neck in a neutral position. - Hold for 1 second and then return to starting position.
3. Oblique Abdominal Crunch 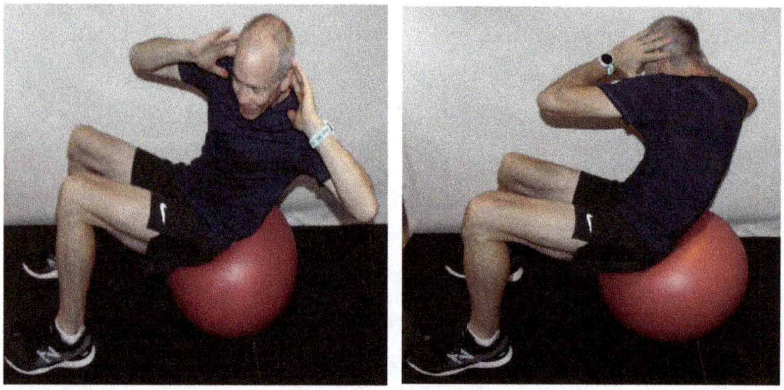	- Start in similar position as the abdominal crunch. - When you lift your chest up angle diagonally toward the outside of one knee. - Return to starting position and lift diagonally toward the other knee.
4. Abdominal Crunch with lower legs on Stability Ball 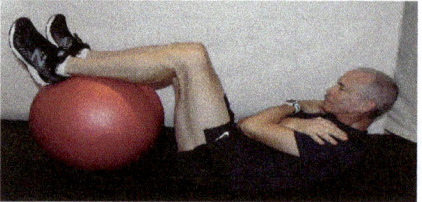	- Lying flat on a mat with hips bent 90° and lower legs resting on SB. - Hands across your chest of at ear level. - Lift chest and shoulder blades off the mat and hold for 1 second. Keep neck in neutral position.
5. Oblique Abdominal Crunch with lower legs on Stability Ball 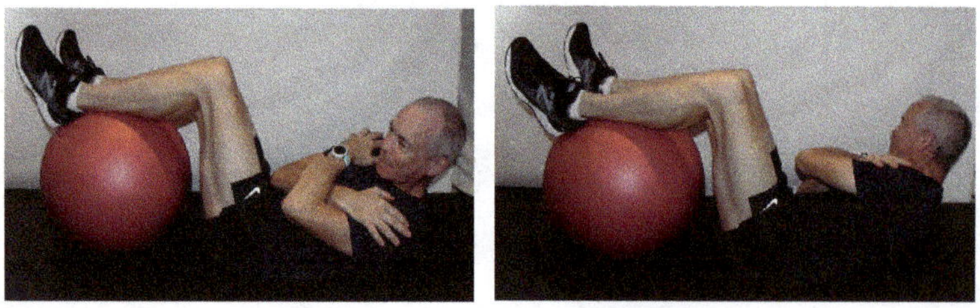	- Lying flat on a mat with hips bent 90° and lower legs resting on SB. - Hands across your chest of at ear level. - Diagonally lift chest and shoulder blades off the mat toward one knee and hold for 1 second. Keep neck in neutral position. - Return to starting position and repeat the chest lift to the opposite side.

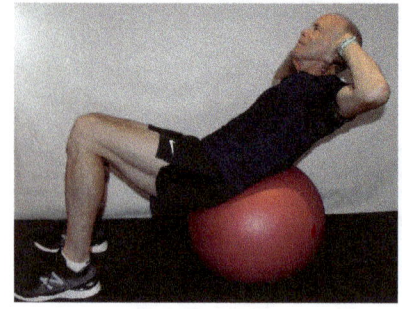

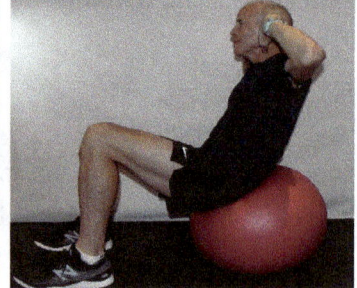

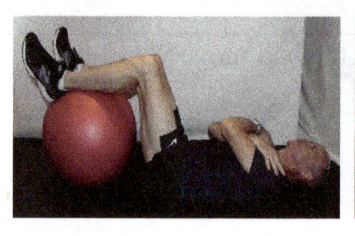

Oblique Abdominal Crunch with Legs in Figure-4 Position **Straight Crunch** **Obliques Crunch** 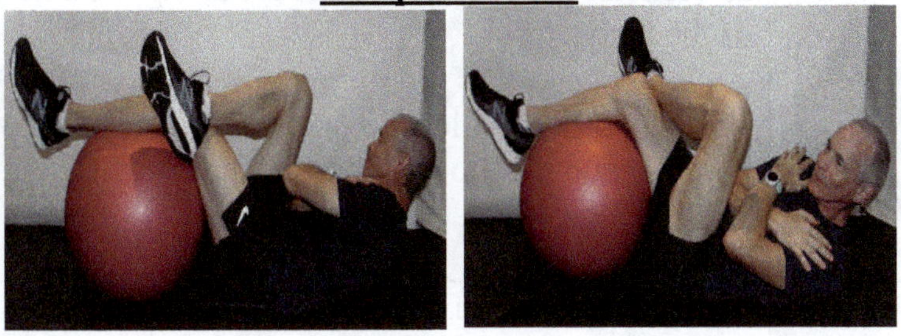	- Lying flat on a mat with hips bent 90º and lower legs resting on SB. - Cross one leg over the other so they make a figure-4 design. - Hands are across your chest, at ear level. - Diagonally lift chest and shoulder blades off the mat toward the one knee that is bent across the other leg and hold for 1 second. Keep neck in neutral position. - Return to starting position and repeat the chest lift to the same side again. - After repeated number of repetitions, change leg position and repeat chest lift to the opposite side.
7. Supine Reverse Abdominal Crunch with SB Between the Legs 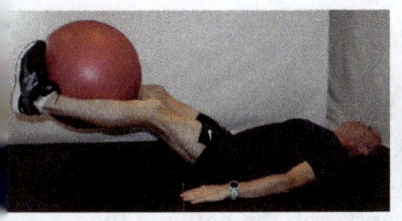	- Laying flat on a mat with legs straight and ball squeezed between your ankles. - Bend the knees and move them toward your chest. - Hold for one second and then straighten knees and return to starting position (Try not to have the ball touch the ground before repeating the reverse crunch).
8. Prone Reverse Abdominal Crunch (Jackknife) 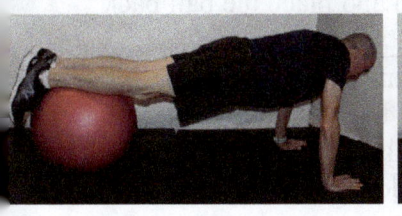	- Lying Prone (face down) on the mat place both feet/ankles on the ball and extend the knees so legs are straight. - Lift your chest off the mat by supporting yourself with your forward arms or hands. You are now in a plank position. - Slowly bend the knees towards your chest. The ball will move from the ankles to the top of the feet. - Hold for 1 second and then straight the knees and return to starting plank position.

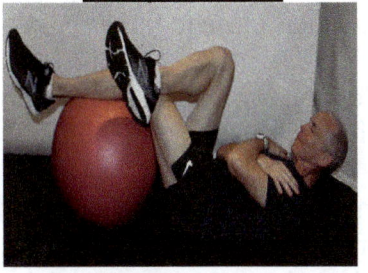

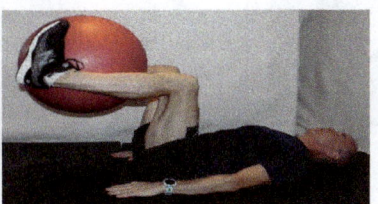

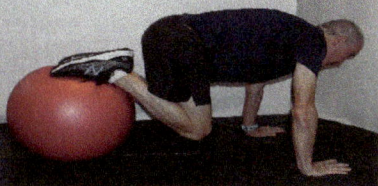

9. Straight Leg Raise		- Supine – legs extended and arms along the side of your body.
		- Keep the knees as straight as possible and lift the legs up to as close to 90º as possible.
		- Hold for 1 second and then return to starting position.
		- Don't let the heels touch the ground before repeating the exercise.
10. Abdominal Twist		- Supine – keep the knees straight and lift the legs as vertically as you can. Arms are along the side of the body.
		- Slowly rotate the legs to one side as far as possible and then to the opposite side
11. "V" Sit-up and Grab Ball		- Lying supine with knees extended and arms extended over your head or in front of your chest (advanced).
		- Place ball between the ankles.
		Simultaneously:
		1. Lift the legs and ball as vertical as possible while keeping the knees as straight as possible.
		2. Lift the chest up and grab the ball and then lower the legs and chest.
		- Repeat the motion and place the ball back between the ankles.
12. Bridge with Hip Drop (Shoulders on SB)		- From an erect sitting position, slowly roll forward so only the back of your shoulders are supported on the ball. Your heels should be on the mat supporting the legs.
		- Lift the hips up so you are in a "bridge" position.
		- Slowly drop your hips down toward the mat and then lift the hips up back to the "bridge" position.

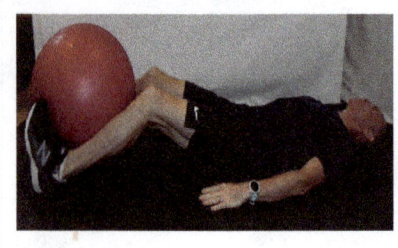

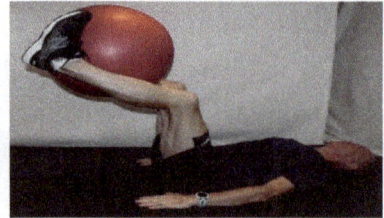

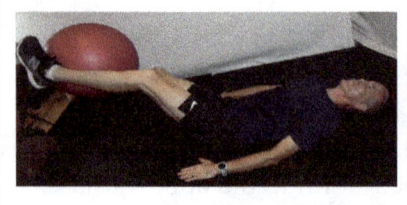

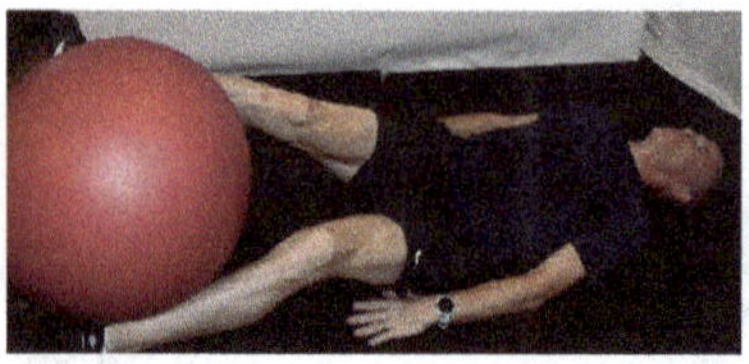

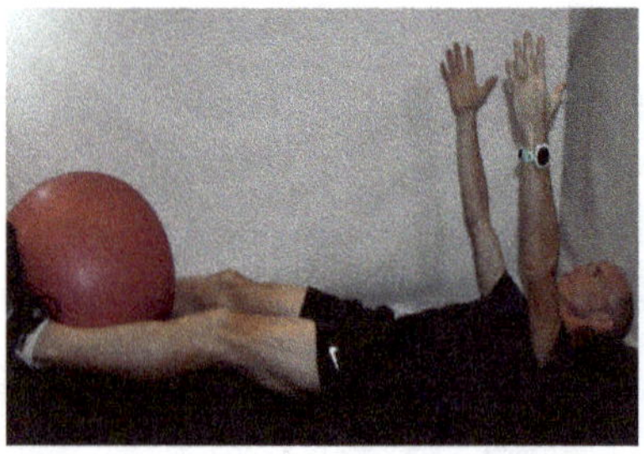

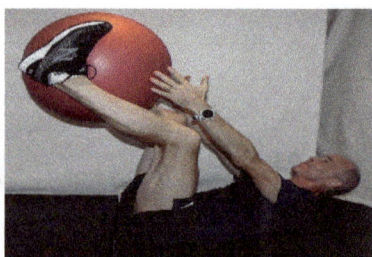

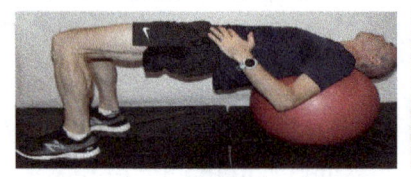

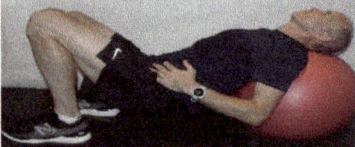

3. Reverse Bridge with Hip Drop (Heels on SB) 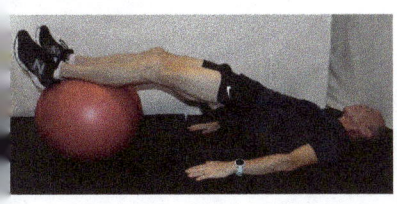 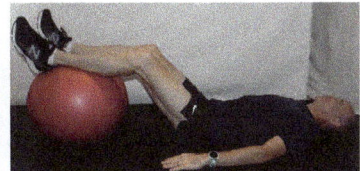	- Lying supine on mat with both heels on the ball. - Lift the hips off the mat into a "bridge" position (Back of the shoulders are on the mat and heels/ankles on the ball). - From "bridge" position drop the hips toward the floor and then raise them back to "bridge" position.
4. Back Extensions 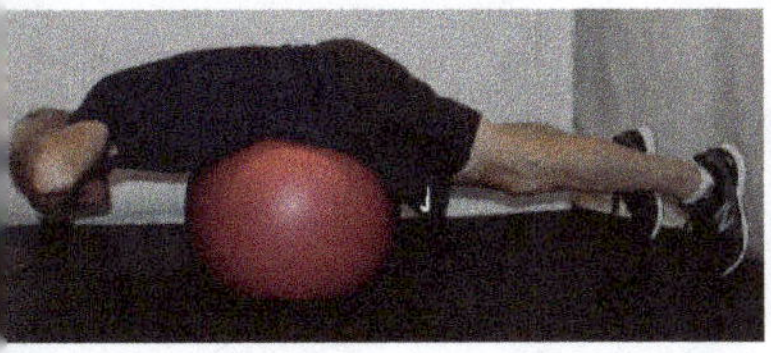 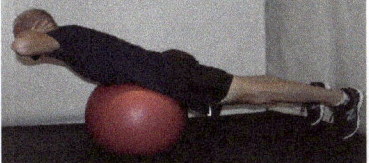	- Lie prone with the lower waist supported on the ball and chest low toward the ground. - Place your hands beside your ears or in the small of the back. - Lift your chest up as high as possible. (Keep your neck in a neutral position) and then lower to starting position. Advanced – When the back is in a fully extended position do small (6") oscillations up and down.
5. Planks (on hands (high planks) or forearms (low planks):	- Upper body supported by hands or forearms on the SB - Lower body supported by toes on the mat Key – keep the abdominal muscles tight. (Abdominal bracing - squeeze in the belly button)
4. Prone 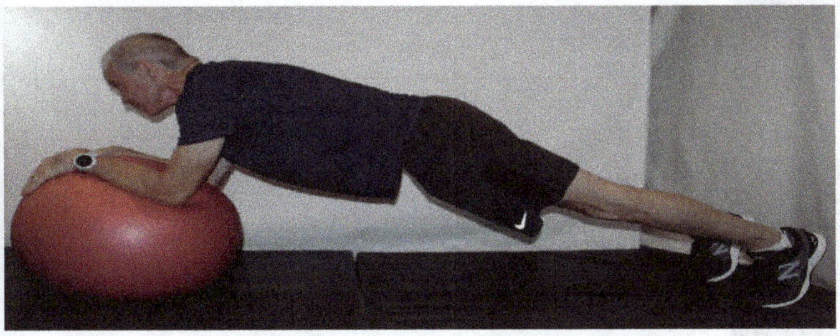	- Lying face down.

789

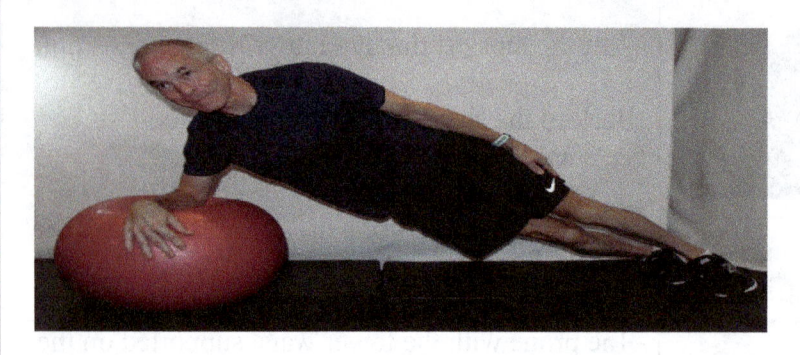

2. Lateral	- Lying sideways.
3. Supine (Bridge) 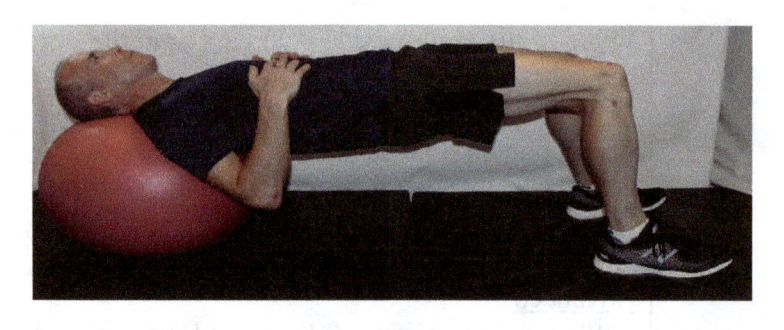	- Lying face up.
16. Bird **Starting** 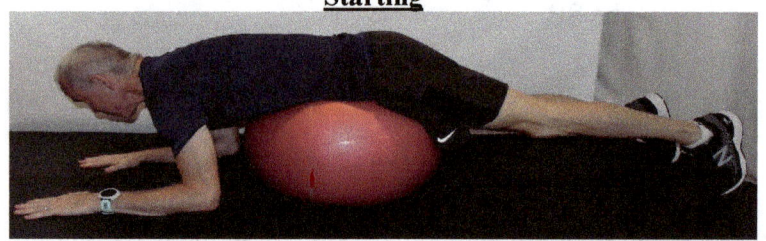 **Right Arm & Leg** 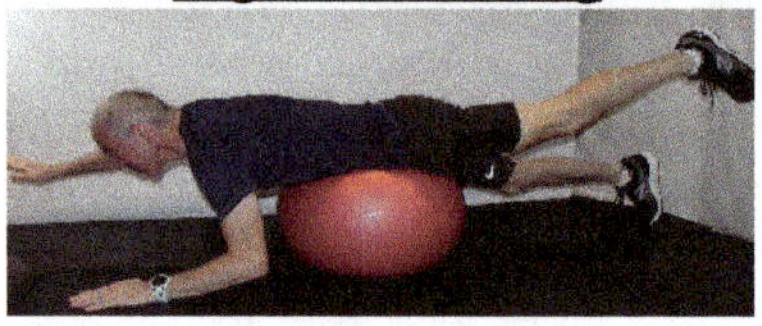 **Left Arm and Leg** 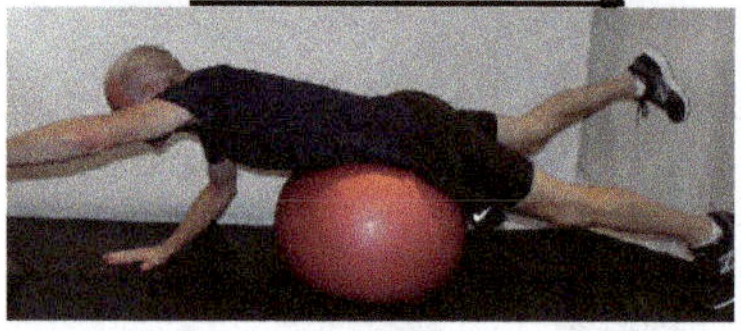	- Start in prone position on your hands and knees. - Simultaneously, extend one arm out in front of the head and opposite leg backwards. - Hold for 3-5 seconds. - Repeat with opposite arm and leg. Beginner: 1. Extend only an arm or a leg at one time.
17. Front Rollouts 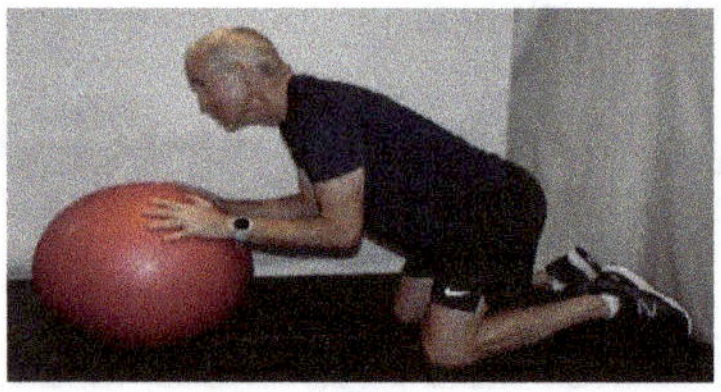 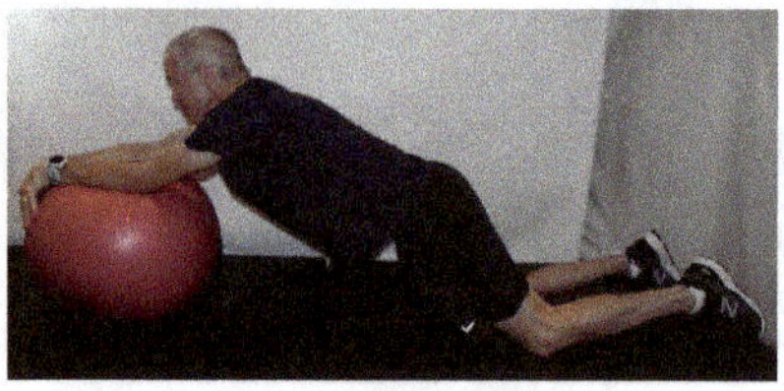	- Lying prone, place forearms on the ball. - Support lower body by kneeling knees or toes on the mat. - Roll the ball out in front of you along the forearms one foot and then roll back. Key – Keep the abdominal muscles tight. Do not let the belly sag down. (Abdominal bracing)

Upper Body:
Upper Back:

1. Sitting Bent Over Rows

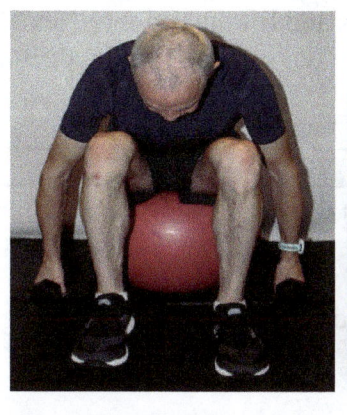

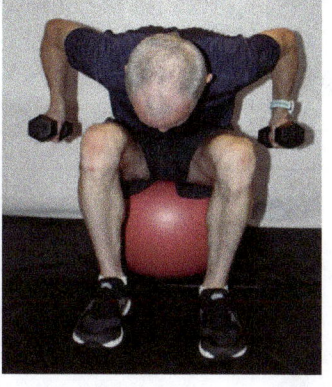

- From a sitting erect position bend forward at the hips as far as possible.

- Hold the weights on both sides of your feet.

- Lift the weight up towards your ribs and keep the elbows as close to ribs as possible during the lift. (Feel your shoulder blades squeeze together)

- Hold for 1 second and then return to starting position.

2. Sitting Bent over Flies

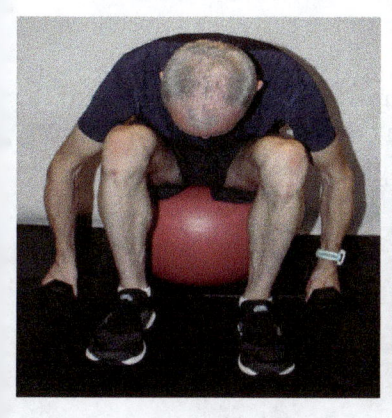

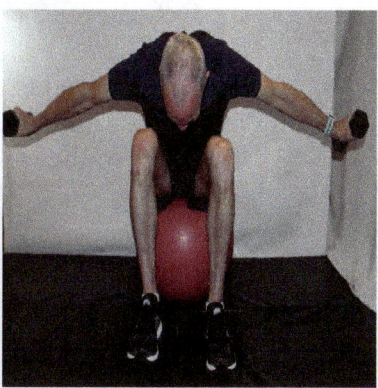

- From a sitting erect position bend forward at the hips as far as possible.

- Hold the weights on both sides of your feet.

- Lift the arms up to shoulder level with elbows straight of bent 90º.

(Feel the shoulder blades squeeze together)

3. Sitting Two Angle Shoulder Flies

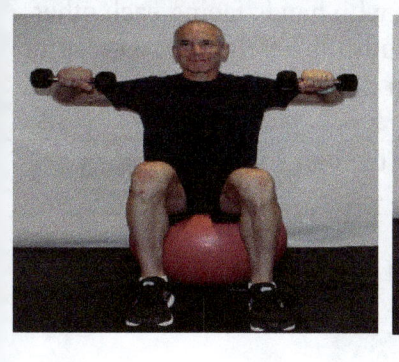

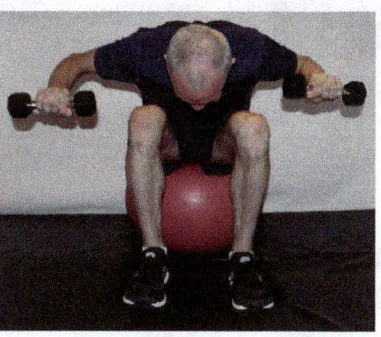

1. Sitting erect and arms extended to the floor.

- Bend the elbows 90º and lift the weight laterally to shoulder height. (Feels like you are shrugging your shoulders)

- Return the weights to starting position.

2. Bend forward as far as possible.

- Lift the weights laterally to shoulder height with the elbows bent 90º. (feel the shoulder blades squeeze together)

- Lower the weights to starting position and return to erect posture and repeat.

4. Prone Reverse Flies	- Lying prone on the ball at waist level. - Keep the head and chest down. - Extend the elbows and lift the weight to shoulder height (feel the shoulder blades squeeze together).
Chest:	
1. Supine Chest Press **Standard Press** **Alternating Arm Press** **Swimmers Press**	- Lying supine with the ball supporting the upper back. - The hips are raised so upper body, hips and upper legs are flat. - Hold the weights just above the chest, shoulder width apart. The hands are facing forward toward the feet. - Lift both weights upward and slightly toward the mid-line so almost a complete elbow extension. The sides of the weights may touch. - Hold for 1 second and then lower weights to starting position. Modifications: 1. <u>Alternating</u> - lifting one weight up at a time. 2. <u>Swimmers</u> - start with hands facing each other (inwards) and as you lift the weights you twist the arms so at extension the weights are facing outwards.
2. Supine Chest Fly	- Lying supine with the ball supporting the upper back. - The hips are raised so upper body, hips and upper legs are flat. - Start with arms extended vertically and weight facing each other (medially). - Lower the weights to shoulder height. Try to keep the elbows as straight as possible. - Hold for1 second and then left the arms back to starting position.

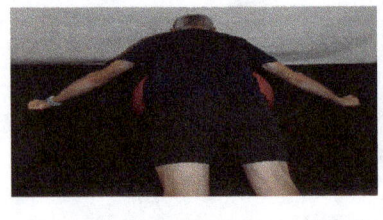

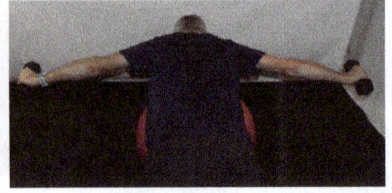

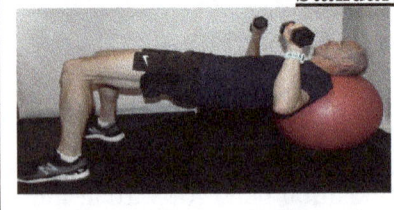

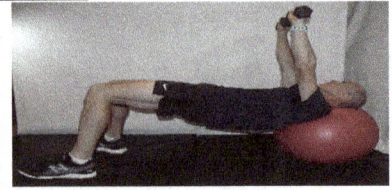

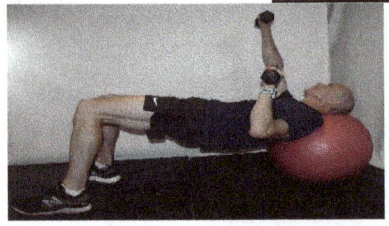

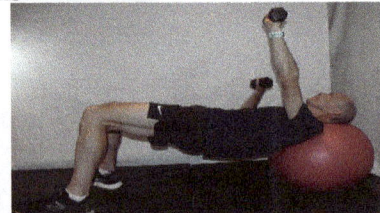

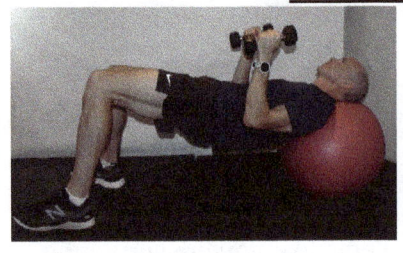

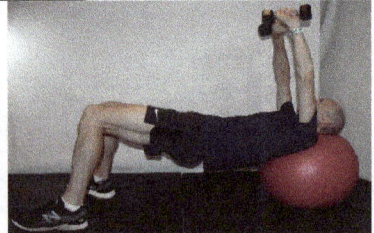

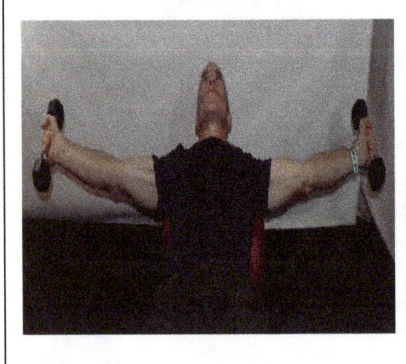

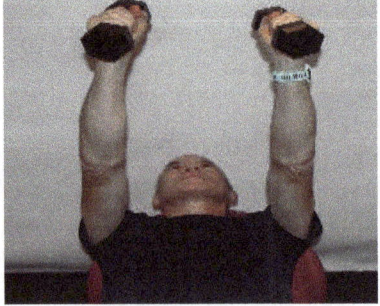

3. Push-ups (Hands on SB)	- Start in a prone plank position with the hands on the ball and toes or knees (modified) can be supporting the lower body)
Modified (on knees)	- Do a push-up on the ball by lowering your chest towards the ball.
4. Decline Push-ups (Feet on SB)	- Start in a prone plank position and then place your feet onto the ball. - The body is extended and supported by the hands. - Do a push-up from this position (feet are supported on the ball).

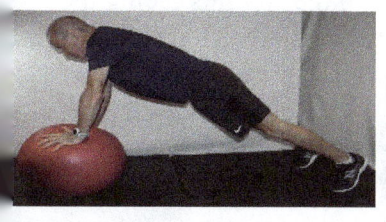

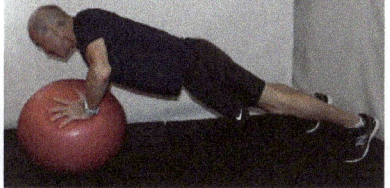

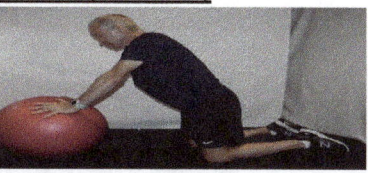

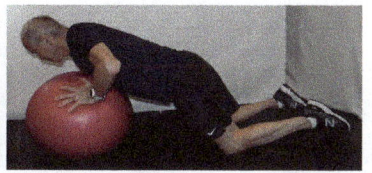

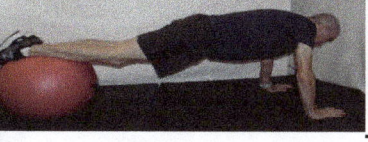

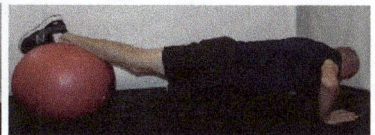

Shoulders:

| 1. Sitting Overhead Press (I's, Y's, Alternating, Swimmers)

Starting   I's   Y's

Alternating | - Sitting erect on the ball and holding the weights at ear level and shoulder width. Weights/hands are facing forward.

- "I's" – lift the weights straight upwards. The insides of the weight can touch at almost complete extension

- "Y's" – lift the weights up at a slight outward angle so at almost complete extension the arms make a "Y" or 'V' shape

- Alternating – lift one weight up at a time |

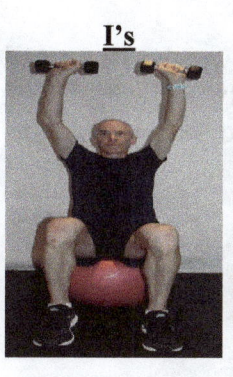

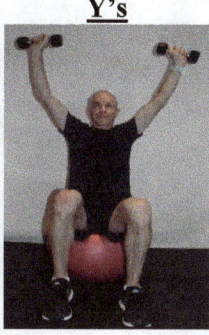

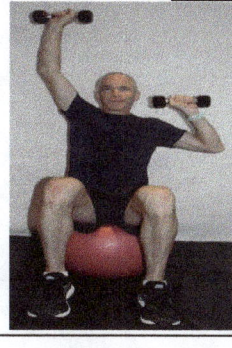

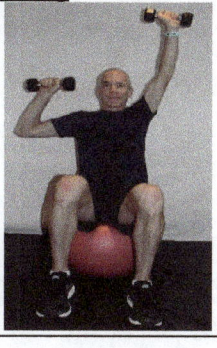

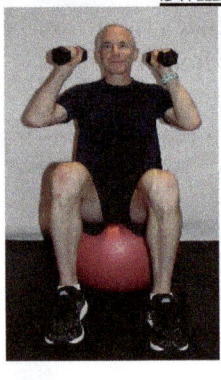

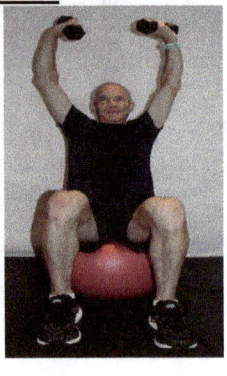

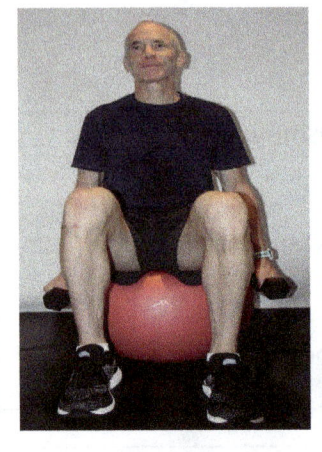

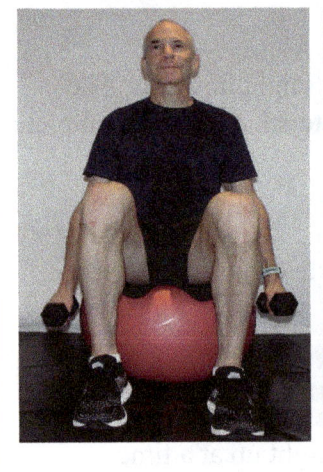

Swimmers	- <u>Swimmers</u> – start with the weights facing the ears (medially) and at complete extension the arms have rotated and the weights are facing outwards (laterally).
2. Sitting Lateral Raises	- Sitting erect with weight along the side of the body. - Lift the weights up laterally to shoulder height.
3. Sitting Pours	- Sitting erect with weight along the side of the body. - Lift the weights up laterally to shoulder height and then twist the hands so the weights point downward (pretend you are pouring a bottle of wine).

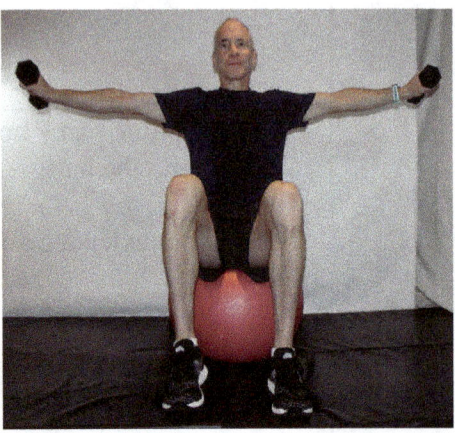

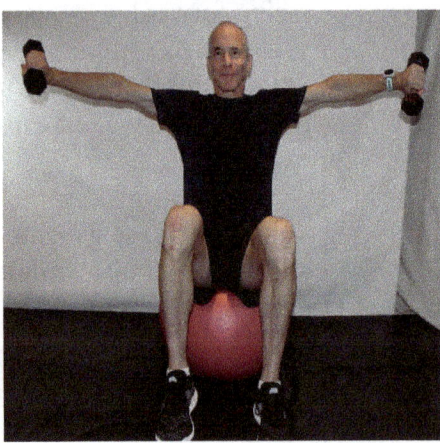

4. Sitting Scarecrows	- Sitting erect, lift the weights laterally (lateral raise) and then bend the elbows 90° and rotate weights and lower arms upward so they are pointing vertical. - Rotate the lower arms down/forward so they are horizontal. - Rotate the arms back to vertical.
5. Anterior Raise	- Sitting erect with weights along the side of the body and facing inward (medially). - Lift the weights up to shoulder level.
6. Sitting In's and Out's In's Out's	- Sitting erect, do the following: 1. Anterior Raise (In's) 2. Lateral Raise (Out's)

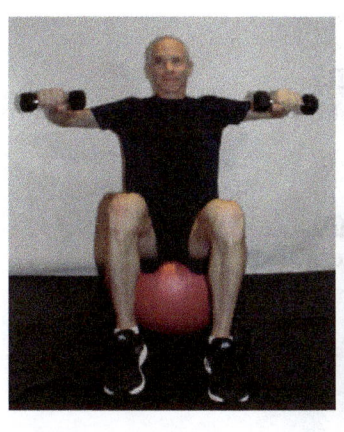

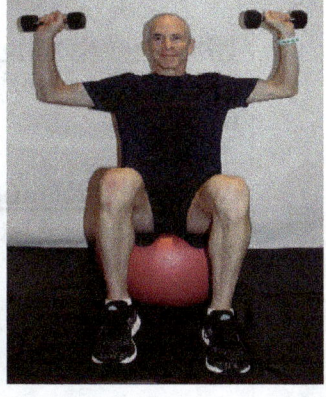

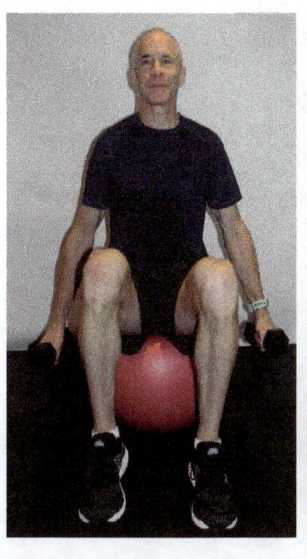

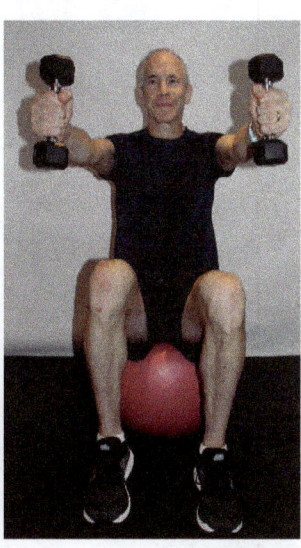

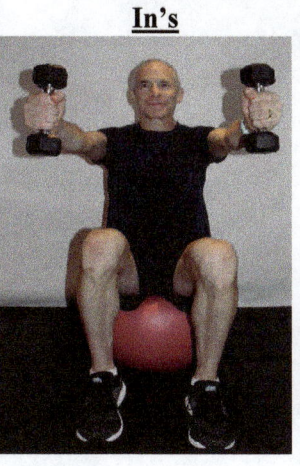

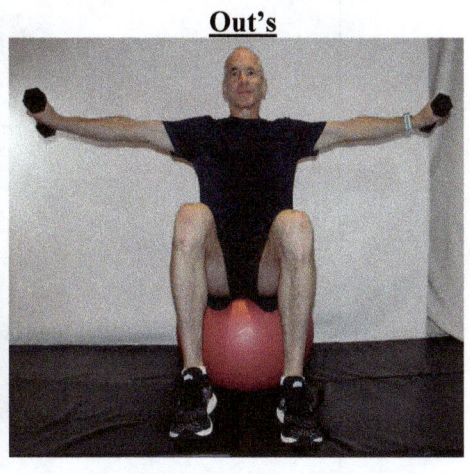

7. Sitting Horizontal Rotations (One arm at a time)

Starting　　**Internal Rotation**

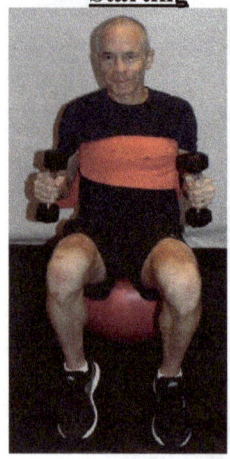

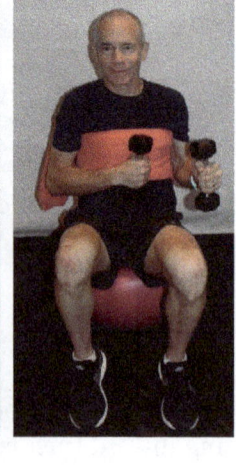

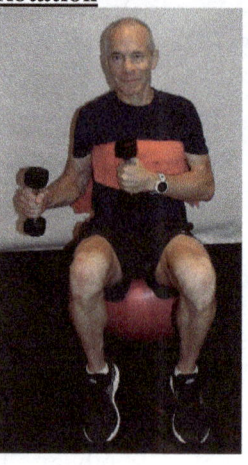

External Rotation

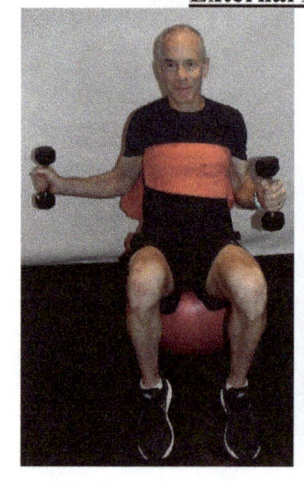

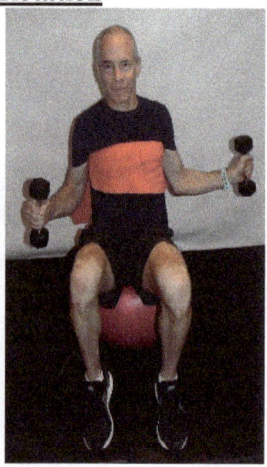

- Sitting erect with a towel between the ribs and upper arm.

1. Internal Rotation
- Elbow is bent 90º and rotated medially against the chest.

2. External Rotation
- Rotate the arm laterally as far as possible

Arms:

Biceps (Sitting):
Key – don't sway the body or move the elbows forwards when you lift the weights.

1. Regular Curls	- Sitting erect and arms with weights at your side. - Weights are facing forward. - Bend elbows and lift the weights to the top
2. Hammer Curls	- Sitting erect and arms with weights at your side. - Weights are facing inward (medially). - Bend elbows and lift the weights to the top
3. In's and Out's (Regular or hammers) In's Out's	- Sitting erect and arms with weights at your side. - Weights are facing forward. **1. In's** - Bend elbows and lift the weights so they squeeze against the forearm. **2. Out's** - Rotate the arms outward 45° and bend the elbows and lift the weights so they squeeze against the forearms.

4. Twenty Ones 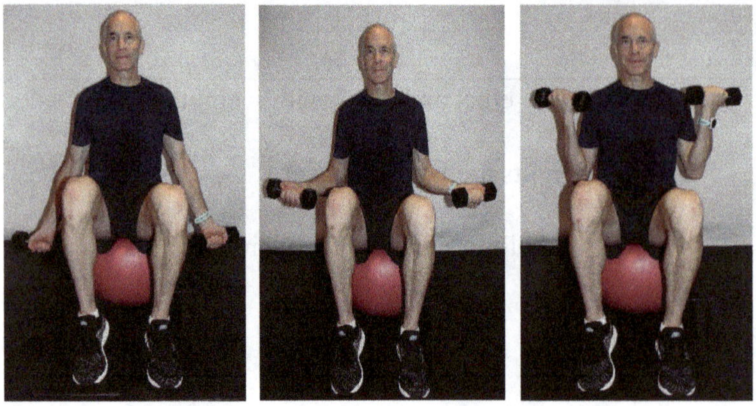	- Sitting erect and arms with weights at your side. - Weights are facing forward: 1. Lift weights to 90º 7x's. 2. Lift weights from 90º to top 7x's. 3. Do a full regular curl 7x's.
5. Static Curls **Left Arm Static** 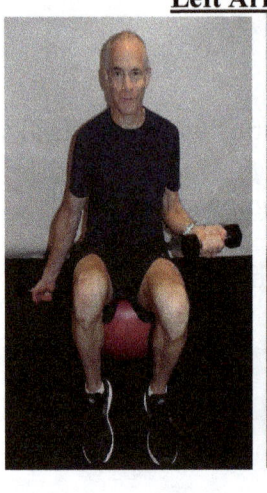 **Right Arm Static**	- Sitting erect and holding one arm static at 90º. - Do a full regular curl with the opposite arm 8x's. - Repeat with opposite arm.

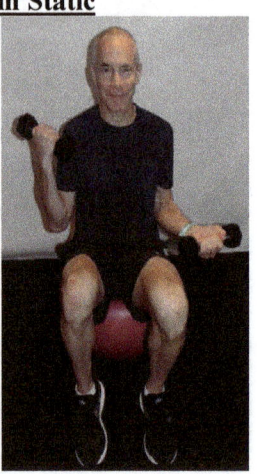

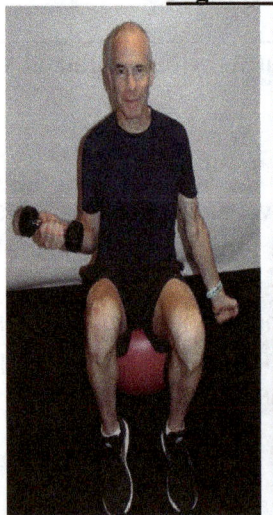

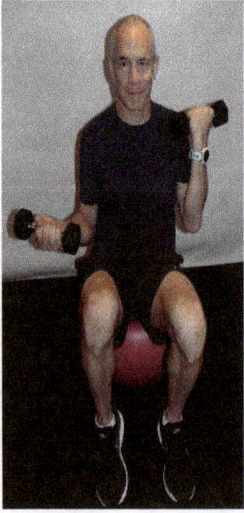

Triceps:

1. Sitting Overhead Triceps Extensions:

1. Double Arm

- Sitting erect, lift both arms over your head and fully bend the elbows. (The elbows should be pointing close to vertical).

- Weights are pointing inward (medially).

- Extend the elbows so arms are almost completely extended above your head.

- Do not sway the elbows as they are extended.

(<u>Note</u> – do not arch your back and focus on getting complete flexion and extension of the elbows)

2. Single Arm

- Sitting erect, lift one arms over your head and fully bend the elbow. (The elbows should be pointing close to vertical).

- Weight is pointing inward (medially)

- Support the raised elbow with the opposite hand so it does not sway.

- Extend the elbow so arm is almost completely extended above your head.

(<u>Note</u> – do not arch your back and focus on getting complete flexion and extension of the elbow)

2. Lying Overhead Triceps Extensions:

1. Double Arm

- Lying supine with only the shoulders supported by the ball.

- Hips are raised so upper body, hips and upper legs are in a horizontal position.

- Lift both arms so elbows are pointing vertical.

- Weights are pointing inward (medially)

- Bend the elbows so weights are beside the head.

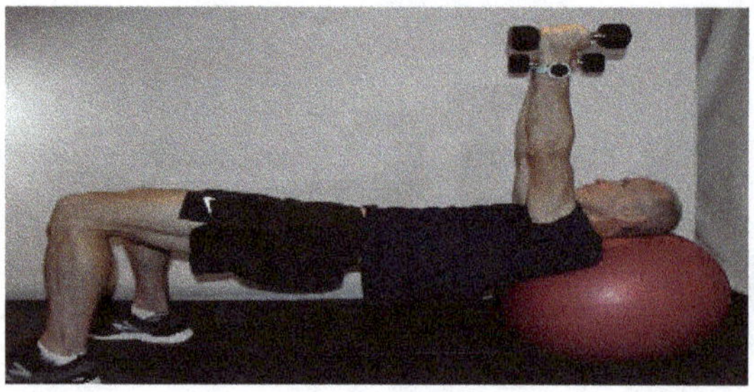

- Extend both elbows almost completely so arms are vertical.

- Lower the weights to starting position

Note:

1. Don't sway the elbows as you extend them.

2. Focus on complete flexion and almost complete extension of the elbows

2. Single Arm

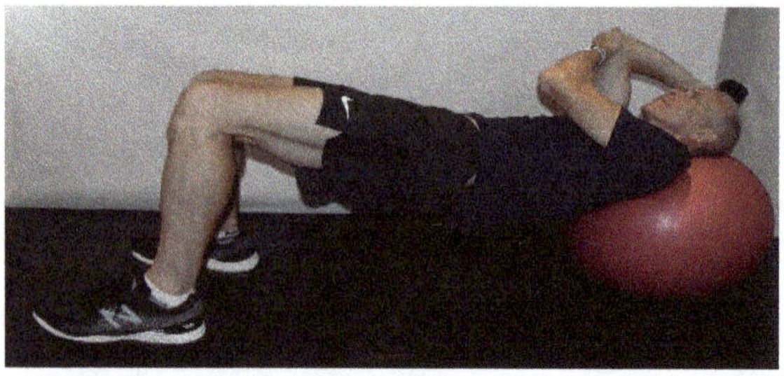

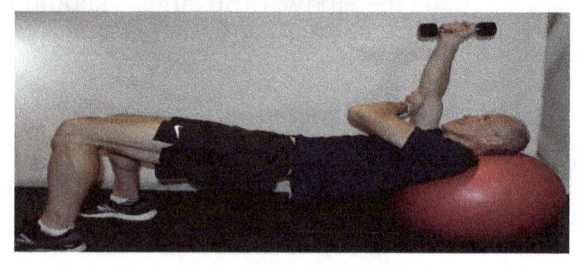

- Lying supine with only the shoulders supported by the ball.

- Hips are raised so upper body, hips and upper legs are in a horizontal position.

- Lift one arm so elbow is pointing vertical.

- Weight is pointing inward (medially).

- Bend the elbow so weight is beside the head.

- Extend the elbow almost completely so arm is vertical.

- Lower the weights to starting position.

Keys:

1. Don't sway the elbow as you extend it.

2. Focus on complete flexion and almost complete extension of the elbow.

Lower Body:

Quadriceps:

1. Wall Squats

- Stand erect with ball in the small of the back and pressed against a wall.

- The feet are shoulder width apart.

- Bend the knees and squat no deeper than 90°. (Pretend you are going to sit in a chair)

<u>Note</u> – don't let your knees go past your toes as you squat.

Hamstrings:

2. Reverse Double Leg Curls

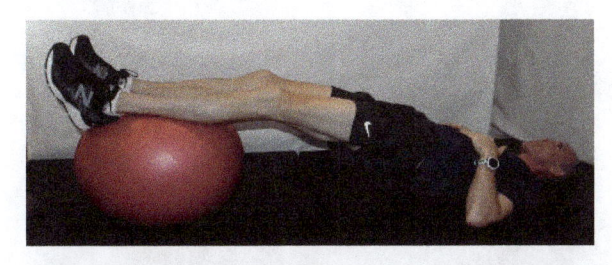

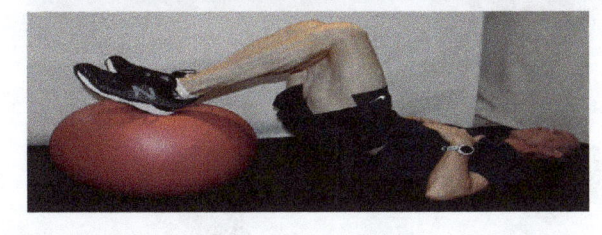

- Lying on the mat with legs extended and lower calves resting on the ball.

- Lift hips up into a bridge position.

- Bend the knees so they go high into the air and roll the ball closer to your buttocks.

- Straighten the knees and return the ball to its starting position.

<u>Note</u> – keep the hips high in a bridged position.

Groins:

3. Lying Ball Squeeze

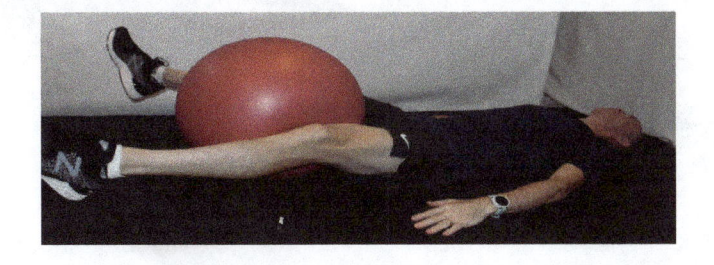

- Lying supine with the ball in between the knees.

- Squeeze the ball with your knees.

2. Sitting Ball Squeeze	- Sitting on a bench and place the ball between the knees. - Squeeze the ball with your knees.

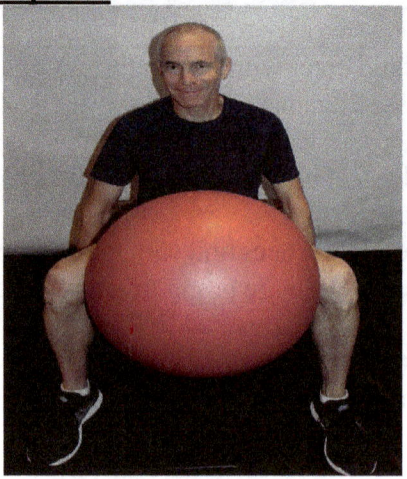

Reference

Jespersen, Michael., Potvin, Andre Noel. (2000). *The Great Body Ball Handbook*. Productive Fitness Products Inc.

Appendix 9.1.7. BOSU Exercises Described and Illustrated

Introduction

The BOSU Balance Trainer is standard exercise equipment in modern fitness facilities. It can augment cardio vascular, strength, and flexibility training for the older adult, but its real value is helping to improve agility, balance, and coordination.

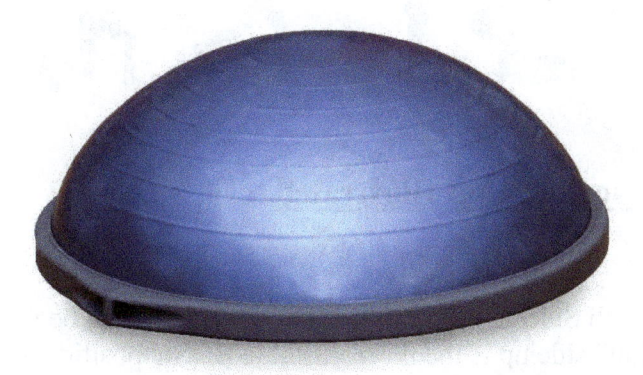

Balance is the foundation of all movement and athletic performance. It requires not only muscular strength but also strong neurologic input called proprioception. The body relies on its eyes (visual), the middle ear (vestibular), and muscles and joints (somatic) for its proprioceptive input. The instability created by the BOSU challenges and stimulates the muscles and joints to help train their proprioceptive reflexes to "kick in" more effectively for better and safer movements. More responsive proprioceptive reflexes allow the high-caliber athlete to perform more efficiently, thus saving energy and performance time. For the older adult, more responsive proprioceptive reflexes mean better protection against falling.

When used properly, the BOSU is a safe way of introducing instability into a person's exercise routine. It can be used as a stand-alone piece of exercise equipment for body weight exercises or used in conjunction with dumbbells, medicine balls, and resistance bands to stimulate muscles and reflexes.

The BOSU introduces instability into the exercise so for safety, it is important to follow illustrations and descriptions for each exercise in this appendix.

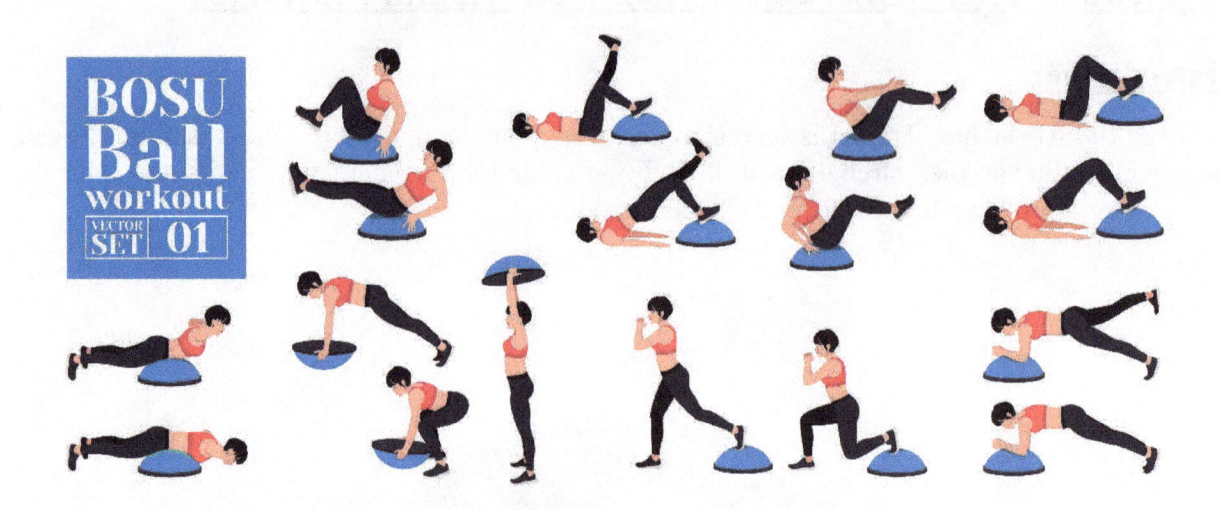

BOSU Exercises Described and Illustrated

Notes:

1. BOSU stands for "Both Sides UP." Both sides of the BOSU can be used to improve strength and balance. The "flat" side up is the more unstable BOSU position and should be used only by those that are more experienced, well trained and have no compromising issues with respect to balance.

2. Sitting and Standing on Dome Side - The higher or more on top a person sits or stands on the "dome" side, the more unstable the position becomes.

3. Most of the exercises that were described under Core Strengthening (appendix 9.1.2.1.1) and Whole Body Strengthening (appendix 9.1.2.2.1) can be performed with the BOSU and are illustrated and described below.

1. Isolate Lower Abdominal Muscles (Hip Flexors will be engaged as well):

1. Flutter kicks

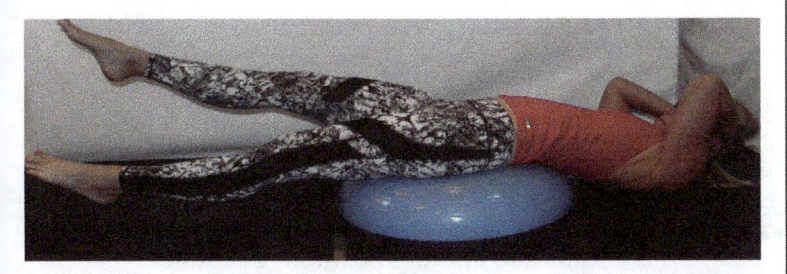

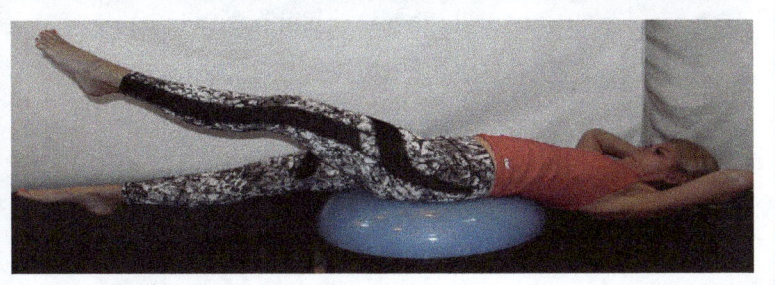

Lying Supine with BOSU supporting the lower back

- Head, shoulders and legs are off mat and you are lying in a horizontal position

- Hands behind neck for support

- Alternatively, and repetitively, flutter kick (lift the legs up and down 1-2 feet without touching the floor.

2. Heel Taps

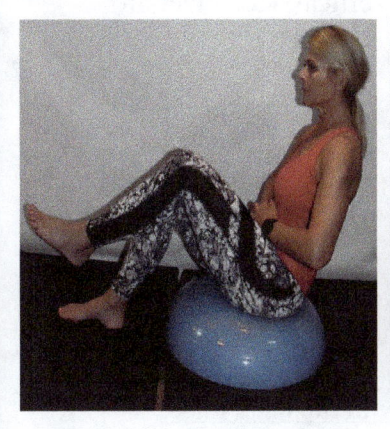

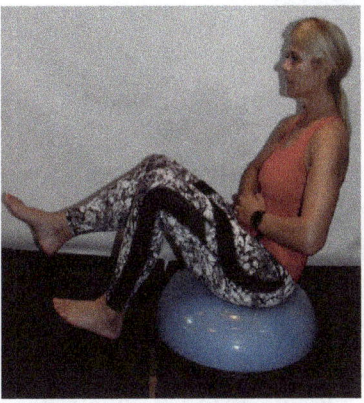

Sitting on BOSU with hips and knees bent 90° and feet off mat 1-2 feet

- Hands resting on lower abdominal area.

- Slowly lower one bent knee so heel touches the floor and then squeeze your abdominals to help raise your foot back to top

- Then repeat with opposite leg.

3. Supine Reverse Crunch

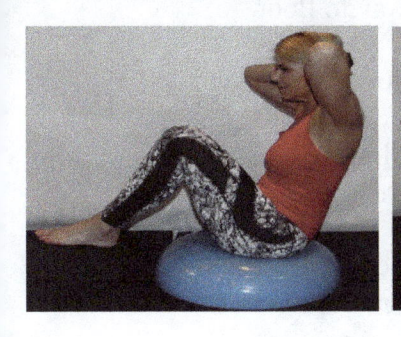

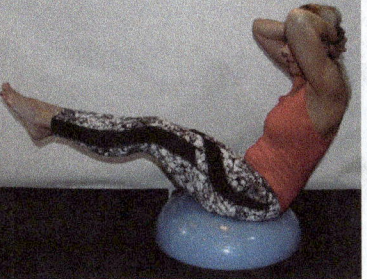

Sitting on BOSU with hips and knees bent 90° and feet off mat 1-2 feet.

- Lower upper back ¼ to ½ way to floor and straighten hips to 30°.

- Slowly straighten and then slowly return to starting position. The upper back does not move.

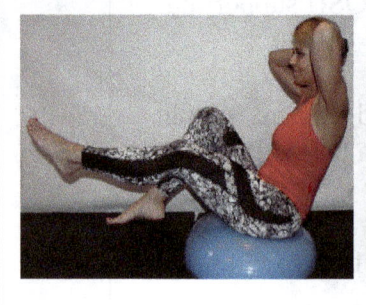

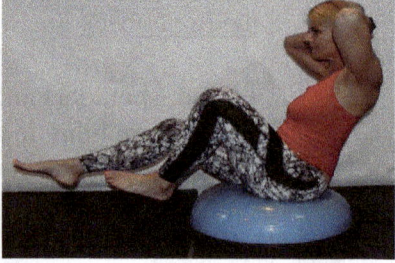

4. 1/2 Bicycles	Sitting on BOSU with hips and knees bent 90º and feet off mat 1-2 feet. - Lower back ¼ to ½ way to floor and straighten hips to 30º. - Keeping back stable straighten one knee - Return to starting position (bent knee position) and repeat with opposite knee.

2. Crunch/Sit-ups (trying to isolate Rectus abdominus and abdominal obliques):

Crunches:

1. Abdominal Crunch	Sitting on BOSU with hips and knees bent 90º and feet on ground. - Lower upper back 2/3 way to floor. - Keep neck in neutral position and lift chest up to almost vertical. Keep feet on floor. Modifications: 1. Keep one foot lifted off ground 45º and crunch. 2. Cross one leg over the other in a Fig 4 position and crunch.
2. Supine Double Crunch	Sitting on BOSU with hips and knees bent 90º and feet on ground. - Lower back 2/3 way to floor. - Keep neck in neutral position and simultaneously lift chest up to almost vertical while bending the hips and raising knees towards chest. - Lower chest and legs but don't let feet touch the floor before repeating the crunch.

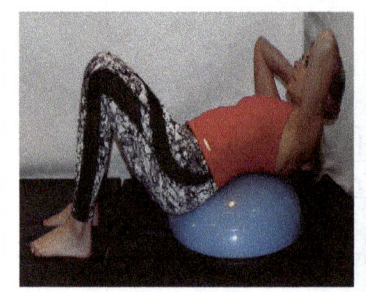

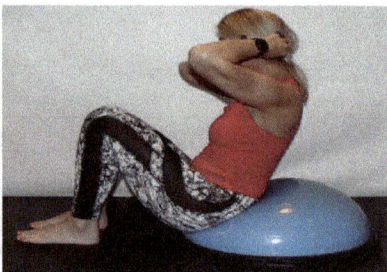

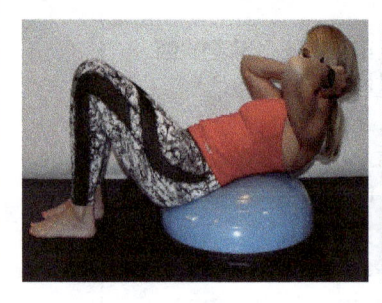

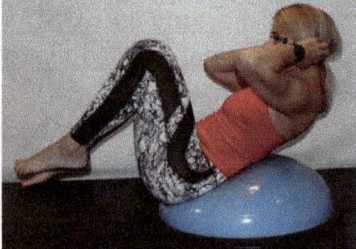

3. Supine Oblique Crunch

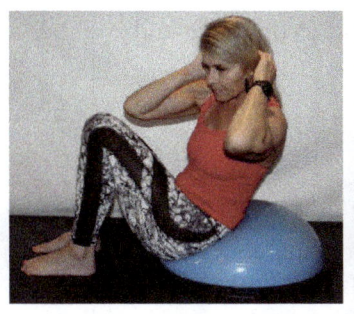

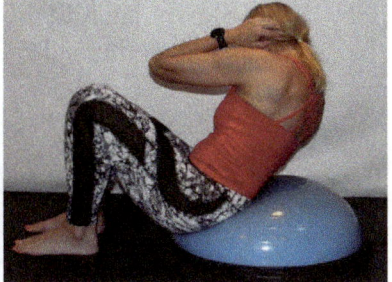

Sitting on BOSU with hips and knees bent 90º and feet on ground.

- Lower back 2/3 way to floor.

- Keep neck in neutral position and diagonally lift chest up towards one knee.

- Return to starting position repeat oblique crunch to opposite knee.

4. Supine Figure 4 Oblique Crunch

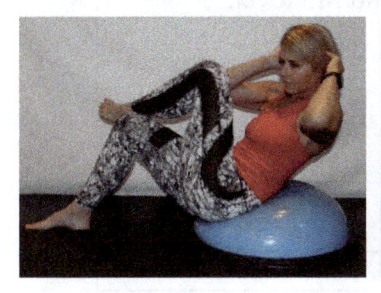

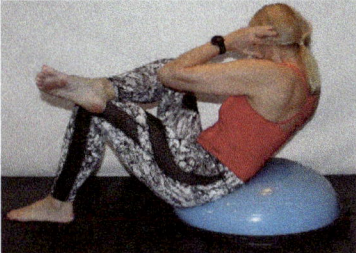

Sitting on BOSU with hips and knees bent 90º and feet on ground.

- Lower back 2/3 way to floor.

- Cross one leg over the other so they are in a figure 4 position.

- Keep neck in neutral position and raise chest towards the bent knee that is crossed over the opposite leg.

- Repeat to the same side for target number of repetitions and then change leg position and repeat.

5. Lateral Crunch on BOSU

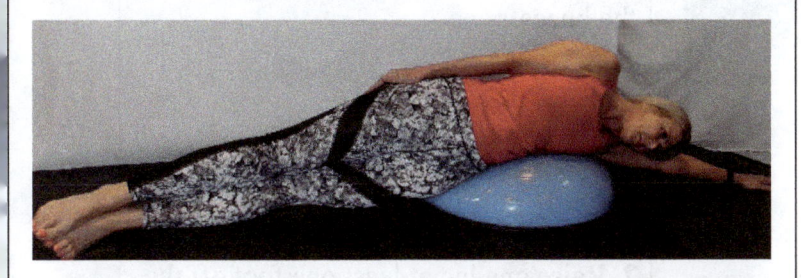

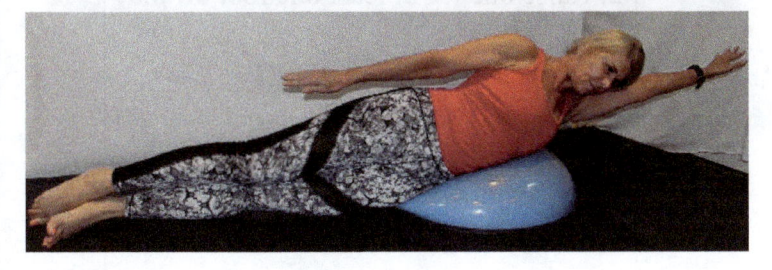

Lying on the side of your hips on the BOSU

- Bottom arm extended along the floor and top arm extended along the side of the body.

- Lift trunk and bottom arm off floor as high as possible and then lower to just above mat level and repeat.

Notes:

1. Avoid your hips rotating backwards. Your hips needs to be vertical on the BOSU.

2. The higher up on the BOSU the hips are, the harder the exercise (more unstable).

6. Standing Lateral Crunch	Stand erect on BOSU - Slowly laterally bend to one side and then the other side. Advanced; 1. Hand weights in your hands. 2. Hands behind head and raise one knee as you laterally bend to the side and have the same side elbow touch the raised knee at around hip level.

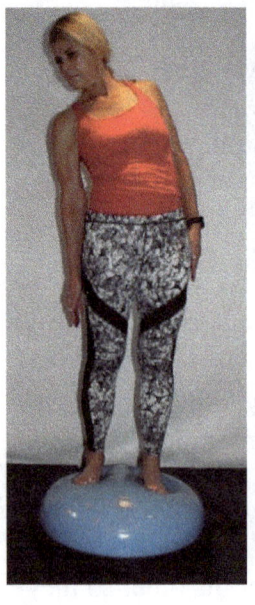

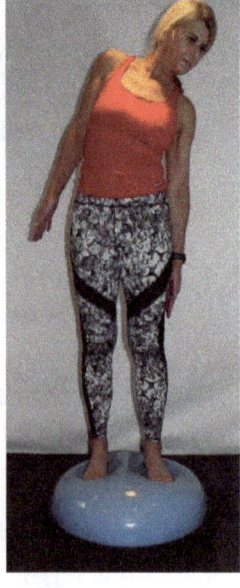

Sit-ups:	
1. Full sit-ups	Sitting on BOSU - hands in front of chest or behind neck, knees bent and feet on ground or anchored under something or held. - Lean back until back is 30° off floor. - Raise chest as far as possible toward the knees. Advanced: 1. Try with no anchor of feet or feet in butterfly position. 2. Raise one leg at least one foot off the floor.

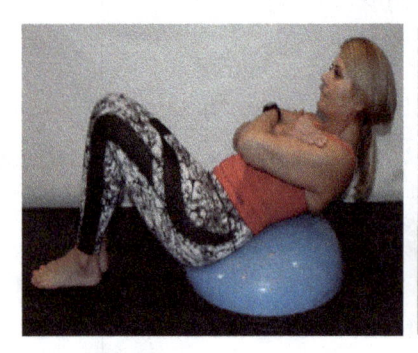

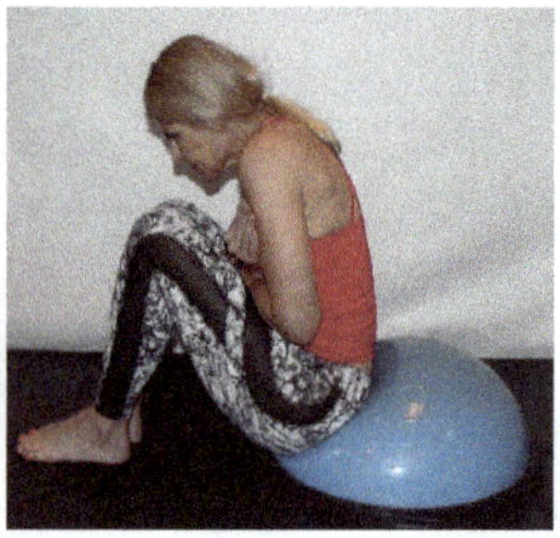

2. Oblique Full Sit-ups

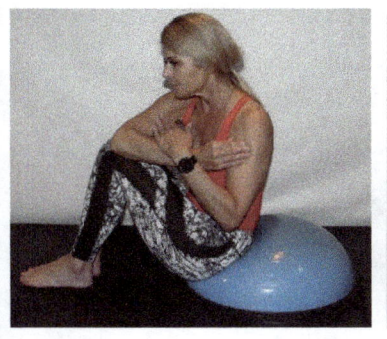

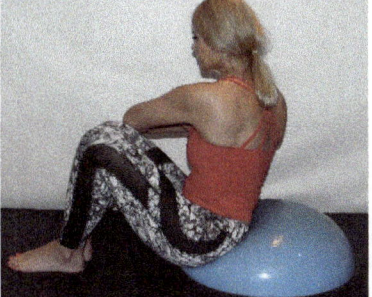

Sitting on BOSU - hands in front of chest or behind neck, knees bent and feet on ground or anchored under something or held.

- Lean back until back is 30º off floor.

- Raise chest diagonally toward one knee as far as possible. Try to get elbow to outside of knee.

Advanced:

1. Try with no anchor of feet or feet in butterfly position

2. Raise one leg at least one foot off the floor

3. Twisting Exercises to Isolate the Abdominal Obliques:

1. Russian Twist

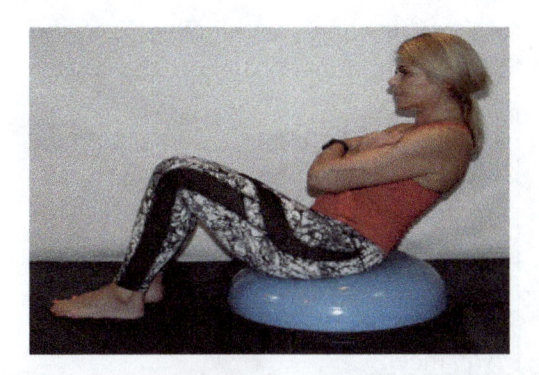

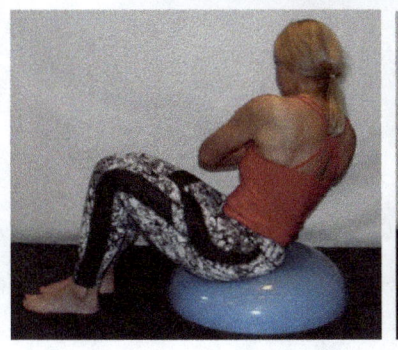

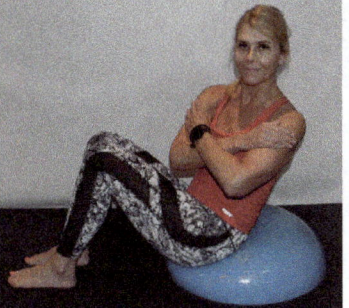

Sitting on BOSU with feet on or off (advanced) the ground

- Rotate shoulders and chest to one side and then the opposite side.

Note - Keep hands tight in front of your chest (small rotations of shoulders) or extended in front of the chest so you can swing the arms to touch the floor behind you (big rotation of shoulders).

Advanced:

1. Hold medicine ball tight in front of chest and do small shoulder rotations.

2. Hold MB with arms extended in front of chest and as you rotate the shoulders swing MB to touch mat behind.

Small rotation with Medicine Ball

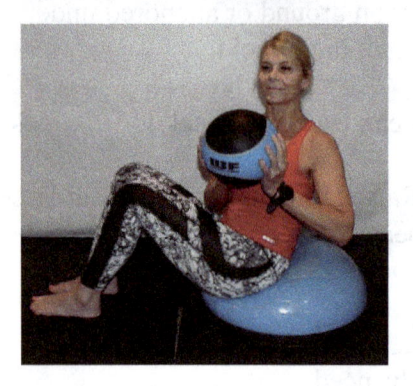

2. Woodchopper

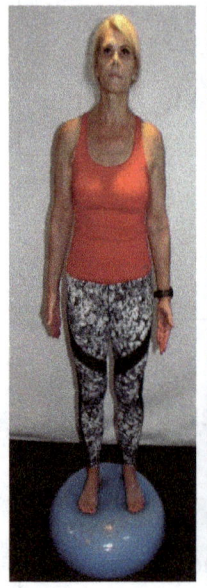

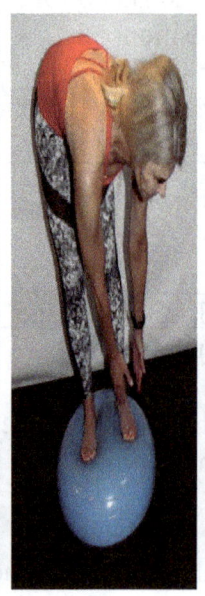

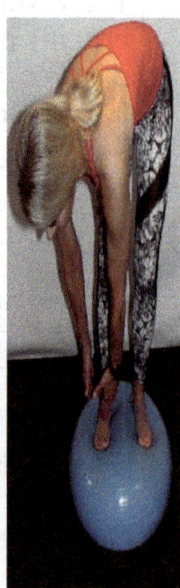

Sitting or kneeling

– Start with arms at your side or extended above your head and hips and shoulders slightly twisted to one side.

- Uncoil your hips and shoulders and bring your hands down diagonally toward the floor outside the opposite hip (if sitting) or knee (if kneeling).

- Your hips and shoulders will now be pointing in the opposite direction.

- Return to starting position and repeat

- After you completed a set number of repetitions in one direction repeat the "chop" toward the opposite hip or knee.

Advanced:

1. Medicine Ball for resistance.

3. Cross Body Twist (Standing Russian Twist)

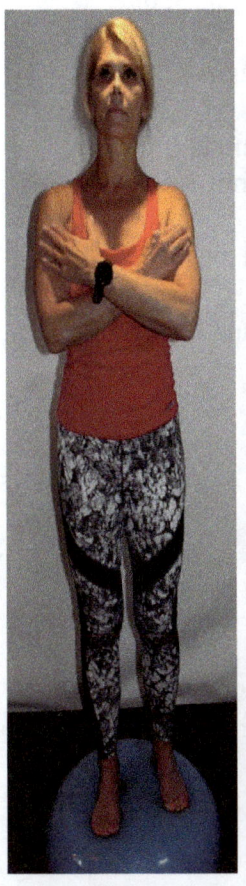

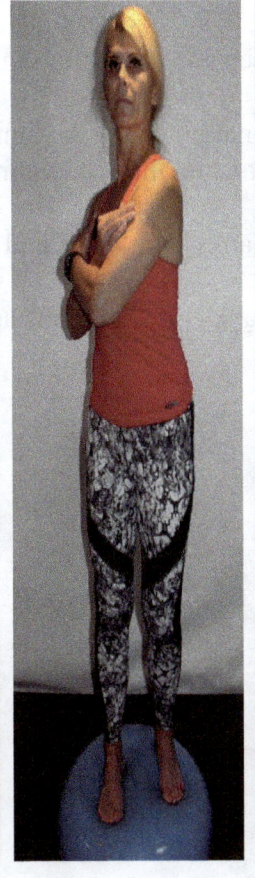

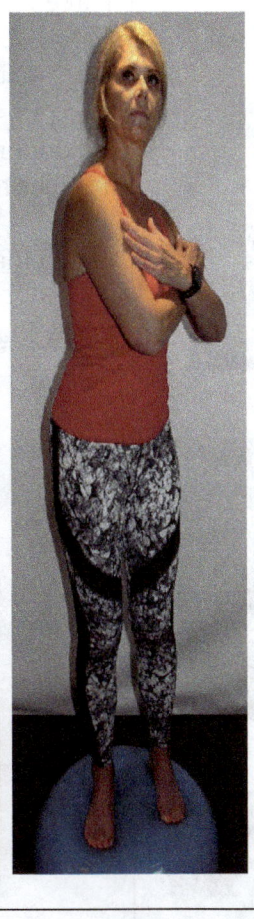

Standing or Kneeling

- Start with shoulders and hips rotated to one side and arms crossed in front of the chest.

- Uncoil and twist so the hips and shoulder are now facing the opposite direction.

- completely twist back in the other direction to return to starting position.

Advanced - Medicine Ball for resistance.

4. Pendulum

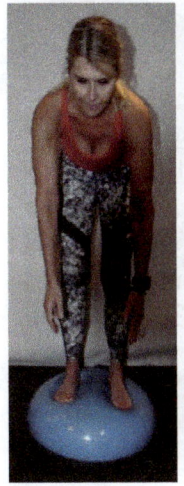

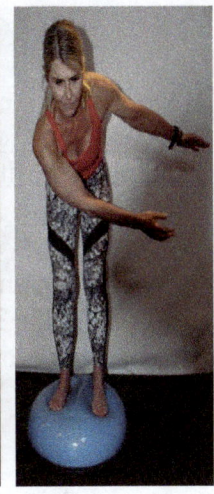

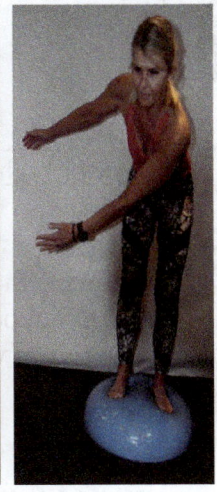

Standing on BOSU in a slight squat position (Knees slightly bent)

- Bend forward at the hips 45° and with arms extended down in front of your knees.

- Laterally raise shoulders and arms to one side up to shoulder height. Repeat motion to opposite side.

Advanced – Medicine Ball for resistance.

4. Planks and Variations (Isolates Arms, Shoulders, Chest, Core, Hips and Legs

1. Standard Planks

Prone Low Plank

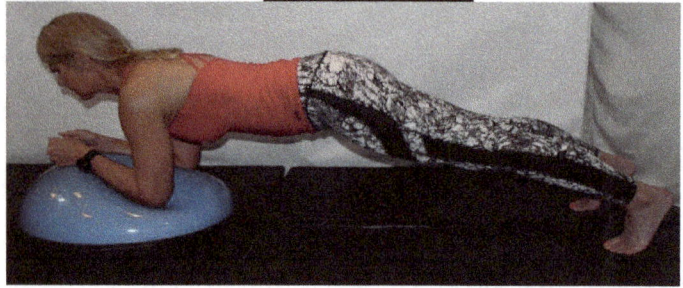

Lateral Low Plank

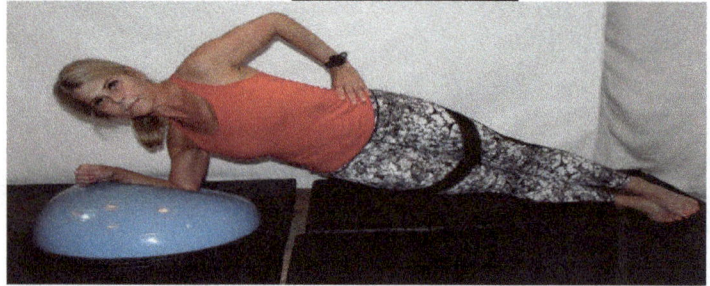

Supine Low Plank

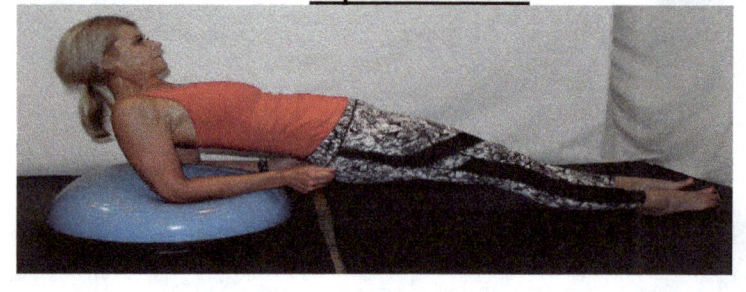

Three Positions - Prone, Lateral, Supine

Key – keep core tight, no sagging.

(Abdominal bracing - Abdominal muscles tucked into your spine)

- High Planks - on hands and toes.

- Low Planks - on forearms and toes.

2. Bird

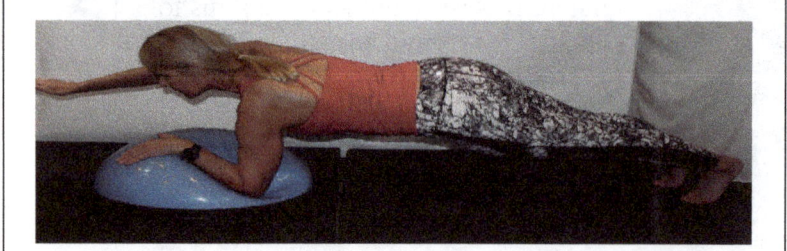

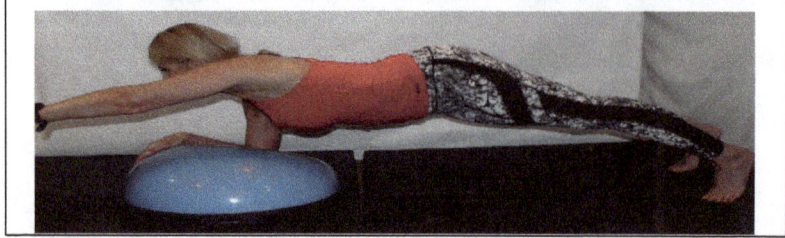

Low or high hand plank position on BOSU

- Elevate the opposite arm and leg to horizontal position, hold for 3-5 sec and then repeat with the other arm and leg.

Easier Modifications - Extend only one arm or one leg at a time.

3. Mountain Climber

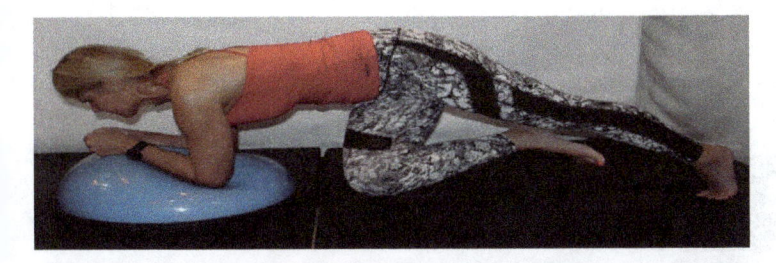

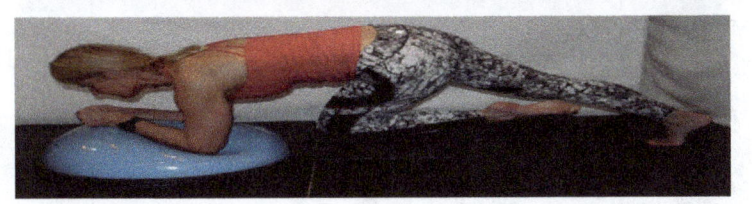

High plank position (Hands on BOSU)

- Draw one knee between your hands to same side chest and then alternate quickly with opposite knee.

Advanced
– draw knee to outside of arms vs. inside of arm on the same side.

4. Cross-Body Mountain Climber

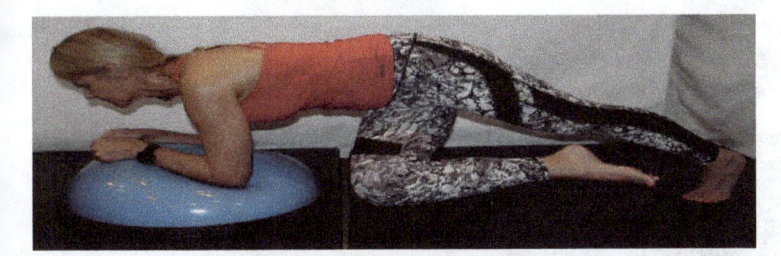

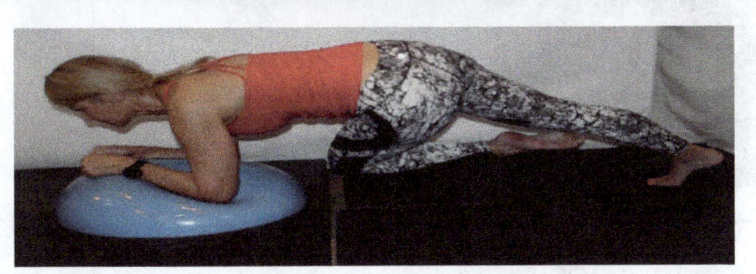

High Plank Position (Hands on BOSU)

- Draw one knee to opposite chest and the alternate quickly with opposite knee.

Advanced
knee to the outside of the opposite arm.

5. Plank with Alternating Shoulder Touches

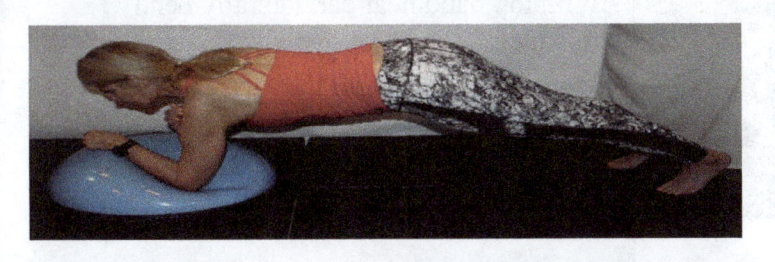

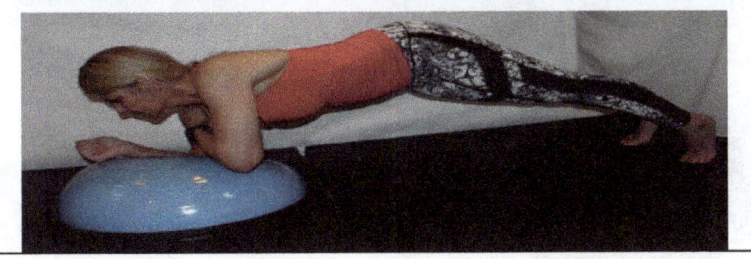

High or low plank position

- Alternate one hand touching opposite shoulder.

Beginner – Start with hands on BOSU, knees and toes on mat and then do alternating shoulder taps.

6. Lateral Plank with Top Leg abduction	High or Low Side plank position on BOSU. Support your balance with top hand if necessary. - Slowly lift the top leg as high as possible. - Hold 3 sec and then return to starting side plank position and repeat.
7. Lateral Plank Hip Dip 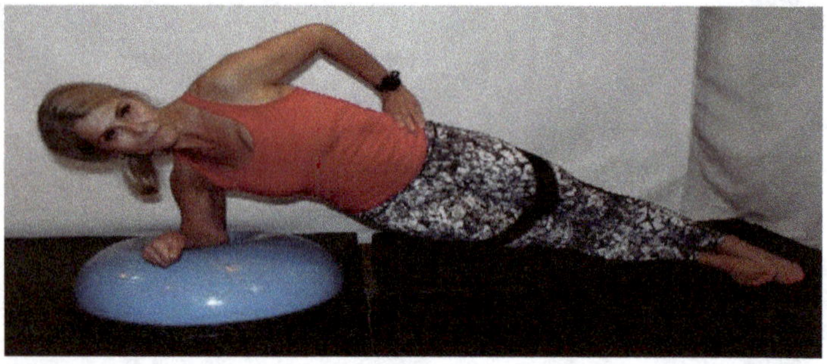 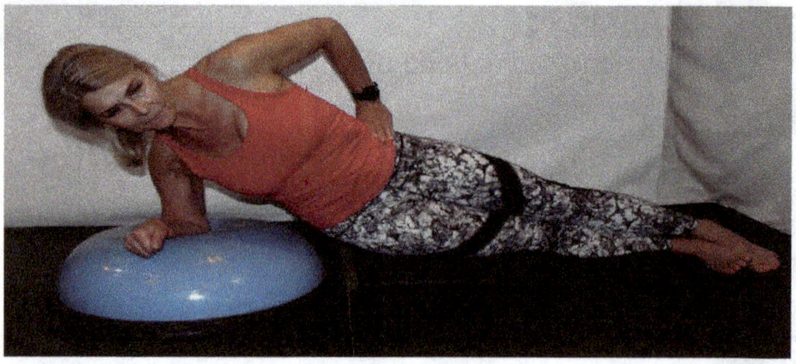	High or low side plank position on BOSU - Lower your hips to just above the mat and raise hips up again.
8. Double Lateral Plank Crunch 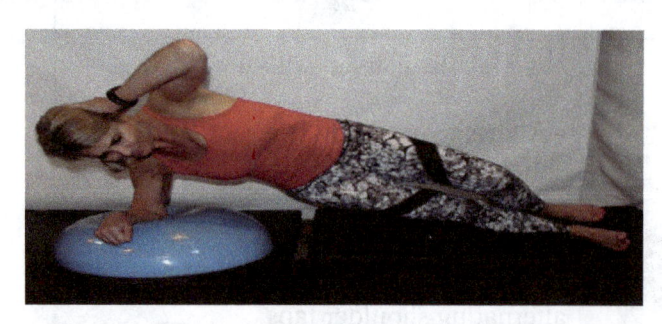 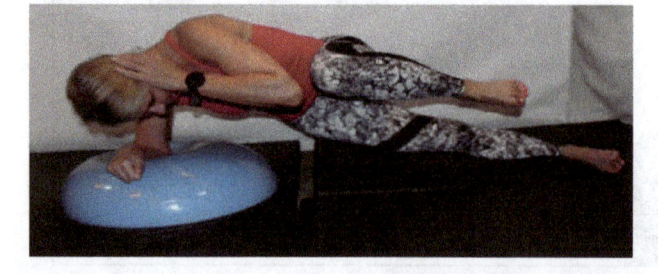	High or Low side plank position on BOSU - With top hand near ear, laterally bend and tap elbow to knee that has been moving toward the elbow.

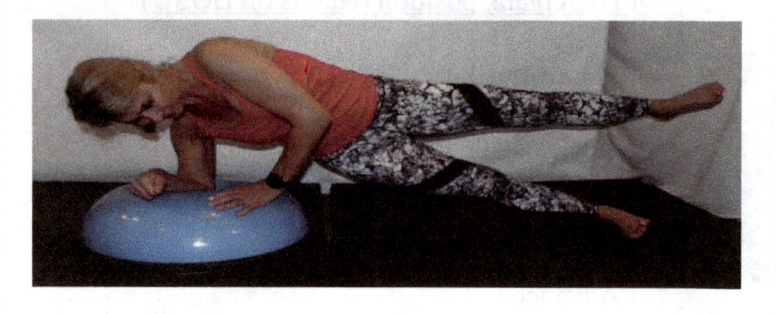

9. Forward Rolling Plank 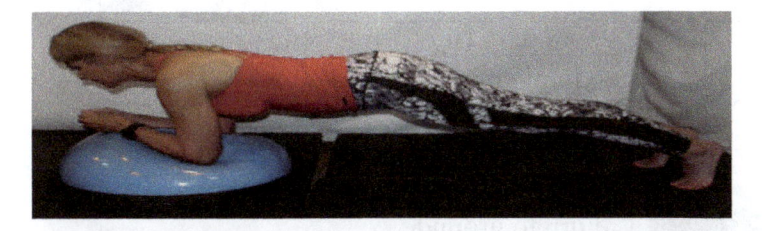 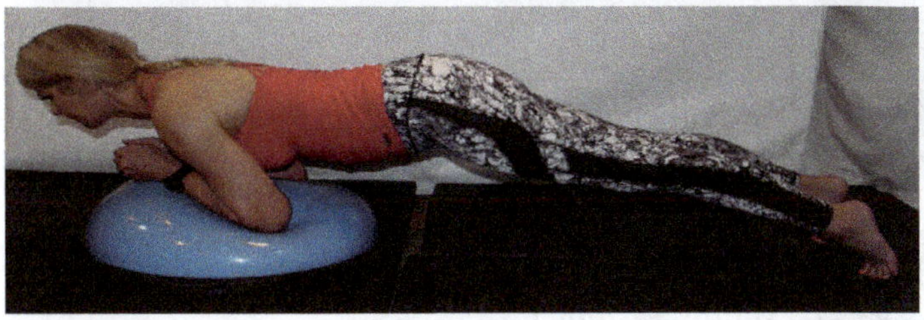	<ins>High or low plank position on BOSU</ins> - Slightly roll forward so shoulders move in front of hands (high plank) or elbows (low plank). - Then return to starting plank position.
10. Plank Jacks 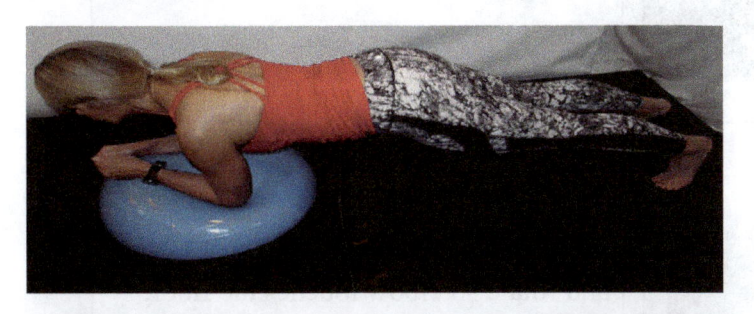 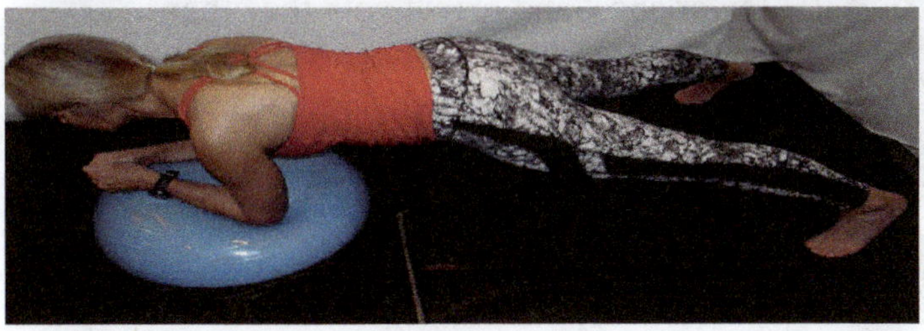	<ins>High or low plank position on BOSU</ins> - Hop (abduct) legs/feet out wide and then back to original position.
11. Abdominal wheel 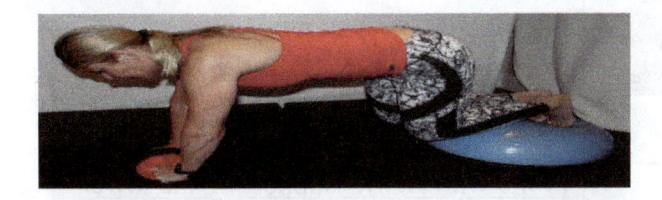 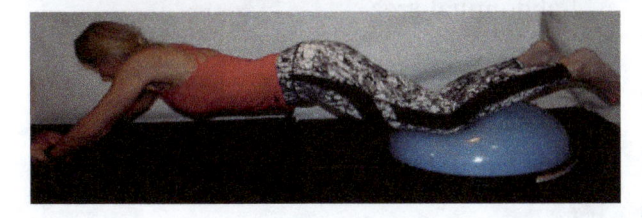	<ins>Sitting with your knees on BOSU both hands on the abdominal roller in front of you</ins> - Roll slowly out to an extended position and then roll back. <ins>Note</ins> - Only rollout and extend as far as you feel comfortable.

5. Back Extensions (Isolate the Back Erector Spinae muscles)

1. Back extensions	Prone with BOSU supporting the lower abdominal area
	- With hands behind head or resting on lower back, lift chest off ground and return to ground. Advanced; 1. Oscillate with chest off the ground. 2. Lift legs off ground (chest stays flat on the ground).
2. Back Extensions with small Rotation	Prone with BOSU supporting the lower abdominal area
	- With hands behind the head. Lift chest and rotate so elbow touches the floor, lower chest and repeat with the other elbow.
3. Superman's	Prone with BOSU supporting the lower abdominal area
	- With hands extended out in front of head, behind the head or on small of back. Lift chest & thighs off ground and return to ground.

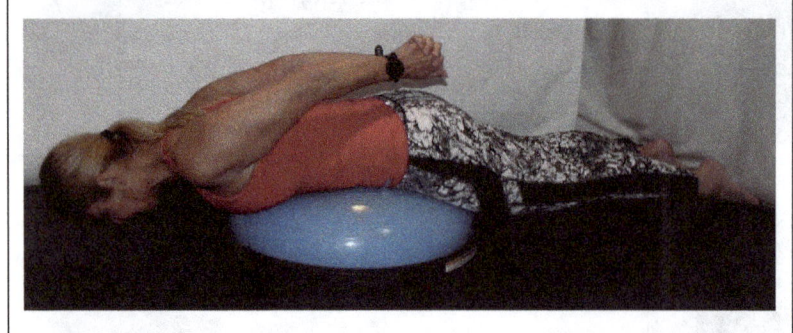

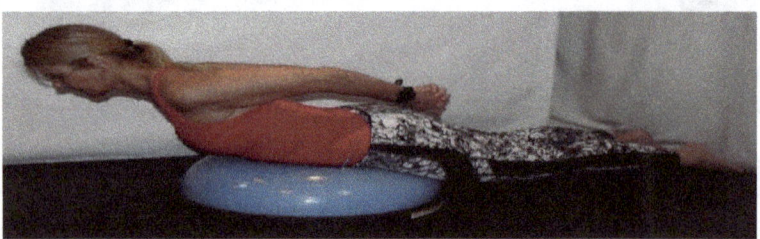

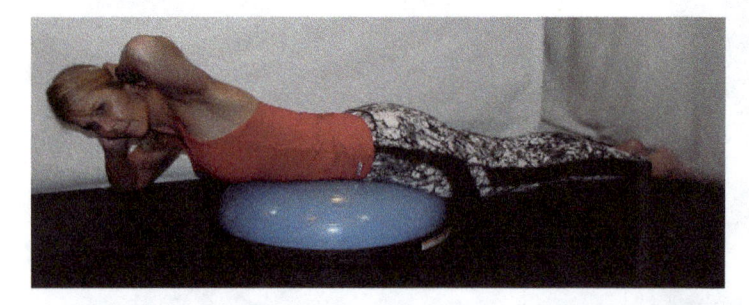

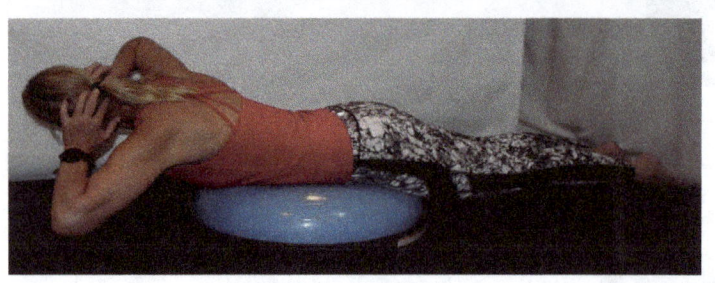

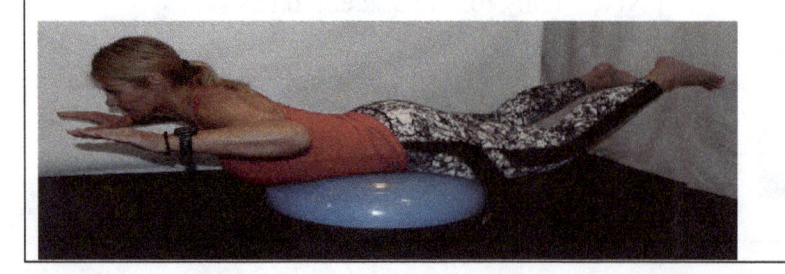

	<u>Advanced</u> - Oscillate with chest & thighs off the ground.
4. Bridges (Upper shoulders on BOSU or Feet on BOSU) **Neck and Shoulders on BOSU** 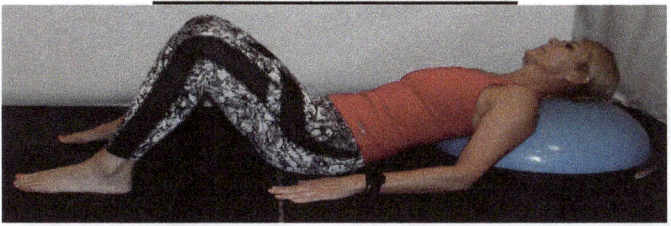 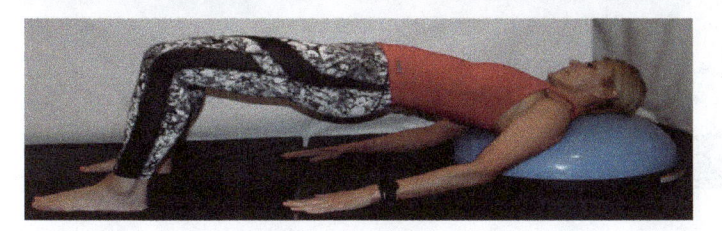 **Feet on BOSU** 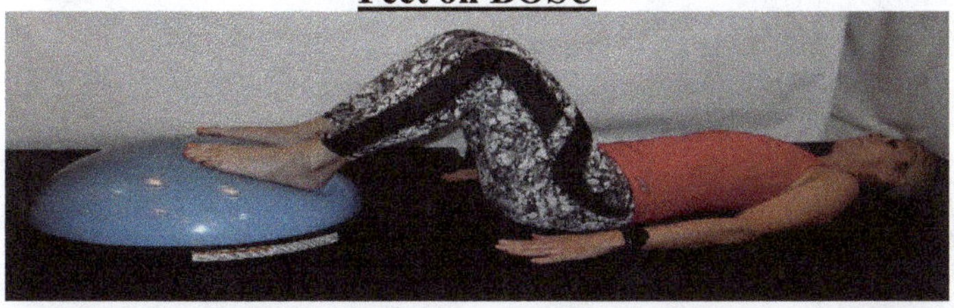 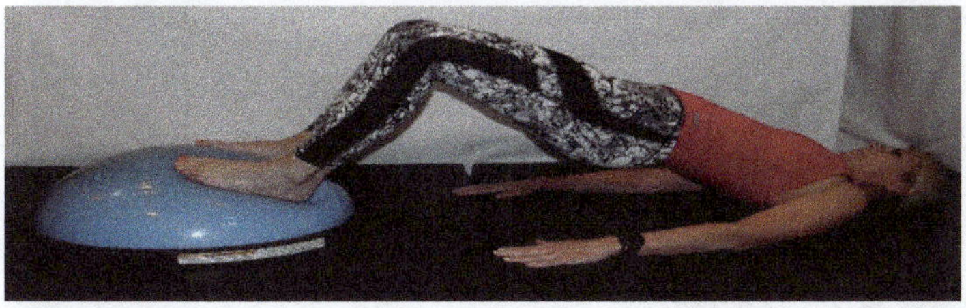	1. <u>Supine with BOSU supporting the upper shoulders</u> - Both feet on ground, hands resting on lower abdominal. - Lift buttocks off mat and hold 5 – 10 sec. 2. <u>Heels on BOSU and upper back resting on mat</u> - Lift buttocks off mat and hold 5 – 10 sec. <u>Advanced;</u> 1. Oscillate hips up and down while in bridge position 2. Extend one leg while in bridge. 3. One leg bridge (other leg in figure 4 position)

6. Push-ups (hands at shoulder level) -strength exercises in a plank position

<u>Notes:</u>
1. Can use "dome (Blue side)" or "flat (Black side)" of BOSU
2. Can do push-ups with hands on BOSU or Toes or Knees on BOSU (Decline Push-ups)
3. All push-ups can be done on hands and toes or modified by being on your knees

1.<u>Regular</u> 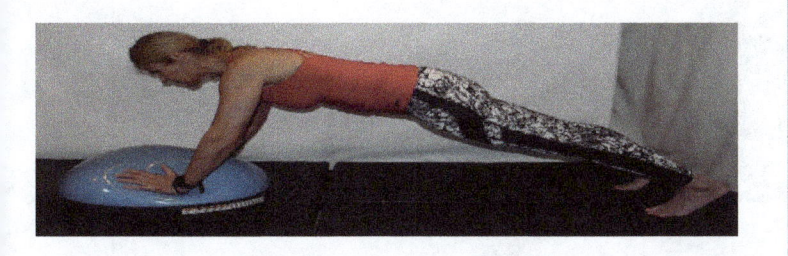	- Hands shoulder width

817

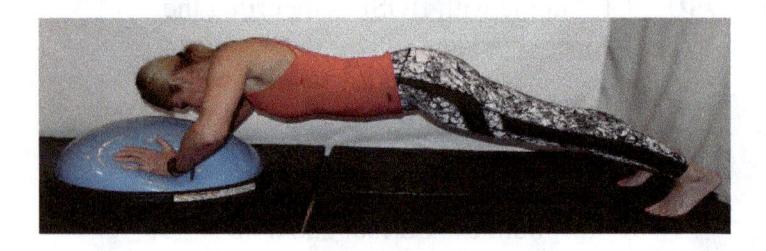

Modified - Knees on ground

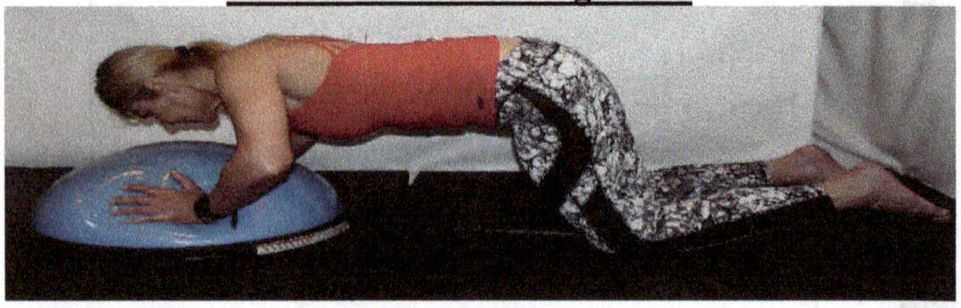

Black side up

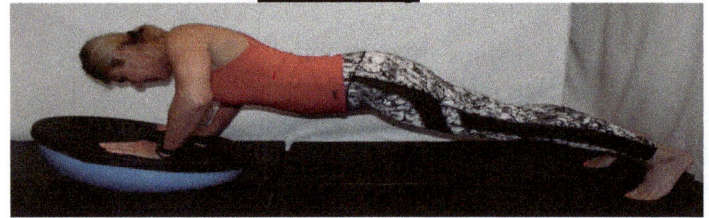

2. Military 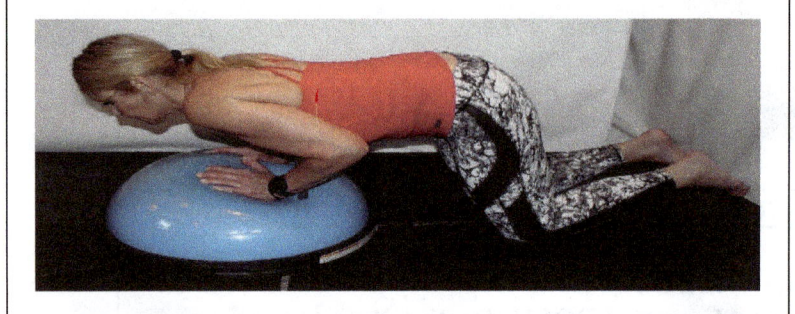	- Hands along sides of your ribs (narrow) and slightly behind shoulders
3. Diamond 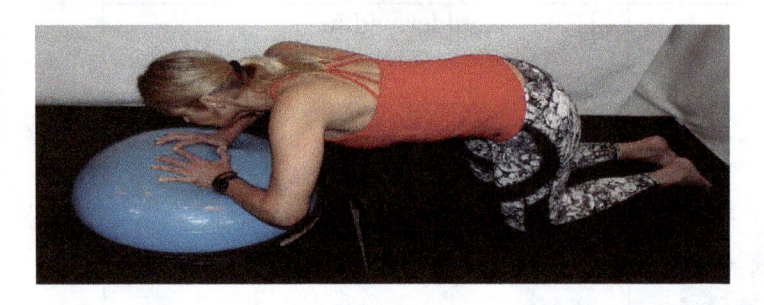	- Hands with index and thumbs of each hand touching to make shape of a diamond.

818

4. Under the fence

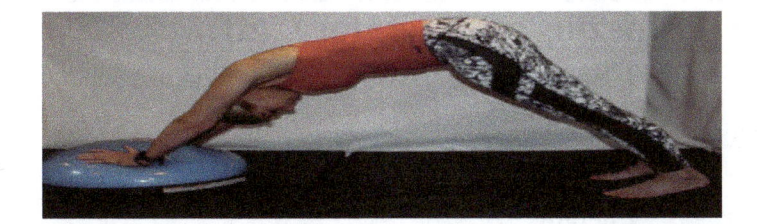

Going Forward under the Fence

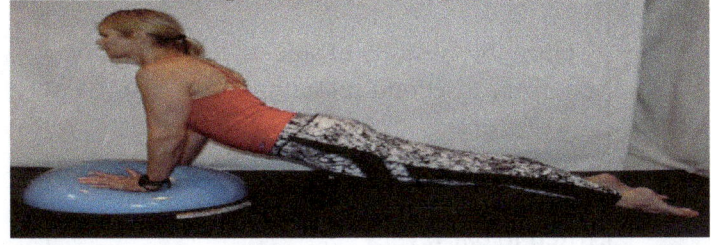

- As you do your push-up pretend you are crawling forward under a fence and then backward under the fence.

5. Decline

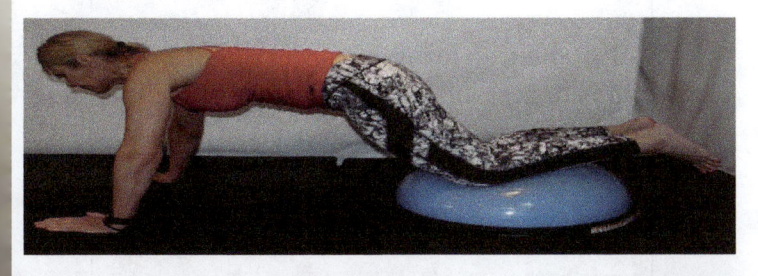

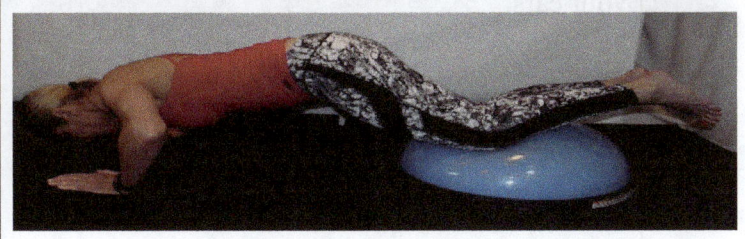

- Feet are elevated on BOSU.

Whole Body Exercises with BOSU

1. Shoulder Exercises (Deltoids, Upper Trapezius and Rotator Cuff)

1. Weighted Circles with Dumbbells	Stand erect on BOSU with weights at your side. - Lift the weights laterally to shoulder height. - Rotate the arms forward in a small circle 8- 10 times and then repeat in opposite (backward) direction. - Drop the weights to side of 10 sec rest or continue a second set without any rest.
2. Straight Overhead Shoulder Press with Dumbbells (I's) **Straight Overhead Press (I's)** 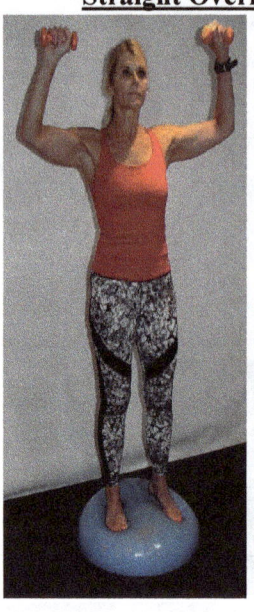 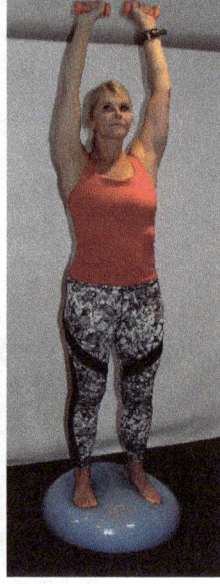	Standing erect on BOSU with weights lifted to ear level. - The weights face forward. - Lift the weights up vertical as high as you comfortably can. Don't full extend the elbows. - The inside of each weight can touch at the top and the arms should be felt against your ears.

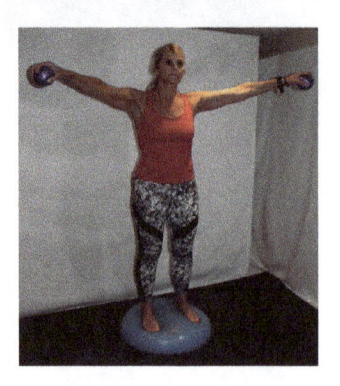

(Y's)

Alternating

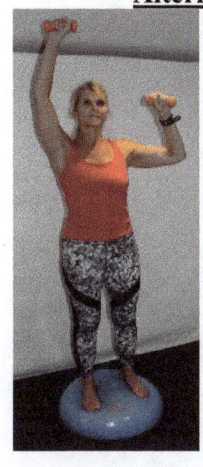

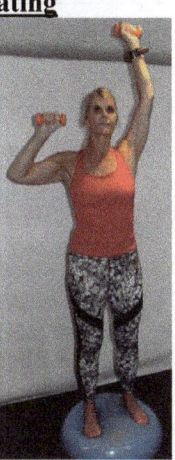

Swimmer's

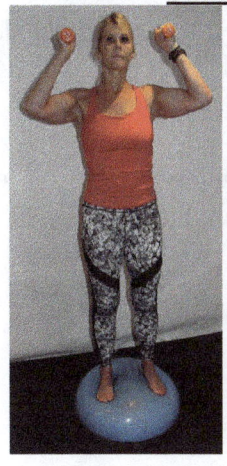

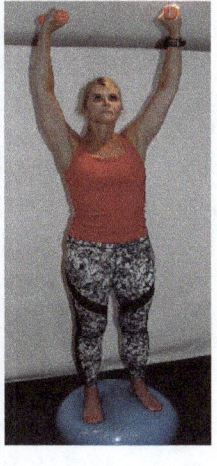

Modifications:

1. <u>Y's</u> - lift weights so arms are 60-70⁰ from horizontal at the top

2. <u>Alternating Overhead Press</u> - alternate lifting arms up over your head to "I" position

3. <u>Swimmers</u> – weights start facing your ears and as your lift them up vertically the arms twist so at the top they face outward (180⁰ rotation)

3. Lateral Raises with Dumbbells	Standing erect on BOSU with weights at your side facing toward your body. - Lift the weights up laterally with arms extended to shoulder height. Modification - Start with elbows bent 90º and lift the arms up laterally to shoulder height with elbows still at 90º.
4. Single Arm Angle Raise with Dumbbell 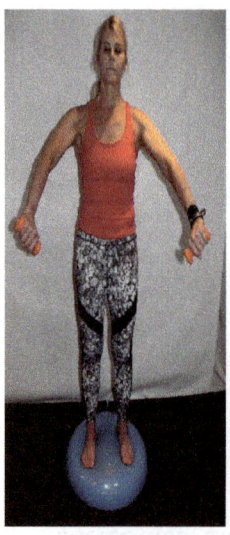 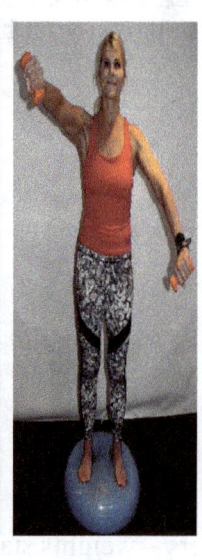 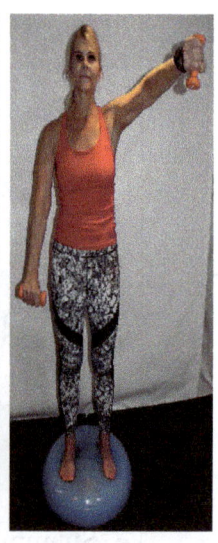	Stand erect on BOSU with arms ½ between the side and front of your bodies. - Turn your hands so thumbs are pointing toward your legs. - Keep the arms in this position as you lift one arm outward diagonally to shoulder level. - Return to starting position and repeat with opposite arm.
5. Anterior Raise with Dumbbells (Hands positioned two ways) **Hands facing backward** 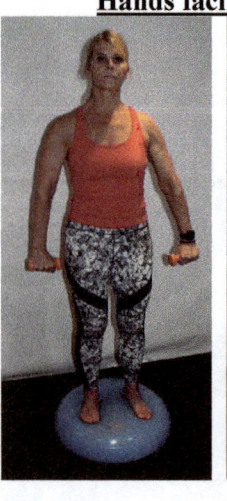 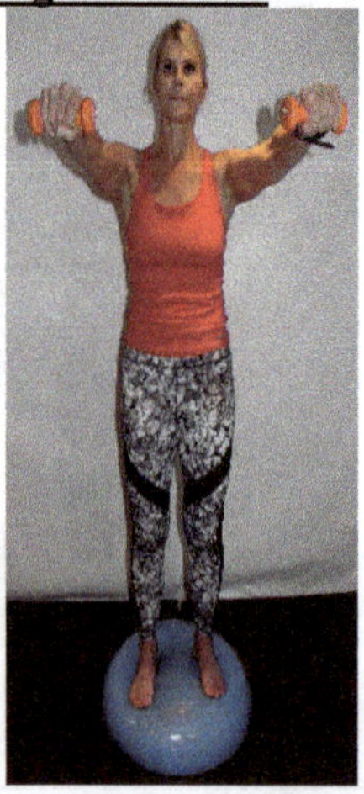	Stand erect on BOSU with arms at side of body with weights facing backwards or toward body (medially). - Lift the arms up anteriorly in front of the body to shoulder height.

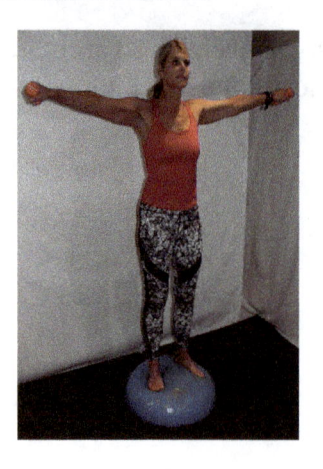

Hands facing inward

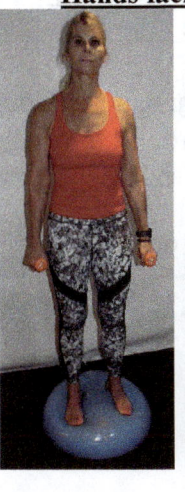

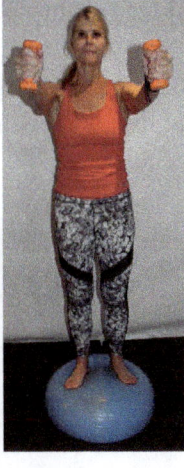

6. In's and Out's with Dumbbells

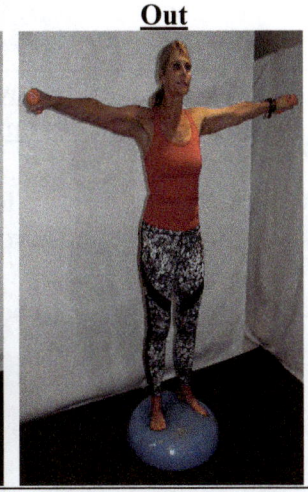

In   Out

Stand erect on BOSU with weight facing your body at your side.

1. In's - Lift the weights to the front of you to shoulder height (Anterior Raise) and then return the weights to your side.

2. Out's - Lift the weights laterally (Lateral Raise) to shoulder height and then return to starting position.

7. Pours with Dumbbells

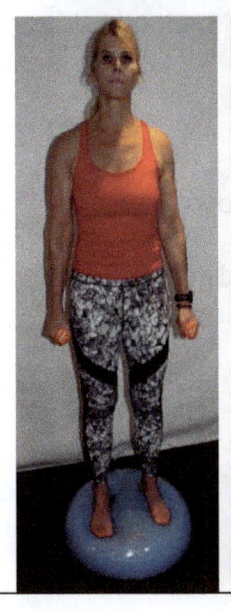

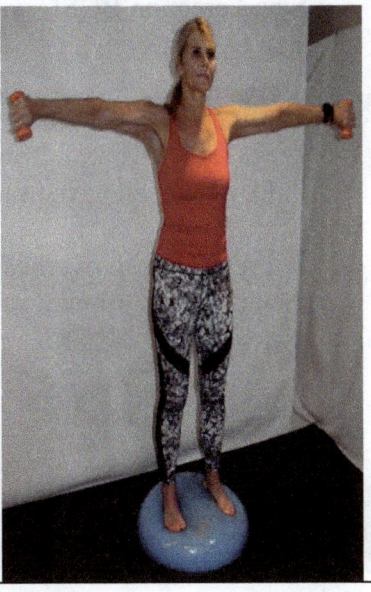

Stand erect on BOSU with weights at your sides.

- Laterally lift weights to shoulder height (Lateral raise)

- rotate the arms so the weights point down.

(The motion is like you are pouring a bottle of wine).

8. Scarecrows with Dumbbells	Stand erect on BOSU and lift weights to shoulder height with the elbows at 90°.

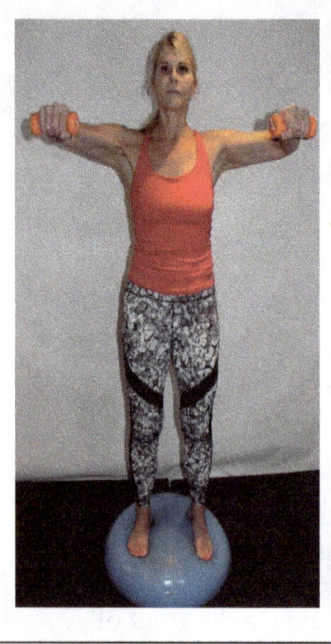

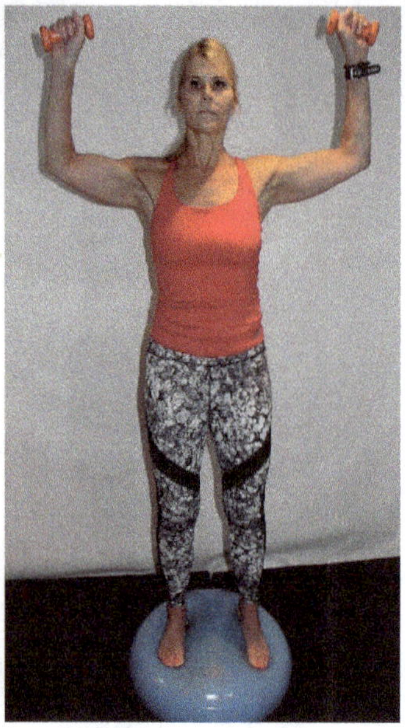

- With arms remaining at shoulder height rotate hands forward 90° so they are at the same height as the shoulders.

- Rotate arms back 90° to vertical and repeat. |
| **9. Upright Rows with Dumbbells** | Stand erect on BOSU with weights together in front of your waist.

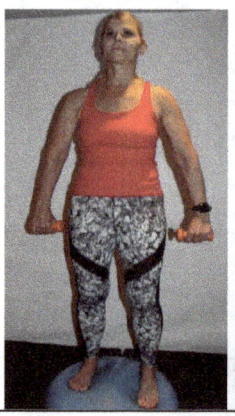

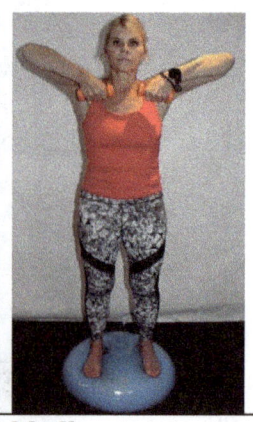

- Keeping the weights together lift the weights to just under your chin.

(Your elbows should be higher than the height of the weights) |
| **10. Fly-Row-Press with Dumbbells**

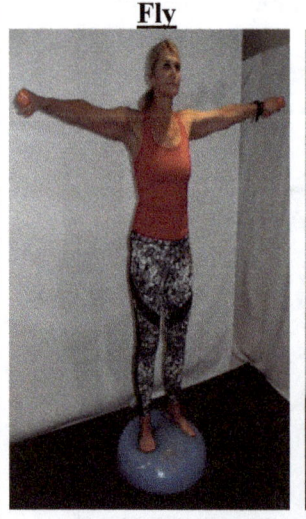

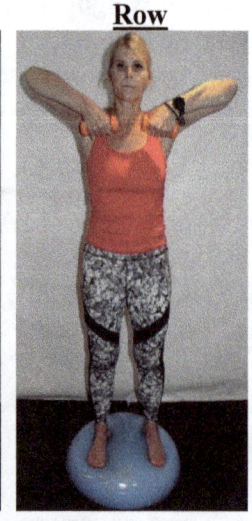

Fly — Row — Press | Stand erect on BOSU with weights at the side of your body.

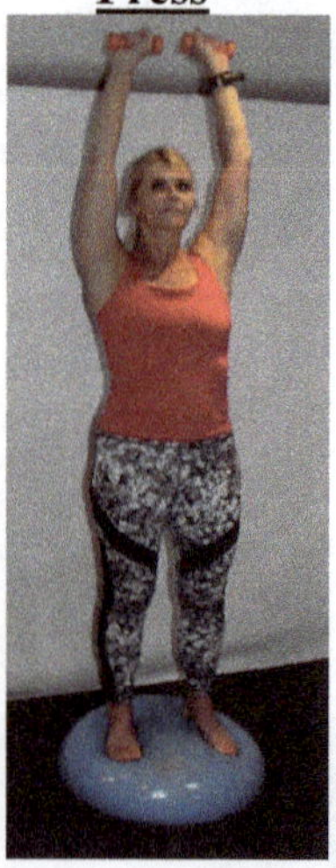

1. Fly - Do a lateral raise

2. Row - Do an upright row

3. Press - Do an overhead "I" press and then return to original starting position and

-Repeat the three lifts. |

11. External and Internal Rotation of Arm 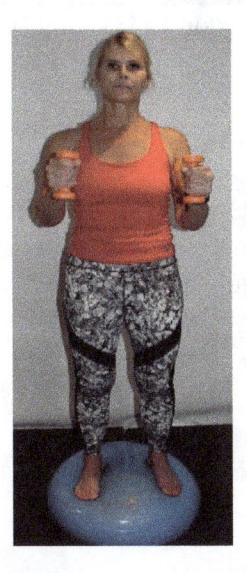 **External Rotation** **Internal Rotation** 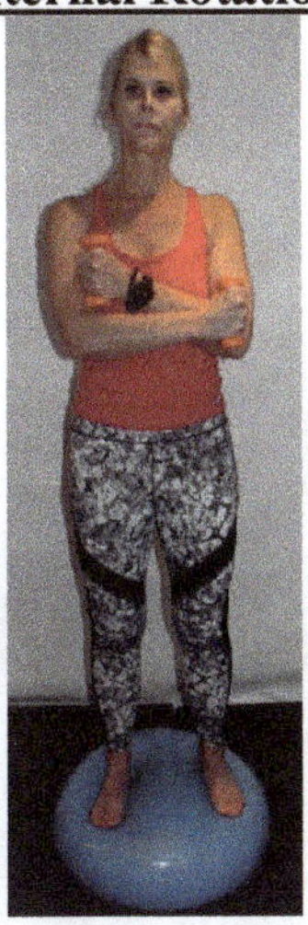	Stand erect on BOSU with elbow bent 90º and weight facing inwards. - Keep your wrist in neutral position and elbows at 90º and tight against your ribs. **External Rotation** - Rotate arm laterally 60-80º. **Internal Rotation** - Rotate arms across the body.
12. Shoulder Shrugs 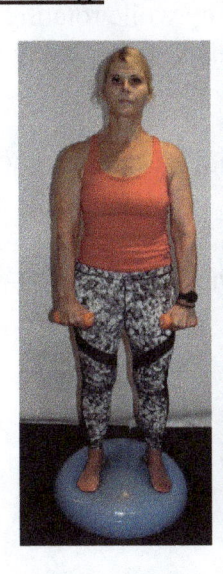	Stand erect on BOSU and weight at side of body. - Squeeze or lift the top of your shoulders (Upper Trapezius) toward your ears and hold 3 seconds.

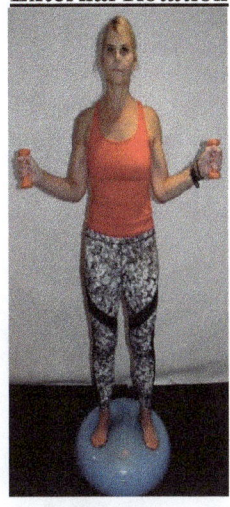

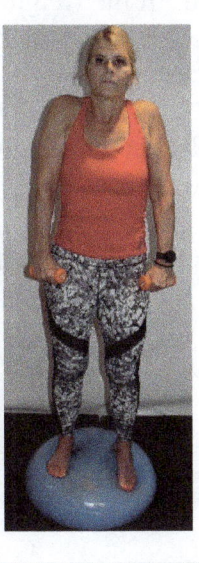

2. Upper Back (Rhomboids and Middle to Lower Trapezius and Latissimus Dorsi)

1. Locomotives

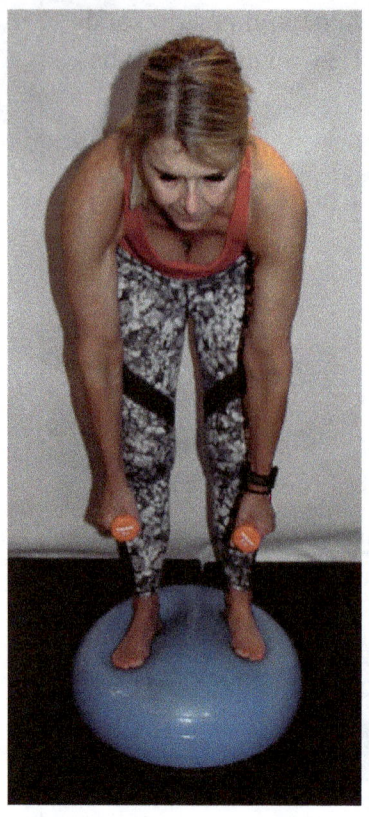

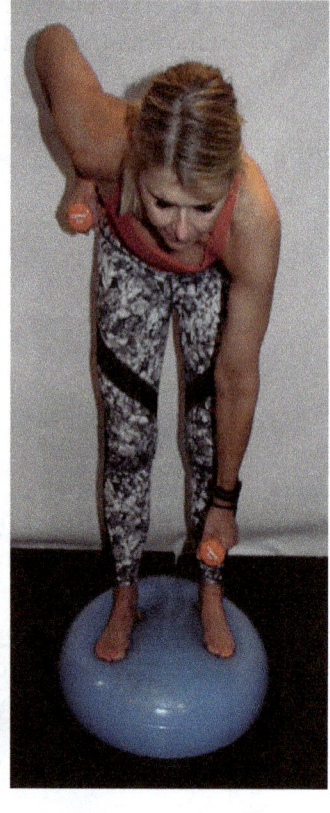

Stand erect on BOSU and bend forward at the waist.

- Reach down for both weights.

- Bend the elbow, keep it close to the body and alternatively lift the weights up to rib level in quick succession for 20 times each arm.

2. Lawnmowers

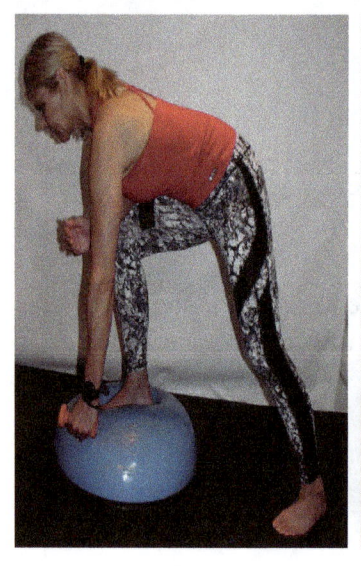

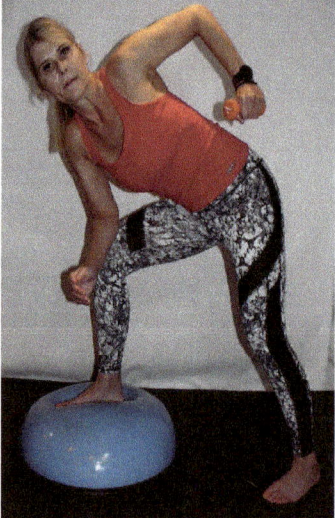

Place one foot on BOSU and then bend forward at the waist and rest elbow on knee.

- Reach down for the weight.

- Bend the elbow, keep it close to the body and lift the weight up while rotating your trunk to the side that you are lifting the weigh on.

- Return the weight to just above the floor and repeat.

- Repeat set with opposite foot on BOSU

3. Bent Over Rows 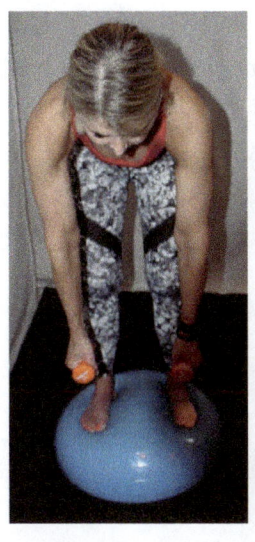 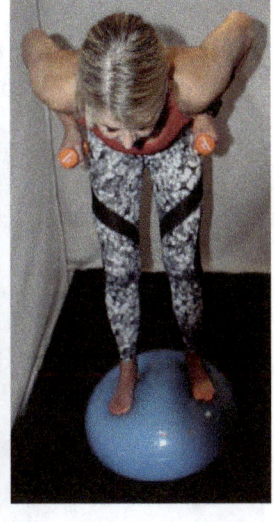	<u>Stand erect on BOSU and bend forward 90º at the waist.</u> - With a slight bend of the knees reach for the weight on the floor. - Bend your elbows, keep the elbows close to your ribs and lift both weights to rib level. (You should feel your shoulder blades squeeze together).
4. Bent Over Flies 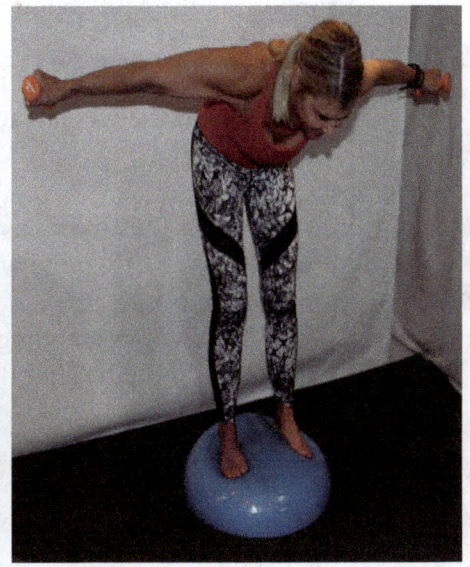	<u>Stand erect on BOSU and bend forward 90º at the waist.</u> - With a slight bend of the knees reach for the weight on the floor. - Lift both arms laterally while in bent over position. The elbows may bend a bit. (Feel the shoulder blades squeezing together). <u>Note</u>- Don't let arms drift back towards ribs when lifting. They should lift straight laterally.
5. Two Angle Shoulder Flies	<u>Standing erect on BOSU with weights are at the side of your body.</u> 1. <u>While standing erect</u> - lift both weights laterally to shoulder level. Your elbows may bend a bit. - Return to starting position. 2. <u>Bend forward 90º</u> - at the waist and laterally lift weights to shoulder level. Elbows can be extended or bent 90º

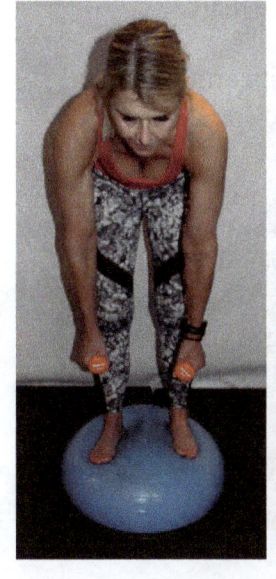

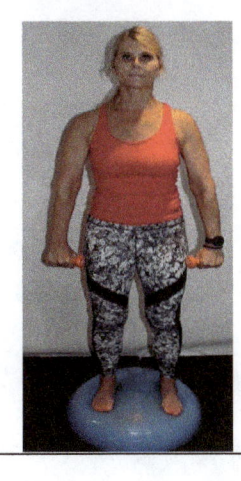

Standing Erect   **Bent Over**

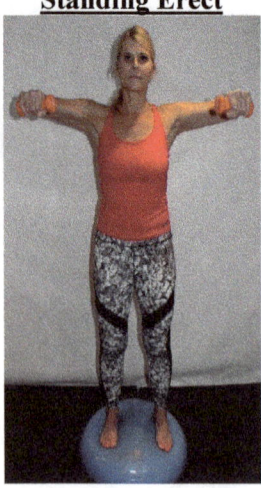

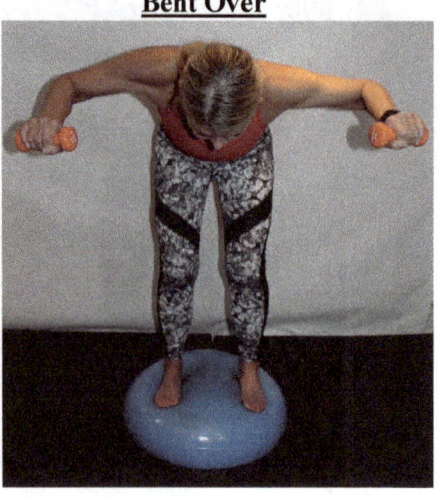

(Feel the shoulder blades squeeze together)

- Return to starting position and get back into erect posture to repeat the exercise.

6. Reverse Flies (Prone "T's")

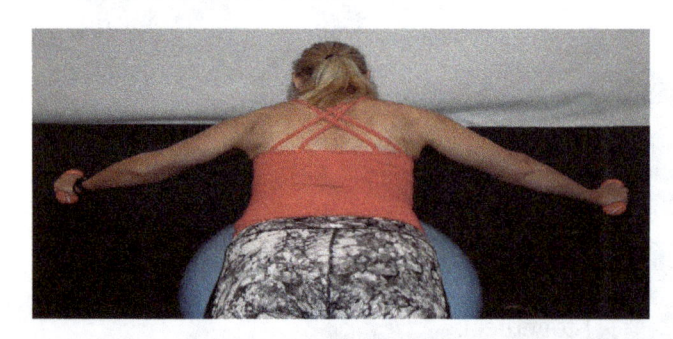

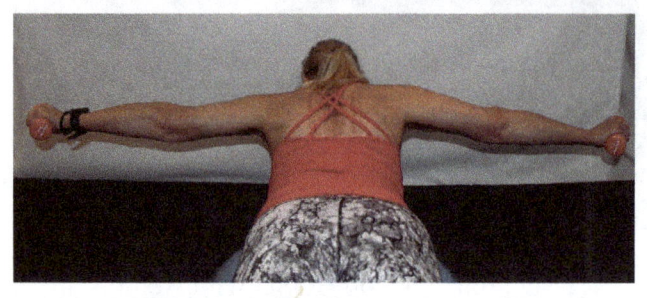

Lying prone (face down) with BOSU supporting the Mid abdominal area.

- Grab both weights and with arms extended, lift the weights to shoulder level.

- Try to keep the elbows as straight as possible while lifting the weights.

- Avoid lifting or extending your neck. Your chin should be slightly tucked into your chest.

- Lower the weights but do not let the weights touch the ground before repeating the exercise.

3. Chest

1. Push-ups (strength exercises in a plank position) - Reviewed under BOSU Core Strengthening Exercises

Notes:
1. Can use "dome" or "flat" side of BOSU
2. Can do push-ups with hands on BOSU or Toes or Knees on BOSU (Decline push-ups)
3. All push-ups can be done on hands and toes or modified by being on your knees)

1. Regular Push-ups

- Hands on BOSU shoulder width apart

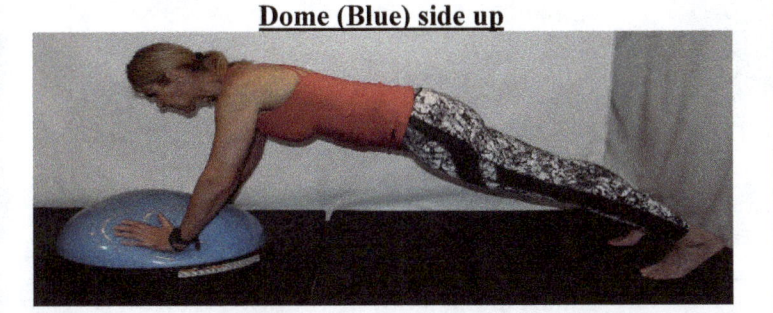

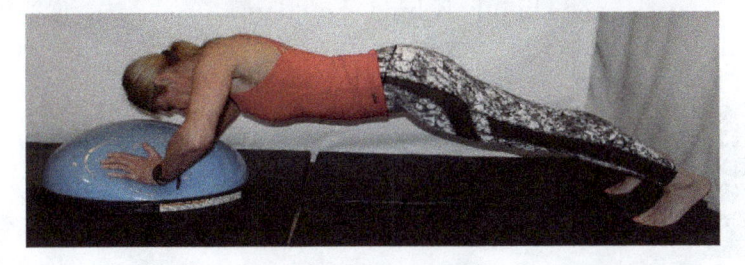

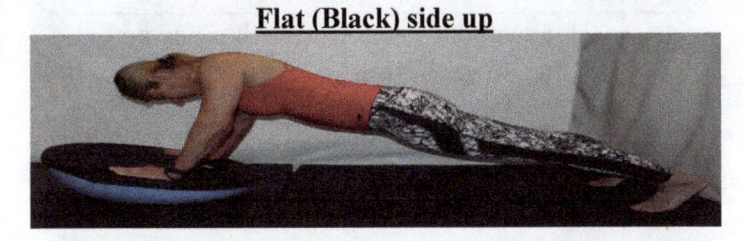

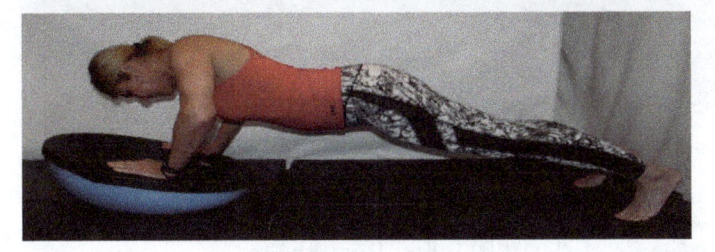

Dome (Blue) side up

Flat (Black) side up

Modified (on knees)

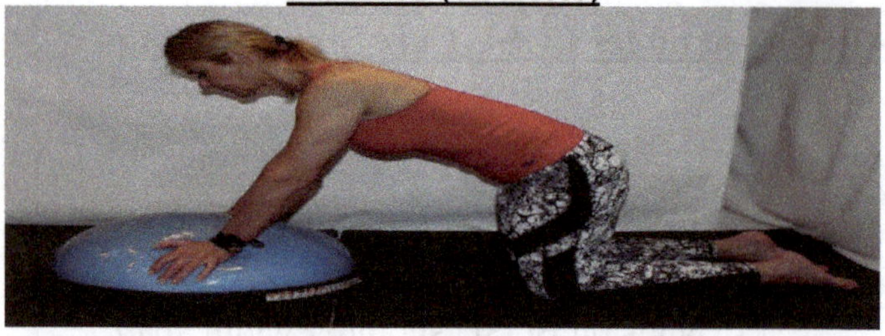

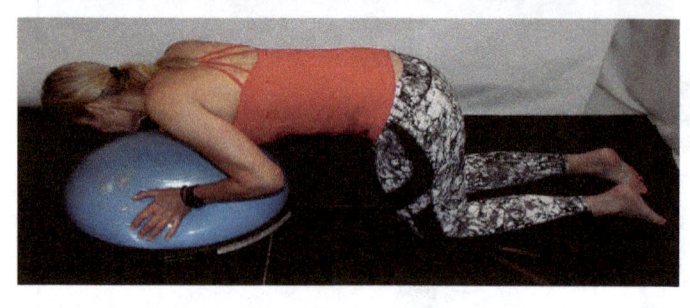

2. Military Push-ups 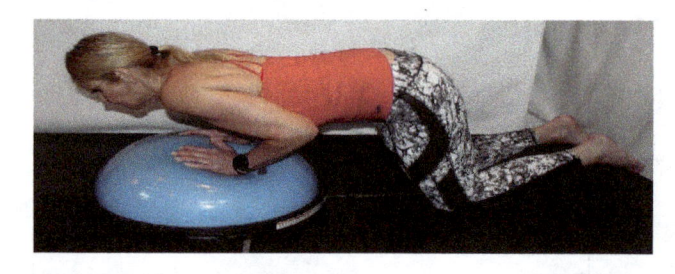	- Hands along sides of your ribs (narrow) and slightly behind shoulders
3. Diamond Push-ups	- Hands under your chest with index and thumbs of each hand touching to make shape of a diamond
4. Under the fence Push-ups 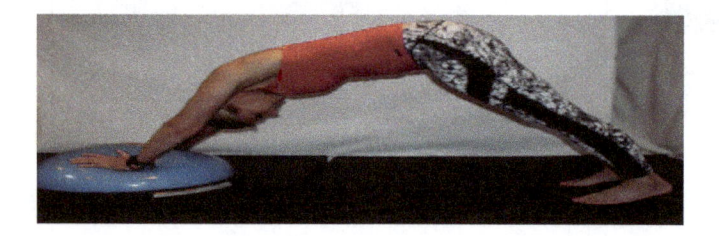	- As you do your push-up pretend you are crawling forward under a fence and backward under the fence

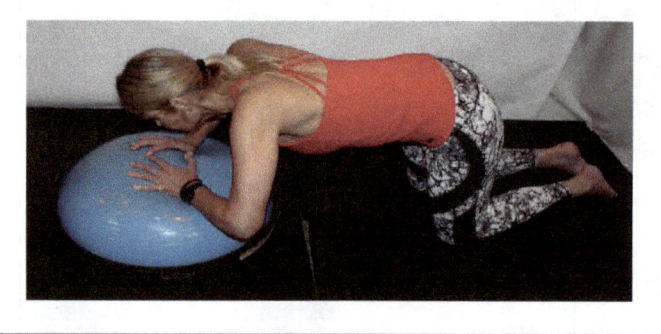

Going Forward Under the Fence

Going Backward Under the Fence

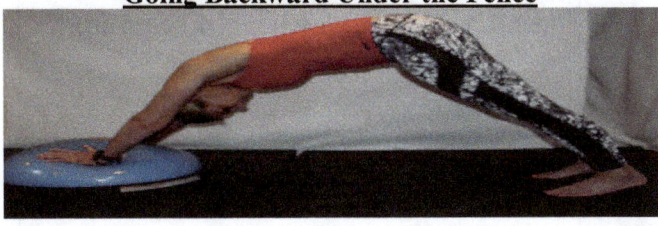

5. Decline Push-ups

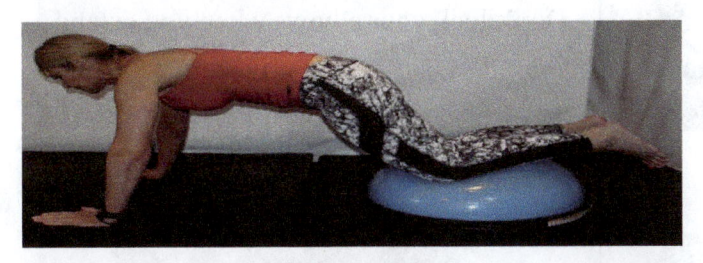

- Feet are elevated on BOSU.

6. Plange Push-ups

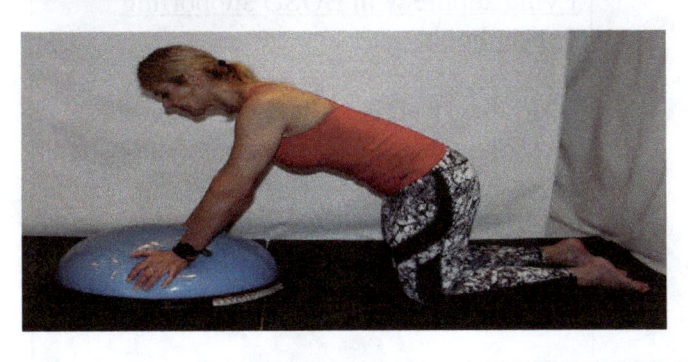

- Hands next to ribs and face outward.

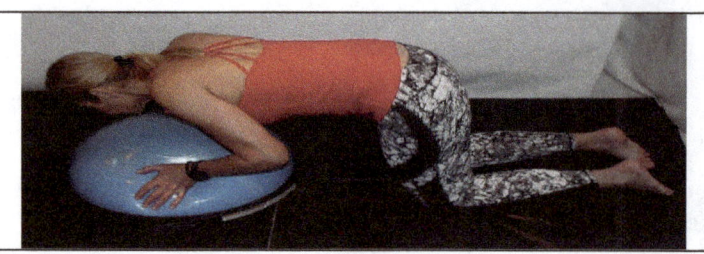 **7. Two-twitch Speed push-ups**	- Do 4 fast regular push-ups (1 beat down and 1 beat up) and then 4 slow regular push-ups (4 beats down and 4 beats up).
2. Chest Press 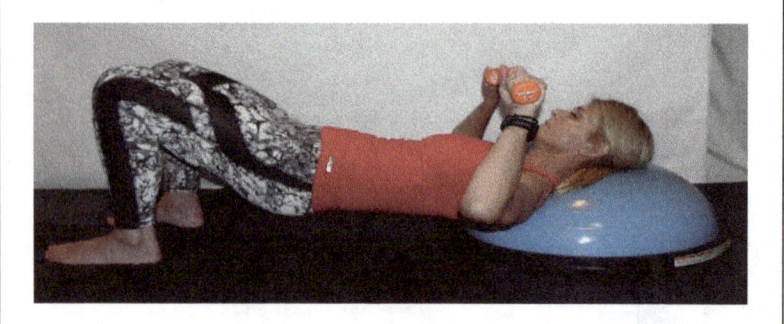 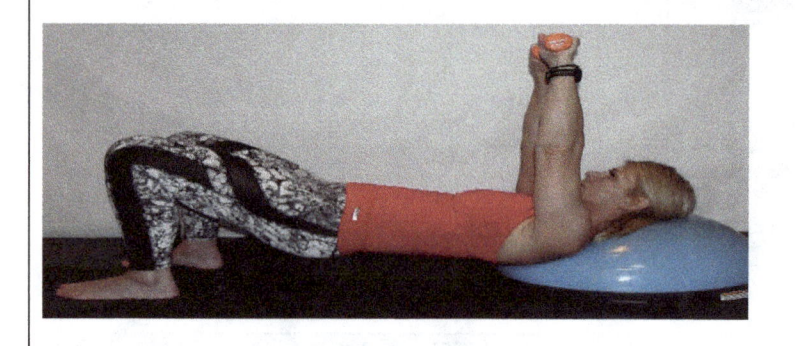	<u>Lying supine with BOSU supporting upper shoulders.</u> - Holding weights just above your chest press upwards. - Don't lock your elbows when you extend your arms.
3. Cross Body Chest Press 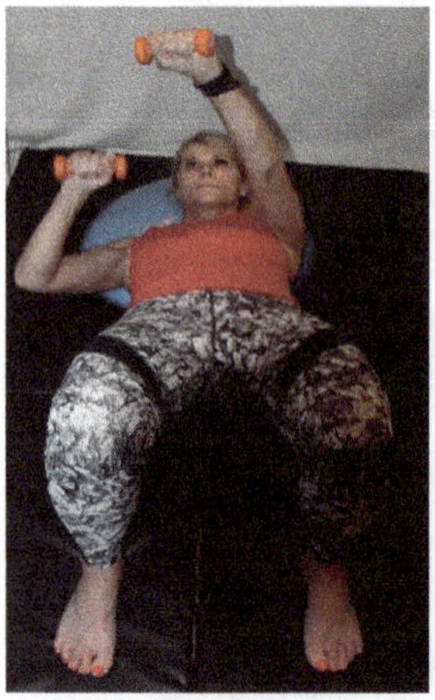 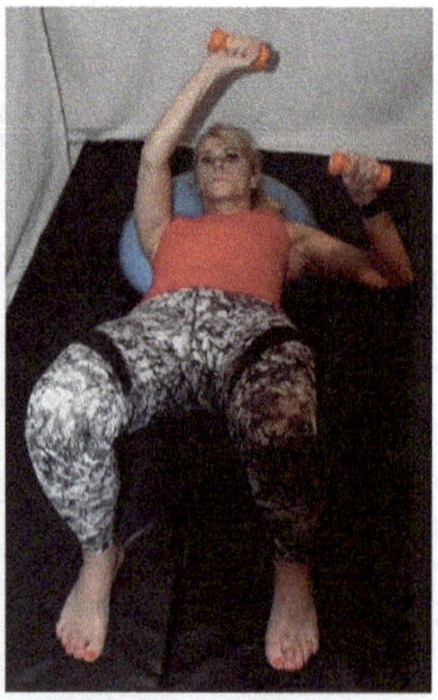	<u>Lying supine with BOSU supporting upper shoulders.</u> - Holding weights just above your chest press diagonally upwards above opposite chest. - Don't lock your elbows when you extend your arms.

4. Chest Flies

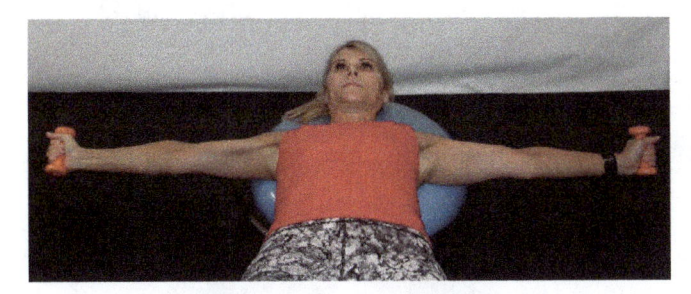

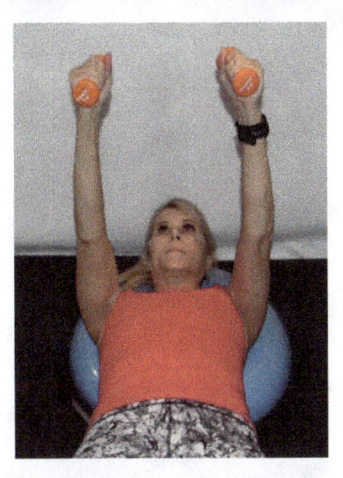

Lying supine with BOSU supporting neck and upper shoulders

- Arms extended out to the sides in a horizontal position.

- Raise arms up to vertical position (Try to keep elbows as straight as possible).

4. Arm Exercises (Biceps, Triceps)

Biceps:

1. Regular Curls

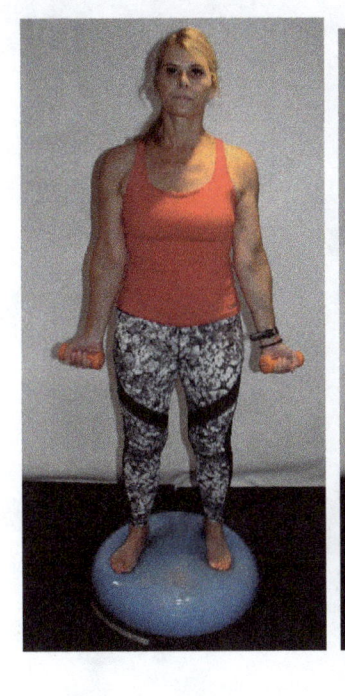

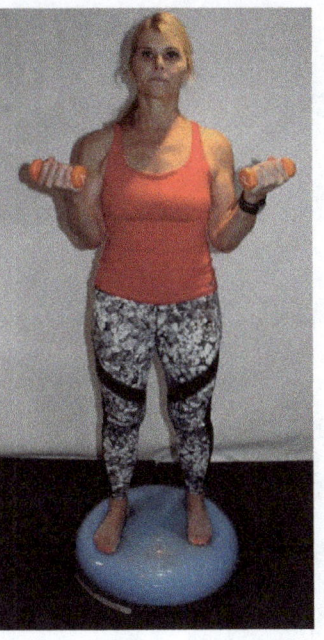

Stand erect on BOSU with resistance at side of body. Hands are facing forward.

- Without swaying the body or swinging the elbows forward, bend the elbows and raise the resistance to shoulder level and against the upper arm.

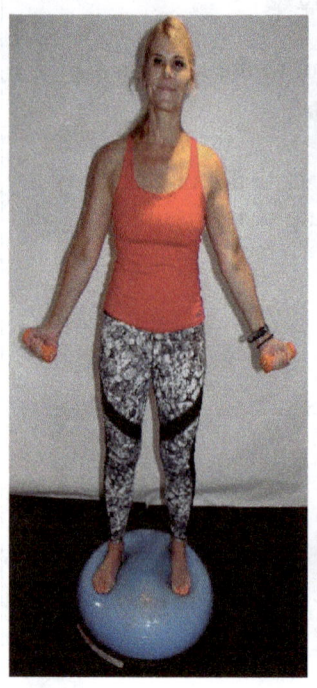

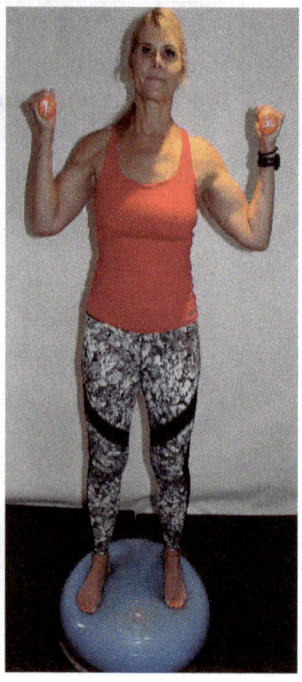

2. Out Curls	Standing erect on BOSU with resistance at side of body but arms are turned out 45º.
	- Without swaying the body or swinging the elbows, bend the elbows and raise the resistance to shoulder level and against the upper arm.
3. In's and Out's In Out	Standing erect on BOSU - do a Regular Curl and an Out Curl.

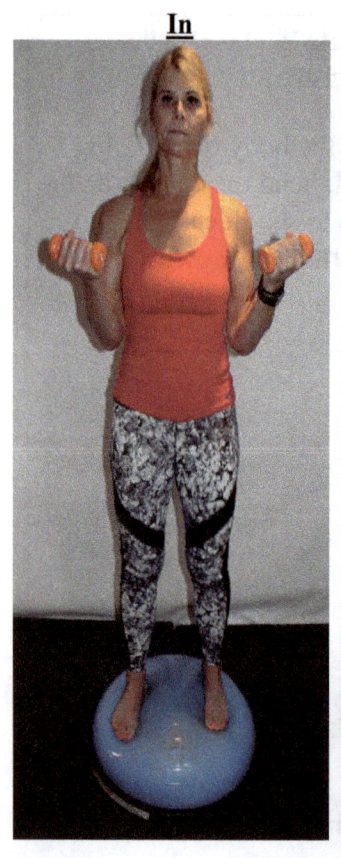

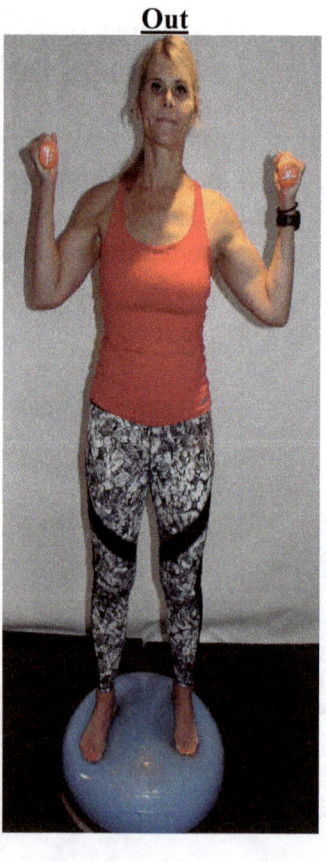

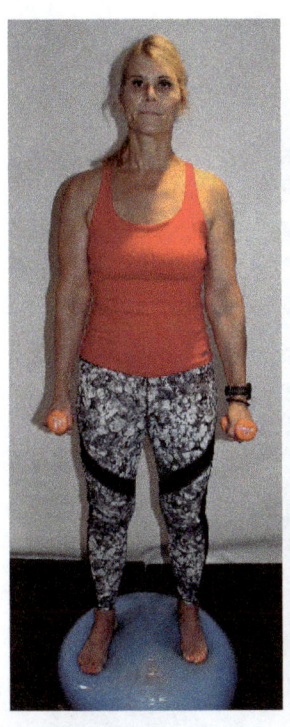

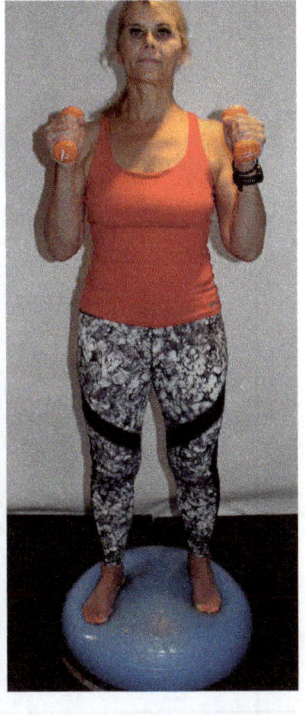

4. Hammer Curls	<u>Standing on BOSU with resistance at side of body.</u> - Turn the hands so they are facing toward the body. - Without swaying the body or swinging the elbows forward, bend the elbows and raise the resistance to shoulder level and against the upper arm.
5. Out Hammer Curls	<u>Standing erect on BOSU with resistance at side of body and the hands are facing the body.</u> - Now turn the arms out 45°. Resistance will now be pointing up and down. - Without swaying the body or swinging the elbows, bend the elbows and raise the resistance to shoulder level and against the upper arm.

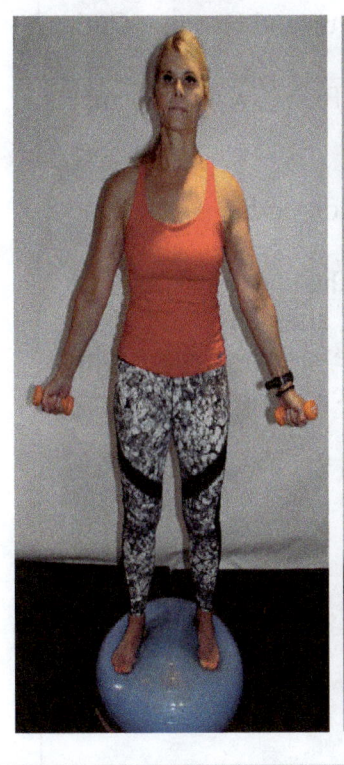

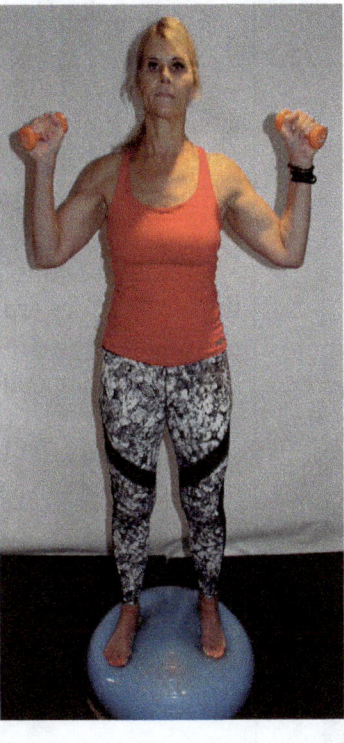

6. In's and Out's Hammer Curls	Standing erect on BOSU
	- do a In Hammer Curls and Out Hammer Curls.
7. Curl Up and Hammer Down	Standing erect on BOSU
	- do a Regular Curl up and Hammer Curl down.
8. Cross Body Curls	- Standing erect on BOSU with resistance at side of body.
	- Hands are facing forward.
	- Without swaying the body or swinging the elbows forward, alternate bending one elbows and raise the resistance across the chest to the opposite shoulder.

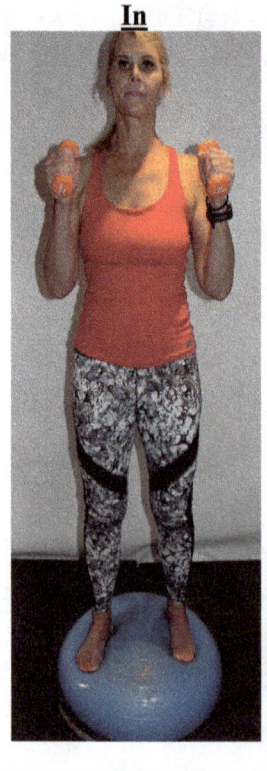

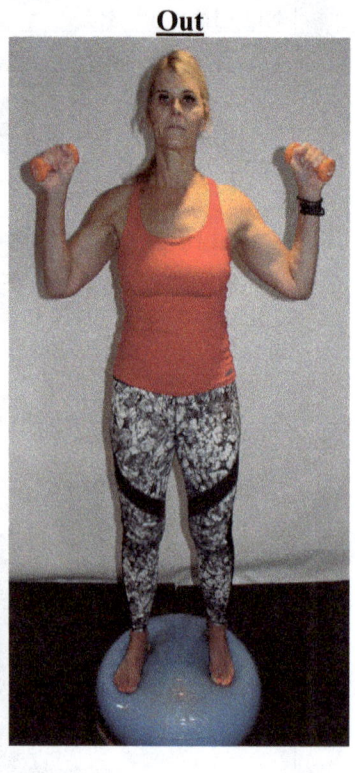

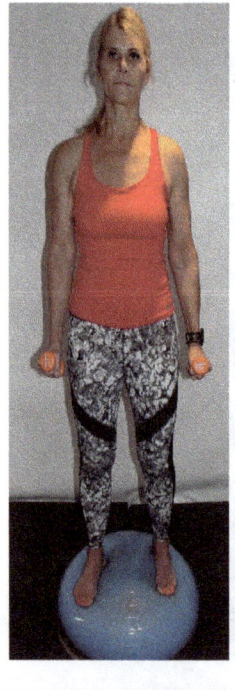

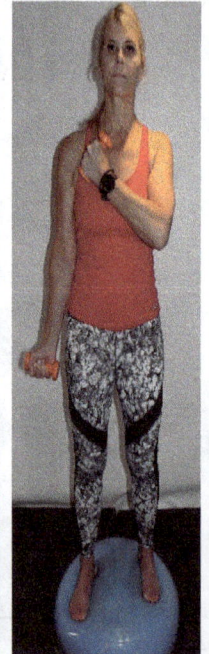

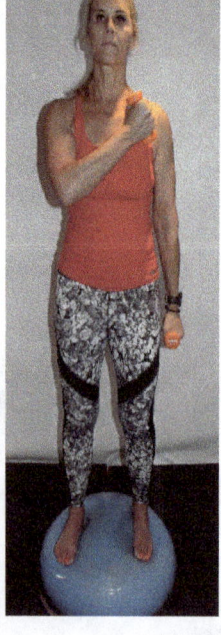

9. Alternating Arm Corkscrew Curl

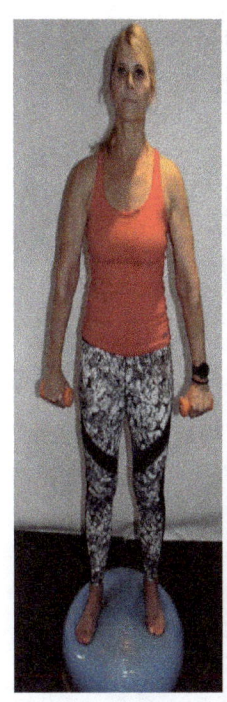

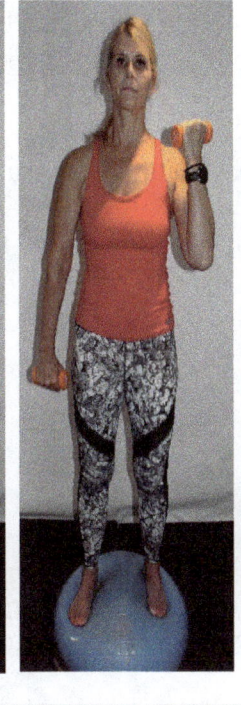

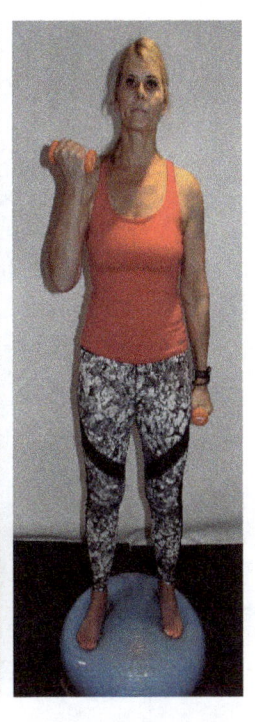

Standing erect on BOSU with resistance at side of body.

- Turn the hands so that they are facing backwards. Without swaying the body or swinging the elbows forward, simultaneously bend the elbows and raise the resistance to shoulder level while twisting the arm so resistance ends up finishing like a Regular Curl against the upper arm.

10. Twenty-ones

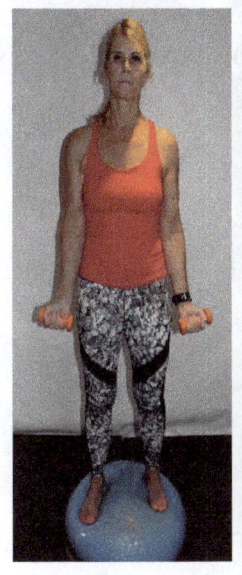

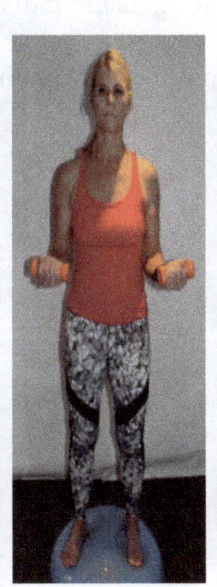

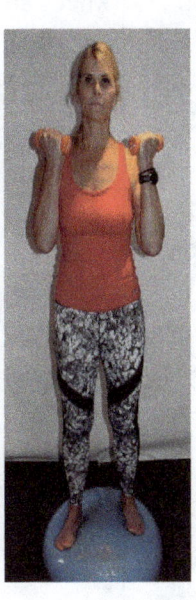

Standing erect on BOSU

- do 7 lower ½ regular curls, 7 upper ½ regular curls and 7 full regular curls

11. Static Arm Curls	Standing erect on BOSU
	- Holding weight in one hand at mid curl position do 8 regular curls with the other arm.
	- Then repeat with the opposite arm.
	- Repeat this sequence twice for a total of 32 repetitions.
12. Crouching Curls	Standing erect on BOSU, spread your legs and knees wide and do ¾ squat.
	- Place the elbows inside the top of the knees so weights are in the middle.
	- Do a regular curl from this position.

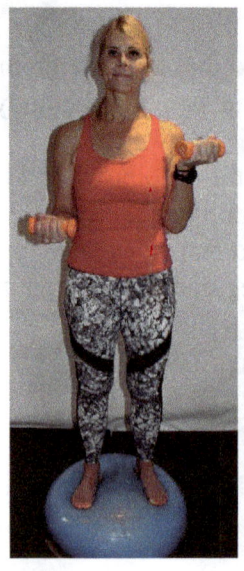

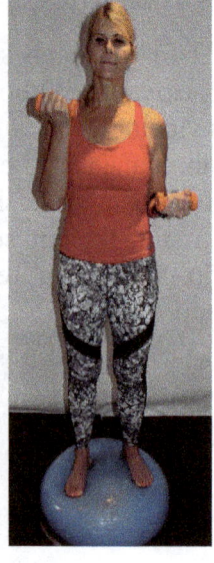

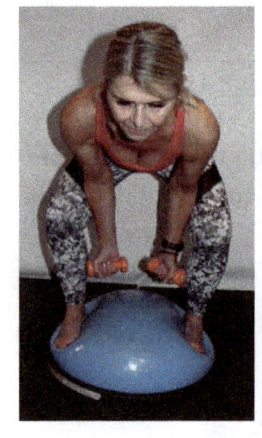

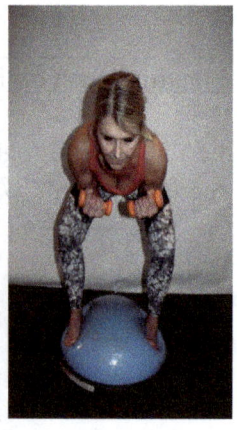

Triceps: **1. Two Arm Triceps Kick Backs** 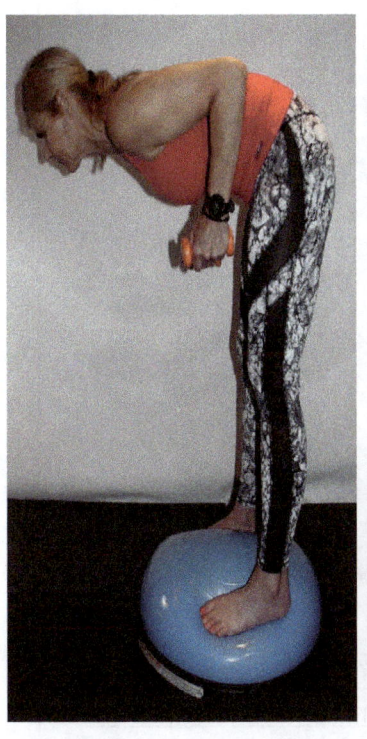 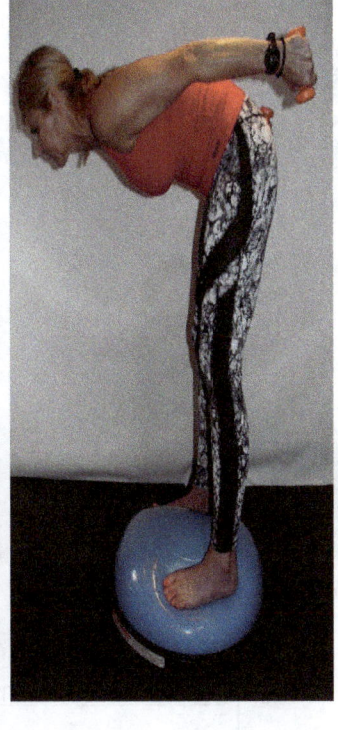	Standing erect on BOSU, bend at the waist and lift elbows up so they are level with the trunk. - Hands are pointing toward the body. - Keep the elbows high as you extend the elbows (kick back).
2. Flip Grip Triceps Kick Backs **Hands pointing backward** 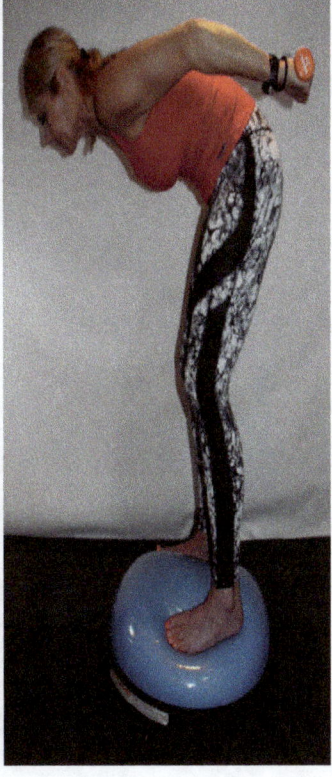	Standing erect on BOSU, bend at the waist and lift elbows up so they are level with the trunk. Arms are pointing downward and hands are pointing backwards. - Keep the elbows high as you extend the elbows (kick back). - When you return to the starting position, you flip the hands over so hands are forward - Keeping the elbows high, extend the elbows again (flip gripped kick back).

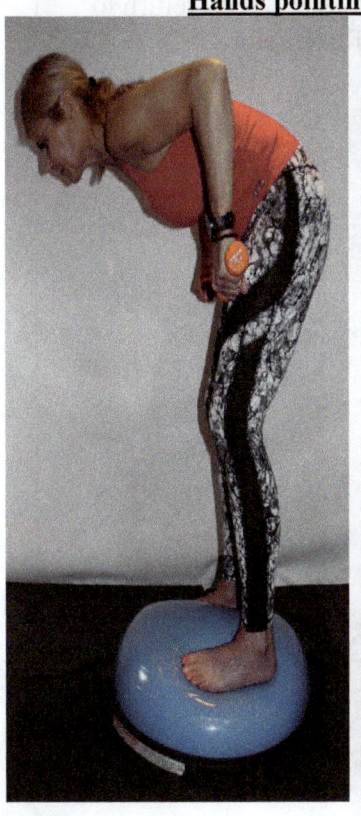

Hands are pointing forward

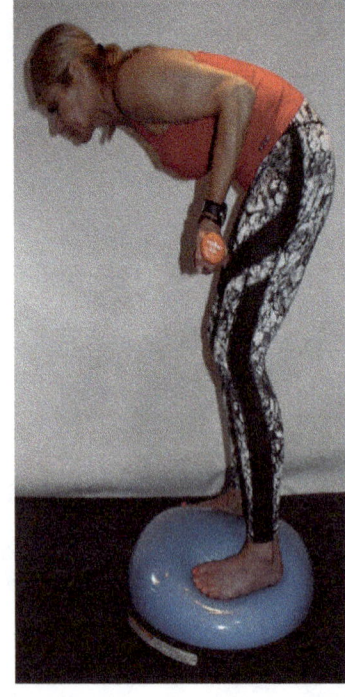

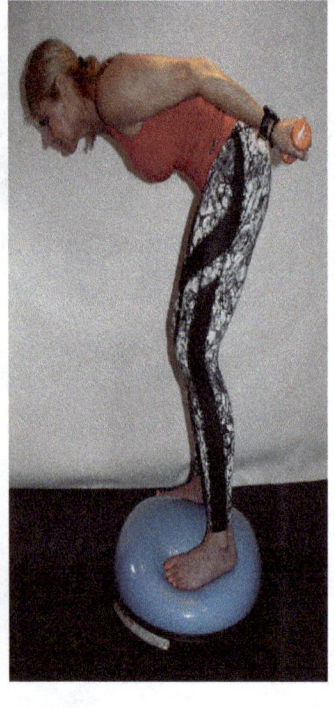

3. Standing Two Arm Overhead Triceps Extension

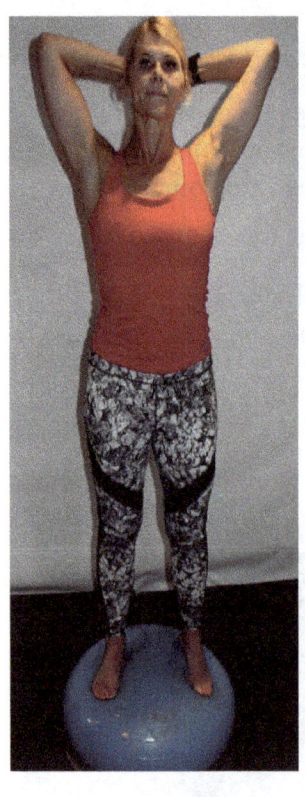

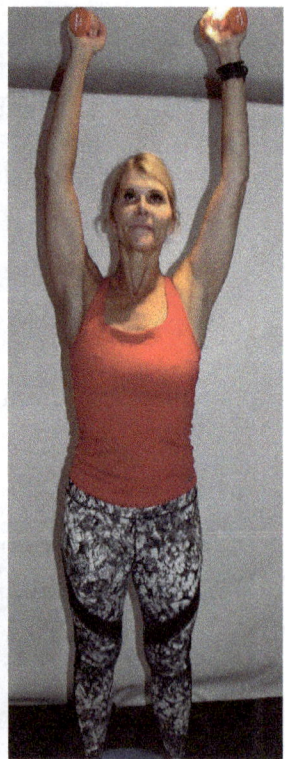

Sitting erect on BOSU place both arms over your head with elbows bent/flexed.

- Both Elbows are pointing straight up.

- Extend both elbows and then return to starting position (flexed elbow).

4. Standing One Arm Overhead Triceps Extension 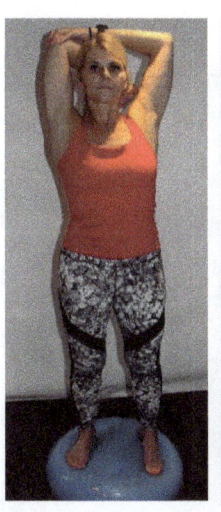 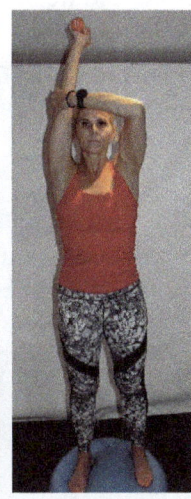 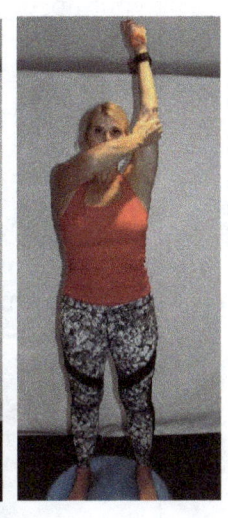	Sitting erect on BOSU position one arms over your head with elbows bent/flexed. - The raised elbow is pointing straight up and supported by the opposite hand. - Extend the elbow and then return to starting position (flexed elbow).
5. Lying Two Arm Triceps Extension 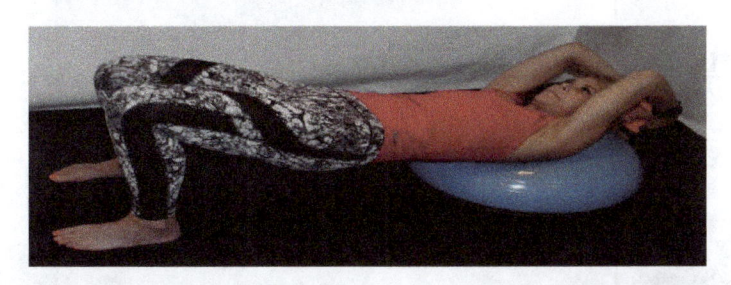 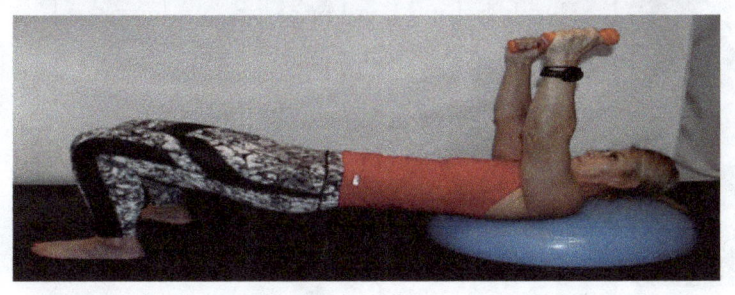	Lying supine (flat) with BOSU supporting your upper back and neck, place both arms over your head so elbows are bend and pointing vertical at your head level. - Extend both elbows and then return to flexed elbow position keeping the elbow pointing vertical.

6. Lying One Arm Triceps Extension 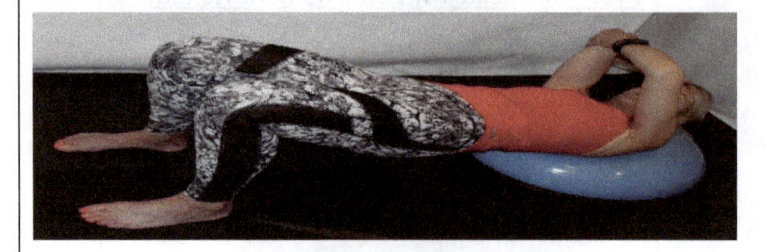 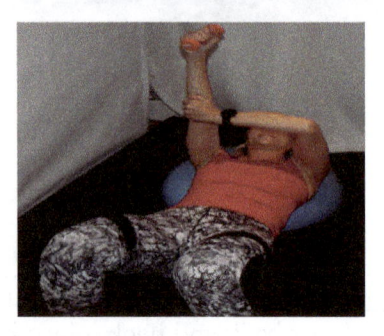	Lying supine (flat) with BOSU supporting your upper back and neck. - place one arm over your head so elbow is bent and pointing vertical at your head level. - Extend the elbow and then return to flexed elbow starting position keeping the elbow pointing vertical.

5. Lower Back Exercises (Also Covered under Core Exercises)

1. Back Extensions (Isolate the back Erector Spinae muscles)

1. Back Extension 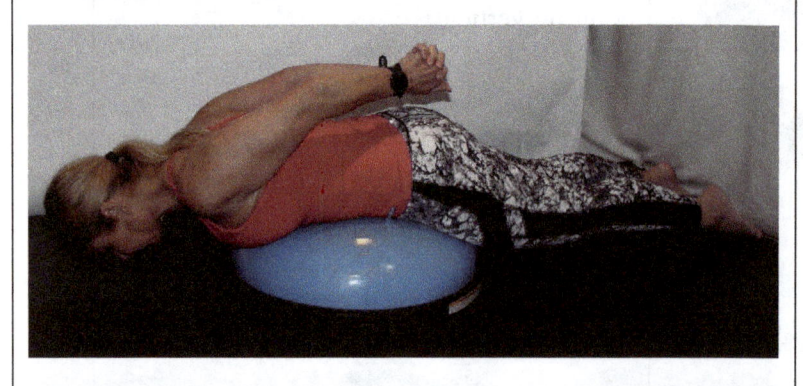 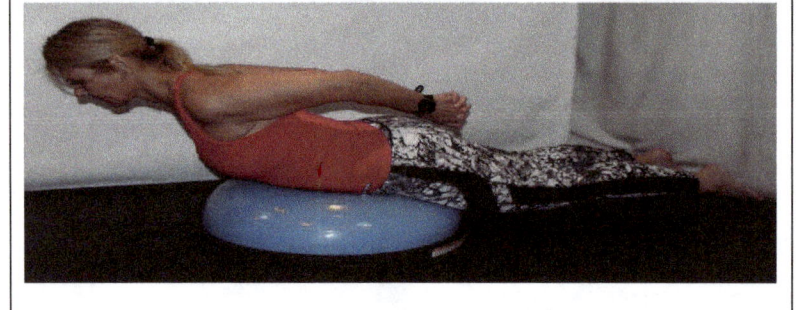	Prone with BOSU supporting your abdominal area. - Hands behind head or resting on lower back. - Lift chest off ground and return to ground. Advanced; 1. Oscillate with chest off the ground. 2. Lift legs off ground (chest stays flat)

2. Back Extensions with Small Rotation 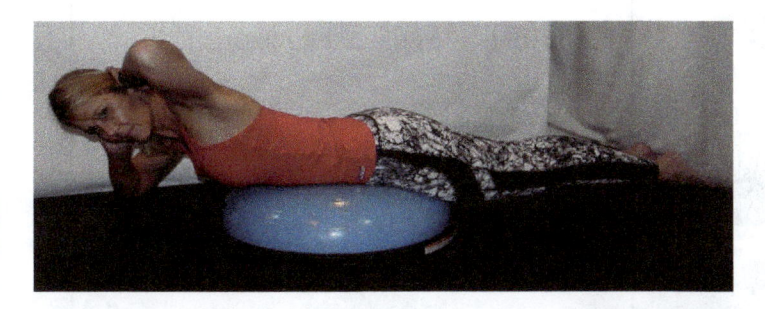 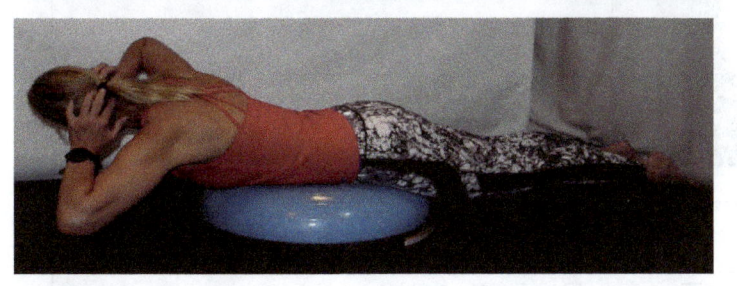	Prone with BOSU supporting your abdominal area - Lift chest and rotate so elbow touches the floor, lower chest and repeat with opposite elbow.
3. Superman's 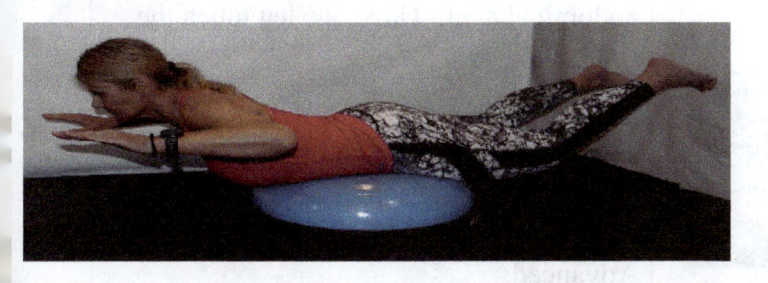	Prone with BOSU supporting your abdominal area - Hands extended out in front of head, behind the head or on small of back. - Lift chest & thighs off ground and return to ground. (Advanced - oscillate with chest & thighs off the ground)
4. Bridges (Upper back or heels on BOSU) **Neck and Upper Back on BOSU** 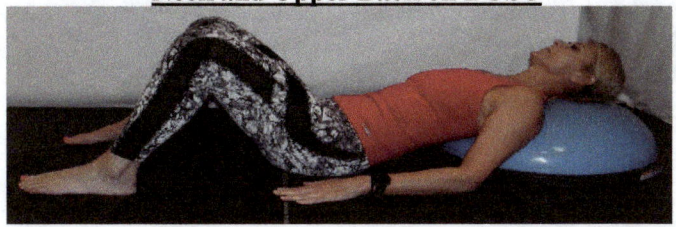 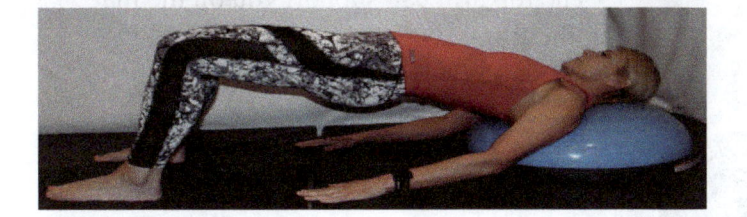	Supine 1. BOSU supporting upper back and neck, body extended, knees bent 90° with both feet on ground, hands resting on lower abdominal. - Lift buttocks off mat and hold 5-10 sec. (Can put feet on SB, BOSU to perform the bridge) Or 2. Heels on BOSU and upper back on mat - Lift buttocks off the mat and hold 5-10 sec

Feet on BOSU

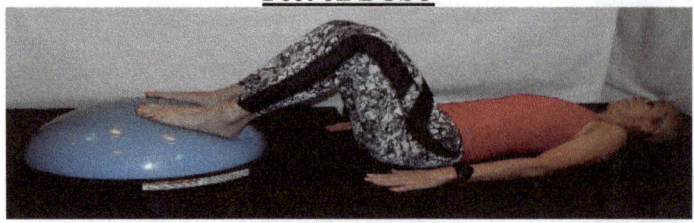

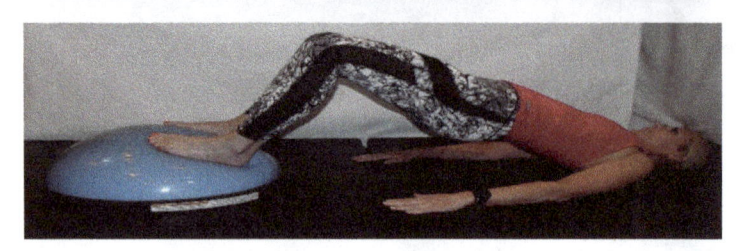

Advanced:

1. Oscillate hips up and down while in bridge position.

2. Extend one leg while in bridge.

3. One leg bridge (other leg in figure 4 position)

6. Hips (Gluteus Medius, Gluteus Maximus, Tensor Facia Lata)

1. Prone Hip Extensions

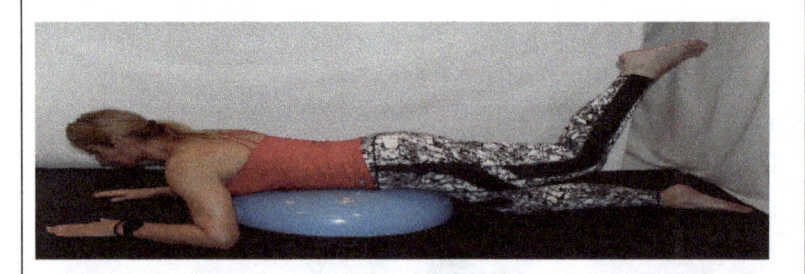

Lying prone with BOSU supporting lower abdominal area - Have one leg touch the floor for stability.

- Bend the opposite leg knee to 90° and lift knee just past horizontal. - Lower the bent knee and repeat.

Advanced:

1. The elevated leg oscillates 4-6".

2. Use ankle weights for additional resistance when lifting the bent knee.

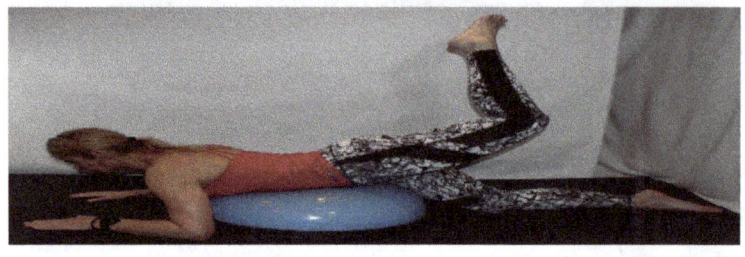

2. Side Lying Hip Abductions

Top arm supports the body

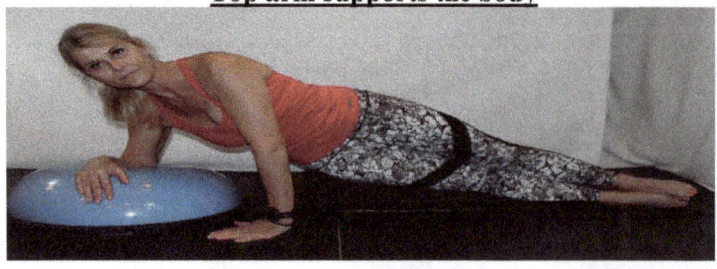

Lying on the side of your ribs on a BOSU or on your bottom arm as shown in the image.
- The top arm can support you on the mat in the front of chest or the arm lies along the side of the body.

- The legs are stacked one on top of the other.

- The bottom leg can be bent at 45° for additional stability.

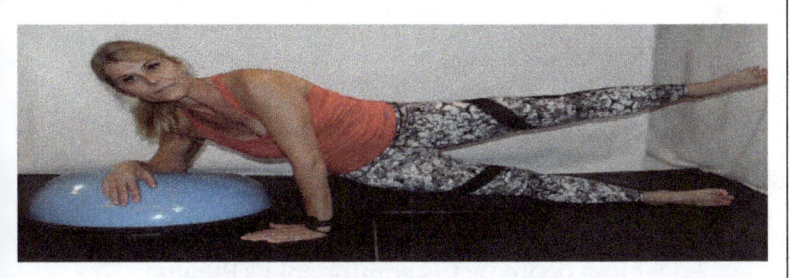

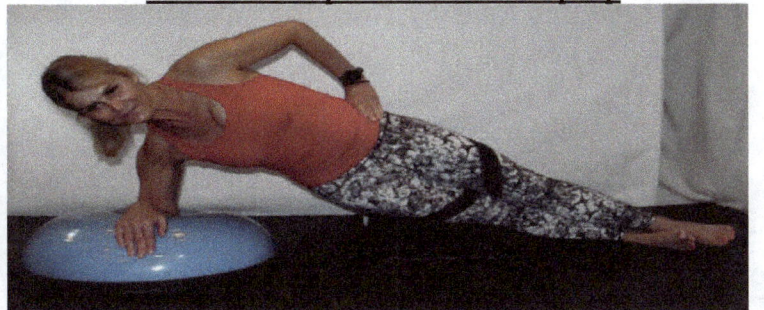

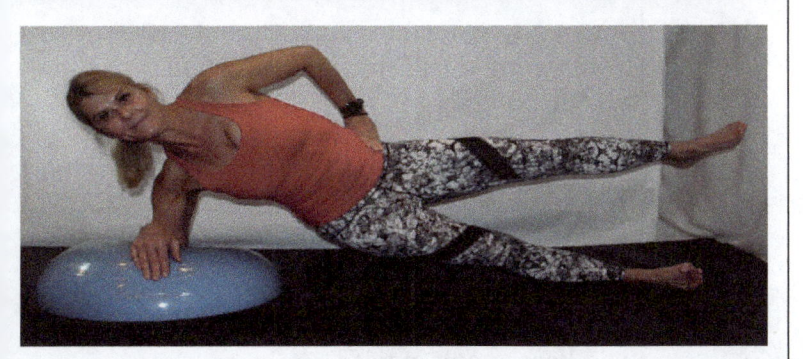

- The top extended leg is lifted up as high as comfortable.

- Lower the raised leg to just above the bottom leg and repeat.

Advanced - Top arm lies on the top hip

3. Fire Hydrant

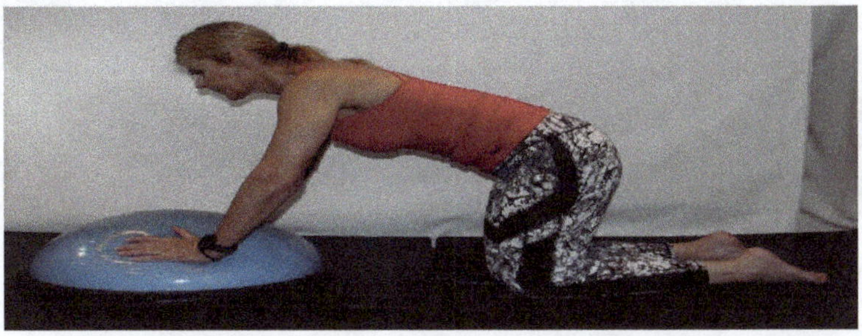

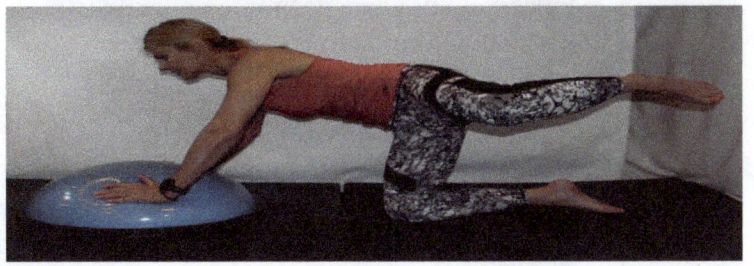

Start with hands on BOSU or knees on BOSU

- abduct (lift sideways) one leg to horizontal position. Knee is bent 90º.

4. Squats

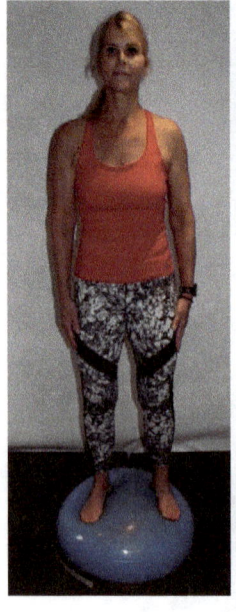

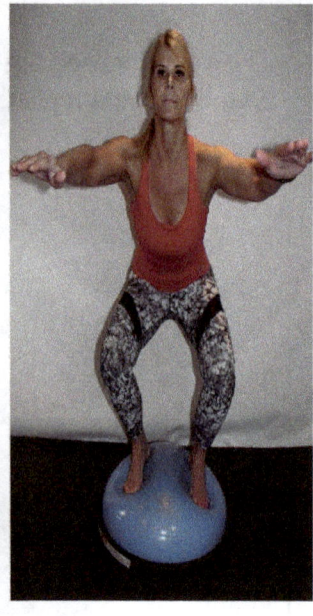

Sumo Squat

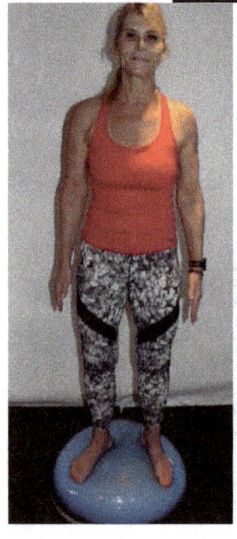

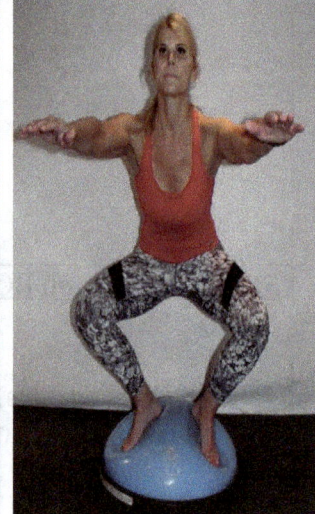

Stand erect on BOSU and feet shoulder width apart.

- The knees can be pointing straight or can be rotated out slightly.

- Begin the exercise by bending the knees to a depth that is comfortable. (Pretend you are sitting in a chair).

- Do not bend the knees past 90º.

- The knees should not go forward past your toes.

- Your chest will lean forward slightly for balance as you move into the squat.

- You may extend the arms out in front of you for additional stability. Return to erect position and repeat.

Advanced:
1. Weights in your hands

Variations of standard Squat:
1. Sumo Squat - Feet are wider and feet and knees point out 45º.

2. Single Leg Squats - non supporting leg is off the ground and knee bent, wrapped around the supporting leg, in a figure four position across the supporting leg or extended out in front of you (Pistol squat) and it does not touch the ground.

- Can touch a chair or wall for balance.

3. Pulse Squat - Once deep into your squat rather than returning to erect position you go up and down about 2-4 inches. Do not do the pulses too fast.

5. Lunges

Forward Lunge

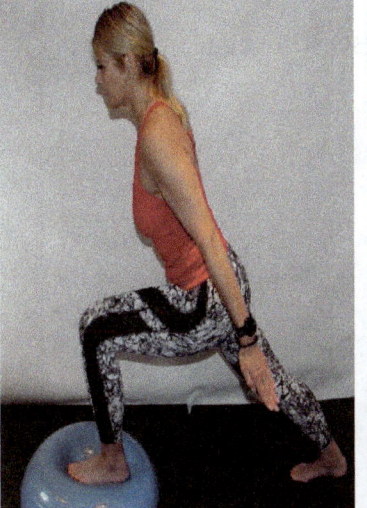

Vertical Twist

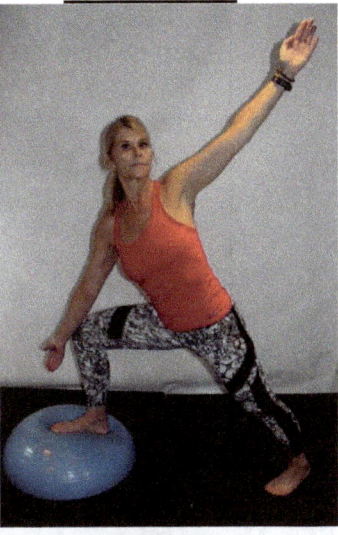

Arms Elevated Over Your Head

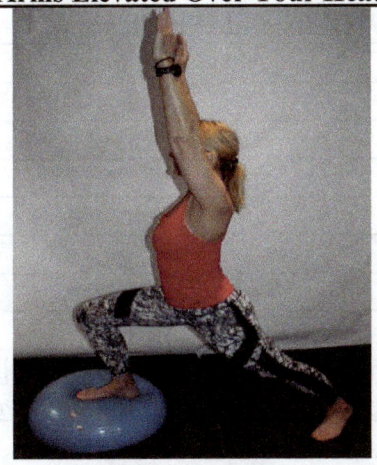

Lateral Lunge

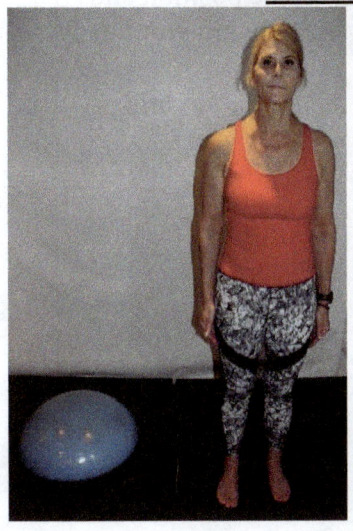

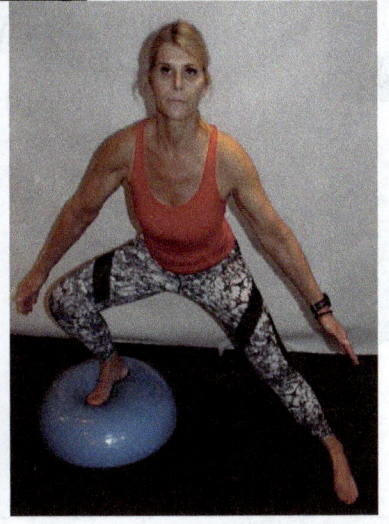

Stand erect and feet shoulder width apart.

- Step forward with one leg onto the BOSU and bend that knee no farther than 90º.

- The knee should not go forward pass the toes.

- Your back should stay erect as you go deep into the lunge.

- Step back to original position and repeat with opposite foot

Advanced:

1. Weights in your hands.

2. Horizontal twist to either side as you lunge. You can twist both ways during one lunge.

3. Vertical twist so one arm reaches to the sky. You can twist both ways during one lunge.

4. Elevating both arms above the head.

Variations of Standard Lunge:

1. Pulse Lunge

- Once in lunge position go up and down about 2-4 inches rather than returning to erect position immediately. Do not do the pulses fast.

2. Lateral Lunge

- Facing forward step laterally onto a BOSU and bend either the lunging knee or the non-lunge knee. The foot and knee should be angled out about 45º.

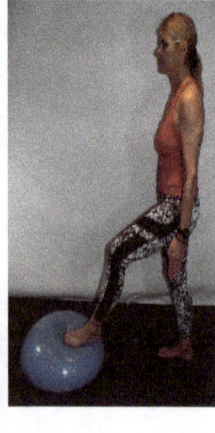

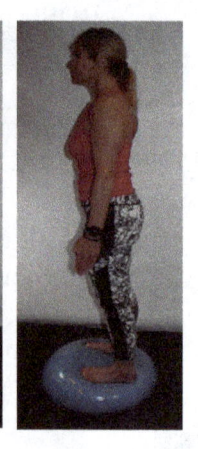

6. Alternating Leg Step ups	Stand erect beside the BOSU -step up onto the BOSU one leg at a time.

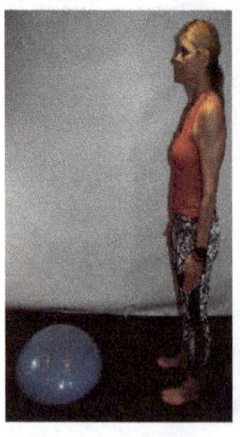

7. Legs (Quadriceps, Hamstrings, Calves, Tibialis Anterior)

Please Note - **Squats, Lunges,** and **Alternating Leg Step Ups** are covered under hip exercises (because they are multi leg muscle exercises and therefore activate the leg muscles (Quads, Hamstrings, Gastroc and Soleus) as well as the hip musculature (Gluts and Hip Flexors)

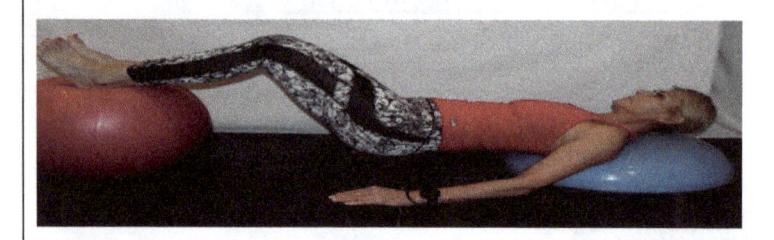

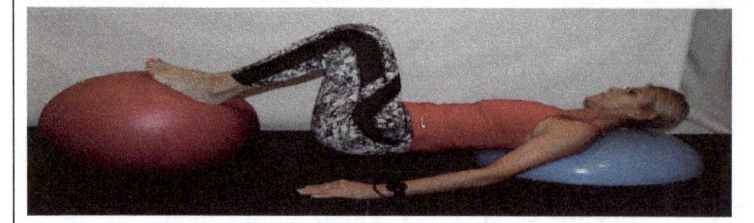

1. Quadriceps:	
1. **Squats**	
2. **Lunges**	
3. **Alternating Leg Step ups**	
2. Hamstrings:	
1. **Squats**	
2. **Lunges**	
3. **Alternating Leg Step ups**	
4. Stability Ball Hamstring Curl	Lying supine with BOSU supporting upper back- place your lower calves and heels on a stability ball. - Lift your hips into a bridge position and then roll the stability ball toward you. - Hold for 1 sec and then return to bridge position and repeat.

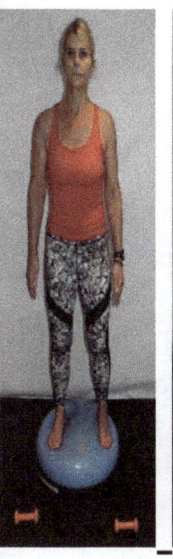

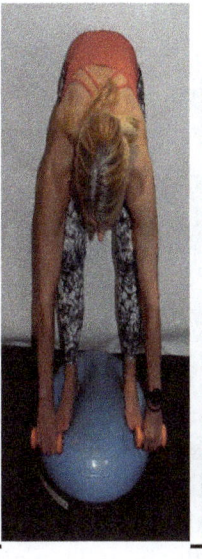

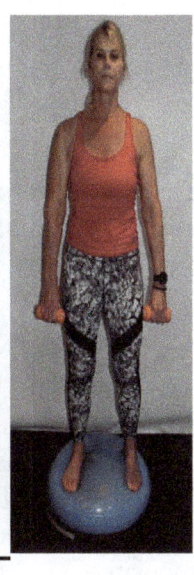

5. Dead Lifts	Stand erect on BOSU and bend over 90º with dumbbells or barbells - Straighten your hips and lift your chest up and straighten your lower back. **Note - Do not hold your breath as you are lifting the weight** - Hold the weight for a second at the top, with locked hips and knees. - Return the weight to the floor by moving your hips back while bending your legs. - Avoid bending at the waist which leaves your lower back vulnerable to strain **Note - It is important that your lower back stay in neutral position to avoid injury.**
3. Calves	
1. Standing Heel Raise Dome Side Up 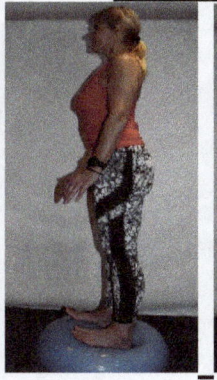 — Flat Side Up 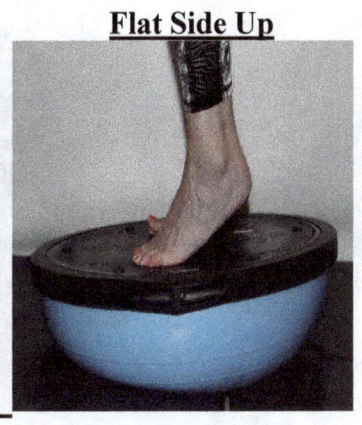	Stand erect on BOSU - Stand on your toes, hold for 1-2 sec and return to starting position.
4. Tibialis Anterior 1. **Standing Toe Raises** Dome Side Up — Flat Side Up	Stand erect. Use wall or chair for stability. - Raise your toes as high off the BOSU as possible for 1- 2 sec and then return to starting position.

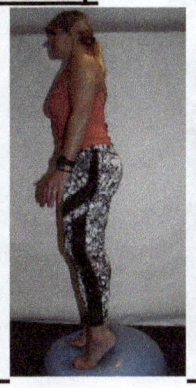

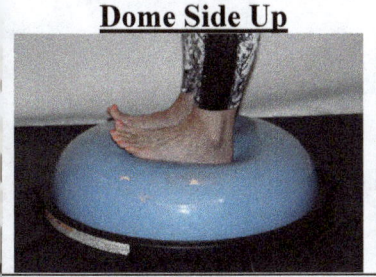

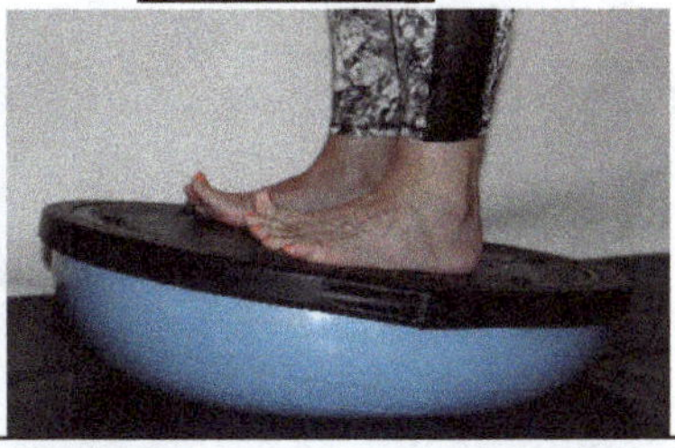

References

www.BOSU.com

Appendix 9.1.8. TRX Exercises Described and Illustrated

(TRX: Total Body Resistance Suspension Training)

Introduction

TRX is an acronym for "Total Body Resistance Exercise" and has become an extremely popular exercise apparatus in mainstream exercise facilities and is excellent for home use. It is relatively inexpensive, very portable and easy to use. It is an effective way for older adults to get a good muscle resistance workout.

The TRX training system was born out of necessity by US Navy Seals, who needed a way to stay in excellent condition when deployed, and traditional exercise equipment was not available. TRX training is body resistance suspension training. Body resistance means that the user's bodyweight is the resistance that must be overcome vs. traditional dumbbells or machine weights. Suspension training implies that with each exercise, the user's hands or feet are placed in a strap and supported by a single anchor point while the opposite end of the body is in contact with the ground.

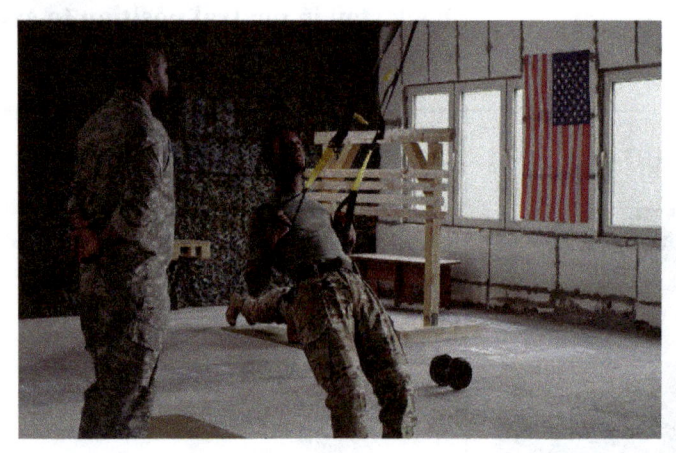

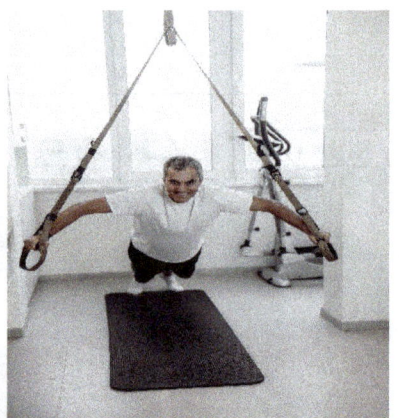

The TRX can be used safely by the older adult. You can modify the intensity or difficulty level of each TRX exercise to meet their needs and capabilities safely. Varying the intensity and difficulty is accomplished in three ways:

1. By changing the size of the base of support. The smaller the support base, the more unstable and challenging the exercise becomes.

2. Modifying the suspension angle from more vertical to horizontal makes the exercise more challenging.

3. Moving farther away from the anchor makes floor exercises more challenging.

The TRX is a stand-alone piece of exercise equipment. The single point of attachment utilized by the TRX provides the ideal mix of support and mobility to improve strength, endurance, balance, coordination, flexibility, power, and core stability.

Follow the illustrations and descriptions below to make safe and effective use of this revolutionary exercise tool. The TRX is an excellent way of introducing variety into a person's exercise routine. Try it; you will like it and, better yet, love the results.

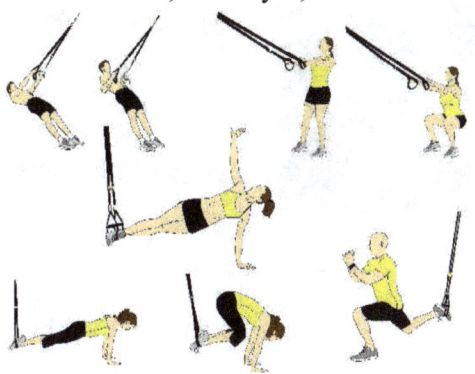

TRX Exercises Described and Illustrated

Note:
- **Pronated hand position** = palms facing down
- **Supinated hand position** = palms facing up
- **Prone position** = face down
- **Supine position** = face up

Core	
Back Extensors:	
1. Standing Overhead Back Extension (Mid Length)	Start - Facing anchor, hands pronated & extended over your head. Movement - Lean back keeping back straight and bend 90° at hip & wt. shifts to heels/tailbone. - Return to starting position (standing straight up with hands over head) by engaging back extensors.
Rectus Abdominus:	
1. Kneeling Roll Out (Mid Calf Length)	Start - Kneeling toward anchor, arms extended & hands in front of hips. Movement - Lean forward & extended arms move away from body to shoulder level or more. Note - Keep strong/straight core alignment (Don't flex at the hips).

2. Supine Bent Knee Full Sit-Up (Mid Calf Length)	Start – Supine and arms extended and holding onto straps in front of hips.

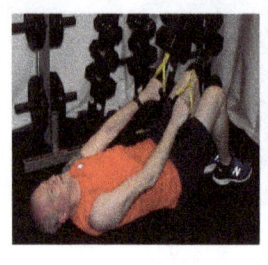

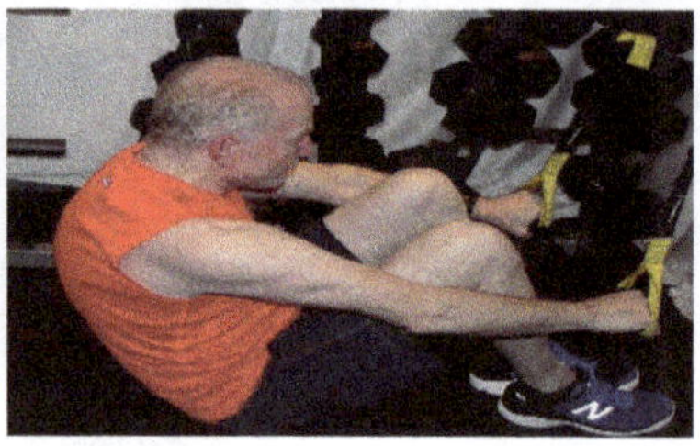

Movement - Press down on handles as move chest up. Keep arms extended and hands will move from one side of knees to other.

Note - Press down on handles (don't grip them). |
| **3. Supine Straight Leg Sit-ups (Mid Calf length)**

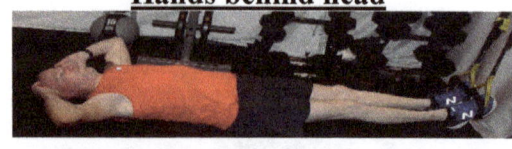

Hands behind head

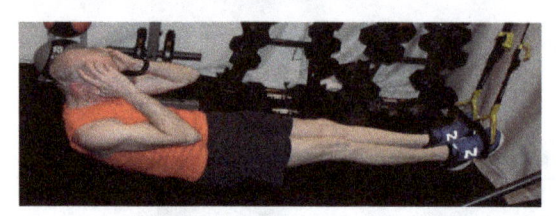

Arms extended in front of chest | Start – Supine with heels in straps, knee's straight & hands behind head or arms extended in front of chest

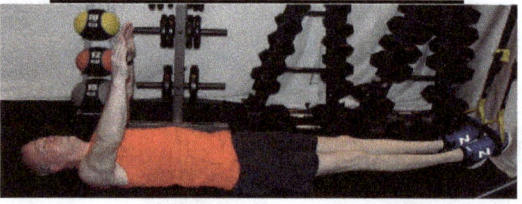

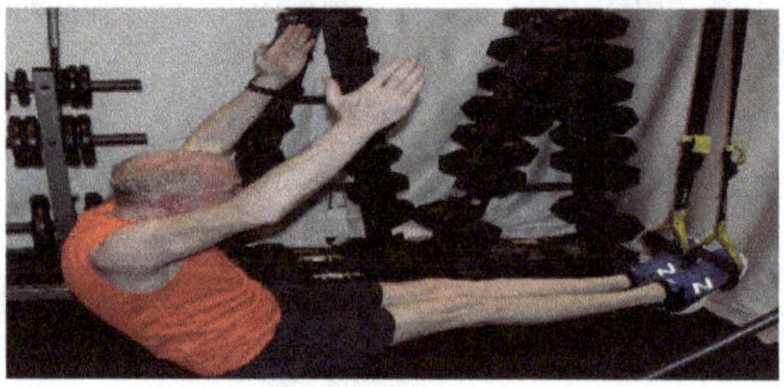

Movement - drive heels down into straps as lift chest up Extended arms move over your head as chest comes up.

Note - SLOW controlled movement as you move back to the floor. |

4. Supine Double Bent Knee Leg Raise (Mid Calf Length) 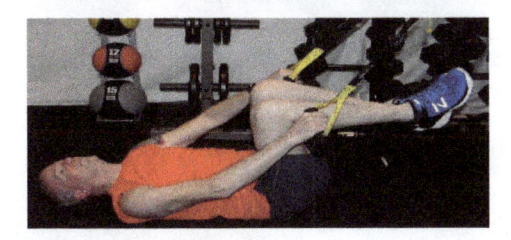	Start - Keep feet and knees together & lift feet 12" off ground. Arms are extended and holding onto straps in front of hips Movement - Bend hips to 90° so legs are in table top position (lower legs are parallel to ground) & slowly lower feet to starting position (12" off ground). Note - Keep knees & feet together.
5. Prone Reverse Crunch (Mid Calf Length) 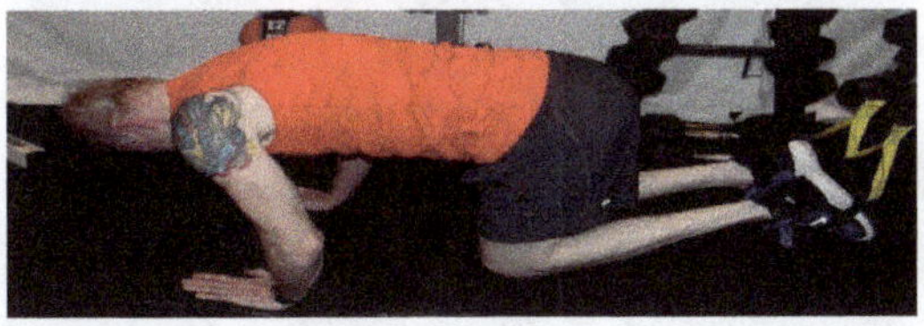	Start - Prone position with feet in the straps Movement - Contract abdominals & lift hips up slightly to allow FULL knee tuck. - Hips are always slightly elevated. Note - Never let abdomen sag toward floor.
6. Prone Pike Crunch (Mid Calf Length) 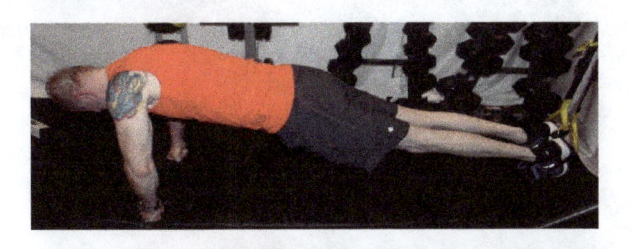 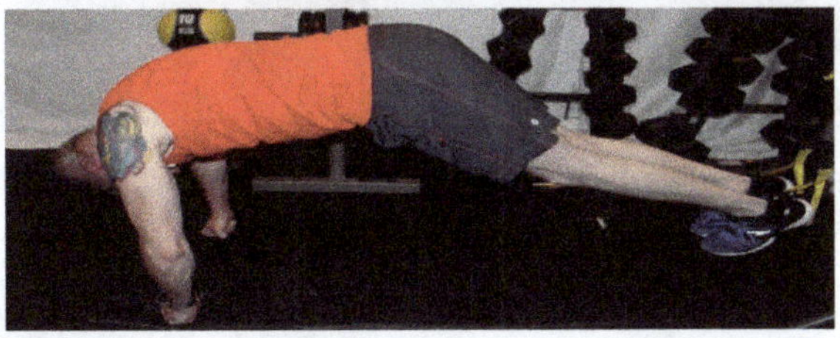	Start - Prone position with feet in the straps Movement - Keep knee's straight as lift hips up into pike position

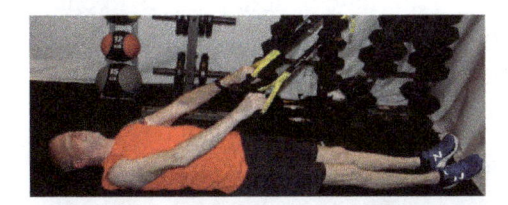

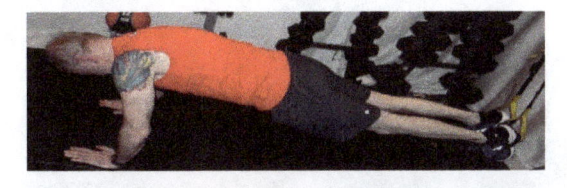

7. Prone Mountain Climber (Mid Calf Length)	Start - Prone position with feet in the straps Movement - Alternate bringing knees to chest Note - Keep even tension on the cradles
Obliques:	
1. Standing Torso Rotations (Mid Length)	Start - Arms extended in front of chest. Movement - Keep hands in front of chest & rotate chest. Hands stay at chest height or rotate up to above the head Note - Focus movement on chest not arms.

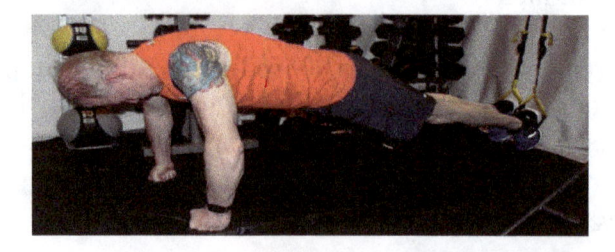

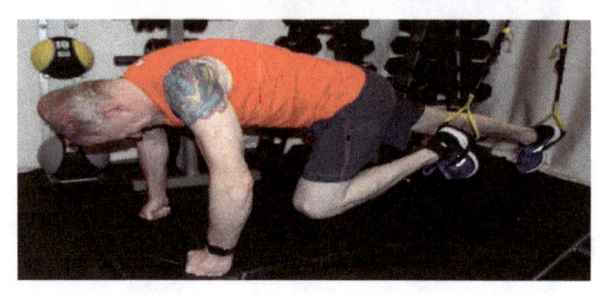

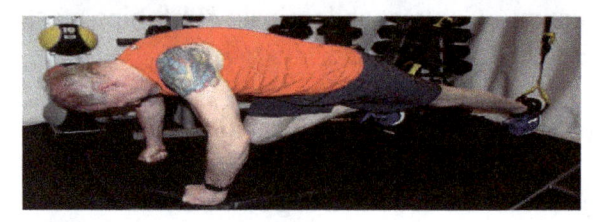

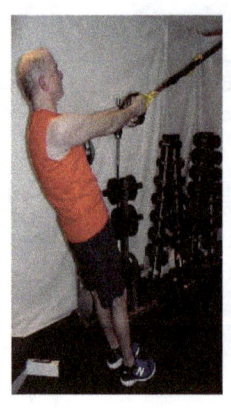

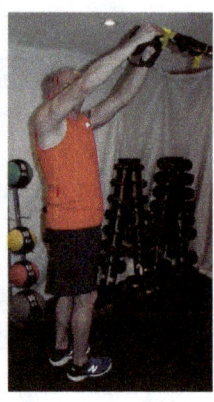

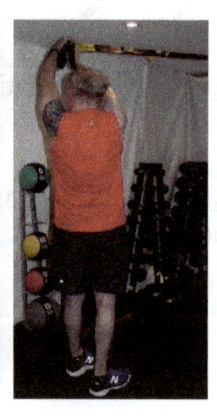

2. Kneeling Oblique Roll Outs **(Mid Calf Length)**	<u>Start</u> - Kneel sideways to anchor, twist trunk toward anchor, arms extended & hands at hip level. - Shoulders are square to anchor & hips are perpendicular to shoulders <u>Movement</u> – Rotate away from anchor & arms move up towards head level or beyond.
Lateral Abdominals: **1. Standing Lateral Hip Drop** **(Mid Length)**	<u>Start</u> - Stand sideways to anchor. Arms on top of head & feet together. <u>Movement</u> - Hips move/drop away from anchor and then return to starting position <u>Note</u> - Don't twist out of alignment
Planks: **(Mid Calf Length):** **1. Prone Plank** **On Forearms** **On Hands**	<u>Start</u> - Prone position with feet in the straps. Upper body supported by forearms (lower plank position) or hands (upper plank position) <u>Movement</u> – Hold the position <u>Note</u> - Keep hips and shoulders square to the ground.
2. Supine Plank **On Forearms** **On Hands**	<u>Start</u> – supine with heels in straps and upper body supported by forearms or hands <u>Movement</u> – hold the position <u>Note</u> - Keep chin off chest, look straight ahead & Keep hips up (don't sag).

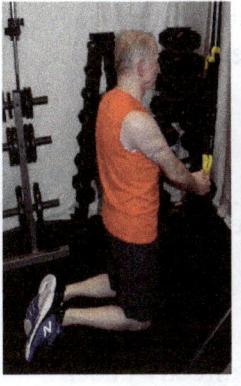

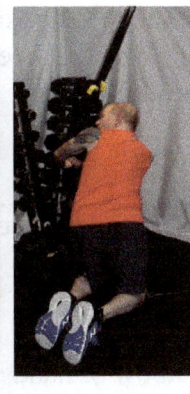

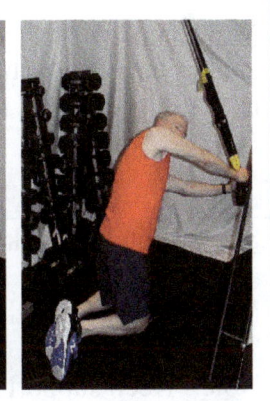

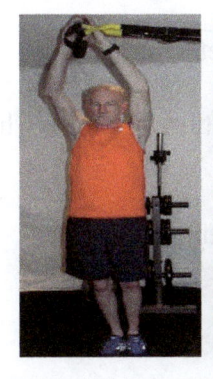

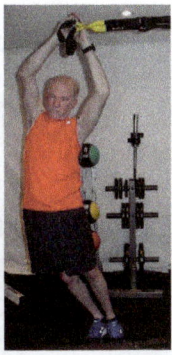

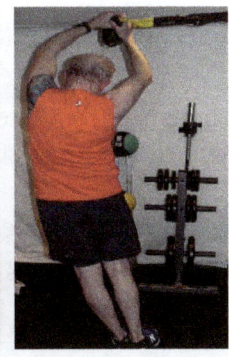

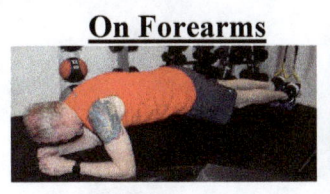

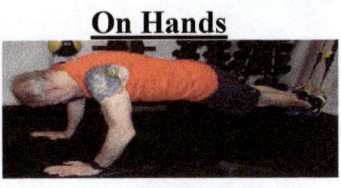

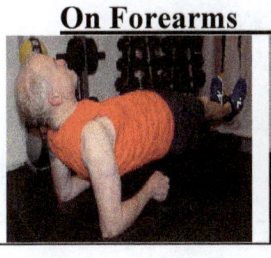

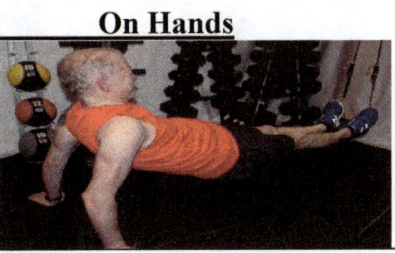

3. Supine Pull Throughs 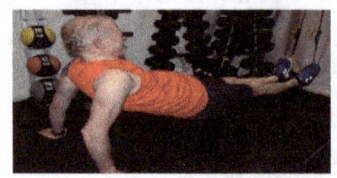 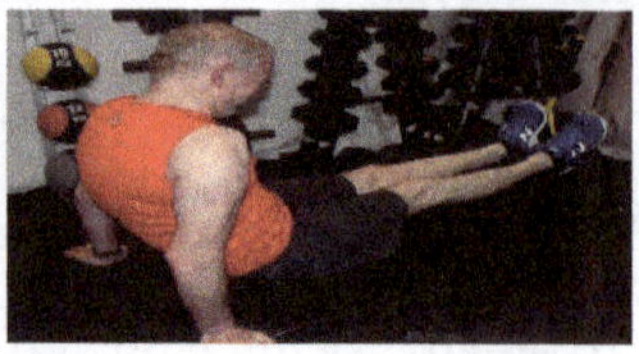	<u>Start</u> - supine with heels in straps and upper body supported by forearms or hands <u>Movement</u> - From supine plank position, contract abdominals & pull hips back between arms, so hips get to 90° & press head towards knees.
4. Lateral Plank (On Forearms or Hands) **On Forearms** 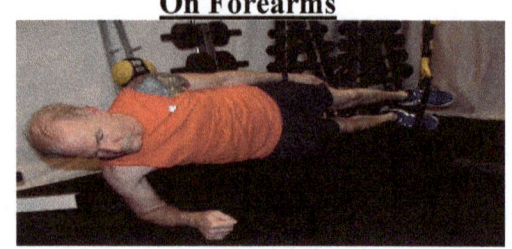	<u>Start</u> – Lateral plank with side of feet in straps <u>Movement</u> – Hold the position <u>Note</u> - Keep support elbow or hand directly under shoulder & maintain alignment (don't let hips sag).
5. Lateral Hip Drop on Elbows or Hands	<u>Start</u> – Lateral plank with side of feet in straps <u>Movement</u> - From lateral plank position drop lower hip & then lift hip up to start position. <u>Note</u> - Keep core & legs tight at all times to avoid involuntary leg swing.

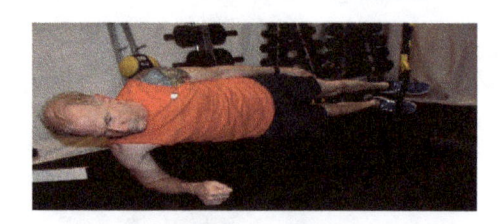

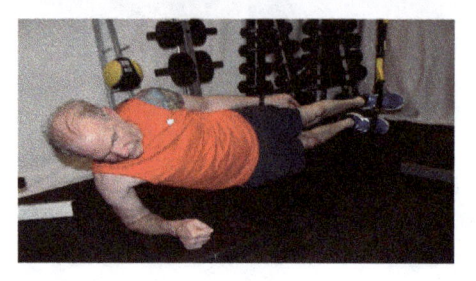

6. Lateral Floor Tap (Supported by elbow or hand)

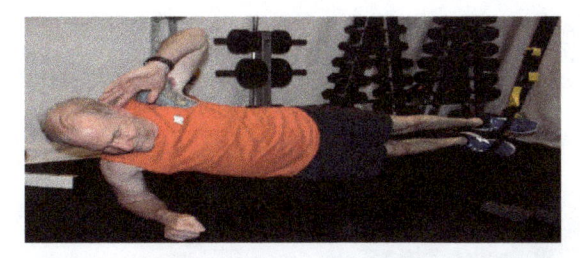

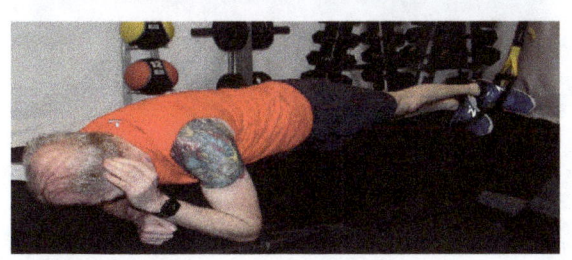

Start - Lateral plank position with top arm flexed and hand touching top ear.

Movement - Slowly lower arm & reach under the body as far as possible to tap the floor with elbow & then return to start position.

Upper Body

Chest: (pectoralis Major)

1. Chess Press (Long Length)

Feet Shoulder Width Apart (Wide Stance)

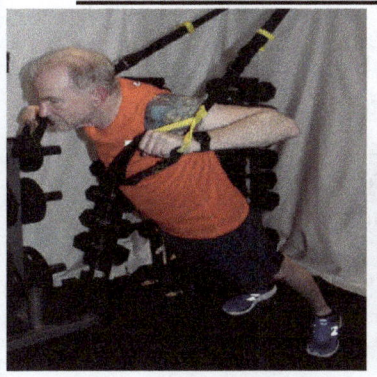

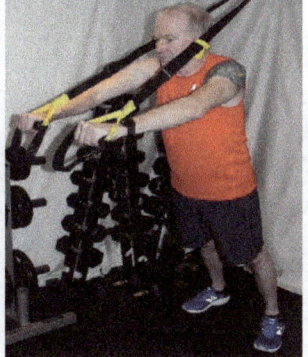

Feet Together (Narrow Stance)

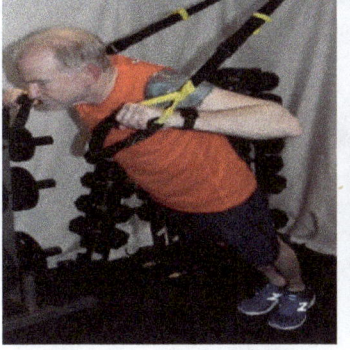

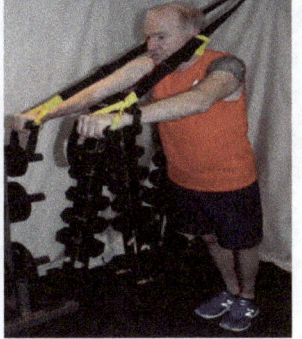

Start – Standing erect with hands in straps and arms extended in front of chest. Face away from anchor.

Movement - Lower chest towards extended hands (Similar to a push-ups).

- Position hands higher or slightly wider to avoid straps rubbing against arms.

Note - Resist rotational movement of chest.

Single Leg Stance

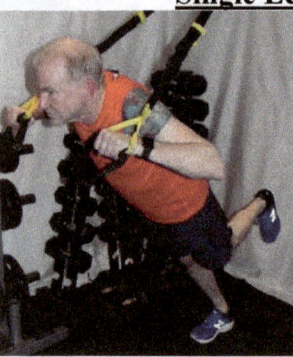

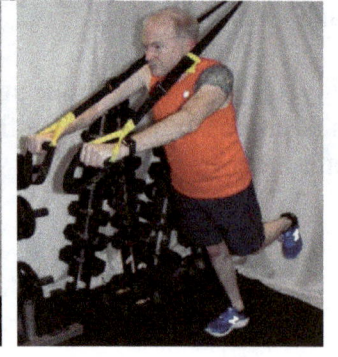

Single Arm and Wide Stance

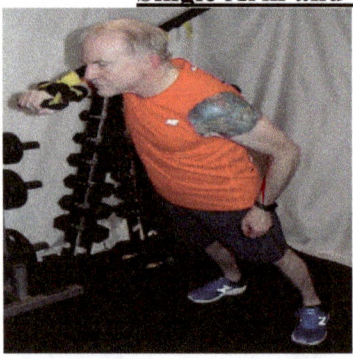

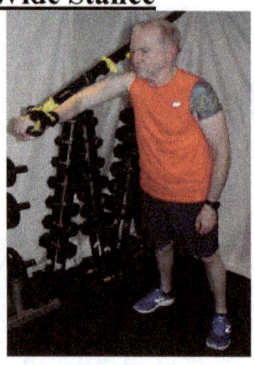

2. Chest Flies (Long length)
Feet can be staggered or shoulder width apart

Wide Stance

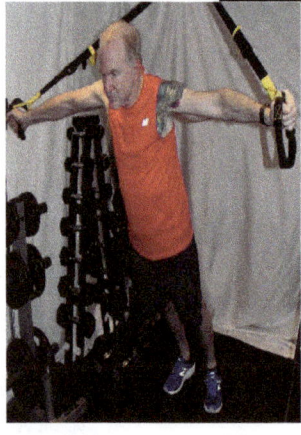

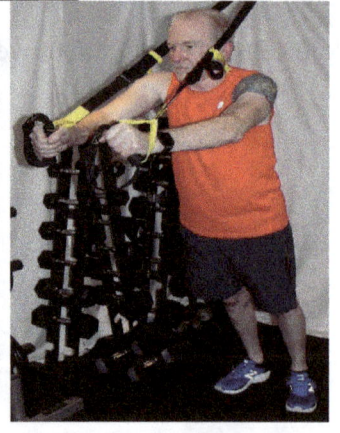

Staggered Stance

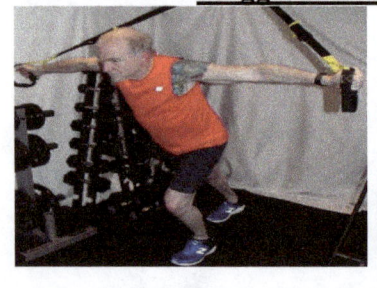

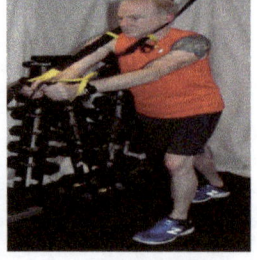

Start – Standing erect with hands in straps and arms extended in front of chest. Face away from anchor.

Movement - Lean forward as arms move laterally at chest height. Hands are facing forward.

- Return arms to front of body with elbows extended.

3. Standard Push-Ups (Mid Calf Length) **Standard Hand Position**	Start – Prone with feet in straps and hands on floor shoulder width Movement – lower chest to ground and then return to staring position Can do with various hand positions; 1. Standard (As shown) 2. Military (Hands close to ribs) 3. Wide (Hands much wider than shoulder width) 4. Diamond (Hands together (Thumbs and index fingers touch) under chest)
4. Combination – Push-up followed by Reverse Crunch **1. Push-up** **2. Reverse Crunch**	Start – Prone with feet in straps and hands on floor shoulder width Movement – Do push-up first and then reverse crunch (both knees move to chest.) Advanced – Reverse crunch in pike position (hips elevated and knees straight.)

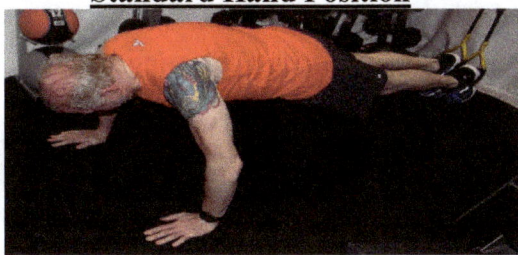

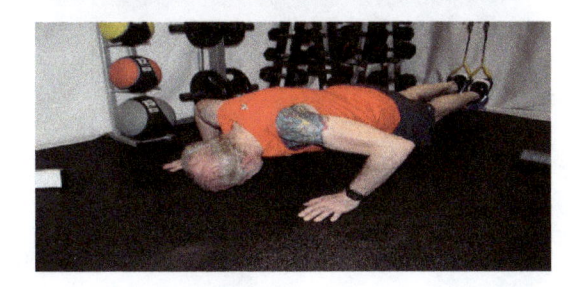

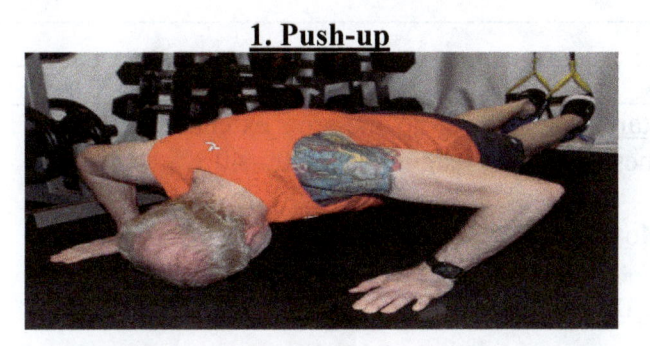

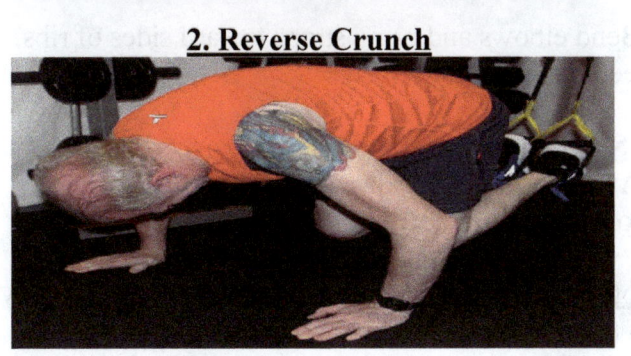

5. Combination Push-up and Oblique Crunch **1. Push-up** **2. Oblique Reverse Crunch**	<u>Start</u> - Prone with feet in straps and hands on floor shoulder width <u>Movement</u> - Bring knees to alternating sides of chest after each push-up
Upper Back	
Rhomboids:	
1. Mid Row **Double Arm** **Single arm**	<u>Start</u> – Hands in strap and arms extended in front of chest and body leaning back 30 – 40 º <u>Movement</u> **1. Double Arms** - Bend elbows and bring straps toward sides of ribs. Keep hands tight to ribs. 2. **Single Arm** - As bring straps to sides of ribs don't rotate the shoulders or hips. Keep them square to the anchor <u>Note</u> - Don't sway the hips forward or backward as you do the movement. The core must stay tight.

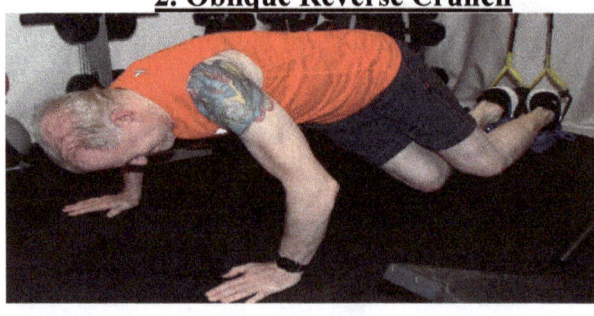

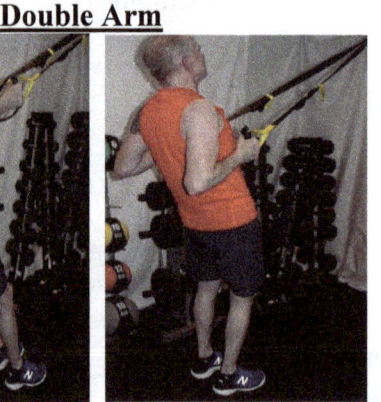

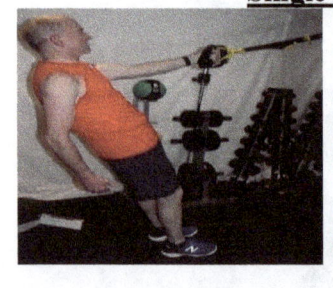

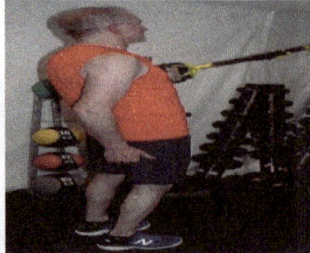

Latissimus Dorsi: **1. Standing Swimmers Pull-Down (Mid Length)**	<u>Starting</u> - Leaning back and arms fully extended, hands pronated <u>Movement</u> - Pull straight down on handles to move body upwards. MUST keep elbows extended as hands move down to hip level.
Shoulders: (Mid Length) **1. Low Deltoid Flies**	<u>Start</u> - Hands supinated and arms extended in front of chest <u>Movement</u> - Pull hands down to hips to a reverse "Y" position. <u>Note</u> - Drive movement from back of arms/shoulder and core.
2. "L" Deltoid Fly	<u>Start</u> - Hands facing each other and arms extended in front of chest <u>Movement</u> - Hands and arms move laterally. The elbows stay tucked close to side of body.

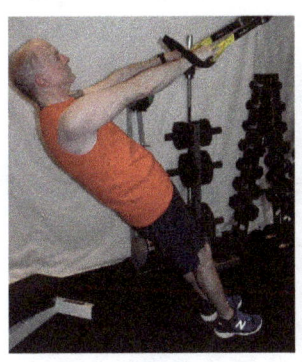

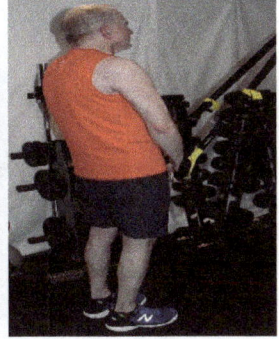

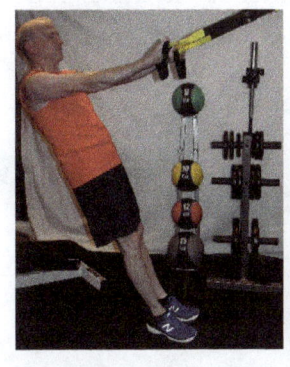

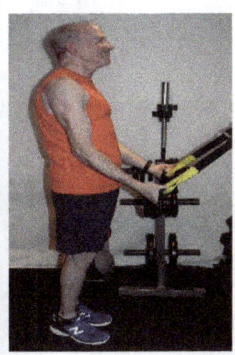

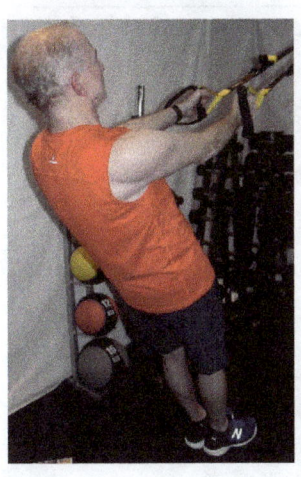

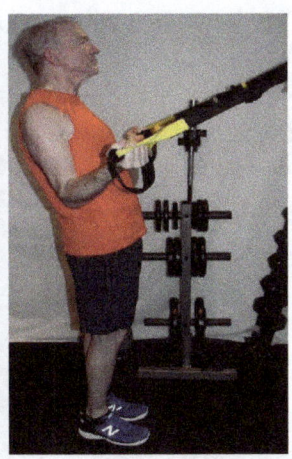

3. "W" Deltoid Flies	<u>Start</u> - Hands pronated and arms extended in front of chest
	<u>Movement</u> – elbows bend 90º and arms and hands rotate up to ear level. Forearms are pointing vertical at end of rotation
4. "T" Deltoid Flies	<u>Start</u> - Hands face each other and arms extended in front of chest
	<u>Movement</u> - elbows stay extended as hands move out laterally to a horizontal position at shoulder height.
	Keep elbows straight as possible
5. "Y" Deltoid Flies	<u>Start</u> - Hands pronated and arms extended in front of chest
	<u>Movement</u> - Lift hands and arms up at 45º angle to a vertical position. Keep elbows straight as possible.

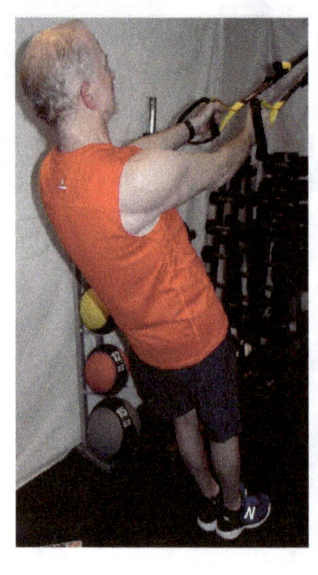

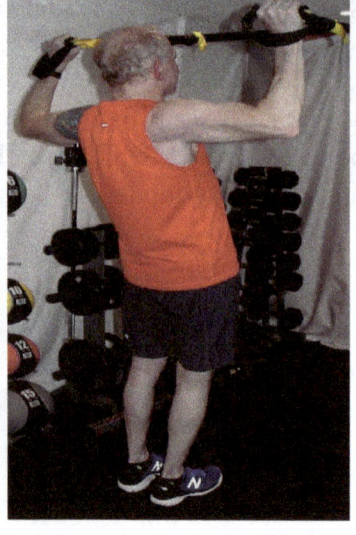

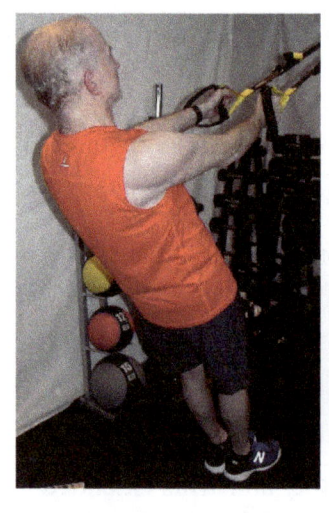

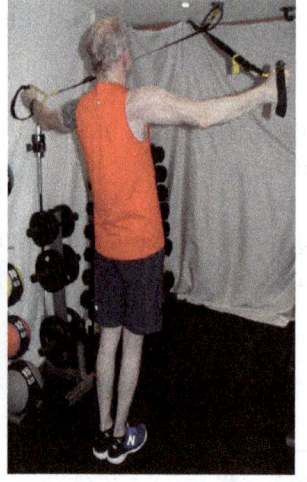

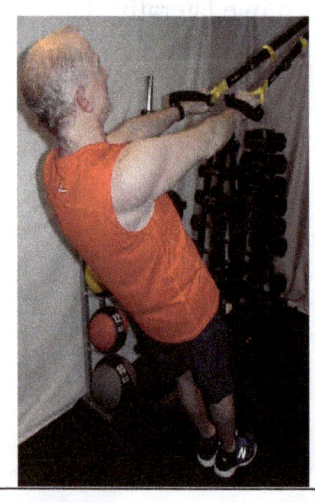

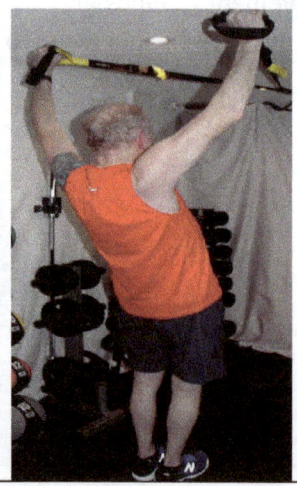

6. "I" Deltoid Flies	Start - Hands pronated and arms extended in front of chest

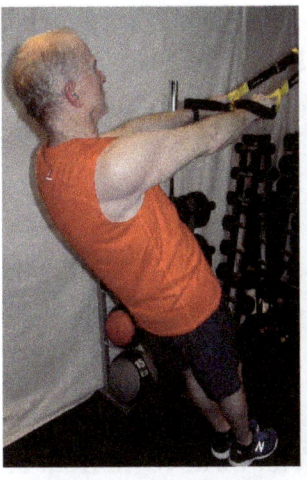

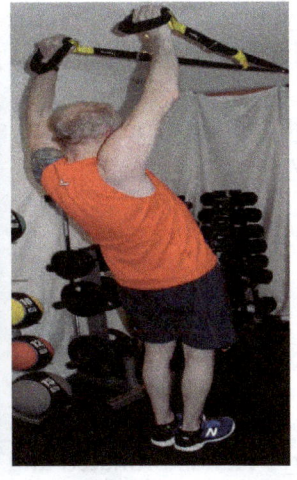

Movement - Lift hands/arms directly over the head to a vertical position. Keep elbows as straight as possible. |
| **7. Split "I" Deltoid Flies** | Start - Hands pronated and arms extended in front of chest

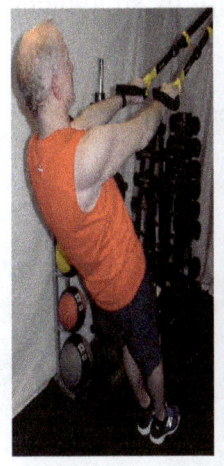

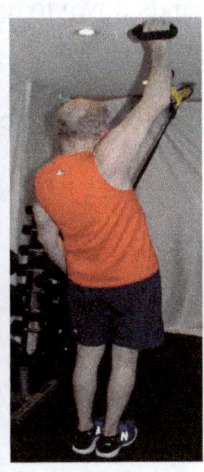

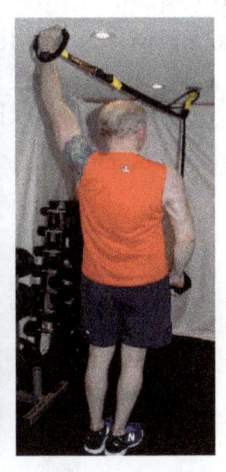

Movement – One arm raises directly over the head and the other moves downward to hip level. Keep the elbows as straight as possible. |
| **Arms:** | |
| **Triceps: (Mid Length) – Keep elbows high** | |
| **1. Pronated or Supinated Double Arm Overhead Triceps Extensions** | Start – Lift arms up to ear level. Elbows flexed and pointing forward and hands facing upward.

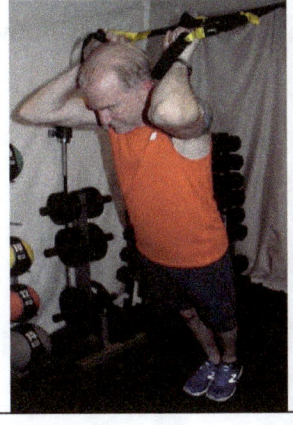

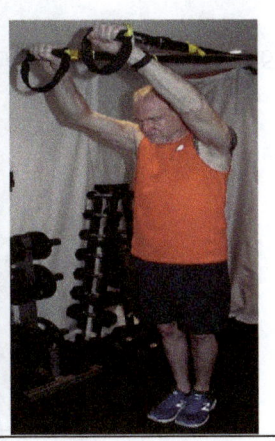

Movement – Straighten the elbows while keeping elbows high (shoulder height) and pointing straight ahead. |

2. Pronated Single Arm Overhead Triceps Extensions	<u>Start</u> - Lift one arm up to ear level. Elbow flexed and pointing forward and hand facing upward. <u>Movement</u> - Straighten the elbow while keeping elbow high (shoulder height) and pointing straight ahead. <u>Note</u> - Do not torque your shoulders or hips. They must stay square.
3. Pronated Triceps Kickbacks	<u>Start</u> - Hands pronated and elbows at 90° in front of chest. <u>Movement</u> - Move hands down to hips by straightening the elbows and shifting wt. back. <u>Note</u> - Keep arms close to side of body.
Biceps: (Mid Length) - Keep elbows High	
1. Supinated Bicep Curls	<u>Start</u> – Hands supinated and arms extended in front of shoulder. Body is leaning backwards 40°. <u>Movement</u> – Bend the elbows while keeping elbows as high as possible.

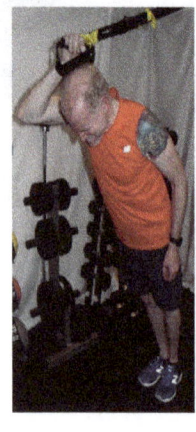

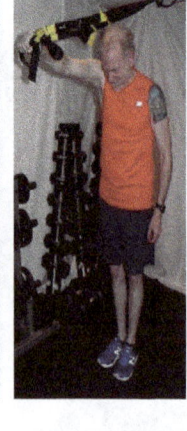

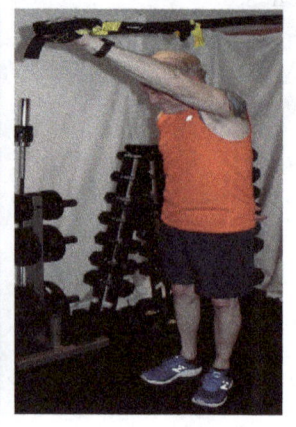

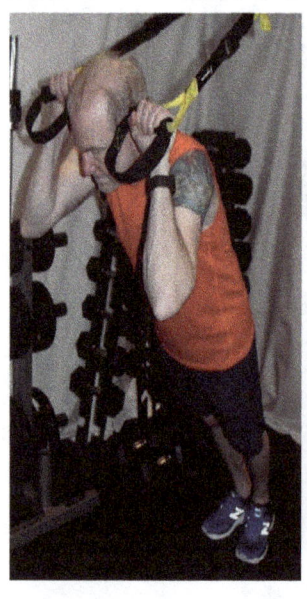

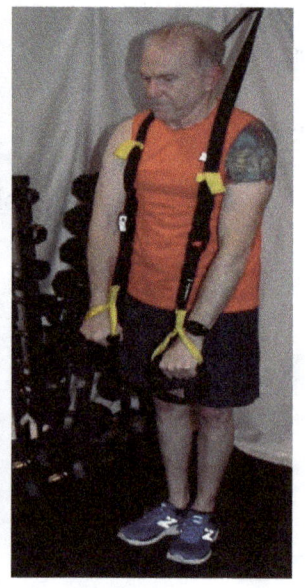

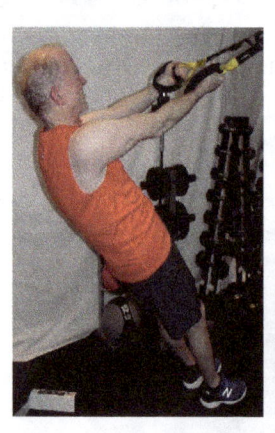

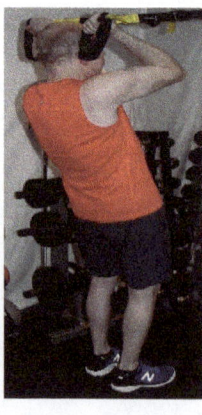

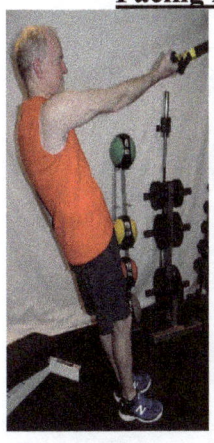

2. Single Arm Bicep Curls **Facing Anchor** 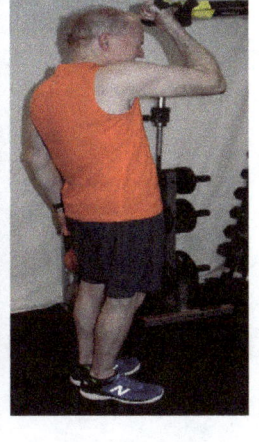	Start – One hand is supinated and arm is extended in front of shoulder. Body is leaning backwards 40º. Movement - Bend the elbow while keeping elbow as high as possible. Avoid torquing the body.

Lower Body:

Quadriceps: (Mid Length)

1. Standard Double Leg Squat	Start – Hands pronated and arms extended in front of chest. Lean backwards 40º. Movement – Bend the knees to 90º. Keep back straight & avoid leaning or rounding forward. - Keep heels on the ground. - Limit arm involvement in pulling body back to standing position. Focus on your legs doing the work.
2. Single Leg Squat	Start - Hands pronated and arms extended in front of chest. Lean backwards 40º. Lift one leg off floor. Movement - Bend the knees to 90º. Keep back straight & avoid leaning or rounding forward. - Keep heels on the ground. - Limit arm involvement in pulling body back to standing position. Focus on your legs doing the work.

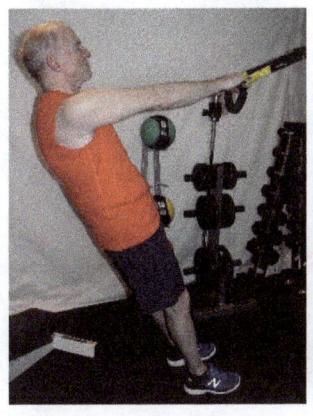

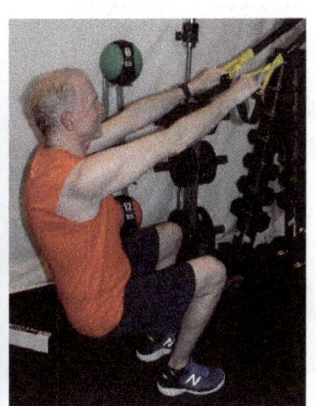

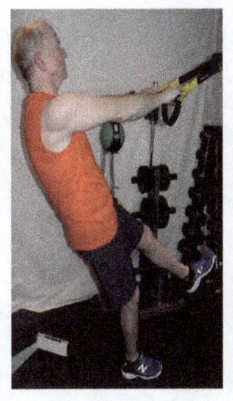

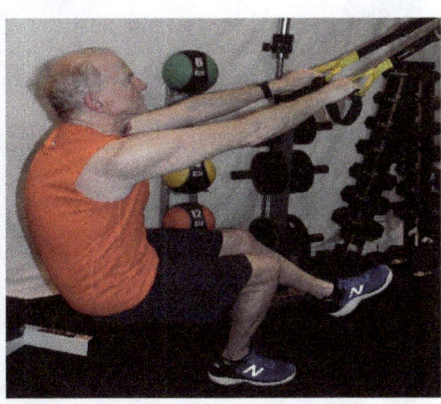

3. Lunges (Hands holding the straps)

1. Assisted Forward Lunge

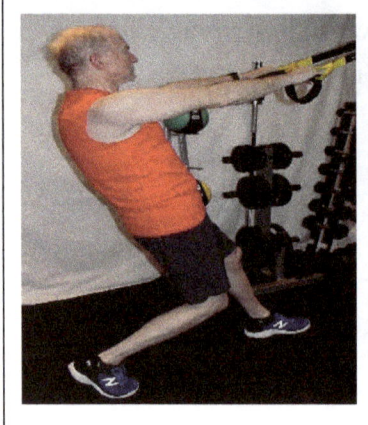

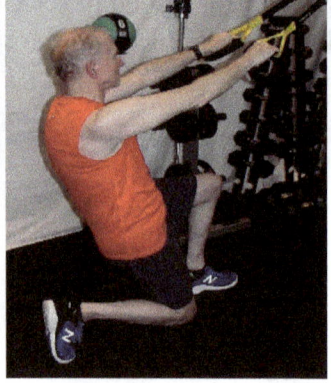

Start - Hands pronated and arms extended in front of chest. Lean backwards 40º.

Movement – Step forward and bend front knee 90º. Keep tension on strap.

2. Step Back Lunge

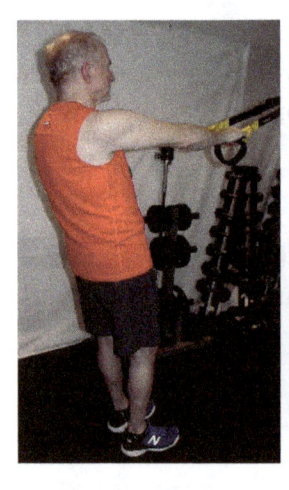

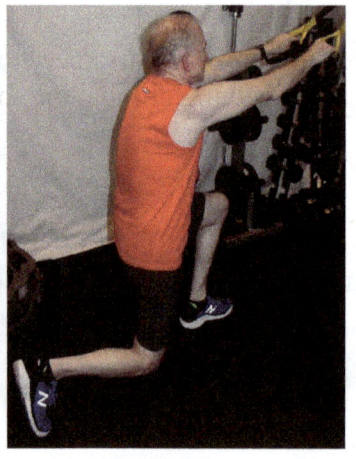

Start - Hands pronated and arms extended in front of chest. Lean backwards 40º.

Movement – Step backwards and bend front knee 90º. Keep tension on strap.

3. Balance Lunge

Leg Supported on a Bench

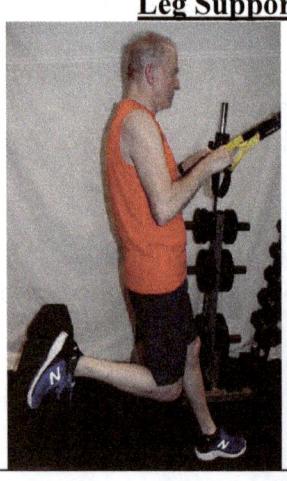

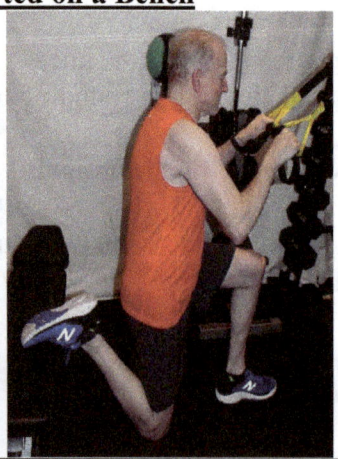

Start - Hands pronated and arms extended in front of chest. Lean backwards 40º.

Movement – Step backwards but back leg does not touch the ground. Bend front knee 90º. Keep tension on strap

Easier Modification
- The back leg can be supported on a bench.

4. Lateral Lunge	<u>Start</u> - Hands pronated and arms extended in front of chest. Lean backwards 40º. <u>Movement</u> – Step laterally (abduction) and drop down over the lateral/abducted leg. Knee bends 90º. Keep tension on strap
5. Curtsey (Back Leg Crossover) Lunge	<u>Start</u> - Hands pronated and arms extended in front of chest. Lean backwards 40º. <u>Movement</u> - Cross one leg behind the stabilizing leg and bend the front stabilizing 90º. The leg may touch the ground. Keep tension on straps for balance.
Lunges with One Foot In the Strap	
1. Standard lunge	<u>Start</u> – Stand erect with back foot in the strap <u>Movement</u> - Move leg in strap backward as you drop down on supported leg 90º.

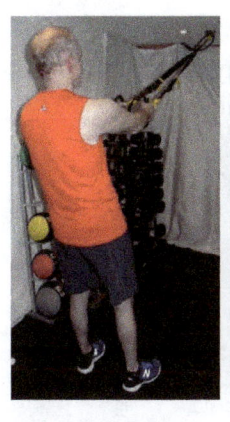

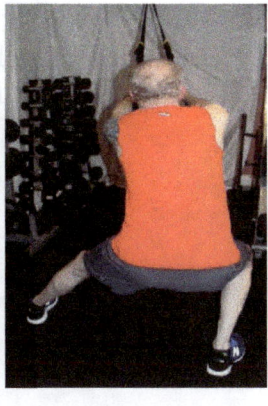

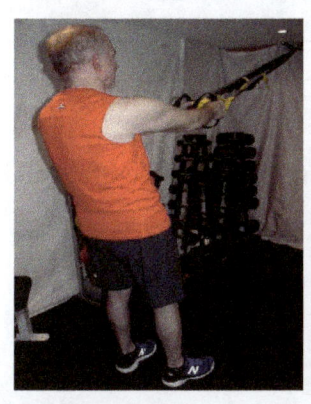

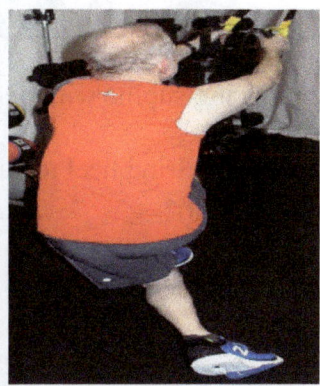

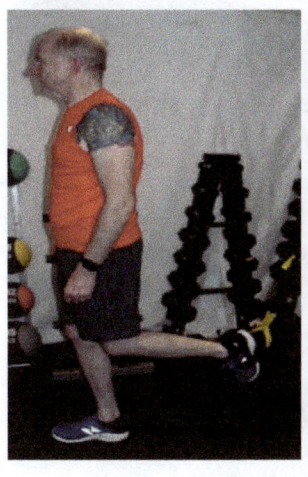

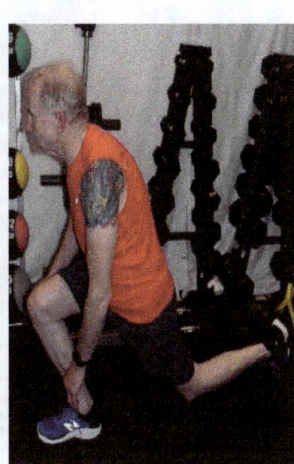

2. Lateral Lunge	Start – Face side ways to the strap and place foot in the strap
	Movement - Move leg laterally toward the anchor as you drop down on supported leg 90°.
Hamstrings: (Mid Calf Length)	
1. Hamstring Curl with Hips on Ground	Start – Lying supine with heels in the straps
	Movement - Bring heel towards glutes. Keep feet and heels together.
2. Hamstring Curl with Hips off Ground	Start – Lying supine with heels in the straps and lift hips off ground.
	Movement - Bring heel towards glutes. Keep feet and heels together. Keep hips elevated as heels move toward glutes.

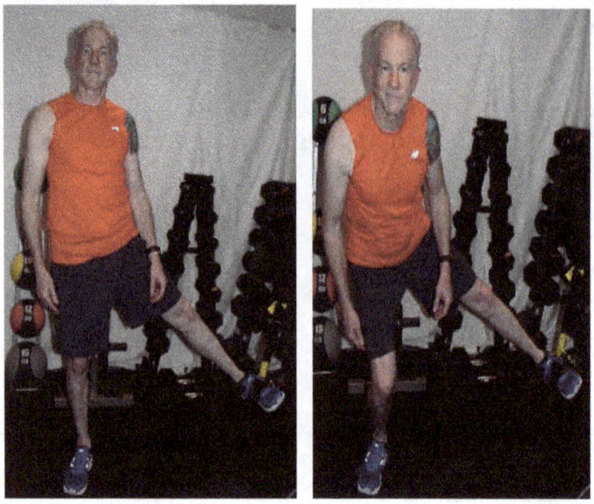

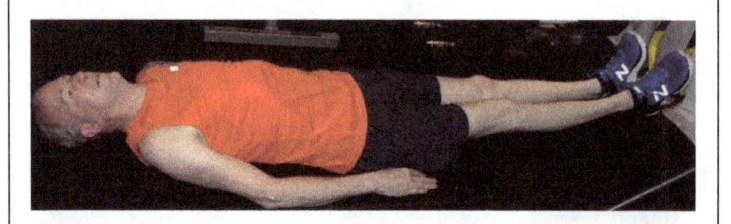

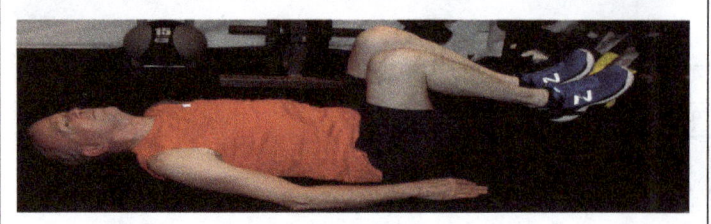

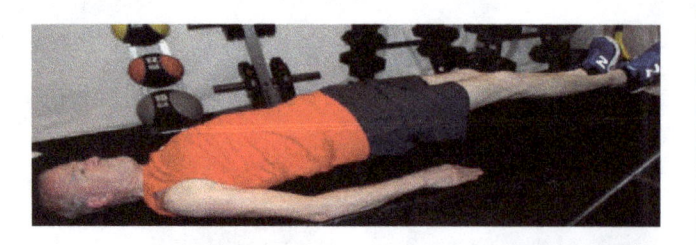

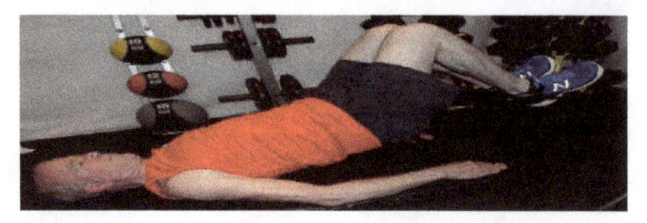

3. Hamstring Runner

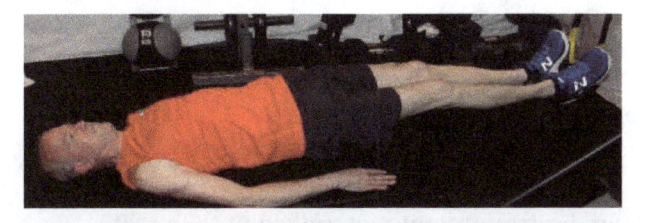

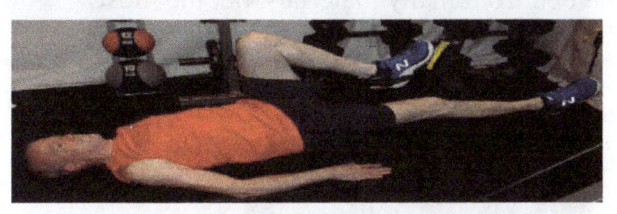

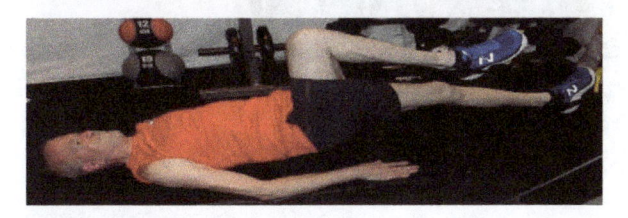

	Start – lying supine with heels in the straps and lift hips off ground. Movement – Bend one knee and bring one heel towards glutes.

Abductors: (Mid Calf Length)
1. Supine Hip Abduction

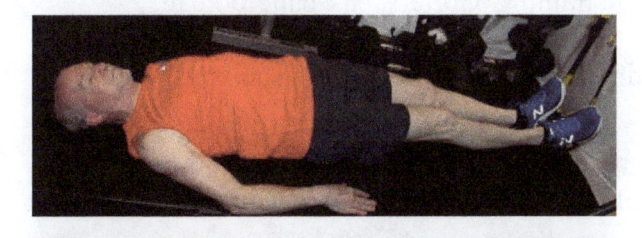

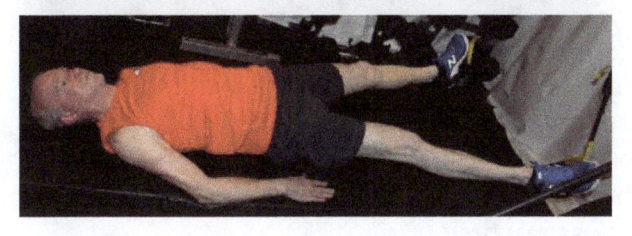

	Start - Hips off ground & hands on ground or folded over chest. Movement – Laterally move/abduct legs as wide as possible but keeps hips up off floor.

Reference

www.trxtraining.com

Appendix 9.1.9. Medicine Ball Exercises Described and Illustrated

Introduction

The medicine ball is one of the oldest and most used pieces of muscle resistance equipment. Hippocrates is said to have stuffed animal skins for patients to toss for "medicinal" purposes. Today, medicine balls come in many sizes and weights to accommodate their versatile use. There are bounce and non-bounce types and the outer shell can be from many materials, but the most common are dense rubber or polyurethane, and the insides are often stuffed with sand, gel, or just inflated with air.

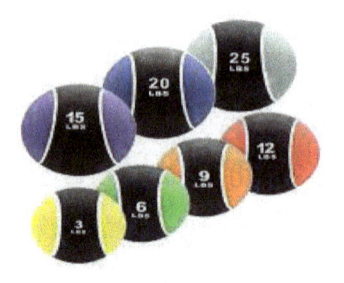

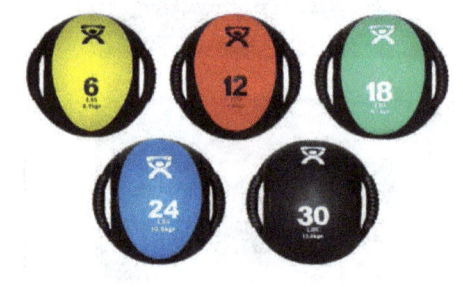

Image source: valorfitness.com   Image source: ballsnbands.com

One of the great benefits of the medicine ball is its versatility. Medicine balls are utilized for physical rehabilitation purposes and fitness and athletic training. Golfers, baseball, football, basketball, and hockey players, use medicine balls in their training because it is an excellent tool for developing the strength, power, and speed needed to excel in their respective sports.

The older adult can use the medicine balls safely because they come in various weights and are easy to hold. The outer material is usually made of non-slip material. Some medicine balls even come with handles to facilitate ease of use.

A large variety of exercises can be done to accommodate a whole-body workout with the medicine ball. A person can do many of these exercises with a partner to enhance agility, balance, and coordination training. Pick a medicine ball that's heavy enough to slow the motion (slower than if you weren't using any weight at all), but the medicine ball can not be so heavy to compromise control and range of motion. Always think safety first!
Utilizing a medicine ball is a great way to enhance fitness training and add variety to a person's workout routine.

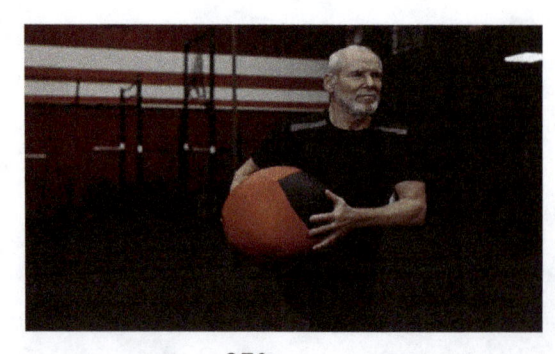

Medicine Ball Exercises Described and Illustrated

Core

1. Abdominal Crunch 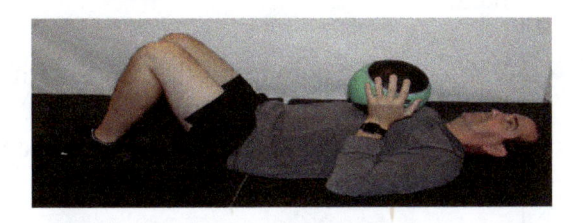 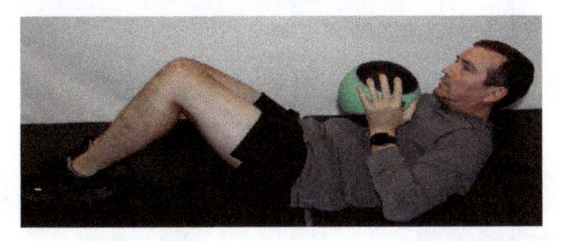	1. Lying on mat with knees bent 90º. 2. Medicine ball is close and in front of chest or extended out in front of chest (advanced). 3. Lift shoulder blades off mat to perform a crunch. 4. Return shoulder blades back to mat and repeat.
2. Arms Extended in Front of Chest Full Sit-Up 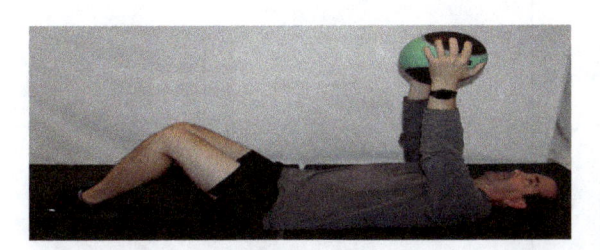 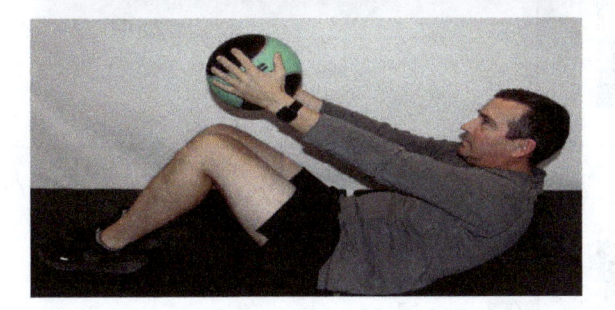	1. Lie on mat with knees bent 90º. 2. Extend your arms and hold medicine ball over your head. 3. Lift shoulders off mat as far as possible and lift/move medicine ball to touch the knees. Try to keep the arms as extended as best as possible. 4. Return shoulder blades back to mat and medicine to position above the head with arms extended.

3. "V" Sit-ups **Knees Bent** **Knees Straight**	1. Lie flat on your back, legs extended. 2. Reach the arms in front of chest or overhead with a medicine ball in both hands. 3. Engage the core to lift the hands with the medicine ball and feet at the same time so the body forms a "V". Try to keep the knees as straight as possible. 4. Return to starting position.
4. Oblique Crunch	1. Lying on mat with knees bent 90º. 2. Medicine ball is close and in front of chest or extended out in front of chest (advanced) 3. Lift shoulder blades off mat at a diagonal to perform an oblique crunch. 4. Return shoulder blades back to mat and repeat in the opposite direction.

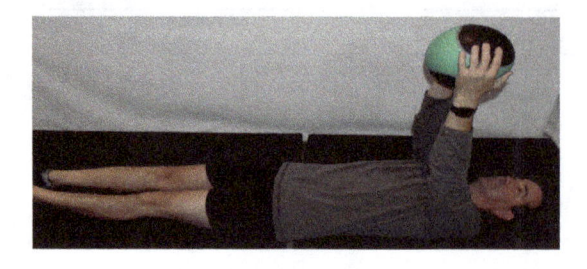

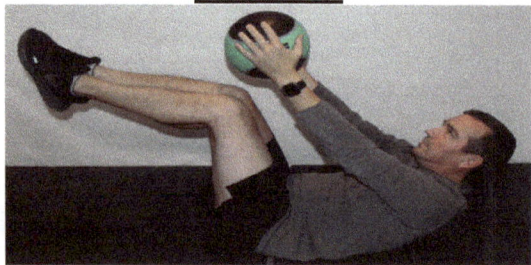

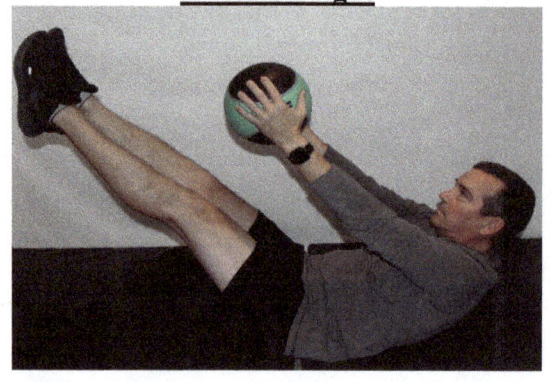

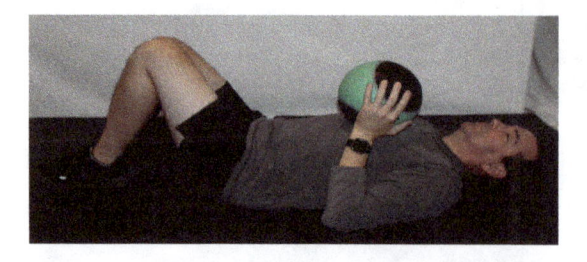

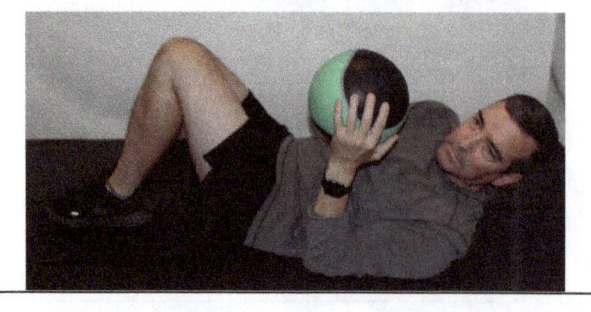

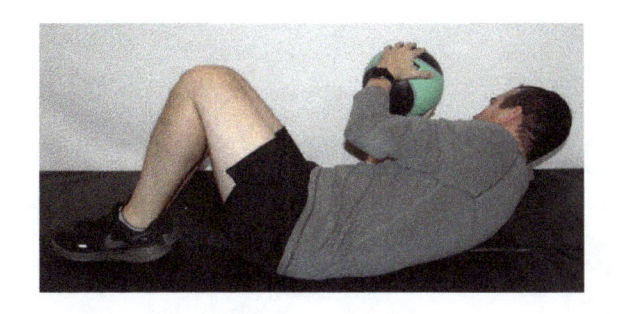

5. Sitting Russian Twist

Arms Bent

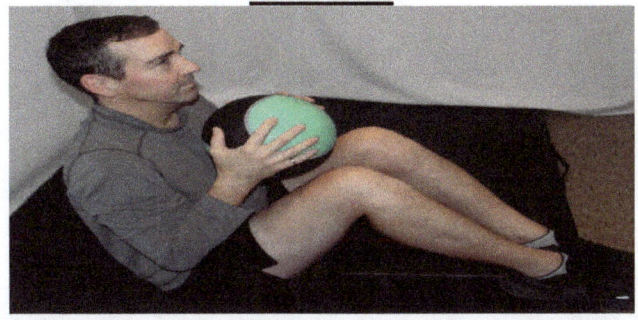

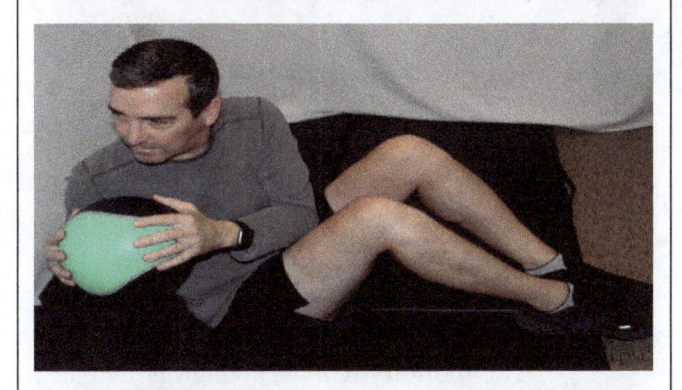

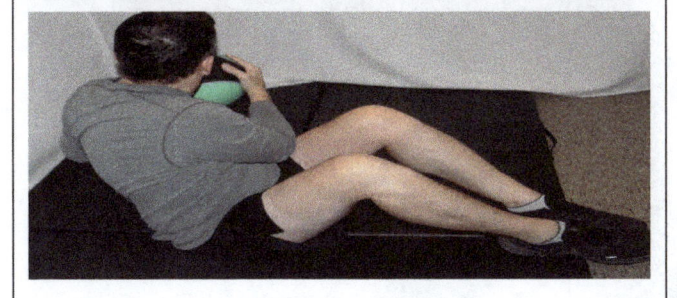

1. Sit with the knees bent 45º and legs together. The medicine ball is held in front of the chest.

2. Keep the head in line with the spine, engage the core and lean back at a 45-degree angle.

3. Rotate shoulders to one side and then the other while keeping the medicine ball close to the chest.
or
rotate the chest and shoulders and touch the medicine ball to the floor beside your hips (large rotation) by extending the medicine ball out slightly from the chest

4. Repeat by rotating to the other side.

Arms Extended

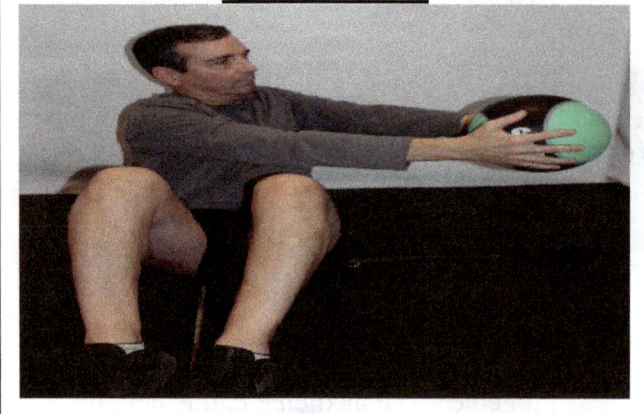

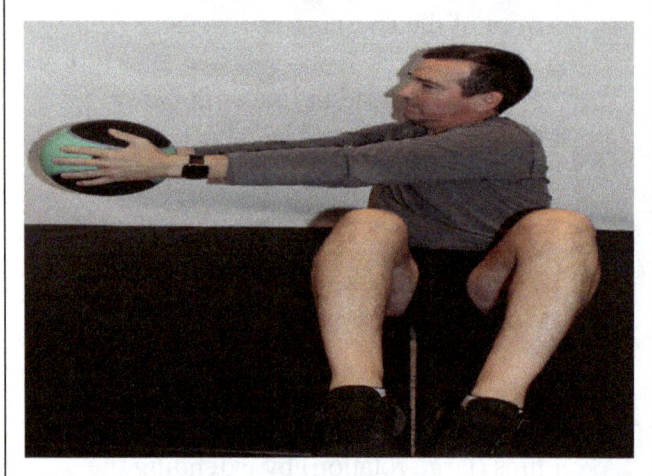

6. Standing Russian Twist

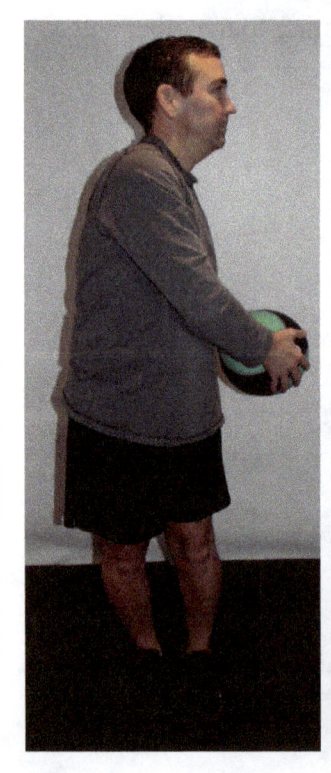

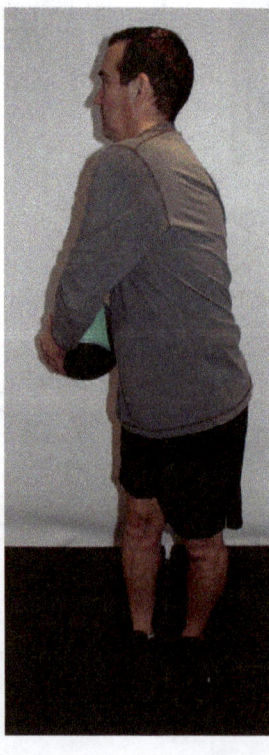

1. Standing with your feet shoulder width apart.

2. The ball is held at waist level just behind your left hip.

3. The motion involves swinging the ball across your body to the opposite side.

4. The move is then repeated in the opposite direction.

5. The abdominals are engaged and tight throughout the movement.

7. Standing, Kneeling or Sitting Woodchopper **Kneeling** **Sitting**	1. Standing or kneeling upright or sitting on stability ball. 2. Start with ball on the floor beside you. 3. Bend over to lift the ball diagonally to chest level or above the head on the opposite side (advanced). 4. Return to starting position and repeat all reps on same side before doing the exercise on the opposite side or diagonally drop ball down to opposite side and repeat.

8. Standing Figure 8's **Start** **Down to left knee**	- Stand upright the ball is held above your left shoulder at approximately the same level as your ear with arms extended.
	
	- The ball is moved in a figure eight motion by:
	
	  1. Taking the ball from the right ear diagonally across the body toward your left knee (similar to the diagonal wood chop)
	
	  2. Move ball up to your right ear
	
	  3. Move ball across to left ear
	
	  4. Diagonally move ball down toward your right knee/foot.

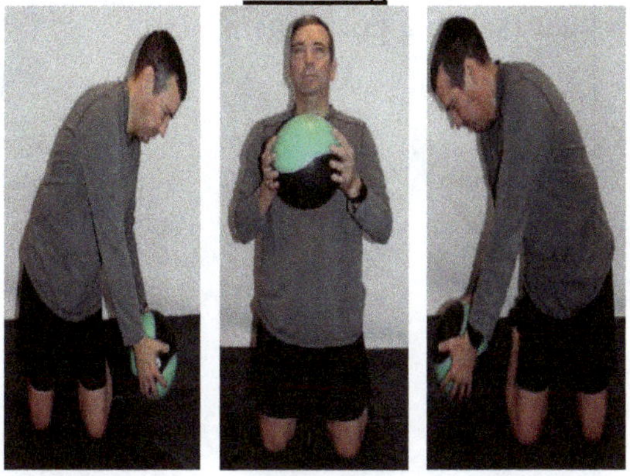

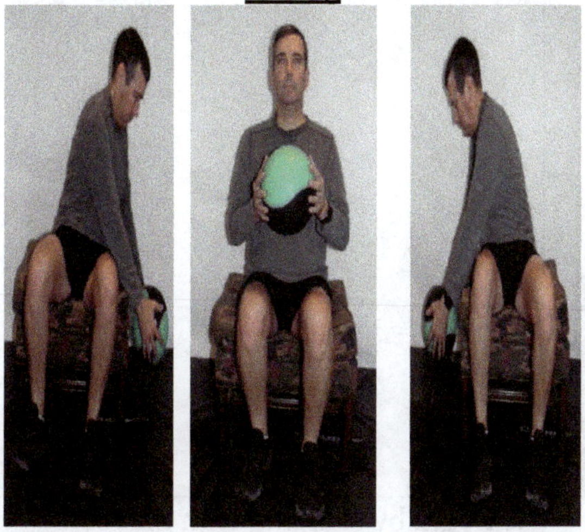

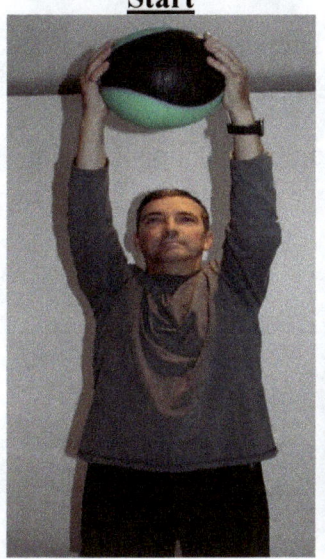

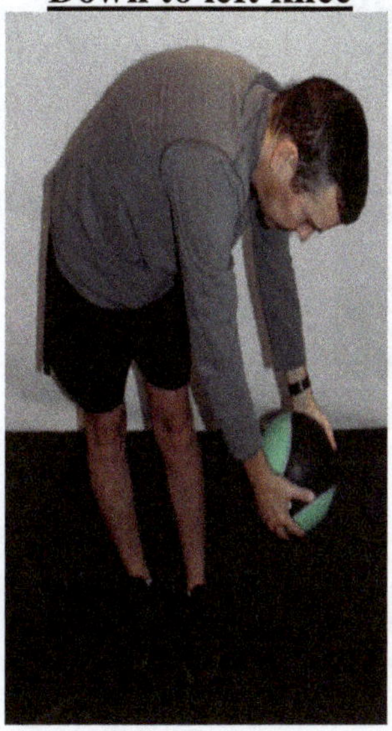

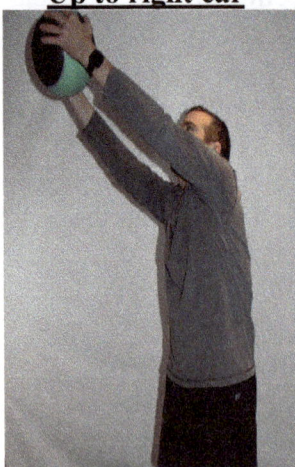

Up to right ear | **Over to left ear**

Down to right knee | **Over to left knee**

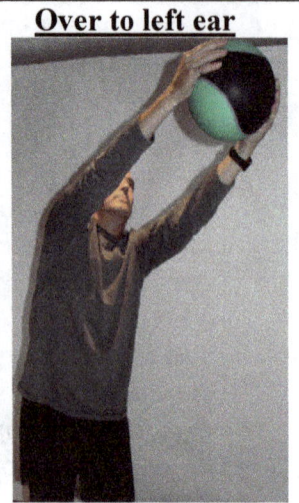

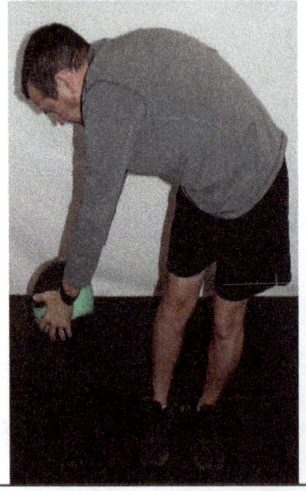

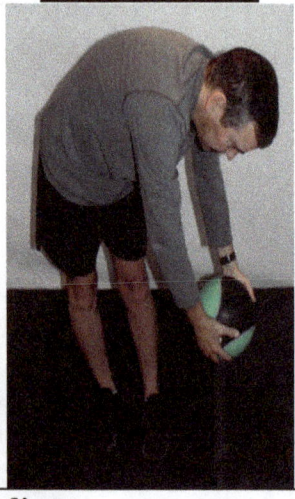

5. Move ball across to left knee/foot.

6. Diagonally move ball back to right ear (starting position)

9. Standing Lateral Bending

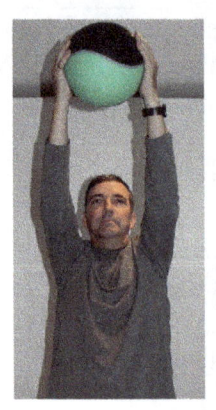

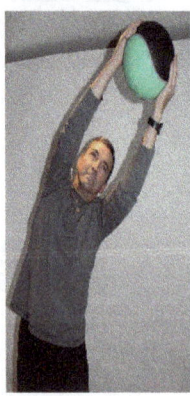

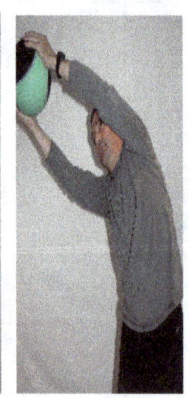

1. Begin by standing with the feet shoulder width apart. The medicine ball held over head with the elbows nearly locked.

2. Move the ball laterally to one side with the waist bending slightly.

3. Repeat by bending to the opposite side.

10. Back Extension Pass	1. Lie face down with your arms and legs extended.
	2. Spread the arms out wide into a "Y" position.
	3. Place the medicine ball close to one hand.
	4. Lift your chest off the floor. (<u>Advanced</u> - lift thighs off floor at same time)
	5. Roll the ball from one hand to the other and then pass it back again.
	6. Repeat passing the ball from one hand to the other while keeping the back in an extended position (chest or chest and legs) off the floor)

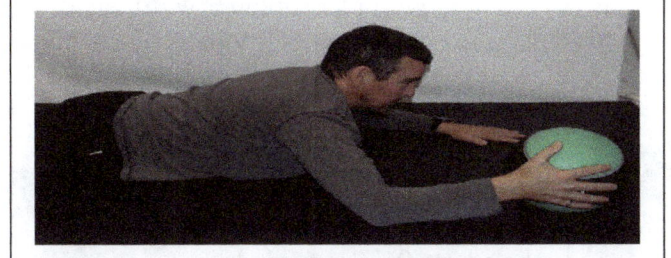

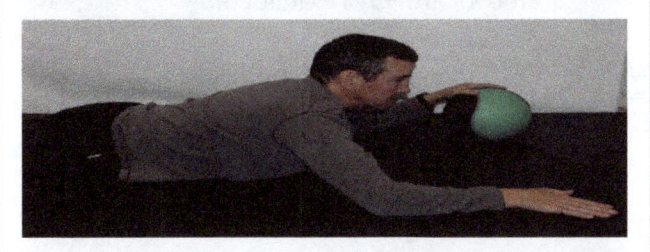

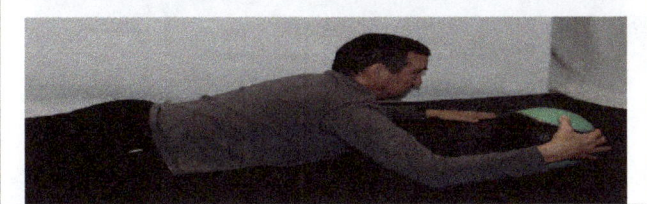

Shoulders

1. Standing or Sitting Overhead Chest Press	1. Standing or sitting on stability ball.
	2. Hold medicine ball in front of face.
	3. Extend arms straight above the head until arms are 95% extended.
	4. Return medicine ball to starting position.
2. Anterior Raise	1. Standing with medicine ball at waist level. Arms extended.
	2. While the arms are extended, the medicine ball is lifted to chest level.
	3. Return medicine ball to start position.

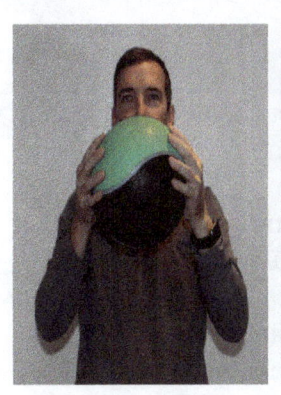

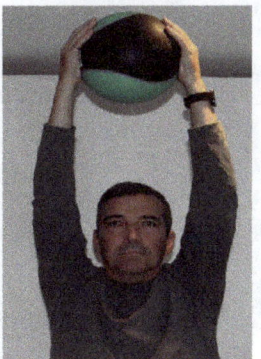

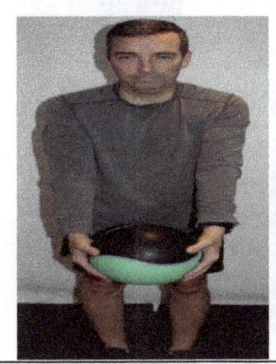

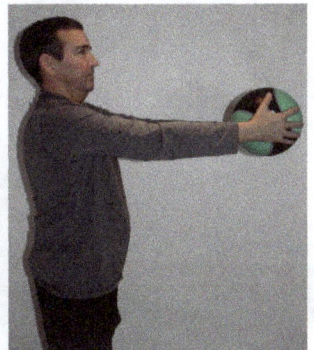

Chest

1. Standing, Sitting or Lying Chest Press

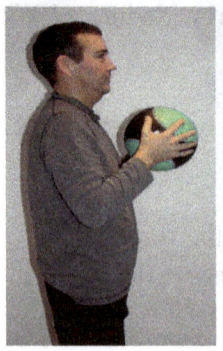

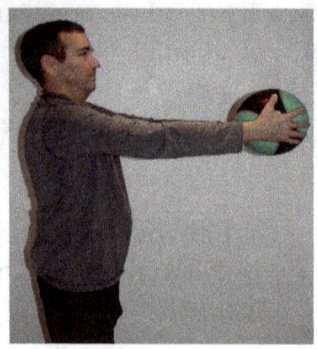

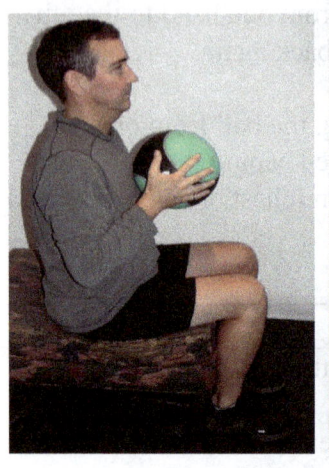

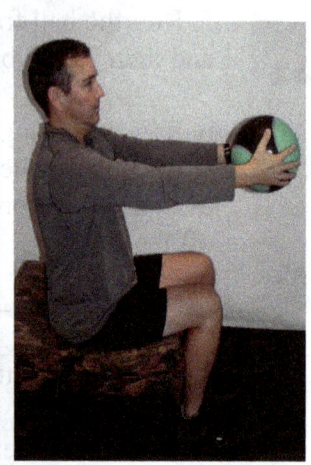

1. Stand with feet shoulder width apart or lying down on stability ball or bench.

2. Hold a medicine ball at chest level with the elbows flexed.

3. The ball is pushed straight ahead until elbows are 95% extended.

4. Return ball back to the chest.

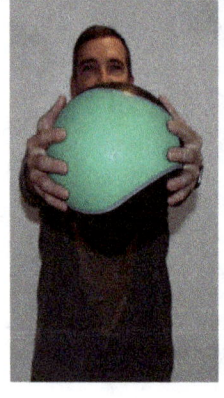

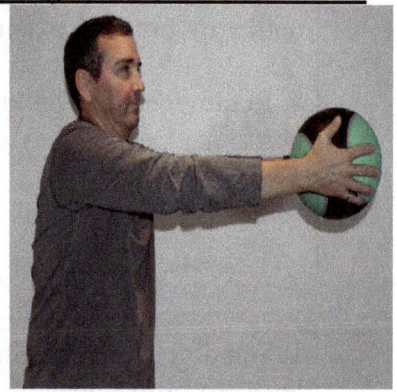

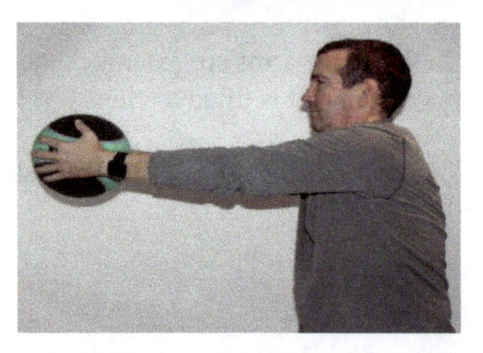

2. Standing or Sitting Rotational Chest Press

1. Stand with feet shoulder width apart or lying down on stability ball or bench.

2. Hold a medicine ball with both hands, elbows flexed at chest level.

3. Push the ball straight ahead until elbows are 95% extended.

4. Rotate to one side with arms extended

5. Return to centre and return ball to chest.

6. Push ball straight ahead a second time and then rotate the opposite direction.

7. Return to centre and repeat.

3. Lying Alternating Chest Fly	1. Lying on stability ball or bench. 2. Hold medicine ball in one hand as you extend arms out to side at shoulder height. 3. Keep the arm extended and raise the ball vertically to above the chest. 4. Let the opposite hand take the ball and it then drops vertically to a horizontal position at head level. 5. Repeat.
4. Push-ups (One hand on Medicine Ball) 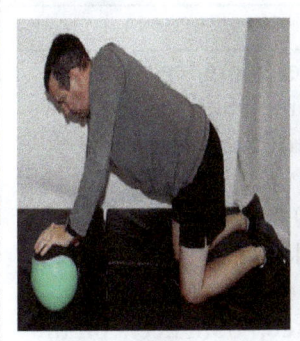 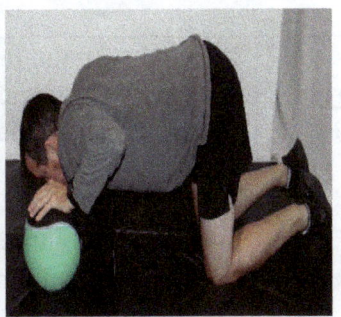 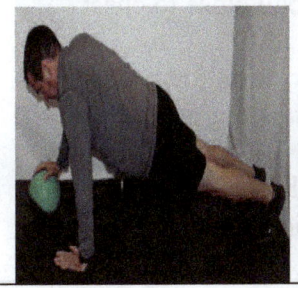 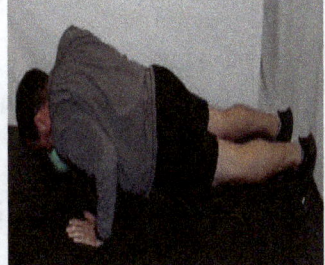	1. Begin in the Push-Up position (on your knees or toes) with one hand on the floor and the medicine beneath the other hand. 2. With one hand on the medicine ball, perform a push-up.

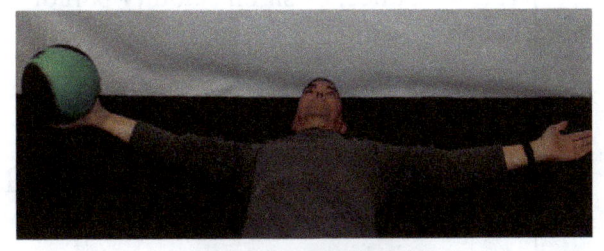

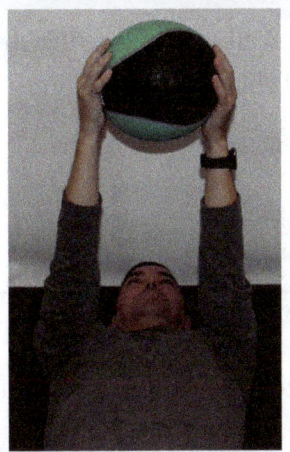

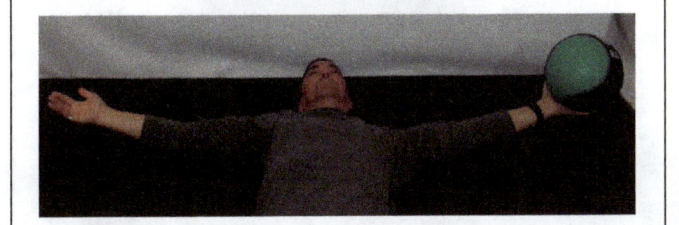

Arms	
1. Standing, kneeling or sitting Triceps Extensions	1. Stand, kneel or sit on stability ball or bench. 2. Hold medicine ball behind your head. 3. Extend the elbows so the medicine ball is raised directly over your head. 4. Bend elbows and return the medicine ball to starting position
2. Standing Biceps Curls 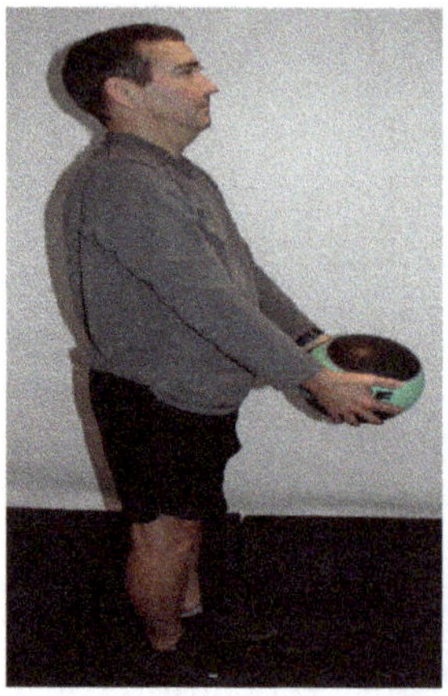 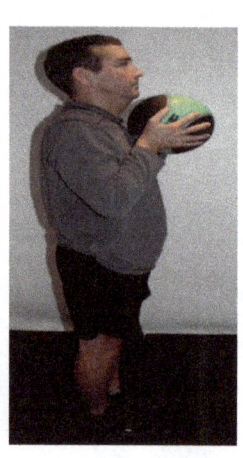	1. Stand upright. 2. Hold the medicine ball in front of the hips. 3. Bend the elbows and lift the medicine ball to chest level. 4. Extend the elbows and return the medicine ball to starting position
Legs and Hips	
1. Squat **Squat with Chest Press** 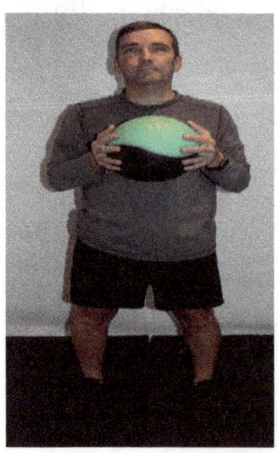 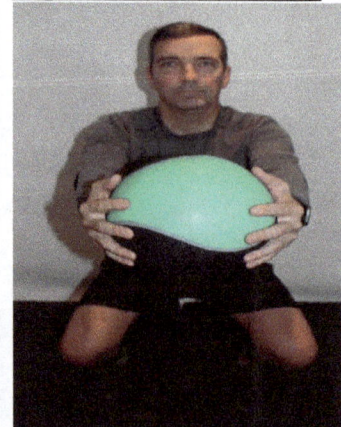	1. Stand with the feet shoulder width apart. Hold a medicine ball close (elbows flexed) and in front of the chest. 2. Flex the knees 90 degree while lowering the buttocks. (Pretend you are sitting down onto a chair). - It is important to keep both heels on the floor and keep the ball close to chest. 3. Hold the squat position for 1-2 seconds, then return to the standing position. Advanced – Do a chest press or overhead press with the medicine ball as you do a squat.

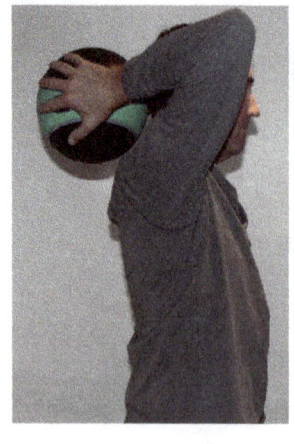

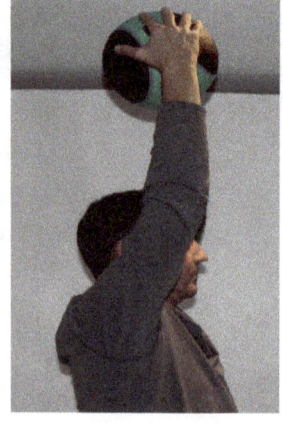

2. Lunges
1. Forward Lunge

Lunge with Chess Press

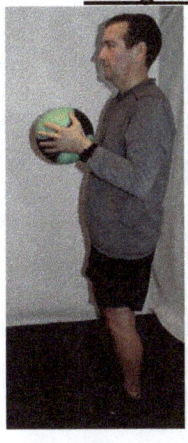

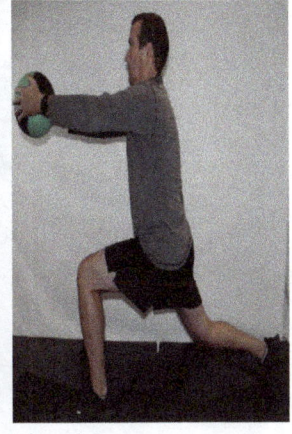

2. Backward Lunge

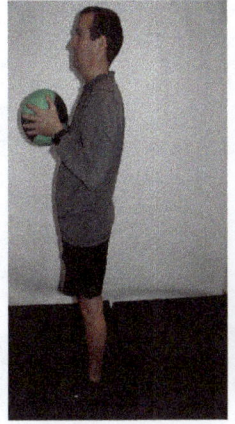

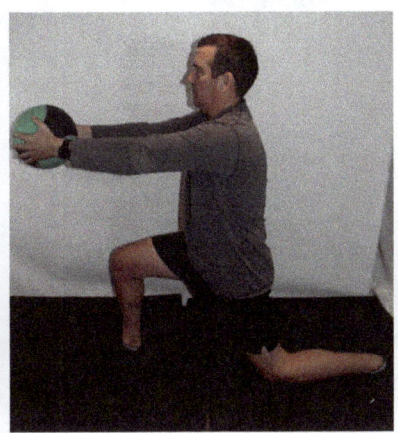

3. Lateral Lunge

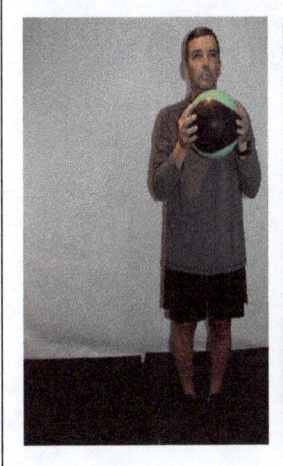

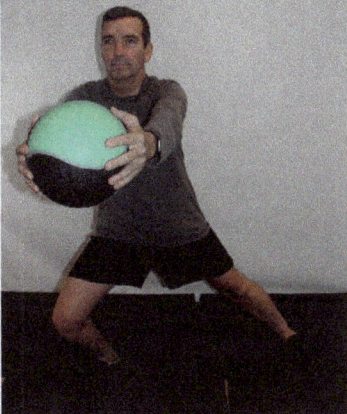

Forward Lunge:

1. Begin with the medicine ball held at chest level.

2. Step forward with one leg and lower yourself until the top of the front leg (thigh) is parallel to the floor (Knee bent 90º).
- Do not allow your lead knee to extend past the toes of the lead foot to avoid injury to the knee.

3. Repeat the movement with the opposite leg.

Advanced – when in a lunged position you incorporate a chest press, overhead press or twist to the lunge leg side

Backward Step Lunge

1. Start with the medicine ball held at chest level.

2. Take a step backward with one leg and lower yourself until the top of your leg (thigh) is parallel to the floor (Knee bent 90º). Do not allow the knee to extend pass the toes to avoid injury.

Advanced – when in a lunged position you incorporate a chest press, overhead press or twist to the lunge leg side

3. Repeat the movement with the opposite leg.

Lateral Lunge

1. The medicine ball held chest level.

2. One leg is moved laterally with its foot pointing out at a 45º angle. Lower yourself until the top of your leg (thigh) is parallel to the floor (Knee bent 90º). Do not allow your knee to extend past your toes to avoid injury to the knee.

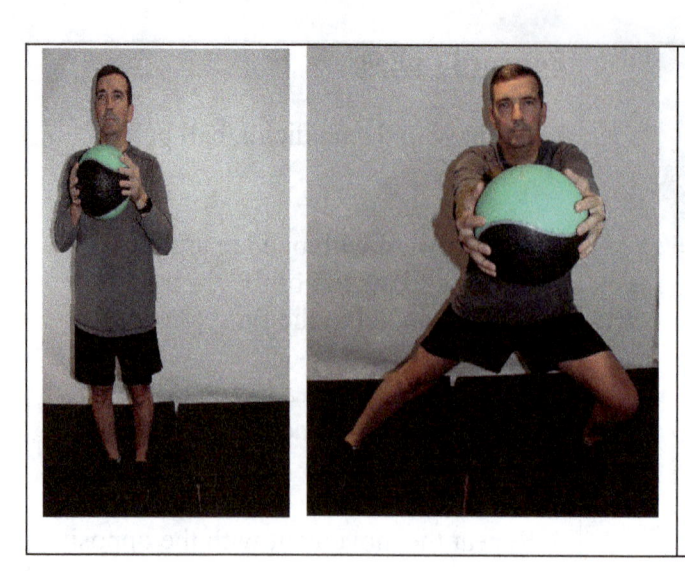

Advanced – when in a lunged position you incorporate a chest press, overhead press or twist to the lunge leg side

3. Repeat the movement with the opposite leg.

Reference

www.nfpt.com/blog/the-power-of-medicine-ball-training

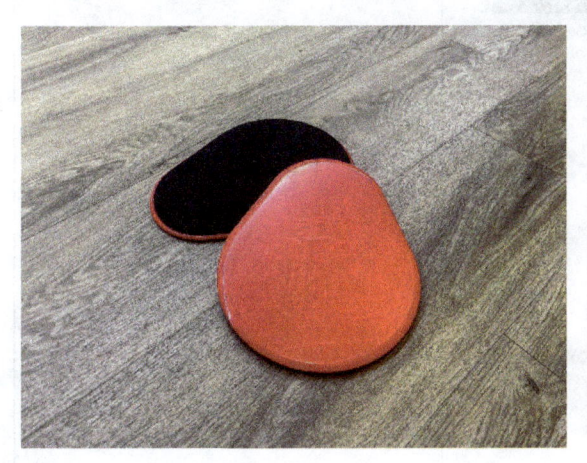

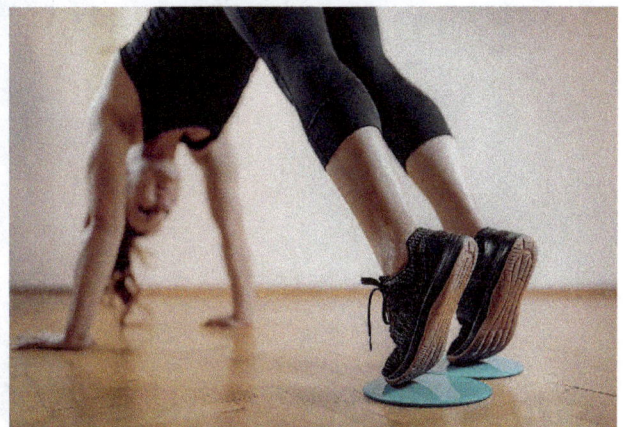

Appendix 9.1.10. Floor Slider Exercises Described and Illustrated

Introduction

Floor slider exercises are an advanced and intense type of movement/resistance exercises. To perform these exercises safely and correctly requires a moderate level of pre-existing strength, agility, balance and coordination. For anyone, and especially the older adult, who has this level of fitness, floor slider exercises are excellent at stimulating the musculature and neurological systems to improve a person's strength, agility, balance and coordination even further. For the older adult, this is important for fall prevention.

Floor slider exercises introduce instability into each movement and a person's body weight is the resistance stimulus. Floor slider exercises work the core and glutes/buttocks muscles during every move.

For safety, the floor slider movements need to be done slowly and under control. Because floor slider exercises are an advanced exercise, once a person feels fatigued, they should stop the exercise. Floor slider exercises are a dynamic type and once fatigue sets in, the proprioceptive system will not be as responsive to movement, which creates a higher probability of injury.

Once a person becomes proficient at using floor sliders, they can increase the speed of performing the exercise to increase intensity of the exercise and the cardiovascular training associated with the exercise.

Because of the increased difficulty of doing these exercises, performing them as illustrated and described in the table below is very important. Progressing "slow and easy" is necessary for safe performance and to obtain optimal results.

Floor Slider Exercises Described and Illustrated

Core	
1. Double Knee Tuck	1. Begin in the high plank position (on hands and toes) with both feet on sliders. 2. <u>Motion</u> - Pull knees in to touch chest and then back to extended high plank position. 3. The core is engaged and tight though out the movement. 4. The hips stay relatively flat.
2. Single-Leg Tuck (Mountain Climber)	1. Begin in high plank position. 2. <u>Motion</u> - Pull one knee into chest and return to extended leg position 3. Slide opposite leg to chest, then push back to extended position.

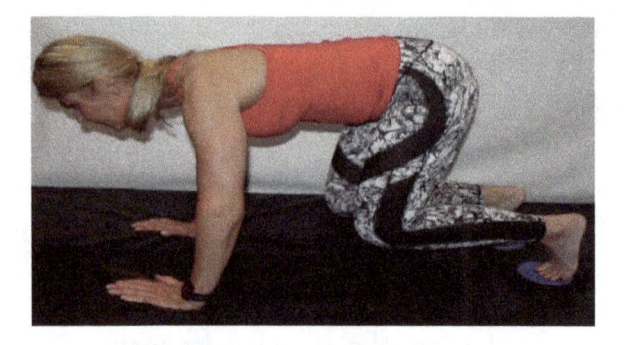

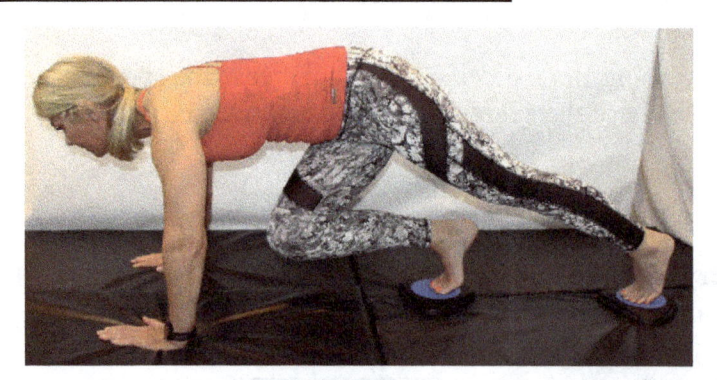

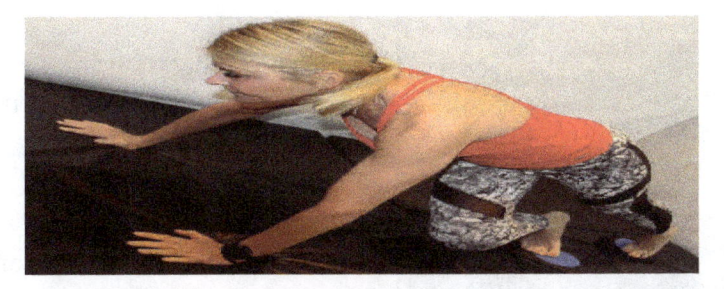

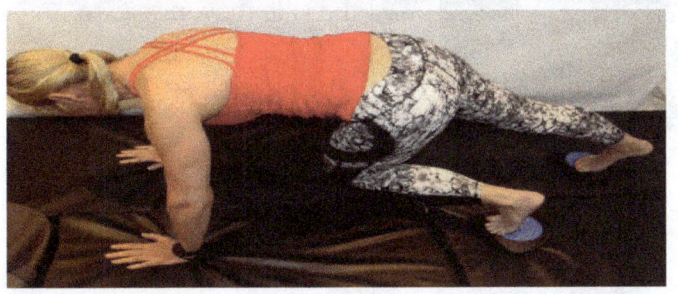

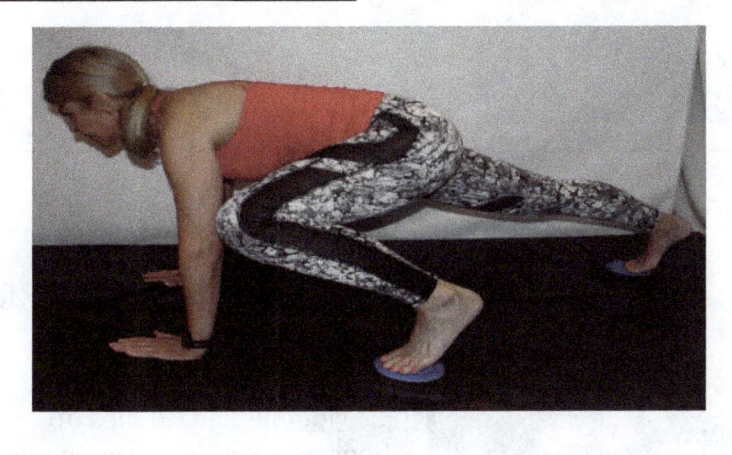

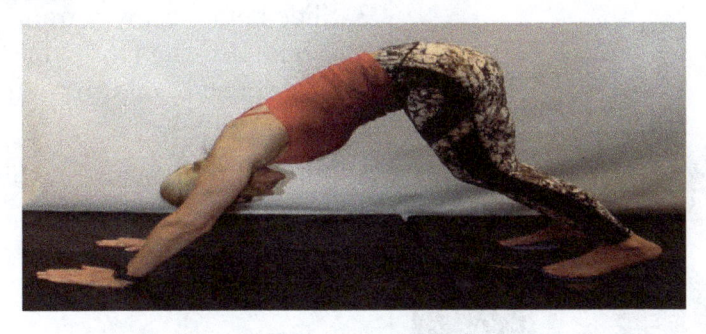

3. Cross Mountain Climber	1. Begin in high plank position.
	2. <u>Motion</u> - Pull one knee across the body into the opposite side chest.
	3. Return to starting position and repeat with the opposite leg.
4. Wide Mountain Climber	1. Begin in high plank position.
	2. <u>Motion</u> - Pull one leg straight forward and to the outside of the same side arm.
	3. Push leg back to starting position, and repeat on other side.
	4. It is important to keep the core engaged
	5. This movement is useful in opening the hips.
5. Pike	1. Begin in the high plank.
	2. <u>Motion</u> - Pike/lift hips toward the ceiling, pulling feet in toward hand,
	3. Slide feet back to return to high plank position and repeat.
	4. To do this motion properly the core must be fully engaged.

| **6 Side to Side Knee Tuck** | 1. Begin in high plank position.

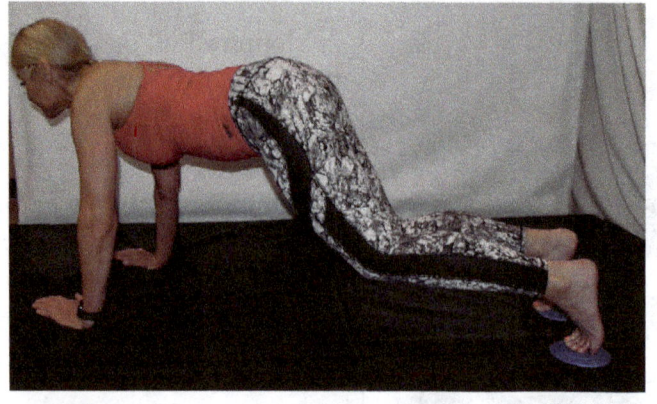

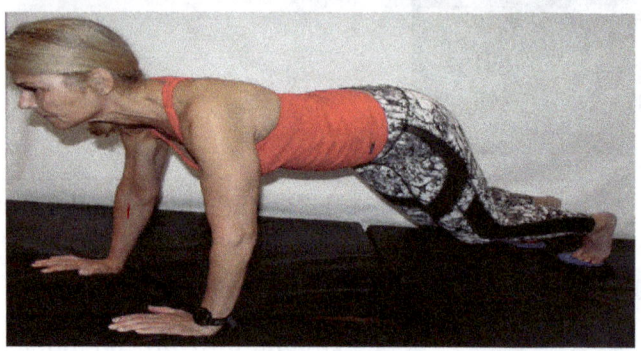

2. <u>Motion</u> - Slightly bring knees in toward chest and then slide both feet to one side.

3. The goal is to finish with both feet outside of the hand on the side they moved to.

4. Slide feet to opposite side. |
|---|---|
| **Lower Body** | |
| **1. Supine Reverse Tuck** | 1. Begin by lying face up (supine) with both feet/heels on sliders and knees bent 45º.

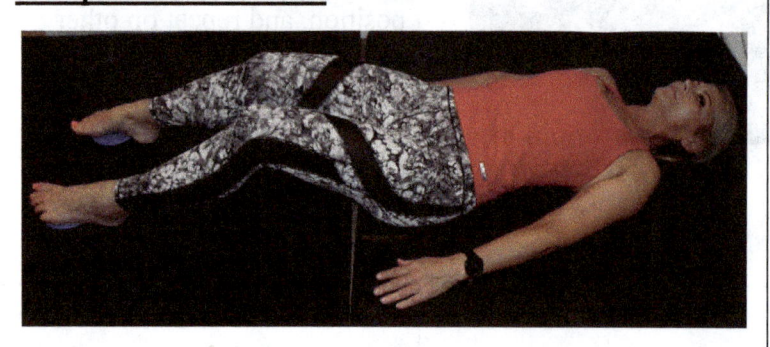

2. <u>Motion</u> - and lift hips off floor into a bridge position by engaging the glutes (buttocks) and hamstrings.

3. Slide both feet away from your butt, keeping hips in the same elevated bridge position.

3. Pull feet back in to 45º while keeping the hips lifted in the bridge position throughout.

4. Repeat.

(<u>Easier Modification</u> – One foot slides forward at a time) |

2. Backward Step Lunge

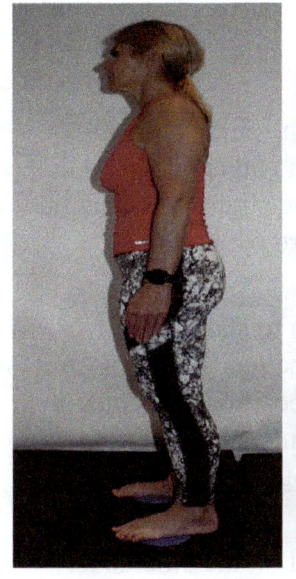

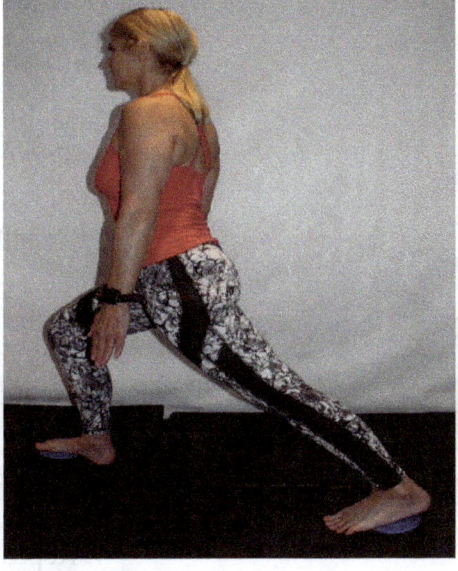

1. Begin by standing with both feet on sliders.

2. <u>Motion</u> - Slide one leg back while the opposite knee bends into a low lunge position.

3. Push down and straighten the forward bent knee while pulling the opposite back leg to the starting position.

4. Repeat on the other side.

(<u>Easier Modification</u> – No slider from under the foot of forward foot that is bending. This will increase your stability).

3. Lateral Lunge

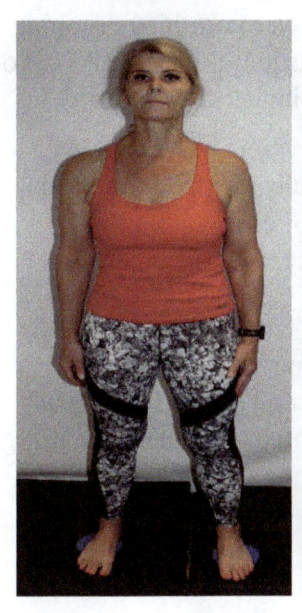

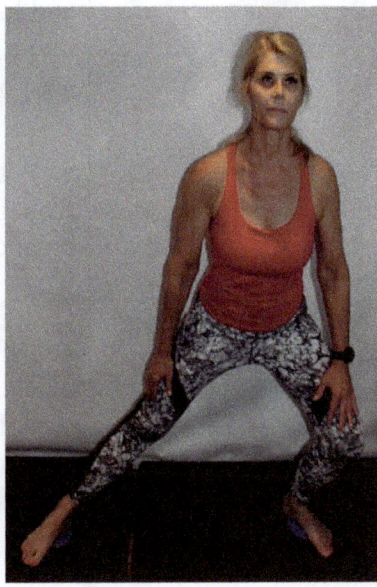

1. Begin by standing, with both feet on sliders.

2. <u>Motion</u> - Slide one foot laterally while keeping the lateral moving leg extended

3. The opposite knee slightly bends into a lunge position

<u>Note</u> - Move the one leg as far lateral as you can while balancing most of your weight on the opposite (slightly bent) leg.

4. Straighten by pulling the lateral foot back toward you to the starting standing position. The opposite knee straightens as you pull the lateral leg back.

5. Repeat on the other side.

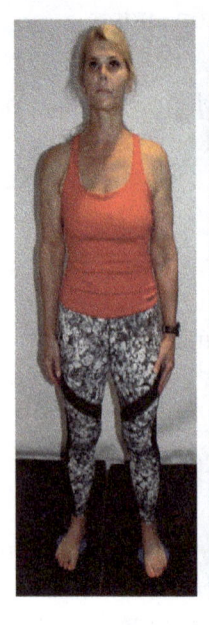

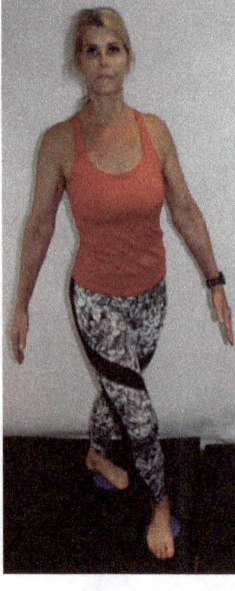

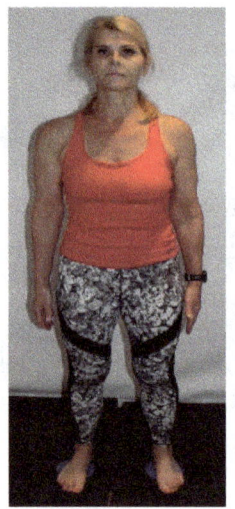

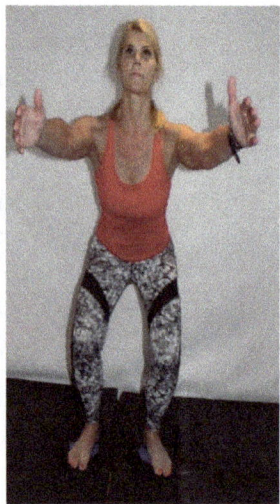

4. Curtsy Lunge	1. Begin with both feet on sliders, knees slightly bent and hips slightly flexed (as if you were just starting to lower into a squat). 2. <u>Motion</u> - Slide one foot behind the other and bend the front knee slightly. (Come into a low curtsy lunge.) 3. Return to start position by sliding the rear foot back so it is starting position. (Keeping the knees bent and hip flexed throughout this motion). 4. Repeat on the other side.
5. Squat	1. Begin by standing with both feet on the sliders. 2. <u>Motion</u> - Bend your knees and lower your hips dropping into a squat position. (As if you are going to sit in a chair). 3. You can extend your arms in front of chest to help with balance. 4. Using your hamstrings, quads and glutes (buttocks), straighten your legs to starting position.

Upper Body	
1. Arm Forward Slide	1. Begin in a kneeling position with both hands on the sliders. (If there is any knee sensitivity, use a towel or mat under your knees). 2. <u>Motion</u> - Slide both arms forward at once, trying to get your chest as close to the ground as possible. (The core must be fully engaged to support this movement) 3. Slide the arms back toward the chest and repeat. <u>Harder modification</u> – Start from a high plank position (on your toes rather than on your knees). <u>Easier Modification</u> –Slide each arm forward separately.

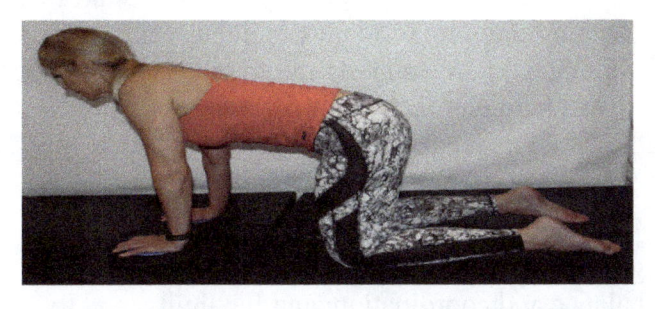

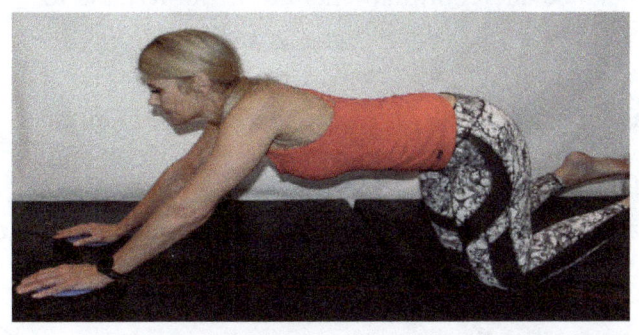

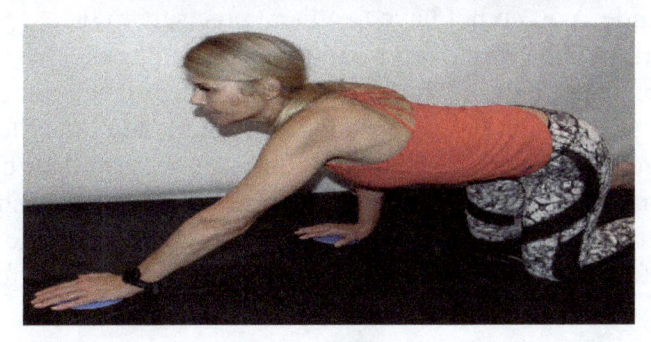

Sample Workout

Each movement is done for 45 seconds, followed by a rest of 15 seconds. Start by completing one round of the entire circuit and then as your fitness improves complete 2 and then 3 sets.

1. Double Knee Tuck
2. Wide Mountain Climber
3. Supine Reverse Tuck
4. Lateral Lunge
5. Squat
6. Double Arm Forward slide
7. Single Arm Forward Slide

Reference
www.greatise.com/move/sliders-workout

9.2.0. Introduction: Workout Sheets

The workout sheets included in this chapter are to assist and guide you to kick start their fitness and health program. The most challenging thing to do when wanting to make a change in life is taking that first step to get started. Often uncertainty and insecurity cloud a person's best intentions to change. These workout sheets will help eliminate, or at least minimize, the uncertainty a person may have regarding how they go about starting to re-introduce exercise and fitness into their daily routine.

Everything that you need to set your goals, start improving your cardiovascular fitness, increase your muscular strength, agility, balance and coordination, and flexibility, and to evaluate your progress is in this chapter.

The workouts are in chart form to make it easy to follow, record efforts, and monitor progress. Monitoring progress after 5-6 weeks is a great way to maintain motivation and reinforce that your new routine is headed in the right direction to achieve your stated goals. If your workouts are not recorded, you cannot measure your progress, so it's essential to utilize the workout sheets.

The workout sheets are meant as a guide. You do not have to adhere precisely to the exercises listed. With experience, you will modify your exercise routines by adding or eliminating certain exercises to meet your specific needs. Refer to the appendices listed under 9.1.0 to help you decide which exercises are best for you. For example, an older adult may feel they need to exercise their shoulders more due to a previous injury than strengthening their chest and upper back. However, it is recommended that you maintain the template format established. This template format will ensure that sufficient recovery between exercising specific muscle groups occurs. The type of exercises performed may change, but the template format to perform these exercises should stay the same.

9.2.1. Goal Setting Worksheet (S.M.A.R.T.)

Reference in Text – Chapter 3.3: The Importance and Art of Goal Setting

Identifying your Health and Fitness Goals:

Over the next _____ months, I want to achieve the following (choose 3 and number by priority);

Exercise more (commit to a regular exercise routine)	
Increase muscle strength/endurance	
Increase cardiovascular endurance	
Increase flexibility	
Reduce muscle/joint stiffness	
Lose weight	
Reduce blood pressure	
Improve my eating habits (follow 80/20 rule)	
Drink 8 glasses of water per day	
Reduce the amount of alcohol i drink	
Reduce and Better Manage Stress	
Have a happier and healthier outlook on life	
Live an active lifestyle	
Have more energy	
Feel healthier	

First Goal:

Specific	
Measurable	
Action	
Realistic	
Time lined	

Second Goal:

Specific	
Measurable	
Action	
Realistic	
Time lined	

Third Goal:

Specific	
Measurable	
Action	
Realistic	
Time lined	

9.2.2. Cardiovascular Exercise and Daily Activity Recording Sheet

Reference in Text – Chapter 4.1.1

9.2.2 Cardiovascular Exercise and Daily Activity Recording Sheet
Warning: You should consult your medical doctor before starting any exercise program
Note: Record Daily Your Activities. Every activity you do trains the heart to a certain degree. The More Intense and longer the activity the better the training effect

Notes:
 If you are exercising and experiences any of the following symptoms, you should stop exercising and immediately consult your doctor or go to the hospital.
  1. Pain and discomfort in the chest, lower jaw or left shoulder.
  2. Feeling of rapid, throbbing heart rate.
  3. Sever pain in leg muscles when walking, running or cycling.
  4. Shortness of breath or difficulty breathing.
  5. Feelings of dizziness or fainting.

Notes:
 When doing dedicated cardio vascular exercise it is important to:
 1. Start Low and Slow. Getting fit and maintaining fitness is a marathon, not a sprint. Start low and progress slowly.
 2. Keep your heart rate within the determined HR Training Zone for a minimum of 20 minutes.
 3. Monitor the intensity of effort by either;
   1. Monitoring your Heart Rate
   2. Estimating your Perceived Effort
   3. Utilizing the Talk Test.
   (Reference chapter 4.1.1)

Month: Date	**Cardiovascular Exercise and Daily Activities and Comments**
1	
2	
3	
4	
5	
6	
7	
8	
9	

10	
11	
12	
13	
14	
15	
16	
17	
18	
19	
20	
21	
22	
23	
24	
25	
26	
27	
28	
29	
30	
31	

9.2.3. Muscle Resistance Workout Sheets

- Core Workout Sheets 896
  - 45 Minute Core Workout #1 896
  - 45 Minute Core Workout #2 898
  - 10 Minute Core Workout #1 900
  - 10 Minute Core Workout #2 901
  - 10 Minute Core Workout #3 902
  - 10 Minute Core Workout #4 903
  - 10 Minute Core Workout #5 904
- Core and Whole-Body Workout Sheets 905
  - Core and Whole-Body Muscle Resistance Routine #1 905
  - Core and Whole-Body Muscle Resistance Routine #2 908
  - Core and Whole-Body Muscle Resistance Routine #3 911
  - Core and Whole-Body Muscle Resistance Routine #4 914
  - Core and Whole-Body Muscle Resistance Routine #5 917
- Core and Upper-Body Workout Sheets 920
  - Core and Upper-Body Muscle Resistance Routine #1 920
  - Core and Upper-Body Muscle Resistance Routine #2 922
  - Core and Upper-Body Muscle Resistance Routine #3 925
  - Core and Upper-Body Muscle Resistance Routine #4 928
- Core and Lower-Body Workout Sheets 932
  - Core and Lower-Body Muscle Resistance Routine #1 932
  - Core and Lower-Body Muscle Resistance Routine #2 934
  - Core and Lower-Body Muscle Resistance Routine #3 936
  - Core and Lower-Body Muscle Resistance Routine #4 938
  - Core and Lower-Body Muscle Resistance Routine #5 940
- Core and Bodyweight Workout Sheets 942
  - Core and Bodyweight Muscle Resistance Routine #1 942
  - Core and Bodyweight Muscle Resistance Routine #2 945

Core Workout Sheets

	45 Minute Core Workout #1									
	Notes: 1. Do all the core exercises in the order presented 2. From Appendix 9.1.2.1.1: Core Exercises Described and Illustrated, you can substitute different core exercises for the different target muscle groups areas 3. Never hold your breath while performing core exercises 4. The slower you perform the core exercises the more effective the exercise will be 5. Based on your fitness level determine the number of repetitions you should do per set. Initially you may only do 1 set of each core exercise. This can increase to 2 or 3 sets over time									
	Date:									
	Lower Abdominal Muscles (Hip Flexors will be engaged)									
1	**Flutter kicks** (Lift shoulders to look at feet)	R-	R-	R-	R-	R-	R-	R-	R-	R-
2	**Mat Supine Reverse Crunch** (<u>Advanced</u> - put SB between knees or ankles)	R-	R-	R-	R-	R-	R-	R-	R-	R-
3	**Scissors** (Hover heels above mat to start and raise legs alternatively to 90°)	R-	R-	R-	R-	R-	R-	R-	R-	R-
4	**Heel Taps** (TT and lower one heel at time to floor)	R-	R-	R-	R-	R-	R-	R-	R-	R-
5	**SB or TRX - Reverse Crunch**	R-	R-	R-	R-	R-	R-	R-	R-	R-
	Upper Abdominals **(Rectus Abdominus, Abdominal Obliques & Lateral Abdominal Muscles)**									
1	**Abdominal Crunch** (Mat, SB, BOSU)	R-	R-	R-	R-	R-	R-	R-	R-	R-
2	**Oblique Abd. Crunch** (Mat, SB, BOSU)	R-	R-	R-	R-	R-	R-	R-	R-	R-
3	**1/2 lateral Oblique Crunch**	R-	R-	R-	R-	R-	R-	R-	R-	R-
4	**Twisting Lateral Plank** **(Eye of the needle)**	R-	R-	R-	R-	R-	R-	R-	R-	R-
5	**RB - Standing Lateral Twist (Mid-level anchor) or Russian Twist** (<u>Advanced</u> - with Medicine ball)	R-	R-	R-	R-	R-	R-	R-	R-	R-

Back Extensors (Prone) (Erector Spinae Musculature)

1	**Upper Back Extensions** (Mat, SB, BOSU)	R-	R-	R-	R-	R-	R-	R-	R-	R-
2	**Upper Back Extension with Twist of shoulders** (SB or BOSU)	R-	R-	R-	R-	R-	R-	R-	R-	R-
3	**Leg Extension** (Mat, SB, BOSU)	R-	R-	R-	R-	R-	R-	R-	R-	R-
4	**Superman's** (Mat, SB, BOSU)	R-	R-	R-	R-	R-	R-	R-	R-	R-
5	**Bridges** - single or double leg (Mat, SB, BOSU)	R-	R-	R-	R-	R-	R-	R-	R-	R-

Planks

6	**Standard** (Mat, SB, BOSU)	T-	T-	T-	T-	T-	T-	T-	T-	T-
7	**Bird** (Mat, SB, BOSU)	T-	T-	T-	T-	T-	T-	T-	T-	T-
8	**Standard Plank** (Mat, SB, BOSU)	T-	T-	T-	T-	T-	T-	T-	T-	T-
9	**Lateral Plank Hip Dip**	R-	R-	R-	R-	R-	R-	R-	R-	R-

Standing

10	**Standing Bent Over Twist** (bend 90° at waist and rotate to one side and then the other) (Hands behind head or extended as you rotate)	R-	R-	R-	R-	R-	R-	R-	R-	R-

45 Minute Core Workout #2

Notes:
1. Do all the core exercises in the order presented
2. From Appendix 9.1.2.1.1: Core Exercises Described and Illustrated, you can substitute different core exercises for the different target muscle groups areas
3. Never hold your breath while performing core exercises
4. The slower you perform the core exercises the more effective the exercise will be
5. Based on your fitness level determine the number of repetitions you should do per set. Initially you may only do 1 set of each core exercise. This can increase to 2 or 3 sets over time

		Date:								
Lower Abdominal Muscles (Hip Flexors will be engaged)									
1	**Pilates 100's** (Feet 30° - 60° off floor)	R-	R-	R-	R-	R-	R-	R-	R-	R-
2	**Double Straight Leg Raise to 90°** (Advanced - SB between knees or ankles)	R-	R-	R-	R-	R-	R-	R-	R-	R-
3	**Pendulum** (Legs lifted 90° and rotate to each side)	R-	R-	R-	R-	R-	R-	R-	R-	R-
4	**Mat or TRX - Mountain Climber** (On all fours and bring knee to same or opposite chest)	R-	R-	R-	R-	R-	R-	R-	R-	R-
5	**Figure 4 and SB Reverse Crunch**	R-	R-	R-	R-	R-	R-	R-	R-	R-
Upper Abdominals (Rectus Abdominus, Abdominal Obliques, Lateral Abdominal Muscles)									
6	**Double Crunch** (Wrap arms around knees)	R-	R-	R-	R-	R-	R-	R-	R-	R-
7	**Double Oblique Crunch (Bicycles)** (Opposite elbow and knee meet)	R-	R-	R-	R-	R-	R-	R-	R-	R-
8	**Lateral Crunch on BOSU** (Advanced – weight held in lower hand)	R-	R-	R-	R-	R-	R-	R-	R-	R-
9	**Russian Twist** (Small or large rotation)	R-	R-	R-	R-	R-	R-	R-	R-	R-
10	**RB - Standing or Kneeling Oblique Twist** (From high anchor)	R-	R-	R-	R-	R-	R-	R-	R-	R-

Back Extensors (Prone) (Erector Spinae Musculature)

11	**Upper Back Extensions** (Mat, SB, BOSU)	R-	R-	R-	R-	R-	R-	R-	R-	R-	R-
12	**Upper Back Extension with Twist of Shoulders** (SB or BOSU)	R-	R-	R-	R-	R-	R-	R-	R-	R-	R-
13	**Leg Extension** (Mat, SB, BOSU)	R-	R-	R-	R-	R-	R-	R-	R-	R-	R-
14	**Superman's** (Mat, SB, BOSU)	R-	R-	R-	R-	R-	R-	R-	R-	R-	R-
15	**Bridges** - single or double leg (Mat, SB, BOSU)	R-	R-	R-	R-	R-	R-	R-	R-	R-	R-

Planks

16	**Standard** (Mat, SB, BOSU)	T-	T-	T-	T-	T-	T-	T-	T-	T-	T-
17	**Standard with Twist of Bent Elbow Down** (Eye of the needle)	R-	R-	R-	R-	R-	R-	R-	R-	R-	R-
18	**Standard** (Mat, SB, BOSU)	T-	T-	T-	T-	T-	T-	T-	T-	T-	T-
19	**Lateral** (Mat, SB, BOSU)	T-	T-	T-	T-	T-	T-	T-	T-	T-	T-

Standing

20	**Bent Over Twist** (Bend 90° at waist and rotate to one side and then the other) (Hands behind head or extended as you rotate)	R-	R-	R-	R-	R-	R-	R-	R-	R-	

10 Minute Core Workout #1

Notes:
1. Do all the core exercises in the order presented
2. From Appendix 9.1.2.1.1: Core Exercises Described and Illustrated, you can substitute different core exercises for the different target muscle groups areas
3. Never hold your breath while performing core exercises
4. The slower you perform the core exercises the more effective the exercise will be
5. Based on your fitness level determine the number of repetitions you should do per set. Initially you may only do 1 set of each core exercise. This can increase to 2 or 3 sets over time

	Date:									

Lower Abdominal Muscles (Hip Flexors will be engaged)

1	**Pilates 100's** (Feet 30° - 60° off floor)	R-	R-	R-	R-	R-	R-	R-	R-	R-	R-

Upper Abdominals
(Rectus Abdominus, Abdominal Obliques, Lateral Abdominal Muscles)

2	**Double Crunch** (Wrap arms around knees)	R-	R-	R-	R-	R-	R-	R-	R-	R-	R-
3	**Oblique Crunch (Bicycles)** (Opposite elbow & knee meet)	R-	R-	R-	R-	R-	R-	R-	R-	R-	R-
4	**Lateral Crunch on BOSU**	R-	R-	R-	R-	R-	R-	R-	R-	R-	R-

Back Extensors (Prone) (Erector Spinae Musculature)

5	**Upper Back Extensions** (Mat, SB, BOSU)	R-	R-	R-	R-	R-	R-	R-	R-	R-	R-
6	**Leg Extension** (Mat, SB, BOSU)	R-	R-	R-	R-	R-	R-	R-	R-	R-	R-

Planks

7	**Standard** (Mat, SB, BOSU)	T-	T-	T-	T-	T-	T-	T-	T-	T-	T-
8	**Lateral** (Mat, SB, BOSU)	T-	T-	T-	T-	T-	T-	T-	T-	T-	T-

10 Minute Core Workout #2

Notes:
1. Do all the core exercises in the order presented
2. From Appendix 9.1.2.1.1: Core Exercises Described and Illustrated, you can substitute different core exercises for the different target muscle groups areas
3. Never hold your breath while performing core exercises
4. The slower you perform the core exercises the more effective the exercise will be
5. Based on your fitness level determine the number of repetitions you should do per set. Initially you may only do 1 set of each core exercise. This can increase to 2 or 3 sets over time

Date:

Lower Abdominal Muscles (Hip Flexors will be engaged)

1	**Double Straight Leg Raise to 90°** (<u>Advanced</u> - SB between knees or ankles)	R-	R-	R-	R-	R-	R-	R-	R-	R-
2	**Pendulum** (Legs 90° and rotate to each side)	R-	R-	R-	R-	R-	R-	R-	R-	R-

Upper Abdominals
(Rectus Abdominus, Abdominal Obliques, Lateral Abdominal Muscles)

3	**Standard Crunch**	R-	R-	R-	R-	R-	R-	R-	R-	R-
4	**Russian Twist** (Small or large rotation)	R-	R-	R-	R-	R-	R-	R-	R-	R-

Back Extensors (Prone) (Erector Spinae Musculature)

5	**Upper Back Extension with Twist of shoulders** (SB or BOSU)	R-	R-	R-	R-	R-	R-	R-	R-	R-
6	**Leg Extension** (Mat, SB, BOSU)	R-	R-	R-	R-	R-	R-	R-	R-	R-
7	**Superman's** (Mat, SB, BOSU)	R-	R-	R-	R-	R-	R-	R-	R-	R-

Planks

8	**Standard** (Mat, SB, BOSU)	T-	T-	T-	T-	T-	T-	T-	T-	T-
9	**Standard with twist of bent elbow down** (Eye of the needle)	R-	R-	R-	R-	R-	R-	R-	R-	R-

10 Minute Core Workout #3

Notes:
1. Do all the core exercises in the order presented
2. From Appendix 9.1.2.1.1: Core Exercises Described and Illustrated, you can substitute different core exercises for the different target muscle groups areas
3. Never hold your breath while performing core exercises
4. The slower you perform the core exercises the more effective the exercise will be
5. Based on your fitness level determine the number of repetitions you should do per set. Initially you may only do 1 set of each core exercise. This can increase to 2 or 3 sets over time

	Date:									
	Lower Abdominal Muscles (Hip flexors will be engaged)									
1	Mat or TRX - Mountain Climber - (On all fours and bring knee to same or opposite chest)	R-	R-	R-	R-	R-	R-	R-	R-	R-
2	SB Reverse Crunch	R-	R-	R-	R-	R-	R-	R-	R-	R-
	Upper Abdominals (Rectus Abdominus, Abdominal Obliques, Lateral Abdominal Muscles)									
3	Standard Crunch (Wrap arms around knees)	R-	R-	R-	R-	R-	R-	R-	R-	R-
4	Lateral Crunch on BOSU	R-	R-	R-	R-	R-	R-	R-	R-	R-
5	Russian Twist (Small or large rotation)	R-	R-	R-	R-	R-	R-	R-	R-	R-
	Back Extensors (Prone) (Erector Spinae Musculature)									
6	Upper Back Extensions (Mat, SB, BOSU)	R-	R-	R-	R-	R-	R-	R-	R-	R-
7	Superman's (Mat, SB, BOSU)	R-	R-	R-	R-	R-	R-	R-	R-	R-
8	Bridges - single or double leg (Mat, SB, BOSU)	R-	R-	R-	R-	R-	R-	R-	R-	R-
	Planks									
9	Standard (Mat, SB, BOSU)	T-	T-	T-	T-	T-	T-	T-	T-	T-
10	Lateral - Left and Right side (Mat, SB, BOSU)	T-	T-	T-	T-	T-	T-	T-	T-	T-
11	Standard (Mat, SB, BOSU)	T-	T-	T-	T-	T-	T-	T-	T-	T-

10 Minute Core Workout #4

Notes:
1. Do all the core exercises in the order presented
2. From Appendix 9.1.2.1.1: Core Exercises Described and Illustrated, you can substitute different core exercises for the different target muscle groups areas
3. Never hold your breath while performing core exercises
4. The slower you perform the core exercises the more effective the exercise will be
5. Based on your fitness level determine the number of repetitions you should do per set. Initially you may only do 1 set of each core exercise. This can increase to 2 or 3 sets.

	Date:									
	Lower Abdominal Muscles (Hip Flexors will be engaged)									
1	**Scissors** (Raise legs alternatively to 90°)	R-	R-	R-	R-	R-	R-	R-	R-	R-
2	**Heel Taps** (TT and lower one heel at time to floor)	R-	R-	R-	R-	R-	R-	R-	R-	R-
3	**SB or TRX - Reverse Crunch**	R-	R-	R-	R-	R-	R-	R-	R-	R-
	Upper Abdominals (Rectus Abdominus, Abdominal Obliques & Lateral Abdominal Muscles)									
4	**Abdominal Crunch** (Mat, SB, BOSU)	R-	R-	R-	R-	R-	R-	R-	R-	R-
5	**1/2 Lateral Oblique Crunch**	R-	R-	R-	R-	R-	R-	R-	R-	R-
6	**Twisting Lateral Plank** (Eye of the needle)	R-	R-	R-	R-	R-	R-	R-	R-	R-
	Back Extensors (Prone) (Erector Spinae Musculature)									
7	**Upper Back Extensions** (Mat, SB, BOSU)	R-	R-	R-	R-	R-	R-	R-	R-	R-
8	**Upper Back Extension with Twist of shoulders** (SB or BOSU)	R-	R-	R-	R-	R-	R-	R-	R-	R-
9	**Superman's** (Mat, SB, BOSU)	R-	R-	R-	R-	R-	R-	R-	R-	R-
	Planks									
10	**Bird** (Mat, SB, BOSU)	T-	T-	T-	T-	T-	T-	T-	T-	T-
11	**Standard Plank** (Mat, SB, BOSU)	T-	T-	T-	T-	T-	T-	T-	T-	T-
12	**Lateral Plank Hip Dip**	R-	R-	R-	R-	R-	R-	R-	R-	R-

10 Minute Core Workout #5

Notes:
1. Do all the core exercises in the order presented
2. From Appendix 9.1.2.1.1: Core Exercises Described and Illustrated, you can substitute different core exercises for the different target muscle groups areas
3. Never hold your breath while performing core exercises
4. The slower you perform the core exercises the more effective the exercise will be
5. Based on your fitness level determine the number of repetitions you should do per set. Initially you may only do 1 set of each core exercise. This can increase to 2 or 3 sets over time

	Date:									

Lower Abdominal Muscles (Hip Flexors will be engaged)

#	Exercise									
1	**Flutter Kicks** (Lift shoulders to look at feet)	R-	R-	R-	R-	R-	R-	R-	R-	R-
2	**Mat Supine Reverse Crunch** (Advanced- put SB between knees or ankles)	R-	R-	R-	R-	R-	R-	R-	R-	R-

Upper Abdominals
(Rectus Abdominus, Abdominal Obliques & Lateral Abdominal Muscles)

#	Exercise									
3	**Abdominal Crunch** (Mat, SB, BOSU)	R-	R-	R-	R-	R-	R-	R-	R-	R-
4	**Oblique Abd. Crunch** (Mat, SB, BOSU)	R-	R-	R-	R-	R-	R-	R-	R-	R-

Back Extensors (Prone) (Erector Spinae Muscular)

#	Exercise									
5	**Upper Back Extensions** (Mat, SB, BOSU)	R-	R-	R-	R-	R-	R-	R-	R-	R-
6	**Leg Extension** (Mat, SB, BOSU)	R-	R-	R-	R-	R-	R-	R-	R-	R-
7	**Superman's** (Mat, SB, BOSU)	R-	R-	R-	R-	R-	R-	R-	R-	R-

Planks

#	Exercise									
8	**Standard** (Mat, SB, BOSU)	T-	T-	T-	T-	T-	T-	T-	T-	T-
9	**Lateral Plank Hip Dip**	R-	R-	R-	R-	R-	R-	R-	R-	R-

Standing

#	Exercise									
10	**Standing Bent Over Twist** (Bend 90° at waist and rotate to one side and then the other) (hands behind head or extended as you rotate)	R-	R-	R-	R-	R-	R-	R-	R-	R-

Core and Whole-Body Workout Sheets

	Core and Whole-Body Muscle Resistance Routine #1					
	Core					
	Notes: 1. Do all the core exercises in the order presented 2. From Appendix 9.1.2.1.1: Core Exercises Described and Illustrated, you can substitute different core exercises for the different target muscle groups areas 3. Never hold your breath while performing core exercises 4. The slower you perform the core exercises the more effective the exercise will be 5. Based on your fitness level determine the number of repetitions you should do per set. Initially you may only do 1 set of each core exercise. This can increase to 2 or 3 sets over time					
	Date:					
1	Mat - Pilates 100's	R- 2 x 100	R- 2 x 100	R- 2 x 100	R- 2 x 100	R- 2 x 100
2	SB - Crunch	R- 2 x	R- 2 x	R- 2 x	R- 2 x	R- 2 x
3	Mat - Straight leg raises (<u>Advanced</u> - SB ball between ankles or knees)	R- 2 x	R- 2 x	R- 2 x	R- 2 x	R- 2 x
4	SB - Oblique Crunch	R- 2 x	R- 2 x	R- 2 x	R- 2 x	R- 2 x
5	BOSU - Lateral Crunch	R- 2 x	R- 2 x	R- 2 x	R- 2 x	R- 2 x
6	SB - Back extensions	R- 2 x	R- 2 x	R- 2 x	R- 2 x	R- 2 x
	Resistance					
	Notes: 1. Do all odd numbered resistance exercises first and then the even numbered resistance exercises (Exercise 1, 3, 5 etc. and then Exercise 2, 4, 6, etc.) 2. From Appendix 9.1.2.2.1: Whole-Body Exercise described and illustrated you can substitute different exercises for the same muscle group 3. NEVER hold your breath as you lift a weight 4. Lift at a pace of 2 beats up and 2 beats down 5. Based on your fitness level you can start with 8, 10, 12, 15 reps					
1	**Chest** Push-up's - Regular	R-	R-	R-	R-	R-
2	Machine 30° - Chest press	R- W-	R- W-	R- W-	R- W-	R- W-

#	Exercise										
3	**Upper Back** Machine - Regular Lats Pull downs	R-	W-	R-	W-	R-	W-	R-	W-	R-	W-
4	SB - Two-way shoulder flies	R-	W-	R-	W-	R-	W-	R-	W-	R-	W-
5	**Chest** Push-ups - Military (M) or Wide (W)	(M) R-	(W) R-	(M) R-	(W) R-	(M) R-	(W) R-	(M) R-	(W) R-	(M) R-	(W) R-
6	TRX - Chest Flies	R-		R-		R-		R-		R-	
7	**Upper Back** Machine - Closed Lats pull downs	R-	W-	R-	W-	R-	W-	R-	W-	R-	W-
8	SB - Reverse Flies	R-	W-	R-	W-	R-	W-	R-	W-	R-	W-
9	**Shoulders** Dumbbells - "Y's"	R-	W-	R-	W-	R-	W-	R-	W-	R-	W-
10	RB - Lateral Raise	R-	RB-	R-	RB-	R-	RB-	R-	RB-	R-	RB-
11	**Legs** Standing -Dead Lifts	R-	W-	R-	W-	R-	W-	R-	W-	R-	W-
12	BOSU -Lateral/side step	R-		R-		R-		R-		R-	
13	**Shoulders** Dumbbells - "I's"	R-	W-	R-	W-	R-	W-	R-	W-	R-	W-
14	TRX - Alternating "I's"	R-		R-		R-		R-		R-	
15	**Legs** Machine - Single leg extensions	R-	W-	R-	W-	R-	W-	R-	W-	R-	W-
16	Machine - Single or double leg curls	R-	W-	R-	W-	R-	W-	R-	W-	R-	W-

17	**Biceps** SB - Concentration Curls	R-	W-	R-	W-	R-	W-	R-	W-	R-	W-
18	Standing -Regular Curls	R-	W-	R-	W-	R-	W-	R-	W-	R-	W-
19	**Triceps** SB - Lying down double arm	R-	W-	R-	W-	R-	W-	R-	W-	R-	W-
20	Dips	R-		R-		R-		R-		R-	

Core and Whole-Body Muscle Resistance Routine #2

	Date					

Core

Notes:
1. Do all the core exercises in the order presented
2. From Appendix 9.1.2.1.1: Core Exercises Described and Illustrated, you can substitute different core exercises for the different target muscle groups areas
3. Never hold your breath while performing core exercises
4. The slower you perform the core exercises the more effective the exercise will be
5. Based on your fitness level determine the number of repetitions you should do per set. Initially you may only do 1 set of each core exercise. This can increase to 2 or 3 sets over time.

#	Exercise					
1	Mat - Crunch	R- 2 x	R- 2 x	R- 2 x	R- 2 x	R- 2 x
2	Mat - Oblique crunch with lower legs on SB	R- 2 x	R- 2 x	R- 2 x	R- 2 x	R- 2 x
3	Mat - Flutters	R- 2 x	R- 2 x	R- 2 x	R- 2 x	R- 2 x
4	SB - Prone (face down) Reverse crunch	R- 2 x	R- 2 x	R- 2 x	R- 2 x	R- 2 x
5	BOSU - Lateral Crunch	R- 2 x	R- 2 x	R- 2 x	R- 2 x	R- 2 x
6	Mat - Standard Plank (Prone - face down)	T-	T-	T-	T-	T-

Resistance

Notes:
1. Do all odd numbered resistance exercises first and then the even numbered resistance exercises (Exercise 1, 3, 5 etc. and then Exercise 2, 4, 6, etc..)
2. From Appendix 9.1.2.2.1: Whole-Body Exercise described and illustrated you can substitute different exercises for the same muscle group
3. NEVER hold your breath as you lift a weight
4. Lift at a pace of 2 beats up and 2 beats down
5. Based on your fitness level you can start with 8, 10, 12, 15 reps

Chest

#	Exercise					
1	Push-up - Phalange	R-	R-	R-	R-	R-
2	Push-ups - Under the fence	R-	R-	R-	R-	R-

3	**Upper Back** Machine - Lats pull downs- regular grip	R-	W-	R-	W-	R-	W-	R-	W-	R-	W-
4	Machine - Lats pull downs - reverse grip	R-	W-	R-	W-	R-	W-	R-	W-	R-	W-
5	**Chest** SB – Swimmer's chest press	R-	R-	R-	R-	R-	R-	R-	R-	R-	R-
6	SB -Alternating one arm flies	R-	W-	R-	W-	R-	W-	R-	W-	R-	W-
7	**Upper Back** SB - Bent over flies	R-	W-	R-	W-	R-	W-	R-	W-	R-	W-
8	SB - Bent over rows	R-	W-	R-	W-	R-	W-	R-	W-	R-	W-
9	**Shoulders** SB - overhead shoulder press	R-	W-	R-	W-	R-	W-	R-	W-	R-	W-
10	SB - "Y" overhead press	R-	W-	R-	W-	R-	W-	R-	W-	R-	W-
11	**Legs** Standing - Lateral Lunge	R-		R-		R-		R-		R-	
12	Standing - Squat	R-		R-		R-		R-		R-	
13	**Shoulders** Dumbbells - Standing lateral abduction	R-	W-	R-	W-	R-	W-	R-	W-	R-	W-
14	TRX - Alternating "I's"	R-		R-		R-		R-		R-	
15	**Legs** Machine - Single or double leg extensions	R-	W-	R-	W-	R-	W-	R-	W-	R-	W-
16	Machine - Single or double leg curls	R-	W-	R-	W-	R-	W-	R-	W-	R-	W-

	Biceps										
17	Standing -21's	R-	W-	R-	W-	R-	W-	R-	W-	R-	W-
18	Standing - Out curls	R-	W-	R-	W-	R-	W-	R-	W-	R-	W-
	Triceps										
19	Standing - Flip grip kick backs	R-	W-	R-	W-	R-	W-	R-	W-	R-	W-
20	- Dips	R-		R-		R-		R-		R-	

Core and Whole-Body Muscle Resistance Routine #3

		Date				
	\multicolumn{6}{c}{**Core**}
	Notes: 1. Do all the core exercises in the order presented 2. From Appendix 9.1.2.1.1: Core Exercises Described and Illustrated, you can substitute different core exercises for the different target muscle groups areas 3. Never hold your breath while performing core exercises 4. The slower you perform the core exercises the more effective the exercise will be 5. Based on your fitness level determine the number of repetitions you should do per set. Initially you may only do 1 set of each core exercise. This can increase to 2 or 3 sets over time					
1	Mat - full sit-up (stabilize the feet)	R- 2 x	R- 2 x	R- 2 x	R- 2 x	R- 2 x
2	Mat -Lateral plank (eye of the needle)	R- 2 x	R- 2 x	R- 2 x	R- 2 x	R- 2 x
3	Mat - Bicycles	R- 2 x	R- 2 x	R- 2 x	R- 2 x	R- 2 x
4	Mat - Supine (face up) Reverse crunch (advanced SB between ankles or knees)	R- 2 x	R- 2 x	R- 2 x	R- 2 x	R- 2 x
5	BOSU – Superman's	R- 2 x	R- 2 x	R- 2 x	R- 2 x	R- 2 x
6	Mat - Standard Plank (Prone - face down)	T-	T-	T-	T-	T-
	\multicolumn{6}{c}{**Resistance**}
	Notes: 1. Do all odd numbered resistance exercises first and then the even numbered resistance exercises (Exercise 1, 3, 5 etc. and then Exercise 2, 4, 6, etc..) 2. From Appendix 9.1.2.2.1: Whole-Body Exercise described and illustrated you can substitute different exercises for the same muscle group 3. NEVER hold your breath as you lift a weight 4. Lift at a pace of 2 beats up and 2 beats down 5. Based on your fitness level you can start with 8, 10, 12, 15 reps					
	Chest					
1	Push-up - wide arm	R-	R-	R-	R-	R-
2	Push-ups - regular to lateral plank	R-	R-	R-	R-	R-
	Upper Back					
3	Machine - Lats pull downs- regular grip	R- W-	R- W-	R- W-	R- W-	R- W-

4	Machine - Lats pull downs - closed grip	R-	W-	R-	W-	R-	W-	R-	W-	R-	W-
	Chest-										
5	Push-ups - Floor fly	R-		R-		R-		R-		R-	
6	Machine - chest press	R-	W-	R-	W-	R-	W-	R-	W-	R-	W-
	Upper Back										
7	RB - "T's"	R-	RB-	R-	RB-	R-	RB-	R-	RB-	R-	RB-
8	TRX - one arm rows	R-		R-		R-		R-		R-	
	Shoulders										
9	SB - "I's" overhead shoulder press	R-	W-	R-	W-	R-	W-	R-	W-	R-	W-
10	TRX - "W's"	R-		R-		R-		R-		R-	
	Legs										
11	Standing - Forward lunge with twist away from lunge leg	R-		R-		R-		R-		R-	
12	Standing - Step up onto BOSU and Squat	R-		R-		R-		R-		R-	
	Shoulders										
13	RB - Lateral raises	R-	RB-	R-	RB-	R-	RB-	R-	RB-	R-	RB-
14	Machine - overhead press	R-	W-	R-	W-	R-	W-	R-	W-	R-	W-
	Legs										
15	Machine - double leg extensions	R-	W-	R-	W-	R-	W-	R-	W-	R-	W-
16	Machine - Single or double leg curls	R-	W-	R-	W-	R-	W-	R-	W-	R-	W-
	Biceps										
17	SB - Single arm concentration Curls	R-	W-	R-	W-	R-	W-	R-	W-	R-	W-
18	SB - Single arm concentration Curls	R-	W-	R-	W-	R-	W-	R-	W-	R-	W-

19	**Triceps** Sitting - Overhead triceps extension	R-	W-	R-	W-	R-	W-	R-	W-	R-	W-
20	Dips	R-		R-		R-		R-		R-	

Core and Whole-Body Muscle Resistance Routine #4

		Date					
	Core							

Notes:
1. Do all the core exercises in the order presented
2. From Appendix 9.1.2.1.1: Core Exercises Described and Illustrated, you can substitute different core exercises for the different target muscle groups' areas
3. Never hold your breath while performing core exercises
4. The slower you perform the core exercises the more effective the exercise will be
5. Based on your fitness level determine the number of repetitions you should do per set. Initially you may only do 1 set of each core exercise. This can increase to 2 or 3 sets over time

#	Exercise					
1	Mat - 3/4 sit-up (stabilize the feet)	R- 2 x	R- 2 x	R- 2 x	R- 2 x	R- 2 x
2	BOSU -Lateral crunch (<u>Advanced</u> - weight in outstretched arm)	R-2x W-	R-2x W-	R-2x W-	R-2x W-	R-2x W-
3	SB - Figure 4 Obliques	R- 2 x	R- 2 x	R- 2 x	R- 2 x	R- 2 x
4	Mat - Russian Twist (<u>Advanced</u>- hold medicine ball or weight in hands)	R-2x W-	R-2x W-	R-2x W-	R-2x W-	R-2x W-
5	SB - Bridges	R- 2 x	R- 2 x	R- 2 x	R- 2 x	R- 2 x
6	Mat - Standard Plank	T-	T-	T-	T-	T-

Resistance

Notes:
1. Do all odd numbered resistance exercises first and then the even numbered resistance exercises (Exercise 1, 3, 5 etc. and then Exercise 2, 4, 6, etc..)
2. From Appendix 9.1.2.2.1: Whole-Body Exercise described and illustrated you can substitute different exercises for the same muscle group
3. NEVER hold your breath as you lift a weight
4. Lift at a pace of 2 beats up and 2 beats down
5. Based on your fitness level you can start with 8, 10, 12, 15 reps

Chest

#	Exercise					
1	Push-up -Decline	R-	R-	R-	R-	R-
2	Push-ups - on black side of BOSU	R-	R-	R-	R-	R-

3	**Upper Back** Machine - Lats pull downs- regular grip	R-	W-	R-	W-	R-	W-	R-	W-	R-	W-
4	Machine - Lats pull downs - reverse grip	R-	W-	R-	W-	R-	W-	R-	W-	R-	W-
5	**Chest-** Push-ups - Military	R-		R-		R-		R-		R-	
6	SB or Bench - Dumbbell chest press	R-	W-	R-	W-	R-	W-	R-	W-	R-	W-
7	**Upper Back** Machine - Lats pull downs - close grip	R-	W-	R-	W-	R-	W-	R-	W-	R-	W-
8	SB - Prone flies	R-	W-	R-	W-	R-	W-	R-	W-	R-	W-
9	**Shoulders** Machine - overhead shoulder press	R-	W-	R-	W-	R-	W-	R-	W-	R-	W-
10	TRX - "I's"	R-		R-		R-		R-		R-	
11	**Legs** Bench - Balanced lunge	R-		R-		R-		R-		R-	
12	Standing - Monster lateral walk	R-		R-		R-		R-		R-	
13	**Shoulders** Push-up - Pike	R-		R-		R-		R-		R-	
14	Dumbbells - In and outs	R-	W-	R-	W-	R-	W-	R-	W-	R-	W-
15	**Legs** Machine - Single or double leg extensions	R-	W-	R-	W-	R-	W-	R-	W-	R-	W-
16	Machine - Single or double leg curls	R-	W-	R-	W-	R-	W-	R-	W-	R-	W-
17	**Biceps** Standing - Hammer Curls	R-	W-	R-	W-	R-	W-	R-	W-	R-	W-
18	Standing - Regular Curls	R-	W-	R-	W-	R-	W-	R-	W-	R-	W-

	Triceps									
19	TRX - Triceps extensions	R-	W-	R-	W-	R-	W-	R-	W-	R-	W-
20	Dips	R-		R-		R-		R-		R-	

Core and Whole-Body Muscle Resistance Routine #5

	Date					
	Core					
	Notes: 1. Do all the core exercises in the order presented 2. From Appendix 9.1.2.1.1: Core Exercises Described and Illustrated, you can substitute different core exercises for the different target muscle groups' areas 3. Never hold your breath while performing core exercises 4. The slower you perform the core exercises the more effective the exercise will be 5. Based on your fitness level determine the number of repetitions you should do per set. Initially you may only do 1 set of each core exercise. This can increase to 2 or 3 sets over time					
1	Mat – Double Crunch	R- 2 x	R- 2 x	R- 2 x	R- 2 x	R- 2 x
2	BOSU – Lateral crunch (advanced- weight in outstretched arm)	R- 2 x W -	R- x W -	R- x W -	R- x W -	R- x W -
3	Mat – Oblique crunch (lower legs rest on SB)	R- 2 x	R- 2 x	R- 2 x	R- 2 x	R- 2 x
4	Mat – Pendulum	R- 2 x	R- x	R- x	R- x	R- x
5	BOSU – Superman's	R- 2 x	R- 2 x	R- 2 x	R- 2 x	R- 2 x
6	Mat – Standard Plank	T-	T-	T-	T-	T-
	Resistance					
	Notes: 1. Do all odd numbered resistance exercises first and then the even numbered resistance exercises (Exercise 1, 3, 5 etc. and then Exercise 2, 4, 6, etc..) 2. From Appendix 9.1.2.2.1: Whole-Body Exercise described and illustrated you can substitute different exercises for the same muscle group 3. NEVER hold your breath as you lift a weight 4. Lift at a pace of 2 beats up and 2 beats down 5. Based on your fitness level you can start with 8, 10, 12, 15 reps.					

	Chest									
1	Push-up - side-to-side	R-		R-		R-		R-		R-	
2	Machine 30º - Incline chest press	R-	W-	R-	W-	R-	W-	R-	W-	R-	W-
	Upper Back										
3	Machine - Lats pull downs - regular grip	R-	W-	R-	W-	R-	W-	R-	W-	R-	W-
4	SB - Bent over rows	R-	W-	R-	W-	R-	W-	R-	W-	R-	W-
	Chest										
5	Push-ups - Regular	R-		R-		R-		R-		R-	
6	Machine - flies	R-	W-	R-	W-	R-	W-	R-	W-	R-	W-
	Upper Back										
7	Machine - Lats pull downs - close grip	R-	W-	R-	W-	R-	W-	R-	W-	R-	W-
8	SB - Two angle shoulder flies	R-	W-	R-	W-	R-	W-	R-	W-	R-	W-
	Shoulders										
9	Dumbbells - "I's" overhead press	R-	W-	R-	W-	R-	W-	R-	W-	R-	W-
10	TRX - "L's"	R-		R-		R-		R-		R-	
	Legs										
11	BOSU - Lunge	R-		R-		R-		R-		R-	
12	BOSU - Squats (Advanced - hold weight in hands)	R-	W-	R-	W-	R-	W-	R-	W-	R-	W-

	Shoulders										
13	Standing - Upright rows	R-	W-	R-	W-	R-	W-	R-	W-	R-	W-
14	Dumbbells - Lateral raises	R-	W-	R-	W-	R-	W-	R-	W-	R-	W-
	Legs-										
15	Machine - Single or double leg extensions	R-	W-	R-	W-	R-	W-	R-	W-	R-	W-
16	Machine - Single or double leg curls	R-	W-	R-	W-	R-	W-	R-	W-	R-	W-
	Biceps										
17	TRX - Biceps	R-		R-		R-		R-		R-	
18	Standing - Regular Curls	R-	W-	R-	W-	R-	W-	R-	W-	R-	W-
	Triceps										
19	SB - Lying single triceps extensions	R-	W-	R-	W-	R-	W-	R-	W-	R-	W-
20	Dips	R-		R-		R-		R-		R-	

Core and Upper-Body Workout Sheets

Core and Upper-Body Muscle Resistance Routine #1

	Date					

Core

Notes:
1. Do all the core exercises in the order presented
2. From Appendix 9.1.2.1.1.: Core Exercises described and illustrated you can substitute different core exercises for the different target muscle groups' areas
3. Never hold your breath while performing core exercises
4. The slower you perform the core exercises the more effective the exercise will be
5. Based on your fitness level determine the number of repetitions you should do per set. Initially you may only do 1 set of each core exercise. This can increase to 2 or 3 sets over time

#	Exercise						
1	SB - Abdominal Crunch	R-	R-	R-	R-	R-	R-
2	SB - Oblique Crunch- Fig 4	R-	R-	R-	R-	R-	R-
3	Mat - Straight leg raises 90º (Advanced - SB between ankles of knees)	R-	R-	R-	R-	R-	R-
4	Mat - Mountain Climber	R-	R-	R-	R-	R-	R-
5	BOSU - Lateral Raise	R-	R-	R-	R-	R-	R-
6	Mat - Russian Twist	R-	R-	R-	R-	R-	R-
7	Mat - Planks- Prone	T-	T-	T-	T-	T-	T-

Resistance

Notes:
1. Do all odd numbered resistance exercises first and then the even numbered resistance exercises (Exercise 1, 3, 5 etc. and then Exercise 2, 4, 6, etc.). Then repeat for set #2 and 3.
2. From Appendix 9.1.2.2.1: Whole-Body Exercise described and illustrated you can substitute different exercises for the same muscle group
3. NEVER hold your breath as you lift a weight
4. Lift at a pace of 2 beats up and 2 beats down
5. Based on your fitness level you can start with 8, 10, 12, 15 reps and 1, 2 or 3 sets

#	Exercise										
1	Machine – Chess Press	R-	W-	R-	W-	R-	W-	R-	W-	R-	W-
		R-	W-	R-	W-	R-	W-	R-	W-	R-	W-
		R-	W-	R-	W-	R-	W-	R-	W-	R-	W-

2	Machine – Chess Fly	R-	W-	R-	W-	R-	W-	R-	W-	R-	W-	R-	W-
		R-	W-	R-	W-	R-	W-	R-	W-	R-	W-	R-	W-
		R-	W-	R-	W-	R-	W-	R-	W-	R-	W-	R-	W-
3	Machine – Regular Lats Pull Down	R-	W-	R-	W-	R-	W-	R-	W-	R-	W-	R-	W-
		R-	W-	R-	W-	R-	W-	R-	W-	R-	W-	R-	W-
		R-	W-	R-	W-	R-	W-	R-	W-	R-	W-	R-	W-
4	Machine - Lower Rows (Rhomboids)	R-	W-	R-	W-	R-	W-	R-	W-	R-	W-	R-	W-
		R-	W-	R-	W-	R-	W-	R-	W-	R-	W-	R-	W-
		R-	W-	R-	W-	R-	W-	R-	W-	R-	W-	R-	W-
5	SB – Dumbbells - Over Head press (Shoulders- Upper Trapezius)	R-	W-	R-	W-	R-	W-	R-	W-	R-	W-	R-	W-
		R-	W-	R-	W-	R-	W-	R-	W-	R-	W-	R-	W-
		R-	W-	R-	W-	R-	W-	R-	W-	R-	W-	R-	W-
6	Standing - Lateral Raise (Shoulders- Lateral Deltoids)	R-	W-	R-	W-	R-	W-	R-	W-	R-	W-	R-	W-
		R-	W-	R-	W-	R-	W-	R-	W-	R-	W-	R-	W-
		R-	W-	R-	W-	R-	W-	R-	W-	R-	W-	R-	W-
7	Seated - Bicep Concentration Curl (Arms- Biceps)	R-	W-	R-	W-	R-	W-	R-	W-	R-	W-	R-	W-
		R-	W-	R-	W-	R-	W-	R-	W-	R-	W-	R-	W-
		R-	W-	R-	W-	R-	W-	R-	W-	R-	W-	R-	W-
8	Machine - Triceps Extensions (Arms - Triceps)	R-	W-	R-	W-	R-	W-	R-	W-	R-	W-	R-	W-
		R-	W-	R-	W-	R-	W-	R-	W-	R-	W-	R-	W-
		R-	W-	R-	W-	R-	W-	R-	W-	R-	W-	R-	W-

Core and Upper-Body Muscle Resistance Routine #2

	Date:						

Core

Notes:
1. Do all the core exercises in the order presented
2. From Appendix 9.1.2.1.1.: Core Exercises described and illustrated you can substitute different core exercises for the different target muscle groups' areas
3. Never hold your breath while performing core exercises
4. The slower you perform the core exercises the more effective the exercise will be
5. Based on your fitness level determine the number of repetitions you should do per set. Initially you may only do 1 set of each core exercise. This can increase to 2 or 3 sets over time

#	Exercise						
1	Mat - Double Crunch	R-	R-	R-	R-	R-	R-
2	Mat - Bicycle - Oblique Crunch	R-	R-	R-	R-	R-	R-
3	SB - Prone Reverse Crunch	R-	R-	R-	R-	R-	R-
4	Mat - Supine Reverse Crunch (Advanced - SB between ankles of knees)	R-	R-	R-	R-	R-	R-
5	Mat - Twisting Lateral Plank (Eye of the Needle)	R-	R-	R-	R-	R-	R-
6	Mat - Heel taps	R-	R-	R-	R-	R-	R-
7	Mat - Standard Plank (Prone - Face down)	T-	T-	T-	T-	T-	T-

Resistance

Notes:
1. Do all odd numbered resistance exercises first and then the even numbered resistance exercises (Exercise 1, 3, 5 etc. and then Exercise 2, 4, 6, etc.). Then repeat for set #2 and 3.
2. From Appendix 9.1.2.2.1: Whole-Body Exercise described and illustrated you can substitute different exercises for the same muscle group
3. NEVER hold your breath as you lift a weight
4. Lift at a pace of 2 beats up and 2 beats down
5. Based on your fitness level you can start with 8, 10, 12, 15 reps and 1, 2 or 3 set.

1	SB or Bench - Dumbbell Chest Press (Chest)	R-	W-	R-	W-	R-	W-	R-	W-	R-	W-	R-	W-
		R-	W-	R-	W-	R-	W-	R-	W-	R-	W-	R-	W-
		R-	W-	R-	W-	R-	W-	R-	W-	R-	W-	R-	W-
2	SB or Bench - Dumbbell Chest Fly (Chest)	R-	W-	R-	W-	R-	W-	R-	W-	R-	W-	R-	W-
		R-	W-	R-	W-	R-	W-	R-	W-	R-	W-	R-	W-
		R-	W-	R-	W-	R-	W-	R-	W-	R-	W-	R-	W-
3	Standing - Dumbbells - Lawnmowers (Upper Back)	R-	W-	R-	W-	R-	W-	R-	W-	R-	W-	R-	W-
		R-	W-	R-	W-	R-	W-	R-	W-	R-	W-	R-	W-
		R-	W-	R-	W-	R-	W-	R-	W-	R-	W-	R-	W-
4	SB or Bench -Dumbbells - Two Angle Shoulder Flies sitting (Upper Back)	R-	W-	R-	W-	R-	W-	R-	W-	R-	W-	R-	W-
		R-	W-	R-	W-	R-	W-	R-	W-	R-	W-	R-	W-
		R-	W-	R-	W-	R-	W-	R-	W-	R-	W-	R-	W-
5	SB or Bench - Dumbbells Over Head press - (Shoulders- Upper Traps)	R-	W-	R-	W-	R-	W-	R-	W-	R-	W-	R-	W-
		R-	W-	R-	W-	R-	W-	R-	W-	R-	W-	R-	W-
		R-	W-	R-	W-	R-	W-	R-	W-	R-	W-	R-	W-
6	Standing - Dumbbells In's and Out's (Shoulders- Ant. & Lateral Deltoids)	R-	W-	R-	W-	R-	W-	R-	W-	R-	W-	R-	W-
		R-	W-	R-	W-	R-	W-	R-	W-	R-	W-	R-	W-
		R-	W-	R-	W-	R-	W-	R-	W-	R-	W-	R-	W-

7	Standing - Dumbbells - Regular Bicep Curl (Arms- Biceps)	R-	W-	R-	W-	R-	W-	R-	W-	R-	W-	R-	W-
		R-	W-	R-	W-	R-	W-	R-	W-	R-	W-	R-	W-
		R-	W-	R-	W-	R-	W-	R-	W-	R-	W-	R-	W-
8	SB or Bench - Dumbbells - Lying Triceps Ext.	R-	W-	R-	W-	R-	W-	R-	W-	R-	W-	R-	W-
		R-	W-	R-	W-	R-	W-	R-	W-	R-	W-	R-	W-
		R-	W-	R-	W-	R-	W-	R-	W-	R-	W-	R-	W-

Core and Upper-Body Muscle Resistance Routine #3

		Date:					
		Core					

Notes:
1. Do all the core exercises in the order presented
2. From Appendix 9.1.2.1.1.: Core Exercises described and illustrated you can substitute different core exercises for the different target muscle groups' areas
3. Never hold your breath while performing core exercises
4. The slower you perform the core exercises the more effective the exercise will be
5. Based on your fitness level determine the number of repetitions you should do per set. Initially you may only do 1 set of each core exercise. This can increase to 2 or 3 sets over time.

#	Exercise						
1	Mat - Abdominal Crunch	R-	R-	R-	R-	R-	R-
2	Mat - 1/2 Lateral Oblique Crunch	R-	R-	R-	R-	R-	R-
3	Mat - Scissors	R-	R-	R-	R-	R-	R-
4	Mat - Pendulum	R-	R-	R-	R-	R-	R-
5	Mat - Lateral Plank- Elbow to Mat	R-	R-	R-	R-	R-	R-
6	Mat - Standard Plank – Prone (Face down)	R-	R-	R-	R-	R-	R-
7	Mat - Lateral Plank	T-	T-	T-	T-	T-	T-

	Resistance						

Notes:
1. Do all odd numbered resistance exercises first and then the even numbered resistance exercises (Exercise 1, 3, 5, etc. and then Exercise 2, 4, 6, etc.). Then repeat for set #2 and 3.
2. From Appendix 9.1.2.2.1: Whole-Body Exercise described and illustrated you can substitute different exercises for the same muscle group
3. NEVER hold your breath as you lift a weight
4. Lift at a pace of 2 beats up and 2 beats down
5. Based on your fitness level you can start with 8, 10, 12, 15 reps and 1, 2 or 3 set

#	Exercise						
1	Mat - Push-ups (Standard or Modified)	R- W-	R- W-	R- W-	R- W-	R- W-	R- W-
		R- W-	R- W-	R- W-	R- W-	R- W-	R- W-
		R- W-	R- W-	R- W-	R- W-	R- W-	R- W-

2	<u>SB or Bench</u> - Dumbbell - Cross body chest press (Chest)	R-	W-	R-	W-	R-	W-	R-	W-	R-	W-	R-	W-
		R-	W-	R-	W-	R-	W-	R-	W-	R-	W-	R-	W-
		R-	W-	R-	W-	R-	W-	R-	W-	R-	W-	R-	W-
3	<u>Standing</u> - Dumbbells - Bent over rows (Upper Back)	R-	W-	R-	W-	R-	W-	R-	W-	R-	W-	R-	W-
		R-	W-	R-	W-	R-	W-	R-	W-	R-	W-	R-	W-
		R-	W-	R-	W-	R-	W-	R-	W-	R-	W-	R-	W-
4	<u>SB</u> - Dumbbells- Bent over flies (Upper Back)	R-	W-	R-	W-	R-	W-	R-	W-	R-	W-	R-	W-
		R-	W-	R-	W-	R-	W-	R-	W-	R-	W-	R-	W-
		R-	W-	R-	W-	R-	W-	R-	W-	R-	W-	R-	W-
5	<u>SB</u> - Dumbbells - Swimmers Over Head Press (Shoulders- Upper Trapezius)	R-	W-	R-	W-	R-	W-	R-	W-	R-	W-	R-	W-
		R-	W-	R-	W-	R-	W-	R-	W-	R-	W-	R-	W-
		R-	W-	R-	W-	R-	W-	R-	W-	R-	W-	R-	W-
6	<u>SB</u> - Dumbbells Lateral Raise and Pour - (Shoulders- Lateral Deltoids and Rotator Cuff)	R-	W-	R-	W-	R-	W-	R-	W-	R-	W-	R-	W-
		R-	W-	R-	W-	R-	W-	R-	W-	R-	W-	R-	W-
		R-	W-	R-	W-	R-	W-	R-	W-	R-	W-	R-	W-
7	<u>Standing</u> - Dumbbells – Biceps Curl In's and Out's (Arms- Biceps)	R-	W-	R-	W-	R-	W-	R-	W-	R-	W-	R-	W-
		R-	W-	R-	W-	R-	W-	R-	W-	R-	W-	R-	W-
		R-	W-	R-	W-	R-	W-	R-	W-	R-	W-	R-	W-

8	SB or Bench - Dumbbells - Lying Overhead Triceps Extensions (Arms - Triceps)	R- W-	R- W-	R- W-	R- W-	R- W-	R- W-
		R- W-	R- W-	R- W-	R- W-	R- W-	R- W-
		R- W-	R- W-	R- W-	R- W-	R- W-	R- W-

Core and Upper-Body Muscle Resistance Routine #4

Note: Focus on SLOW, DELIBERATE & COMPLETE movements

	Date:					

Core

Notes:
1. Do all the core exercises in the order presented
2. From Appendix 9.1.2.1.1: Core Exercises described and illustrated you can substitute different core exercises for the different target muscle groups' areas
3. Never hold your breath while performing core exercises
4. The slower you perform the core exercises the more effective the exercise will be
5. Based on your fitness level determine the number of repetitions you should do per set. Initially you may only do 1 set of each core exercise. This can increase to 2 or 3 sets over time

#	Exercise						
1	Mat - Double Crunch	R-	R-	R-	R-	R-	R-
2	Mat - Pendulum	R-	R-	R-	R-	R-	R-
3	Mat - Flutter Kick	R-	R-	R-	R-	R-	R-
4	SB - Oblique Reverse Crunch (Prone- Face down)	R-	R-	R-	R-	R-	R-
5	Mat - Russian Twist	R-	R-	R-	R-	R-	R-
	Advanced- use Medicine ball	W-	W-	W-	W-	W-	W-
6	Mat - Standard Plank - Prone (Face down)	T-	T-	T-	T-	T-	T-
7	Mat - Lateral Plank Hip Dips	R-	R-	R-	R-	R-	R-

Resistance

Notes:
1. Do all odd numbered resistance exercises first and then the even numbered resistance exercises (Exercise 1, 3, 5 etc. and then Exercise 2, 4, 6, etc.). Then repeat for set #2 and 3.
2. From Appendix 9.1.2.2.1: Whole-Body Exercise described and illustrated you can substitute different exercises for the same muscle group
3. NEVER hold your breath as you lift a weight
4. Lift at a pace of 2 beats up and 2 beats down
5. Based on your fitness level you can start with 8, 10, 12, 15 reps and 1, 2 or 3 set.

#	Exercise												
1	Push-ups - Wide Arm (Standard or Modified)	R-	W-	R-	W-	R-	W-	R-	W-	R-	W-	R-	W-
		R-	W-	R-	W-	R-	W-	R-	W-	R-	W-	R-	W-
		R-	W-	R-	W-	R-	W-	R-	W-	R-	W-	R-	W-

2	SB - Dumbbell - Alternating arm Chest Press (Chest)	R-	W-	R-	W-	R-	W-	R-	W-	R-	W-	R-	W-
		R-	W-	R-	W-	R-	W-	R-	W-	R-	W-	R-	W-
		R-	W-	R-	W-	R-	W-	R-	W-	R-	W-	R-	W-
3	SB - Dumbbells - Locomotives (Upper Back)	R-	W-	R-	W-	R-	W-	R-	W-	R-	W-	R-	W-
		R-	W-	R-	W-	R-	W-	R-	W-	R-	W-	R-	W-
		R-	W-	R-	W-	R-	W-	R-	W-	R-	W-	R-	W-
4	SB – Dumbbells - Elbow out Lawnmowers (Upper Back)	R-	W-	R-	W-	R-	W-	R-	W-	R-	W-	R-	W-
		R-	W-	R-	W-	R-	W-	R-	W-	R-	W-	R-	W-
		R-	W-	R-	W-	R-	W-	R-	W-	R-	W-	R-	W-
5	SB - Dumbbells - Alternating Over Head Press (Shoulders and Upper Traps)	R-	W-	R-	W-	R-	W-	R-	W-	R-	W-	R-	W-
		R-	W-	R-	W-	R-	W-	R-	W-	R-	W-	R-	W-
		R-	W-	R-	W-	R-	W-	R-	W-	R-	W-	R-	W-
6	Standing - Dumbbells - Circles - (Shoulders- Lateral Deltoids and Rotator Cuff))	R-	W-	R-	W-	R-	W-	R-	W-	R-	W-	R-	W-
		R-	W-	R-	W-	R-	W-	R-	W-	R-	W-	R-	W-
		R-	W-	R-	W-	R-	W-	R-	W-	R-	W-	R-	W-
7	Standing - Dumbbells - Hammer Curls (Arms- Biceps)	R-	W-	R-	W-	R-	W-	R-	W-	R-	W-	R-	W-
		R-	W-	R-	W-	R-	W-	R-	W-	R-	W-	R-	W-
		R-	W-	R-	W-	R-	W-	R-	W-	R-	W-	R-	W-
8	Bench - Dumbbells - Triceps Dips (Arms - Triceps)	R-	W-	R-	W-	R-	W-	R-	W-	R-	W-	R-	W-
		R-	W-	R-	W-	R-	W-	R-	W-	R-	W-	R-	W-
		R-	W-	R-	W-	R-	W-	R-	W-	R-	W-	R-	W-

	Core and Upper-Body Muscle Resistance Routine #5							
Note: Focus on <u>**SLOW, DELIBERATE & COMPLETE**</u> movements							
		Date:						
	<u>Core</u>							
	<u>Notes:</u> 1. Do all the core exercises in the order presented 2. From Appendix 9.1.2.1.1.: Core Exercises described and illustrated you can substitute different core exercises for the different target muscle groups' areas 3. Never hold your breath while performing core exercises 4. The slower you perform the core exercises the more effective the exercise will be 5. Based on your fitness level determine the number of repetitions you should do per set. Initially you may only do 1 set of each core exercise. This can increase to 2 or 3 sets over time							
1	<u>BOSU</u> - Double Crunch	R-	R-	R-	R-	R-	R-
2	<u>Mat</u> - Double Straight Leg Raise 90º (Advanced - use SB between ankles of knees)	R-	R-	R-	R-	R-	R-
3	<u>Mat</u> - Pilates 100's	R-	R-	R-	R-	R-	R-
4	<u>SB</u> - Oblique Reverse Crunch	R-	R-	R-	R-	R-	R-
5	<u>BOSU</u> - Lateral Crunch (<u>Advanced</u> – use weight)	R- W-	R- W-	R- W-	R- W-	R- W-	R- W-
6	<u>Mat</u> - Standard Plank - Prone (Face down)	T-	T-	T-	T-	T-	T-
7	<u>Mat</u> - Lateral Plank Elbow to Mat	R-	R-	R-	R-	R-	R-
	<u>Resistance</u>							
	<u>Notes:</u> 1. Do all odd numbered resistance exercises first and then the even numbered resistance exercises (Exercise 1, 3, 5 etc. and then Exercise 2, 4, 6, etc.). Then repeat for set #2 and 3. 2. From Appendix 9.1.2.2.1: Whole-Body Exercise described and illustrated you can substitute different exercises for the same muscle group 3. NEVER hold your breath as you lift a weight 4. Lift at a pace of 2 beats up and 2 beats down 5. Based on your fitness level you can start with 8, 10, 12, 15 reps and 1, 2 or 3 set							

	Exercise												
1	Push-ups - Under the Fence (Standard or Modified (on knees))	R-	W-	R-	W-	R-	W-	R-	W-	R-	W-	R-	W-
		R-	W-	R-	W-	R-	W-	R-	W-	R-	W-	R-	W-
		R-	W-	R-	W-	R-	W-	R-	W-	R-	W-	R-	W-
2	Machine – Lat. Pull Downs (Upper Back)	R-	W-	R-	W-	R-	W-	R-	W-	R-	W-	R-	W-
		R-	W-	R-	W-	R-	W-	R-	W-	R-	W-	R-	W-
		R-	W-	R-	W-	R-	W-	R-	W-	R-	W-	R-	W-
3	Dumbbell - Alternating arm Chest Flies	R-	W-	R-	W-	R-	W-	R-	W-	R-	W-	R-	W-
		R-	W-	R-	W-	R-	W-	R-	W-	R-	W-	R-	W-
		R-	W-	R-	W-	R-	W-	R-	W-	R-	W-	R-	W-
4	Machine - Reverse Grip Lat. Pull Downs	R-	W-	R-	W-	R-	W-	R-	W-	R-	W-	R-	W-
		R-	W-	R-	W-	R-	W-	R-	W-	R-	W-	R-	W-
		R-	W-	R-	W-	R-	W-	R-	W-	R-	W-	R-	W-
5	Machine - Over Head Press (Shoulders- Upper Trapezius)	R-	W-	R-	W-	R-	W-	R-	W-	R-	W-	R-	W-
		R-	W-	R-	W-	R-	W-	R-	W-	R-	W-	R-	W-
		R-	W-	R-	W-	R-	W-	R-	W-	R-	W-	R-	W-
6	Standing - Dumbbells - Scarecrows - (Shoulders- Lateral Deltoids and Rotator Cuff))	R-	W-	R-	W-	R-	W-	R-	W-	R-	W-	R-	W-
		R-	W-	R-	W-	R-	W-	R-	W-	R-	W-	R-	W-
		R-	W-	R-	W-	R-	W-	R-	W-	R-	W-	R-	W-
7	Standing - Dumbbells - Hammer Curls (Arms- Biceps)	R-	W-	R-	W-	R-	W-	R-	W-	R-	W-	R-	W-
		R-	W-	R-	W-	R-	W-	R-	W-	R-	W-	R-	W-
		R-	W-	R-	W-	R-	W-	R-	W-	R-	W-	R-	W-
8	Standing - Dumbbells - Triceps Kick Backs (Arms - Triceps)	R-	W-	R-	W-	R-	W-	R-	W-	R-	W-	R-	W-
		R-	W-	R-	W-	R-	W-	R-	W-	R-	W-	R-	W-
		R-	W-	R-	W-	R-	W-	R-	W-	R-	W-	R-	W-

Core and Lower-Body Workout Sheets

Core and Lower-Body Muscle Resistance Routine #1

Note: Focus on **SLOW, DELIBERATE & COMPLETE** movements

	Date:					
	Core						

Notes:
1. Do all the core exercises in the order presented
2. From Appendix 9.1.2.1.1.: Core Exercises described and illustrated you can substitute different core exercises for the different target muscle groups' areas
3. Never hold your breath while performing core exercises
4. The slower you perform the core exercises the more effective the exercise will be
5. Based on your fitness level determine the number of repetitions you should do per set. Initially you may only do 1 set of each core exercise. This can increase to 2 or 3 sets over time

#	Exercise						
1	Mat - Crunch with Knee's at TT on SB (get shoulders off floor)	R-	R-	R-	R-	R-	R-
2	Mat - Russian Twist (Advanced - hold medicine ball or weight in hands)	R- W-	R- W-	R- W-	R- W-	R- W-	R- W-
3	SB - Back Extensions	R-	R-	R-	R-	R-	R-
4	Mat - Oblique Crunch with Knee's at TT on SB	R-	R-	R-	R-	R-	R-
5	Mat - Pendulum	R-	R-	R-	R-	R-	R-
6	BOUS – Superman's	R-	R-	R-	R-	R-	R-

Resistance

Notes:
1. Do all odd numbered resistance exercises first and then the even numbered resistance exercises (Exercise 1, 3, 5 etc. and then Exercise 2, 4, 6, etc.). Then repeat for set #2 and 3.
2. From Appendix 9.1.2.2.1: Whole-Body Exercise described and illustrated you can substitute different exercises for the same muscle group
3. NEVER hold your breath as you lift a weight
4. Lift at a pace of 2 beats up and 2 beats down
5. Based on your fitness level you can start with 8, 10, 12, 15 reps and 1, 2 or 3 set

1	Standing - Squat (Advance - hold medicine ball or weight in hands)	R-	W-	R-	W-	R-	W-	R-	W-	R-	W-	R-	W-
		R-	W-	R-	W-	R-	W-	R-	W-	R-	W-	R-	W-
		R-	W-	R-	W-	R-	W-	R-	W-	R-	W-	R-	W-
2	Standing - Balance Lunge (Put back foot on bench or chair)	R-	W-	R-	W-	R-	W-	R-	W-	R-	W-	R-	W-
		R-	W-	R-	W-	R-	W-	R-	W-	R-	W-	R-	W-
		R-	W-	R-	W-	R-	W-	R-	W-	R-	W-	R-	W-
3	Machine – Double or single Leg Press	R-	W-	R-	W-	R-	W-	R-	W-	R-	W-	R-	W-
		R-	W-	R-	W-	R-	W-	R-	W-	R-	W-	R-	W-
		R-	W-	R-	W-	R-	W-	R-	W-	R-	W-	R-	W-
4	Machine- Single or double Leg Hamstring Curl	R-	W-	R-	W-	R-	W-	R-	W-	R-	W-	R-	W-
		R-	W-	R-	W-	R-	W-	R-	W-	R-	W-	R-	W-
		R-	W-	R-	W-	R-	W-	R-	W-	R-	W-	R-	W-
5	Machine- Single or double Leg Knee Extension	R-	W-	R-	W-	R-	W-	R-	W-	R-	W-	R-	W-
		R-	W-	R-	W-	R-	W-	R-	W-	R-	W-	R-	W-
		R-	W-	R-	W-	R-	W-	R-	W-	R-	W-	R-	W-
6	Machine- Lateral Hip Abductors-Abduct Leg	R-	W-	R-	W-	R-	W-	R-	W-	R-	W-	R-	W-
		R-	W-	R-	W-	R-	W-	R-	W-	R-	W-	R-	W-
		R-	W-	R-	W-	R-	W-	R-	W-	R-	W-	R-	W-
7	Machine- Gluteus Medius - Abduction of Leg 45°	R-	W-	R-	W-	R-	W-	R-	W-	R-	W-	R-	W-
		R-	W-	R-	W-	R-	W-	R-	W-	R-	W-	R-	W-
		R-	W-	R-	W-	R-	W-	R-	W-	R-	W-	R-	W-

Core and Lower-Body Muscle Resistance Routine #2

Note: Focus on **SLOW, DELIBERATE & COMPLETE** movements

		Date:					
	**Core**						

Notes:
1. Do all the core exercises in the order presented
2. From Appendix 9.1.2.1.1.: Core Exercises described and illustrated you can substitute different core exercises for the different target muscle groups' areas
3. Never hold your breath while performing core exercises
4. The slower you perform the core exercises the more effective the exercise will be
5. Based on your fitness level determine the number of repetitions you should do per set. Initially you may only do 1 set of each core exercise. This can increase to 2 or 3 sets over time

#	Exercise						
1	Mat- Pilates 100's	R- 2 x 100	R- 2 x 100	R- 2 x 100	R- 2 x 100	R- 2 x 100	R- 2 x 100
2	Mat -crunch with lower legs on SB	R- 2 x	R- 2 x	R- 2 x	R- 2 x	R- 2 x	R- 2 x
3	Mat - Straight leg raise (Advanced - with SB ball between ankles or knees)	R- 2 x	R- 2 x	R- 2 x	R- 2 x	R- 2 x	R- 2 x
4	Mat - Oblique Crunch	R- 2 x	R- 2 x	R- 2 x	R- 2 x	R- 2 x	R- 2 x
5	BOSU - Lateral Crunch	R- 2 x	R- 2 x	R- 2 x	R- 2 x	R- 2 x	R- 2 x
6	SB- Back extensions with twist	R- 2 x	R- 2 x	R- 2 x	R- 2 x	R- 2 x	R- 2 x

Resistance

Notes:
1. Do all odd numbered resistance exercises first and then the even numbered resistance exercises (Exercise 1, 3, 5 etc. and then Exercise 2, 4, 6, etc.). Then repeat for set #2 and 3.
2. From Appendix 9.1.2.2.1: Whole-Body Exercise described and illustrated you can substitute different exercises for the same muscle group
3. NEVER hold your breath as you lift a weight
4. Lift at a pace of 2 beats up and 2 beats down
5. Based on your fitness level you can start with 8, 10, 12, 15 reps and 1, 2 or 3 set

#	Exercise												
1	Standing - Forward walking Squat (take 5 steps and reverse direction) (Advance - hold weight in hands)	R-	W-	R-	W-	R-	W-	R-	W-	R-	W-	R-	W-
		R-	W-	R-	W-	R-	W-	R-	W-	R-	W-	R-	W-
		R-	W-	R-	W-	R-	W-	R-	W-	R-	W-	R-	W-

#	Exercise												
2	Standing - Lateral Lunge (Advanced - put rubber band around ankles and hold weight in hands)	R-	W-	R-	W-	R-	W-	R-	W-	R-	W-	R-	W-
		R-	W-	R-	W-	R-	W-	R-	W-	R-	W-	R-	W-
		R-	W-	R-	W-	R-	W-	R-	W-	R-	W-	R-	W-
3	Standing - Dead Lifts (Dumbbells or Barbells)	R-	W-	R-	W-	R-	W-	R-	W-	R-	W-	R-	W-
		R-	W-	R-	W-	R-	W-	R-	W-	R-	W-	R-	W-
		R-	W-	R-	W-	R-	W-	R-	W-	R-	W-	R-	W-
4	Machine- Single or double Leg Hamstring Curl	R-	W-	R-	W-	R-	W-	R-	W-	R-	W-	R-	W-
		R-	W-	R-	W-	R-	W-	R-	W-	R-	W-	R-	W-
		R-	W-	R-	W-	R-	W-	R-	W-	R-	W-	R-	W-
5	Machine- Single or double Leg Knee Extension	R-	W-	R-	W-	R-	W-	R-	W-	R-	W-	R-	W-
		R-	W-	R-	W-	R-	W-	R-	W-	R-	W-	R-	W-
		R-	W-	R-	W-	R-	W-	R-	W-	R-	W-	R-	W-
6	Standing - Lateral Monster Walk (Advanced - put rubber band around ankles and hold weight in hands)	R-	W-	R-	W-	R-	W-	R-	W-	R-	W-	R-	W-
		R-	W-	R-	W-	R-	W-	R-	W-	R-	W-	R-	W-
		R-	W-	R-	W-	R-	W-	R-	W-	R-	W-	R-	W-
7	SB - Hip abductions (prone) (Advanced - put ankle weights on)	R-	W-	R-	W-	R-	W-	R-	W-	R-	W-	R-	W-
		R-	W-	R-	W-	R-	W-	R-	W-	R-	W-	R-	W-
		R-	W-	R-	W-	R-	W-	R-	W-	R-	W-	R-	W-

Core and Lower-Body Muscle Resistance Routine #3

Note: Focus on **SLOW, DELIBERATE & COMPLETE** movements

		Date:					

Core

Notes:
1. Do all the core exercises in the order presented
2. From Appendix 9.1.2.1.1.: Core Exercises described and illustrated you can substitute different core exercise for the different target muscle groups' areas
3. Never hold your breath while performing core exercises
4. The slower you perform the core exercises the more effective the exercise will be
5. Based on your fitness level determine the number of repetitions you should do per set. Initially you may only do 1 set of each core exercise. This can increase to 2 or 3 sets over time

#	Exercise						
1	Mat- Crunch	R- 2 x	R- 2 x	R- 2 x	R- 2 x	R- 2 x	R- 2 x
2	Mat -crunch with lower legs on SB	R- 2 x	R- 2 x	R- 2 x	R- 2 x	R- 2 x	R- 2 x
3	Mat - Flutters	R- 2 x	R- 2 x	R- 2 x	R- 2 x	R- 2 x	R- 2 x
4	SB- Prone (face down) Reverse Crunch	R- 2 x	R- 2 x	R- 2 x	R- 2 x	R- 2 x	R- 2 x
5	BOSU - Lateral Crunch	R- 2 x	R- 2 x	R- 2 x	R- 2 x	R- 2 x	R- 2 x
6	Mat - Standard Plank (Prone face down)	T-	T-	T-	T-	T-	T-

Resistance

Notes:
1. Do all odd numbered resistance exercises first and then the even numbered resistance exercises (Exercise 1, 3, 5 etc. and then Exercise 2, 4, 6, etc.). Then repeat for set #2 and 3.
2. From Appendix 9.1.2.2.1: Whole-Body Exercise described and illustrated you can substitute different exercises for the same muscle group
3. NEVER hold your breath as you lift a weight
4. Lift at a pace of 2 beats up and 2 beats down
5. Based on your fitness level you can start with 8, 10, 12, 15 reps and 1, 2 or 3 set

#	Exercise												
1	BOSU - Step onto BOSU and Squat and then step off (Advanced - Hold weight)	R-	W-	R-	W-	R-	W-	R-	W-	R-	W-	R-	W-
		R-	W-	R-	W-	R-	W-	R-	W-	R-	W-	R-	W-
		R-	W-	R-	W-	R-	W-	R-	W-	R-	W-	R-	W-
2	Standing - Back step Lunge (Advanced - hold weight in hands)	R-	W-	R-	W-	R-	W-	R-	W-	R-	W-	R-	W-
		R-	W-	R-	W-	R-	W-	R-	W-	R-	W-	R-	W-
		R-	W-	R-	W-	R-	W-	R-	W-	R-	W-	R-	W-
3	Standing - Dead Lifts (Dumbbells or Barbells)	R-	W-	R-	W-	R-	W-	R-	W-	R-	W-	R-	W-
		R-	W-	R-	W-	R-	W-	R-	W-	R-	W-	R-	W-
		R-	W-	R-	W-	R-	W-	R-	W-	R-	W-	R-	W-
4	Machine - Single or double leg hamstring curl	R-	W-	R-	W-	R-	W-	R-	W-	R-	W-	R-	W-
		R-	W-	R-	W-	R-	W-	R-	W-	R-	W-	R-	W-
		R-	W-	R-	W-	R-	W-	R-	W-	R-	W-	R-	W-
5	Machine - Single or double leg knee extension	R-	W-	R-	W-	R-	W-	R-	W-	R-	W-	R-	W-
		R-	W-	R-	W-	R-	W-	R-	W-	R-	W-	R-	W-
		R-	W-	R-	W-	R-	W-	R-	W-	R-	W-	R-	W-
6	Mat - Clam shell (Advanced - Use ankle weights)	R-	W-	R-	W-	R-	W-	R-	W-	R-	W-	R-	W-
		R-	W-	R-	W-	R-	W-	R-	W-	R-	W-	R-	W-
		R-	W-	R-	W-	R-	W-	R-	W-	R-	W-	R-	W-
7	Standing - Heel and Toe walk (10 steps forward and reverse) (Advanced - Hold weight)	R-	W-	R-	W-	R-	W-	R-	W-	R-	W-	R-	W-
		R-	W-	R-	W-	R-	W-	R-	W-	R-	W-	R-	W-
		R-	W-	R-	W-	R-	W-	R-	W-	R-	W-	R-	W-

Core and Lower-Body Muscle Resistance Routine #4

Note: Focus on **SLOW, DELIBERATE & COMPLETE** movements

	Date:						
	\multicolumn{7}{c}{**Core**}

Notes:
1. Do all the core exercises in the order presented
2. From Appendix 9.1.2.1.1: Core Exercises described and illustrated you can substitute different core exercises for the different target muscle groups' areas
3. Never hold your breath while performing core exercises
4. The slower you perform the core exercises the more effective the exercise will be
5. Based on your fitness level determine the number of repetitions you should do per set. Initially you may only do 1 set of each core exercise. This can increase to 2 or 3 sets over time

#	Exercise						
1	Mat - Full Sit-up (Stabilize the feet)	R- 2 x	R- 2 x	R- 2 x	R- 2 x	R- 2 x	R- 2 x
2	Mat - lateral plank eye of the needle	R- 2 x	R- 2 x	R- 2 x	R- 2 x	R- 2 x	R- 2 x
3	Mat - Bicycles	R- 2 x	R- 2 x	R- 2 x	R- 2 x	R- 2 x	R- 2 x
4	Mat - Supine (face up) Reverse crunch (Advanced - SB between ankles or knees)	R- 2 x	R- 2 x	R- 2 x	R- 2 x	R- 2 x	R- 2 x
5	BOSU – Superman's	R- 2 x	R- 2 x	R- 2 x	R- 2 x	R- 2 x	R- 2 x
6	Mat - Standard Plank (Prone face down)	T-	T-	T-	T-	T-	T-

Resistance

Notes:
1. Do all odd numbered resistance exercises first and then the even numbered resistance exercises (Exercise 1, 5 etc. and then Exercise 2, 4, 6, etc.). Then repeat for set #2 and 3.
2. From Appendix 9.1.2.2.1: Whole-Body Exercise described and illustrated you can substitute different exercises for the same muscle group
3. NEVER hold your breath as you lift a weight
4. Lift at a pace of 2 beats up and 2 beats down
5. Based on your fitness level you can start with 8, 10, 12, 15 reps and 1, 2 or 3 set

1	Standing - Sumo Squat - (feet pointing out 45°)	R-	W-	R-	W-	R-	W-	R-	W-	R-	W-	R-	W-
		R-	W-	R-	W-	R-	W-	R-	W-	R-	W-	R-	W-
		R-	W-	R-	W-	R-	W-	R-	W-	R-	W-	R-	W-
2	Standing - Lunge with twist (Twist toward lunge side)	R-	W-	R-	W-	R-	W-	R-	W-	R-	W-	R-	W-
		R-	W-	R-	W-	R-	W-	R-	W-	R-	W-	R-	W-
		R-	W-	R-	W-	R-	W-	R-	W-	R-	W-	R-	W-
3	Standing - Dead Lifts (Dumbbells or Barbells)	R-	W-	R-	W-	R-	W-	R-	W-	R-	W-	R-	W-
		R-	W-	R-	W-	R-	W-	R-	W-	R-	W-	R-	W-
		R-	W-	R-	W-	R-	W-	R-	W-	R-	W-	R-	W-
4	Machine- Single or double leg hamstring curl	R-	W-	R-	W-	R-	W-	R-	W-	R-	W-	R-	W-
		R-	W-	R-	W-	R-	W-	R-	W-	R-	W-	R-	W-
		R-	W-	R-	W-	R-	W-	R-	W-	R-	W-	R-	W-
5	Machine- Single or double knee ext.	R-	W-	R-	W-	R-	W-	R-	W-	R-	W-	R-	W-
		R-	W-	R-	W-	R-	W-	R-	W-	R-	W-	R-	W-
		R-	W-	R-	W-	R-	W-	R-	W-	R-	W-	R-	W-
6	Mat - Side lying hip abduction	R-	W-	R-	W-	R-	W-	R-	W-	R-	W-	R-	W-
		R-	W-	R-	W-	R-	W-	R-	W-	R-	W-	R-	W-
		R-	W-	R-	W-	R-	W-	R-	W-	R-	W-	R-	W-
7	Standing - RB leg abductions	R-	RBC-	R-	RBC-	R-	RBC-	R-	RBC-	R-	RBC-	R-	RBC-
		R-	RBC-	R-	RBC-	R-	RBC-	R-	RBC-	R-	RBC-	R-	RBC-
		R-	RBC-	R-	RBC-	R-	RBC-	R-	RBC-	R-	RBC-	R-	RBC-

Core and Lower-Body Muscle Resistance Routine #5

Note: Focus on SLOW, DELIBERATE & COMPLETE movements

		Date:					
	\multicolumn{7}{c}{**Core**}

Notes:
1. Do all the core exercises in the order presented
2. From Appendix 9.1.2.1.1.: Core Exercises described and illustrated you can substitute different core exercises for the different target muscle groups' areas
3. Never hold your breath while performing core exercises
4. The slower you perform the core exercises the more effective the exercise will be
5. Based on your fitness level determine the number of repetitions you should do per set. Initially you may only 1 set of each core exercise. This can increase to 2 or 3 sets over time

#	Exercise						
1	Mat -3/4 Sit-up (Stabilize the feet)	R- 2 x	R- 2 x	R- 2 x	R- 2 x	R- 2 x	R- 2 x
2	BOSU - Lateral crunch	R- 2 x	R- 2 x	R- 2 x	R- 2 x	R- 2 x	R- 2 x
3	Mat - Figure 4 Obliques (lower legs on SB)	R- 2 x	R- 2 x	R- 2 x	R- 2 x	R- 2 x	R- 2 x
4	Mat - Russian twist (advanced - hold medicine ball or weight)	R- 2 x	R- 2 x	R- 2 x	R- 2 x	R- 2 x	R- 2 x
5	Mat - Bridges	R- 2 x	R- 2 x	R- 2 x	R- 2 x	R- 2 x	R- 2 x
6	Mat - Lateral Plank (facing sideways)	T-	T-	T-	T-	T-	T-

Resistance

Notes:
1. Do all odd numbered resistance exercises first and then the even numbered resistance exercises (Exercise 1, 3 etc. and then Exercise 2, 4, 6, etc.). Then repeat for set #2 and 3.
2. From Appendix 9.1.2.2.1: Whole-Body Exercise described and illustrated you can substitute different exercises for the same muscle group
3. NEVER hold your breath as you lift a weight
4. Lift at a pace of 2 beats up and 2 beats down
5. Based on your fitness level you can start with 8, 10, 12, 15 reps and 1, 2 or 3 set.

#	Exercise												
1	SB - against wall Squat (Advanced - hold weight)	R-	W-	R-	W-	R-	W-	R-	W-	R-	W-	R-	W-
		R-	W-	R-	W-	R-	W-	R-	W-	R-	W-	R-	W-
		R-	W-	R-	W-	R-	W-	R-	W-	R-	W-	R-	W-

#	Exercise												
2	Standing - Curtsey Lunge (one leg crosses behind) (Advanced - hold weight)	R-	W-	R-	W-	R-	W-	R-	W-	R-	W-	R-	W-
		R-	W-	R-	W-	R-	W-	R-	W-	R-	W-	R-	W-
		R-	W-	R-	W-	R-	W-	R-	W-	R-	W-	R-	W-
3	Standing - Dead Lifts (Dumbbells or Barbells)	R-	W-	R-	W-	R-	W-	R-	W-	R-	W-	R-	W-
		R-	W-	R-	W-	R-	W-	R-	W-	R-	W-	R-	W-
		R-	W-	R-	W-	R-	W-	R-	W-	R-	W-	R-	W-
4	Machine - Single or double leg hamstring curl	R-	W-	R-	W-	R-	W-	R-	W-	R-	W-	R-	W-
		R-	W-	R-	W-	R-	W-	R-	W-	R-	W-	R-	W-
		R-	W-	R-	W-	R-	W-	R-	W-	R-	W-	R-	W-
5	Machine - Single or double leg knee extension	R-	W-	R-	W-	R-	W-	R-	W-	R-	W-	R-	W-
		R-	W-	R-	W-	R-	W-	R-	W-	R-	W-	R-	W-
		R-	W-	R-	W-	R-	W-	R-	W-	R-	W-	R-	W-
6	Mat - Fire hydrant (advanced - use ankle weight)	R-	W-	R-	W-	R-	W-	R-	W-	R-	W-	R-	W-
		R-	W-	R-	W-	R-	W-	R-	W-	R-	W-	R-	W-
		R-	W-	R-	W-	R-	W-	R-	W-	R-	W-	R-	W-
7	Standing against wall or chair - hip extensions and 45° hip abduction (Advanced - use ankle weight or RB)	R-	W-	R-	W-	R-	W-	R-	W-	R-	W-	R-	W-
		R-	W-	R-	W-	R-	W-	R-	W-	R-	W-	R-	W-
		R-	W-	R-	W-	R-	W-	R-	W-	R-	W-	R-	W-

Core and Bodyweight Workout Sheets

Core and Bodyweight Muscle Resistance Routine #1

Note: Focus on SLOW, DELIBERATE & COMPLETE movements

	Date:						
	\multicolumn{7}{c}{**Core**}

Notes:
1. Do all the core exercises in the order presented
2. From Appendix 9.1.2.1.1.: Core Exercises described and illustrated you can substitute different core exercises for the different target muscle groups' areas
3. Never hold your breath while performing core exercises
4. The slower you perform the core exercises the more effective the exercise will be
5. Based on your fitness level determine the number of repetitions you should do per set. Initially you may only do 1 set of each core exercise. This can increase to 2 or 3 sets over time

1	Mat - Flutter Kicks	R- 2 x	R- 2 x	R- 2 x	R- 2 x	R- 2 x	R- 2 x
2	Mat - Supine Reverse Crunch (Advanced - Put SB between ankles or knees)	R- 2 x	R- 2 x	R- 2 x	R- 2 x	R- 2 x	R- 2 x
3	Mat - Double Crunch	R- 2 x	R- 2 x	R- 2 x	R- 2 x	R- 2 x	R- 2 x
4	Mat - Oblique Crunch	R- 2 x	R- 2 x	R- 2 x	R- 2 x	R- 2 x	R- 2 x
5	SB or BOSU - Back Extensions	R- 2 x	R- 2 x	R- 2 x	R- 2 x	R- 2 x	R- 2 x
6	Mat - Standard Plank (Prone - Face down)	T-	T-	T-	T-	T-	T-

Resistance

Notes:
1. Do Resistance Exercises in Pairs (Exercise 1 & 2 then Exercise 3 & 4, etc.)
2. From Appendix 9.1.2.3.1 -Bodyweight exercise described and illustrated you can substitute different exercises for the same muscle group
3. NEVER hold your breath as you lift a weight
4. Perform exercise at a pace of 2 beats up and 2 beats down
5. Based on your fitness level you can start with 8, 10, 12, 15 reps and 1, 2 or 3 sets.

Chest:

1	Mat - Military Push-ups (Modification- Knee or Wall Assisted)	R-	R-	R-	R-	R-	R-
2	Mat - Regular Push-up to side Plank (Modification - Knee or Wall Assisted)	R-	R-	R-	R-	R-	R-

Upper Back and Biceps:

3	Standing - Pull-ups using high cross bar (Modification – stand on Bench or Chair for assistance)	R-	R-	R-	R-	R-	R-
4	Standing - Chin-ups using high cross bar. (Modification – stand on Bench or Chair for assistance)	R-	R-	R-	R-	R-	R-

Triceps

5	Bench - Dips	R-	R-	R-	R-	R-	R-
6	**Bench** - Dips	R-	R-	R-	R-	R-	R-

Hips:

7	Mat - Clam Shell (Advanced - Wear rubber band around knees)	R-	R-	R-	R-	R-	R-
8	Standing - Hip Extensions and 45º Hip Abduction (Advanced - Wear ankle weights or rubber band around ankles)	R-	R-	R-	R-	R-	R-

	Legs:						
9	Standing - Squats (Advanced - hold a weight in hands or do on BOSU or another unstable surface)	R-	R-	R-	R-	R-	R-
10	Standing - Lateral Lunge (Advanced - hold a weight in hands)	R-	R-	R-	R-	R-	R-
	Combined Exercise:						
11	Standing - Burpee with Push-up and/or Jumping Jack	R-	R-	R-	R-	R-	R-
	Plyometrics:						
12	Standing - Double Leg lateral Jump (Advanced- Double Leg Lateral Jump onto an elevated surface 6-12-18 inches high)	R-	R-	R-	R-	R-	R-

Core and Bodyweight Muscle Resistance Routine #2

Note: Focus on **SLOW, DELIBERATE & COMPLETE** movements

	Date:						
\multicolumn{8}{c}{**Core**}							

Notes:
1. Do all the core exercises in the order presented
2. From Appendix 9.1.2.1.1: Core Exercises described and illustrated you can substitute different core exercises for the different target muscle groups' areas
3. Never hold your breath while performing core exercises
4. The slower you perform the core exercises the more effective the exercise will be
5. Based on your fitness level determine the number of repetitions you should do per set. Initially you may only do 1 set of each core exercise. This can increase to 2 or 3 sets over time

1	Mat -3/4 Sit-up (Stabilize the feet)	R- 2 x	R- 2 x	R- 2 x	R- 2 x	R- 2 x	R- 2 x
2	BOSU - Lateral crunch	R- 2 x	R- 2 x	R- 2 x	R- 2 x	R- 2 x	R- 2 x
3	Mat - Figure 4 Obliques (lower legs on SB)	R- 2 x	R- 2 x	R- 2 x	R- 2 x	R- 2 x	R- 2 x
4	Mat - Russian twist (Advanced - hold medicine ball or weight)	R- 2 x	R- 2 x	R- 2 x	R- 2 x	R- 2 x	R- 2 x
5	Mat or SB - Bridges	R- 2 x	R- 2 x	R- 2 x	R- 2 x	R- 2 x	R- 2 x
6	Mat - Lateral Plank (facing sideways)	T-	T-	T-	T-	T-	T-

Resistance

Notes:
1. Do Resistance Exercises in Pairs (Exercise 1 & 2 then Exercise 3 & 4, etc.)
2. From Appendix 9.1.2.3.1 Bodyweight exercise described and illustrated you can substitute different exercises for the same muscle group
3. NEVER hold your breath as you lift a weight
4. Perform exercise at a pace of 2 beats up and 2 beats down
5. Based on your fitness level you can start with 8, 10, 12, 15 reps and 1, 2 or 3 sets

Chest

1	Mat - Regular Push-ups (Modification- Knee or Wall Assisted)	R-	R-	R-	R-	R-	R-
2	Mat - Wide-Fly Push-ups (Modification - Knee or Wall Assisted)	R-	R-	R-	R-	R-	R-

	Upper Back and Biceps:						
3	Standing -Pull-ups using high cross bar. (Modification – Stand on Bench or Chair)	R-	R-	R-	R-	R-	R-
4	Standing - Chin-ups using high cross bar. (Modification – Stand on Bench or Chair)	R-	R-	R-	R-	R-	R-
	Triceps:						
5	Bench - Dips	R-	R-	R-	R-	R-	R-
6	Bench - Dips	R-	R-	R-	R-	R-	R-
	Hips:						
7	Mat - Side Lying Lateral Leg Raise (Advanced - ankle weights or rubber band around ankles)	R-	R-	R-	R-	R-	R-
8	Standing - Hip Extensions (Advanced - Wear ankle weights)	R-	R-	R-	R-	R-	R-
	Legs:						
9	Standing - Squats (Advanced - hold a weight in hands or on BOSU or another unstable surface)	R-	R-	R-	R-	R-	R-
10	Standing - Forward Lunge (Advanced - hold a weight in hands and/or twist to the lunge (forward) leg side)	R-	R-	R-	R-	R-	R-
	Combined Exercise:						
11	Standing - Burpee	R-	R-	R-	R-	R-	R-
	Plyometrics:						
12	Standing - Double Leg Forward Jump (Advanced- Double Leg Forward Jump onto an elevated surface 6-12-18 inches high)	R-	R-	R-	R-	R-	R-

9.2.4. Agility, Balance and Coordination Workout Sheets

Core, Leg Strengthening and Agility, Balance and Coordination Exercise Routine 948

Core and Leg Strengthening Exercise Routine To Improve Agility, Balance and Coordination (Illustrated) 952

Core and Leg Strengthening Exercise Routine to Improve Agility, Balance and Coordination 956

Agility and Coordination Exercise Routine 957

Balance Exercise Routine (Illustrated) 959

Balance Exercise Routine 962

Core, Leg Strengthening and Agility, Balance and Coordination Exercise Routine

Remember - To improve agility, balance and coordination, a person needs to strengthen their leg and hip muscular and perform the agility and balance exercises frequently. It is recommended a minimum of 2x/week.
All exercises listed are full described in Appendix 9.1.3.1

Date:							
Leg Strengthening Exercises:							
Core:							
1. Abdominal Crunches	R-	R-	R-	R-	R-	R-	R-
2. Back Extensions (Superman's)	R-	R-	R-	R-	R-	R-	R-
3. Lateral Hip Raises/dips	R-	R-	R-	R-	R-	R-	R-
4. Regular (face down) Planks	T-	T-	T-	T-	T-	T-	T-
5. Side Planks	T-	T-	T-	T-	T-	T-	T-
Hip Exercises:							
1. Hip Abductions (side lying and standing)	R-	R-	R-	R-	R-	R-	R-
2. 45º Hip Abduction	R-	R-	R-	R-	R-	R-	R-
3. Hip Extensions	R-	R-	R-	R-	R-	R-	R-
Leg Exercises:							
1. Regular Squats	R-	R-	R-	R-	R-	R-	R-
2. Forward Lunges	R-	R-	R-	R-	R-	R-	R-
3. Heel and Toe Raises	R-	R-	R-	R-	R-	R-	R-

Balance Exercise:
Open the following link for instructional video:
http://www.youtube.com/watch?v=AWuKEt96Jjs

Progressions:

Progress SLOWLY and have a chair or wall close by to help if there is a loss of balance

6 Stages of progression for increase difficulty:
1. Feet shoulder or hip width apart
2. Stagger step Position - one foot takes a step forward
3. Split position 1 - one foot is one step ahead but directly in front of back foot
4. Split position 2 - same as split position one but heel of forward foot is touching the tow of the back foot
5. Stand on single leg
6. Stand on unstable surface (inflatable disc, wobble board, BOSU)

Inflatable Disc   **Wobble Board**   **BOSU**   **Agility Ladder**

(Rate as: no problem, mild, moderate or significant hesitation)

1. Standing on Both Legs:							
1. Move both arms over your head and hold							
2. Raise a finger in front of your eye and follow it with your eyes as you move it up and down and to the sides							
Standing on One leg:							
1. Swing leg forward and back with the opposite arm swinging opposite direction of the leg							
2. Swing leg out to the side and then across the body. The opposite arm swings in the opposite direction of the leg							

3. Swing leg out to the side and then across in front of the body and then across the back of the body. The opposite arm swings in the opposite direction of the leg.							
Agility and Coordination Exercises: **(Rate as: no problem, mild, moderate or significant hesitation)**							
1. Walking Drills (Forward, sideways and cross over):							
1. Forward walking:							
1. Regular walking							
2. Take one step forward and then opposite foot catches up before you take the next step							
2. Sideways Walking:							
1. One foot walking sideways and then the other foot catches up. (Return to start position with other leg leading the sideway walk)							
2. Front Cross-over moving sideways. (Return to start position with other leg leading the crossover walk)							
3. Carioca - Outside foot is the leading crossover foot and alternate going in front and then behind the other leg. (Return to start position with opposite leg leading cross over)							

Hop Drills:							
1. Forward Hop Drill:							
1. Both feet hop forward at same time							
2. One leg hop forward							
3. Two feet narrow and then wide hop Scotch							
2. Sideways Hop Drills:							
1. Both feet hop sideways							
2. One foot hop sideways							
3. Scissor Hop Drills:							
1. Scissor Hop- as hop forward the legs split and land with one leg in front of the other. On the next hop the opposite leg lands in front.							
4. Diagonal Hop:							
1. Double foot diagonal hop together							
2. Alternating single leg diagonal hop (hop to right and then to left alternating the feet)							
5. Rotational Hop Drill:							
1. 90° two-legged hop rotation. Do the rotation in both directions.							
2. 180° two-legged hop rotation. Do the rotation in both directions.							

Core and Leg Strengthening Exercise Routine To Improve Agility, Balance and Coordination (Illustrated)

Remember - To improve agility, balance and coordination a person needs to strengthen their leg and hip muscular and perform the agility and balance exercises frequently. It is recommended a minimum of 2x/week.
All exercises listed are fully described in Appendix 9.1.3.1

Key Points:
1. Focus on **SLOW, DELIBERATE & COMPLETE** movements
2. Breathe normally as you do each movement
3. All movements must be done within a pain free range of movement
4. Avoid any movement if they are painful.

	Date:							
	Core							
1. Abdominal Crunch		R-	R-	R-	R-	R-	R-	R-
2. Back Extensions (Superman)		R-	R-	R-	R-	R-	R-	R-
3. Lateral Hip Dips		R-	R-	R-	R-	R-	R-	R-

952

4. Planks (Face down)	T-	T-	T-	T-	T-	T-	T-
5. Side Planks	T-	T-	T-	T-	T-	T-	T-

Leg Strengthening Exercises

Hip Exercises

1. Lateral Hip Raise (Hip Abductions) **Side lying** **Chair Assisted**	R-	R-	R-	R-	R-	R-	R-
2. 45° Hip Abduction	R-	R-	R-	R-	R-	R-	R-

3. Hip Extensions **On Hands and Knees** **Lying flat on Mat**	R-	R-	R-	R-	R-	R-	R-
Leg Exercises:							
1. Squats **Chair Assisted**	R-	R-	R-	R-	R-	R-	R-

2. Lunges **Forward** **Backward** **Chair Assisted Lunges** **Lateral Lunge**	R-	R-	R-	R-	R-	R-	R-
3. Toe and Heel Raises **Toe Raise** **Heel Raise**	R-	R-	R-	R-	R-	R-	R-

Core and Leg Strengthening Exercise Routine to Improve Agility, Balance and Coordination

Remember - To improve agility, balance and coordination a person needs to strengthen their leg and hip muscular and perform the agility and balance exercises frequently. It is recommended a minimum of 2x/week.
All exercises listed are full described in Appendix 9.1.3.1

Date:									
Core									
1. Abdominal Crunches	R-	R-	R-	R-	R-	R-	R-	R-	R-
2. Back Extensions (Superman's)	R-	R-	R-	R-	R-	R-	R-	R-	R-
3. Lateral Hip Raises/dips	R-	R-	R-	R-	R-	R-	R-	R-	R-
4. Regular (face down) Planks	T-	T-	T-	T-	T-	T-	T-	T-	T-
5. Side Planks	T-	T-	T-	T-	T-	T-	T-	T-	T-
Leg Strengthening Exercises									
Hip Exercises:									
1. Hip Abductions (side lying and standing)	R-	R-	R-	R-	R-	R-	R-	R-	R-
2. 45° Hip Abduction	R-	R-	R-	R-	R-	R-	R-	R-	R-
3. Hip Extensions	R-	R-	R-	R-	R-	R-	R-	R-	R-
Leg Exercises:									
1. Squats	R-	R-	R-	R-	R-	R-	R-	R-	R-
2. Lunges	R-	R-	R-	R-	R-	R-	R-	R-	R-
3. Calf Raises	R-	R-	R-	R-	R-	R-	R-	R-	R-

Agility and Coordination Exercise Routine

Remember - To improve agility, balance and coordination a person needs to strengthen their leg and hip muscular and perform the agility and balance exercises frequently. It is recommended a minimum of 2x/week.
All exercises listed are full described in Appendix 9.1.3.1

Date:										

Agility and Coordination Exercises:
(Rate as no, moderate or significant hesitation)

1. Walking Drills (Forward, sideways and cross over):

1. Forward walking:

1. Regular walking										
2. Take one step forward and then opposite foot catches up before you take the next step										

2. Sideways Walking:

1. One foot walking sideways and then the other foot catches up. (Return to start position with other leg leading the sideway walk)										
2. Front Cross-over moving sideways. (Return to start position with other leg leading the crossover walk)										
3. Carioca - Outside foot is the leading crossover foot and alternate going in front and then behind the other leg.(Return to start position with opposite leg leading cross over)										

Hop Drills:

1. Forward Hop Drill:

1. Both feet hop forward at same time									
2. One leg hop forward									
3. Two feet narrow and then wide hop Scotch									

2. Sideways Hop Drills:

1. Both feet hop sideways									
2. One foot hop sideways									

3. Scissor Hop Drills:

1. Scissor Hop- as hop forward the legs split and land with one leg in front of the other. On the next hop the opposite leg lands in front.									

4. Diagonal Hop:

1. Double foot diagonal hop together									
2. Alternating single leg diagonal hop (hop to right and then to left alternating the feet)									

5. Rotational Hop Drill:

1. 90° two-legged hop rotation									
2. 180° two-legged hop rotation									

Balance Exercise Routine (Illustrated)

Remember - To improve agility, balance and coordination a person needs to strengthen their leg and hip muscular and perform the agility and balance exercises frequently. It is recommended a minimum of 2x/week.
All exercises listed are full described in Appendix 9.1.3.1

Date:							

Balance Exercise:
Open the following link for instructional video:
http://www.youtube.com/watch?v=AWuKEt96Jjs

Progressions:

6 Stages of progression for increase difficulty:

1. Feet shoulder or hip width apart

2. Stagger step Position - one foot takes a step forward

3. Split position 1 - one foot is one step ahead but directly in front of back foot

4. Split position 2 - same as split position one but heel of forward foot is touching the tow of the back foot

5. Stand on single leg

6. Stand on unstable surface (inflatable disc, wobble board, BOSU) or us agility ladder.

Progress SLOWLY and have a chair or wall close by to help if there is a loss of balance.

Inflatable Disc

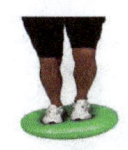

Wobble Board

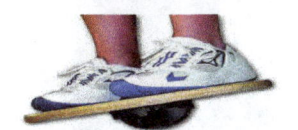

BOSU

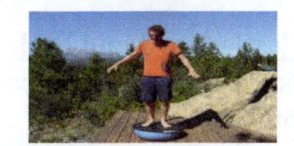

Agility Ladder

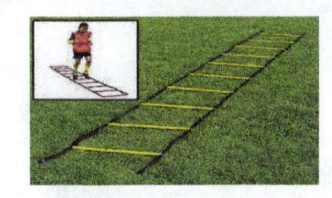

Do each exercise 3 to 5 times and rate as no, little, moderate or unable to do

1. Standing on Both Legs: 1. Move both arms over your head and hold.								
2. Raise a finger in front of your eyes - follow it with your eyes as you move it up and down and to the sides								
Standing on One leg: **1. Swing leg forward and back** - the opposite arm swinging opposite direction of the leg. **Forward Swing** **Backward Swing**								

2. Front Leg Swing leg

- swing leg out to the side and then across the body.

-The opposite arm swings in the opposite direction of the leg

3. Front and Back Leg Swing

- swing leg out to the side and then across in front of the body and then out to the side and then across the back of the body.

- The opposite arm swings in the opposite direction of the leg.

Balance Exercise Routine

Remember - To improve agility, balance and coordination a person needs to strengthen their leg and hip muscular and perform the agility and balance exercises frequently. It is recommended a minimum of 2x/week.
All exercises listed are full described in Appendix 9.1.3.1

Date:									

Core:

Balance Exercise:
Open the following link for instructional video:
http://www.youtube.com/watch?v=AWuKEt96Jjs

Progressions:

Progress SLOWLY and have a chair or wall close by to help if there is a loss of balance

6 Stages of progression for increase difficulty:
1. Feet shoulder or hip width apart
2. Stagger step Position - one foot takes a step forward
3. Split position 1 - one foot is one step ahead but directly in front of back foot
4. Split position 2 - same as split position one but heel of forward foot is touching the tow of the back foot
5. Stand on single leg
6. Stand on unstable surface (inflatable disc, wobble board, BOSU) or use agility ladder

Inflatable Disc	**Wobble Board**	**BOSU**	**Agility Ladder**

Do each exercise 3 to 5 times and rate as no, little, moderate or unable to do

1. Move both arms over your head and hold					
2. Raise a finger in front of your eye and follow it with your eyes as you move it up and down and to the sides					

Balance on One Leg:

1. Swing leg forward and back with the opposite arm swinging opposite direction of the leg					
2. Swing leg out to the side and then across the body. The opposite arm swings in the opposite direction of the leg					
3. Swing leg out to the side and then across in front of the body and then across the back of the body. The opposite arm swings in the opposite direction of the leg.					

9.2.5. Stretching to Improve Flexibility Workout Sheets

45 Minute Dynamic and Static Stretching Routine 964

10 Minute Dynamic and Static Stretching Routine (Illustrated) …..………………...976

10 Minute Dynamic Stretching Routine (Illustrated) 973

10 Minute Static Stretching Routine (Illustrated) 976

Yin Yoga - Upper Back, Chest and Shoulders (Illustrated) 980

Yin Yoga - Lower Back, Hips and Legs Routine (Illustrated).................................... 983

Myofascial Self Massage Utilizing a Roller (Illustrated) ……...………………......987

45 Minute Dynamic and Static Stretching Routine

Reference - Chapter 5.1 and Appendix 9.1.4.1

(You do not have to do each of these stretching exercises each time you stretch. Do some one day and others the next)

Remember - To improve your flexibility you need to stretch frequently. It is better to stretch 3 x/day for 5 minutes each than 1 x/day for 15 minutes.

Frequency and consistency are the keys

Dynamic

Key Points:
1. Focus on SLOW, DELIBERATE & COMPLETE movements
2. Breathe normally as you do each movement
3. All movements must be done within a pain free range of movement
4. Avoid any stretch movements if they are painful

#	Date:									
1	Semi-circle head rolls (3 - 5+ reps)	R-	R-	R-	R-	R-	R-	R-	R-	R-
2	Wide stance trunk rotations (3 - 5+ reps)	R-	R-	R-	R-	R-	R-	R-	R-	R-
3	Wide stance side stretch (3 - 5+ reps)	R-	R-	R-	R-	R-	R-	R-	R-	R-
4	Shoulder rolls (3 - 5+ reps)	R-	R-	R-	R-	R-	R-	R-	R-	R-
5	Arm Circles (3 - 5+ reps forward and backward)	R-	R-	R-	R-	R-	R-	R-	R-	R-
6	Huggers (3 - 5+ reps)	R-	R-	R-	R-	R-	R-	R-	R-	R-
7	Marching (10 reps each leg)	R-	R-	R-	R-	R-	R-	R-	R-	R-
8	Leg Swings (10 reps forward and backward, side to side)	R-	R-	R-	R-	R-	R-	R-	R-	R-

Static

Key Points:
1. All movements must be done within a pain free range of movement
2. Initially hold each stretch for 5 to 20 sec. You can progress to hold each stretch from 30 seconds to one minute.
3. Never hold your breath as you hold the stretch. Breathe normally.

	Date:											
Neck:												
1	Side/Lateral head pulls (hold 5 - 20 seconds)											
1	Single arm reach across your chest (hold 5 - 20 seconds)											
2	Hands behind your head and squeeze your shoulder blades together (hold 5 - 20 seconds)											
3	Single arm adduction facing the wall (hold 5 - 20 seconds)											
4	Single arm adduction facing the wall (hold 5 - 20 seconds)											
5	Single arm over shoulder and scratch upper back (hold 5 - 20 seconds)											
6	Underneath lower back stretch (hold 5 - 20 seconds)											
Lower Back:												
1	Rag doll (hold 5 - 20 seconds)											
2	Child Pose with or without blocks (hold 5 - 20 seconds)											
3	Cat/Cow Pose (hold 5 - 20 seconds)											

4	Upward dog (hold 5 - 20 seconds)											
5	Sitting butterfly (hold 5 - 20 seconds)											
6	Supine (lying down) twist (hold 5 - 20 seconds)											
7	Seated spinal twist (hold 5 - 20 seconds)											

Hips:

1	Knee to chest (hold 5 - 20 seconds)											
2	Knee to Opposite chest (hold 5 - 20 seconds)											
3	Thread the needle (hold 5 - 20 seconds)											
4	Sitting pose with or without block (hold 5 - 20 seconds)											

Legs:

1	Supported standing heel to buttocks (hold 5 - 20 seconds)											
2	Bent over at hips 90° and touch wall (hold 5 - 20 seconds)											
3	Modified standing toe touch (hold 5 - 20 seconds)											
4	Standing foot on bench (hold 5 - 20 seconds)											
5	Sitting single leg extension (hold 5 - 20 seconds)											
6	Gastroc and Soleus/Achilles tendon (hold 5 - 20 seconds)											

10 Minute Dynamic and Static Stretching Routine (Illustrated)

Reference - Chapter 5.1 and Appendix 9.1.4.1

Remember - To improve your flexibility you need to stretch frequently. It is better to stretch 3 x/day for 5 minutes each than 1 x/day for 15 minutes.

Frequency and consistency are the keys

Dynamic

Key Points:
1. Focus on SLOW, DELIBERATE & COMPLETE movements
2. Breathe normally as you do each movement
3. All movements must be done within a pain free range of movement
4. Avoid any stretch movements if they are painful.

	Date:						

Neck:

1. Semi-circle head rolls (3 - 5 reps)

	R-	R-	R-	R-	R-	R-	R-

Shoulders:

2. Shoulder Rolls (10 x forward and backward)

	R-	R-	R-	R-	R-	R-	R-

3. Standing Arm Circles (10 x forward and backward)

	R-	R-	R-	R-	R-	R-	R-

4. Huggers (3 - 5+ reps)	R-	R-	R-	R-	R-	R-	R-

Trunk:

5. Wide stance trunk rotations (3 - 5+ reps)	R-	R-	R-	R-	R-	R-	R-
6. Wide stance side stretch (3 - 5+ reps)	R-	R-	R-	R-	R-	R-	R-

Legs and Hips:

7. Marching (10 reps each leg)	R-	R-	R-	R-	R-	R-	R-

	R-	R-	R-	R-	R-	R-	R-
8. Leg Swings (10 reps forward and backwards & 10 reps sideways)							

Static

Key Points:
1. All movements must be done within a pain free range of movement
2. Initially hold each stretch for 5 to 20 sec. You can progress to hold each stretch from 30 seconds to one minute.
3. Never hold your breath as you hold the stretch. Breathe normally.

	Date:						
Neck: 1. **Side/Lateral head pulls** (hold 5 - 20 seconds)							
Shoulders: 2. **Single arm reach across your chest** (Hold 5 - 20 seconds)							

3. Single arm over shoulder and scratch upper back (Hold 5 - 20 seconds)								
4. Underneath lower back stretch (Hold 5 - 20 seconds)								

Lower Back:

5. Child Pose with or without blocks (Hold 5 - 20 seconds)								
6. Upward dog (Hold 5 - 20 seconds)								

Hips:

7. Knee to chest
   (Hold 5 - 20 seconds)

8. Knee to Opposite chest
   (Hold 5 - 20 seconds)

9. Sitting Butterfly
   With or Without Block
   (Hold 5-20 seconds)

Using block to support head

Legs:

10. Supported standing heel to buttocks
(hold 5 - 20 seconds)

11. Modified standing toe touch
(hold 5 - 20 seconds)

12. Sitting single leg Bench extension (hold 5 - 20 seconds)

13. Gastroc and Soleus/ Achilles Tendon
(hold 5 - 20 seconds)

Gastroc   Soleus

10 Minute Dynamic Stretching Routine (Illustrated)

Reference - Chapter 5.1 and Appendix 9.1.4.1

Remember - To improve your flexibility you need to stretch frequently. It is better to stretch 3 x/day for 5 minutes each than 1 x/day for 15 minutes.

Frequency and consistency are the keys

Dynamic Stretching

Key Points:
1. Focus on **SLOW, DELIBERATE & COMPLETE** movements
2. Breathe normally as you do each movement
3. All movements must be done within a pain free range of movement
4. Avoid any stretch movements if they are painful

Date:							

Neck:

1. **Semi-circle head rolls (3 - 5+ reps)**	R-	R-	R-	R-	R-	R-	R-

Shoulders:

2. **Shoulder Rolls (10 x forward and Backward)**	R-	R-	R-	R-	R-	R-	R-

3. Standing Arm Circles (10 x forward and backward)	R-	R-	R-	R-	R-	R-	R-
4. Huggers (3 - 5+ reps)	R-	R-	R-	R-	R-	R-	R-

Trunk:

5. Wide stance trunk rotations (3 - 5+ reps)	R-	R-	R-	R-	R-	R-	R-

6. Wide stance side stretch (3 - 5+ reps)	R-	R-	R-	R-	R-	R-	R-

Legs and Hips:

7. Marching (10 reps each leg)	R-	R-	R-	R-	R-	R-	R-
8. Leg Swings (10 reps) **Forward and backwards swings** **Sideway swings**	R-	R-	R-	R-	R-	R-	R-

10 Minute Static Stretching Routine (Illustrated)

Reference Chapter 5.1 and Appendix 9.1.4.1
Remember - To improve your flexibility you need to stretch frequently. It is better to stretch 3 x/day for 5 minutes each than 1 x / day for 15 minutes.

Frequency and consistency are the keys

Static Stretching

Key Points:
1. All movements must be done within a pain free range of movement
2. Initially hold each stretch for 5 to 20 sec. You can progress to hold each stretch for 30 seconds to one minute.
3. Never hold your breath as you hold the stretch. Breathe normally.

Date:							

Neck:

1. Side / Lateral head pulls
(hold 5 - 20 seconds)

Shoulders:

2. Single arm reach across your chest
(Hold 5 - 20 seconds)

3. Single arm over shoulder and scratch upper back (hold 5 - 20 seconds)						
4. Underneath lower back stretch (hold 5 - 20 seconds)						
Lower Back:						
5. Child Pose with or without blocks (hold 5 - 20 seconds)						
6. Upward dog (hold 5 - 20 seconds)						

Hips:							
7. Knee to chest (hold 5 - 20 seconds)							
8. Knee to Opposite chest (hold 5 - 20 seconds)							
9. Sitting Butterfly with or Without Block (Hold 5-20 seconds) **Using Block to Support Head**							

Legs:							
10. Supported standing heel to buttocks (hold 5 - 20 seconds)							
11. Modified standing toe touch (hold 5 - 20 seconds)							
12. Sitting single leg Bench extension (hold 5 - 20 seconds)							
13. Gastroc and Soleous / Achilles Tendon (hold 5 - 20 seconds) **Gastroc** **Soleus**							

Yin Yoga - Upper Back, Chest and Shoulders (Illustrated)

Reference - Chapter 5.1.3 and Appendix 9.1.4.3

(You do not have to do each of these poses each time you do your Yin Practice. Do some one day and others the next)

Remember - To improve your flexibility you need to stretch frequently. Doing Yin Yoga is an excellent way of complementing a traditional stretching program

Frequency and consistency are the keys

Key Points:
1. Focus on SLOW, DELIBERATE & COMPLETE movements as you move into each pose
2. Breathe normally as you do each pose
3. All poses must be done within a pain free range of movement
4. Avoid any pose if they are painful
5. Initially, each pose should be held for at least one minute and over time increased to 3 to 4 minutes

	Date:						

Upper Back :

1. Bow Tie	T-	T-	T-	T-	T-	T-	T-

Chest Openers:

2. Sphinx	T-	T-	T-	T-	T-	T-	T-

3. <u>**Supportive Fish**</u>	T-	T-	T-	T-	T-	T-	T-

Shoulders:

4. <u>**Child Pose**</u>	T-	T-	T-	T-	T-	T-	T-
5. <u>**Side Lying Chest Opener**</u>	T-	T-	T-	T-	T-	T-	T-
6. <u>**Tread the Needle**</u>	T-	T-	T-	T-	T-	T-	T-

7. Cow Face Arms Towel Assisted	T-	T-	T-	T-	T-	T-	T-

Yin Yoga - Lower Back, Hips and Legs Routine (Illustrated)

Reference - Chapter 5.1.3 and Appendix 9.1.4.3

(You do not have to do each of these poses each time you do your Yin Practice. Do some one day and others the next)

Remember - To improve your flexibility you need to stretch frequently. Doing Yin Yoga is an excellent way of complementing a traditional stretching program

Frequency and Consistency are the keys

Key Points:
1. Focus on **SLOW, DELIBERATE & COMPLETE movements** as you move into each pose
2. Breathe normally as you do each pose
3. All poses must be done within a pain free range of movement
4. Avoid any pose if they are painful
5. Initially, each pose should be held for at least one minute and over time increased to 3 to 4 minutes

Date:							

Lower Back :

1. **Butterfly**
Sitting

Bent over

	T-	T-	T-	T-	T-	T-	T-

2. Half Butterfly Pose	T-	T-	T-	T-	T-	T-	T-
3. Dragonfly **Booster Supported**	T-	T-	T-	T-	T-	T-	T-
4. Caterpillar	T-	T-	T-	T-	T-	T-	T-
5. Child Pose	T-	T-	T-	T-	T-	T-	T-

6. Seal Pose	T-	T-	T-	T-	T-	T-	T-
7. Sitting Spiral Twist Pose	T-	T-	T-	T-	T-	T-	T-

Hips:

8. Dragon Pose **Block Supported**	T-	T-	T-	T-	T-	T-	T-
9. Sleeping Swan Pose	T-	T-	T-	T-	T-	T-	T-

		T-	T-	T-	T-	T-	T-	T-
10. Swan Pose								

Quads, Shins and Ankle :

		T-	T-	T-	T-	T-	T-	T-
11. Saddle Pose **Booster Support**								
12. Half Saddle Pose		T-	T-	T-	T-	T-	T-	T-

Myofascial Self Massage Utilizing a Roller (Illustrated)

Reference - Chapter 5.1.4 and Appendix 9.1.4.4

(You do not have to do each of these massage positions each time you use the Roller. Do some one day and others the next)

Remember - Myofascial massage is an excellent way of complementing your stretching routine to improve your flexibility and health of your muscles.

Frequency and consistency is the key.

Key Points:
1. Never us a roller over joints or bony prominences or inside of the upper arms.
2. All movements (rolling) are done slowly with gentle to deep pressure for a count of 10.
3. Focus on deep controlled breathing which is in rhythm with your rolling.
3. If you find a sensitive spot you may apply pressure with the grid over this spot for 10 to 30 sec.
4. Correct posture and positioning of the roller is necessary for effective results.
5. It will take practice to learn how to perform each movement correctly.

Date:						

Supine (Face up) Position:

1. Calf (posterior lower leg)

(Hips off Mat)

2. Hamstring (posterior upper leg)

3. Glutes (buttocks)							
4. Piriformis (posterior lateral aspect of buttocks)							
5. Mid to upper back							
Side Lying:							
1. Peroneal (lateral aspects of lower legs)							

2. IT Band & Vastus Lateralis (Angled Side Plank) (lateral and anterior lateral aspect of upper leg)							
3. Tensor Fascia Lata (lateral hip)							
4. Latissimus Dorsi (lateral aspect of upper chest)							
Prone (Face down):							
1. Tibialis Anterior (anterior lateral lower leg)							

2. Quadriceps (anterior aspect of upper leg)							
3. Adductors (Groins) and Vastus Medialis (medial and medial anterior upper leg)							
4. Pectoralis Major and Minor (anterior /front of chest)							

9.2.6. Re-Evaluation Worksheets

Physical Activity Re-Evaluation 992
Nutritional Balance Re-Evaluation 993
Holistic Wellness Re-Evaluation 994
Physical Fitness Re-Evaluation 995
Goal Setting Re-Evaluation 1020

Physical Activity Re-Evaluation

<u>Reference – Chapter 8.0</u>

Date: _____

(Assessment of Current Physical Condition and Activity Level)

Physical condition or physical activity is best described as the ability to maintain a physically active lifestyle. Listed below are 20 statements that refer to physical activity. Use the scale, and respond to each question by circling the number that best describes your current lifestyle.

Description	Great	Good	Fair	Needs Attention
2. Amount of energy every day.	4	3	2	1
2. Cardiovascular endurance.	4	3	2	1
3. Ability to perform continuous activity for 30 minutes.	4	3	2	1
4. Accumulate at least 30 minutes of physical activity most days of the week.	4	3	2	1
5. Muscular strength and endurance.	4	3	2	1
6. Upper-body strength.	4	3	2	1
7. Ability to lift and carry heavy objects.	4	3	2	1
8. Perform resistance exercise regularly.	4	3	2	1
9. The range of motion in joints.	4	3	2	1
10. Ability to move arms and legs with minimal pain and limitations.	4	3	2	1
11. Participation in stretching and flexibility activities regularly.	4	3	2	1
12. Posture and low back strength.	4	3	2	1
13. Physical appearance.	4	3	2	1
14. Body weight.	4	3	2	1
15. Amount of body fat versus muscle.	4	3	2	1
16. Live an active lifestyle.	4	3	2	1
17. Ability to engage in activities with a moderate amount of effort or intensity.	4	3	2	1
18. Level of current physical fitness.	4	3	2	1
19. Physical condition for age.	4	3	2	1
20. Overall assessment of my health/wellbeing.	4	3	2	1
Totals				

Total Physical Activity SCORE _____ /80

Score	Physical Activity Category
70 - 80	Excellent
60 - 69	Good
50 - 59	Average
< 49	Needs Improvement

(<u>Reference</u>: Can-Fit-Pro - Nutrition and Wellness Specialist Certification Manual, March 2007)

Nutritional Balance Re-Evaluation

<u>Reference</u> – Chapter 8.0

Date: _____

(Assessment of Current Nutritional Choices and Health)

Nutritional balance is the ability to make intelligent and beneficial dietary choices. Listed below are 25 statements that refer to nutritional balance. Use the scale, and respond to each question by circling the number that best describes your current lifestyle.

Description	Great		Good	Fair	Needs Attention
3. Amount of energy every day.	4		3	2	1
2. I enjoy eating a diet with lots of variety.	4		3	2	1
3. I eat at least 3.5 to 5 servings of vegetables daily.	4		3	2	1
4. I eat a variety of vegetables (lots of different colours).	4		3	2	1
5. I eat at least 3.5 to 5 servings of fruit each day.	4		3	2	1
6. I eat a variety of fruit.	4		3	2	1
7. I eat 6 to 8 servings of grain products each day.	4		3	2	1
8. I attempt to eat whole grain products and avoid refined (white flour) grain products.	4		3	2	1
9. I am careful to eat appropriate serving sizes of grain products.	4		3	2	1
10. I consume 2 to 3 servings of milk products daily.	4		3	2	1
11. I avoid milk products that are high in fat.	4		3	2	1
12. I eat 2 to 3 servings of meat and alternatives each day.	4		3	2	1
13. I have reduced my consumption of red meat.	4		3	2	1
14. I eat beans and legumes.	4		3	2	1
15. I eat seafood / fish at least once a week.	4		3	2	1
16. I choose healthy snacks and avoid snacks that have low nutritional value.	4		3	2	1
17. I drink at least 8 to 12 glasses of water daily.	4		3	2	1
18. I take supplements to balance my diet.	4		3	2	1
19. I read labels and am careful about the food I serve.	4		3	2	1
20. I am happy with my body weight.	4		3	2	1
21. My body's ratio of fat versus muscle is appropriate.	4		3	2	1
22. I avoid eating fast food.	4		3	2	1
23. I am pleased with my physical appearance.	4		3	2	1
24. Generally, my diet is balanced.	4		3	2	1
25. Overall assessment of my health/wellbeing.	4		3	2	1
Totals					

Total Nutritional Balance SCORE _____ /100

Score	Nutrition Balance Category
85 - 100	Excellent
75 - 84	Good
65 - 74	Average
< 64	Needs Improvement

(<u>Reference:</u> Can-Fit-Pro - Nutrition and Wellness Specialist Certification Manual, March 2007

Holistic Wellness Re-Evaluation

<u>Reference</u> – Chapter 8.0

Date: _____

(Assessment of Current Holistic Wellness Health)

Holistic wellness is the ability to develop balance and harmony in life. Listed below are 25 statements that refer to holistic wellness. Use the scale, and respond to each question by circling the number that best describes your current lifestyle.

Description	Most of the Time	Frequently	Sometimes	Rarely or Never
4. I have a good relationship with my family	4	3	2	1
2. I am involved in my community	4	3	2	1
3. I do something for fun and for myself every week.	4	3	2	1
4. I provide support for others.	4	3	2	1
5. My life has meaning and direction.	4	3	2	1
6. I have life goals and I strive to achieve them.	4	3	2	1
7. I look forward to the future.	4	3	2	1
8. I have a sense of peace in my life.	4	3	2	1
9. I feel positive about myself and my life.	4	3	2	1
10. I learn from my mistakes.	4	3	2	1
11. I can say no without feeling guilty.	4	3	2	1
12. I find it easy to laugh	4	3	2	1
13. I cope with life's changes in a healthy way.	4	3	2	1
14. I prepare ahead of time for events that may cause stress.	4	3	2	1
15. I schedule enough time to accomplish what I need to get done.	4	3	2	1
16. I participate in activities that relieve stress.	4	3	2	1
17. I stay calm and patient under pressure.	4	3	2	1
18. I know what my values and beliefs are.	4	3	2	1
19. I have interest outside my work.	4	3	2	1
20. I am interested in learning new things.	4	3	2	1
21. I make time to relax regularly	4	3	2	1
22. I cope well with changes in my life.	4	3	2	1
23. I feel that things often go my way.	4	3	2	1
24. I get enough sleep and have little trouble going to sleep.	4	3	2	1
25. I am happy and enjoy life.	4	3	2	1
Totals				

Total Holistic Wellness SCORE _____ /100

Score	Holistic Wellness Category
85 - 100	Excellent
70 - 84	Good
55 - 69	Average
< 54	Needs Improvement

(Reference: Can-Fit-Pro - Nutrition and Wellness Specialist Certification Manual, March 2007

Physical Fitness Re-Evaluation

Reference – Chapter 8.0

Note - When assessing your Re-evaluation look for trends rather than actual numbers

1. Resting Heart Rate

Take your radial (wrist) or carotid (neck) pulse for 10 sec and multiply by 6.

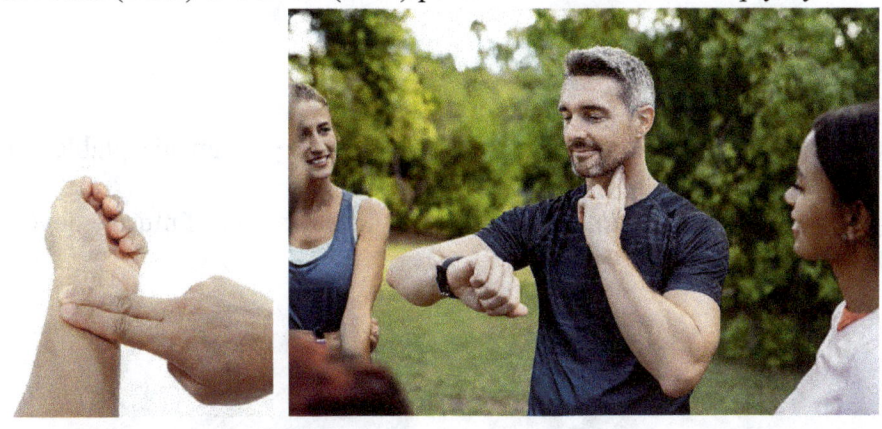

	Initial			
Date				
Resting Heart Rate				

Comment: Even though the reading of a resting heart rate can vary by about 10%, a lowering in resting heart rate is a positive sign because it is usually an early indication of improved fitness. On the other hand, a high resting heart rate could be an indication of infection, chronic stress or a heart condition, and would warrant further investigation.

(A person should take their heart rate just before they get out of bed in the morning three to five days in a row to get an accurate reading of your resting heart rate).

2. Resting Blood Pressure

Everyone should have a self-administered blood pressure monitor at home.

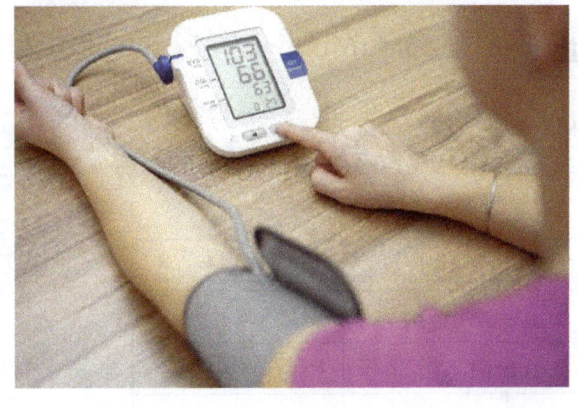

	Initial			
Date:				
Resting Blood Pressure				

Comment: 120/80 is considered a normal resting BP. The systolic pressure (the top value) can vary quite a bit (i.e. - 180) due to excitement, anxiety and exertion, however the diastolic pressure (the bottom value) remains relatively constant. A diastolic pressure over 90 would indicate borderline hypertension and require further investigation and possible medication.

3. Body Composition
1. Body Mass Index

Purpose: Use as a guideline to determine if you are carrying an acceptable amount of weight for your height.

(Major Limitation – It does not take into account the amount of muscle development of a person)

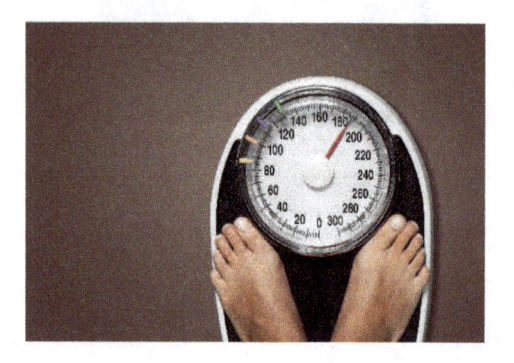

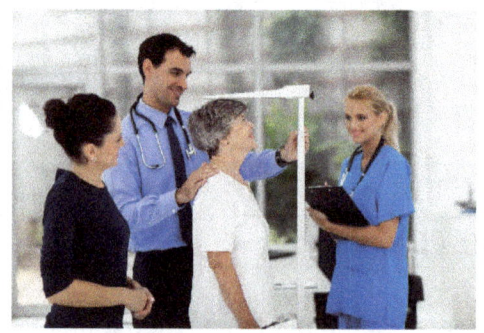

	Initial			
Date				
1. Weight (Kg.)				
2. Height (M)				
BMI (wt/ht²)				

Example Calculation – Ht 1.55M (6'1"), wt. 91 kg (200 lbs)

Formula BMI = wt (Kg)/Ht²(M)
= $91/(1.55)^2$ = 91/2.4 = 37.9 (Obese 2)

Category	BMI
Underweight	<18.5
Normal	18.5 – 24.9
Overweight	25.0 – 29.9

Evaluation of BMI

Obese 1	30.0 – 34.9
Obese 2	35.0 – 39.9
Extreme Obesity	>40.0

2. Waist-to-Hip Ratio

Purpose – Recent research indicates that it is the distribution/areas of fat on the body and not the amount of body fat that determines the cardio-vascular health risk of obesity. Fat carried internally in the abdominal area carries the greatest risk.

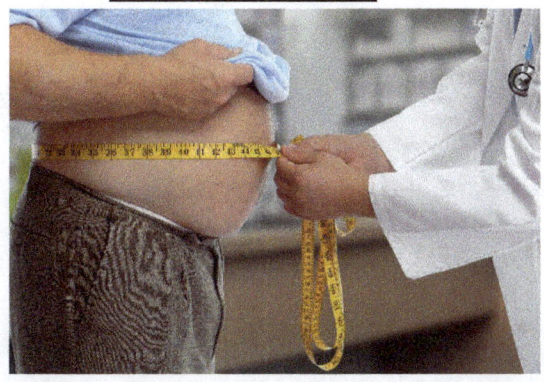

Waist Measurement   **Hip Measurement**

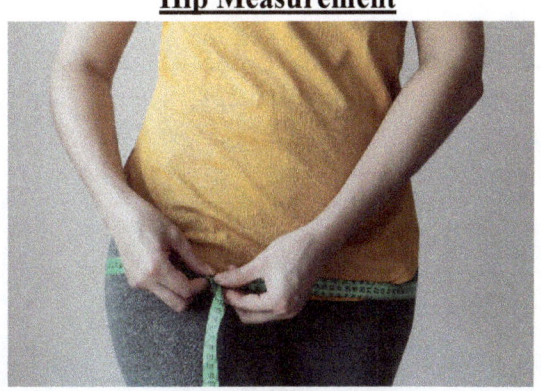

Initial

Date				
1. Waist Girth (Measure around your belly button) (inches)				
2. Hip Girth (Measure 2" below iliac crest) (inches)				
Waist/Hip Ratio				

Example calculation – waist 40" & Hip 38" (50 year old male)

Formula – waist measurement (inches)/hip measurement (inches)
= 40/38 = 1.05 (very high risk of heart disease)

| | Risk for Heart Disease ||||||||
| | Low || Moderate || High || Very High ||
Age	Men	Women	Men	Women	Men	Women	Men	Women
20-29	< 0.83	< 0.71	0.83 - 0.88	0.71 - 0.77	0.89 - 0.94	0.78 - 0.82	> 0.94	> 0.82
30-39	< 0.84	< 0.72	0.84 - 0.91	0.72 - 0.78	0.92 - 0.96	.79 - 0.84	> 0.96	> 0.84
40-49	< 0.88	< 0.73	0.88 - 0.95	0.73 - 0.79	0.96 - 1.00	0.80 - 0.87	> 1.00	> 0.87
50-59	< 0.90	< 0.74	0.90 - 0.96	0.74 - 0.81	0.97 - 1.02	0.82 - 0.88	> 1.02	> 0.88
60-69	< 0.91	< 0.76	0.91 - 0.98	0.76 - 0.83	0.99 - 1.03	0.84 - 0.90	> 1.03	> 0.90

4. Flexibility Evaluation

Purpose – To detect muscle imbalances (one side of body less flexible than the other side) and joint instabilities (excessive mobility).

1. Upper Body Flexibility Evaluation

Evaluation – do you feel/notice one arm is stiffer (can't scratch as far on the back as the other side)

Initial

Date:				
1. External Rotation (Upper back scratch)				
2. Internal Rotation (Lower back scratch)				

3. Abduction **(Lifting arms over your head)**					

2. Lower Body Flexibility Evaluation

Initial

Date:				
1. LB Forward Flexion (Inches/cm from to toes/floor) (Standing and touch toes without bending your knees)				

2. LB Extension (Do you feel restricted) (Standing and lean back at the waist)				
3. Quadriceps (Inches/cm from heel to buttocks) (Lie on stomach and bend heel to buttocks)				
4. Groin (Inches/cm from bottom of knee to floor) (Sit on mat with heels touching)				

5. Ankle and Calf (Does one ankle feel more restricted than the other) (Extension/Flexion) **Extension** **Flexion**				
6. Hip extensors **1. Gluteus Medius** (Inches/cm from knee to chest) (Lie on floor and bring knee to opposite side chest) **2. Gluteus Maximus)** (Inches/cm from knee to chest) (Lie on floor and bring knee to same sided chest)				

7. Hip Flexors (Observe if opposite leg raises off the floor/table) (Lie on floor and bring one knee to chest)				
8. Trunk Rotation (Observe if there is restriction on rotation in either direction) (Sitting, arms crossed against the chest and rotate shoulders in both directions)				

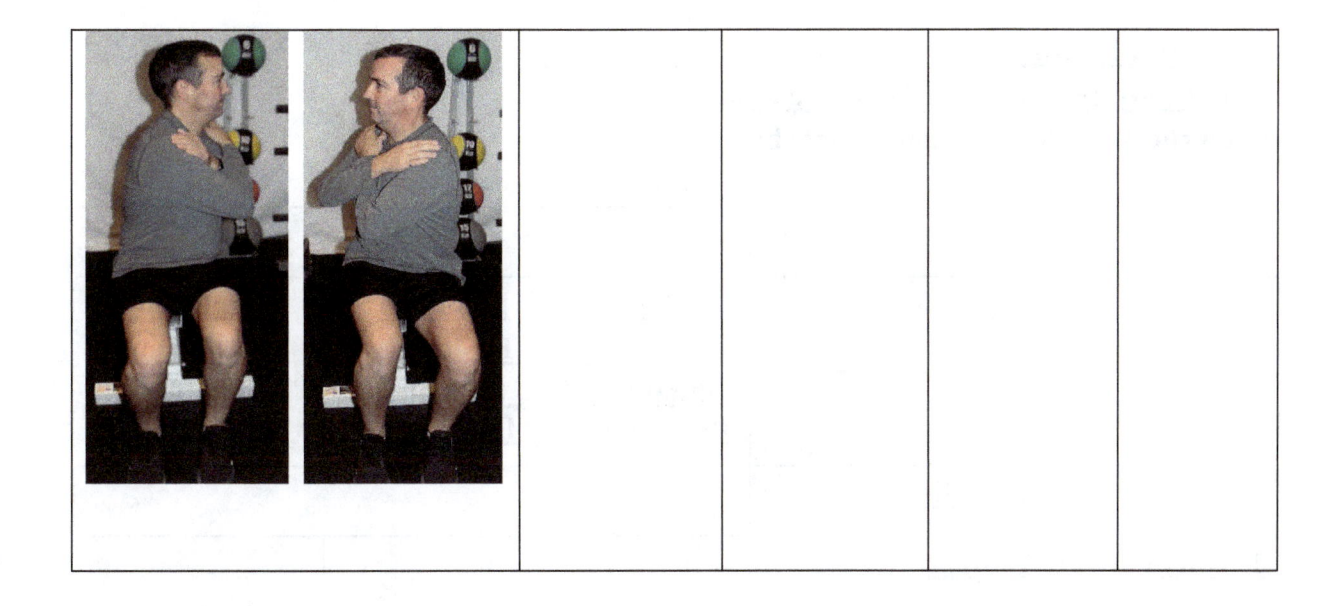

5. Agility, Balance and Coordination Evaluation
1. Agility and Coordination Evaluation
(Put a check mark in the appropriate box)

Initial

Date:			
Test	**No Hesitation/ Stumbles/ Difficulties**	**Moderate Hesitation/ Stumbles/ Difficulties**	**Significant Hesitation/ Stumbles/ Difficulties**
Walking Drills:			
1. Walk Forward 10 steps			
2. Walk Backward 10 steps			
3. Walk Sideways 10 steps			

4. Walk sideways crossing your legs 5 steps (Alternate the crossing leg going in front and then behind the other leg.) (Do a second time with the opposite leg crossing over)			
Hop Drills:			
1. Forward Hop Drills:			
1. Double leg forward hop 5 x's			
2. Single leg forward hop 5 x's (Repeat with opposite leg 5 x's)			

3. Feet wide then narrow hop scotch			
4. Scissor hop in a stationary position			
2. Sideways Hop Drills:			
1. Double leg hop sideways			

2. Single foot hop sideways			
3. Rotational Hop Drills			
1. 90° rotation hop			

Reference: Rose, Debra J. (2010), *Fall Proof: A Comprehensive Balance and Mobility Training Program*, Human Kinetics, 2nd Edition

2. Static Balance Test – Eyes Open and then Closed
(Stand on an unsupported leg for maximum of 10 seconds)

Eyes Closed

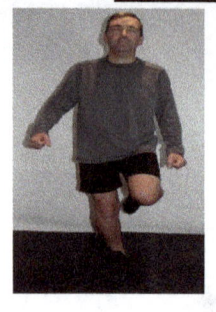

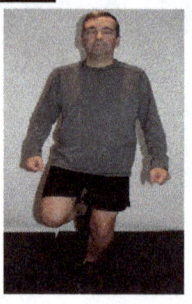

Initial

Date:				
Eyes Open (sec.)	R- - L -	R- L -	R- L-	R- L-
Eyes Closed (sec.)	R- L-	R- L-	R-. L-	R- L-

6. Muscular Strength and Endurance Evaluation

(<u>Note</u> - **All exercises listed below are described in detail and illustrated in Appendix 9.1.2.2.1)**

1. Muscle Strength Evaluation

<u>Initial</u>

Date:							
<u>Exercise</u>		<u>Weight Lifted (lbs.)</u>	<u>Reps</u>	<u>Weight Lifted (lbs.)</u>	<u>Reps</u>	<u>Weights Lifted (lbs.)</u>	<u>Reps</u>
1. Leg Extensions (Quadriceps) **Machine** - Single or Double Leg Extension or **Bench Balance Lunge**	**Machine:** <u>Single Leg</u> <u>Double Leg</u>		R- L-		R- L-		R- L-

	Balance Lunge:						
2. Leg Curls (Hamstrings) **Machine** - Single or Double Leg Curl or **Stability Ball Leg Curl**	**Machine:** **Single Leg** **Double Leg**		R- L-		R- L-		R- L-

	Stability Ball Single Leg Curl:		R- L-		R- L-		R- L-
3. Chest Press (Pectoralis Major) **Machine** Chest Press or **Dumbbell** Chest Press	**Machine:** **Dumbbells**						

4. Machine Pull Down (Latissimus Dorsi)

Machine
Lat. Pull Down

or

Dumbbells
Lying Down Overhead Two-Handed Vertical Raise

Machine:

Dumbbells:

5. Overhead Press (Trapezius) **Machine** Overhead Shoulder Press or **Dumbbells** Overhead Press	**Machine** **Dumbbells**						
6. Rows (Rhomboids) **Machine** Cable Rows or **Dumbbells** Bent Over Rows	**Machine:** **Cable Rows**						

	Dumbbells **Bent Over Rows:**						
7. Lateral Raises **(Deltoids)** **Dumbbells** **Or** **Resistance bands**	**Dumbbells**						

8. Arm Curls
(Biceps)

Machine
Arm Curls

or

Dumbbells
Arm Curls

Machine:

Dumbbells:

9. Arm Extensions (Triceps) Machine Triceps Arm Extensions or **Lying or sitting** Double Triceps Extensions	**Machine** **Standing Double Arm Extensions**						

2. Muscle Endurance Evaluation

Initial

Date:				
1. Push-ups **Regular** **Wall** **Modified (on knees)**				
Number completed				

3. Core Strength Evaluation

Initial

Date				
1. Full Sit-ups **Stabilize the feet**				
Number Completed				

7. Cardiovascular Fitness Evaluation
1. Walking Fitness Test

	Initial			
Date:				
Heartrate at end of a one-mile walk				
Time it took to complete the walk				

Rate of Perceived Effort
    7 – very, very light
    9 – very light
    11 – light
    13 – somewhat hard
    15 – hard
    17 – very hard				

Goal Setting Re-Evaluation

First Goal:

Specific	
Measurable	
Action	
Realistic	
Time lined	
Evaluation (If not accomplished why? What can I do better to be more successful)	

Second Goal:

Specific	
Measurable	
Action	
Realistic	
Time lined	
Evaluation (If not accomplished why? What can I do better to be more successful)	

Third Goal:

Specific	
Measurable	
Action	
Realistic	
Time lined	
Evaluation (If not accomplished why? What can I do better to be more successful)	

9.3.0. Online Support

Online resources are becoming the norm in our high-tech information "I want it now" society. Forever Active's website is available to recognize this trend and the need for Older Adult Forever-Active Playbook readers to have access to continually evolving information concerning their fitness, nutrition, mental health, and an easy way to ask questions.

The website will be updated regularly with new educational and motivational material to help individuals' health and fitness journeys become more enjoyable and successful.

Additionally, all your inquiries will be responded to within 24 hours.

For online support visit;

www.forever-active.com

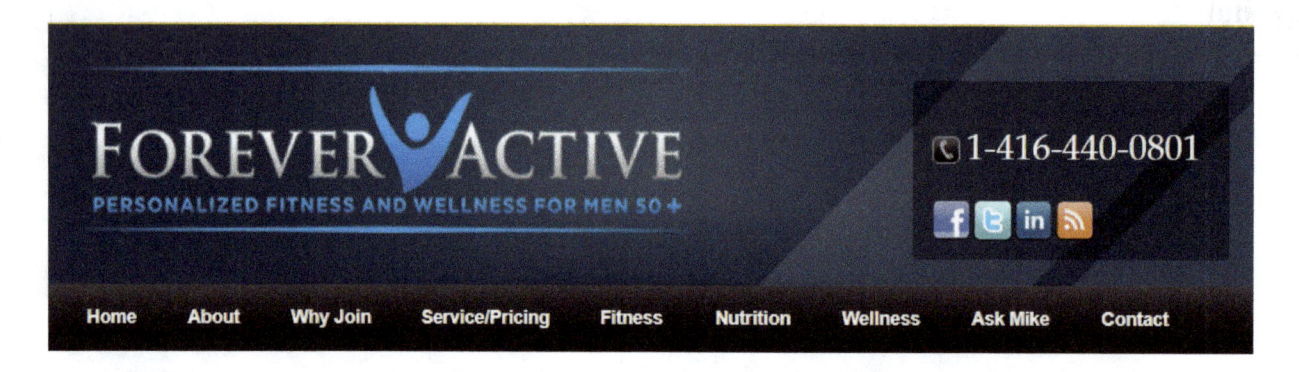

9.4.0. Introduction: Reference Library

Continuing education is the key to one's intellectual growth. A person must never be satisfied with the status quo and never say that they know enough. In today's information age, the body of knowledge available is growing and constantly changing.

Information presented in hard copy books, is the traditional way of learning. However, online resources are now becoming the norm to access information. This section presents health and fitness resources both ways; hard copy books (many of which are available as eBooks) and online links.

Forever Active Older Adult health and Fitness Playbook is a tremendous resource for you to use to improve your health and fitness. However, it should not be your only resource. There will be topics touched upon in this book that you will want to know more about. Use this reference library as a starting point to access traditional books and online links that specialize in the areas you want additional information.

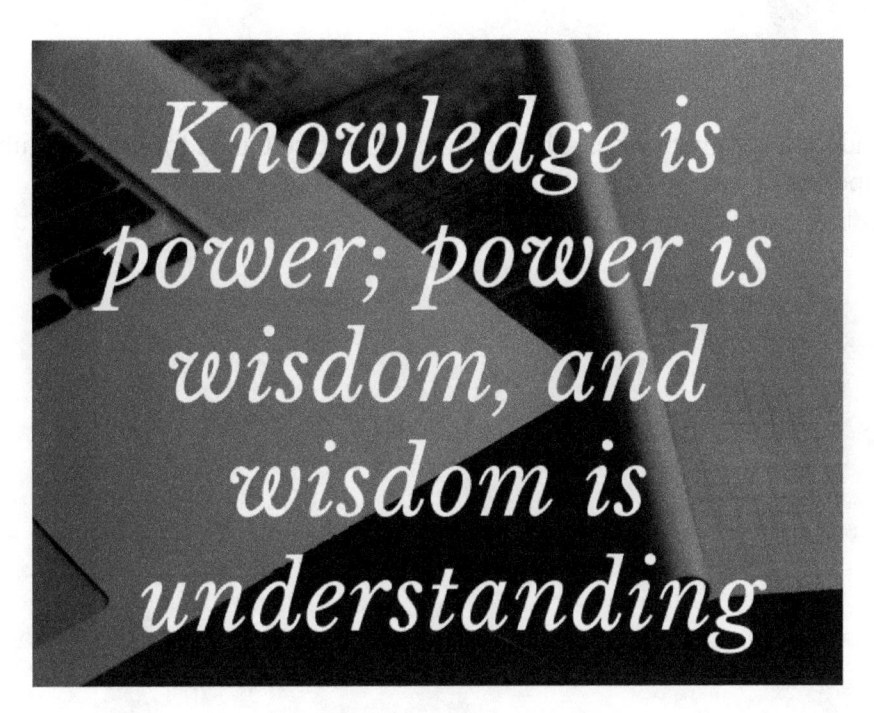

Knowledge is power; power is wisdom, and wisdom is understanding

Image source: careergrade.com

9.4.1. Hard Copy Reference Library

(1) Exercise and the Older Adult

1. Exercise and Wellness for Older Adults - 2nd Edition: Practical Programming Strategies [Paperback]
Kay Van Norman (Author)

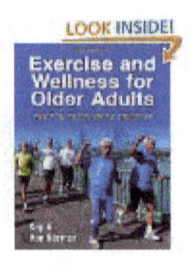

2. Bending the Aging Curve: The Complete Exercise Guide for Older Adults [Paperback]
Joseph Signorile (Author)

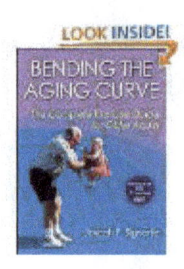

1. The Yoga Workout: Honoring Exercise for Older Adults [Paperback]
Rita M. Joseph (Author)

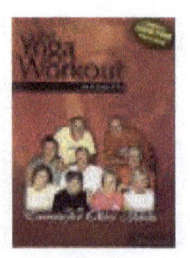

(2) Wellness

1. The Wellness Workbook, 3rd ed: How to Achieve Enduring Health and Vitality [Paperback]

   John W. Travis (Author), Regina Sara Ryan (Author)

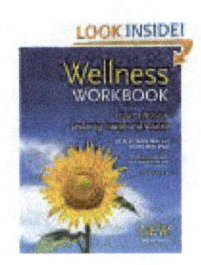

2. An Invitation to Health: Choosing to Change, Brief Edition (with Personal Wellness Guide) [Paperback]

   Dianne Hales (Author)

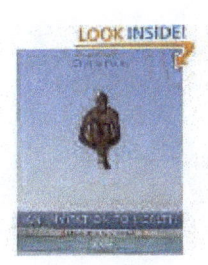

(3) Mindfulness

1. Full Catastrophe Living: Using the Wisdom of Your Body and Mind to Face Stress, Pain, and Illness [Paperback]

   Jon Kabat-Zinn (Author)

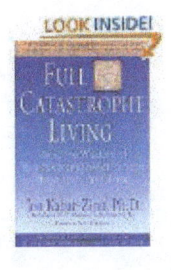

2. Guided Mindfulness Meditation [Audiobook] [Audio CD]
Jon Kabat-Zinn (Author)

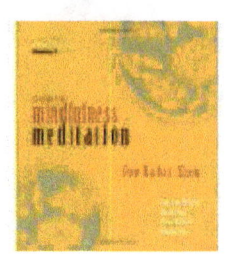

3. Wherever You Go There You Are [Paperback]
Jon Kabat-Zinn (Author)

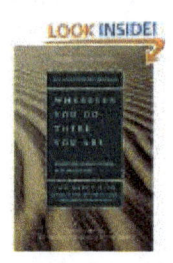

(4) General

1. Younger Next Year: A Guide to Living Like 50 Until You're 80 and Beyond [Hardcover]
Chris Crowley (Author), Henry S. Lodge (Author)

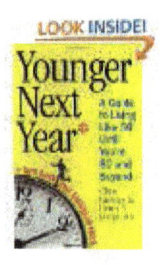

2. Younger Next Year for Women [Paperback]
Chris Crowley (Author), Henry S. Lodge (Author)

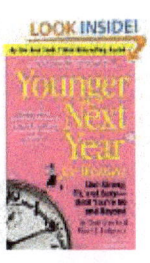

3. Younger Next Year: The Book & Journal Gift Set for Men [Paperback]
Henry Lodge (Author), Chris Crowley (Author)

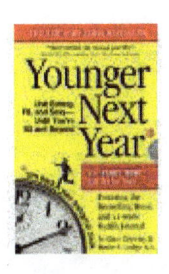

(5) Men's Health and Fitness

1. Men's Health Best: Weight-Free Workout [Paperback]
Men's Health Magazine (Author)

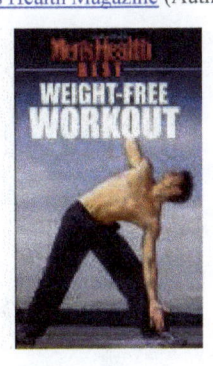

2. 50+ Looking and Feeling Great! Fitness Is a Lifestyle, Not a Fad!: Book 1: Let's Get Started [Paperback]
Steven P. McNair (Author)

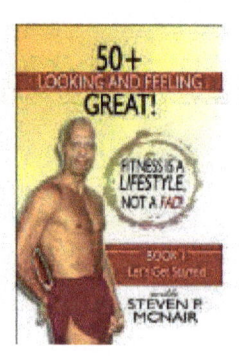

3. Pilates Plus: Grown-Up Pilates for 50+ [Paperback]
Alan Herdman (Author), Gill Paul (Author)

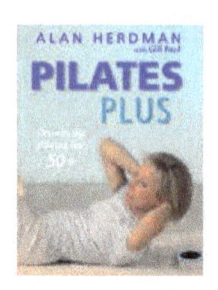

4. Fit for 50+ Men [Paperback]
Greg Chappell (Author)

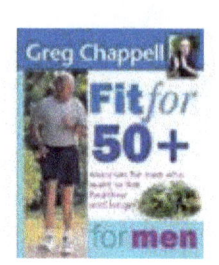

(6) Nutrition

1. Natural Health at 50+ [Paperback]
C Scott-Moncrieff (Author)

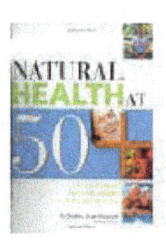

2. Nutrition For Canadians For Dummies [Paperback]
Carol Ann Rinzler (Author), Doug Cook (Author)

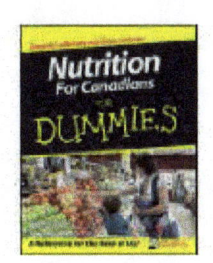

9.4.2 Online Reference Library: Healthy Links

Canadian Centre for Activity and Aging (www.uwo.ca/actage/)

Active Living Coalition for Older Adults (www.alcoa.ca)

International Council on Active Aging (www.icaa.cc)

Canadian Association of Fifty Plus (www.carp.ca)

Canadian Physical Activity Guide for Older Adults (http://www.phac-aspc.gc.ca/hp-ps/hl-mvs/pa-ap/index-eng.php)

Canada's Health Food Guide (http://www.hc-sc.gc.ca/fn-an/food-guide-aliment/index-eng.php)

Canadian Arthritis Society (http://www.arthritis.ca/tips%20for%20living/exercise/default.asp?s=1&province=ca)

Canadian Cancer Society (Exercise used to help cope with Cancer) (http://www.cancer.ca/Ontario/About%20cancer/Coping%20with%20cancer/Exercise%20can%20help%20you%20cope%20with%20side%20effects.aspx?sc_lang=en)

Canadian Diabetic Association (Exercise and Diabetes) (http://www.diabetes.ca/diabetes-and-you/healthy-guidelines/physical-activity-and-exercise/)

Canadian Orthopaedic Foundation (www.canorth.org)

Heart and Stroke Foundation (Exercise and heart and Stroke patients) (http://www.heartandstroke.com/site/apps/nlnet/content2.aspx?c=ikIQLcMWJtE&b=5552717&ct=7608693)

Osteoporosis Society of Canada (Exercise and Osteoporosis – what type of activities are best) (http://www.osteoporosis.ca/index.php/ci_id/5524/la_id/1.htm)

Baycrest – Smart Aging (http://www.baycrest.org/smartaging-201202-06.php)

American Association of Retired Person (AARP) (https://www.aarp.org/)

McMaster Optimal Aging Portal (https://www.mcmasteroptimalaging.org/)

Section 10
Epilogue

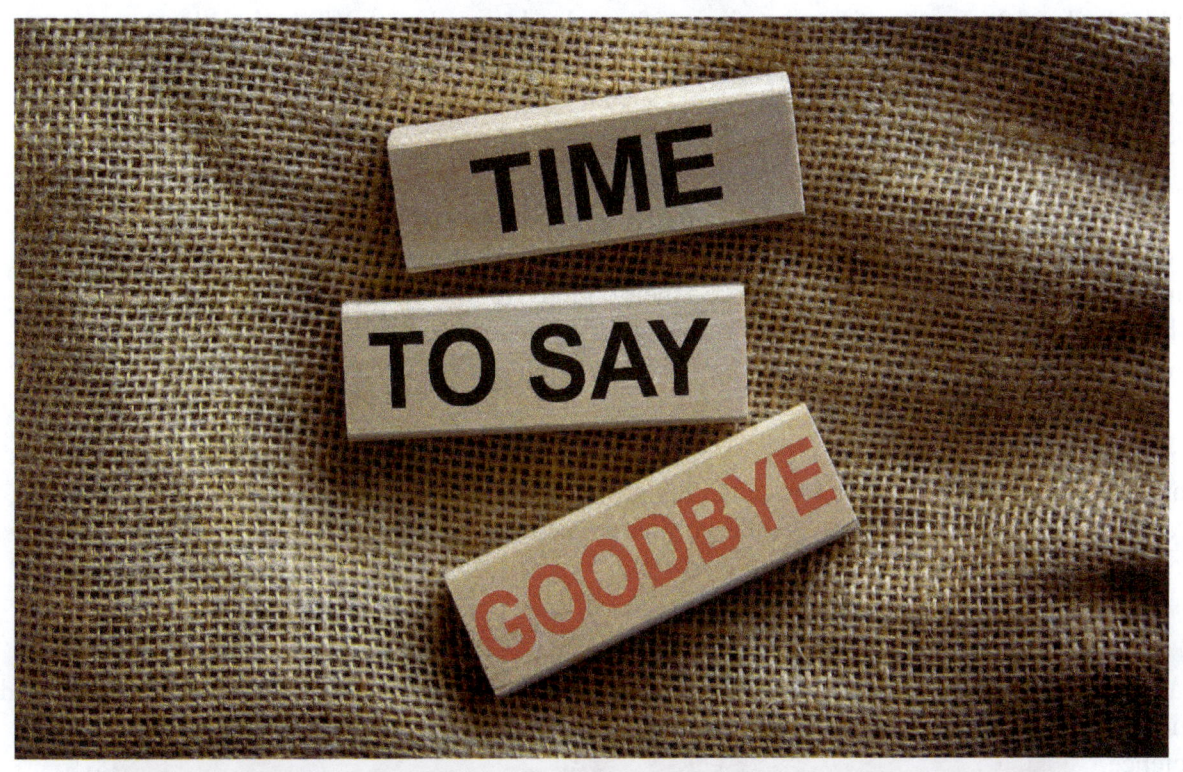

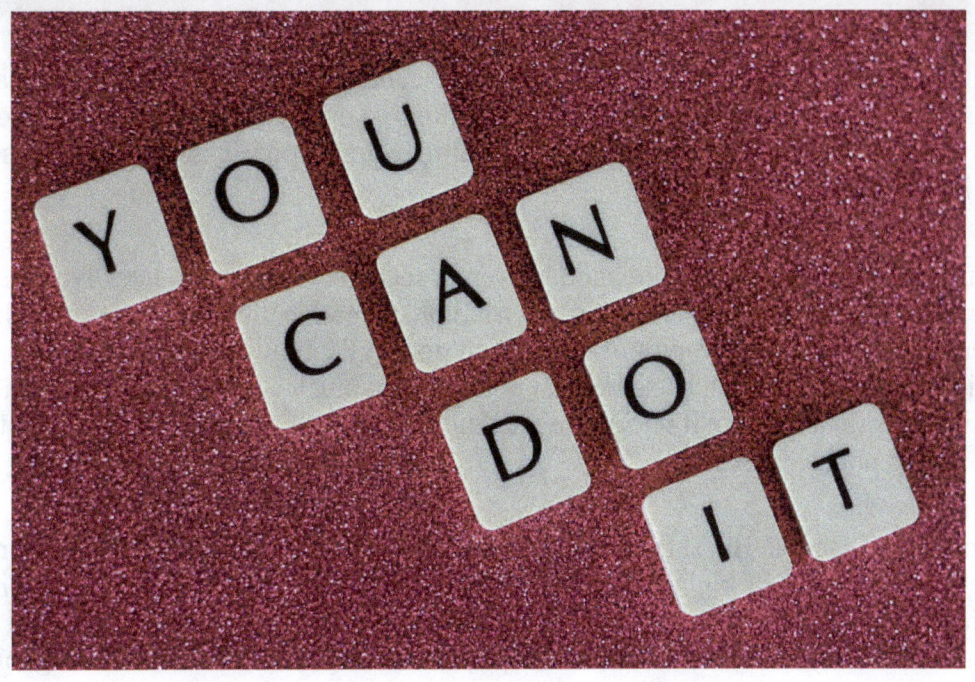

10. Epilogue

It is now January 1, 2022, oh what a 65th year it has been. Covid continues to rage its ugly head with the Delta and Omicron variant infecting young and old alike but especially those individuals unvaccinated.

This past summer has seen an unprecedented number of severe wildfires in Canada resulting in hundreds of thousands of square miles of forest land being burnt. While there has been drought and fires in one part of the country there has been severe flooding in other parts. The polar ice cap is melting at an unfathomable speed. Unfortunately, there are some who still discount the reality of global warming??

On the world stage, Afghanistan has fallen into the hands of the Taliban. It makes you question the worth of 158 Canadians dying and thousands more who came home suffering physical and mental injury as they served their country in this theater of war. My friend Brian, who served two tours in Afghanistan and who is one of five people to whom I dedicated this book, wonders this very thing every day. This situation has not helped his suffering.

Politically, another federal election has come and gone. The election was called two years early, in the middle of the pandemic and the growing crisis in Afghanistan. Over $610 million was spent and nothing changed. Could not that money be spent in better places like feeding and housing the poor?

Ok, that was some of the tough stuff that has happened this year, but a lot of good stuff has happened too. Despite peaks in infection rates, the world is a safer place because of the early and successful development of the Covid vaccine. This is an unprecedented success for modern science.

Globally, climate change is slowly starting to take center stage on politicians' agendas. Unfortunately, it has taken much suffering and the threat of even greater suffering but politicians are finally noticing and implementing action to minimize greenhouse gases. The scientists say it is not too late. My fingers are crossed.

The fan-less Olympics, against great odds, were a success. Once again, the Olympics showed the power of personal dedication, sacrifice and triumph over adversity. If this was not illustrated strongly enough during the Olympics, it was on full display 10 times more during the Paralympics. The Olympics can be somewhat political, but much can be learned from the athletes who perform and make it one of the great human performance spectacles every two years and should not be missed.

The courage of Simone Biles, the world's greatest gymnast, to recognize and confront her mental frailty on the world's biggest stage, cannot go unmentioned. A tremendous lesson for all, but especially for young boys and girls and older adults who are so vulnerable to mental health issues. "I am Listening" and "Let's talk" are important messages that should not be ignored. Mental health is such an important part of a person's overall health and fitness and the specific reason why a whole section in this book, Section 6: Special Teams: Mental Health (14 chapters), was dedicated to it.

Though we all experience tough times, and the 22 months of the Covid pandemic has pushed many to their limits, there is much to be thankful for. Family, friends, community our health and our health care system all make our life easier and more enjoyable. It is important to celebrate all the little things that bring us joy because those celebrations make us stronger to withstand the more challenging times.

It is my hope that this book has accomplished its goal and helped educate and inspire everyone, but especially older adults, to improve their physical and mental health fitness so they can engage and enjoy a longer and enhanced quality of life.

"We don't stop playing because we grow old, we grow old because we stop playing."
George Bernard Shaw

I would like to conclude with a quote from Michael J. Fox who has been suffering from Parkinson's disease for over 30 years, "with gratitude, optimism becomes sustainable." I am extremely grateful to all the people who have touched and enhanced my life these past 65 years. I am optimistic for the future, and I hope this book has helped others become optimistic for their future as well.

Cheers, Peace, Love.
Mike

PS – In my introduction, I discussed that I planned to complete an Ironman race this past year. I also mentioned that you would have to read the epilogue to see how I did. Hopefully, you have read some of this book and are on your way to improved health and fitness before reading this epilogue.

I was originally supposed to do my Ironman in Penticton BC in August, and then it got pushed back to the end of September, and then finally it was cancelled. I was fortunate to find Cozumel Ironman still accepting registrants for its November 21st race. Cozumel's Ironman was going to present a different challenge than Penticton. Whereas Penticton was at the end of the summer when I was acclimatized to the heat, with a hilly ride and run course, Cozumel had a flat ride and run course but strong winds, heat and humidity, which I would have to confront after I was no longer acclimatized to running and riding in the heat.

Fortunately, the weather was not too severe (28 Celsius) but I did ride though a BIG thunderstorm. The race went well with a strong swim (with the current) and bike ride, and for 36 kilometers, the marathon run. I was slowing down but doing ok. With 6 kilometers to go I asked a spectator what time it was and they said 10:15 pm. I got into the water to start my swim at 8 am so I knew I had until 1 am to complete the race. With 6 kilometers to go I said, "I've got this," or I thought I "had this." Shortly after I knew I was in good shape time wise, my body shut down.

My pace in the run had been slowing down but with 6 kilometers remaining, there was nothing left in the tank.

I started to walk and my pace slowed from 8–9-minute kilometers to 11 and then 15 and then 20-minute kilometers. I was forcing myself to walk 10 steps and then bend over to try to relieve the exhaustion and discomfort. After previously running 25 marathons, I thought I had experienced all the pain and exhaustion that one could feel from physical exertion. I was wrong.

With 4 kilometers remaining, I was unsure if I could or would finish. In fact, even today I am unsure how I finished, but I did finish, and with 19 minutes to spare. My official finishing time was 16:41:42. It took me over 2 hours to complete the last 6 kilometers of the race. But I made it, and heard the announcer say, "Michael Bedard, you are an Ironman." That is all I wanted to hear. Goals, the power of setting goals, is immense.

The Swim **The Bike** **The Finish**

PSS – The week prior to my Ironman, I read a beautiful book recommended to me by my wife Ann titled, *The Happiest Man on Earth: The Beautiful Life of an Auschwitz Survivor*. He ends his book with these three lines which I love and wanted to share with you.

May you always have lots of love to share,

Lots of good health to spare,

And lots of good friends who care.

Jaku, Eddie. The Happiest Man on Earth, HarperCollins, 2021

CPSIA information can be obtained
at www.ICGtesting.com
Printed in the USA
BVHW090803180422
634463BV00003B/10

9 781915 424228